NURSING INFORMATICS:
AN INTERNATIONAL OVERVIEW FOR
NURSING IN A TECHNOLOGICAL ERA

NURSING INFORMATICS: AN INTERNATIONAL OVERVIEW FOR NURSING IN A TECHNOLOGICAL ERA

Proceedings of the Fifth IMIA International Conference on Nursing Use of Computers and Information Science, San Antonio, Texas, USA, June 17-22, 1994

Editors:

Susan J. Grobe
Center for Health Care Research and Evaluation
The University of Texas at Austin
School of Nursing
Austin, Texas, USA

Elly S.P. Pluyter-Wenting
Bazis Foundation
Central Development- and Support Group
Hospital Information System
Leiden, The Netherlands

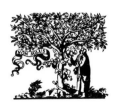 1994

ELSEVIER, Amsterdam, London, New York, Tokyo

TABLE OF CONTENTS

B. Workload, acuity, staffing and rostering

C. Benefits and realization

*Due to circumstances beyond our control, this article has been placed at the end of
  the volume*

D. Nursing minimum dataset

Section II. Nursing health information systems
A. Development, implementation and evaluation

B. Bedside systems; point-of-care systems

C. Order management; care plans; computerized care record

D. Expertise/expert systems; decision support systems

E. Gerontology; community health; patient education

Section III. Research

Section IV: Education
A. Informatics education

* Due to circumstances beyond our control, this article has been placed at the end of
this volume

B. Technology for education

C. Attitudes toward computerization

Section V: Standards
A. Standards; terminology

B. Quality improvement

C. Classifications

D. Technology assessments; guideline development

Panels

Posters

Graduate students posters

Demonstrations

FOREWORD

Today, many nurses enjoy the use and support of computer systems in daily practice. Increasingly, the use of information technology has become a normal occurence in health care and nursing. The title of this international symposium is 'Nursing in a Technological Era'. Nurses have traditionally used and appreciated technology that enhances the quality of their care of individuals. Accurate and timely communication of information is an essential condition for good care. Well designed care, based on current information through appropriate technology, together with an individualized approach to patients, is most important to give the best possible nursing care.

In 1985, Maureen Scholes, founder of Working Group 8 'Nursing Informatics' of IMIA, identified that the application of information technology is a challenge for nursing practice, management, education and research in the 21st century. Since 1985, the nursing profession has made significant progress in informatics. This Fifth International Symposium on Nursing Informatics is clear evidence that the nursing profession is well aware of the potential that computer technology holds for improving the quality and efficiency of health care if information systems are well designed, integrated and professionally managed.

At present, the nursing profession is not only aware of the enormous power of computers used in health care, but has also been confronted with practical problems. The lack of uniform terminology makes communication about care between institutional caregivers very difficult to accomplish in information systems. Provisions for security and confidentiality are a necessity that is often underestimated or not well understood. The unforeseen risks of poorly managed databases can result in loss of essential data and presentation of unreliable information.

Nevertheless, if we examine the progress made during the last two decades we see that many hospitals and health care settings are using computers in one way or another. Remarkably, the computer has found its place in health care. Unfortunately, less progress than expected has been made in the field of decision support systems and artificial intelligence, believed to be the two areas to have potential of supporting the professional practice of nursing. To carry out intellectual functions seems to be the challenge of the first decades in the next century.

Susan J. Grobe
Elly S.P. Pluyter-Wenting

FROM THE EDITORS

The contents of this book represent the present state-of-the-art on nursing informatics. The editors are proud to have had the opportunity to construct these proceedings following the style of presentation of earlier international nursing informatics symposia of 1982 (UK), 1985 (Canada), 1988 (Ireland) and 1991 (Australia). We believe the current volume continues to be of high quality and very worthy as an international publication. Importantly, this volume contributes to describing the developing science of nursing informatics.

The editors have worked closely with the members of the Scientific Program Committee and a large number of reviewers from nursing and other health disciplines. Each paper in the volume was reviewed by 2 individuals and a member of the Scientific Program Committee. We are most grateful for these reviewers' input, energy and knowledge. Authors responded graciously to suggestions and comments. These combined efforts resulted in approximately 150 high quality paper contributions from many countries.

The structure of the Symposium and the organization of the papers in this volume represent the work of the Scientific Program Committee and the editors. In addition to the scientific papers, the editors have also included authors' descriptions of panels, posters and scientific demonstrations, giving readers an excellent overview of the current state-of-the-art of nursing informatics. For the first time, in order to encourage young colleagues to publish, graduate students in nursing informatics submitted poster abstracts that are also included in the volume. We trust that this volume contributes to the description of the developing science of nursing informatics.

Susan J. Grobe
Elly S.P. Pluyter-Wenting

ACKNOWLEDGEMENTS

Working Group 8, "Nursing Informatics" of the International Medical Informatics Association, the Scientific Program Committee and the Organizing Committee of Nursing Informatics 1994 wish to express their sincere gratitude to Dean Dolores Sands of the School of Nursing of the University of Texas at Austin for all the support in making this Symposium possible. We also wish to thank our IMIA colleagues and the USA nursing cosponsors: The Council for Nursing Informatics of the National League for Nursing (NLN) and The Council on Computer Applications in Nursing of the American Nurses' Association (ANA).

We also recognize the endorsement by the Nursing Professional Specialty Group of the American Medical Informatics Association (AMIA) and the World Health Organization (WHO). We acknowledge the early and ongoing support of the Symposium by the Texas Nurses' Education and Research Foundation, as well as the encouragement and enthusiastic support from nursing colleagues internationally.

Excellent technical and support services were provided by the Continuing Education Department of the School of Nursing, under the direction of Marilyn Pattillo, and the staff of the Center for Health Care Research and Evaluation, Kaye Abikhaled and Julia Bedrich. Helpful editorial guidance was kindly provided by the staff of Elsevier.

SCIENTIFIC PROGRAM COMMITTEE

Elly S. P. Pluyter-Wenting, Chair (The Netherlands)
Ulla Gerdin (Sweden)
Susan J. Grobe (USA)
Evelyn J. Hovenga (Australia)
Kathleen A. McCormick (USA)
Marianne Tallberg (Finland)

USA ORGANIZING COMMITTEE

Susan J. Grobe, Chair
Virginia K. Saba, Vice-Chair
William L. Holzemer
Carole I. Hudgings
Judith G. Ozbolt
Judith S. Ronald
Harriet H. Werley
Rita D. Zielstorff

PROCEEDINGS EDITORIAL BOARD

Susan J. Grobe (USA)
Elly S. P. Pluyter-Wenting (The Netherlands)

KEYNOTE ADDRESS

Open Systems; perspective or fata morgana ?

Bakker A R

BAZIS Foundation, Schipholweg 97, 2316XA Leiden, The Netherlands

First the term "open systems" is discussed; various aspects of openness are considered. It is observed that there is in general a positive appreciation of the term, however, its meaning is vague, leading to confusion. For five aspects the stage of realisation is analysed.

The development of information systems is briefly reviewed. Until now developments have been realized mainly by progress in hardware, communication facilities and system software. For systems to be "open" major developments in standardization are required. Such standardization is by nature a slow process, where too early standardization might hamper the progress in functionality.

The paper concludes that efforts to gradually realize fully open systems are needed and worthwhile. However, for the coming decade we should live with severe restrictions on openness.

1. Introduction

While in the past decade integration of an information system was considered to be its most important characteristic, nowadays the most important characteristic seems to be "openess".

When the term "open" is used one should always ask what is meant; the following meanings are found:
- the possibility to communicate with other systems,
- the possibility to extract data for external use,
- the possibility to import data from external systems in the database,
- the possibility to run the system on different hardware platforms,
- the possibility to extend an information system with modules from an other supplier.

For each of these five meanings it will be discussed in this paper to what extent they can be realized and what the principle problems and limitations are.

First the developments in information technology are considered, it will be found that most major steps forward were based on mere progress in technology. For some of the essential aspects of openess however non-technical ingredients like concensus of users and standardization will turn out to be indispensable.

Anyhow the term "open" has very positive associations when used in relation to health information systems. Such a positive association is not obvious when comparing with other appearances of the word "open" in our vocabulary. The following examples demonstrate that the adjective open may have both positive and negative meanings: open mind, open gate, open dike, open wound.

2. Developments in Information Technology

2.1 Operating systems, functionality

Initially computers were organized to carry out one task (program) from begin to end. Soon it turned out that the control of input/output devices was complicated and could not be left to each programmer, so the idea "operating system" arose: software that could carry out a number of management tasks for the programmer and in particular could act as an intermediary in dealing with peripheral devices. The operating system was in general supplied by the manufacturer of the computer and specific for each type of computer.

To ease the handling of computer tasks the concept batch programming was developed: a collection of tasks was offered to the computer to be handled consecutively without human intervention, the next program was started (by the operating system) when its predecessor was finished. Already in that phase of development the word "open" was introduced: a distinction was made between so-called "closed shops", where users had to submit their computer tasks at a desk, and "open shops", where users could feed the tasks into the computer themselves.

The jobs in a batch could have quite different requirements for the computer resources. This meant initially that if a heavy task had to be carried out all easy tasks behind it had to wait until the heavy task was finished. The introduction of the principle of multiprogramming brought a significant improvement. This principle means that more tasks are loaded in the computer besides each other, each competing for the computer resources. When the task being executed has to wait for a peripheral device another task could get the CPU at its disposal. To prevent monopolization of the computer by a heavy task the mechanism was introduced that after consuming a certain amount of resource capacity the other tasks were given a chance to get this resource. The consequence of this principle is that light tasks will finish quicker. Also by utilizing the waiting time for resources the efficiency could be improved. Although the principle is simple, its application lead to a significant increase of the complexity of the operating system.

In section 2.3 the further developments of operating systems, triggered by datacommunication facilities will be presented

2.2 Programming languages

Initially each developer/manufacturer of a computer invented its own set of instructions that that specific computer could carry out. This is still the case, different computers have different instruction sets. The major development in this respect has been that this specific internal instruction set has become hidden for the users (in almost all situations).

An important step to reduce the dependency on a specific type of computer was the introduction of symbolic high level programming languages for the formulation of the task that had to be carried out. These were initially developed to make programming easier and less error prone, however by standardization of the languages the programs could in principle after compilation (by a computer-specific translation program that converted the symbolic description into computer instructions) be run on different computers. The main so-called third generation programming languages like COBOL, FORTRAN, PASCAL (and to a lesser extent BASIC and MUMPS) have achieved a reasonable level of standardization, be it that vendors are tempted to add additional facilities, in that way reducing the portability of the programs.

It is surprising to see that for the so-called fourth generation languages (that claim to reduce the programming effort, at least for applications of limited complexity) no standardization exists at all ! Software described in such languages is dependent on the supplier of the system software that can transform the programs to executable code. Several vendors offer their fourth generation languages for more than one computer platform, so the dependency on the computer manufacturer is not so much a point of concern.

2.3 Data communication facilities

Another important development is the posssibility to connect peripheral devices at distance using datacommunication techniques. Initially keyboard/printer terminals were introduced, followed later by keyboard/display combinations. Nowadays a wide range of remote devices is available. With such terminals remote access became possible, another aspect of "openess". Users did not have to go to the computer centre, the computer could be accessed from a remote location.

Although remote batch facilities were already attractive, the idea interactive processing, combined with the principle of time-sharing was another major step forward. Interactive means that the computer program asks input from the user at his terminal/workstation and reacts to this input quickly. The principle of timesharing is to assign in a cyclic way small amounts of resources to those users who need it. The principle works when users are a significant percentage of the time in a waitstate, either because they are preparing new input or are receiving output and in addition to that ask in general only for limited amounts of the computer resources (in particular the CPU). By taking account of their previous use of the resources, many users can be served simultaneously with a fast response for users that require only limited amounts of capacity.

Most hospital information systems in practical use are based on the principle of a central configuration maintaining a large database to which a large number of interactive terminals/workstations are connected via datacommunication facilities. The central configuration may consist of several computers sharing the workload; the datacommunication facilities may extend beyond the borders of one hospital.

With the appearance of PC networks an approach to system set-up has come up where an application is split-up in three parts: user communication, processing, database handling. The three parts can be implemented on different computers. This approach is often described as client/server architecture. It increases the possibilities to add capacity when needed. When the interfaces between the parts are standardized it leads to increased flexibility with respect to the computer equipment used, another aspect of openess.

2.4 Standardization in system software

System software and in particular operating systems were until recently manufacturer and computer specific. Since the system software offers the application programs access to computer facilities the construction of the programs is influenced by the operating system used. By consequence even programs formulated in standardized third generation programming languages are not easily portable to another computer. In addition to that the operating system determines the working methods around the computer configuration of both operators and system managers. Changing the operating system and other system software has turned out to be a major operation. The UNIX operating system, initiated by Bell labs [1] lead to a quite different scene. UNIX is intended to be an operating system that can be used on a wide variety of computers. Although it has taken a long time since the initiation of the UNIX development in the early seventies, nowadays most vendors offer a UNIX operating system for their computers. Siginificant progress has been made in standardization of UNIX, unfortunately there are still small but significant differences between the UNIX versions offered. Nevertheless when UNIX is used the porting of applications from one computer to another has become much easier. For porting of applications standards are required that describe the interfaces between applications and the system software, until now UNIX is the best (be it not an ideal) example of such standardisation. For other system software still a lot of standardization work has to be done.

2.5 System interconnection

In communication several pieces of equipment play a part, for a harmonious cooperation standardization is a must. For telephone communication the importance of such standardization was recognized long ago. The international organisation CCITT took care of the standards. The results achieved in this field are impressive, reliable telephone communication all around the world is a well accepted and appreciated reality.

In the informatics field besides communication between terminals and computers we need also the mutual communication of computers. For such communication the ISO developed its Open Systems Interconnection model (ISO 7498) [2]. This model distinguishes seven levels in the comunication (see fig 1). Nowadays this is a well-known and widely standard, it is important to bear in mind that it has taken considerable time to arrive at this stage of acceptance. The first draft was produced in 1978, the standard was internationally accepted in 1984, in the mean time standards have been developed for the lower levels (like TCP/IP for level 2 and 3), standardization at the application layer (level 7) is still rudimentary. For health care aplications HL7 (health level 7) [3] made a significant contribution to standardization especially in the USA, in Europe CEN TC251 is involved in standardization.

Nowadays technical interconnection of computers is possible and standardized to a large extent, so *data* can be exchanged. To allow for *information* exchange a mutual understanding of the meaning of the data is required, the problems involved will be discussed in the next chapter.

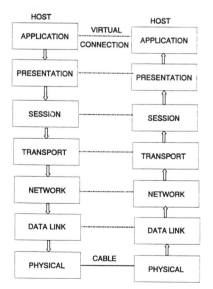

Figure 1: *The ISO reference model, which reduces the communication problem to seven sub-*

2.6 Assessment of the developments in information technology

This brief overview of developments in information technology makes clear that significant progress has been achieved, the general tendency is that by standardization the dependency on the supplier of a specific piece of technology has been reduced considerably. Standardization is at hand for third generation programming languages, a database query language (SQL) and the UNIX operating system; for fourth generation languages no such standardization is available, use of such tools implies dependency on the supplier of the tool.

For interconnection of systems standardisation is available at the technical level.

Standardisation in system software has taken a tremendous effort and the result is far from complete, there are competing standards ,for several aspects the standards are missing. Some standards are formally approved and public, others are de facto and proprietory.

For almost all available standards holds that they deal with the technical level and have been developed with involvement of large industries that can afford to invest in this activity. In the sequel of this paper we will find that open applications will require standards at a different level. Looking at the difficulty to arrive at standards for system software the question arises how and at what speed the additional standards needed can be developed, accepted and implemented.

3. Aspects of openess, level of realization

3.1 Approach to openess

In chapter 1 five aspects of openess have been mentioned. Taking account of the developments in information technology as briefly described in chapter 2 in this chapter each of the aspects will be discussed, problems will be identified.

3.2 Possibility to communicate with other systems

Thanks to the OSI model a lot of progress has been made in the interconnection of systems. Exchange of data, especially at file level is technically possible. This does not necessarily mean that in practice such data exchange is easy to realize, however the technical problems can be overcome.

In concrete information systems the coupling is not intended for the exchange of *data* but for the exchange of *information*. To exchange information a common meaning has to be assigned to the data, this is a non-trivial requirement. This may be illustrated by a comparison with the telephone communication. Even a perfect reproduction of the sounds produced at the other side of the connection is not sufficient to be able to understand each other; the persons using the telephone connection need to understand each others language. Telephone calls to Japan are no technical problem at all, however for me English as a common language is required (non-trivial !). In addition to that for communication a shared base of background knowledge is required; for me for instance messages on antique Chinese porcelain do not convey information, even when formulated in the English language.

So in principle communication between systems is possible (the technology is there) however to be able to use it effectively a number of boundary conditions need to be satisfied. These boundary conditions are not so much in the domain of information technology but rather in the application domain: standards for messages and standard data definitions are missing.

Because our health care was and is in general supplied by institutions that work almost completely in isolation the need to fulfil these crucial conditions was not there until recently, so no effort was made in this respect. If we look at the long delivery time of standards in the field of information technology, where standardization is an important aspect in the minds of the main players, one should not be too optimistic about the time it will take to create the necessary climate for fruitful information exchange between health care information systems.

3.3 The possibility to extract data for external use

A system can also be considered closed if the data contained in its database can only be accessed via its own programs, so in the way precooked by the designers of the system.

In most systems we find nowadays facilities for flexible querying of the database. In that sense the systems are opening. Storing the data retrieved in a file and exporting the data is technically possible and opens the gate to external processing. However, to be able to ask for the data one should know what data are stored in the system and what their meaning is; for this a data dictionary system can be of great help. To be able to process the query a directory system that keeps track of the way the data is stored internally can reduce the effort involved considerably. Such data dictionary/directory systems (DD/DS) [4] are not yet widely available. Without a good data description the risk for misinterpretation of the data retrieved is high.

Even when a data dictionary is available one should be very careful with the use of the data outside the context of the information system where they were recorded. The data have been collected in a certain context and should be analysed with this context in mind.

Information stored in health information systems very often is of a confidential nature. The data should be accessible only to authorized users who have a need to know. In most western countries there is a Dataprotection Law. Although there are differences in detail the general principles of the Recommendation R(81) Council of Europe Regulation for Automated Medical Data Banks [5] are in general taken as guiding principle.

The present information systems in health care have facilities for authentication of users. Based on the access rights of the users and their involvement in the care/cure of the patient it is checked whether a requested access is allowed. General query facilities are a potential danger to the privacy of the patients, the authentication of the user of the facility may still be carried out, however only very global checks on the authorization can be performed. When the extracted data are transported as a file to an external system the further processing of the data is outside the control of the system where the data were initially registered. By refined analysis facilities privacy threatening information might be derived even from data that are at first sight anonymous. Rules should be defined how query facilities and export of files has to be controlled. Confidentiality sets limits to openess.

The conclusion of this section is that extraction of data is becoming possible and technically easier, there are however many pitfalls in the interpretation of the data outside the context in which they were generated/collected. When personal data are stored in the system the confidentiality of the data should be taken into account when answering queries to the database. From the point of view of confidentiality the systems should not be fully "open" there should be a gatekeeper controlling access.

3.4 The possibility to import data from external systems in the database

An organisation will often have more than one information system. Even when the organisation is committed to the concept of an integrated system there will be or will come other systems with specific functions. Because the systems are supporting the same organisation there will be a need to use data collected by one system within an other. This may be illustrated by the example of a hospital using a dedicated ECG analysis system besides an integrated HIS, the latter having the objective to gradually include an Electronic Patient Record (EPR). The results of the ECG analysis should be contained in such an EPR. So there is a need to import the ECG analysis outcome in the HIS database and offer these results as a component of the EPR.

With present day database management systems the definition of a new record type "Result of ECG analysis" should not be too difficult. In addition, most software systems have file import/export facilities, so it seems easy to export a file with ECG analysis results and load the records to the database of the other system. The following details may illustrate that even for this simple case the realization is not obvious although the technology in the system software is assumed to be available:

- first of all it should be clear what is meant by each data item recorded; it turns out that even for entities that at first sight seem to be trivial an accurate definition is missing leading to confusion; e.g. diagnosis, location, address, etc.
- the ECG results should refer to a patient, so the patient should be uniquely identified. If the HIS uses a unique patient identification number this number should be recorded within the ECG system when the analysis is carried out. If the ECG analysis system uses a different way of identification the mapping is far from trivial;
- it should be guaranteed that all new results recorded in the ECG system are really received and stored in the HIS, also when the system might go down during the transmission of the results file; if the result in the ECG system is updated/modified, this modification should be transmitted as well;
- if the record not only consists of plain text, but also holds coded fields, e.g. for requesting departments, specialists or diagnoses, the code tables in both systems should be kept compatible, mutations in such reference files should also be communicated. This situation becomes more complex if the codes are also used by other applications;
- the records not only have to be stored, they also have to be presented (as part of the EPR), for ECG analysis this may be simple; for laboratory results this is less obvious, especially when they are to be presented in relation to other test results (cumulative reporting).

The situation becomes principally more complicated if the same type of record or even data item may be recorded in different systems and the data are afterwards collected in one database. Although each of the systems can be expected to carry out tests for validity and consistency, these tests will not be identical, so when the data are imported the

consistency and validity of the data in the receiving database is at stake. In principle this might be solved by chanelling the data from the external system through the same tests as the receiving system usually carries out. Although this sounds logical it is not easy:
- most systems are not organised to carry out these tests on records received from external sources, the tests being interwoven with the conversational recording of the data;
- if the tests can be carried out, what to do if the tests lead to an error message that is expected to be handled conversationally ?

3.5 The possibility to run the system on different hardware platforms

With the increasing functionality of health care information systems the importance for the functioning of the organisation is increasing. Already now or in the near future the system will be vital for the organisation. This vital dependency on the system leads to the question how dependent the organisation is on a specific supplier. In case the system can only run on specific computers there is such a dependency on the supplier of those computers. The possibility to run the same software on different computers is called "portability". Although such portability is seldom found in practise it is realizable at the moment if in the design and management of the system a consistent and sufficiently wide set of standards is strictly applied. Standards have to cover system software such as operating system, programming languages and database management system.

This type of openess will be facilitated by the progressing standardization in system software, especially the UNIX developments have brought portability much closer to reality. Unfortunately there are still a number of UNIX "standards".

At the application side for this portability no new standards are needed, only a strict management of the development activity. This opposed to the aspect discussed in the next section.

3.6 The possibility to extend an information system with modules from an other supplier

Within health care institutions there are significant benefits in integration of the information system [6],[7] integration has several dimensions:
- *data integration*; data recorded within one application are stored in a database and used by other applications; this requires a common data definition;
- *functional integration*; towards users functions belonging to different applications can be offered as a coherent service;
- *technical integration*; all services can be accessed through a coherent technical infrastructure; one terminal/workstation being the gate to the services.

Health information systems are complex and large. The development of an integrated HIS requires several hundreds of manyears. To be able to deal with its complexity the system is divided in subsystems, e.g. laboratory system, pharmacy system, appointment system, order management, stock control, etc. There are three reasons why it would be attractive to be able to combine modules from different suppliers:
- complete systems for large institutions don't exist, there are always applications missing that one would like to add,
- in the market an other supplier may offer software for a certain application that would be preferred over the one offered by the main supplier of the system;
- when introducing a new information system one might want to maintain some existing applications, e.g. the laboratory information system.

Building a coherent system from modules of different suppliers is at the moment an illusion, this would require a widely accepted agreement on the allocation of functions to the different subsystems. Such an agreement does not exist, there even is no proposal. This seems surprising and some consultants and suppliers suggest the opposite, however considering a concrete mature application like a laboratory system demonstrates that even for such a well established application there is no common interpretation of its main functionality as can be illustrated bu the following questions:
- is billing a function within this application or is it to be carried out by the billing subsystem ?
- is result reporting a part of this subsystem or is it to be carried out by the reporting subsystem ?
- is order registration a function within this subsystem or is it to be carried out by the order management subsystem, or by the nursing subsystem ?

For application software from different suppliers, even when they are based on the same system software environment and run on the same computer our expectations for combining modules should be modest. With significant efforts we might manage to couple, however integration is an illusion unless in the design of the modules the future integration has been foreseen.

Of course the possibility to be able to combine modules would be marvellous, however bear in mind that in the automobile industry (that is much more mature) the possibilities for such combination of modules from different suppliers is still very limited. First a tremendous amount of effort has to be invested in producing a sensible proposal for standards of decomposition of systems in subsystems with well-defined interfaces and with a standard data definition. Next it will require even more effort to get such standards implemented. Such efforts definitely are worthwhile on the long run and should be given a high priority by the organisations of health care professionals, however don't expect the possibility to flexibly combine software modules of different suppliers, leading to an integrated system, before the year 2005.

4. Discussion

It was found that there are different aspects of openess. This often leads to confusion in discussions on the realization of openess. The stage of realization for these aspects was found to be different, in this chapter an overview is given of the findings from chapters two and three.

The development of information technology has lead to a situation where systems are accessible from the working location, they can be directly integrated in the daily activities. Interconnection of systems has become technically feasible, however to exchange information in a useful way still a lot has to be done; here considerable efforts will be needed to arrive at standard data definitions for the data items used in health care and to get those standards implemented.

Extracting data for further processing by other systems not only requires these standards but also requires provisions to be able to cope in a responsible manner with the confidential nature of the information.

Importing in the database data collected by external systems is still confronted with significant complications partly of a technical nature, but more importantly in the field of quality and consistency of the data.

Porting application software from one platform to another is feasible only if in the design and management of the system standards for system software interfaces are carefully selected and maintained. So a certain level of openess can be achieved here. One should realise that the dependency on the supplier of the application software is not reduced by such openess.

For the time being it is an illusion to expect to be able to build an integrated system by combining modules of different suppliers. This would require not only standards on data definition but also a widely accepted standard for decomposition of an integrated system into subsystems, with well-defined interfaces between the modules. If such standard will ever come it will take many years to get it approved and again many years to get it implemented in the products of the suppliers of health information systems.

5.Conclusion

If all aspects of openess were realized such open systems would compare to the present situation as an oasis to a desert. We all would like to be in the oasis.

However, one should not have too high expectations as to openess. In some respects it can be realized. For other aspects we know that it is somewhere, like the oasis seen in a fata morgana, it seems closer than it really is. It is a perspective but our view is distorted, we don't know how to reach it.

Like in the desert the fata morgana gives hope to the traveller, however, like in the desert it is dangerous to change the route. We better can be on the safe side and use available resources in a responsible manner. In the meantime trying to check whether the palm trees we see in the distance are really reachable.

References

[1]   Ritchie DM and Thompson K. The UNIX Time-Sharing System. *Communications of the ACM* 1974, 17: 365-375.

[2]   Information Processing Systems-Open Systems Interconnection- Basic Reference Model ISO 7498-1984; International Organization for Standardization, 1984.

[3]   Health Level Seven, an application protocol for electronic data exchange in healthcare environments. Health Level Seven Inc, Ann Arbor, Michigan, 1991.

[4]   Hooymans M and Liefkes H. Meta information management for a large, integrated HIS. In: MIE 93. Reichert A, Sadan, BA, Bengtsson S, Bryant J and Piccolo U (eds). London: Freund Publishing House, 1993:698-702.

[5]   Council of Europe Regulations for Automated Medical Data Banks. Recommendations R(81). Strasbourg, 1981.

[6]   Leguit FA. The Case: Leiden University Hospital Information Systems. In: PROCS of the IFIP IMIA Working Conference Towards New Hospital Information Systems, Nijmegen The Netherlands. Bakker AR, Ball M, Scherrer JR and Willems JL (Eds.) North Holland, Amsterdam, 1988, 59-64.

[7]   Leguit FA. Interfacing Integration. In: PROCS of the IMIA Working Conference Trends in Modern Hospital Information Systems: Scope-Design-Architecture. Bakker AR, Ehlers C, Bryant JR and Hammond WE (eds). North Holland, Amsterdam, 1991, 141-148.

Section I

ADMINISTRATION

A. General topics

Nursing Informatics: An International Overview for Nursing in a Technological Era
S.J. Grobe and E.S.P. Pluyter-Wenting, eds.

Information Technology Developments: Issues for Nursing

Nagle LM[a] Shamian J[a] Catford P[b]

[a]*Gerald P. Turner Department of Nursing, Mount Sinai Hospital,*
 600 University Avenue, Toronto, Ontario CANADA M5G 1X5

[b]*Information Services Department, Mount Sinai Hospital,*
 600 University Avenue, Toronto, Ontario CANADA M5G 1X5

This paper will focus on issues related to the need for increased sophistication in the development of comprehensive, integrated clinical information systems. Critical issues for future system developments are described and include those which are informational, technical, and organizational in nature. The need to develop a corporate view to the advancement of wholly integrated hospital/clinical information systems is crucial in moving systems into the future. Moreover, the notion of re-engineering existing practice expands the possibilities for integrating multi-dimensional technological applications and truly add value to the sphere of nursing practice.

1. Introduction

In literature of recent years, nurse authors have used the term *"information technology"* synonymously with automation and computerization. The phrase "nursing information system" has been used by many to generically describe systems which support nursing activities in administration, practice, research, and education. According to Saba and McCormick [1], a nursing information system is:

"a computer system that collects, stores, processes, retrieves, displays, and communicates timely information needed to do the following: administer the nursing services and resources in a health care facility; manage standardized patient care information for the delivery of nursing care; link the research resources and educational applications to nursing practice" (p. 120).

The conceptual elements of a nursing information system have been described by several nurse authors [2,3,4] Moreover, models have been proposed to assist organizations in defining their nursing information system requirements [5,6]. Although these conceptualizations and designs have served nursing well in advancing an understanding of nursing's needs for informational support, the time has come to move into a new era of technological possibilities.

Health care has lagged behind other industries in the adoption of new information technologies, but hospital administrators and government officials have demonstrated an increased interest in having access to quality clinical and financial information. In fact, the demands of current and future health care delivery models are dictating a new era of information management support.

These authors advance the notion that striving for a "nursing" information system per se will not be sufficient to carry nurses into the 21st century. Indeed, we need to redefine nursing's informational requirements within the contexts of: future health care delivery, the notion of integrated systems, and innovative applications of available technologies. For the purposes of this paper, information technology refers to all manner of data and information management, manual and automated systems, and communication devices as used by nurses in the performance of their work.

2. Nurses and Information Technology

Information technology is being used daily by nurses working in diverse roles and settings. Nurse administrators use information technology to capture and measure nursing workload, to support the management of human and fiscal resources, and for the purposes of quality assurance monitoring. The specific tools employed range from a simple adaption of a spreadsheet application (e.g. LOTUS 1-2-3) to the purchase of a sophisticated standalone or integrated system application (e.g. unit-based nursing workload linked to staffing and patient costing).

Information technology has been incorporated into the provision of patient care through the automation of clinical activities including: order entry, nursing care planning, and documentation. Although such systems are increasingly desirable, a very small percentage of health care organizations in North America had implemented a clinical information repository system.

Additional benefits of information technology are being realized in meeting the learning needs of nurses and patients. Nursing research activities such as data retrieval and statistical analyses have also been expedited through the use of information technology.

Historically, a majority of hospitals made the decision to purchase and implement *clinical* information systems because of the need to improve the timeliness and accuracy of documentation and the efficiency of inter-departmental communication. It would appear that these goals have been achieved within most organizations that have implemented hospital-wide systems.

3. Outcomes Realized

Based upon interviews with nurse administrators (n = 12) from Canadian and U.S. hospitals, there are some common perceptions of the benefits derived from clinical information systems to date [7]. The most consistently cited outcomes include: (a) the standardization of practice by providing clear guidelines for documentation and an up-to-date policy and procedure reference, (b) more attention to accountability for practice, (c) increased precision of documentation, and most commonly, (d) decreased clerical tasks performed by nursing staff. Some administrators also reported a reduction in medication errors and a decrease in disputes between individuals (e.g. between nurses and physicians with regard to physician orders) and departments (e.g. the system provides confirmation of specimens being received in the labs).

Changes relevant to nursing administration were reported to include: (a) a decrease in costs related to overtime - because of less time being spent charting at the end of shifts, (b) the ability to assign cost of nursing services per case type, (c) the ability to satisfy accreditation requirements, and (d) improved legibility and completeness of patient records.

Several attitude changes were reported as a direct result of introducing a clinical information system. Nurses became more acutely aware of the need to preserve "hands on care"; the humanistic components of practice. Some staff became more acutely aware of confidentiality issues relevant to patient information. Whether fully computerized or not, most reported the development of a dependency on the system; this had become most evident during system downtime. For some administrators, this dependency translated into a need for staff education about the system's fallibility. Others reported that in some instances nurses were overly confident in the accuracy of system inputs and outputs (e.g. physician orders). In these situations, the need to scrutinize computerized data was stressed as being no different than in the world of manual systems. Despite these changes and improvements in the efficiency of information flow, administrators reported that nurses were experiencing information overload worse than in pre-system days. In many ways more documentation was being required, resulting in more paper and more information to process on a daily basis.

Disappointments with the limitations of existing systems and a demand for more technology and specific applications has begun to surface in institutions with a relatively long system history (greater than 10 years). The results reported by the administrators in these institutions suggests that the original purpose of systems dictated the outcomes. There were improvements in documentation and communication, and the processing of certain kinds of information had become more efficient. Enhancements to clinical practice and improved patient outcomes were not identified as part of the benefits realization.

Nurses have indicated that they want to see system developments which: (a) increase the focus on clinical practice, (b) increase the meaningfulness of clinical data, and (c) support clinical decision-making. Fully exploiting the possibilities of information technology for nursing, necessitates moving beyond the traditional conceptualizations of a nursing information system to that of an integrated clinical information system.

4. Integrated Clinical Information System

The term "nursing information system" is limiting in a hospital environment with a multi-disciplinary, multi-departmental patient care focus. A hospital information system in its entirety will be comprised of many inter- and intra-departmental applications designed to supply necessary patient-related information to serve corporate administrative and clinical patient-care functions. A clinical information system is integral to the overall hospital information system, has applications which are unique to nursing and others which derive data elements from complementary applications in other departments/disciplines.

The concept of "integrated systems" is becoming a familiar phrase in the health informatics literature [8,9]. Many existing hospital systems are comprised of several different systems supporting patient care and typically require several entries of the same data. The principle of integration implies that each patient data element is entered into a system with minimal replication and is accessible to all health care providers as necessary.

Ideally, nursing applications should be developed as components of an integrated clinical information system. Patient specific data are the focal point of integrated systems. Considering the multiple sources and users of patient data such a system would provide a common database accessible to all care providers. An integrated system would also support the recent trend of a case management approach to patient care. Clearly there is much patient data which is not exclusive to nursing. There is, however, a need to ascertain those components which are the exclusive responsibility of nursing. Such identification will expedite a more efficient and non-redundant collection of patient information. An integrated patient care system needs to accommodate various levels of users. Not only are the users of an integrated system professionally diverse, they may also be practising at varying levels of expertise, from the in-house trained technician or aide to the clinical specialist in nursing, medicine, pharmacy, etc. Clinical information systems should: (a) make expert knowledge accessible to the practitioner, (b) provide cues to enhance practice and optimize patient care outcomes, and (c) assimilate practice and research findings to guide the nurse in day to day practice.

5. Critical Issues for Informatization

"Informatization" is the synergistic integration of computer, nursing, and information science which facilitates the generation of new knowledge for nursing practice [10]. Clinical information system developments should be driven by the ultimate goal of informatization: the management of outcomes. The successful attainment of informatization in clinical care delivery settings will be contingent upon an understanding of the informational requirements of care providers and the possibilities for meeting those needs given existing technology. Issues of an informational, technological, and organizational nature will need to be addressed in order to achieve such an understanding. The central leadership role of nursing in addressing these issues and the application of state of the art technology to clinical settings are identified as focal to realizing the epitome of an integrated clinical information system.

5.1 Informational

With increasing sophistication and insight, nurse researchers are attempting to disentangle and understand the complex processes of nurses' clinical decision-making [11,12]. Several nurses have addressed the relative value of computerized decision support tools for nursing practice [13,14,15,16]. Although there is a plethora of literature on decision-making, an understanding of the elements of information processing, clinical inference, and intuitive knowledge in nursing remains somewhat elusive. In the future, systems modelled on these processes will indeed simplify the tasks of organizing and interpreting clinical data, and hopefully result in more efficient and efficacious patient outcomes.

5.2 Technical

For many organizations, no matter which generation or configuration of information system was selected, the technology seemed to be outmoded within a few short months of implementation, if not purchase. The occurrence of premature obsolescence has been largely due to a propensity to under-resource these projects. Anticipating future technological advances and strategically designing a system infrastructure to allow for the integration of new technologies has been and continues to be a major challenge for information systems personnel and health care providers. The technical elements of data capture, processing, storage, and retrieval capacities will likely continue to evolve, becoming less costly with increased capabilities in multiple orders of magnitude. In the future, we can expect a clinical information system with the technical flexibility which allows for non-sequential/multi-dimensional access to data.

Health care administrators are demanding increased system efficiency and immediate access to quality information. Care providers are seeking system support to ease the burden of increased clinical complexity in environments of declining human resources. Therefore, clinical information systems need to be designed such that meaningful information is accessible by whoever needs it, whenever they need it, and where ever they need it. The key elements of clinical information for technical consideration are accessibility, portability, and user-defined data.

5.2.1 Accessibility

Evaluations of automated systems to support nursing information management have yet to provide a convincing argument for either central or bedside as a preferred location of access. We advance the notion of a compact, wholly portable device, with two-way communication for data entry, retrieval, and management. Moreover, as bio-technical research continues to develop improved, non-invasive, cost-effective patient monitoring/assist devices, increasing volumes of clinical data will be readily available to care providers.

5.2.2 Portability

System interaction should be possible from where ever the care provider legitimately requires access without impeding the delivery of patient care. The user interface should allow for multiple devices and modes of data entry, retrieval, and manipulation. The incorporation of multi-media capabilities (e.g. voice and image) and the accommodation of mouse, bar code, pen-based, and radio-frequency technologies will provide unprecedented opportunities in health care computing.

5.2.3 User defined data

A majority of clinical information systems have been designed on the basis of existing manual systems. Automating previous practice without evaluating re-engineering requirements adds limited value to the practice of care providers. Care providers must still sift through the volumes of data collected on individual patients and ensure that they have considered all data elements in the process of making a clinical judgement. However, if a system presented patient data and information to care providers in a manner not only unique to the scope of their practice, but also within the limits of their clinical expertise, the potential for added value would be tremendous.

5.3 Organizational

An organization's mission, philosophy, and goals should provide the foundation for the development of a philosophy of information management. Requisite to the operationalization an innovative information management philosophy is a clearly articulated strategic direction with unmitigated corporate support. A critical element of that support will be the acceptance and encouragement of process re-engineering to move the organization to successful informatization.

6. Directions for the Future

- Need for a corporate view to advance the development of wholly integrated clinical information systems.

- Need for a collaborative model between health professionals, information services, and vendors.

- Need for increased sophistication in the development of decision support tools for practice and administration. Systems should be designed to make decision support available to practitioners at all levels and incorporate current clinical data and research findings on a continuous basis.

- Need to apply new technology including multimedia and portable devices for the input, retrieval, monitoring and manipulation of data. The use of robotics should begin to provide more consistent data/information while assisting in the delivery of patient care and providing opportunities for improved process re-engineering.

7. References

[1]   Saba V K and McCormick K A. *Essentials of Computers for Nurses*. Philadelphia:J.B. Lippincott, 1986.

[2]   Gassert C A. Defining nursing information system requirements: A linked model. Proceedings: *The Thirteenth Annual Symposium on Computer Applications in Medical Care*. Washington, D.C.: IEEE Society Press, 1989:779-783.

[3]   Graves J R and Corcoran S. Design of nursing information systems: Conceptual and practice elements. *J Prof Nurs* 1988, 4:168-177.

[4]   Miller E. A conceptual model of the information requirements of nursing organizations. Proceedings: *The Thirteenth Annual Symposium on Computer Applications in Medical Care*. Washington, D.C.:IEEE Computer Society, 1989:784-788.

[5]   Rieder K A and Norton D A. An integrated nursing information system - A planning model. *Comput Nurs* 1984, 2:73-79.

[6]   Powell N. Designing and developing a computerized hospital information system. *Nursing Management* 1982, 13:40-45.

[7]   Nagle L M. The impact of computerization on nurses' thinking. *Unpublished manuscript*, 1990.

[8]   Ball M J and Douglas J V. Integration of systems for patient care. *Proceedings of Fourth International Conference on Nursing Use of Computers and Information Science*. New York: Springer-Verlag, 1991:110-114.

[9]   Korpman R A. Integrated nursing systems: The future is now. Proceedings of Fourth International Conference on Nursing Use of Computers and Information Science. New York: Springer-Verlag, 1991: Addendum.

[10] Shamian J, Nagle L M, and Hannah K J. Optimizing outcomes of nursing informatization. In *MEDINFO 92* Lun K C, Degoulet P, Piemme T E, and Rienhoff O (eds.). Amsterdam: North Holland, 1992:976-980.

[11] Corcoran S, Narayan S, and Moreland H. "Thinking aloud" as a strategy to improve clinical decision making. *Heart Lung* 1988, 17:463-468.

[12] Thiele J E, Baldwin J H, Hyde R S, Sloan B, and Strandquist G A. An investigation of decision theory: What are the effects of teaching clue recognition? *J Nurs Educ* 1986, 25:319-324.

[13] Brennan P F and McHugh M J. Clinical decision-making and computer support. *App Nurs Res* 1988, 1:89-93.

[14] Cuddigan J E, Logan S, Evans S, Hoesing H. Evaluation of an artificial-intelligence-based nursing decision support system in a clinical setting. Proceedings: Third International Symposium on Nursing Use of Computers and Information Science. St. Louis: C.V. Mosby, 1988:629-636.

[15] Henry S B, LeBreck D B, and Holzemer W L. The use of computer simulations to measure clinical decision making in nursing. Proceedings: Third International Symposium on Nursing Use of Computers and Information Science. St.Louis: C.V. Mosby, 1988:485-491.

[16] Sinclair V G. Potential effects of decision support systems on the role of the nurse. *Comput Nurs* 1990, 8:60-65.

Nursing Informatics: An International Overview for Nursing in a Technological Era
S.J. Grobe and E.S.P. Pluyter-Wenting, eds.

Organizational Priorities for the
Nursing Informatics Specialist

Mills M E[a] and Braun R[a]

[a]University of Maryland School of Nursing, 655 W. Lombard Street, Baltimore, Maryland 21201.

As tertiary care institutions invest major financial and human resources in computer support systems, the challenge for the nurse administrator is how to best identify organization wide and nursing specific information and technology needs and how to best organize, coordinate and develop information system management. Due to the rapid increase with which nurses are using information technology to assist them in performing more sophisticated and complex duties, many institutions have developed a Nursing Informatics Specialist position or Nursing Information System Coordinator role.

This paper reports the results of a national study which was conducted to identify the most effective organizational placement and use of the Nursing Informatics Specialist (NIS), the perceived needs of nurses relative to information technology as identified by Vice Presidents of Nursing (VPN) and the relationship of current and future organizational priorities for NIS activities.

The study was based on responses of VPNs at more than one hundred (100) tertiary care hospitals over 500 beds in size located across the United States. Results have indications for the establishment of organizational placement and role expectations for the NIS and directions for the further development of nursing staff with regard to information systems.

1. Nursing Information System Specialist

Healthcare computing is increasingly being developed to support clinical and administrative nursing information requirements. The challenge for the nurse administrator is how to best organize, coordinate and develop information system management. At this point in time, nursing departments are being asked to examine the potential of automating information processing functions related to patient care on nursing units and to assist with hospitalwide information system development, education, implementation, evaluation and upgrading [1, 2].

Hannah [3] has defined nursing informatics as the use of information technologies in relation to the functions which are within the purview of nursing and are carried out by the nurse in the care of patients or in the educational preparation of individuals to practice the disciplines. As described by Schwirian [4], nursing informatics includes the use of information management technologies to facilitate nursing practice, education, administration and research. Graves and Corcoran [5] further identified nursing informatics as the combination of computer science, information science and nursing science to assist in the management and processing or transformation of nursing data, information and knowledge. The role activities of practicing nurses, educators, researchers, and administrators were described by Grobe [6] in relation to informatics competencies.

Due to the rapid increase with which nurses are using information technology to assist them in performing more sophisticated and complex duties, many nurses have been placed in the role of nursing information system coordinator [7]. This role was specifically developed to create and support information systems for use in health care settings which will meet the needs of users [8].

Romano and Heller [9] cited four activities as being basic functions to the NIS role:

1. Identification of the properties, structure, use, and flow of clinical and management information from the patient, to the health care provider, and subsequently throughout the health care organization.
2. Assessment of real and potential problems related to the communication, accessibility, availability, and use of information for clinical and administrative decision-making.
3. Determination of alternative methods of information handling and of system design options.
4. Evaluation of the cost/risks in relation to the benefits or effectiveness of information technologies.

The conceptual framework (Figure 1) driving the NIS Organizational Priority study includes the influences of NIS educational level and organizational position, available information systems applications and use by nursing staff, and organizational priorities for the NIS on perceived system effectiveness and NIS role activities.

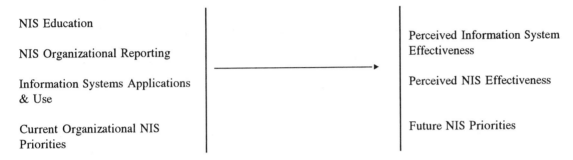

Figure 1. NIS Organizational Priorities and Effectiveness

2. Survey of NIS Organizational Priorities

In an effort to identify how nursing information management functions are currently structured in large tertiary care hospitals, Vice Presidents of Nursing in tertiary care hospitals over 500 beds in size were surveyed by mailed questionnaire. The objectives of the survey were three fold. First, to examine organizational placement, use and perceived effectiveness of the organizational placement, use and perceived effectiveness of the NIS. Second, to identify information systems applications and the level of their use by nursing staff and managers. And third, to explore current and future organizational priorities for the NIS.

Surveys were organized into five sections: demographics of NIS' and VPNs; actual use of time by the NIS; current and future organizational priorities for NIS role functions; NIS organizational reporting relationships and perceived effectiveness, and information systems status.

Surveys were mailed to all tertiary care hospitals over 500 beds in size located in the United States. It was felt that this group of hospitals would have more resources to invest in information systems, be more complex in structure and have a greater diversity of information system applications to drive the identification of organizational priorities.

The American Hospital Association identified a total of 302 tertiary care hospitals, over 500 beds in size. These hospitals were surveyed by mailed questionnaire in February, 1993. The questionnaire included 17 items and took approximately 15 to 20 minutes to complete. It was composed of 10 personal and organizational demographic questions, 3 NIS organizational priorities scales, 3 information system/NIS effectiveness scales and 1 scale measuring availability and multidisciplinary use of specific information system applications. Survey questions were based on the results of a pilot study conducted using a national expert panel in 1992 for this purpose. Confidentiality of study data was guaranteed by not collecting identifying information as to the name of respondents or their hospitals.

3. Results

Responses were received from 111 individuals holding top leadership responsibilities for nursing services. This represented a response rate of 37 per cent. Although the response rate was modest, the number of responses was sufficient to conduct data analysis based on 15 items per predictor variable [10]. Analysis was conducted using descriptive and correlational statistics, analysis of variance and t-tests.

Responses were received from all 9 geographic areas of the United States The greatest response was received from the Middle Atlantic (24.3%, n=27), South Atlantic (21.6% n=24), East North Central (20.7%, n=23) and East South Central (10.8%, n=12) regions. This can be attributed to the time frame within which survey returns were requested and the date of receipt due to postal delivery distance.

Of the responding hospitals, 66.7 per cent (n=74) were classified as teaching hospitals, 22.5 per cent (n=25) were classified as community hospitals, and 9.9 per cent (n=11) were classified as other - such as federal or county owned hospitals. Hospitals ranged in size from 500 to 1600 beds with a median of 644 beds.

Positions for Nursing Information Specialists were reported in 79.3 per cent (n=88) of the responding hospitals. These positions had been in place for between 1 and 16 years with a mean of 5.5 years. Most positions (65.8%), n=73) had been in place 5 years or less. Of the persons occupying positions responsible for nursing information systems, 94.2 per cent (n=104) were registered nurses. Most were educated at the Master of Science level (48.8%, n=54) with the next most common preparation at the Baccalaureate level (34.7, n=39). Education specific to the field of informatics or computer systems most frequently occurred in the form of Continuing Education workshops and conferences (65.3%, n=72). Most (64.5%, n=71) of the respondents also had some background in computers via personal use. Less than half of the respondents (47.1%, n=52) had obtained college credits in the field of computers and of these 75 per cent indicated they had achieved 12 credits (approximately 4 courses) or less.

Position titles for persons responsible for nursing information systems were widely varied. Examples of titles included: Nursing Systems Analyst; Director of Nursing Systems; Program Director Nursing Informatics; Nursing Automated Data Processing Coordinator; and, Coordinator of Information Systems. Only a few of the NIS (35.5%, n=32) had top level responsibility for organizationwide information system management. Organizationally, the NIS position most commonly reported within the Nursing Department. The Vice President for Nursing or Vice President for Nursing/Patient Care was cited most often (38.8%, n=43). Other individuals within Nursing to whom the NIS reported included the Education Director, Assistant Administrator for Nursing, and Director of Nursing Resources. Less often (23%), respondents reported outside of Nursing to positions such as the Clinical Systems Manager, Vice President for Information Services and Associate Director for Hospital Information Systems. Analysis of variance revealed no specific effect of organizational reporting relationships on perceived effectiveness of the NIS

Nursing Information Specialists were reported to be most heavily engaged in the areas of project management, staff training, implementation of clinical systems, and advisory and coordinating capacities. The top four organizational priorities listed by Chief Nurses were systems implementation, systems development, advisory and coordinating capacity and project management. Respondents indicated that the NIS works with a number of information systems applications - some of which are displayed in Table 1 along with the level of use of these systems by nursing staff

Perceived needs for additional development of information systems and related work with nursing staff by the NIS were especially focused on nursing applications. Nursing Progress Notes, Nursing Assessment, Quality Improvement, Scheduling and Care Planning had the lowest implementation rates and the lowest level of use by nursing staff.

Communication between the Chief Nurse Administrator and Nursing Information Specialist appeared to be least well developed surrounding the areas of systems planning (r = .4397; p< .01), implementation of clinical nursing systems (r = .3374; p< .01), and strategic planning (r= .3333; p< . 01). Five year future priorities were focused on systems implementation, strategic planning, systems development and coordinating capacity.

Chief Nurses specifically rated the extent to which they perceived the NIS as effectively impacting the use of information systems (IS) by clinical nurses, nursing management and physicians. The NIS was evaluated by responding Chief Nurses as having a moderate or strong influence on the use of IS by clinical nurse: 'h a frequency of 82.6 per cent (n=81). The impact of the NIS on nursing management use of IS was rated as moderate or strong by 75.2 per cent (n=73) and on physicians by 41.0 per cent (n=39) of Chief Nurse respondents.

Table 1
Systems Use by Nursing Staff

Systems	%	n	Level of Mean*	Systems SD	Use n
Adm/Discharge/Transfer	88.3	98	4.0	1.3	97
Laboratory	87.4	97	4.2	1.2	95
Radiology	75.7	84	4.1	1.3	83
Order Entry/Results	72.1	80	4.4	1.2	74
Progress Notes	18.9	21	2.0	1.5	28
Care Planning	45.0	50	3.5	1.6	53
Nurse Assessment	30.6	34	2.5	1.8	34
Nurse Scheduling	51.4	57	3.1	1.7	58
Patient Classification	73.0	81	4.0	1.5	81
Quality Improvement	31.5	35	2.5	1.5	34

*Range 1-5

4. Discussion

As a relatively new field of emphasis with broad organizational impact, Nursing Informatics positions have been adopted (albeit in different forms) by a majority of large tertiary care hospitals responding to this study. The organizational placement, position title and education of nurses responsible for nursing information systems varies widely. Based on data analysis, there does not appear to be a significant difference in job function as a direct result of organizational placement. However, the majority of respondents in the present survey reported to someone within the Nursing Department.

The actual amount of time spent in specific job functions was a reasonable, although not exact, match to current organizational priorities. While the NIS spent the greatest number of working hours in project management and staff training, the organizational priorities were focused on systems implementation and systems development. In a sense, there appears to be a process orientation on the part of the NIS and an outcome orientation on the part of the Chief Nurse Administrator. This discordance may be a source of frustration for both the NIS and CNA. There are implications for the need to increase the level of understanding of the CNA regarding the realities of informatics practice and of the NIS regarding organizational development.

Future priorities for the next five years indicated that while systems implementation would remain a focus, strategic planning will over take systems development in the order of priority. Increased attention will be placed on the planning and development of nursing information systems such as patient assessment and care planning. An investment in the education of the NIS as a key member of the nursing organization, along with careful organizational placement, clearly articulated priorities and resource support will be increasingly important.

Study respondents indicated that, at this time, the NIS is perceived as most effectively impacting the use of Information Systems by clinical nurses while having slightly less impact on nurse managers. Considering the growing emphasis of strategic planning identified within future priorities, the utilization of the NIS role to facilitate nurse manager access and use of information supportive of managerial decision making should also increase as a role priority.

12

5. References

[1]   Ball M, Hannah NJ, Jelger G and Peterson H. *Nursing Informatics Where Caring and Technology Meet*. New York: Springer-Verlag, 1988.

[2]   Behrenbeck J, Davitt P, Ironside P, Mangan D, O'Shaughnessy D, and Steele S. Strategic Planning for a Nursing Information System (NIS) in the Hospital Setting. *Computers in Nursing* 1990, 8:6 - 236-242

[3]   Hannah K J, Guillemin E J and Conklin D N. *Nursing Uses of Computers and Information Sciences*. Amsterdam: North Holland, 1985.

[4]   Schwirian P. The NI Pyramid - A Model for Research in Nursing Informatics. *Computers in Nursing* 1986, 4:3 - 134-136.

[5]   Graves, J R, & Corcoran, S (1989). The study of nursing informatics. 21:4-227-231. Image J Nurs Sch.

[6]   Grobe, S J (1989). Nursing informatics competencies. Methods Ins Med, 28:4-267-269.

[7]   Hannah NJ. Using Computers to Educate Nurses. In: *Nursing Informatics Where Caring and Technology Meet*. Ball M, Hannah NJ, Jelger G and Peterson H. (eds). New York: Springer-Verlag, 1988.

[8]   Ball M J and Hannah N. *Using Computers in Nursing*. Reston: Prentice-Hall, 1984.

[9]   Romano C and Heller B. Nursing Informatics: A Model Curriculum for an Emerging Role. *Nurse Educator* 1990, 15:2 - 16-19.

[10]   Stevens J. *Applied Multivariate Statistics for the Social Sciences*. Hillsdale, New Jersey: Lawrence Erlbaum Associates, 1986.

Nursing Informatics: An International Overview for Nursing in a Technological Era
S.J. Grobe and E.S.P. Pluyter-Wenting, eds.

13

Nursing Informatics Program in the Hospital Setting: A Model for Success

Shamian J[a] and Nagle LM[b]

[a]Vice-President, Nursing, Gerald P. Turner Department of Nursing, Mount Sinai Hospital,
  600 University Avenue, Toronto, Ontario CANADA M5G 1X5

[b]Program Director, Nursing, Nursing Informatics Program, Mount Sinai Hospital,
  600 University Avenue, Toronto, Ontario CANADA M5G 1X5

This paper describes Nursing Informatics as a key professional program in a Nursing Department's vision and structure. The Nursing Informatics Program has been focal to the achievement of the corporate vision for information systems in this organization. Leadership for the Nursing Informatics Program is provided by senior nursing personnel. The program is positioned within the corporate structure such that synergy is attained for the Nursing Department and the organization as a whole. In conjunction with other professional nursing and clinical programs, Nursing Informatics has become highly instrumental in the achievement of clinical excellence in this organization. Converging expertise from all areas of nursing practice provides the Nursing Informatics Program with a richness and diversity which reaps multiple benefits for the department.

1. Introduction

Building organizational structures to support automation is a very important component of successful automation. This paper will address the process and the factors that go into successful organizational structure for automation. Organizations need to take into account their vision, mission, and philosophy in designing their informatics organizational structure. The organization needs to articulate expectations of information processing. When these factors are carefully examined, organizations will be in a position to determine how extensive, participatory, and broad their informatics organizational structure should be. In this presentation we will describe how we structured a nursing informatics program within a complex teaching organizational structure.

2. Optimizing Informatization

An organization's vision, mission, and philosophy provide a fundamental understanding of organizational values and are pivotal in designing the informatics structure. From these elements arise the expectations of information processing within the organization. These two building blocks (1) vision, mission and philosophy, and (2) expectations of information processing can provide the foundation for articulating the optimal corporate and departmental informatics related structures for an organization.

In this paper, we use Mount Sinai Hospital in Toronto, Canada as a case in point. We will concentrate primarily on the structure of the Nursing Department with some reference to the corporate structure. The basic framework that is recommended in this paper is transferable to other departments and relevant to other corporate structures.

2.1 Organizational Structure

Mount Sinai Hospital (MSH) is a university teaching hospital with a mission to achieve excellence in practice, education and research:

> *"Mount Sinai Hospital dedicates its resources to the service of the Community for the attainment of health through compassionate high quality care. This is achieved by the integrated application of the triad of excellent patient care, education and research"*[1]

The Nursing Department does not have a separate mission statement because of the belief that the organizational mission and the Nursing Department mission are the same. The Nursing Department has a responsibility to further the organizational mission. The Nursing Department is committed to advancing a professional, academic department that shares the organization's commitment to excellence in practice, education and research.
Some principles from the Nursing Department's Vision and Philosophy are:

- A high level of staff participation at the unit and department level

- Every patient will receive excellent, knowledge-based care every time

- Practice is based on current knowledge

- Collaborative practice with other disciplines and within the discipline

- High level partnership among staff, clinical teachers, clinical nurse specialist, nurse scientist and nursing management.

Our Philosophy of Nursing Excellence positions the department to succeed in the attainment of high quality patient care by creating an atmosphere of and for excellence. Success in achieving this goal is facilitated by values which include:

- Accepting that change is a certainty and an opportunity

- Encouraging professional initiative

- Providing human, financial, physical and technological resources

- Strengthening pride and ownership in patient care

In order to understand the second key component, the expectations of information processing, it is important to understand the internal organizational structure. The corporate organizational structure is comprised of two major components: (a) a clinical program structure, and (b) departments organized under central vice presidents. This matrix structure enhances multidisciplinary partnership by allowing for cohesive corporate planning without destroying professional identities.

The Nursing Department's Structure is organized under nursing programs, and clinical programs. **Nursing Programs** include the *Professional Practice, Decentralization, Nursing Informatics, and Conceptualization programs*. **Clinical Programs** include the *Oncology/Palliative Care, Perinatology, Gastrointestinal/Perioperative Care, Clinical Specialties/Respiratory/Thoracic, and Musculoskeletal/Psychiatry* programs. The clinical nursing programs are consistent with the corporate clinical programs. Moreover, each clinical nursing program chair is an active participant if not the chair of the hospital clinical program.

2.2 Expectations of Information Processing

In examining both the vision, mission, and philosophy and the structure of the organization, it becomes apparent that within this organization we need information processing which provides:

- Both central and decentralized access to data

- Data organization by clinical programs, corporate and nursing

- Data organization by department

- Support for advanced nursing practice

- Support for the measurement of outcomes

- Decision support which is discipline specific and multidisciplinary

- Educational support

3. Role of the Nursing Informatics Program

A Nursing Informatics Program was established because of our belief that achieving a high level integration of our vision, mission, and philosophy could be facilitated by informatics expertise. Furthermore, meeting the information processing requirements of our administrative and academic commitments within the department necessitates a major emphasis on nursing informatics. *We believe that the Nursing Informatics Program will facilitate and enhance the integration and synthesis of existing and required data and information and turn it into the type of knowledge we need to meet our vision of excellence in practice, education and research.*

Within the context of our particular environment the Nursing Informatics Program is one of four professional nursing programs which guide departmental activities. As such the program is administered by a Program Director of Nursing. A large program committee provides a forum for decision-making, discussion of issues, and the dissemination and receipt of information. The members, primarily staff nurses, provide representation from all clinical programs and the other nursing programs. The principal Function of the program is to:

"Facilitate and provide leadership for the identification, development, implementation, and evaluation of information technologies which have the potential to increase the effectiveness and efficiency of nursing's clinical, administrative, educational, and research activities"

The basic assumptions which underpin the Nursing Informatics Program initiatives are as follows:

1) The notion of a Hospital Minimum Data set is fundamental to the implementation of the corporate administrative and clinical components of the hospital information system.

2) A Nursing Minimum Data Set will have administrative and clinical components and be directly linked to a Hospital Minimum Data set.

3) Nursing activities are performed in conjunction with and independent of other professional disciplines and ancillary departments. Thus, it is recognized that data exists at intra and interdepartmental levels.

4) All nursing informatics program initiatives will acknowledge, incorporate, and support each of the clinical programs and the other nursing programs.

5) Information technology will be used to support and enhance the efficiency and effectiveness of all nursing activities including those of a clinical, administrative, research, and educational nature.

6) The use of information technologies in nursing will be evolutionary.

7) When appropriate and possible, decision support will be integral to nursing system components.

The Nursing Informatics Program activities and resources are directed to support and advance the Hospital Strategic foci [1], the Nursing Department Vision and Structure and the specific initiatives related to information management within Mount Sinai Hospital (MSH). The Nursing Informatics Program advocates the adoption of information technologies which support client-focused care and the practice of nursing and optimize outcomes of patient care delivery in a cost-effective manner.

4. Nursing Informatics and Information Services

The introduction of personal computers has revolutionized the relationship between computer departments and users of the technology. The computer expert no longer controls the data and report generation; users manipulate their own data and decide how, when, and what reports will be generated. Furthermore, many nursing departments have recruited individuals with expertise in nursing and clinical computerization. What were once considered computer departments are beginning to evolve as providers of information services, not limited to computer support. Increasingly, information services departments and end-user groups such as nursing are beginning to establish collaborative partnerships in order to maximize the benefits of information technologies in health care settings.

In MSH, nursing personnel work very closely with the information services department (ISD). However, the nursing department is largely responsible for identifying priorities for informatization within the department. Priorities most commonly encompass clinical applications, but extend to the management of information in the conduct of administrative, educational, and research tasks. Nursing identifies the process and sets priorities which are congruent with the department's philosophy and goals and objectives. The Nursing Informatics Program offers a cadre of personnel with nursing and informatics expertise and these individuals are called upon to provide the leadership for project management. The support and expertise of information services is solicited for the purpose of identifying appropriate system options, evaluation for compatibility with an integrated systems approach, interface programming, and final contract negotiations. (For further discussion ISD-Nursing structures see [1]). Information services personnel are also permanent members of the Nursing Informatics Program Committee and fully participate in our regular monthly meetings. Appropriate support personnel such as the PC and Mainframe system managers and programmers are also members of specific nursing project committees. Similarly, ISD frequently calls upon the Nursing Informatics Program staff to participate in hospital-wide or other departmental information management projects.

5. Conclusion

The MSH structure for informatization has begun to demonstrate a significant impact by improving our ability to effectively achieve our information processing requirements. The effects are being experienced at the corporate and departmental level and demonstrate congruence with our goals for academic and clinical excellence. In our experience, a careful examination of the vision, mission, philosophy, and expectations of information processing will provide organizational direction for the articulation of an effective informatics structure.

6. References

[1] Board of Directors, Mount Sinai Hospital. Strategic focus 1990's. Toronto, ONT:Mount Sinai Hospital, 1990.

[2] Shamian J, Nagle L M, and Hannah K J. Optimizing outcomes of nursing informatization. In *MEDINFO 92* Lun K C, Degoulet P, Piemme T E, and Rienhoff O (eds.). Amsterdam: North Holland, 1992:976-980.

Nursing Informatics: An International Overview for Nursing in a Technological Era
S.J. Grobe and E.S.P. Pluyter-Wenting, eds.

A Methodological Approach for Determining Information Needs of Chief Nurse Executives

Barton AJ

Shands Hospital at the University of Florida, Gainesville, Florida, USA

The specific purposes of this research were to (a) prioritize issues for strategic planning decisions that are expected to involve chief nurse executives during the next 10 years and (b) determine the information required to reduce uncertainty in making strategic decisions. The methodology employed was a modification of the Policy Delphi using two rounds with a national sample of 240 nurse executives. Responses were obtained form 121 chief nurse executive (50.4%). As a result of this study, prioritized topics of concern to chief nurse executives for the next 10 years were identified. In addition, analysis of the information required for decision support revealed a greater proportion of financial information items to be of concern when compared with prioritized items from the clinical, human resource, and environmental categories.

1. Introduction

Nurse executives in acute care hospitals make decision in rapidly changing internal and external (to the institution) environments and require timely information concerned with (a) epidemiology/demography, referral patterns, and case mix of patients; (b) resource availability, allocation, and utilization; (c) performance measures, including output, outcome, quality, and consumer feedback; (d) skill maintenance of staff; (e) monitoring and maintenance of morale; and (f) shaping and maintenance of organizational culture [1]. Progress in the field of information systems has enhanced the amount and quality of information available for executive decision making. Unfortunately, even though much information is available, it is often not retrievable in a format useful for decision making by nurse executives (i.e., a decision support system to support strategic decision making). The specific purposes of this research were to (a) prioritize issues for strategic planning decisions that are expected to involve chief nurse executives during the next 10 years and (b) determine the information required to reduce uncertainty in making strategic decisions.

2. Methods

2.1 Design

Numerous methods for delineating information requirements have been reported in the information systems literature: (a) analyzing tasks and developing data flow diagrams [2], (b) interviewing the decision maker [3], (c) deriving requirements from an existing system [4], (d) combining normative and descriptive decision making models [5], and (e) identifying strategic goals and concerns [6]. Cats-Baril and Gustafson [7] identified several weaknesses that may potentially limit the applicability of these methods in developing decision support systems. First, some of the methods focus on present and past information needs and issues. For a DSS, information needs for the future must be derived. Second, other methods focus on a single issue, task, or decision. Support for strategic decision making requires the ability to address a broad range of problems. Third, some of the methods direct attention to the information currently transmitted between workers and not to the pertinent issues. Finally, some methods focus on the personal goals of the decision makers, without considering organizational context .

To overcome these weaknesses, two methods have emerged. The first is the critical success factors approach developed by Rockart [8]. The second is the use of the Delphi technique, as proposed by Cats-Baril and Gustafson [7] to solicit future issues of importance and to generate a prioritized list of information needs.

The critical success factors (CSF) method includes a series of interviews to help executives identify their information needs [8]. The focus of the first interview is on the identification of the CSFs, a limited number of areas in which satisfactory results will ensure successful organizational performance [8]. Subsequent interviews are used to provide feedback on the development of the CSFs and to verify these with the executive.

An alternate method was proposed by Cats-Baril and Gustafson [7]. They suggested the Delphi technique as a method in which important future issues were first identified, and information requirements were subsequently developed based on those future issues. Cats-Baril and Gustafson [7] surveyed 48 experts in mental health policy across the United States in order to determine the important issues and information requirements. They concluded that the identification of a small core of information items could support the analysis of a wide variety of issues.

The specific method used for this research was a modification of the policy Delphi. The policy Delphi is an organized method for presenting viewpoints regarding a specific policy area that allows the respondents the opportunity to react to the various views [9]. This method was appropriate for the present study because the document that results from the strategic planning process is foundational to the formulation of policies. Furthermore, this method has been used in a variety of nursing administration studies pertaining to strategic planning [10,11], workload planning [12], determining research priorities [13,14] and determining policy [15].

The strengths of this method include anonymity, iteration with controlled feedback, and statistical group response [16]. Anonymity allowed participants to respond to items without pressure from others in the group. Iteration with controlled feedback informed participants about the collective group's opinion. Statistical group response provided participants with a gauge of how their responses were similar to or different from others in the group. The weaknesses of this method, which were related to content validity of the questionnaire and use of experts [17], were overcome in this study through content validity testing and random sampling.

2.2 Sample

The population of interest was the 5,067 chief nurse executives of nonfederal, acute care hospitals that held membership in the American Hospital Association [18]. Those individuals with the title of Vice President for Nursing and Patient Services or the equivalent were assumed to be experts by virtue of their decision authority.

A stratified random sample was compiled from a computerized version of the AHA directory and these nurse executives constituted the expert panel for the Delphi. Hospitals were stratified according to four regions of the country (northeast, north central, south and west; [19]) and three levels of hospital size (less than 300 beds, 300-499 beds, over 500 beds). A stratified random sample was used to insure a cross-section of the entire group of chief nurse executives and avoid generation of an elitist "expert" sample [17]. Stratification also assisted in preventing bias due to geographic region and hospital size. A power analysis was computed based on four independent groups for region, using an alpha level of .05 and beta of .10 following the methodology outlined by Yarandi [20] and revealed that a minimum of 30 chief nurse executives were needed for each region. The indicated sample size was doubled to accommodate non-respondents and drop-outs.

A sample of 240 chief nurse executives received a cover letter explaining the nature of the study and an invitation to participate, a questionnaire booklet, and a stamped, addressed envelope for return of the completed questionnaire. Postcards were sent as a reminder to the participants at two weeks and four weeks after the questionnaires were mailed.

2.3 Questionnaire Development

The contents of the three refereed nursing administration journals (Journal of Nursing Administration, Nursing Administration Quarterly, and Nursing Economics) from 1990 and 1991 were evaluated to determine an appropriate framework for scenario development. A total of 235 titles were initially categorized into 78 themes. The themes were then matched to the categories within each of the four frameworks analyzed in order to determine the framework that best represented the factors of concern to nurse executives. Seventy-five percent of the themes from the content analysis of the literature were matched to the framework that included the following domains: social, economic, political, technologic, and environmental [21].

In order to develop specific scenarios, articles dealing with strategic planning in health care and nursing administration were reviewed. The growth of the aging population was a consistent theme in the literature [22,23]. Current projections suggest that one third of all Americans will be 65 years of age or older by the year 2050. Furthermore, five percent of the population will be 85 years of age or older. It is expected that the demand for service will change, but the overall impact of the aging population is unclear [24]. A second theme related to patient populations was the increasing numbers of AIDS patients and their impact on resource utilization in acute care [23,24].

Several themes related to health care organizations emerged. First, an increase in the intensity of competition among health care organizations was projected [23-25]. It was speculated that increased competition will be primarily due to the prevalence of managed care. Related to competition, then, a second theme was the proliferation of integrated health plans [22,23]. A third theme described the more educated consumer who is keenly interested in how and where health care services are provided [22,23].

The delivery of health care services was another theme consistently identified in the literature [22,23]. Coile [25] characterized the future delivery of health care services as a series of shifts with money moving from the inpatient to outpatient setting, from fee-for-service to capitation, from the public realm to the private realm, and from an emphasis on acute care to an emphasis on long-term care and health promotion. In addition, the transition from quality assurance to quality improvement was cited as a future trend [26,27]. Two related themes were the growth of multi-hospital systems and the need for increased accountability within health care settings [24,25].

A fourth theme focused on technological innovations. Coile [25] computerization, artificial intelligence, office automation, genetic engineering, super drugs, and bioreplacement technology as technologic revolutions. The decreasing cost and increasing portability of technology make it possible for many more services to be offered outside of the hospital.

The final theme mentioned throughout the literature concerned ethical issues [22,23]. Specific issues included rights to live or die and access to health care for the indigent and uninsured.

The resulting questionnaire consisted of a series of two-part sections. The first section in each series described strategic planning factors pertaining to one of the scenario domains. The second section in each series provided descriptions of information that may be used to enhance the strategic planning process. Chief nurse executives were requested to rate scenarios on a 5-point Likert scale addressing the impact each issue would likely have on the nursing profession in the next 10 years. Similarly, respondents rated the information items on a 5-point Likert scale indicating the importance of each item in reducing uncertainty when making strategic decisions. Specific questions versus open-ended questions were used to insure that forecasts were relevant to the research objective and to enhance participation of subjects [16].

2.4 Content Validity Testing and Pilot Study

The content validity phase involved testing the scenarios and information items with an expert panel. A sample of 10 nurses with experience as a vice president or associate vice president for nursing service (and not included in the study sample) rated the questionnaire for content validity. During the content validity testing, the subjects were asked to rate each item for relevance, using a 4-point scale (a score of 1 indicating low relevance and a score of 4 indicating high relevance). All items were rated as 3 or 4 by all judges and were retained [28]. A pilot study was conducted with a randomly selected sample of 48 chief nurse executives. The purpose of the pilot study was to refine the data collection procedure and the questionnaire. Completed questionnaires were received from 23 chief nurse executives. No scenarios were added or deleted based on the pilot study.

3 . Results & Discussion

Responses were obtained form 121 chief nurse executive (50.4%). Analysis of respondents and nonrespondents revealed no statistically significant differences with regard to organizational factors such as average daily census, occupancy rate, number of full-time equivalents employed, total expenses, hospital ownership, geographic location, or hospital size. The knowledge chief nurse executives will require for decision support was determined by rank ordering the scenario items by mean score.

The top ten scenarios (those with a mean score of 4.5 or higher) represented a broad range of issues. Within the social domain, the impact of the growing elderly population, retention of registered nurses, and the advanced preparation of nurse managers were ranked within the top 10. The highest ranked scenario dealt with the increasing numbers of elderly. This finding was not surprising since this issue was raised by several authors [22,23]. Retention of registered nurses was identified as a priority for the 21st century by Corcoran, Meyer, & Magliaro [29]. The need for advanced preparation of nurse managers was not identified as a major issue in the literature, but was contributed by respondents during the round one of data collection.

The four scenarios from the economic domain that were ranked within the top 10 pertained to (a) cost containment necessitating the reallocation and redesign of work, (b) accountability through development of a standardized method for measuring and controlling quality, (c) health care purchasers dictating the services and locations in which they are required, and (d) managed care as the predominant reimbursement mechanism.

Only one scenario from the political domain was ranked among the top 10. This scenario referred to pressure from accrediting agencies continuing to emphasize quality improvements.

Two scenarios from the technologic domain completed the top ten. One scenario pertained to information technology and dealt with the use of information systems [23,24]. The second scenario pertained to managerial technology and dealt with continuous quality improvement [19,20].

The information chief nurse executives would require for decision support was determined by rank ordering the information items by mean value. The largest proportion of the priority information items was financial (40%), followed by clinical (24%), environmental (20%), and human resource (16%) items.

The priority clinical information items for decision support included (a) patient's satisfaction with care given by individual nurses; (b) indicators that measure quality outcomes; (c) patient information tracking across inpatient, outpatient, and home care settings; (d) quality of care related to patient outcomes; (e) clinical protocols that facilitate patient care for populations of interest; and (f) summary of treatments, procedures, and outcomes by DRG. Only one item, the summary of treatments by DRG, is most amenable to retrieval at this time since this information is provided on the patient's discharge summary.

The priority information items within the financial category pertained to various trends and cost accounting information. The priority trends pertained to (a) the methods of reimbursement for services; (b) wage, health care, and expense benefits; (c) the cost of technology; (d) the amount of uncompensated care; and (e) the availability and cost of technology in the market area. The priority cost accounting items included the cost of providing nursing care, supplies and equipment, and facility operations.

Finally, the priority information items within the human resource category comprised staffing need forecasts, employee satisfaction assessment, internal harmony within and between departments, and trends in productivity indicators. Yet again, qualitative information items concerning employee satisfaction and internal harmony were included.

The priority information items within the environmental category were predominantly concerned with the institution's reputation or consumer satisfaction. Specific information items were (a) the institution's reputation among consumers, (b) the expectations of patients regarding services offered, and (c) consumer satisfaction with the availability of and access to services. In addition, one item pertaining to state or federal requirements was also among the top 25. Several of the priority environmental information items are either qualitative in nature or remain to be defined, posing problems for DSS development.

4. References

[1] Halloran EJ, Sermeus W, Barber B, et al. Decision support systems for nursing management and administration. In: Ozbolt JG, Vandewal D, Hannah KJ. eds. *Decision support systems in nursing*. St. Louis: Mosby, 1990:29-40.

[2] Ellis HC. A refined model for definition of system requirements. *Database Journal* 1982, 12(3):2-9.

[3] Gustafson DH, Thesen A. Are traditional information systems adequate for policy makers? *Health Care Management Review* 1981, 6:51-63.

[4] Munro MC, Davis GB. Determining management information needs: A comparison of methods. *MIS Quarterly* 1977, 1:55-67.

[5] Stabell CB. A decision-oriented approach to building DSS. In: Bennett JL. ed. *Building decision support systems*. Reading, MA: Addison-Wesley, 1983:221-260.

[6] Battiste JL, Jung JT. Requirements, needs, and priorities: A structured approach for determining MIS project definition. *MIS Quarterly* 1984, 8:215-228.

[7] Cats-Baril WL, Gustafson DH. Determining information requirements: A methodology for providing cost-effective support of policy issues. In: Lee RM, McCosh AM, Migliarese P. eds. *Organizational decision support systems*. Amsterdam: North-Holland Elsevier Science, 1988:199-212.

[8] Rockart JF. Chief executives define their own data needs. *HBR* 1979, 57:81-93.

[9] Turoff M. The policy Delphi. In: Linstone HA, Turoff M. eds. *The Delphi method: Techniques and applications*. Reading, MA: Addison-Wesley, 1975:84-101.

[10] McKnight J, Edwards N, Pickard L, et al. The Delphi approach to strategic planning. *Nurs Manage* 1991, 22(4):55-57.

[11] Synowiez BB, Synowiez PM. Delphi forecasting as a planning tool. *Nurs Manage* 1990, 21(4):18-19.

[12] Henney CR, Chrissafis I, McFarlance J, et al. A method of estimating nursing workload. *J Adv Nurs* 1985, 7:319-325.

[13] Lindeman CA. *Delphi survey of clinical nursing research priorities*. Boulder: Western Interstate Commission for Higher Education, 1975.

[14] Henry B, Moody LE, Pendergast JF, et al. Delineation of nursing administration research priorities. *Nurs Res* 1987, 36:309-314.

[15] Snyder Hill BA. A Delphi application: Health care, practice, education and education administration, *circa* 1992. *Image: J Nurs Sch* 1984, 16:7-8.

[16] Couper MR. The Delphi technique: Characteristics and sequence model. *ANS* 1984, 7:72-77.

[17] Sackman H. *Delphi critique.* Lexington, MA: Lexington Books, 1975.

[18] American Hospital Association . *AHA directory on diskette.* Chicago: Author, 1991.

[19] Stockwell EG. *The methods and materials of demography.* Orlando, FL: Academic Press, 1979.

[20] Yarandi HN. Planning sample sizes: Comparison of factor level means. *Nurs Res* 1991, 40:57-58.

[21] Zentner RD, Gelb BD. Scenarios: A planning tool for health care organizations. *Hospital and Health Services Administration* 1991, 36:211-222.

[22] American Nurses Association . *Nursing's agenda for health care reform.* Kansas City, MO: Author, 1991.

[23] Pierskalla WP, Woods D. Computers in hospital management and improvements in patient care: New trends in the United States. *J Med Syst* 1988, 12:411-428.

[24] Christman L, Count MA. The changing health care environment: Challenges for the executive team. *Nurs Adm Q* 1989, 13(2):67-76.

[25] Coile RC. *The new hospital: Future strategies for a changing industry.* Rockville, MD: Aspen, 1986.

[26] Roberts JS, Schyve PM. From QA to QI: The views and role of the Joint Commission. *The Quality Letter for Healthcare Leaders* 1990, May:9-12.

[27] Tilbury MS. From QA to CQI: A retrospective review. In: Dienemann J. ed. *C.Q.I.: Continuous Quality Improvement in Nursing.* Washington, DC: American Nurses Association, 1992:3-13.

[28] Waltz CW, Bausell RB. *Nursing research: Design, statistics and computer analysis.* Philadelphia: F.A. Davis, 1981.

[29] Corcoran NM, Meyer LA, Magliaro BL. Retention: The key to the 21st century for health care institutions. *Nurs Adm Q* 1990, 14(4):23-31.

Nursing Informatics: An International Overview for Nursing in a Technological Era
S.J. Grobe and E.S.P. Pluyter-Wenting, eds.

Pediatric Informatics: Managing Information Within a Professional Practice Model

Reske T[a], Rucki S[b] and Sheehan S[c]

[a] Department of Information Services, Patient Care Information Systems, Baystate Health Systems, 3300 Main Street, Springfield, Massachusetts 01107, United States of America

[b] Baystate Medical Center Children's' Hospital, 759 Chestnut Street, Springfield, Massachusetts 01199, United States of America

[c] Nursing Information Services, Baystate Medical Center, 759 Chestnut Street, Springfield, Massachusetts 01199, United States of America

Computers have become integral to the management of patient care in the tertiary care setting. Yet to date, computerized patient information systems have not satisfactorily reflected the unique needs of pediatric patients. A development team at one alpha site in the private sector for TDS 7800 designed the model for the pediatric population. Initially, the Research and Development team designed and incorporated strategies to make an adult system "user friendly." Following the achievement of this goal, physician ordering pathways and nursing order screens were developed. The second phase presently underway is to develop a documentation system which organizes nursing information according to nursing diagnoses and standards of care. The team is presently designing total quality management applications for the system. The model developed by this team will be discussed and representative examples of the components of this system will be presented. Finally, outcomes and issues as future goals related to the project will be examined.

1. Introduction

The rapid expansion of the knowledge base for pediatric clinical nursing practice far exceeds the capacity of practitioners to "know-it-all" or "have -it-all" available for use at any one time. The sheer quantity of raw data collected on a single pediatric patient can be overwhelming as it is categorized, processed and applied to patient care [1].

Information System vendors are assuming the role of "transformational leaders" as they develop computerized systems for patient care applications. In their quest for applications which are user-friendly and representative of advanced models of technology, vendors are deciding what nurses need to have available for documentation and care planning. These critical decisions are being made without the benefit of first hand discussion with direct care providers about trends in patient care. In other words, vendors are designing generic, packaged applications for clinical nursing practice; therefore, the models are able to be marketed to a wide variety of user communities. While nurses are not expected to contribute expert advice when issues related to system applications are debated, they need to be sensitive to a system's performance, and understand the importance of performance in eliciting staff acceptance [2]. The authors would agree that effective communication related to patient needs require effective information management. The vendor without a clinical "grassroots perspective" cannot articulate what the system requires in the "real world." In turn, the nurse without input from professional colleagues on the health care team cannot develop an individualized plan of care that represents the complexity of today's pediatric patient. This perception is supported by the literature that suggests the need for multidisciplinary collaboration to design an integrated plan of care. It is, as a result of this collaboration, that patient outcomes are achieved.

2. Review of Literature

Imperatives for computerized documentation and patient care, albeit limited in pediatrics, can be found throughout nursing and informatics literature. Mathews and Zadak outlined the results of a recent poll of computer professionals. They suggested that the greatest investment in computer systems over the next two years will be directed toward patient care applications [3]. Edmunds predicts that the use of computerized systems to guide patient care is just beginning [4]. For the successful integration of computerization with nursing services, attention must be directed toward the unique requirements of individual nurse user groups who care for unique patient groups. In one sense, progress towards this end will result in an information system which will improve nursing's ability to effectively plan and deliver nursing care services.

Literature suggests that nurses are required to translate requisite information into reliable and measurable units of care. With the advent of advanced nursing applications, staff nurses supported by administration need to examine unit business operations and professional values that influence care. They need to critically explore their daily work environment including the process for recording, storing, and accessing patient data. The methodologies used to communicate that data with ancillary and support areas, physicians, colleagues, and finally between patient and family are instrumental in structuring and defining guidelines for practice.

The Joint Commission of the Accreditation of Healthcare Organizations' (JCAHO) agenda for change stresses the development of an outcome as well as a process orientation. At the same time, the American Nurse's Association is linking quality management with patient attainment of specified and predetermined outcomes. [5]. As the Clinton Administration turns its attention towards health care reform, computerization will capture physician and nurse practice guidelines, care modalities by all health team members and provide a repository for all health data on any specific individual. International leaders are awaiting the emergence of this new model.

Fagin contends that comprehensive health care today requires the broad spectrum of knowledge that no one practitioner can solely provide. Costs of health and medical care have been reduced by the appropriate utilization of nurses working in teams or in consultative relationships with physicians [6]. Regardless of the financial climate, the American Organization of Nurse Executives (AONE) endorses the need to deliver patient-centered, holistic and less episodic care which in turn, will compel system reform [7]. With this in mind, nurses must take initiative in developing systems that work toward strong relationships with patient, family, and significant others . If we envision the knowledge and activities of nurses and the knowledge and activities of physicians as occupying two different yet partly intersecting spheres, we then agree with Fagin that neither profession can function without the other [8].

To summarize, the essential ingredient for change in the 90's is teamwork. A hospital wide, mission-driven effort has been demanded in the nurse-physician relationship to provide the highest quality of care in the most economical manner.

3. Building Upon Success

American Medical Association Board of Trustees, supportive of Fagin's concept, report that the independent patient-centered nursing models and protocols must be a cooperative effort between physicians and nurses. Herein lies the real challenge of breaking new ground in the care of the pediatric patient, physically and psychosocially.
Nurses and physicians at the Baystate Medical Center Children's Hospital (BMCCH) previously participated on collaborative planning teams. The Department of Information Systems and the Children's Hospital administration believed that active and well-informed nurses and physicians will contribute to the system development and design. Nurses were trained to the "hands on" practice computer application to basically understand how to data entry orders, retrieve data results and to increase learning experience in their pediatric nurse trainer's role. Data collection procedures included a comprehensive patient medical record review, clinical observations of patients during an admission, previous files of nursing care plans and review of pediatric literature. Extensive pre-implementation data collection identified key factors: the most common pediatric DRG's (diagnosis related groups), the most commonly admitted diagnosis by age-group, the similarities within physician practice models, the nursing care plans developed for age-group specific patients by diagnoses, the outcomes of frequently admitted chronic patients and nursing practice models.

The role of the nursing informatics specialist was threefold: to ensure that the incorporation of technology into nursing and medical practice met the collaborative team's needs, to promote the clinical system's strengths and minimize its limitations, and to analyze data elements by translating information into "user-friendly" applications [9]. Hendrickson further supports the role of the nursing informatics specialist through measurement of a quality information system that can meet the needs of the user [10].

4. The Process

The Baystate Medical Center (BMC), an 800 bed tertiary care facility, uses a transaction - based computer system which links clinical ordering, ancillary ordering and resulting departments as well as admitting, discharge and transfer information. The distinguishing feature of this software is the computerized Permanent Patient Record. In our system, the Permanent Patient Record is a longitudinal patient record from birth until death. The work satisfiers elicited from this institution's implementation of the clinical system were a well-designed pediatric application programmed from collaborative planning team recommendations and a well-defined installation plan.

One year ago, the BMCCH implemented a computerized clinical application. Early in the implementation process, it was recognized by the nurse implementation team that the computerized system increased physician awareness and interest in further developing pediatric applications. If the nursing teams could link meaningful application to the pediatric patient's plan of care then the decision to manage information would be demonstrated by a process of accurate diagnosis, appropriate interventions and predicted outcomes. The Standard of Care framework designed by the Pediatric Standards Committee, and led by the Clinical Specialist, would be a manual tool trialed prior to the computerization of nursing documentation.

As mentioned previously, software vendors have developed applications automating the plan of patient care. Vendors are competing to create nursing applications which are solution-oriented and capture critical elements in the documentation process all by integrating the multidisciplinary approaches. The BMC is currently collaborating with a software vendor to develop a computer-supported documentation system. As a result of strategic planning, standards of care and care planning were identified as the most time consuming nurse activities. Nurses reported sporadic compliance with care planning. In fact, many nurses believe that care planning activities were merely written exercises that were often developed by colleagues. It was agreed that the standard of care format required more nurse-specific documentation development. By encouraging creativity, the pediatric nurses assumed ownership in revising and changing their documentation practice to simulate the physician and nurse order sets. To support these changes a manual simulation was developed.

This perception is supported by Rundell who writes that the nursing care plan should be a dynamic almost real-time representation of nursing therapy [11]. Prior to computerization, pediatricians would elicit information but rarely requested documentation of the nursing plan of care and evaluation of that plan of care.

5. Prototype and Discussion

Standards of care were developed for the pediatric patient with a view toward automation. There guidelines provided direction for nursing care interventions and flow from a framework commonly understood by all team members. Nursing's contribution to care is uniquely explicit yet related to and supportive of the medical regime.

The standards consist of four patient components: 1) Standard - the overview of the desired goal(s) of care by age group 2) Process criteria - nursing actions and responses to meet the standard, 3) Nurse Documentation - all nurse actions are uniform and elicit patient family responses, 4) Outcome Criteria - measure patient goals achieved as a result of nursing care. Assisting the pediatric staff nurses to change their focus from monitoring nursing process to monitoring patient outcomes posed challenges to the nurse implementation team.

Physician department ordering sets (DOS) which are automated to capture those medical ordering elements particular to a diagnosis are programmed and standardized by design in the physician pathways. An example of a physician department order set would include standardized orders, a medical plan of care, and a comprehensive integrated plan of care. For example the pediatric oncology patient qualifies for three of the defined physician ordering sets, namely, the DEHYDRATION DOS, the HEMATOLOGY/ONCOLOGY DOS and the CHEMOTHERAPY PROTOCOL DOS.

```
MD     HEM/ONC:     NEUTROPENIA  DOS

>ADMIT DIAGNOSIS AND CONDITION
VITAL SIGNS:          Q2H    Q4H    Q _ _ H
ACTIVITY:     AS TOLERATED FOR AGE
-- _ _ _
I&O: STRICT  RECORD Q _ _ H
HEMATEST ALL STOOLS & RECORD RESULTS
DIPSTICK ALL URINES & RECORD RESULTS
NOTIFY H.O. FOR:
TEMP > _ _ _._ F
URINE OUTPUT < _ _ _ _ ML/HR
URINE PH LESS THAN OR EQUAL TO 7
URINE SPECIFIC GRAVITY > _ _ _ _ _
URINE SPECIFIC GRAVITY < _ _ _ _ _
OTHER:-- _ _ _
> LAB ORDERS        > NEXT        > CONSULT
> BLOOD CULTURES                  > PEDI IV'S
> DIET          >XRAY > PLAY > PEDI DOS INDEX
```

Figure 1 is representative of a pediatric department order set (DOS) designed by and programmed for physician order entry. Physician light-pen selection of medical staff approved orders eliminates potential clerical errors on the nursing units.

Figure 1

Each child received a regime of chemotherapy which is developmentally specific and encourages interdisciplinary involvement among physicians, nurses and pharmacists assuring error free medication orders and administration.

```
P           CYTOXAN/MESNA PROTOCOL
                        F5 = CALCULATIONS

HYDRATE:
IV LINE:  START, D5.45NACL, _ _ _ _ML W/KCL _ _
MEQ, AT _ _ _ ML/HR, CONT TIL DC'D
PRE-CHEMO HYDRATION:  WEIGHT _ _ _ _
IF URINE SP.GR. >1.010 AFTER 2HRS, INCREASE IV
RATE TO _ _ _ ML/HR


CHEMOTHERAPY:  START STEP 2 WHEN URINE
SP. GR. IS LESS THAN/EQUAL TO 1.010.
(STEP 2)
CYTOXAN _ _ _ _MG/MESNA _ _ _ _MG, IVPB IN
D5W, _ _ _ _ML TO INFUSE OVER 30 MIN
(STEP 3)
MESNA _ _ _ _MG, IVPB IN D5.45NACL, _ _ _ _ML
TO INFUSE W/KCL _ _ _MEQ, TO RUN OVER 3HR
(STEP 4)
MESNA _ _ _ _MG, IVPB, IN D5W, _ _ _ _ML TO
INFUSE OVER 10 MIN, Q3H
                              > NEXT
```

Figure 2 displays the first computer screen in a series of four screens. It was designed and programmed by the nursing informatics specialist who understands how physicians write medical orders and how nurses implement them.

Figure 2

```
┌─────────────────────────────────────────────┐
│ N      PEDI   CHEMO  NURSE ORDER SET         │
│                                              │
│ CENTRAL LINE CARE: PORTACATH, HUBER NEEDLE,  │
│ GAUGE 22, LENGTH 0.5  IN                     │
│ MONITOR INFECTION                            │
│ EMLA PRIOR TO PORTACATH ACCESS               │
│ RECORD I&O AT EACH POTTY TRAINING            │
│ AGE GROUP:   INFANT            PRE-SCHOOL    │
│              TODDLER           SCHOOL AGE     │
│ CHILD'S NICKNAME:  CHELLIE _ _ _ _ _         │
│ CHILD'S FLUID OF CHOICE:   KOOL-AID_ _ _ _   │
│ CHILD LIFE CONSULT: TREATMENT RELATED        │
│ SUPPORT WITH PARENTS DURING LINE CARE        │
│ RN TO DIETARY:       CYTOXAN/MESNA  THERAPY, │
│ SEND  FREQUENT  SNACKS  AND  STRAWBERRY       │
│ MILKSHAKES                                   │
└─────────────────────────────────────────────┘
```

Figure 3

Based upon the admission assessment and physician orders, the nurse creates the initial plan of care. Computerized nurse order sets (NOS) provide a foundation of nursing comfort measures, safety parameters, feeding guidelines and psychosocial developmental milestones. Nurses within their practice guidelines can order nurse order sets to support their patient's plan of care. Nurse order sets (NOS) are patient-specific nursing actions designed by the patient's nurse to meet individual care needs. A NOS is created, changed and added to frequently during the patient's admission. The child's primary nurse is responsible for assuring that nursing orders are discussed during multidisciplinary rounds. Nurses light-pen select from a pediatric nurse order set menu to create the actions and interventions specific to the child's diagnosis. The computer generates a hard copy road map of the patient's current orders on a "Clinical Worksheet," our facility's acronym for the Kardex. Physician utilization of the ordering criteria in the physician DOS provides a foundation for the correlating standard of care. A standard of care simulating a future computer application is then manually created.

From the nursing informatic specialist's point-of-view, the ability to mirror a computer application provides the user the opportunity to work with a tool prior to tailoring the software. Progress will result in an information system which will improve nurses' ability to plan care effectively and to deliver nursing care services [12].

The nurses and physicians report at their implementation and development meetings that they have begun to develop prototypes and working standards of care models. Physicians participate in formal multidisciplinary patient rounds whereby the process criteria and documentation of those actions are reviewed and evaluated. Pediatric nurses report that the computer application designed should include both developmentally based, age-specific standards and process oriented standards. Requirements have been incorporated in the DOS and NOS for ordering purposes. Standards being developed include physiological, psychosocial and behavioral variables consistent with the child's diagnosis.

6. Summary

It is clear that pediatric nurses, members of the multidisciplinary team, and informatics specialists must accept the challenge and become proactive in the design of a documentation and care planning model which captures the essence of the pediatric patient. Any computer application installed will have some technical limitations related to hardware or software capabilities. However, key to the overall institution success for managing information flow is the nurse, physician, and end-user attitude that several of the installed applications should provide a more efficient method of accomplishing previous manual functions and assist with innovative clinical, administrative and educational applications.

7. References

[1] Milholland K. Patient Data Management Systems (PDMS) Computer Technology for Critical Care Nurses. *Comput Nurse* 1988 2, 237-243.

[2] Edmunds L. Computers for Inpatient Nursing Care What Can Be Accomplished. *Comput Nurs* 1984, 2: 102-108.

[3] Mathews J[a] and Zadak K[b]. Managerial Decisions for Computerized Patient Care Planning. *Nurs Manage* 1993,
24 (7): 54-56.

[4] Edmunds L. Computers for Inpatient Nursing Care What Can be Accomplished, *Comput Nurs* 1984, 2:
102-108.

[5] Holzemer WL[a] and Henry SB[b]. Computer-Supported Versus Manually-Generated Nursing Care Plans: A Comparison of Patient Problems, Nursing Interventions and AIDS Patient Outcomes. *Comput Nurs* 1992, 10: 19-24.

[6] Fagin C. Collaboration Between Nurses & Physicians No Longer A Choice. *Nurs Health Care* 1992, 13: 354-363.

[7] American Organization of Nurse Executives. Cross-Utilization of Nursing Staff. *Nurs Manage* 1993, 24 (7): 38-39.

[8] Fagin C. Collaboration Between Nurses & Physicians No Longer A Choice. *Nurs Health Care* 1992, 13: 354-363.

[9] Rucki SQ[a] Reske TR[b] and Barbeau LA[c]. Developing the Pediatric Data Base: A User Initiative. *1993 HIMSS proceedings* 1993, 2: 117-126.

[10] Hendrickson MF. The Nurse Engineer: A Way to Better Nursing Information Systems. *Comput Nurs* 1993, 11, 67-71.

[11] Rundell S. A Model for the Future. *Nurs Times* 1993, 89 (18): 52-53.

[12] Edmunds L. Computers for Inpatient Nursing Care What Can Be Accomplished. *Comput Nurs* 1984, 2: 102-108.

© *1994 Elsevier Science B.V. All rights reserved.*
Nursing Informatics: An International Overview for Nursing in a Technological Era
S.J. Grobe and E.S.P. Pluyter-Wenting, eds.

Developing Nursing Care Profiles For
Diagnosis Related Groups

McKechnie S

Nursing Branch, South Australian Health Commission, Citi Centre Building, 11 Hindmarsh Square, Adelaide SA 5000, Australia.

Nursing care delivered to patients is held to be the same for particular medical diagnoses. The assumption is that a set of particular nursing activities and interventions can be attached to particular medical diagnoses. Increasingly this has been questioned by nurses who have presented other theories and models for the practice of nursing.

The purpose of the study was to identify the profile of nursing care delivered to groups of patients in particular Diagnosis Related Groups (DRG's). The findings of this survey support the belief in nursing, that medical diagnosis may not be a good predictor of nursing resource use. There are significant implications for these findings in relation to the use and application of DRG models of funding and resource allocation.

1.   Introduction

The development and implementation of sophisticated nursing information systems has created the opportunity to review the costs and practices of nursing. The information has become a powerful tool to assist in the analysis of nursing service provision, support nursing research functions and most significantly, facilitate the delivery of quality nursing care in a constantly changing and financially pressured environment.

Casemix has become a phenomenon around which much activity and discussion occurs in our hospitals but frequently this has been at a level of financial reporting and gross patient activity statistics. Considerable work has been undertaken by nurses across Australia to determine reasonable nursing weighting components of Diagnosis Related Groups (DRGs). However the benefits have reached beyond this validation of nursing inputs to patient care. Access to ongoing nursing clinical information via a standards based care planning and dependency system has provided many insights into nursing practice.

In the course of these studies the details of the nursing care delivered to groups of patients were collected over a two year period in 1991-92. This data was then sorted by DRG and analysed to prepare nursing profiles of care delivered. The profiles detailed all the components of nursing care identified on the nursing care plan for an individual patient. In addition to the nursing care requirements, the hours and costs of nursing care for each patient were examined within the DRG groupings. This paper concentrates on the nursing profile of patients reviewed under DRG 209 "Major Joint and Limb Reattachment Procedures".

The findings of this survey support the belief in nursing, that medical diagnosis may not be a good predictor of nursing resource use. There are significant implications for these findings in relation to the use and application of DRG models of funding and resource allocation.

2.   Study Objective

The purpose of the study was to identify the profile of nursing care delivered to groups of patients classified in particular Diagnosis Related Groups. It was determined to review a group of patients classified in DRG 209 "Major Joint and Limb Reattachment Procedures" in order to examine the nursing resource required to care for these patients.

3.   DRG 209

Before proceeding to the discoveries, it may be useful to put DRG 209 into perspective. Within the structure of DRGs, 209 "Major Joint and Limb Reattachment Procedures", is derived from Major Diagnostic Category (MDC) 8, "Disorders of the Musculoskeletal System and Connective Tissue". Using the International Classification of Diseases Index, procedures are coded and then allocated to the DRG. It is assumed that DRG's represent an homogenous cluster in terms of resource utilisation and as such patient activity within the classification is statistically comparable [1].

It is further held that homogeneity within DRG groups allows for review of effectiveness of care which can be quantified through such variables as:
- length of stay, preoperative length of stay, cost of care (by type of cost), surgical time, severity level, hospital acquired infection, complications of anaesthesia, transfusion error, medication error, death, unscheduled return to operating room, unplanned removal/repair of normal organ and patient satisfaction. [2].

4.   Data Collection

A computerised nursing care planning system was used to collect the details of nursing care delivered to groups of patients over a two year period. The data was then sorted by DRG and analysed to prepare nursing profiles of care delivered. The information is presented in terms of the components of nursing care identified in the care plan throughout the patients' stay and in terms of nursing resource required represented by time and cost.

5.   Results

In all, information was available for 134 patients who had been classified on discharge to DRG 209. Data was incomplete for 22 patients whose records were then excluded. Records for the remaining 112 patients were analysed and are discussed in this paper.

6.   Homogeneity

In the review of DRG 209, 17 procedures were identified as having been included in the coding during the period under review. These ranged from a cluster of orthopaedic surgical procedures, as might have been reasonably expected, but also included such items as rigid proctosigmoidoscopy, arteriography and phlebography of femoral and other lower extremity arteries and veins, pulmonary scans and teleradiotherapy (Table 1).

Table 1
Procedures Classified In DRG 209

- Rigid Proctosigmoidoscopy
- Internal Fixation of Bone without Fracture Reduction
- Removal of Internal Fixation Device
- Closed Reduction of Fracture with Internal Fixation
- Open Reduction of Fracture with Internal Fixation
- Incisions & Excision of Joint Structures - Hip
- Incision & Excision of Joint Structures - Knee/Total Knee Replacement
- Total Hip Replacement with Use of Methyl Methacrylate
- Other Total Hip Replacement
- Other Replacement of Head of Femur
- Other Replacement of Acetabulum
- Arteriography of Femoral & other Lower Extremity Arteries
- Phlebography of Femoral & other Lower Extremity Veins using contrast material
- Other Radioisotope Scan - Pulmonary Scan
- Teleradiotherapy of 1 to 25 MEV Protons
- Osteopathic Manipulative Treatment - other specified Osteopathic Manipulative Treatment

In an analysis of the number of treatments for each procedure, it was identified that Total Knee Replacement, Total Hip Replacement and Repair of Head of Femur accounted for 94% of all procedures (Table 2).

Table 2
DRG 209 Major Joint & Limb Reattachment Procedures

Total Knee Replacement	23% cases
Total Hip Replacement (with methyl methacrylate)	15% cases
Other Total Hip Replacement	15% cases
Other Replacement of Head of Femur	41% cases
Other 209 Procedures	6% cases
	100% cases

Early concerns about homogeneity based on knowledge of different nursing resources required for such a diversity of patients was confirmed through analysis of length of stay (ALOS), nursing time (NHPPD) and nursing cost ($PPD) (Table 3). Total Hip Replacements which comprised 30% of the patients had a 12 day average length of stay compared with the average 10 days for the whole group and therefore used considerably higher nursing hours and cost. However, on a per unit basis 6% of patients, those in the "other" category consumed the highest resources.

Table 3
Length of Stay, Nursing Time & Nursing Cost: Average Length of Stay; Dollars per Patient Day, Nursing Hours per Patient Day

	DRG 209112 patients		
	ALOS	$PPD	NHPPD
All Patients	10 days	$89	5.19
Total Knee Replacement	10 days	$85	5.23
Total Hip Replacement	12 days	$84	4.97
Other Replacement of Head of Femur	10 days	$76	4.35
Other 209 Procedures	9 days	$95	6.44

7.   Length Of Stay

As a variable, length of stay can provide much information about resource utilisation. In particular, mapping of nursing time by day of stay is interesting. It becomes possible to identify patterns of peaks and troughs in nursing care requirement, to isolate the impact of complications on both length of stay and resource requirement and to identify key indicators of nursing resource use. Examples of time variation are illustrated in Table 4 below.

Table 4
DRG 209 Total Knee Replacement Sample: Nursing Time (Minutes) by Day of Stay

	Day of Stay												
	1	2	3	4	5	6	7	8	9	10	11	12	13
Patient	Time (Minutes)												
1	17	367	305	225	215	215	215	215	117				
2	92	456	291	286	264	289	221	303	403	360	355	257	138
3	88	257	323	299	246	183	162	159	171	77			
4	213	185	411	332	243	214	223	229	229	172	90		
5	17	367	305	225	215	215	215	215	117				

Patients 1 and 5 display the same pattern of resource use, while the Patients 2, 3 and 4 in the sample show variations. Examination of the nursing care plans show the impact of complications of deep vein thrombosis (Patient 2). Patients 3 and 4 reflect differing requirements in assistance with activities of daily living.

8. Managed Care Protocols

One of the approaches to quality management is the managed care protocol [3]. The model suggests that it is possible to identify a critical path for decision making and management of patient care. The mapping of nursing time presented in Table 4 shows that it is possible to identify patterns of identical resource, and indeed components of care and progress throughout the length of stay. This was able to be repeated throughout the sample of 112 patients, but only within groupings of specific procedures.

Within the context of this information, it was then decided to review the nursing care data base of the clinical information system and it was possible to identify components of nursing care (resource) which could occur for the length of patient stay and irrespective of medical diagnosis. Such components included sensory deficits (deafness, blindness), communication barriers (speech or language) and functional deficits (physical or intellectual) to name but a few.

9. Conclusion

The work presented in this paper is preliminary but shows, through the use of a nursing clinical information system that nursing resource utilization is not constant within the DRG 209. Assumptions about homogeneity within the DRG may need to be verified when it can be seen that the range of procedures coded to the DRG are so diverse. In the sample reviewed, 94% of patients were accounted for by 3 of the 17 procedures included. This represents a very skewed cluster within the DRG which may not be consistent with aggregated data across the health system.

Further analysis shows patterns of resource use more closely associated with specific nursing care protocols for specific procedures. Additionally variation occurs related to the development of complications, but also in association with particular patient needs for nursing care over that which is directly associated with the medical procedure.

Within the DRG model used, no distinction is made for comorbidities, complications or age on Major Limb and Limb Reattachment Procedures, yet the indications are that these are factors which impact on nursing resource utilization. Additionally there is evidence that nursing measures associated with differing levels of physical, communication or psychological support are relevant predictions of resource use and are independent of medical diagnosis. The implication of these findings is that it is important for nurse administrators to be familiar with the nursing profiles within individual DRGs. Variations to nursing resource use will be driven by the particular clusters of procedures and diagnoses classified to DRGs and by other indicators not necessarily associated with any specific procedure or diagnosis.

It would seem that the natural process could now be to extend this analysis to other DRGs and to isolate actual nursing care components which could be identified as indicators of resource use for any medical diagnosis.

10. References

[1] Fetter R & Freeman R (1986) Diagnosis Related Groups: Product Line Management Within Hospitals. *Academy of Management Review*, 11 (1): 41-54.

[2] Fetter R & Hines H (1992) DRG's and Quality Assurance. *Proceedings of Fourth National Casemix Conference*, Commonwealth Department of Health, Housing and Community Services; Canberra AGPS.

[3] Zander, K (1988) Nursing Case Management: Strategic Management of Cost and Quality Outcomes. J.Nurs.Admin., May 1988.

Nursing Informatics: An International Overview for Nursing in a Technological Era
S.J. Grobe and E.S.P. Pluyter-Wenting, eds.

Managed Care: Outcomes and Automation

Nadler G [a] and Gibson L [b]

[a] *The Medical Center at Princeton, 253 Witherspoon Street, Princeton, NJ 08540*

[b] *Health Data Sciences Corporation®, 268 W. Hospitality Lane, San Bernardino, CA 92408*

At The Medical Center at Princeton, we are well ahead of the insatiable information dragon -- and yet we are behind. The rush for patient care data on clinical and service outcomes that are emerging as the epitome of clinical validation are within our grasp and already we realize we need more. This database must expand to provide patient-focused pathways over the continuum of care. Our emphasis must now move from managing care to measuring and evaluating outcomes through computerization, in order to achieve the sophisticated analysis of patient data that will provide the information needed to improve quality of care while optimizing operational efficiency throughout the health care enterprise.

1. Introduction to Critical Paths at The Medical Center at Princeton

In recognition of the need to measure and evaluate outcomes in order to successfully improve quality while simultaneously increasing efficiency and retaining costs, The Medical Center at Princeton adopted a managed care approach to care delivery. In April of 1990, The Medical Center at Princeton implemented a managed care program utilizing five critical paths on our most common diagnosis related groups (DRGs). We refer to all of our critical paths as "clinical paths," emphasizing the clinical application of the critical pathway analysis approach in the health care industry. Initially, staff nurses were assigned the role of managing care for the chosen DRGs with these five clinical paths. The staff nurses were provided hospital-wide educational sessions on DRG reimbursement and an overview of managed care. Gradually, these clinical paths have increased to 63 DRGs with corresponding teaching plans. The clinical path was developed by staff nurses in conjunction with physicians and appropriate disciplines. The nurse and physician names appear on the clinical path to convey credit to the authors and credibility to the process. Patient brochures were created to explain this concept to patients and families.

Advantages of the clinical path approach are: the approach is patient-centered and allows multiple disciplines to coordinate care effectively; it allows patients to benefit by understanding and participating in their own plan of care; it encourages collaboration; and it develops leadership skills in the nursing staff. Furthermore, the approach supports quality improvement activities by incorporating concurrent and retrospective review of patient care variances. These activities may result in a decreased length of stay, which in turn can help to decrease or maintain staffing levels - both of which will reduce cost.

2. Implementation of Clinical Paths

The initial results of the implementation of clinical paths at The Medical Center at Princeton have been very positive. Nurses and patients are very enthusiastic. A few physicians remain resistant to the clinical path concept, referring to it as "cookbook medicine." Gradually, as physicians have developed their own clinical paths, they have seen the positive results in patient care in terms of collaboration and communication. Many physicians at this point are very involved. The average length of stay on the DRGs that have clinical paths has decreased by 0.4: the average length of stay is now 5.4 days. Trends have been identified through variance analysis and have been addressed through quality improvement. However, medical patients with multiple diagnoses continue to be difficult to manage with separate clinical paths. In addition, managed care is extremely paper intensive and variance analysis needs to be facilitated through computerization. During 1994 we will begin to utilize automated clinical paths on the ULTICARE® System, an integrated hospital-wide patient care information system by Health Data Sciences Corporation® (HDS®). This system is a multidisciplinary, integrated clinical information system that is 100 percent point-of-care. As nursing care documentation, care planning, and clinical paths are brought on-line, we will have tremendous facility in looking at and comparing practice patterns and outcomes for the acute care patient. Outcomes have become the "bottom line" and are the positive proof requested by payors and consumers of the quality of patient care.

According to Edward Geehr, M.D. [1] outcomes management "involves the collection and analysis of the results of medical processes and performances according to agreed upon specifications and the use of this information to optimize health care provision through collaborative efforts of patients, payors, and providers." Outcomes management is clearly dependent on the integration of patient data and care plans with facilities, information systems, and health care professionals.

The Outcomes Management System has four components: the outcomes measurement instrument; the outcomes specification process; the ULTICARE clinical information system by HDS; and Continuous Quality Improvement (CQI).

2.1 Outcomes Measurement Instrument

The outcomes measurement instrument is the clinical path. Staff nurses direct case management of patients and use the clinical paths as a tangible method to coordinate care concurrently and can produce retrospective outcome information. Point-of-care technology integrates interdisciplinary care and promotes CQI at the patient care level. Through case management, clinical paths can be used as templates in a computerized system to analyze care for patient groups, episodes, and practitioners. By differentiating patients by diagnosis related groups, conformance to collaboratively developed standards can be compared for reliability and consistency of delivery. Outcome results can be used for peer review, privileging, and credentialing to improve care. To enhance continuity of care, patient history, physicals, and problem lists stemming from physicians' offices and clinics and interdisciplinary acute care, documentation must be combined to provide a complete overview of the patient's care plan. This is achieved more efficiently on-line.

2.2 Outcomes Specification Process

The outcomes specification process indicates which outcomes are desirable and provides a cogent process for measurement, analysis, and action. Clinical paths demonstrate negative and positive characteristics so that variance analysis can be meaningful. Clinical, service, and resource outcomes are identified by episode of care. Negative characteristics include mortality, morbidity, readmission, claims, and cost. Positive characteristics include functional status, patient satisfaction, goals, loss-prevention, or effectiveness. Any outcomes specifications process must have feedback to close the loop and provide opportunities to enhance the appropriateness, effectiveness, and efficiency of care.

2.3 ULTICARE Clinical Information System by IIDS

At The Medical Center at Princeton, each clinical path has a specific outcome that is desirable, and each of the characteristics are reported on the reverse side of the clinical path worksheet (in the manual approach) as positive or negative progress. In the automated method, as a negative or positive characteristic or opportunity to improve care occurs based on documentation and variances to the clinical path, the nurse will concurrently be prompted by the ULTICARE System to identify the reasons for this variance and queried to advise what action needs to be taken as a result of the variance. In terms of retrospective review, all clinical information in the ULTICARE System is coded so that reports can be generated based on any type of information and grouped according to episode of care or type of patient. This measurement by practitioner will be available to hospital departments and clinical chairs to review outcomes in terms of clinical service, resources, and quality.

2.4 Continuous Quality Improvement (CQI)

Continuous Quality Improvement is the mechanism for not only measurement but feedback to all parties on criteria that influence outcomes. In terms of measurement in our current manual approach, we continuously expand our database for high volume DRGs that present as resource or clinical problems. In addition, we review existing clinical paths for areas requiring revision. In terms of feedback, variance reports on clinical and service outcomes are distributed to clinical chairs and management. Outcomes-based feedback strategies are provided to all practitioners, nursing, and physicians to look at ways of improving care in the future. Outcomes-based education is provided to physicians and all practitioners to orient staff to more of a patient-focused, outcomes-based critical thinking process. Any indicators or measurement can be rolled into the Continuous Quality Improvement program to improve care. The availability of this information grouped by diagnosis or service is a major benefit in planning a continuous quality improvement plan and looking at care retrospectively. Prospectively, as each individual patient has variances occur, their care is effected moment-to-moment, shift-to-shift as it is occurring and everyone is aware of the ongoing patient problem list and what actions need to be taken. Currently, parameters used for outcomes monitoring are: mortality, morbidity, length of stay, cost, structure, and process. In the future, the patient's functional status on discharge at six months, one year, and three years will be an essential component of the outcomes monitoring plan. In addition, quality of life, burden of care on family, patient/family satisfaction, cost of care on the community, readmission, and effective and efficient use of high-tech care are important parameters that will be examined in outcomes monitoring.

3. The Role of Information Systems

To be effective in supporting the managed care process, it is imperative that the management information system contain specific features and functions; most importantly: system integration; on-line longitudinal medical record; and variance identification and analysis.

3.1 System Integration

System integration provides a common patient database and allows the system to present all patient information in a patient-centered way. Consequently, every process of care from every provider is continuously consolidated into a current and accurate reflection of each patient's status. Thus, the managed care process, which is highly multidisciplinary in nature, is effectively supported by merging all activities into a single, patient-centered world view. Furthermore, system integration significantly improves communication among all providers and enhances the case manager's ability to coordinate care among multiple disciplines.

Another important design feature is the ability to retrieve data in provider-specific ways. All providers have different data world views and need rapid access to patient results in data flows and formats that meet their individual needs. System integration eliminates the departmental barriers that all too commonly restrict the flow of accurate, timely information to the appropriate providers.

3.2 On-line Longitudinal Medical Record

Increasing requirements for continuity of care across institutions, requirements for rapid retrieval of clinical data upon repeat visits, and increasing demands for retrospective individual and aggregate data by a variety of parties indicate a need for the on-line longitudinal medical record. As the managed care process at The Medical Center at Princeton evolves from a unit based implementation toward managing the continuum of care, the on-line longitudinal medical record will be a crucial element in providing a patient-centered view. Moreover, as the focal point of the managed care process changes from managing care to managing outcomes and identifying and evaluating variances, the database must include accurate patient information from all venues of care such as extended care facilities, home care, rehabilitation centers and other community-based facilities.

3.3 Variance Identification and Analysis

Critical to the success of any managed care program is the capability to accurately and concurrently identify patient outcome variances and clinical path variances. This is also the most difficult and time-consuming task associated with managed care. The nurse managers at The Medical Center at Princeton spend at least eight hours per month aggregating data from each of their individual units. The time that each staff nurse spends identifiying individual patient variances fluctuates widely. With the automation of the managed care process utilizing the clinical path as the outcomes measurement instrument, variance identification and data collection time will be cut to a fraction of the time currently spent completing these processes. The ULTICARE System will provide on-line concurrent and prospective variance identification with the ability to triage variances. This means that key interventions and/or patient outcomes may be identified for urgent processing with the ability to automatically alert the appropriate provider or provider groups as variances occur or even if they are predicted to occur. This will allow all providers more time to actually manage outcomes rather than managing the process.

At The Medical Center at Princeton, information systems are a critical component of effective outcomes management and variance analysis. The information presented must be patient-focused, integrated, and measurable. Real time decision support for care decisions and risk benefit analysis is an important component of any MIS design. The patient data must extend beyond the acute hospital and examine the patient in the continuum from primary care provider through patient episodes, such as home care, longterm care, rehabilitation, and other community referrals. The ULTICARE System supports multiple facilities including many care provider offices, and maintains a central repository for patient data. The ULTICARE System standardizes information and documentation and will allow for the transmission of data, voice, and image. It provides the most current patient data on-line including problems lists to be evaluated in the continuum of care. In addition, with the availability of financial and acuity information integrated with clinical information such as physician order entry, resource utilization can be predicted and monitored. Automation allows the health care enterprise to predefine clinical paths that are embedded in the order entry system. Alternatively, usage of clinical paths may be restricted to monitoring practice patterns for the purposes of determining best practice and providing feedback. As care is rendered, variances from both the clinical path and defined outcomes will be identified and the appropriate providers will be notified automatically. With this system there is improved tracking of actual patterns of care within a DRG along with improved identification and measurement of clinical patient outcomes.

4. The Role of Nursing Informatics

The director of nursing informatics will perform a crucial role in the automation of clinical paths: that of champion, coach, and coordinator. Many important aspects of implementing managed care are within the domain of nursing: helping to define clinical paths; providing and documenting care as defined by the clinical path; monitoring progress on the clinical path concurrently and initiating action to address variances; and retrospective analysis of outcomes to improve clinical paths for future use. The role of nursing becomes even more crucial as clinical paths are automated, because nursing documentation provides the bulk of the data needed to extract both concurrent and retrospective information about variances and outcomes. Therefore, the director of nursing informatics should ideally drive the automation of clinical paths, providing both clinical and technical expertise and bridging the gap between the I.S. department and the range of care providers.

5. Conclusion

The Medical Center at Princeton has recognized the need to focus on outcomes in order to improve quality while reducing cost and optimizing operations. Thus, we have implemented a managed care program which includes extensive use of clinical paths. To fully achieve the benefits of this program, plans are in place to implement clinical paths on the ULTICARE System patient care information system during 1994.

Managed care and the use of clinical paths will be increasingly utilized by health care enterprises in the years ahead. Karen Zander RN, MS [2] states that "Unless outcomes are defined, managed, and evaluated at the detailed patient-clinician level, there is no quality for the patient currently under your care. There can be caring, there can even be satisfaction, but quality entails precision of interventions as measured by their results." The success of a managed care program cannot be assessed without the ability to define, measure, and evaluate patient outcomes, both individually and in aggregate. To do so effectively and efficiently, management information systems must be utilized to support the evolution from managing care to managing cost, quality, and outcomes.

6. References

[1] Geehr E, The Search for What Works. *Healthcare Forum Journal* 1992, 29-33.

[2] Zander K, Quantifying, Managing, and Improving Quality, Part I: How CareMaps Link CQI to the Patient. *The New Definition* Spring 1992, 1-3.

Nursing Informatics: An International Overview for Nursing in a Technological Era
S.J. Grobe and E.S.P. Pluyter-Wenting, eds.

Identification of information and technology needs of nurses in preventing the development of cumulative trauma disorders

Gordon DG

ADP Coordinator, Nursing Service, Department of Veterans Affairs Medical Center 4100 West Third Street, Dayton, Ohio 45428

Technological changes in the area of information management are creating injuries accumulating over time. The reaction of individuals to these dangers is comparable to the individuals who worked with asbestos. There is a latent period between the exposure to the problem and the development of signs and symptoms. The injuries are caused by the interaction between the user and the machine. These are known as Cumulative Trauma Disorders (CTDs). CTDs involve musculoskeletal disorders, tendon disorders, nerve disorders and neurovascular disorders. These disorders are preventable[1] (Ergonomics, Summit Training Sources, 1991, video tape). Charles J. Austin[2](1989) states, "No industry is more information intensive than the health care industry where timely and accurate information is essential for high-quality patient care and strategic management".

1.0 Problem Statement

Nursing personnel and other allied health care employees are at risk for developing acute and chronic illnesses related to the introduction of computer systems and personal computers in their work environment. These health problems are known as Cumulative Trauma Disorders (CTDs). They affect the upper extremities and torso. There is a long latent period between exposure to the environmental problems and the actual development of signs and symptoms by the employees.

2.0 Purpose Statement

The purpose of this project was to try out a program to help nurses in hospitals and other health care facilities identify the potential environmental risk factors in the development of Cumulative Trauma Disorders (CTDs). Guidelines for changing the environment using some practical cost effective means were developed. The project also included education for the employees in preventing the development of CTDs.

3.0 Significance and Justification

Cumulative Trauma Disorders have been studied in various industries for years. They were described as related to the crafts workers pursued by Ramazzini[3](1713) over two hundred eighty years ago. He described the problems as being caused by "...the harmful character of the materials they handled..." and by "...certain violent and irregular motions and unnatural posture of the body, by reason of which, the natural structure of the vital machine is so impaired that serious diseases gradually develop therefrom". During the last ten years the explosion of information management technology has created an "...epidemic of repetitive strain injury affecting Video Display Terminal (VDT) operators".[4] Since the rapid expansion of information technologies is continuing in the health care industry, high technology workers are an at-risk population in this milieu.

3.1 Cumulative Trauma Disorders are injuries to soft tissues. "Although they can occur in nearly all tissues, the nerves, tendon, tendon sheaths, and muscles of the upper extremity are the most frequently reported sites".[5] CTDs are caused by excessive repetitive movements, high force, mechanical stress, poor posture, vibrations, noise, and unusual work activities.[4] Heilbroner[6] (1993) further describes them as "...gradual onset work related illnesses...".

The National Safety Council[7] (1981) reported more than 400,000 hand and arm injuries occur each year. These account for 16 million lost days annually and are second only to back injuries in the United States. The costs of these injuries are skyrocketing. Including hospital, medical, and wage compensation, workers' compensation costs were 1.3 billion dollars annually[7]. "Related worker's compensation and absenteeism cost U.S. employers upwards of $20 billion in 1990".[6]

Health care facilities and various health care providers are delivering care to many clients suffering from CTDs. "However, the need for workplace evaluation may be as close as our own backyards. We often neglect to critically analyze our own workspaces".[8] Thomas Armstrong[9] (1992) says, "An important component of an ergonomics program is some kind of surveillance. That can either be a passive surveillance - where you wait for workers to come to you with a complaint - or it can be an active surveillance - where you go out and do some kind of surveys and interviews of your workers". In order to determine the potential for cumulative trauma disorders development, the choice of active surveillance was made.

Based on the experience of the writer, if an observational survey is conducted of health care facilities, the survey will show Personal Computers or Video Display Terminals (VDTs) sitting on charting surfaces and desks. Most of them are semi-stationary and cannot be adjusted to the various workers who use them in retrieving or entering data. These are prime areas for the development of CTDs, although they often are not recognized as an environmental threat.

4.0 Definitions

4.1 Ergonomics
As defined by Grandjean[10](1980), is the process of fitting the task to the person. It is the adaptation of the environment, work methods and design of necessary equipment involved in producing the product while protecting the worker from excessive risk or injury or illness. For the purpose of this paper, ergonomics will refer to the interaction between the health care worker, data entry tasks, and the work area where the tasks are performed.

4.2 High technology health care workers
For the purpose of this project, high technology health care workers are defined as those individuals spending two or more hours per day entering data into a Video Display Terminal (VDT) or a Personal Computer (PC) in a health care setting.

5.0 Project Steps

In conjunction with the Employee Health Department Nurse, or other designee, the following task activities were performed to assess potential for the development of Cumulative Trauma Disorders for the defined data entry personnel:

5.1 Observational Survey of work site
Can PC/VDT height be adjusted? Can keyboard height be adjusted? Can the chair be adjusted for height and back support? Does the task require repetitive motion? Does the task require awkward body movements? How many hours per day does the task require?

5.2 Employee Survey
Questions designed to elicit information concerning: Headaches, Blurred Vision, Upper Extremity (eg. pain, numbness, tingling, "pins & needles feelings"); Pain or discomfort after duty hours, etc.

5.3 If potential is identified, temporarily modify environment
Raise height of PC/VDT with phone books/boxes, rolled towels to protect wrists or support backs, train staff in importance of adjusting chair height to fit the person and design cardboard hoods to decrease glare from overhead lighting.

5.4 Educate managers concerning signs and symptoms of CTDs and alert them to potential environmental problem areas.

5.5 Provide executive summary of analyzed results with suggestions for change.

5.6 Demonstration training for employees in preventative stretching exercises and proper body mechanics.

6.0 Assumptions

6.1 Computer system Video Display Terminals are placed in the hospital/health care environment on normal charting surfaces.

6.2 Personal Computers are placed in the hospital/health care environment on space available surfaces in the various offices.

6.3 Staff have reported vague symptoms of "headaches", "wrist hurts", "back aches" to their supervisors or employee health department. They are unable to pinpoint the cause of their discomfort.

6.4 Management is unaware of the potential problems for lost time injuries of their employees related to the introduction of computer systems and personal computers into their facility.

7.0 Limitations

7.1 Number of employees willing to participate in the project may not provide an adequate number to create change.

7.2 The developed assessment research tool may have limited validity and reliability.

7.3 Funding may be unavailable for environmental changes in the institution.

8.0 Pilot Project

A **pilot project** concerning the potential for development of Cumulative Trauma Disorders by hospital employees while working with a computer system was proposed and accepted by the Director of Medical Information Systems (MIS) and Director of Nursing for a small (150 bed) urban hospital in January, 1992. The project began in January, 1992 and was completed in March, 1992.

Staff who used the computer system or personal computers in their daily work routine were asked to participate. The personnel considered at risk were designated as those staff who spent a minimum of two consecutive hours at data entry on a daily basis. The total number of employees fitting the criteria was 60. Ninety percent of the staff involved in this type of work were female. This included Unit Clerks, Programmers, Software Package Coordinators, and Systems Analysts. Employee participation in the study was on a volunteer basis. A formal presentation at the monthly Unit Clerks meeting was requested by the participating hospital. The Medical Information Systems service also requested a formal presentation at their scheduled weekly meeting. A total of 26 employees (43% participation rate) volunteered to take part in the project.

Blattner[11] (1981) defines preventive nursing as those activities which maintain and promote health and prevent health disruption. This would include helping a business and its employees manage their environment. These consist of such activities as health hazard appraisal, enforcing environmental safety programs, conducting wellness inventories, and teaching clients about preventative techniques. In order to **identify a potential problem an assessment must be accomplished**. This includes **looking at the environment, the individuals, and the interaction between the individuals and the environment**. **Observational surveys** of both facilities were scheduled and conducted during the last two weeks of January, 1992.

8.1Findings - Observational Surveys
The **Medical Information Systems** personnel's environment was a single building designated for their use. Personal Computers or VDTs were placed on desks or at work stations for the MIS staff. The keyboards at the computer

workstations were adjustable for height or tilt. The **PC monitors only had one height setting**. Height adjustable swivel chairs were used. The **VDTs used by MIS staff were placed on desk tops. No adjustments were available to accommodate the employees**. This caused awkward body posture during data entry by MIS staff. The employees were unable to maintain a neutral position: elbows were bent at greater than 90 degree angles, shoulders were rotated forward with head and neck flexed, and the low back was not supported by the chairs.

The **observational survey of the 7 nursing units at the Urban Hospital** also revealed **all VDTs on charting surfaces. None had adjustable keyboards. The terminals could not be adjusted.** Chair height could be adjusted, but no back support adjustments were available. A PC in use in the Head Pain Clinic did have the keyboard on an adjustable arm. The PC monitor screen could not be adjusted. **Direct lighting, placement of equipment in front of windows, or beneath fans contributed to excess glare on VDT screens.**

8.2 Follow up - Observational Surveys

After reviewing the information provided through analysis of the Observational Survey, the Director of Nursing and the Medical Information Systems Director **both requested a formal presentation be made to their employees.** The first presentation took place during the monthly morning Unit Clerk's meeting on February 4, 1992. A demonstration of a proper workstation/site setup through the use of a poster from Krames communications was given. The **Employee Survey** with a cover letter explaining the project, requesting volunteers, and guarantee of Rights of Human subjects was distributed. A second presentation for the MIS staff, duplicating the morning meeting, was given on the afternoon of February 4, 1992. Employees at both facilities were given 1 week to fill out and return the surveys.

8.3 Findings - Employee Survey

Surveys were collected and analyzed with the following results: **50% of the staff experienced frequent headaches, blurred vision, or burning eyes; 44% experienced elbow pain** and **38% reported neck pain.** These discomforts occurred in the afternoon (42%) and were followed closely (39%) during evening and nights. These discomforts affected the daily living of 23% of the staff. **Repetitive motions were required by 96% of the staff in performing their job tasks. Sitting for longer than two hours at a time was reported by 87% of the staff.** The raw data from the Employee Survey and the Observational Survey was shared with the Directors of both facilities and their managers. The indications of potential employee health problems related to the development of cumulative trauma disorders while entering data in the corporate computer system was obtained by the raw data collected. Frequency ratio was used in analyzing the Employee Survey. **The complaint of headaches, blurred vision, burning eyes, neck pain and elbow pain correlated with the Observational Survey.** Inability to adjust the height of the VDTs and keyboards relates to neck and elbow pain, and possibly to stimulating headaches. Overhead glare could also be a contributing factor.

8.4 Follow up - Employee Survey

Meetings with managers and employees were scheduled during March, 1992. Managers requested and received a form created to assist them in recognizing signs and symptoms in the development of CTDs in their employees. A presentation of Preventative Stretching Techniques and Proper Body Mechanics for Data Entry was given during the March Unit Clerks meeting at the participating hospital. A second training session was presented at the MIS monthly staff meeting. Posters showing these techniques were distributed to all data entry personnel.

9.0 Summary and Recommendations

A definite potential for developing cumulative trauma disorders was discovered at the participating facilities. Recommendations and suggestions to correct the environmental problem areas include: purchasing ergo arms for raising and lowering VDTs and keyboards on the busiest units; raising the height of VDTs in offices with individual user with phone books, boxes, etc.; rolling towels to use as wrist supports in helping employees maintain proper alignment; make cardboard hoods to be place over the tops of the VDTs or PCs affected by overhead glare. Management will need to review their budget to plan for more permanent adjustments.

The method necessary to reduce or eliminate the problem potential for CTDs involves educating the manager to ergonomic hazards. The Urban Hospital Nurse Managers are responsible for budget planning for their units. Salary expense is based on productive time (time actually worked) and non-productive time (benefit time-sick leave, vacation, etc.). These non-productive expenses are a significant portion of the acute care budget[12]. The nursing strategy used for health promotion with the nurse managers is to decrease costs through prevention of CTDs. Shearn and Armstrong[9] (1992) relate managers need to be "sensitized to ergonomic hazards so they don't shrug off their employees' upper extremity complaints. They need to understand that early identification and treatment are important". Depending on the extent of the ergonomic refinements that will be supported, the costs to the corporate medical facilities could be a few hundred dollars upwards to several thousands of dollars.

The rationale for the recommended ergonomic changes and health care promotion is cost containment and education in the prevention of some painful disorders. "Employee health care costs are one of the most crucial management issues facing American corporations today...the average company spends $2,000 per employee per year on health benefits...costs are escalating at 10% to 30% per year for many employers"[13]. The employees themselves are feeling the increase as more of the insurance costs are being transferred to them.

There are two target populations that the prevention plan was designed to influence: management and employees. The employees will be able to have individual control over some preventative and rehabilitative techniques. Management, however, has the responsibility to provide a safe work environment.

Recommendations for the future include replication of this project in other health care settings. Movements toward electronic patient records will increase the potential for development of Cumulative Trauma Disorders in health care workers. The scope of future studies should include all areas of health care where data entry will become a daily performance task.

10.0 References

[1]Summit Training Sources. *Ergonomics, Video Cassette Recording*, 1991. Grand Rapids, MI.

[2]Austin G. Information Technology and the Future of Health Services Delivery. *Hosp Health Serv Adm* 1989, 34 (20):158-165

[3]Ramazzini B. *Diseases of Workers (1713)*. Translation and notes: Wright W. Chicago: University of Chicago Press:1940

[4]Sauter S, and Schleifer L. Workstation design, and Musculoskeletal Discomfort in a VDT Data Entry Task. *Hum Factors* 1991, 33(2):151-167.

[5]Armstrong T. Ergonomics and Cumulative Trauma Disorders of the Hand and Wrist. In: *Rehabilitation of the Hand:Surgery and Therapy*. Hunter J, Scheider L, Mackin E, Callahan A (eds). St. Louis: CV Mosby, 1990:1175-1190.

[6]Heilbroner D. The Handling of an Epidemic. *Working Woman*, Feb. 1993:60-65.

[7]*National Safety Council*: Accident Facts. 1981: (ed).

[8]Lear C, and Pomeroy S. Better way-Workplace Modification in Your Facility. *Occ Therap Forum* 1992, Feb:4-6.

[9]Shearn W, and Armstrong T. Ergonomics for VDT Users: Maintaining Healthy Workers. *Hosp Employee Health* 1992, 11:64-66.

[10]Grandjean E. *Fitting the Task To the Man: an Ergonomic Approach*. London: Taylor and Francis Ltd, 1988.

[11]Blattner B. *Holistic Nursing*. Englewood Cliffs, New Jersey: Prentice-Hall, 1981.

[12]Stassen L. *Key Business Skills for Nurse Managers*. Philadelphia: JB Lippincott Company, 1986.

[13]Stasics E. Wellness and the Sickness Benefits to Health Benefits Transformation of the 90s. In: *National Wellness Institute's National Wellness Conference*, (eds). 1991:339-343.

© 1994 Elsevier Science B.V. All rights reserved.
Nursing Informatics: An International Overview for Nursing in a Technological Era
S.J. Grobe and E.S.P. Pluyter-Wenting, eds.

Strategic Plan on Health Care Technology

Caloren H [a] and Salois-Swallow D [b]

[a] Nursing Consultant, Health Issues, Canadian Nurses Association, 50 The Driveway, Ottawa, Ontario, Canada

[b] Nursing Systems Coordinator, York Central Hospital, 10 Trench Street, Richmond Hill, Ontario, Canada

The use of technology in health care has profound implications for providers and consumers of services. Science has advanced quickly and some health care technology has been put into use with seemingly little understanding of the possible impact on clients, families, health care professionals and the health care delivery system. Recognizing an urgent need, The Board of the Canadian Nurses Association (CNA) instructed its Special Committee on Clinical Practice Issues (CPIC) to develop a Strategic Plan on Health Care Technology which could give guidance and support to nurses in addressing the issues raised by the use of technology in health care. This presentation will describe the process used by the Committee for gathering nurses' input regarding how the use of technology in health care affects their practice and how this information was used to develop a framework for the CNA to plan specific activities which will address technology related issues in nursing management, practice, education and research.

1. Background

The Canadian Nurses Association (CNA) recognizes the many benefits resulting from the use of health care technologies and their potential to improve the care given by nurses. However, to realize the optimum positive effect of technology use in health care, nurses must be involved in the decision processes by which specific technologies are developed, selected, incorporated into treatment programs and evaluated. There must also be provision for input from clients/patients and family members regarding their experiences with technology in the health care setting. Conversely, nurses are often required to use technology with little or no training and with little technical or other assistance. In such situations there is significant potential for negative outcomes. In order to provide direction and support for nurses faced with such situations the Board of CNA commissioned a literature review on Technology and Nursing [1] and directed its' Clinical Practice Issues Committee (CPIC) to develop a strategic plan on technology as a first step in addressing some of the issues.

2. The Special Committee on Clinical Practice Issues

This is a fourteen member committee composed of nurses with designated clinical expertise, including three members who also sit on the Board in specified capacities. The committee terms of reference include the identification of emerging clinical practice issues of concern to Canadian nurses; the recommendation of priorities, positions and strategic actions to the Board; and specified action on practice issues referred from the Board. The ultimate purpose is to increase responsiveness to the clinical practice concerns of registered nurses in Canada and to increase visibility and accountability of the professional association.

3. Committee Response

Committee members shared the concern that implementation of technological advances has potential to affect the role of nurses and content of nursing practice in the future and agreed that vigilance is needed to ensure that nursing has appropriate input to developments. Thus Board's action was timely.

4. Definition and Framework for Analysis

The committee reviewed background documentation and in, keeping with CNA's primary health care approach to issues, adopted a definition of technology which is broad and by which technology is understood to include much more than technical equipment (hardware). Such things as work organization, placement of services and computerization of records are understood to be part of technology. The framework which was accepted for analysis of the impact of technology is adapted from Jacox, Pillar and Redman [2], and includes the following three categories (1) cost benefit and effectiveness, (2) safety, and (3) social impact.

4.1 Data Gathering

The Committee reviewed a package of background documentation and the literature review. It was decided to circulate a questionnaire to nurses practising in a variety of settings in order to obtain further information. The Committee designed a survey to ask individual nurses what aspects of technology affecting nursing practice should be dealt with in CNA's strategic plan under the three categories identified in the framework. For purposes of clarification the survey preamble briefly defined the three areas under investigation- costs and benefits/effectiveness, safety and social impact.

4.2 Responses

Approximately eighty responses were received and in many instances these consolidated input from sizable groups of nurses. The areas of practice represented in the responses included, community, long term care, rehabilitation, acute care, maternity, paediatrics, education, nursing informatics and supervision/management. National nursing interest groups responded at the Advisory Council (annual meeting - June, 1991) as well as individually. Government nurse consultants and the member associations of CNA also responded. This rate of response indicates the importance for nurses generally, of issues related to the use of health care technology.

In addition to the recognition that technology use in health care can provide enormous benefits, questionnaire responses indicated that there is a high degree of concern among nurses in all areas of practice about the effect of technology use, not only on the client, but also on the health care providers and on the overall care system. The major areas of consensus identified are reflected in the goals and objectives of the strategic plan which was developed.

5. Process

A synthesis was developed based on survey information. This was used by the committee in developing a grid which served to ensure that all the concerns could be included under one of four categories (practice, education, research and management) which are identified in the Mission of CNA as areas in which excellence is to be fostered. The grid was used by the CPIC in developing the draft Strategic Plan on Technology which was presented to the CNA Board (March, 1992) and approved.

6. The Strategic Plan

The overall goal was to develop a strategic plan on health care technology that addresses issues related to costs and benefits, safety, and social impact and to provide a framework to guide nursing administration, practice, education and research in addressing technology related issues in those areas. Thus the Strategic Plan on Health Care Technology provides a framework for identifying specific activities on an annual basis to address issues raised for nurses by the use of technology in a variety of practice settings. The goals and objectives and selected sample activities follow.

6.1 Goal One

The first goal of the plan is to promote the selection of cost effective and efficient health care technology that supports patients by involving nurses from administration, practice, education and research in the processes for technology development, acquisition and assessment. Three objectives flow from this goal:

1. To encourage development and accessability to, educational opportunities for nurses that enable their participation in technology development, assessment and acquisition processes.
   Sample activities:
   a) Encourage provinces that hold conferences such as *Nursing Practice Conference* to consider profiling issues related to the costs and benefits of technology in developing their programs
   b) Approach the *Canadian Association of University Schools of Nursing* (CAUSN) regarding collaborative initiatives to encourage the introduction of courses on the impact of technology in all nursing programs

2. To encourage individual nurses at the national, provincial/jurisdictional and local levels to seek to participate in technology assessment and acquisition processes and in the development of technology that supports nursing administration, practice, education and research.

3. To encourage the development and evaluation of comprehensive frameworks to guide nurses in their role in technology development, acquisition and assessment processes, eg., total costs, outcome measurement, benefit realization for individuals vs groups.

6.2 Goal Two

The second goal is to identify and address safety implications of the use of health care technology for clients, families, nurses and other health care personnel. The related objectives are:

1. To promote the development of, and accessibility to, educational opportunities that foster the safe and appropriate utilization of health care technology by clients and families, nurses and other health care professionals.

2. To promote the importance of nursing practice standards to provide client/family centred care in the health care technology context.
   Sample activity:
   a) Invite readers to submit statements or brief articles to CNA*Today* detailing the ethical and safety issues related to the use of technology which they have experienced, with emphasis on the role of nursing.

3. To encourage the development of policies and guidelines at all levels to minimise and address potential hazards in the use of health care technology, eg., infection control, conservation of the environment, security and confidentiality of health records.
   Sample activity:
   a) Request *Nurse Administrator Interest Group* to take initiatives to encourage nurses in administration to work for the safe use of technology in the workplace by establishing product evaluation and technology assessment committees, and introducing policies and guidelines regarding informed consent and confidentiality of information.

6.3 Goal Three

The third major goal outlined by the plan is to identify and address social implications of the use of health care technology for clients, families, nurses and other health care professionals and society. Objectives outlined for this goal are:

1. To encourage ongoing assessment of the impact of health care technology on the quality of life of individuals, families and communities eg., informed consent, living wills, ongoing supportive services, effects of client displacement for treatment (isolated areas), legal status of automated charting and electronic signatures and security of clients records.
   Sample activity:
   a) Support initiatives which could lead to the development of a framework/model for the assessment of the social impact of technology in health care.

2. To promote the use of current research findings in developing strategies to address work life issues related to the use of technology eg., role conflict, work related stress and workload levels.

3. To encourage the establishment of mechanisms to facilitate the resolution of ethical and legal dilemmas raised by the use of health care technology eg., multidisciplinary ethics committees, legal and ethical advisors, involvement of clients/community representatives in the decision making process, use of ethical decision making models.
   Sample activity:
   a) CNA to use all available opportunities to stress the need to use multidisciplinary committees with representation from nursing to review the implications of technology on the delivery of care, eg. discuss related issues during the annual lobby of Members of Parliament by CNA Board members.

7. Position Statement

The CPIC brought a recommendation to the CNA Board (November, 1992) for the development of a position statement on the *Role of the Nurse in Relation to the Use of Technology in Health Care.* The statement was published in 1993 and circulated to member groups of the CNA. One of the issues discussed by the Board and which received approval for inclusion, was the notion that in addition to playing a key role in decision making about technology design, selection and acquisition, utilization and evaluation, nurses should be encouraged to identify the need for and conceptualize new technologies which would benefit patient care.

8. Summary

The increasing requirement and opportunity for nurses to use technology in the provision of health care has resulted in the development of a Strategic Plan on Health Care Technology and a Position Statement on the Role of the Nurse in Relation to the Use of Technology in Health Care. The availability of these documents, provides support and direction for nurses in practice, education, research and management with regard to their responsibilities and the opportunities afforded them for input to the development, selection, use and evaluation of health care technologies. This increases the potential for health care providers to make wise decisions about technology use. The end result should be reflected in the quality of care available to clients of the health care system thus helping to ensure that technology provides positive support for patients in whose care it is used.

9. References

[1] Campbell M., McCaskell L, *Technology and Nursing. A Review and Analysis of Selected Literature*, prepared for CNA.,(1990) Ottawa, Non published

[2] Pillar B., Jacox A.K., and Redman B.K. Technology, Its Assessment, and Nursing. *Nurs Outlook,* 1990,38:1 16-19

Nursing Informatics: An International Overview for Nursing in a Technological Era
S.J. Grobe and E.S.P. Pluyter-Wenting, eds.

New South Wales Information Technology Strategy:
a description

Van der Weegen L[a] Morris S[b] and Cook R[c]

Information Management Division, NSW Health Department, LMB 961, North Sydney, 2059

In 1989 the Australian state of New South Wales developed an information strategy aimed at bringing the Health system into the 21st century with systems capable of providing relevant decision support information to clinicians and managers and promoting an environment for change to a more patient focused health system. Minimal resources had been allocated to Information Technology (IT) prior to this and it was decided to invest in a *patient focused, integrated hospital information system in hospitals across the state.*

This paper outlines the scope of the NSW IT strategy, the methodology devised for system selection, and unique lessons learned during the implementation on such a wide scale.

1. Background to the Australian Health Care System

In Australia, *the provision and funding of health is a dual responsibility* shared by both the Commonwealth and State Governments, the Commonwealth regulating and administering Medicare, our universal health insurance scheme and each state administering the provision of health services.

The Department of Health is responsible for the provision of health services to the state of New South Wales (NSW). This is accomplished via a central policy and planning body and Area (10) and District (23) Health Services, each responsible for the provision of health services via a number of Public Hospitals ranging from major teaching hospitals (16 in total) to small district/country hospitals (total public hospital 250), plus Community Health Services. The annual Health Budget is $AUS 4 Billion, and comprises 80,000 employees statewide.

Like many countries, Australia is under pressure to improve the quality of our services, better meet the needs of the health care consumer and achieve productivity gains, while simultaneously containing costs. It is within this framework that the government realised the need for a new information systems strategy that would envisage a progressive upgrading of the quality of systems available in public hospitals and provide a catalyst for change, via process innovation and re-engineering, within the health system. The focus is the provision of an information framework for all health professionals, clinicians and managers, which is patient focused and results in improvements in patient services and outcomes, plus improved management of resources.

2. Key elements of NSW IT Strategy

The following points summarise the major strategic direction:
- Recognition of the differing business needs of each market segment;
- Provide the infrastructure to allow decentralisation of Information System delivery and support;

- Provide the bulk of one-off implementation costs to each site;
- Maintain the Strategy focus and momentum via user participation in Steering Committee guidance;
- Facilitate day to day management from a Central consulting body;
- Involve expert users in all stages of the system selection processes;
- Selection of <u>developed</u> software products on current hardware where possible;
- Evaluate systems within pilot implementations prior to general release of software statewide;
- Focus on operational support to clinicians with aggregated information for management including Casemix and Clinical costing analysis; and
- Phased implementation of sophisticated technology as this becomes feasible both on operational and financial grounds.

3. Selection of systems

System selection has been approached in *two main phases*. The first addressed selection of the "base" elements (financial, laboratory and core patient administration/order communications systems), the second addressed specialised systems selection including nursing, pharmacy, dietary, radiology, critical care and operating theatre systems. A *consistent approach* to selection was achieved by following a generic Acquisition Methodology which included the following steps:

- *Problem Identification & Definition* (identification of business needs per market segment);
- *Identification of Solutions* (analysis of currently available products and their suitability to resolve or support the business needs identified in previous step, followed by options analysis which may or may not recommend continuing to the following steps);
- *Pre-qualification* (high level formal analysis via Expression of Interest or Request for Information of currently available systems);
- *Selective Request for Tender* (more detailed evaluation of functional, technical and vendor support capabilities from book response);
- *Detailed Product Evaluation* (the use of scripted demonstrations as a method of confirming the book responses of the most appropriate responses from the Selective Tender); and
- *Contract Negotiations and Pilot Implementation* (negotiations with the most suitable vendor to implement their product for further pilot evaluations at a range of hospitals to confirm their suitability to the NSW Health environment. Addition of further customers to the contract hinges on a successful pilot report).

In each case a group of expert users was gathered from around the state to identify and prioritise functional requirements in consultation with key players. This team were also involved in the evaluation of products *promoting user ownership* of the systems. Other evaluation criteria including systems integration were assessed by a team of Department of Health Information Management Division (IMD) staff with relevant skills.

3.1. Nursing System selection

As an example, for selection of the nursing systems, a group of twelve nurses covering a wide range of experience and skills was gathered to define the desired scope, develop functional, security and user interface requirements, weighted criteria and demonstration scripts. The functional requirements were packaged as three distinct entities, listed in order of priority, with the following broad requirements:

- ▸ Patient Management
  - Assess, Plan, Document and Evaluate collaborative patient care delivery
  - Focus on achievement of desired patient outcomes
  - Feasible for multidisciplinary use in clinical setting
  - Calculate cost of care and number and skill of staff required to provide care;
- ▸ Staff Scheduling to budget
  - Flexibility of scheduling methods incorporating patient demand input
  - Provide modelling on shift, staff number and skill parameters
  - Provide costs for all schedules generated whether planned or actual; and

▸ Staff Management
  • Provide reporting & query access on employee database
  • Maintain all facets of employee details
  • Model organisational positions against available budget
  • Maintain professional development paths & course attendance.

At the time of preparing this paper, discussions are taking place regarding the development of the Patient Management component, available products have been identified and a tender for the Staff Scheduling & Budgeting component is due to close in late September 1993. The Staff Management component will be incorporated within the Human Resource/Payroll Strategy in the long term, with short term resolution of access to currently held information addressed during the implementation of the Staff Scheduling & Budgeting system.

4. Implementation

To date, the current implementations have been:
  • Oracle (Oracle Financials)   - Financial System
  • Cerner (Pathnet)   - Laboratory System
  • First Data Corporation (Precision Alternative)   - Clinical System

4.1 Clinical Systems

Prior to the implementation of the clinical systems, a *formal process of localisation* was undertaken by the IRMC, the three pilot sites and the vendor to "localise" the software to suit the NSW environment. It involved a process of workshops over a period of 3 months, with each pilot site identifying specific changes to the software, depending on the differing complexities of their organisations. A negotiation process then followed to rationalise and prioritise the number of changes requested. The outcome was a *comprehensive list of changes* required to satisfy both the Department of Health reporting requirements and state regulatory requirements in addition to those at the local level.

Many of the changes identified through localisation, especially those relating to security and audit, highlighted the differing methods of practice between Australian and the United States. Current legislation requirements in NSW, state that orders for pathology, radiology and pharmaceutical be placed and signed by a doctor in their own hand writing for the purpose of reimbursement and clinical accountability. At a state level, much negotiation has taken place between the Health Insurance Commission, a Commonwealth regulatory body responsible for Medicare and the NSW Pharmacy Branch to accept electronic signatures. Although the legislation will be changed to include electronic signatures as a valid and accepted form of identification, it is not foreseen that the current practice of doctors placing their own orders will be changed.

The major difficulty during the implementation phase was and still is, to *gain the clinicians acceptance of using the computer as a means of communicating orders and retrieving results at the ward level*. This has required a major undertaking in training at individual hospitals, regular communication and consultation between professional groups, relevant unions and the tertiary education sector.

The process of achieving benefits from the implementation of the systems has followed a continuous quality improvement framework. Small cross-functional teams, comprised of end users, have reviewed current processes and developed *new and innovative processes* to take advantage and gain maximum leverage of the new information systems, as well as simultaneously making quality improvements to linked processes within the organisation. The *use of small teams* has been beneficial in managing the change process, gaining user acceptance of the new system, and ownership of the new "way of doing things". *The key to the success has proven to be the education of management and staff to ensure their commitment.*

5. So why a State Strategy, not individual areas/regions/hospitals selecting systems to meet their needs?

5.1 A state strategy has the advantages of:
- Providing an integrated/interfaced complete HIS;
- Reducing the overall costs of the system and ensuring the system can "communicate" with each other;
- Providing consistent comparable information throughout the state;
- Achieving of economies of scale through the sharing of information and resources for implementation and less duplication of work;
- An improved bargaining position for purchasing and modifications to the software to meet NSW Health needs;
- Consistent software for staff training and transportability of skills;
- Reducing implementation time through less software modifications and customisation at each hospital; and
- Provision of state standards for data sets and information collection.

5.2 Disadvantages of a state strategy:
- Obtaining consensus on changes during the negotiation phase of localisation;
- Underlying risk of not identifying the needs of those hospitals not involved in the pilot localisation;
- Potential for decreased commitment to the strategy from other hospitals not involved in the pilot studies;
- That the strategy will not meet the needs of all market segments;
- Purchasing proven "off the shelf" products has the potential to limit Australian participation in product development; and
- Purchasing "off the shelf" products can potentially reduce functional fit to 60%.

6. Conclusions

The selection and implementation of a state wide solution for IT requires the contribution of, and consultation with, a wide variety of health professionals in the determination of their baseline requirements and selection of systems. The systems that provide these *requirements*, and the *flexibility* to be modified at *minimal cost* to meet the individual facility's needs, are one of the best matches you will find, without the timely task of developing systems in house.

The challenge still remaining however is the *acceptance of computerisation* by our health professionals. This involves working closely with staff and gaining their participation in all implementation activities thus ensuring maximum benefits are gained. In conclusion, a perfect match in health information technology, is as difficult to find as the perfect human relationship.

7. References

[1] Touche Ross Consultants and Office of Public Management. NSW Information Technology Strategy, 1989.

[2] NSW Public Health System. Acquisition Methodology for Information Systems, July 1990.

Nursing Informatics: An International Overview for Nursing in a Technological Era
S.J. Grobe and E.S.P. Pluyter-Wenting, eds.
51

A process for introducing a Hospital Information System in a Greek cardiac surgery hospital-nursing's integral role

Papadandonaki A[a] Papathanassoglou E[b] Tsirintani M[c]

[a]Adjunct Professor of Nursing, University of Athens, Department of Nursing, Nursing Education Councelor, Onassis Cardiac Surgery Center.

[b]Nurse-Instructor/councelor for the HIS applications, ICU Staff-Nurse, Onassis Cardiac Surgery Center, Athens.

[c]Nurse-Instructor/councelor for the HIS applications, Onassis Cardiac Surgery Center, Athens.

This study represents the first attempt to implement a Hospital Information System in Greece and to standardize essential Nursing Data. The Hospital involved is the Onassis Cardiac Surgery Center (OCSC) which is a new, relatively small (150 beds), high acuity hospital in Athens.
The purpose of this study is two fold: 1) To describe the process undertaken to implement a Hospital Information System in Greece to meet, primarily, the nurses' needs, and 2) To identify the Nursing's integral contribution to the success of the system.

1. Introduction

Hospital Information Systems (HIS) are rapidly evolving within the health care arena in an effort to improve communication and curtail spiraling health care costs. Vast amounts of patient data, as well as departmental communication are collected, stored, retrieved, and transmitted through automated means. These technological advances have the capabilities of enhancing Nursing efficiency and increasing productivity [1]. Nursing personnel; often accounting for over one half of hospital's work force, are typically the most frequent users of an automated HIS. Unfortunately, input from professional nurses is seldom provided when the commitment to automate occurs within a health-care setting. One possible explanation is that computer specialists intimidate and distance the nursing staff from contributing to automated systems by using language that is very specific to data processing environments, or perhaps, nurses feel threatened because traditionally they have not been educated in basic computer literacy skills [2].

Nurses can be involved from the earliest stages of the selection of technology, the initial planning, and throughout the implementation acting as the "bridge" between the systems staff and clinical users [3]. As the primary users of clinical data systems, nurses are the ones most affected by them. The acceptance and full use of such systems depends on the extent to which the clinical nursing staff is helped as the result of a Patient Data Management System implementation.

Nursing input into the planning and tailoring of a clinical computer system can range from involvement in the number and placement of computer terminals, printers, and other equipment to designing the clinical component of the database [4].

Nurses compose the largest group of health professionals providing direct service to patients on a daily basis. No other profession has more involvement with hospital information systems that touch all aspects of patient care. Nursing's challenge is to use computer technology to innovate and to transform the manner in which nursing care is delivered [5].

2. The Hospital Information System implementation effort at the OCSC-Nursing's contribution

The Hospital Information System was purchased by the Hospital Administrators to obtain automation to support administrative, nursing, and medical needs. Automation was considered to be a criterion of quality and thus it was desirable by the Board of Directors, since the Onassion Institution was represented by its delineates to the Board, and was committed to set off the OCSC as a paragon for Greek Hospitals and cardiac surgery. So omitting any problem analysis phase the Board proceeded to the selection of contract services, long before the OCSC started to function. Since there was no previous experience, analysis, or design the system suppliers selection depended mainly on the cost factor. No actual requirements were at this time set by the hospital to check the feasibility and the cost of their fulfillment. However, the Hospital Administration was committed to purchase an Integrated System with a high degree of automation and between departments communication, with the objective to eventually eliminate all paper-sheet documentation. Their sight was that the Onassis Hospital would become one of the four "paperless" hospitals in Europe.

At the system selection phase there was no nursing input on either contract selection procedures, or development for various reasons. Apart from the fact that there was no final decision about the members of the nursing personnel, the key reason was that the Board lacked sufficient understanding of the nursing role and thus nurse's needs. To their perception nurses were at the most executing orders, and as far as their practice was mostly defined by other health-care professionals they had no actual needs for the information system support.

So when finally the OCSC concluded to a computer systems vendor the implementation of nursing care modules was considered of low priority and was not included in the contract signed. The system vendors, however, offered a few nursing applications, whose the use was for months jeopardised in a circle of contradicted opinions and several nursing job descriptions, failing to capture expertise knowledge.

We will now describe the modules offered by the original Hospital Information System to prove them insufficient for the nursing tasks management. The overall system included the following options:

1. Patient Admission   2. Nursing care module   3. Laboratory module
4. Operating Room Module   5. Pharmacy module   6. Medical records

From the above only the Patient Admission and Nursing care module were active. Nursing care menu included the following options:

1. Lab-tests and Medications ordering and billing   2. Materials billing
3. Care of patient with IV infusion   4. Nurses' notes
5. Vital Signs diagram   6. Pre-operative assessment
7. Dietary Information

It is worth noticing that the Hospital Administration focused on the need to manage the first two options, that is Lab-tests, medications, and materials billing. Their prime concern was to eliminate all unjustified expanses. Although this was obviously a non nursing activity nurses were forced to perform these tasks. In the meantime there was no planning for physicians' involvement with the system, and the surprisingly limited number of ward secretaries, was at the most performing bed-management, and typing tasks. Furthermore, two days per week and during all evening and night shifts, nurses had to take over all clerical responsibilities, since no such personnel was available.

Nursing Administrators alerted by the concern that basic Nursing Standards would be ignored, in a process aiming to use nursing staff to diminish costs, insisted that nurses; end-shift report should be documented via the Information System for every patient. At this time nurses, being understaffed and already under an immense workload, failed to conceive the real motivations of their administrators and interpreted this requirement as unjustified and unrealistic. They claimed that data entry through a keyboard using one single working station per ward and having no previous experience with keyboard and terminal functions was so laborious that there would be no actual time left for direct patient care delivery. And that was the reality.

So the unpredicted outcome of this arbitrary HIS implementation effort was an increasing personnel dissatisfaction, and an immense concern for the patients' well-being. Nurses, having concluded that no benefit for their practice would ever come up from the system, adopted a hostile attitude towards the HIS, in coherence with the physicians who hoped that at last nurses would be available to perform their traditional role.

What had happened was that a supposingly integrated, advanced Hospital Information System, which cost millions of dollars, had finally failed seriously jeopardising the quality of care delivered, and after a long period of professional debates and laborious efforts. Before contract retrieval, Nursing Administrators made a last effort and this time it was successful. They proposed a committee to be formed by nurses to help scrutinize the Hospital Information System pitfalls, to organize activities, and eventually to develop new effective applications. At their majority organization and planning were addressed to nursing personnel and tasks. Despite, this practice was judged insufficient by the Administration, the new Hospital Information System developed was both viable and satisfactory for the users, insinuating that maybe at a HIS designing nurses' needs should be taken into consideration first.

3. Designing the Nursing Applications of the HIS

The design of new applications was inevitably linked with already existing applications modification. Nursing process steps served as a directive for both rationalizing the original ones, and for designing new records and files. The primary objective was to eliminate duplicate and/or repetitive charting, and relieve nurses from the performance of other professionals responsibilities. Big effort was made to conclude to a minimum Nursing Data Set which should be entered for each patient.

The prime concern was to maintain professional standards, but the most intrinsic part was the effort to avoid transferring substandard practice to the computer system. We must notice that nursing practice had not yet focused on the nursing process applications. So building an Information System for the OCSC was actually developing a nursing care system based on care plans and the nursing process, which attempt is innovative for Greece.

Hopingly, data input requirements would define the steps undertaken by the nurse to care for the patients. The computer system was designed to meet the ultimate need: to drive the nurse toward the patient, to the patient's bedside.

For all applications analysis and design the following steps were taken:

During the *analysis phases* data were collected through written documents, paper files, interviews with staff and head-nurses, but mostly by constant observations of the current data flow and the work assignments.

During the *design phase* first step was to design the outputs according to the desirable functionality of the records and files. The outputs would identify the data required as input, and generally judge the success of the information system. Thus extensive reference was considered and experimental outputs were repeatedly tested by the Nurse Administrators and staff members to confirm their accuracy and effectiveness. All outputs would be reports produced on paper.

An important issue at this phase was to assure the consistency of the nursing care process and documentation practices across all units. For this purpose adequate in-service education was conducted.

Second step was the inputs design. The majority of applications inputs were directly defined by the outputs. Inputs forms were designed to be generated directly from the computer, to assist nurses for data collection.

4. Nursing Applications

We will now discuss the new applications developed. All applications were designed by nurses according to the analysis. Software was developed by the system vendor programmers to meet the requirements of the Relational Database Management System. The applications are:

- Nursing Care Plans
- Fluid-Balance Record
- Medications Information Record
- Lab-tests results management
- Nursing History
- Medications Administration Record
- Physicians Orders Record

First application to be considered was the *Patient Progress Documentation Record* . Originally the system offered a S.O.A.P. structure to record the patient status and the delivery of care. The (S) Subjective notes should capture patient's complaints, the (C) Objective section should contain objective findings as resulted from physical assessment and observations, along with the documentation of the care delivered, and of the outcomes. The (A) Assessment field is oriented to documenting assessment and diagnostic tests procedures. The (P) Plan section allows the nurse to document patient care plan, including nursing diagnoses.

However, two were proved to be the disadvantages of the S.O.A.P. record: 1) The nursing process steps were quite obscure and their input was not identified by the record format, being depended on the will of nurses. 2) The record structure was not problem-oriented.

For these reasons efforts were oriented to *Nursing Care Plans Record* design. Nursing care planning is an integral part of the professional nursing practice. The care plan documents the problem-solving process of nursing care and provides for consistent care delivery. However, given the workload and nursing understaffing, care planning tasks seemed to be of low priority to the provision of care. Furthermore, writing care plans often involves reiterations of the same information for several patients. Another concern is the validity of care plans formed by nurses within the limited margins of shift time. Best response to these problems seemed to be the development of pre-structured complete Nursing Care Plans according to the prevalent patient problems.

So there are two options offered to nurses: 1) to use the pre-structure care plans as paradigms, and 2) to activate a selected plan and then to enrich it with new patient problems and nursing interventions (either selected from another plan or written by the nurse), omitting any data irrelevant to the patient needs. This way the Care Plan Record permits the nurse to create a valid, tailored, and individualized plan of care, with minimum key board dated entry.

These care plans also serve as an easy accessible decision support tool, reflecting the Hospital Standard Policy and Procedures as well as an educative tool for new personnel instruction.

Plans were formed for the prevalent patient problems and were entered into the system. This process was largely simplified by the fact that the problems of cardiac surgery or coronary care patients are similar.

At the *Nursing History Record* design we again tried to eliminate the free text format data input aiming to time saving and user satisfaction. The Nursing History format used came up from active nursing research. Information is organized according to current health problems and anamnestic history, and problems as confined at each organ system trying to capture Nursing Assessment information as well. Each field of the History is consisted of several items each related to a problem. Characters are assigned to the items by the nurse: "Y" for YES and "N" for NO. At the end of each field a few scroll lines provide for free text entry, if needed.

One of the major disadvantages of this structure is that since data collection must be done at patient bedside data must be first collected by hand onto paper chart and then entered to the system. A solution for this problem would be the use of bedside terminal.

Nursing History forms are generated by the computer to serve as input data paper forms. Demographic data and all information collected by other departments prior to nursing documentation, appears automatically at this form respectively all information items entered by the nurse (e.g. allergies, medications administered at home, etc.) are automatically transferred to all pertinent files avoiding redundant entry and repetition of the same questions to the patient.

The *Fluid Balance Record* provides for consistent documentation of all intake and output volumes at each shift.

Type of fluid is also recorded, and a relevant Vitals Signs Field allows the nurse to record any alterations, mainly for Critical Care needs (e.g. FFP injected when A.P. fell or pulse rate rose). Following each entry totals are calculated automatically and the net fluid balance appears.

The *Medications Administration Record (MAR)* consists of 8 subsequent fields in a table format, where all medications including IV infusions prescribed for the patient appear. Dosages, route of administrations, frequency, and administration schedule are also recorded, together with the starting date and the solution desired. Following the administration the nurse signs in the exact time and his/her electronic signature appears on the screen at an identification field. At this latter field notifications and observations can be entered, if needed. Inactive drugs appear at the bottom of the screen. The medication field allows the nurse to call a helping record providing information about specific drugs. Administration routes and indicated solutions can be transferred to the MAR using a function key.

The *Physicians Order Record* consists of 4 fields each one followed by a scroll free ward processing text field.

Orders are entered for medications, IV infusions, lab-tests, and treatments. Medications information can also be retrieved from this record. By entering data once information is transferred to all pertinent files.

5. Implementation phase

5a. Users training: The overwhelming majority of the users trained to the HIS applications had no previous experience with computer applications. Only the members of the Nursing and Clerical personnel attended to the programs, since the physicians resistance was already apparent from the beginning. Initial training was provided by the system vendors and was consisting of 25 training hours per each employee. The program included basic computer science concepts, training to specific applications, and hardware management. Following this initial approach, on-the-job training programs were conducted, throughout a period of 6 months. Instructors to these programs were the nurses involved in the system design, who were also specialized to computer applications through an academic program (MSN). The instructor to trainee ratio ranged from 3:1 to 1:1 (most commonly). Instruction is ongoing, since modifications are introduced and new applications are developed. The system was documented by both the nurses-instructors and the system vendors, and detailed users' manuals were prepared.

5b. Implementation of the system. At the implementation phase a "parallel" approach was adopted. The system run parallel to the already existing paper-sheet documentation system till the nurses became adjusted to the new requirements and the instruction was completed.

5c. Evaluation of the system. The evaluation of the system is still ongoing. Preliminary results insinuate that there has been a favorable impact on nursing and other departments (such as laboratories, billing and census services) performance. The effects on performance are judged according to the following parameters:

1) *Decision support capability.* Such capability is provided through the Nursing Care Plans Record and Medications Information Record, as reported by the users. Hopingly the increased consistency and accessibility of nursing documentation will assist clinical decision making.

2) *Improved communication.* The speed of information transfer is greatly improved, as is accuracy. Coordination throughout the hospital appears to be improved, with less waiting time for order and test result transmission and less duplication of effort, as reported by others, too [6].

3) *Enhancement of the quality of nursing practice.* We consider the Computer defined use of the Nursing Care Plans based on the Nursing Process as an ultimate criterion for quality. Furthermore, decreased documentation and communication time releases nursing time for direct care delivery. Another contribution to quality comes throughout he process of defining a minimum nursing documentation data-set, and of standardizing these data.

4) *Documentation efficiency.* Time savings have been reported since the system prevents from redundant entry and provides pre-structured reports. Automated calculations are a great contribution to time saving and information accuracy.

5) *Nurses' satisfaction.* Increased job satisfaction was reported due to decreased communication time and from the fact that a new challenge is faced.

6. Conclusions

Nursings' input to all phases of a Hospital Information System development and implementation is both imperative and challenging. We have learned a great amount through experience. Decisions made, both right and wrong, will be valuable input for the future.

7. References

[1] Jenkins C. Automation improves nursing productivity. *Comput Healthcare* 1988, 2: 40-41.

[2] Lenkman S. Nursing satisfaction and job design. *Comput Healthcare* 1988, 2: 26-30.

[3] Farlee C and Coldstein B. A role for nurses in implementing computerized hospital information systems. *Nursing Forum* 1971, X: 339-357.

[4] Milholland K. Patient Data Management Systems (PDMS)-Compute technology for Critical Care Nurses. *Comput Nurs* 1988, 6: 237-241.

[5] Hersher BS. The job search and information systems opportunities for nurses. *Nurs Clin N Am* 1985, 20(3): 585-594.

[6] Saba VK and McCormick KA. Essentials of Computers for Nurses. Philadelphia: J.B. Lippincott Co.

ADMINISTRATION

B. Workload, acuity, staffing and rostering

© 1994 Elsevier Science B.V. All rights reserved.
Nursing Informatics: An International Overview for Nursing in a Technological Era
S.J. Grobe and E.S.P. Pluyter-Wenting, eds.

Computer Support in the Zebra system : A Neccessity for the Patient

Anna-Karin Levenstam

Department of Information Technology, University Hospital of Lund, S-241 85 Lund, Sweden.

Since the health care field is changing to be more like "the free market for goods and services" it is most urgent that the individual patient's need for nursing care can be expressed in such a way that it can be used for both calculating staff requirements and nursing costs. This is vital for maintaining quality in nursing care in the future. Using the Zebra system, the most used patient classification system in Sweden, makes it possible to do that.

1. Introduction

Today in Sweden there is a total change in the economic systems in health care. Health care organizations will be operating under conditions similar to "the free market for goods and services." In this new situation it is most urgent that an individual patient's need for nursing care can be documented in such a way that the information can be used for both calculating staff requirements and nursing costs. If nursing costs not are related to reality, which can happen if fixed costs are used as in the DRG system, is it difficult to maintain quality in nursing care. One way of describing the patients' need for nursing care so it can be used both for economical purposes and for calculating staff requirements is to use the Zebra system, a patient classification system[1].

The Zebra system consists of two parts, (1) *The Patient Classification method* which was taken from the Hospital Systems Study Group's System, Canada and (2) *The Activity study method* (a time study method) which was taken from the Public Health Service Patient Classification System, USA. Both methods have been developed futher in Sweden. The patient classification categorizes the patients according to their dependency level in direct nursing care activities. From the collected data in the Activity study one can calculate both staffing coefficients (a figure which shows staff requirements per category of care and working shift) and total minutes of nursing care per patient, per category of care and day, which is for calculating nursing cost per day, per patient stay or per diagnosis or DRG. The total minutes include minutes for the direct nursing care activities, indirect nursing care activities, unit related activities, personal time (meal time, coffee break).

2. The computer support for the Zebra system

When the patient classification had been in daily operation for some years and two Activity studies had been conducted in two departments of the University hospital of Lund (a general hospital with 1200 beds), one in 1989 in the Infection department and one in 1990 in the Neurosurgery department, the development of the computer support started. A computer support is a neccessary if the Zebra system shall be used for economical purposes. In September 1991 the computer support was put into operation in the Infection department (three units) and in the Neurosurgery department (three units). In 1992 it was introduced in the Gyneocology department (two units). The computer support is an interactive system built with Oracle's database and running on a workstation connected to both personal computers emulating terminals and to terminals. The program is menu driven with 23 different alternatives. The Main menu has 10 alternatives (figure 1). Under "Reports"(number 8) there are 7 more functions and under "Administration of the system" (number 9) there are 8 more functions.The users have access only to the information of one's own unit, with the exception of using the SQL-function under "Administration of the system", number 9 where information from the whole department can be retrieved.

The alternatives 1, 2, 3, 6 and 10 in the Main menu consist of screen views in which data can be inserted, altered, deleted or searched for. In the alternatives 4, 5 and 7 the users can only ask questions (search) to the database, not change any information. In most cases the answeres can be printed out. Under "Reports" (number 8) are the predesigned reports where the users can choose to get a print out for a certain period. Under

"Administration of the system" (number 9) are functions for setting values of different variables in the computer system, for example minutes per category of care per unit and number of beds in different units.

Main menu
1. Patient classification
2. Staffing situation
3. The individual patient's stay
4. Number of patients per category of care, per day
5. The staffing situation per day
6. Changing the patient's identifaction number
7. Summary of the patients' stay
8. Reports (7 alternatives)
9. Administration of the system(8 alternatives)
10. Changing password

Figure 1. The screen view of Main menu

2.1 The patient classification and staff situation

The patient classifiaction and the staff situation is read daily into the computer by one of the nurses in the unit. There is several validity checks to secure the quality in the information. The screen view for patient classification is very much like the Daily Classification Sheet on which the classification is written down by the staff which has cared for the patient. When the classification is read into the computer, the program starts with making a copy of the last classification so it is just to alter those variables that has changed since last time. This makes it both easier and faster to get the daily classifiaction into the computer.

The staff situation is entered into the database by choosing number 2 and the approriate date on a list on the screen. Then it is just to enter the actual number of staff and the required number of staff as the nurse in charge percieves it, for different working shifts.

In number 4 and 5 of the alternatives in the Main menu it is possible to see the patient and staff situation per day and it is also possible to do searching, for exampel in number 4 which days in January and February where there more than five patients in category 3 and two patients in category 4 or in number 5 how many days in March has two or more staff been absent in the day shift?

2.2 The individual patient's stay

In "The individual patient's stay" (number 3) it is possible to view a patient's dependency level each day in both the components of care and category of care (figure 2).

The individual patient's stay

Id number	Initial	Admission date	Discharge date	Diagnos
4012012345	L.AK	930101	930104	
	Fever			

Date	Unit Smin	Hyg	Nut	Obs	Mob	Un	Ex	Categ	Nmin
930101	81	A		A	B			2	521
930102	81	B		A	B			2	521
930103	81	B		A	A			2	357
930104	81	A		A	A			1	424

								Total:	1823

Figure 2. A print out of the individual patient's stay (a few headings have been left out).

The components of care are: Hygiene (Hyg), Nutrition (Nut), Observation (Obs=medication, information, treatment a.s.o), Mobilization (Mob), Uncontrolled output (Un), and Extra need of nursing care (Ex). The A,B and C:s represent different dependency levels in the components of care. An "A" represents the lowest level of dependency and "C" the highest.The corresponding total minutes of nursing care (Nmin) and minutes of surveillance (Smin) are attached per day to the patient's category of care (Catg) in those departments where Activity studies have been conducted.There are two different numbers of nursing minutes for the same category of care. That depends on that the two first days in category 2 are week days (Monday to Friday) and the third day is a Saturday (Saturday to Sunday). The minutes per day are summarized for the whole stay. The patient in figure 2 did not have any surveillance during this stay.

2.3 The summary of patients' stay

In the "Summary of the patients' stay" (number 7) many different patients' stay can be retrieved. As can be seen in figure 3 the patient's number of days in different catgeories of care is shown as well as the total minutes of nursing care for the whole stay. These summaries of patients' stay can be exported to other programs for calculating the nursing costs by multiplying the nursing minutes with the nursing dollars per minute.

In the screen view it is also possible to search for patients within a certain age group (in Sweden the id number is the year, month and day of birth and the last four numbers are check numbers), admission or discharge date or patients with a certain diagnosis as in the figure 3. It is possible to set one or more conditions in one column or to set conditions in several columns.

Summary of the patients' stay

Id.number	Init.	Adm	Dis.	Diagnos	Catg1	Catg2	Catg 3	Catg 4	Nmin
2005123567	A.B	930105	930121	Pneumonia		1	11	4	12441
7012054578	C.D	930115	930126	Pneumonia			4	8	7154
1510125896	D.E	930125	930130	Pneumonia	6				2406

Figure 3. The screen view of The Summary of patients' stay. (The column of surveillance has been left out).

2.4 Predesigned reports

Under "Reports" (number 8) there are several predesigned reports which makes it easy for the users to print out reports of the patient and staff situation for a certain period. One of these reports shows the daily number of patients per category of care, the number of admissions and discharges, the occupancy rate and the turnover per bed. In an other of these predesigned reports the information is summarized per month and shows also the mean values for the patient distrubution in different categories of care, the number of admissions and discharges, the occupancy rate and the turnover per bed.

The staffing reports are organized in the same way. One report shows the number of staff per working shift and in another the information is summarized per month.

There is also a predesigned report for the "Summary of patients' stay"

2.5 SQL-questions

It is also possibile to ask questions directly to the database by using the SQL language (Standard Query Language) (under alternative 8). There is a preset format for how a question shall be organized and help screens for choosing tables, columns and functions. That gives to the users total freedom to retrieve any information they want from the database. The users are not limited to ask questions just in the predetermined screen views.The answeres on the SQL questions can be printed out.

3. The effects of the computer support

The nurses using the computer support have pointed out as the most immidiate effect is that they do not need to summarize the daily patient classification and staff situation every month, which is time consuming and that the quality in the data is increased. So far the output of reports is done by the Zebra system manager (the author) not because users can not do it, but beacuse the information is transformed to a graph showing the patient distribution and staff situation during the past month. Graphs are designed after each units' requirements. Another reason for the organisation of the print outs is that the quality control of the Zebra information lays upon the system manager.

The main benifit of the Zebra system so far is that the clinical manager and the staff get the same "picture" of the patient and working situation each month. They can discuss the situation and see how changes in the organization of health care affects their workload. The calculated staffing coefficients have not so far been used for calculating the patients' staff requirements. In a near future the Zebra information will be used for economical purposes in those clinics where the Activity study have been conducted.

Another result of the computer support is that it is possible to get a print out of the individual patient's stay which can be attach to the patient's file. A print out which makes it easy to follow a patient's dependency level through a stay or through a whole period of illness.

A third effect of the computer support is that it is possible to calculate mean value, standard deviation and coefficient of variation for nursing care per diagnosis or DRG. Analyzing total minutes of nursing care per patient stay is also important when deciding how well the standard cost for nursing for a diagnosis or DRG will reflect the actual nursing cost for a period of time.

During autumn 1992 and spring 1993 several other clinics in the University hospital of Lund have started vid the Zebra system, the manual version. As son as the data communication in the hospital and the computer capacity is expanded these new clinics will be attached to the computer support.

Today in Sweden the main reason for putting resources into the Zebra system and its' computer support is the possibility to calculate the actual nursing cost per patient stay and compare that with the nursing cost calculated with a standard cost. How to use the Zebra information for calculating staff requirements according to the patients' need for nursing care is disscussed more and more.

4. References

[1] Levenstam A-K. The Zebra - A Patient Classification System which makes it possible to put the the patient's need in focus in planning and converting nursing care to costs. In: *Lecture Notes in Medical Informatics. Nursing Informatics '91.* E.J.S: Hovenga, K.J. Hannah, K.A. McCormick, J.S: Ronalds (eds). Melbourne: Australia. 1991: 242-247.

Nursing Informatics: An International Overview for Nursing in a Technological Era
S.J. Grobe and E.S.P. Pluyter-Wenting, eds.

EDS: A Contemporary Emergency Department System

Carter BE

Information Technology Services, Alfred Hospital, Commercial Road, Prahran, Victoria 3181, Australia.

The introduction of a computerised Emergency Department System (EDS) at a major teaching hospital in Melbourne, has provided nurses with an effective patient management tool. EDS captures patient demographic, acuity and diagnostic details from time of presentation until disposal. This data assists the registration, tracking and monitoring of emergency patients. Staff enter and modify patient details as changes occur providing real-time status of patients and the department. This paper describes the system's development, features, functionality, and benefits for end-users.

1. Introduction

Emergency Department nurses need to have access to real-time information in order to effectively manage patients and resources. It was using this view that a computerised Emergency Department System (EDS) was designed, developed and implemented at Alfred Hospital. Whilst computers have been used in the past to register names and address of emergency patients, this system provides comprehensive information that can be used for departmental management and overall hospital planning. The Emergency Department (ED) consists of a trauma centre, serviced by helicopter and ambulance; a casualty cubicles area serviced by ambulances and a general clinics area where non-urgent patients are seen.

In 1992 total emergency patient attendances were 38,976 (monthly average 3,248), of these 36.3% required admission to the Alfred or to another hospital. Twelve percent of patients were recorded as time-critical requiring medical attention within minutes, 40% were urgent requiring attention within one hour and 44% needed to been seen within 4 hours. Figures recorded for the first half of 1993 demonstrate an increase in attendance and acuity. The introduction of information technology was considered essential for coordinating a smooth ED process and providing a means of capturing necessary information to support resource and funding requests.

2. Nursing Role in System Development and Implementation

Software was designed with collaborative input from nursing, medical and administrative staff, and the application was written by Information Technology Services (ITS) staff. Nurses, being the major user-group, provided a significant contribution which ensured that the system developed actually reflected what was required in the practice environment [1, 2]. The design process took six months. During this time consensus was obtained for determining procedures, defining the interface, selecting code classifications, determining system security and specifying the reporting features.

Once the application was written representative end-users were able to test and critique it. Only minor modifications to screen layout were required prior to system implementation. Education of 169 users (nurses, doctors and clerks) was provided in the 3 weeks prior to go 'live' date. A nurse teacher, seconded to ITS, conducted the education sessions and the prepared the EDS user documentation. All education sessions were attended in duty time and were designed to familiarise users with EDS functionality and provide transferable basic computer literacy.

3. System Design

The EDS network comprises of 9 IBM Compatible microcomputers with connectivity to the hospital mainframe via Telix 3.2 Emulator. The latter provides the necessary integration of EDS with HIS, facilitating access to the Patient Master Index (PMI), inpatient medical systems, radiology, pathology, bedstate and waiting lists. A laser printer (LZR 1200 Series) is connected to the network and produces hard copy reports. Three additional registration terminals are linked directly to the mainframe permitting a rapid retrieval of patient Unit Record (UR) numbers and another provides the admitting officer with bedstate information. A centrally located large colour video monitor is integral to the system as it is from this that staff can easily view the real-time activities of the Department without having to go to a terminal.

3.1 System Features

EDS features many of the system requirements considered necessary to support nursing information needs [3]. These include the use of colour, menu driven selections, coded fields, windowing, on-screen exception reporting and on-line help facilities. All free text fields can be edited with wordprocessing functions.

A major feature is the display of patient data in a manner that makes it 'information'. Colour is used to indicate illness severity and time-critical level of patients so nurses and doctors can see at a glance the status of patients and can prioritise management accordingly.

3.2 Data Elements and Reporting Features

Key data elements are captured, at the source, within the clinical information pathway of the ED process. At time of registration demographic details are collected that will identify the patient with a previous presentation or a new UR number is allocated. Additional details such as triage type, location (within ED), time of arrival, admission problem, name of attending doctor, nursing management, investigations, consultations, ward status, diagnosis and disposal type are also entered. Staff are able to modify data as changes occur and each entry is time-stamped so only current information is displayed. The timing feature is also necessary for calculating the cost of emergency care.

Data collected produces accurate reports of the whole ED process and each activity within it. Standard reports are generated daily and are used for planning, budgetary control, casemix funding and QA purposes. Each week ED data is down loaded from the mainframe to a PC with database facility (Paradox 4). This enables nurses to develop ad hoc reports which provide key statistical information essential for performing nursing audits, nursing research and monitoring nursing resource utilisation.

4. Data Presentation and Using the System

There are two major EDS screens for data display and a number of secondary screens utilised for supporting information.

4.1 The Emergency Department screen (Table 1) is a 'read only' screen with information being entered and edited via the Patient Details Screen (see Table 2). The Emergency Department screen displays by location (cubicle area, trauma centre or general clinics) the details of all patients in colour. The colours represent the triage level of the patient and are based on the National Triage Scale e.g.,

RED	Seconds
YELLOW	< 10 minutes
MAGENTA	Half-hour
GREEN	One hour
BLUE	Two hours

Patients not triaged have their details flashing on the screen in WHITE. This continues until the triage process is completed i.e., nursing assessment of the patient's acuity and time-critical level has been established and the appropriate colour coding has been entered.

Table 1
View of Patients in Cubicle Area (copy of Emergency Department screen).

				CUBICLES				
01	*	1		ANDREWS George	M	CHEST PAIN		08:15
02		2	0	BREHENY Fred	M	SUDDEN COLLAPSE		CITIZE
03	na	3		JONES Freda	F	HEAD INJURY		JONES
04	7A	C5	R	SMITH Angela	F	ABDO PAIN	GS1	SMITH
05	3A	10	W	SHEPHERD Betty	F	BURNS	09:00	CARTER
06	*	C8		LEWIS Edwin	M	EPISTAXIS		08:45
A	B	C	D	E	F	G	H	I

Key to screen details:

A *Number*: identifies patient and permits Patient Details Screen retrieval.

B *Patient Status*: * = not seen by doctor; na (flashing) = needs admission; 7A = ward to which patient is to be admitted.

C *Location*: patient's location in ED, e.g. room, cubicle, or corridor.

D *Admission Status*: O = potential admission (based on nursing diagnosis); R = ward is ready to accept patient; W = waiting for ward to ring.

E *Surname and given name.*

F *Gender.*

G *Admission Problem*: presenting problem as assessed by nurse.

H *Outside Consultation*: unit (other than Emergency) called to see patient.
   Time: admitting ward will ring at this time for patient transfer.

I *Patient Arrival Time*: time patient presented to ED.
   Doctor Code: Name of doctor currently managing patient.

4.2 The Patient Details screen (Table 2) displays the data elements recorded in the process of treating the patient. These items are necessary for ensuring continuity of medical and nursing management and for tracking the location of the patient. Patients may move not only within the ED e.g to Xray, but may also leave ED to have specialised investigations e.g. angiogram, CT scan, Ultrasound and MRI. The times recorded for consultations to occur and for investigations to be complete are critical for monitoring the duration of patients' ED attendance, for improving the ED process, and for increasing productivity.

4.3 Whilst additional information is available, such as previous record search and results (radiology, microbiology, biochemistry, haematology, anatomical pathology and endocrinology), it is accessed via secondary screens.

4.4 Specialised functions are available via the main EDS menu, these include the ability to cancel erroneous disposals, search for current inpatients and print standard departmental status reports.

Table 2
View of Patient Details Screen

```
UR NO:        750148      Title:      MR      Contact:
SURNAME:      BREHENY      Sex:        M       Relationship:
GIVEN:        FRED         Age:        60      Phone:
ADDRESS:                                       DOBirth:      01/01/33
PHONE:                     Mat/Stat:   M       Pat. Type:
LANGUAGE:     ENGLISH      F/Class:    H       Source: Emergency Local
```

1. Admission Problem: SUDDEN COLLAPSE   10/10/93 08:53
2. Nursing Remarks:
3.   Ward: 3C Unit: CARD
4.   *** WAITING ***
5. Triage Code: R   RED see in seconds   6. Time: 08:55
7. Location: 2   Room 2   8. Time: 08.56

9. Doctor: CITIZE   Dr. J. CITIZEN   10. Time: 08.57

11. Management: ECG   12. O/Investigation: ANG 10.45
                     DC Reversion   13. Consultation: CARD 09:15
14. Disposal: 4   Admission   15. Diagnosis: 5 2A 00
16. Disposal time: 11:00

The majority of fields displayed in the Patient Details Screen are self-explanatory, however a number are presented below to ensure clarity of purpose. It should be noted that the patient's home address and next of kin contact details are withheld from view unless specifically requested to be shown, via function key operation.

Each of the following fields can be expanded, via a window, to reveal additional entries:

11.   Management - up to 205 different treatment/management codes can be listed;
12.   Outside Investigations - up to 6 investigations may be listed together with the time of patient leaving and returning to ED;
13.   Consultations - up to 6 different units can be listed together with the time unit called, and the time patient seen;
14.   Disposal - nine disposal types are available, if the disposal code is 'transfer to another institution' this field holds details of the actual hospital; reason for transfer e.g., no CCU (Coronary Care Unit) bed available; transport mode and escort type;
15.   Diagnosis - up to 6 different diagnoses can be listed. These are currently based on an in-house combination of Basic Routine Injury Surveillance (BRIS) and National Injury Surveillance Project (NISP) codes and consist of a disease category, aetiology and anatomy. A change to ICD9-CM coding is anticipated at next revision.

Data entry is mandatory in fields 5 (Triage), 8 (Doctor), 10 (Management) and 14 (Diagnosis) as this key information is required for casemix information, hospital and government reports and research. The system will not permit patient disposal if any one of these fields is left blank. An exception to this is the patient who absconds before these details can be captured. In this case a function key operation will automatically load abscond data into the mandatory fields of Doctor, Management and Diagnosis fields, thus permitting disposal of the patient.

5. Conclusion

Since the introduction of EDS (November 1991), staff have indicated that they have no desire to return to the previous manual system. Reasons include user-friendliness of the system and less stress associated with work because staff are kept informed at all times about the status of their patients. The ED process has also become more fluent as nurses are able to easily locate, schedule and monitor patients from anywhere in the department. Nurses have been diligent regarding data entry and as a result have been able to demonstrate objectively their workload activities and therefore justify changes to the department's staffing profile.

The data captured has also provided nurses with information necessary to maintain budgetary control, cut waiting times for services and produce activities reports for management and the Government Health Department. The system ability to provide precise numbers of patients in various categories has directed clinical teachers to develop inservice education that meets changing patient condition profiles. Research has using EDS data has also been conducted in the areas of asthma, bicycle injuries and cardiac conditions.

EDS has been demonstrated to Charge Nurses and Medical Directors of Emergency Departments of other major teaching hospitals in Melbourne, and to the Health Department of Victoria. Feed back from these demonstrations has been positive and one hospital has implemented the system in August 1992.

Computerising a busy Emergency Department of a major teaching hospital has resulted in better patient care, departmental and resource planning, education and research. The success of EDS can equally be attributed to a well defined and developed system, and to a fully committed and appropriately trained staff.

6. References

[1]   Johnson D. Decisions and Dilemmas in the Development of a Nursing Information System. *Comput Nurs* 1987, 5.3:94-98.

[2]   Palmer B. A Smarter Way of Nursing? *Nurs Times* 1990, 86.9:64-66.

[3]   Kohl S. *HIS Requirements for Effective Nursing Information Management.* Wisconsin: Wi-Can, 1989.

© 1994 Elsevier Science B.V. All rights reserved.
Nursing Informatics: An International Overview for Nursing in a Technological Era
S.J. Grobe and E.S.P. Pluyter-Wenting, eds.

68

Three approaches to predicting workload

Corley M C[a] Satterwhite B[b] Blount M[c] and Hontz C[d]

[a]Dept of Nursing Administration and Information Systems, School of Nursing, Virginia Commonwealth University, Box 567, Richmond, Virginia, USA

[b]Dept of Nursing, Medical College of Virginia Hospitals, Box 73, Richmond, Virginia 23298, USA

[c]Doctoral student, Dept of Nursing Administration and Information Systems, School of Nursing, Virginia Commonwealth University, Box 567, Richmond, Virginia 23298, USA

[d]Masters student, Dept of Nursing Administration and Information Systems, School of Nursing, Virginia Commonwealth University, Box 567, Richmond, Virginia 23298, USA

Identifying approaches that improve the ability to predict workload can facilitate planning and budgeting. The fluctuations in health care policy make workload prediction difficult. Three approaches for predicting workload were assessed in an ambulatory oncology clinic using personal computer software.

1. Research Objectives

The increasing availability of computerized data in a health care organization facilitate its use for planning, predicting workload and anticipating cost. This research was undertaken to compare three approaches to predicting workload in an ambulatory oncology clinic using data from five years of clinic activity. The three approaches were regression, moving average and time series analysis.

Forecasting is based on the assumption that underlying factors affecting utilization in an area change in a consistent fashion and that trends can be identified. The two-stage process of forecasting involves first, identifying appropriate measure of demand and how demand will be used in the decision process; and second, projecting the appropriate measure of demand into the future.[1]

2. Methods

The ambulatory oncology clinic designates specific days for the following clinics: Adjuvant, AIDS, Breast, Hematology, Colposcopy, General Surgery, Gynecology, Head and Neck, Pediatrics. Data for five years for the Head and Neck Clinic were incomplete; they were excluded from analysis. Over 17,000 patients are treated each year in this state-supported medical center.

Data from five years of clinic activity were entered into spreadsheets using the software program, QUATTRO™. These data were then used to predict the sixth year of clinic activity using a single equation regression analysis and the moving average. The program calculates regression as one of its advanced functions. The moving average is calculated by subtracting the predicted from the actual numbers for the five years of data.[2] The percent difference is calculated by dividing the difference by the predicted number. The percent differences for 3-month intervals over 5 years are summed and averaged (N=15/average) and this average percent is then used to adjust the predicted number. These results were compared to evaluate which approach provided the most accurate prediction of activity for each clinic.

The data on clinic visits were also entered into the software program, STORM™ and analyzed using the forecasting function, based on time series analysis. STORM™, an integrated software package consists of quantitative modeling techniques for business and engineering problems; the mathematical models are drawn from operations research/management science, operations management/industrial engineering, and statistics.[3] The time series approach involves a test of the first two years of data to predict the last two years of the data and then selects the best approach to use, i.e. level, trend, seasonal, or random. Level refers to the long-run average of a time series. In the trend approach, the per period change is assessed to determine if it is linear or nonlinear. The seasonal assessment determines if there is a recurring pattern about the level component or level and trend components, possibly related to seasons or some other factor. The random component refers to unexplained period-to-period fluctuations in demand not due to other effects.[4] Time series uses exponential smoothing, a procedure for revising estimates of the forecast model components weighing the most recent events (a certain fixed fraction) more than earlier events. The effect is that if the forecast for the current period appears too low, it will be raised for the next period and vice versa.

The forecasted number of visits using the model of best fit from STORM™ was compared to the actual number of visits in the first 10 months of the 6th year. The average percent difference was calculated for each clinic.

3. Results

Only the AIDS Clinic data showed optimal seasonality and trends when subjected to regression and the moving average analysis. The Hematology, Colposcopy, and General Surgery Clinics showed a trend toward a steady increase. When clinic data were studied by month, the Colposcopy Clinic showed a decline for the 7th month. Although the Pediatric Clinic showed random fluctuations of activity, the trend line predicted little growth in this clinic. A decline in clinic activity was predicted for the Adjuvant, Breast, Genito-Urinary, and Gynecology Clinic.

The variance explained by the regression model ranged from 0 (Adjuvant Clinic) to 69% for the AIDS Clinic. The Hematology Clinic variance was 25% as shown in Table 1. When the percentage of variance explained is low, causes other than trends and seasonality need to be assessed.

The moving average procedure was assessed to determine if it improved the ability to predict workloads. These new data were then compared to the actual number of patients seen in the sixth year. The moving average ranged from zero to 29% (see Table 1). The moving average provided a better approximation of the actual number of visits than did the data predicted from the linear regression for the AIDS Clinic patient load; however, the moving average for the general surgery clinic in 1990 was actually a poorer predictor than the linear regression line.

Using the STORM™ function of time series analysis, the models of best fit for the clinic were as follows: a) Level for Adjuvant, AIDS, Gynecology and Pediatric Clinics; and b) Seasonal for Breast, Colposcopy, General Surgery, and Hematology Clinics. The mean absolute percent error ranged from 11% to 35%: (Adjuvant 35%; AIDS 11%; Breast 20%; Colposcopy 17%; General Surgery 37%; Gynecology 19%; Hematology 19%; and Pediatrics 13%). When forecasted data using time series were compared to actual number of visits in the sixth year, the percentages ranged from 7% to 21% as shown in Table 1.

4.   Tables

Table 1.
Variance explained, moving average, using linear regression, and time series analysis for ambulatory oncology clinics

Clinic	Variance	Moving Average				Time Series
		July/Sept %	Oct/Dec %	Jan/Mar %	Apr/June %	Ave. Diff. %
Adjuvant	.001	.00	-.14	.06	.02	.17
AIDS	.690	.07	.01	.03	.07	.17
Breast	.070	.02	-.03	-.02	.07	.21
Colposcopy	.040	-.20	-.40	-.19	-.23	.07
General Surgery	.010	-.14	-.29	-.05	.26	.11
Gynecology	.090	.00	-.17	-.11	-.05	.07
Hematology	.250	.09	.04	-.08	-.02	.21
Pediatric	.001	.03	-.03	-.01	-.01	.13

5.   Discussion

The forecasting approaches of linear regression and moving average were most effective in predicting future patient visits when clinic activity experienced growth characterized by trend and seasonality. The moving average provided a more accurate prediction than regressions alone. However, most clinics experienced a random pattern of activity. Time series analysis tended to accurately predict the actual workload at least 21% of the time and in some clinics the percent of error was as low as 7%. The rapid growth in the AIDS Clinic and limited past experience with this disease make the data of this study especially valuable for future planning including budgeting.[5] Although a review of the graphs of the actual data seemed to show random activity, STORM™ identified a seasonal influence for four of the clinics. Further review of the activity by seasons, including impact of holidays, in these clinics would be valuable in developing the budget and determining staffing. Each of the three approaches to predicting workload has advantages and given their ease of use, all three should be evaluated for the specific activity under study. Once the approach with the greatest predictive accuracy is identified, it could be used for ongoing forecasting.

When the workload data are entered into the database on a continuous basis, the prediction can be modified by recent or anticipated major advances in treatment to make changes in practice in a timely manner. This modified prediction can be assessed for accuracy once the predicted period has elapsed.

Forecasting has been used extensively in business and in hospital administration to develop a financial feasibility management model to determine future bed needs and to predict the number of AIDS cases expected. [6,7,8]

However Nursing has only recently begun to report the use of forecasting primarily to predict workload. These reports were limited to descriptions of the approaches used [9,10] and to restructure of work for optimal use of staff. [11] Further research using computer programs to predict workload could be used in inpatient settings where acuity as well as census data are available. The findings from the current research demonstrate the value of using regression with longitudinal data to improve predictions of workload. The five-year timeframe provides data on seasonal activity and trend, not available when the previous three months are used as the only source of trend information.

6. References

[1] Warner D, Holloway D and Grazier K. *Decision making and control for health administration.* 2nd ed. Ann Arbor: Health Administration Press. 1984.

[2] Finkler S. *Budgeting concepts for nurse managers.* 2nd Ed. Philadelphia: W.B. Saunders. 1992.

[3] Emmons H, Flowers AD, Khot C and Mathur K. *STORM. Personal version 3.0.* Englewood Cliffs, NJ: Prentice Hall/Allyn & Bacon, 1992.

[4] Stevenson W. *Production/Operations Management.* Homewood, Ill:Irwin, 1990.

[5] Satterwhite B, Settle J, Cushnie P, and Kaplowitz L. Ambulatory care for patients with HIV/AIDS: Creating a specialty clinic. *Oncol Nurs Forum* 1991, 18:555-8.

[6] Page JA. Development and utilization of a microcomputer-based financial feasibility management model in planning for new or expanded ambulatory care programs. In: Scherubel J, Shaffer F (eds). *Patients and purse strings II.* New York: National League for Nursing, 1988:65-84.

[7] Walsh D and Bicknell W. Forecasting the need for hospital beds: A quantitative methodology. *Public Health Rep 1977*, 92:199-210.

[8] Griffith JR and Wellman BT. Forecasting bed needs and recommending facilities plans for community hospitals. *Med Care 1979*, 17:293-303.

[9] Hicks L, Bopp K and Speck R. Forecasting demand for hospital services in an unstable environment. *Nurs Econ* 1987, 5:304-10.

[10] Mills A, Blaesing S and Carter J. Preparing nurses to use microcomputers for the work of management. *Comput Nurs* 1991, 9:179-83.

[11] Golberg M. Super managers need not apply. *Nurs Econ* 1992, 10:155-6.

Nursing Informatics: An International Overview for Nursing in a Technological Era
S.J. Grobe and E.S.P. Pluyter-Wenting, eds.

A quality-driven rostering system for primary care nursing

Richards B and Hardiker N

Department of Computation, UMIST, Sackville Street, Manchester M60 1QD., England

There have been many programs produced which deal with Nurse-scheduling (rostering). However, these concentrate on producing an evenly balanced solution rather than one which gives the optimum result looked-at from the patients' point of view. Also, producing an off-duty rota manually is both time consuming and removes the nurse from those tasks for which he/she is trained, namely caring for patients. In what follows is described a computer program which not only does the off-duty rota but one which produces a solution which maximises the quality of the nursing care available to the patients. Regular use of the system has shown it to be about 30 times faster than the old manual method. This system has been produced by nurses for nurses to use. The users think it is a great success.

1. Introduction

As a result of the move to patient-centred care it is now common practice to adopt the concept of Primary Nursing. What is Primary Nursing? Primary nursing may be seen both as a philosophy which involves planned, individualised care with continuity for both patient and nurse [1], and as an implicit organisational design i.e. the nursing care of a specific patient is under the continuous guidance of one nurse from admission to discharge [2]. Its place has been evaluated [3]. There are many benefits to be had from efficient scheduling, the moreso if the final result is high in the quality of care contained in that schedule. These benefits include the efficient use of scarce staff resources and the benefits to the patient both quantitative and qualitative, this latter covering the psychological aspect of the patient knowing who is going to be the next nurse-face to come on duty to continue the nursing care.

How does Primary Nursing benefit patients? Its aims include less fragmented nursing care, increased professionalisation of nurses, greater quality of care, and increased patient and staff satisfaction [3]. For the above reasons Ward 15 is separated into several disjoint teams where staff crossover is not considered desirable. Each patient has a primary nurse who is responsible (24 hours per day) for assessing, planning and evaluating care. Each primary nurse leads a team of associate nurses who act as surrogate if the primary nurse is absent and who are responsible for implementing the planned care.

2. Previous Work

There are several characteristics inherent in all nurse scheduling systems. These are: (i) Coverage i.e. the number of nurses (of each grade) actually on duty compared with some measure of minimum numbers (ii) Quality, i.e. the measure of a shift pattern's desirability as measured by the nurses who must work it; (iii) Stability, i.e. the extent to which nurses know the shift pattern they will work in the foreseeable future; (iv) Flexibility, i.e. the ability of a scheduling system to respond to changes; (v) Fairness, i.e. the extent to which each nurse has equal influence on the scheduling process; (vi) Cost, i.e. the resources consumed in the scheduling process.

Current research identifies four main approaches to nurse scheduling, all of which include the above characteristics, but to varying degrees. Perhaps the simplest approach uses trial and error in attempting to establish a schedule which maintains coverage whilst taking issues of quality into account. This technique is very flexible but is time consuming and often produces sub-optimal solutions. A variation on this first method, although apparently largely unstructured, is a well recognised system of duty allocation, i.e., computing and assigning days-off before filling in gaps on an ad-hoc basis, and has been shown to be up to four times faster than methods which preceded it [4]

Another approach which follows on from trial and error is that of self planning [5]. This method involves each nurse identifying those shifts he/she is prepared to work, with all members of staff collectively ensuring that coverage is maintained. Optimisation follows with the validation of coverage and the addition or deletion of shifts as required. The main advantages of this technique are the high degrees of flexibility and quality, as each nurse identifies only those shifts he/she is able or willing to work. There are, however, potential problems with fairness and coverage and a real problem of increased use of resources in that all nurses must spend time making the scheduling decision. Despite these disadvantages this approach has been successfully used at several sites.

The third, and probably the most widely used, method for automated rostering is the cyclical approach which establishes a high quality schedule for an initial period and then repeats that schedule, period after period. Although considerable effort is required in the formulation of the initial schedule, this technique is obviously highly stable and fair, given that the initial schedule is fair and the scheduling decision is easily made after the initial work. It is however very inflexible which is probably why so many existing automated rostering systems are seen as inappropriate for general use on wards.

The final approach is also the most complex of those identified [6]. This method has two phases. Initially a set of policy decisions is made by the ward sister concerning coverage, quality etc. Then, for each scheduling period, these decisions, plus recurrent input concerning requests and restrictions, define the parameters for the second phase, a process of mathematical programming. This process associates with each nurse one element from a set of potential schedules, i.e., the scheduling decision is posed as a multiple choice programming problem within a framework of adequate coverage and optimum quality. The intention is to incorporate the flexibility of the trial and error approach while maintaining the stability of the cyclical approach.

High quality schedules are assured in this system, firstly by including only high quality schedules in the set of potential schedules, and secondly by analysing each nurses' aversion to certain shift patterns. Thus nursing preference is used to drive the rostering process. This is the procedure used in the system described in this paper. Upon implementation, this system reduced schedule - making time by approximately 95%, was enthusiastically received by ward sisters, and an increase in schedule quality was perceived.

3. Rostering to provide optimum patient care.

The problem area in question is simply the allocation of duty for a variable number of full and part-time members of nursing staff of various skill-levels. Upon first consideration of this broad area there are conflicting viewpoints concerning the scheduling decision, in that what may be considered desirable for the individual nurse, is actually unrealistic from the viewpoint of the resource manager or the allocation officer. The resource manager has an interest in reducing the staffing level and minimisng unsocial hours payments. The interests of the allocation officer include providing a minimum level of care for each shift, and maintaining a continuity of care for patients. To fulfil these requirements, there is a need not only for a high staffing level, but also for flexibility in work patterns. A key requirement for the individual nurse is, of course, a high-quality schedule. A major conflict arises therefore, as the staffing level largely dictates both the level of care, and the quality of schedules. What is therefore required is a resolution of this conflict to provide an adequate, if not optimal, solution for all users of the system.

4. The Scheduling System

4.1. Outline of the System

In order to be independent of any hospital main-frame computer system, and to aid portability, the Ward Scheduling system has been written to run in a stand-alone PC. It is menu-driven and comprises two sub-systems. The first covers the ward regime for the assignment of staff, eg the number of staff of each grade which are required to match the needs of the patients. The second sub-system does the actual allocation on a weekly basis. The first sub-system, called the Policy sub-system, requires information reflecting ward policy. This information will be changed infrequently and can be input by the Senior Sister or Ward Manager. This information includes (i) a definition of the minimum staffing numbers, both ward-wise and team-wise, (ii) the name, staff grade, and team number of every member of the nursing staff, and (ii) regular requests or constraints appertaining to individual members of staff. It needs to be re-stated that the Primary Care nursing system is based on a small number of teams covering identified groups of patients (areas of the ward). In the example described herein, there are three teams covering the medical ward. It is to the member of his/her own team that the patient will relate.

The second sub-system does the actual schedule for the forthcoming week. It needs to recall from the computer's memory the schedule used previously. It also needs to be given, as input, details of the current staff position, ie staff on holiday, staff ill, staff available, and staff not available because of study days etc.

To produce a schedule for the week ahead, the computer will use both sub-systems. From the first sub-system the scheduler will know which staff (usually the senior sisters) have a fixed pattern of duty and those whose duty patterns are flexible. The scheduling process then begins with the objective of obtaining the maximum quality of patient care in the solution. The process of improvement in the schedule continues whilst ensuring that there is ward coverage at all times. Then attention is turned to the individual teams. However, changes in team make-up are only made if the result produces better coverage within the team without any depreciation in ward coverage.

The scheduler then looks at each individual shift to even out the level of coverage. In an ideal world this would give a solution. However, resources, or lack of them, may intervene and it may be necessary to refine the schedule to produce a sub-optimum solution commensurate with the lower staffing levelThe final solution will ensure that there is adequate ward coverage, this being the first priority. Given that, the solution will then optimise within teams. The solution will also reflect the legal requirements for the presence of staff of certain grades and hence such senior/trained staff will be allocated early in the scheduling process. Thus the final solution will be both quality assured and within the statutory requirements.

4.2. The Initial Schedule

Duty allocation commences with an initial selection of standard duties of the highest possible quality for each staff member working variable shifts. The selection of maximum quality shifts for staff members involves the repeated comparison of shift pattern aversion weightings for duties in the standard duty list. That pattern which displays the lowest aversion weighting is then selected for allocation.

The quality of shifts is determined by minimising aversion weightings which are added in the cases where a shift pattern violates the shift pattern constraints. This is achieved using several trivial functions e.g. adding a weighting of 1 to any shift pattern which has a full shift (early or late) on Saturday. There is a similar process for requests of a high priority (low priority requests do not necessarily exceed this threshold), the difference being that where requests cannot be placed i.e. they do not fit any of the predefined shift patterns, they will be omitted. Restrictions, on the other hand, will always be honoured as they replace rather than match duties.

4.3 Optimising

Following the initial allocation, an attempt is made to cover the ward. This is followed by a similar process for teams. Ward and team optimisations are structured very similarly apart from the fact that with team optimisation, ward coverage levels are fixed whilst attempting to achieve team coverage. They are performed in decreasing order of priority in that higher graded staff are allocated before lower grades. The latter therefore fill in the coverage gaps left by the former. The optimisations together represent the fulcrum of the implementation. They are repetitive processes which run until coverage is achieved, or the ward file is not updated in a single cycle, or a predetermined effort is expended (to remove the possibility of two staff members "thrashing" between duties). A maximum of 3 cycles has been shown to give optimum results.

4.4. Coverage

As actual numbers of staff barely allow coverage it is generally useful to do some fine tuning of the final off-duty produced by the system. Because coverage takes precedence over shift pattern quality, a procedure is added which swaps certain duties without harming the shift type ratios of schedules. This is done only for those shifts which are not covered (i.e. do not appear in the set of covered shifts) where there exists another shift which is overcovered (i.e. appears in a set of shifts for which the number of staff exceeds the predefined minimum number). The ward file is
sequentially read and staff of the appropriate grade group, whose shift pattern is not fixed and who do not have an outstanding request or restriction on either the undercovered or overcovered shifts, are selected. The appropriate shifts are then swapped in an attempt to improve the situation. This process is repeated until a pre-determined effort is expended (the optimum has been shown to be 2 repeats), or no write procedures have been carried out in a complete pass through the ward file.

A further procedure attempts to smooth out uneven staffing numbers (which are not intended by the users) by spreading staff evenly throughout the week. This is achieved by decrementing the predefined minimum numbers for each day of the week and performing fine tuning as described above, until either the ward is covered according to these new numbers or until the number for any shift drops below 2. It has the effect of levelling staff numbers so that each shift is approximately even in terms of coverage. The procedure itself is only used when the ward is not covered and does not, in principle, violate the user definition of minimum numbers as all numbers are decremented at the same time, thus maintaining the desired ratios of staff numbers for all shifts i.e. it is the numbers themselves that are reduced, not the proportion of staff on individual shifts.

5. Results

The results of the usage of the system show firstly that the computer method is so much quicker, saving almost 2 hours of Sister's time. See Figure 1. They show that fewer of the constraints present in an ideal solution have been violated, albeit marginally so. The violation of constraints is very much a function of the staffing level: with an abundance of staff most of the constraints can be observed. The real test of the acceptability of the solution comes in the quality of the result. Increased team coverage allows for greater continuity of care which, in turn, benefits the individual patient. When staffing levels are at the minimum, as they are in UK hospitals at present, the main benefits of the system are the savings in Sister's time, the incorporation of staff preferences into the schedule, and the simplicity of the resulting rotas. However the system always attempts to provide an optimal solution in terms of both ward and team coverage. The computer system will give the most congenial solution for the nurses, commensurate with maintaining adequate patient care.

	Manual	Automated
Planning Time	120 mins	4 mins
Coverage (ward)	45.8%	54.8%
Coverage (teams)	77.8%	78.6%
Constraint violations	31	30

Figure 1. Comparison of the Manual v Computer Systems

6. User Reactions

The authors of this paper have talked at length with the Senior Sister to get her reactions to the system. These are all favourable. Because she is familiar with the system, she feels very much at home. A colleague in the same ward but with less familiarity naturally felt less at ease but agreed that the system had much to commend it and she said she would use it rather than do the job manually.

The reaction from the staff nurses was equally favourable. The shift patterns produced compared even more favourably than those produced by the manual system. For a given nurse, a shift pattern without the day-on, day-off, cycle was very much welcomed. The system adequately picks up any duty planning problems and acts on requests and restrictions.

The system has been installed in several other hospitals. Two reactions can be mentioned. One was that the users preferred black text on a white screen (in line with most Windows software). The program has subsequently been changed (reversed) to accommodate this preference. The second was that the system was very powerful and therefore requires some non-trivial amount of time to learn.

Because the system is so comprehensive it needs time and patience, on the part of the Ward Sister and the staff to write down and think through all the staff preferences, requests, etc. This has made the system less popular with Ward Sisters in those hospitals where the driving force has been higher authority. In the hospitals where the system has been introduced on a Sister-to-Sister basis a more favourable evaluation has been given.

7. Conclusion

The prototype system successfully satisfies the user requirements and as such will replace the existing manual system. It fills a gap in the nurse duty planning systems market by providing a low cost and flexible expert system which maximises quality and coverage through optimal staff deployment. As such it should be an indispensible part of any primary nursing environment.

8. References

[1]   Ersser S and Heenan A. Primary Nursing: *Nursing Times* 1990, 86(7); 27-32

[2]   Hegyvary S T. *The Change to Primary Nursing: a cross cultural view of professional nursing.* St Louis C V Mosby Co. 1982

[3]   MacDonald M. Primary Nursing: Is it worth it? *J. Adv. Nursing* 13; 797-806

[4]   Megeath J D. Successful Hospital Personnel Scheduling: *Interfaces 8; 55-59*

[5]   Cowley M A common-sense duty rota. *Nursing Times* 86: 47; 31

[6]   Warner D M. Scheduling nursing personnel according to nursing preference: a mathematical programming approach: *Operations Research* 24: 5; 842-856

Nursing Informatics: An International Overview for Nursing in a Technological Era
S.J. Grobe and E.S.P. Pluyter-Wenting, eds.

Prospective and Retrospective Patient Nurse Dependency System: Developed, Computerised and Trialled in Australia

Cherryl J A Lowe

Director of Nursing, Mater Misericordiae Hospital, Mackay. Queensland. Australia.

The fully automated Patient Nurse Dependency System "*TREND*" has been developed over a period of eight years. *TREND* accommodates the dynamic nature of nursing practice and the unpredictable elements of patient care. Nurses from a variety of specialties were involved in developing the criteria for the patient classification component, the design of reports for prospective (predicted) and retrospective (actual) variance analysis, the establishment of a data input procedure at ward level, and the development of an educational package for users. The system was initially established on a Lotus 123 Spreadsheet using keyboard operation. The recently developed software modules for the system operate through Windows 3.1 or OS/2. The software has been developed in two separate modules to accommodate Hospitals with varying levels of computerisation (central single PC, PC network or fully integrated systems). Four major private hospitals and three public hospitals in Queensland, Australia, have participated in testing these modules during 1993. This presentation will include initial development methodologies, software design, development and testing, implementation costs, cost savings and other benefits.

1. Patient Classification

The first phase of the development for the Patient Nurse Dependency System involved a study of patient variables, identified as independent variables, and their effect on the nursing hours required to provide quality patient care, identified as the dependent variable. The independent variable, can be thought of as the cause of stimulus for change in the dependent variable [1, p. 327].

Studies in patient care areas in two Mercy Hospitals in Queensland, clearly demonstrated that the timing of specific nursing interventions was not a valid method for categorising patients. Cumulative timing of a wide range of nursing interventions showed that the time taken to do the same procedure on different, or even the same patient varied greatly according to specific patient variables. In cumulative timing the watch runs from when the nurse begins to *set up* for the procedure until the total procedure, including *the clean-up*, is completed. Stopwatch time studies are limited to repetitive work activities which immediately rules out the majority of nursing interventions [2, p. 175].

Categorisation of patients by disease and/or medical procedure was also trialled, however the impact of variances relating to doctors treatment preferences and individual patient differences were found to have a significant impact on nursing interventions on particular shifts for the same diagnosis/medical procedure. [3, p. 243] warns against adopting this approach for determining day to day nursing requirements. The major difficulty in determining the amount of nursing time required to care for a patient in each diagnostic category is the fact that patients generally require different types and amounts of care at different stages of illness.

The independent variables, mobility, hygiene and nutrition, are utilised in many patient classification systems. These proved to be the most critical patient variables, and were adopted as the basic criteria for the categorisation model. TREND is built up around the patient variables/nursing care activities that have shown to be the main consumers of nursing staff resources and hence cause the majority of variance in the nursing time required. These activities, in the main, centre around mobility, hygiene, nutrition, level of orientation, frequency of observations, continence, medications, treatments, teaching/counselling and emotional support, language/communication difficulties, whether the patient requires isolation and whether the patient requires transferring to another area. Specific additional criteria are utilised for speciality units such as Maternity, Paediatrics, Neo-natal Intensive Care, Intensive Care and Geriatrics. The number of critical patient variables were kept to an absolute minimum and defined broadly, so that all factors which significantly increased the time required to care for an individual patient are acknowledged.

2. Weighting of Categories

According to the intensity of nursing care required, four patient categories were identified for general medical/surgical patients. By conducting time and motion studies the nursing time required on each shift to care for a broad cross section of patients from each category was measured. An average time value for each shift was then established. TREND recognises eight hours of nursing care as being a workload that an average Registered Nurse can comfortably complete in one eight hour shift. This includes seven hours of predicted nursing care and approximately one hour for unpredicted activities/contingencies (58.4 minutes). Allowance for any measurable item of delay should be included in the operational work standard [2, p. 182]. Non-productive *downtime*, meal breaks and time spent at ward in-service or doing quality assurance activities or ward administration were not included.

The validation of the time allocated for each patient category for each shift has been through the evaluation of outcomes. High quality patient care and patient satisfaction has been confirmed through quality assurance activities such as patient questionnaires, telephone audits, nursing care audits and incident reviews. Nurse satisfaction has also been confirmed through evaluation questionnaires and compliance to the system standards in rating patient variances (nurses do not attempt to deliberately *load* patient categories). Efficiency statistics for actual hours worked in hours per patient days are in line with hospital targets and efficiency standards for the acute hospital.

3. Computerisation

The initial computerisation of the System was implemented in 1987 and involved the processing of the patient categorisation data to generate variance reports. The software used was Lotus 123 with the programme being developed in-house. This simple acuity system developed in-house, proved to be an accurate and extremely easy to use management tool. It facilitated the implementation of numerous cost saving strategies such as adjustment to staff rosters to meet the peaks and troughs in patient acuity, more appropriate allocation of work to nursing staff and the introduction of zero based budgeting for nursing budgets. Enormous cost savings were achieved using this Patient Nurse Dependency System. The hours per patient day were reduced significantly (1.7 hours per patient day) with no detrimental effects on the quality of patient care provided . In dollar terms this was a saving of approximately 2.8 million dollars for a 250 bed hospital over a twelve month period.

4. Limitations of the Initial System

- It was necessary to retain hard copy files of unit statistics.
- Only clinical nursing hours were accounted for in the calculations with all non-clinical calculations being calculated manually.
- Patient dependency profiles were not able to be retrieved for individual patients for clinical costing.
- The collection of data from the ward and distribution of reports was time consuming and required streamlining.

5. Review of Alternative Systems

During 1991 numerous nurse managers from the private and public sector had viewed the existing patient nurse dependency system and were requesting to trial the system in their own hospitals. The majority of hospitals in Queensland did not have effective patient nurse dependency systems in place, and most did not have computers available to the nursing departments.

In 1992 Nurse Managers from three Mercy Hospitals reviewed a wide range of Patient Nurse Dependency Software Programmes as part of a plan to implement a fully integrated computer system which would include all appropriate nursing modules. However, none of the systems met the minimum criteria set by the nurse managers. Many other hospitals in Queensland had the same experience and were still interested in being involved in further development of the system now known as *TREND*. Serious consideration had to be given to the feasibility of such a development project.

6. Development of Software

The preliminary investigations conducted to judge the feasibility of developing a stand alone programme for the Dependency System involved:
- Discussions and Workshops with a cross section of public and private hospitals in Queensland to identify needs, expectations and benefits of the development.
- Consultation with legal and business planning consultants to protect personal investment.
- Indepth review of the proposed system with a System Analyst to determine the size and cost of the project.
- Review of various financial options for the development in relation to maintaining the integrity of the system and security of personal investment.

The preliminary investigations are aimed at clarifying the technical, operational and economic feasibility of the request [5, p. 87].

Numerous information sessions were held with the System Analyst to determine the system requirements and identify features the new system should have. The details of the existing Patient Nurse Dependency System were demonstrated and its limitations outlined. Calculations and efficiency graphs were explained and examples given for future reference. The needs and expectations of other hospitals were considered together with their user abilities and time restraints. Hardware availability and financial restraints of potential users was also discussed.

After studying the requirement data it was identified that the software should be developed in two modules. The first module (TREND-PNDS I) required manual patient categorisation in the ward area with the patient category data being entered into a central computer. The development of this first module was seen as the priority as very few Queensland hospitals had access to computers in ward areas. The software development for the second module (TREND-PNDS II) enabled patient classification by computer in individual nursing units, and an option for integration into major commercially available hospital information systems such as rostering, payroll, admission/discharge and clinical costing. Data entered at the nursing unit is accessed by Nursing Administration through a shared network system.

The lack of nursing staff computer experience was a major consideration in the development of the software. The software programme was written with a graphical user interface (GUI) to provide end users with ease of use. The Language C++ was used to maximise the object orientated techniques. The platforms for operation are Windows 3.1/or OS/2. The data base files used are Standard D BASE files and indices. The output screens for both modules are uncluttered and logically organised so that information is presented in a form that is easy to read. Readability must be a guiding objective when designing systems output [5, p. 415].

7. Software Features

Some of the main features of the software modules include:
- Patients are categorised by the registered nurse allocated for their care.
- Data entry at the ward level is quick and easy for the operator.
- All nursing hours and changes in patient acuity are accounted for.
- Data entry is minimal and reports are easy to interpret.
- Employee maintenance files provide alphabetical listing of all ward employees including qualifications and experience.
- Ward maintenance files identify type of ward and number of beds in each ward.
- All required nursing hours are predicted, for a 24 hour period, with patient categories being routinely reviewed by registered nurses every eight hours or more frequently if required.
- Prospective reports are produced each shift which identify variances between nursing hours required and nursing hours allocated for the shift.
- Retrospective variance reports are generated at the end of each twenty four hour period, showing variances in nursing hours required by dependency and nursing hours actually worked for each shift.
- Daily efficiency reports are generated for each nursing unit showing variances in hours per patient day, unit occupancy and comparisons between clinical and non-clinical hours worked.
- Daily hospital summary reports are generated to identify the efficiency of each unit and also the total hospital, in hours per patient day for clinical and non-clinical hours worked.
- All efficiency reports identify clinical and non-clinical hours, and nursing and non-nursing hours.
- Non-clinical nursing hours are categorised under Administration, Training and Quality Assurance. Non-nursing hours can be categorised under Clerical or Orderly.
- Ward nursing hours allocated to outpatients and theatre are also collected.
- A variety of monthly and annual efficiency graphs can be produced for all areas comparing nursing hours per patient day, unit occupancy, clinical and non-clinical hours, nursing and non-nursing hours.
- A variety of monthly and annual efficiency graphs can be produced for the total hospital.
- Patient profiles by DRG identifying *actual* dependency hours and ward type can be produced using Module 2 interfacing with the hospital mainframe to enable the development of DRG nurse cost weights.

8. Testing of Software

Module 1 was completed and parallel tested in late 1992. This was an essential test as there are a large number of complex calculations concealed within the programme to produce a variety of statistical reports. A parallel test involves duplicating on paper all functions that are being done using the computer for a specific period of time - usually ten to twenty-four hours [6, p. 234]. To pilot test this module four private hospitals and three public hospitals were utilised. This cross section included one large metropolitan hospital, five provincial hospitals, ranging from 158 beds to 360 beds, and a small 30 bed country hospital. Prior to the pilot test only four hospitals were using an acuity system of which two utilised a computer for calculations. However all four private hospitals plan to have ward terminals installed by January, 1994. Training Workshops were held for all hospitals prior to their pilot testing. The basic concepts of Patient Nurse Dependency, including patient categorisation, allocation of work by dependency, interpretation of variance reports and utilisation of statistical information to improve efficiency were included. The software was demonstrated and explained by the System Analyst who was responsible for the development. Adequate training in patient classification and work allocation by dependency was considered crucial for reliable testing of the software. Many software systems are not used to their full potential because of inadequate management skills and end user training. The most common problems encountered during the initial *live period* fall into two categories: procedure insecurities and people insecurities. Procedure insecurities occurs when training is inadequate [6, p. 235].

All pilot hospitals implemented the software for testing in only one nursing unit for the first month, with further units being utilised in the remaining months. A Co-ordinator was nominated in each hospital so that any problems could be channelled through the Co-ordinator to the Developers. A twenty-four hour hotline was available for any trouble shooting during the trial period. At the end of each month a questionnaire was completed by all users to monitor the degree of user satisfaction through the six month period. After the completion of the Trial in August, 1993, User Meetings were held to evaluate the System and identify technical, training or procedural problems requiring further development.

9. Trial Outcomes Module I

Minor modifications were made to the classification tools to accommodate *outliers* in paediatrics and seriously ill medical/surgical patients. An additional patient category (Category 5) was developed to accommodate these outliers. The number of patient categories for labour ward was increased to accommodate the variations in time spent in the actual birth suite. Approximately 778,000 patient categories were calculated and successfully validated the adjusted category hours. Evaluations at the end of the trial indicated that TREND-PNDS I was well accepted by both clinical and management nurses. The main advantages identified by users were:
- The system was very user friendly
- The system allowed an equitable distribution of human resources.
- The required hours per patient day determined by the system facilitated cost efficient quality care.

During the trial, five of the six hospitals identified actual and/or potential cost savings in nursing wages. One 250 bed public hospital reported a saving of $125,000 in the six month trial period. Thirty hospitals throughout the state have indicated their intention to purchase TREND-PNDS I at an implementation cost of $6,950. This includes the Module I Programme, Training and Maintenance.

10   Conclusion

Although bedside terminals may be common place in some parts of the world, many Queensland Nurses are only beginning to experience computer technology in their environment. This system is, by design, *nurse friendly* as it has been developed *by nurses for nurses*. The development of this system offers encouragement to all nurses to be innovative in the development of new systems in computer technology.

(Module 2 (TREND-PNDS II) will be ready for testing in October, 1993, an overview of this fully automated system will be included in my final submission in January, 1994.)

11   References

Books:
[1]   Abruzzese RS. *Nursing Staff Development - Strategies for Success.* St. Louis: Mosby - Year Book Inc., 1992, p. 327.

[2]   Cabban PT and Caswell JR. *Work Study for Hospitals - Second Edition.* Crows Nest: Community Systems Foundation, 1993, p. 175.

[3]   Gillies DA. *Nursing Management: A System Approach - Second Edition.* Philadelphia: W B Saunders: Harcourt Brace Jovanovich, 1989.

[5]   Senn JA. *Analysis & Design of Information Systems - Second Edition.* Singapore: McGraw-Hill Book Co., 1989.

[6]   Mikuleky MP and Ledford C. *Computers in Nursing - Hospital and Clinical Applications.* Menlo Park, CA: Addison-Wesley Publishing Company, 1987.

An evaluation study of off-the-shelf patient classification systems

Seipp K A and O'Donnell J P

Directorate of Health Care Studies and Clinical Investigation, U.S. Army Medical Department Center and School, Ft. Sam Houston, Texas 78234-6100

Very often, organizations begin testing systems without a clear understanding of their requirements. In addition, marketing information often overstates a system's capabilities and understates its limitations. Conflicting definitions of what should be common terms further complicates making comparisons. All these factors can significantly delay putting a new system into the hands of the nursing staff. This study was conducted to determine if any commercially available, off-the-shelf patient classification systems (PCS) would meet the functional requirements for a federal multi-hospital system's nursing management information needs.

1. Introduction

Although an evaluation of commercial systems can examine many characteristics, functionality is usually given the highest priority. Functionality encompasses not only the range of functions performed, but the specific way the system accomplishes those functions (Pivnicny & Carmody, 1989). Before committing to expensive, time-consuming testing, it is essential to identify the systems that will produce the desired outcomes in a satisfactory manner. The evaluation model used in this study provided a framework for the collection of functional information to identify suitable systems for further consideration.

A 3-phase plan was developed to expedite identification of suitable systems using readily available information. Respectively, the objectives were to: (a) identify and collect information on commercially available, off-the-shelf PCS's, (b) organize pertinent information using an adapted evaluation model, and (c) identify the PCS's meeting predetermined selection criteria.

2. Methodology

Eighty-nine potential PCS sources were identified from lists in nursing administration and hospital automation references ("Software Guide," 1991; Rowland & Rowland, 1989; "Directory of Consultants," 1990). A data collection form guided the telephone interviews. Written materials on PCS methodology were also requested. Information was sorted using an adapted model which organized data according to system content, input, process and product. Pre-established selection criteria identified suitable systems.

The views expressed in this article are those of the authors and do not reflect the official policy or position of the Department of the Army, Department of Defense, or the U.S. Government.

2.1 Phase I

The majority of the PCS sources were consultant or information systems companies. Most firms referred the inquiries to registered nurses on their staff who functioned as members of the design, research and/or implementation teams. Occasionally, questions were answered by marketing personnel. Although the information received from marketing personnel may not be totally accurate or complete, it was not unreasonable to expect them to provide accurate product information to potential clients. This was considered an acceptable limitation, as the purpose of the study was to identify functionally suitable systems for further review, not to make a final selection. Fourteen sources were eliminated due to lack of response from the companies.

Fifty-seven sources were eliminated for various reasons. Some rejected sources did not have a PCS methodology. These included nursing information systems without PCS modules, software programs that automate a hospital's existing PCS, management applications of acuity data, and firms that only provided consultative services. Eight of the eliminated sources had PCS's used in only one specialty area. Other sources eliminated from further evaluation had PCS's that were one module of an extensive automated system and could not function as a stand-alone system.

Product information was provided by fifty-nine of the sources. To reduce selection bias in the event several suitable systems were identified, code numbers were assigned to the information for the remainder of the study.

2.2 Phase II

The context-input-process-product (CIPP) model is an evaluation tool proposed by Stufflebeam (1987) for use with educational programs. Context, input, process and product are the four parameters evaluated in the model (Stufflebeam et al, 1971). Information about objectives, needs and expectations is obtained through context evaluation. Input evaluation yields information regarding procedural designs as well as strengths and limitations. Process evaluation provides information regarding implementation and monitoring. Product evaluation allows decision makers to assess information about results, reactions, and deficiencies.

After synthesizing information from the literature regarding patient classification systems, the researchers constructed a framework comprised of four parameters: operating context, system capabilities, implementation design and outcomes. See Table 1 for an outline of the adaptation.

Table 1
Adaptation of the CIPP Evaluation Tool

I.   PCS Tool Code Number

II.   Operating Context

      a. Purpose
      b. Setting - Size and type of hospitals/clinical units
      c. Historical information - Year developed, length of time in use
      d. Intended and realized information needs generated - Acuity, scheduling, productivity monitoring, audit procedure

III.   Input or System Capabilities

      a. Design
      b. Research
      c. Procedures for use
      d. Resource requirements for implementation

IV.   Process or Implementation Design

      a. Monitoring System - Audit procedures
      b. Program/System Redesign - Customizing, maintenance

Table 1 (continued)

    c. Defects
    d. Cost

V. Evaluation or Outcomes

    a. Customer satisfaction
    b. Changes in patient assignment, staffing, productivity, etc
    c. Problems
    d. Benefits
    e. Additional studies on tool

_____

A CIPP evaluation matrix was completed from the information from each source. PCS sources were eliminated from the study as soon as they were identified as meeting one of the rejection criteria. This occurred at various stages of the study. Some sources remained in the study through Phase III, while others were eliminated after the first telephone call.

2.3 Phase III

Selection criteria for a major system requires clarity about the strategic goals of the organization as well as the needs of customers at all levels. Therefore, selection criteria were developed before data collection to identify systems meeting functional requirements. The predetermineded selection criteria required: (a) reliable & valid tool(s) for seven clinical areas, (b) tool(s) requiring minimal or no adaptation, (c) standardized categories used across clinical specialties, (d) information for rating patients accessible in hospital records, (e) in use in multiple sizes and types of hospitals, (f) an audit, or interrater reliability system, and (g) a predictive daily staffing system.

3. Findings

Eighteen sources were identified as having commercially available PCS's and were evaluated using the CIPP matrix. Four sources were subsequently deleted when they were found to provide duplicate tools. Two of the 14 systems met all selection criteria described earlier. Both are reported by their companies as well-researched, valid and reliable PCS tools reflecting current nursing practice. Developed in the 1970's, both tools are used nationwide in many teaching and nonteaching acute care facilities of various sizes. Factor evaluative, or checklist-type tools, they use standard categories across all units. The acuity values are weights, not time. Interrater reliability is determined from information in the medical record.

The number of patients per acuity category is reported and therefore available for development of acuity-based staffing standards. Translating acuity weights to full-time equivalents by the staffing systems requires some customizing by the companies to identify the needs and philosophy of the facility or multi-hospital system. The staffing systems project staffing requirements as numbers of each skill mix per shift.

Additionally, both companies have other management applications that use the acuity and staffing data. The cost of the two systems is flexible and dependent on the amount and type of support requested from the companies. Implementation time appears about the same for both systems.

Despite the similarities between the two systems and the fact that they both meet the selection criteria, there are significant differences. These differences between the two PCS's provide a mechanism for selecting a system to replace the current system, if an off-the-shelf option is deemed acceptable. The differences are detailed in the following table.

Table 2
Differences Between PCS A and PCS B

Criteria	PCS A	PCS B
Basis of acuity	Amount & complexity of care	Risk, complexity, skill level & time
Number of indicators	36	70
Time/frequency of acuity rating	Daily	Every shift
Tool modification	None required	Minimal
Face validity for nursing staff	Total nursing domain not shown	Total nursing domain is shown
Number of categories	6	7
Staffing system	Projects staffing 3 shifts based on planned care	Projects staffing 1 to 3 shifts based on actual care
Input used to determine staffing	Direct and indirect time, operating constraints	Direct and indirect time, short length of stay patients, outpatients, operating constraints
Number of hospitals using the tool	300	70
Automation	Multiple options available	Currently manual
Access to civilian data base	Yes, annual reports	No
Maintenance of system	Comprehensive support & maintenance	Annual updates

4. Discussion

The sense of urgency felt by users and top management to replace an obsolete system is understandable. "If problems with an existing system are serious enough to justify spending tens of thousands of dollars to find a new system . . . how can a hospital spend years waiting for a new system to be in place?" (Doyle, 1990). The process of identifying a system that meets organizational needs is necessarily time consuming.

However, there are strategies for meeting the goals of the search for a system and reducing time delays. First, senior management must define their expectations. The requirements of the system should be derived from the organization's strategic plans (Doyle, 1990). Selection criteria can then be developed that identify the purpose of the system and set priorities on customers' needs in accomplishing that purpose. The next major step is to identify systems for thorough review and pilot testing. Missteps can result in expensive delays by implementing and testing systems that do not meet functional requirements.

Adapting the Stufflebeam CIPP model resulted in identification of relevant data in a systematic manner, facilitating the judgement process. Clearly identifying systems that meet functionality requirements from readily available information reduced both the time and cost of the selection process. Examining system functionality does not eliminate the need for further evaluation. Other aspects of purchasing a system must be explored to insure valid performance in any practice setting. The differences between systems provide a mechanism for final selection.

5. References

[1] Pivnicny VC and Carmody JG. Criteria Help Hospitals Evaluate Vendor Proposals. *Healthc Financ Manage* 1989, 43:38-47.

[2] Software Guide. *Nurs Manage* 1991, 22:65-92.

[3] Rowland H and Rowland B. *Hospital Software Sourcebook*. Rockville, MD: Aspen Publishing, 1989.

[4] Directory of Consultants to Nursing Administration. *J Nurs Adm* 20:43-81.

[5] Stufflebeam DL. Planning evaluation studies. In: *Handbook in Research and Evaluation*. Isaac S, Michael W (eds). San Diego, CA: Edits Publisher, 1987.

[6] Stufflebeam DL, Foley WJ, Gephart WJ, Guba EG, Hammond RL, Merriman HO, and Provus MM. *Educational Evaluation and Decision Making*. Itasca, IL: Peacock, 1971.

[7] Doyle O. Making the Most of Information System Consultants. *Healthc Financ Manage* 1990, 44:34-44.

© 1994 Elsevier Science B.V. All rights reserved.
Nursing Informatics: An International Overview for Nursing in a Technological Era
S.J. Grobe and E.S.P. Pluyter-Wenting, eds.

Nursing Utilization Review System (NURS) - Rationale and issues associated with the costing of nursing services by DRG

Hovenga EJS[ab] Tims J[b] Skinner J[b]

[a]*Faculty of Health Science, University of Central Queensland , Rockhampton M.C. 4702, Australia*

[b]*Evelyn J.S. Hovenga & Associates Pty Ltd, 12 Sleipner Street, North Rockhampton Queensland 4701 Australia*

Nursing cost variations between hospitals, by DRG, may be due to a number of different factors. This paper identifies and discusses these relative to the capture of nursing resource usage (staffing) and actual cost data. The main issues are those of *terminology, cost allocation methods and the measurement of nursing resource usage*. It then proceeds to discuss how these data may be processed and used as a basis for efficiency review and management decision making. It is concluded that the widespread use of standard methods for resource and cost identification by DRG will provide the most comprehensive and useful information on which to base management and policy decisions regarding nursing resource allocation. A list of questions to assist cost variance analysis is provided.

1. Introduction

The Nursing Utilization Review System (NURS) was designed specifically to process the data obtained from the use of the Patient Assessment and Information System (PAIS) [1], a nursing workload measurement system widely used throughout Australia. PAIS quantifies nursing time required per patient, may be used prospectively to predict staffing needs for the following shift and provides statistical data from which the cause and effect of various staffing situations may be ascertained. PAIS is a factor type patient classification system. NURS was designed to accommodate any type of patient classification system, to provide flexibility and to allow for the inclusion of wards and departments where nursing services are provided but where PAIS is not suited. NURS is sensitive to ward or departmental operating hours and is able to vary the distribution of work between shifts by day of the week. It monitors user defined reasons for staff changes, and relates accidents and incidents with workload and staffing statistics. NURS is PC based and runs on a Novell network.

Nurse staffing budgets in Australia have evolved over time based on a variety of arbitrarily defined criteria. As a result hospitals exibit wide variations both in nurse to bed ratios and the mix of nursing staff. Nurse staffing variations were found to be associated with the hospitals' location, staff mix, rate of sick leave and turnover [2]. As from July 1993 Diagnosis Related Group (DRG) based funding will commence in some States, thus individual hospitals have a need to account for the total nursing resource budget and to effectively relate nursing resource usage to various hospital nursing services, units of work and DRG. Nursing costs are a significant component of any hospital's total expenditure. Therefore, the development of a costing system for hospital output requires considerable attention to be directed to costing nursing usage by tracing nursing costs from admission to discharge. A treated discharged patient (output) includes a number of discrete services, including nursing services provided by more than one ward or department. Some patients are moved between wards during their length of stay. Given that most hospitals already need to use a workload measurement system for staffing purposes, this requires a small extension to current operations within any nursing division. Few hospitals have information systems that enable a quick assessment of nursing staff numbers and expenditure to be made.

2. Nursing resource usage

Nurses perform numerous individual units of activity. It is not cost effective to allocate a cost to each unit as they are too numerous. As a result nursing workload measurement systems either use clusters of activities, critical indicators of dependency (factor type classification) or descriptions of various levels of dependency (prototype classification) to overcome this numerosity problem. In such situations it is appropriate to use a model which represents an approximation of relative resource usage [3]. Relative value unit scales permit the determination of labour resource usage for one level of dependency or activity cluster relative to another. A constant is identified to equal 1 and all others values on the scale are calculated relative to that constant. PAIS can be used as a model to represent relative values. It provides a simplified representation (proxy) of reality. Abernethy et al [4] concluded that the classification of a patient based on expected nursing care predicted at the beginning of a shift can be used as a valid predictor of the actual care received. NURS is designed to distribute actual costs per ward or department to individual patients using relative value units.

Hospitals using the PAIS patient classification system capture actual hours provided for patient services by ward and staff category including non-nursing staff. Some inefficiencies inherent in hospital nursing are due to the industrial award requirement to procure and roster staff to meet a predicted level of service well in advance. If last minute replacements or additional staff are needed on a per shift basis then they may come from another ward, casual staff pool or a nursing agency. The latter two categories of staff are usually more expensive on an hourly basis then permanent staff. PAIS also captures data regarding time spent out of the ward on an ad hoc basis for a variety of purposes, such as out of hospital escorts, accident and emergency services, labour ward, meetings, in-service education etc. These total hours need to be costed by service and patient, using the appropriate hourly rate, for each item and totalled. These hours (costs) are deducted from the ward's cost centre's costs and distributed by patient where possible or included as an overhead cost. This results in a more accurate picture of direct (patient service) costs by service. The use of PAIS supports the making of resource allocation and management decisions, which aim to match as closely as possible resource availability with those required to meet in-patient nursing service needs. Changes resulting from decisions made are reflected in PAIS reports which contain information regarding labour resources rostered, actually used and predicted/required to meet actual service need.

PAIS uses a standard time value to reflect average resource usage for each of six patient categories for three different patient populations. These standard time values include non-nursing ward staff and were obtained from work measurement studies conducted in a number of hospitals and have a high degree of accuracy. The method used ensured that the universe of nursing work was reflected by these time values. The sample was sufficiently large to represent a normal distribution of occurrences in terms of patient population, staff performance, staff availability and nursing activity. The predicted labour resources required to service in-patients are expressed in terms of staff hours and are compared with those actually provided, by staff category, to ascertain staffing adequacy.

To some extent the nursing workload measurement system used to provide the time values to be used as a basis for costing will influence how costs are captured and distributed. For example the PAIS timevalues include nursing and some non nursing ward staff and apply to direct patient care, patient related indirect care, ward related indirect care and include a 15% non-productive (staff related) component. Some nursing workload measurement systems may only provide time values for direct patient care provided by RNs. Variables in nursing costs per DRG between hospitals have been reported in the literature [5, 6, 7, 8]. It was noted by Sherman [9] that studies calculating nursing costs are not comparable for three reasons:

- Patient classification systems, the basis for all these costing studies, include idiosyncracies unique to each organization.
- There is a lack of a uniform definition of nursing costs.
- There is a lack of consideration of variables that affect nursing care in addition to patient care needs and staff mix. p.13

Therefore prior to using any timevalues for costing purposes one needs to ascertain such relationships so that the timevalues are multiplied by the corresponding staff categories hourly cost. This hourly actual cost by staff category, shift and day of the week may be used as a basis for costing future rosters or to establish the nursing salaries and wages budget per ward/unit. If calculated on a pay period basis for a twelve month period then seasonal variations may be identified and an annual average calculated. This cost data may reflect predicted, required, actual (relative) nursing resource usage. This is dependent upon the basis upon which costs were identified or calculated. Length of stay has been shown to be a good predictor of nursing resource usage and hence costs. However as demonstrated by Abernethy et al [10] each patient's dependency best explains variations in nursing resource usage between patients who have identical lengths of stay or who are assigned to the same DRG.

Although many hospitals are using PAIS, unfortunately few hospitals kept individual patient data; nor did they accumulate the daily standard and/or actual staff hours data by patient as generated through the use of PAIS. Their failure to do so was primarily due to the inefficiencies of the information systems in use. Patient data was recorded on a white board or a laminated form and only summary data were batch processed. Thus the opportunity for comparing actual nursing cost with standard nursing costs by DRG between numerous hospitals, Australia wide, was lost. Earlier Thompson [11] had noted that hospital nursing divisions frequently use nurse staffing methodologies, including nursing oriented patient classification systems and suggested that an attempt should be made to use this clinical nursing data for costing purposes. He advocated the use of massive data sets to derive a valid cost allocation statistic at the DRG level and to enable the examinination of the variability within a single DRG. Only those who routinely and continuously collect the required information operationally in a manner that permits such analysis can hope to achieve this aim. If the hospitals currently using PAIS were to standardise the interpretation and application of PAIS as well as [1], use NURS to process their PAIS data and cost their nursing services by DRG, then this requirement would be easily met.

Both patient dependency and hourly nursing costs vary by shift and day of the week. The cost of a patient treated from admission to discharge by patient type/classification, is influenced by medical and nursing treatment/care philosophies, clinical management strategies and resources made available, together or interdependently. DRG's may be used to directly relate resources consumed and costs incurred to patient type or case mix. This enables the development of clinical budgeting and provides a basis for allocating resources and for comparing hospital and department performance [12, 13, 14, 15]. The actual cost per patient may be arrived at retrospectively by distributing the total actual ward nursing costs, using a nursing workload measurement system as a basis for determining relative or weighted values on a per shift basis. Just as the actual hours made available vary from those predicted when using any nursing workload measurement system, so will the standard (predicted) and actual costs vary. These costs are then aggregated over the length of stay and assigned to each patient's DRG. For some patients this will mean aggregating per shift costs from a number of different units including the accident and emergency department, critical care and, for surgical patients, operating room nursing costs. Abernethy et al [16] have demonstrated that the PAIS patient/nurse dependency system can confidently be used in this manner as a proxy to denote actual nursing resource usage.

The widespread use of NURS by hospitals using PAIS will enable them to make comparisons between actual and standard costs by using the PAIS standard time values. They will also be able to calculate their own nursing weights per DRG, both in standard and actual terms, and compare these with any three alternative nursing weights, such as the one used as a basis for funding, one from a hospital with the same casemix as determined by overall DRG weighting and possibly the Region or State average nursing weight. This feature allows the user to focus on and analyse the processes of those DRGs for which the variation in nursing resource is greater than funded. The number of DRGs and total nursing cost for a specified period within each hospital is also identified to ascertain the magnitude of the problem.

3. Nursing Services Costs

Total nursing salary costs are distributed to the nursing division through the general ledger/payroll system. These costs include salary costs associated with actual hours worked, all paid leave, various allowances, on-costs (superannuation, payroll taxes, workcare etc.) including hours paid for in-service education. Not all Australian hospitals are able to identify these costs on a per ward or unit basis, ie by cost centre. Frequently organisational structures determine which staff categories are assigned to individual cost centres. For example Assistant Directors of Nursing or their equivalent may be assigned to the nursing administration cost centre in one hospital or to one or more clinical cost centres in another. Agency and casual staff costs are frequently not allocated to the cost centre where these staff actually worked, the usual practice is to have a cost centre specifically for this category of staff. Thus apparently identical cost centres in various hospitals may include different costs.

---

[1] A review of 21 hospitals using PAIS revealed a number of variations in usage which influenced the actual resources made available to individual wards and hence will influence final costs obtained. Inter-hospital reliability testing against PAIS standards for usage, was recommended.

Some hospitals identify all educational costs seperately, others don't. For some hospitals this is a very significant cost as they provide any number of specialist courses. For example some critical care courses have as many as 500 theory (in class room hours) where the students are part of the workforce and paid their usual salary but are replaced in the clinical setting whilst attending study days. This is an additional educational cost to the cost of the education department (cost centre) which typically includes only the nurse educators and support staff. These educational costs have to date been absorbed within the operational budget and were considered necessary to recruit staff to these specialty areas. Most midwifery educational programs continue to be provided by individual hospitals in the same way, as are operating room nursing courses. There are a number of others, although not all include such a large amount of paid educational (non-service) time. The range is from 80 hours to 600 hours per course per annum.

The total hourly cost will vary by ward, shift, day of the week and hospital as it is dependent upon staff mix, shift and other allowances, the inclusion or exclusion of non-productive (overhead) costs and educational costs. For example the NSW public hospital nurses (State) award (1992) has 95 different staff categories, each with their own pay rate which reflect both position and years of experience. The 1986 Victorian Registered Nurses Award has 29 pay points, the Tasmanian private hospitals award (1988) lists 41 different pay points. All allowances also vary between the States. Individual hospitals are likely to have any combination as their own staff mix usually using a total of around 40 different pay points.

Abernethy et al [17] demonstrated these variations in their matrix of pay rate indices for two different hospital campuses. For example the hourly pay rate for the weekend night shift for a grade 4 RN on one campus was 5 times greater than that for a student enrolled nurse working a week day early shift at the same hospital. The average hourly RN rate per ward varied from $13.28 to $18.52. Clearly staff mix is an important variable and must be noted when cost comparisons are being made. These individual hourly salary costs need to be calculated for a specified period e.g. one month. Due to staff turnover, roster changes and changes in pay rates, the hourly costs will vary over time. Thus for each ward one needs to calculate the average hourly cost by staff category (or staff groups such as NUMs/Charge, all other RNs, all ENs, non-nursing ward staff), day of the week and shift. Frequently ward or unit costs also include the cost of supplies and sundry other items which need to be excluded from the nursing costs.

The total costs need to be seperated into those areas/wards directly concerned with patient care and those departments which support nursing services such as nursing education and nursing administration. These latter costs represent an overhead cost which needs to be distributed on a proportional basis to each patient care area if a total actual nursing cost per ward and patient is to be arrived at. The sum of the costs associated with each ward, unit or department (cost centre) should represent the nursing division's total salaries and wages budget/expenditure for the associated time period. This final total nursing cost divided by the corresponding total nursing hours used for patient care provides an average hourly cost for each ward. Alternatively the total cost is distributed according to the relative weights of each staff category to arrive at an average hourly cost per staff category.

Clearly some modelling of cost relationships is required when identifying actual costs. Such models determine how to distribute overhead costs. Also the use of relative values to distribute costs by patient constitutes cost modelling. Cost modelling identifies relationships between costs, activities and casemix products and models these by making a set of simplifying assumptions about these relationships in order to arrive at the required product cost estimates [18]. This process does not usually require the collection of additional service utilisation data about individual patients. It does require an appropriately weighted measure of utilisation by patients whose costs of care are allocated to a specific cost centre. Service weights are estimated using the best available data on costs for individual patients discharged and are estimates of relative costs per patient discharged. Service weights needed to apply the Yale cost model may be arrived at by using PAIS and NURS.

4. Review of Resources Used

As in industry, once process and total costs are identifiable one can explore the most cost-effective method to be employed to achieve the desired outcome. Through the examination of the production relationships (inputs relative to outputs) one gains an understanding of those elements which can explain cost variations between hospitals. Outputs need to be defined not only in terms of the product as expressed by casemix but also in terms of outcomes. The latter is an essential prerequisite to the evaluation of service cost effectiveness. An understanding of the production relationships is necessary when using cost data as a basis for management decision making aimed at improving both efficiency and effectiveness of services provided.

Currently no standard nursing workload measurement system is recommended in Australia and that may not be necessary. What is required however is an understanding about each system in use, in terms of which aspects of patient care are included in the resultant staff hours which form the basis of costing nursing services by DRG. Strictly speaking only those hospitals using the same workload measurement system and costs allocation method are comparable.

The review of treatment patterns relative to resource usage, outcomes and DRG will reveal the greatest potential for cost savings. A system which reviews nursing utilisation should therefore include the notation of critical events throughout the length of stay and process of care. Critical path standards can be determined to a large extent from the PAIS patient dependency data by examining and critically evaluating the norms regarding dependency indicators throughout the length of stay by DRG over time. This should be done for the top ten (10) volume DRGs in the first instance as these will consume the greatest proportion of all nursing resources. These data can then be used by case managers throughout the length of stay. Efficiences made to the care of these patients will result in the greatest benefits. NURS will track any deviations from the critical path, record actions taken and relate these to actual costs and outcomes.

5. Conclusion

Widespread use of standard methods for resource and cost identification by DRG will provide the most comprehensive and useful information on which to base management and policy decisions regarding nursing resource allocation. However there are a number of issues which need to be addressed by the nursing profession before such systems can be used with confidence for pricing nursing services by DRG, for comparative purposes or for policy decisions regarding resource allocation. These are issues of terminology, cost allocation methods, and how nursing resource usage is best measured. Other issues and questions for consideration are;

    i)   Do all staff allocated to a ward cost centre contribute fully to the services provided by that cost centre?
    ii)   Are educational costs seperated from service costs?
    iii)   Are movements of staff accounted for by the system in use?
    iv)   Is the collection of nursing workload data consistent and reliable?
    v)   Is the system used in accordance with the system's design?
    vi)   Does the workload measurement system use valid time values and produce realistic staff estimates?
    vii) Are all nursing costs accounted for?
    viii) Are the nursing/ward costs in one hospital comparable with those in another?

Once a nursing division is satisfied that the total actual cost centre nursing costs captured by the costing system reflect the actual situation then the distribution of those costs on a per patient basis can proceed.

Variations in nursing/ward costs per patient between hospitals, regions or States may be due to any one or a combination of these variables. In the absence of relevant standards or policies and adherence to same, cost variations may be due to the workload measurement system in use or cost allocation methods employed to arrive at a cost per service or cost per in-patient episode. First cost centre cost data need to be comparable before these costs are distributed, using a standard cost allocation method, on a per patient or DRG basis for meaningful results. Finally when costing nursing services by DRG it is first of all necessary to identify the DRG version used. With the many different DRG versions now in use this is fundamental if one is to compare nursing costs by DRG between hospitals.

References:

[1]   Hovenga E.J.S. 1990 *The Origins of PAIS*. Northcote, Australia

[2]   Health Department of Western Australia 1991 *Nurse Staffing Methodology Report* p.30.

[3] Horngren C.T. and Foster G 1987 (6th Ed) *Cost accounting:A managerial emphasis*. Englewood Cliffs: Prentice-Hall

[4] Abernethy M.A., Magnus A, Stoelwinder J.U. 1990 *Costing Nursing Services*. Monash Medical Centre, Victoria, Australia p.136.

[5] Fosbinder D. 1986 Nursing Costs/DRG: A patient classification system and comparative study. *J Nurs Adm Vol.16, No.11 Nov.pp18-23*

[6] Reschak G., Biords D., Holm K., Santucci N. 1985 Accounting for nursing costs by DRG. *J Nurs Adm Vol 15 (9) pp.15-20, 26*

[7] Lagona T.G. and Stritzel M.M. 1984 Nursing Care Requirements as Measured by DRG. *J Nurs Adm Vol 14 (5) pp.15-18*

[8] Mowry M.M. and Korpman R.A. 1985 Do DRG reimbursement rates reflect nursing costs? *J Nurs Adm Vol 15 pp.29-35*

[9] Sherman J.J. 1990 Costing nursing care: A review. *Nurs Adm Q Vol 14(3) pp.11-17*

[10] Abernethy et al 1990 op.cit.

[11] Thompson J.D. 1984 The Measurement of Nursing Intensity. *Health Care Financing Review Nov. Annual Supplement pp.47-55*

[12] Fetter R., Shin Y., Freeman J.L., Averill R.F., Thompson J.D. 1980 Casemix Definition by DRG. *Supplement Medical Care Vol.18 No.2*

[13] Williams S.V., Finkler S.A., Murphy C.M., Eisenberg J.M. 1982 ?Improved Cost Allocation in Case Mix Accounting. *Medical Care Vol.20, No.5, pp.450-459*

[14] Stoelwinder J.U., Stephenson L.G., Wallace P.G., Abernethy M.A., Putt C.M. 1986 Clinical Costing at the Queen Victoria Medical Centre. *Australian Health Review Vol.9 No.4 pp.372-386*

[15] Horn S.D. and Horn R.A. 1986 The Computerised Severity Index: A new tool for casemix management. *J Med Syst 10:73-78*

[16] Abernethy et al 1990 op.cit.

[17] id ibid

[18] Palmer G., Aisbett C., Fetter R., Winchester L., Reid B., Rigby E. 1991 *Casemix Costs and Casemix Accounting in Seven Major Teaching Hospitals*. Centre for Hospital Management and Information Systems Research and School of Health Services Management, University of New South Wales, Sydney, Australia.

Nursing Informatics: An International Overview for Nursing in a Technological Era
S.J. Grobe and E.S.P. Pluyter-Wenting, eds.

Automated Staffing/Scheduling Systems
Selecting the Right One

Plummer C A

Director of Nursing Education & Research, Al Hada Armed Forces Hospital, P.O Box 1347, Taif, Saudi Arabia.

Automated staffing/ scheduling systems are invaluable tools for the nursing profession. With the ability to process a high number of variables, these systems hold potential as highly advanced decision support tools for management. It is critical, however, that users be cognizant of the functions needed. This is to ensure that the systems not only meet the users' needs, but that their purchase can be cost justified to senior management. The purpose of this paper is to review the critical functions of staffing/scheduling systems based on the identified needs of the nurse managers in a major tertiary care teaching facility in Vancouver Canada. This project did not proceed beyond the requirement's definition phase.

1. Introduction

The major focus of attention in British Columbia Canada since the late1980's has been the need to develop satisfactory nursing staff work schedules for the hospital setting. In February 1989 the Health Labour Relations Association of British Columbia and the British Columbia Nurses' Union joined forces to develop a guide for nursing staff shift rotations. In January 1990 a Nurse Scheduling Committee was established to improve the practice of nurse scheduling in British Columbia hospitals. . This committee was funded by both the Federal and Provincial governments. Due to the stricter scheduling constraints in the Collective Agreements nurse managers found it more and more difficult to develop schedules that were: flexible yet manageable; meeting workload requirements; driven by ever increasing patient acuity; and addressing staffing issues related to quality and continuity of care, budgeting, staff allocation, and utilization [1].

In this highly complex environment consideration of an option for automation was needed. Satisfactory work schedules should be developed which would meet: the objective of fully utilizing existing staff in provision of quality patient care; all provisions of Collective Agreements; both hospital and nursing unit requirements; employee preferences; and job satisfiers. To this end clear statements of requirements were determined and are briefly discussed below.

2. Staffing and Scheduling System Requirements

The components of the system as described when integrated define a data base management system. This system should support decision-making by nursing management resulting in efficient and effective utilization of human resources.

2.1 Nursing Staff Employee Details

Employees are the key components in such a system. Individual employee information is needed such as: name, employee identification number, hire date, category, status, union affiliation, position, primary cost centre, pay rate classification, address, telephone number, education, languages spoken and read, professional memberships, work experience, certified/delegated medical functions, seniority, responsibility experience, and date of certifications. An essential requirement of this staffing and scheduling system is its linkage to the human resources system. Such a linkage would allow basic demographic data to be entered in Human

Resources and passed to the staffing and scheduling system. This data could then be maintained and updated by nurse managers.

2.2 Staffing

Staffing is the process of placing the appropriate number and mix of personnel in a particular unit to provide the desired outcome of high quality care and productivity. The outcome on a nursing unit is the desired level of care as determined by the needs of the patients in their unit [2]. Ensuring that the nursing employees are available to staff a unit on a given shift is affected by a number of variables. For example, what are the contract, hospital, and unit rules that impact staffing levels? What is the patient acuity/workload measurement system requiring in relation to numbers of nurses and their skill mix? In this hospital the patient acuity system was required to be integrated so that the classification data appeared on the staffing screens. A function was needed to allow the alteration of the unit's staffing profile to demonstrate the fiscal impact of a given staffing decision on the unit's staffing budget. An additional requirement was to allow the nurse manager to perform a 'what/if" analysis to determine staffing alternatives and their budgetary impacts. Any alterations to the staffing patterns need to be captured from the time the change is made through to the shift being worked. If an employee is assigned to a shift that violates any hospital, unit, or collective agreement requirement the system should provide an alert. A further function is the ability to track employee availability and actual hours worked in both relief or overtime situations. Other useful information is on-line on call lists with ability to input justification for refusal. To address the continuity of care component of a staffing decision requires a linkage between the patient assignment and the assigned primary nurse for each shift.

2.3 Staffing Budget

Provision of a link from Finance to draw unit staffing budget data allows the nurse manager to assess, before implementing, certain staffing decisions. A crucial component of the system is the ability to test staffing alternatives against postiive or negative budget variances. For the nurse executive to be able to aggregate and survey the status of the divisional or unit staffing budgets would assist in the ability to formulate long and short-term plans. Other management data and its associated costs that needed to be monitored by units and the division included: sick leave, vacation time, turnover, orientation, and workmen's compensation.

2.4 Schedule Creation and Maintenance

Any scheduling system should ensure that the desired level of patient care can be delivered while maintaining productivity and cost efficiency[3]. In Canada our schedules are created according to contractual agreements between unions and hospitals. For example: patterns that address maximum work hours; minimum time off between shifts; number of weekends off; etc. are the rules that need to be input for the building of master schedules. These rules cannot be violated. Other requirements that are rule-based, pertain to the staff mix to meet the unit baseline requirements and any associated responsibilities. Finally a provision for entering and updating employee preferences needs to be provided. Preferences such as employee availability for certain shifts or days of the week needs to be included to allow for the creation of a unit master rotation which meets hospital, unit, and employee needs. In addition to the system being able to create schedules, each time an assignment is made or a requirement changes the reason for the change is noted and stored creating a data base where new rules can be developed and brought on-line. From the creation of the master, the ability to easily edit is required. Employee requests for paid and unpaid leaves, unit closures, statutory holiday assignment will need to be incorporated. The ability to assign staff to lines in the master rotation is needed, for example in the instance of the new employee starting on the unit or returning from maternity leave. These functions of creating, editing, and maintaining a master rotation that meets hospital, unit, collective agreement and employee needs are critical. A function to allow for the testing of 'what/if" analysis would assist the nurse manager to determine the impact of changes in a timely and efficient manner. Prediction abilities of such a system would be extremely useful during labour negotiations to determine the impact to the hospital of proposed contractual changes.

2.5 Information Synthesis

A significant amount of information can be reported from the employee to the division level as a result of the data collected through staffing and scheduling processes. An example would be provision of individual employee attendance to unit and departmental level to provide a synopsis of all types of absences. These statistics can be used for comparison across the division to determine if attendance standards are being met. Further advantages of tracking these attendance trends would be forecasting staffing needs over specific holiday periods that can then be used to assist in formulating institutional policies. Finally, attendance pay data can be generated which will accurately reflect the actual hours of work per staff member over a given pay period including adjustments for pay premiums. From this, nursing resources can be costed including overtime, sick time, inter-unit assignment, and the use of part-time and casual staff.

3. Cost Justification

The cost of such a system must be balanced by the benefits achieved. Quantifiable benefits include: (1) reduced nursing effort required to develop master rotations, (2) automation of the time-keeping function by linking with Payroll, (3) automation and integration of the employee data, (4) reduced number of contract related grievances, (5) improvement in nurse staffing decisions related to skill mix and budgetary impact.

4. Summary

Throughout this paper operational and management requirements have been identified. It is apparent that to fully meet the needs of nursing management, decision support is required to determine the impact of certain decisions on the unit and the department. The above list of functions is intended to be neither exhaustive nor detailed but to present the major components of a staffing/scheduling system which supports successful nursing management decision-making. Such a system could meet the needs of any department required to staff on a 24-hour basis. It would be optimal if this system could be linked to a Human Resource management system so basic nursing employee data could be electronically transferred. The linkage to the financial sub-systems for payroll purposes and budgetary variance reporting is another essential component. Human Resource, Staffing and Scheduling, Financial systems all linked as one defines a system that becomes a major corporate resource!

5. References

[1] Peat Marwick Stevenson & Kellogg. Survey of Nurse Scheduling Practices. Project Report. January 3rd 1991.

[2] Young L, Hayne A. Nursing Administration: From Concepts to Practice. Philadelphia: W. B. Saunders. 1988.

[3] Young L, Hayne A. Nursing Administration: From Concepts to Practice. Philadelphia: W.B. Saunders. 1988.

Nursing Informatics: An International Overview for Nursing in a Technological Era
S.J. Grobe and E.S.P. Pluyter-Wenting, eds.

Review, Selection and Implementation of Software for Automating Staff Scheduling in the Long Term Care Setting

Michael Beebe

Schools of Nursing and Health Information Science
University of Victoria, Victoria, B.C., Canada, V8W 2Y2

Staffing is usually a time consuming and labour intensive manual process with data required in various formats and the work is fraught with potential for error. Scheduling for appropriate levels of staffing as it relates to expected workloads, along with holidays and unexpected events such as illness has long been a difficult challenge. Any such system used in Canada must take into account a multitude of union requirements such as seniority and appropriate staff for "swapping" of shifts and use of relief workers. The task for nurse administrator is to select a software package which will allow scheduling to become an automated process, provide the data from such a system to be used by human resources personnel in calculating hours worked and facilitate generating pay checks. These and other related issues must be considered when reviewing potential products. Long term nursing care facilities have their unique characteristics and culture. Much of the technology developed for hospitals has been brought into the long term care setting without taking into account their special nature. In addition, at one hospital in British Columbia, Canada, having four physically separate facilities under one corporate structure raises additional logistical and technical issues which must be dealt with. The discussion will focus on the above issues and an attempt will be made to offer some insights for those considering the purchase, implementation and training for use of a staff scheduling software package.

1. Introduction

Throughout the modern history of nursing, staff scheduling in most long term care (LTC) settings has been a manual and highly labour intensive process. At our facility nursing staff represent 68% of the almost 900 personnel and the process of scheduling has been decentralized, and is handled by seven directors of nursing units (DNU). All other departments are centralized in their staffing and in all departments managers have primary responsibility for scheduling. For Nursing, staffing clerks/timekeepers are assigned to every resident care unit. An important aspect of their work is that information about staff may be found in as many as six different ring binders containing paper and pencil forms which have been designed over a period of years. Since staff may be shared between any of the four sites, that means information about any given staff member may have to be manually transcribed into 24 different binders to keep all staff information current. This manual process lends itself to errors which could be costly to the facility. Union contracts have become increasingly more complex throughout health care in Canada. While our staff are located on four physically separate care sites within Victoria, British Columbia, there is a great deal of interest in setting up a centralized staffing system for all nursing personnel to facilitate sharing of staff between the four hospitals, with one shared database which can be accessed and updated by authorized users at any site.

Within virtually all Canadian health care settings there is a move towards increasing use of computers. However, it is my observation that long term care has been much slower to become part of this trend. At our own facility, over the last two years all managers have had computers placed in their area, though not necessarily on their own desk. This change along with other issues mentioned above, make it appropriate to examine the possibilities of moving scheduling to the computer to automate this process, as much as possible. After an exhaustive search throughout North America, eight products were identified as possible contenders for adoption.

The enclosed summary will provide a basis for explaining the need for and possible costs of staff scheduling software. From the data currently collected, it is likely that the costs of this implementation could easily be matched by significant savings to any LTC hospital within a two to three year period.

Last, some procedures for implementing the package will be explained. Much evidence indicates that purchase of software which alters how business is conducted requires a significant period of adaptation and implementation. For instance see Richards [1] and Burkes [2]. It is important to consider the cost of this process as part of the formula for determining which software package should be purchased.

2. Purpose

The purpose of this paper will be to discuss issues related to selection, purchase and implementation of an automated staff scheduling system. Information is provided about the current state of scheduling at one long term care facility in British Columbia, Canada and the estimated costs of doing business without an automated scheduler. Eight systems were extensively reviewed and product and training costs were estimated. In addition, some information will be provided relating to possible cost savings or organizational payback after adopting an automated scheduler.

In its initial inception, this project was to be focused on nurse staff scheduling. However, it has been apparent from the outset that all staff might benefit from automated staffing/timekeeping functions. In reviewing products, it was noted that most packages would in fact allow for scheduling of all staff regardless of their respective department. Setting up a system to schedule and timekeep for each department raises a number of policy, as well as hardware and software issues. However, with the technology available today, it seems probable that all these problems have a solution and no major barriers exist to prevent developing a comprehensive staffing/timekeeping system. While this project was carried out in one facility with the nursing units which have decentralized staffing, most of the issues are quite germane to almost any health care setting. As a result, the final selection recommendations must be made based on products which are judged to be adequate for total organizational scheduling needs.

3. The Culture of Long Term Care

When examining issues related to selecting software for a LTC facility, it may be important to attempt to understand what is unique about this particular setting. Hence, I asked staff what was unique about their workplace. They noted the obvious of higher client ages and longer stays. Our particular hospital is "extended care" which means our goal is to make the resident comfortable for the duration of their life, not necessarily to get them "well" for probable discharge back home. Because of the intensity of resident needs, we have lower resident/staff ratios than acute care facilities. Ours is a true multi-disciplinary model of health, one where the social worker, chaplain and physiotherapist work closely with medicine and nursing to help residents live out their lives with dignity. Resident health problems and crises are more likely to be "functional" rather than necessarily biologic in nature. Residents often have a multiplicity of illnesses or system deficits, rather than just one major health problem. Last, there tends to be closer relations between staff and the residents. It is more like family, perhaps, than acute care. This closeness may also be the result of longer stays, but it is also one which is fostered in our facility.

The natural question arises as to how the culture of LTC affects the scheduling process. In our four hospitals, there is a need to share staff between facilities. However, staff often feel very close to their own colleagues and residents and may not want to move between facilities. In any case, while sharing of "casual" staff between facilities is done often, it is severely hampered by the present totally manual scheduling system. Finally, I found a common aversion to computers by some LTC staff which will only be overcome by software which is extremely user-friendly.

4. Need for Software

During a nine month period interviews were conducted with nursing administrators and nursing staff and timekeepers throughout five different health care organizations in Canada and in particular at three of four sites in our own corporate long term care hospital group in Victoria. During these meetings staff were asked their opinions about the current manual scheduling system. It is important to note that these comments were anonymous and voluntary, but represent staff perceptions. Very consistent trends in the comments have been:

- extreme discontent with the current manual scheduling system, mostly among nurse-aides and casual staff;
- allegations of frequent clerical errors in computing hours worked, vacation/holiday hours accumulated, statutory

holidays computations and other related computations;
- discontent over the way "book-offs" and especially holiday time are filled by staffing/ timekeeping personnel;
- difficulty for nursing administration in tracking chronic tardiness, "book-offs" and related information;
- staff distress over the way supervisory and/or switchboard personnel handle locating and booking casuals.

In addition, timekeepers at all four Victoria facilities, and in all five organizations have been interviewed. Their perceptions/comments have been:
- extremely labour intensive and totally manual process for scheduling;
- information about staff members and casuals may be in **six** different binders which must be constantly updated, which can lead to clerical errors;
- inefficient means for alerting other facility or switchboard staff about the need for or availability of casual staff to meet staffing needs. "Casual" information sheets must be photocopied and sent to the main switchboard at least once per week, by all staffing clerks, which is extremely time consuming.
- inefficient mechanisms for planning and securing casuals to cover holiday times.

5. Cost of Business without an Automated Scheduler

For nursing, currently six staff are utilized, four at .8 Full Time Equivalents (FTE) and two at 1.0 FTE, to assist with staff scheduling and timekeeping. As alluded to earlier, most other departmental scheduling is handled by managers with an average time required of .2 FTE per manager. Within the Human Resources Department two individuals devote 1.5 days each per pay period to input time data into the payroll system. Factoring in time costs for managers, DNUs, timekeepers and payroll clerks, the total approximate current yearly costs to our organization is over $300,000. Conversations with managers in other LTC facilities in Canada who had switched to automated schedulers provided estimates of 50% to 75% savings over previous costs of staffing/timekeeping. See also Bergman & Johnson [3 & 4]. Even with a more conservative estimate of 25%, I calculated that our facility could experience a yearly savings of $76,500 once an automated scheduler was in place. One hospital in Ontario estimated that the automatic payroll interface alone would save them over $100,000 per year. With a "worst case scenario", assuming no staff decrements occurred, only about $4,000 per year might be saved in payroll input expenses.

Scheduling of nursing personnel is complicated by the fact that after business hours switchboard (SB) staff are responsible for locating casual help in the event of an unanticipated "book-off". This situation necessitates that SB staff be provided with accurate and current information about available staff and individual nursing unit needs. With the current manual system it is difficult for SB staff to accomplish this task. In interviews with nursing unit directors and staff (especially casuals) this problem was a source of considerable discontent at all levels.

The current human resources/payroll system regularly generates updated lists of personnel by seniority, and reports of same are submitted to timekeepers and the union quarterly. However, incorrect calling of casual staff (by seniority) is estimated to be costing at least two shifts per month which must be paid for but are not actually worked by the casual staff member. This situation results in requiring the facility to pay two people to work the same shift, which is estimated to total approximately $2,500 per year. More than one manager told me that at least one grievance per month results directly or indirectly from alleged errors in scheduling. There is no way to actually estimate this particular cost to the organization in terms of dealing with these grievances. However, considerable Human Resource and administrative time can be taken up for these kinds of problems.

Workload analysis (WA) is a methodology for capturing information about anticipated care needs of residents and using that data for planning care and staffing, and for prospectively costing of care services. Residents are evaluated on a regular basis in terms of their individual specific hands-on and social care requirements. There are a variety of systems and our staff has created their own unique system for evaluating WA. However, effective WA and the process of turning WA values into cost figures is virtually impossible without automation.

In units without significant daily change in client load (numbers and acuity), which is often the case in LTC settings, WA on a daily basis is not as critical. However, it is important for prospective costing of care which has been difficult with current paper and pencil tools. WA can facilitate the prediction of optimal staffing levels and provide data on how well the organization is able to meet those levels. Most scheduler products which have been reviewed have a WA tool within them or are able to be integrated with some kind of WA system and as such, over time, would allow administration much more accurate prospective cost of care data.

6. Possible Characteristics of a Scheduler

Scheduler characteristics have varied considerably with each product reviewed. However, common features usually found in most packages are:
- staff information database:
- demographics, with staff and professional qualifications ;
- usual shift and site location;
- holiday and sick time hour accrual and disbursement;
- automatic seniority calculation (and staff sorted in that order);
- any other special data unique to long term care or a particular facility;
- staff rotations, master as well as probable schedules for casuals/part time staff;
- typical start and stop times and codes for non-standard shits;
- automatic notation of calls of casuals to fill needed shifts;
- automatic alerting staffing clerks if union rules, would be violated by calling in a particular staff member;
- user definable reporting capabilities which can be saved for future use and really are "user-friendly".

An important component of the scheduler is a staff database (DB), containing information mentioned just above. While the scheduler DB may not replace the Human Resources (HR) Department staff DB, any facility will be best served if there is some kind of interface between the HR DB and that which is kept within the scheduler. At this point HR reports are generated by an off-site mainframe system. In the future, with everyone on the same network and total personnel DB available to all with proper access, it should be much easier, less labour intensive and a far more accurate process of communicating between staffing clerks/timekeepers and Human Resources personnel, while facilitating generation of staffing and costing reports by managers and administrators at all levels.

7. Possible Costs of Software

I found a myriad of different ways that vendors price their products. Most use total bed capacity as one criteria. The fact that we are on four physical sites and therefore could use one network linking all sites or one copy of the product at each site is also a cost factor. Having a networked version versus stand-alone copies may cause significant differences in pricing. We are unique in that one of our driving needs is to have one distributive DB where all staff are listed and all data is updatable, regardless of its source. Last, our training costs would be somewhat higher than normal since staffing/timekeeping personnel reside on all four sites.

It is important to remember that virtually all software products undergo frequent revision or are still in development. Therefore, it would be best to re-review "finalists" and price quotes before a contract decision is made. I also found that United States developed products would need some "Canadianization" before purchase. Nurses in the international arena should realize that any software produced outside their own country will likely require changes before it can be used in their hospital. There may also be costs involved in the adaptation process which should be accounted for before a final purchase contract is signed. In our case, the software reviewed ranged in total price from under $5,000 to greater than $70,000.

8. Costs of Training

Training costs are significant. Whatever product is purchased will have significant impact on the staffing/timekeeper personnel, directors of nursing units, Human Resources Department and eventually all staff. Based on my reviews of products, it has become clear that proper training of staff is critical. For instance, I found that two different organizations using the same scheduling package were having completely opposite experiences with the product, based primarily on the abilities and training of the "staffing" personnel. Training estimates from various vendors range from two to five working days for orientation to the system. It may be least expensive to train just a few of the staffing and nursing personnel and have them train the rest. Some vendors do NOT recommend this evolutionary training approach, even though most suggest starting with one or two nursing areas as pilot test sites before going live for the total facility. Most vendors mentioned the need for one on-site person who could become the software expert to train and work with staff and therefore decrease the number of service calls to the vendor. All five health care organizations I visited had one person on-site who had primary responsibility for facilitating use of the scheduling software.

9. Possible Benefits of Software

Possible benefits will vary, based on the software and unique characteristics of the institution. In any case, I believe that if an automated system functions as promised, it should:
- facilitate easy updating and improvement in the accuracy of personnel data;
- facilitate proper calling replacements for staff who "book-off" or take holidays, within contract limitations;
- facilitate movement towards a centralized scheduling system for the total organization;
- decrease staff discontent with the current scheduling process;
- relieve some of the burden on switchboard staff of problems associated with locating casuals after hours.
- minimize manager time reviewing/checking time sheets and decrease miscalculations;
- improve tracking costs of personnel services and reduce overtime payments to staff;
- improve documentation of the scheduling process, especially in relation to the use of casuals, which might assist management when grievances are filed relating to staffing.

10. Implementation Issues

There is a considerable body of literature relating to implementation of software and bringing automation into client care sites, for instance Pulliam & Boettcher [5]. Two main issues relate to actual training of all affected staff and how automation or new software will change the way we do our work. Training has already been discussed in this paper. Both issues must be dealt with effectively for the scheduling products to become utilized to the fullest and for the organization to realize the kind of cost savings which the products inherently promise. Administrators must work out a carefully developed list of the steps in the selection and implementation process, with estimated time lines of how long these events might require. See also Beebe [6].

11. Conclusion

In this paper I have attempted to describe some of the issues related to a current manual staff scheduling system in one long term care setting in Victoria, British Columbia. All hospitals are unique and in our case having four physically separate sites under one corporate roof necessitated that we develop better means of scheduling staff within and between facilities and improve sharing of information about scheduling. Interviews were conducted with staff in a number of different long term care organizations to ascertain their perceptions about their current scheduling processes and what is unique about long term care settings. The results of those interviews made a strong case for selection of an automated scheduler for our hospital. From my research it has become clear that concerns about cost-benefit, characteristics, and implementation of an automated scheduling system should be carefully addressed before making a final decision on one program for adoption. It may also be important for nurse administrators to take into account whether any product selected might be useful to other areas and disciplines besides nursing. It should be clear by now that even though the total dollar investment in a scheduling product may be small relative to a total institutional budget, its eventual impact on the staff can be far reaching.

12. References

[1] Richards J. Implementing a computer system: Issues for nurse administrators. *Comput Nurs* 1992, 10:9-13.

[2] Burkes M. Identifying and relating nurses' attitudes toward computer use. *Comput Nurs 1991*, 9:190-201.

[3] Bergman C & Johnson J. Managing staffing with a personal computer- Part I. *Nurs Manag* 1988a, 19:28-32.

[4] Bergman C & Johnson J. Managing staffing with a personal computer- Part II. *Nurs Manag* 1988b, 19:55-61.

[5] Pulliam L & Boettcher E. A process for introducing computerized information systems into long term care facilities, *Comput Nurs*, 1989, 7:251-257.

[6] Beebe M. "Selecting Staff Scheduling Software". COACH, yearly meeting, Vancouver, 1992, April.

ADMINISTRATION

C. Benefits and realization

Nursing Informatics: An International Overview for Nursing in a Technological Era
S.J. Grobe and E.S.P. Pluyter-Wenting, eds.

Business Process Improvement in Nursing Plus
Benefits Realization . . . The Connection

Nelson R[a] and Stewart P L[b]

[a]*Major, U.S. Army Nurse Corps, Office of the Assistant Secretary of Defense (Health Affairs), 5109 Leesburg Pike, Suite 502, Falls Church, Virginia 22041*

[b]*Principal/Project Manager, Birch and Davis Associates, Inc., 8905 Fairview Road, Silver Spring, Maryland 20910*

The ultimate goal of any business process improvement program is to improve efficiency, increase productivity, and/or decrease costs. In this article, the authors relate actual experience with planning and implementing a program to improve business practices relating to a comprehensive hospital information system. They discuss specific examples of using business process re-engineering and total quality management techniques in the Department of Nursing to implement new approaches to nursing practice. The program uses a comprehensive process review approach and demonstrates how innovative and measurable performance improvements can help organizations to both rapidly improve their performance and sustain that improvement.

1. Introduction

Few tools in the nurse manager's "toolkit" are designed to effect change in critical cross-functional processes. Traditional management approaches typically avoid staff involvement in the decision making process, yet hold them responsible for implementing the process changes. After decades of incremental improvements, or bandaid attempts to improve the health care delivery process, some Department of Defense (DoD) medical facilities are proactively re-engineering the way work is done via a business process improvement (BPI) initiative called the Benefits Realization Improvement Program (BRIP). The BRIP is being implemented in all facilities that have the Composite Health Care System (CHCS).

The CHCS, the largest hospital information system in the history of the DoD, supports the worldwide delivery of health care in facilities ranging from extremely large medical centers to small, stand alone outpatient clinics. When complete, the system will be designed to enhance health care services. It is an interactive system that supports both inpatient and ambulatory care and provides the full benefits of automation to such areas as nursing, laboratory, pharmacy, radiology, and appointment scheduling using an integrated database. Automation of these functions is essential in DoD facilities in order to increase staff productivity and efficiency, improve communication, and, ultimately, improve the quality of health care.

The ultimate goal of any BPI program is to improve efficiency, increase productivity, decrease costs, and reap the benefits resulting from the successful integration of operations with technology. Industry experience reveals that 66% of benefits from automation result from management practice and workflow engineering changes. Only 33% of benefits come directly from "turning-on" the system and eliminating manual data processing steps. This paper will provide documentation of a program designed to improve business practices and discuss specific examples of using BPI concepts and Total Quality Management (TQM) techniques in nursing to realize system benefits and implement new approaches to practice, care delivery and research.

The opinions or assertations in this article are the private views of the authors and are not to be construed as official or representing the views of the Department of the Army or the Department of Defense.

2. The Benefits Realization Improvement Program and Business Process Improvement

The vital role that the CHCS plays in the health care delivery strategy mandates that facilities take full advantage of the benefits the system offers. The BRIP is designed to facilitate the improvement of business processes and enhance workflow at sites with the system. The BRIP creates synergy among workflow, information, and technology by optimally aligning business processes and technology support to meet the needs of the customers - patients, providers, and other staff.

The BRIP initiative is a blend of TQM tools and techniques and the adeptness to re-think current practices or ways of doing business. The program demonstrates how innovative, short-term success on a continual basis, and measurable performance improvements, allow organizations to rapidly upgrade their performance and create the basis for sustained improvement. The program uses a comprehensive process review approach to meet several goals: improve cost, quality, and access for military health care through improved business processes and improved decision making; target process improvement to achieve the forecasted benefits of the CHCS; and train facility staff in process improvement and facilitation skills for ongoing process redesign and change management. The BRIP is a highly interactive effort involving medical treatment facility staff and BRIP team members who challenge the status quo and implement high quality solutions, rather that getting "boxed-in" by the existing structure and systems. The development of process action teams, the empowerment of staff-driven changes, and the shift away from "This is how we have always done it" to "How can we do things better," have resulted in improved business practices, enhanced workflow, and improved productivity.

The BRIP was launched in September 1991 in a effort to improve the business practice in DoD medical facilities where improvement could be attained via maximal use of the capabilities of the CHCS. Since the system is a hospital-wide system, many of the improvements are multidisciplinary, effecting change in other departments as well as nursing.

Each BPI activity involves creation of a multidisciplinary process action team (PAT) which focuses on an urgent and compelling goal that is achievable in a short period of time -- weeks rather than months, is discreet and measurable, and can be achieved with available resources and authority. The life-cycle approach to BPI and concurrent realization of system benefits employs a structured methodology involving a mission statement, a focused approach, immediate feedback, and maximal use of technology. There are five steps in process redesign:

- Define the business goal or improvement opportunity - Customers are identified and the process outcome expectations developed. Baseline data and research into industry standards are deliberated so the organization can assess how much change to the business process is necessary.
- Analyze the business process - What is the current process, how is work being done today? Step two involves documenting the process flow. The flow must be specific enough to enable staff to see how they spend their time, reveal hidden tasks, and identify nonvalue added activities.
- Redesign the process - Redesigning business processes involves three approaches: (1) Simplification, both at the level of job activity (each worker's role in the process), and workflow (link between activity and worker). Work processes are simplified by elimination of nonvalue added activities and revision of the process to respond to current conditions and goals. (2) Integration of the redesigned steps and innovative solutions into the process. This often crosses functional boundaries offering opportunity for eradicating interdepartmental redundancies and restructuring of the activities/process. (3) Integration of technology. Technology support usually accompanies redesign efforts and can be a key solution in eliminating redundancies. Creative application of system capabilities will reap improved processes and realization of system benefits.
- Implement the improved process - Implementation often occurs in incremental steps. An essential part of implementation is monitoring results. If projected results are not achieved, areas where improvement are needed can be precisely pinpointed.
- Measure the improvements - Measurement of change against the baseline continues well after the new process is fully implemented. Redesigned processes are quantified and measured against the baseline established in step 2. Before and after resource assessments can be summarized and considered, so improvements can be made continuously.

Redesign should be viewed as a process in itself; for organizations in pursuit of sustained competitive advantage, redesign initiatives become a management technique, an ongoing effort. As a by-product of the redesign effort, technology support is built into the improvement strategy and system capabilities are used as they were designed. The approach to benefits realization in Australian hospitals is similar in that emphasis is placed on the need to revise practice and standards in the face of technology. Seven of the ten step benefits realization process, outlined by Mackie, used in Australian hospitals, require work redesign initiatives. Mackie states that Australian health care managers view benefits realization as a methodology for continuous quality improvement -- a journey towards achievement of excellence in health care management and delivery, not a one-time only project with a start and end date. Technology is aligned with the work process it supports and benefits of the system are identified. Immediate feedback encourages continuous organizational improvement.

As in any BPI activity, the approach begins with a review and flow charting of the current process, identification of the gaps or breakdowns in the process, identification of solutions that meet customers' expectations, and generation of a tactical plan for implementation of solutions and improvement of the process as illustrated in Figure 1 below. The tactical plan describes how the BPI solutions will actually be accomplished. To answer the question, "how will we know if we have made any improvement?," the PAT identifies expected outcome criteria used to measure the improvement. Examples of measurement criteria include: a 5% increase in the number of patients treated in a clinic, a 15% decrease in the number of surgery cancellations, or an increase in patient satisfaction.

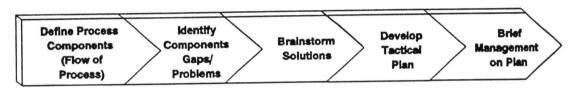

Figure 1: BRIP Activities

The Benefits Realization Improvement Program demonstrates value in five areas:

- **Quality** - The TQM principles help advance the facility's "quality" initiatives by emphasizing the importance of outcome measurement and its role in continuous improvement.
- **Practical Problem Solving** - The program enhances the existing problem solving capability.
- **Consistency** - The business case process ensures consistency and coordination between other initiatives.
- **Focus** - The structured program ensures that efforts at problem identification, problem solving, and benefits realization remain focused on producing value and do not become academic.
- **Connectivity** - The enhanced communication experienced as a by-product of the benefits realization program allows for skill and knowledge transfer among staff.

3. Outcomes of Business Process Improvement Efforts

The CHCS benefits realization program has demonstrated improvement in delivery and patient care in several DoD facilities. Specific examples of improvements realized in nursing practice are discussed below.

3.1 Admitting the Patient to a Ward

At one facility, the process by which patients were admitted to a ward frequently created extended stays in the admissions department. Not only did this create frustration for both the staff and the patients, but, at times, also delayed the initiation of care. Using brainstorming, flow charting, and multi-voting techniques, the process action team identified breakdowns in the workflow which created the delays, and recommended innovative solutions. One solution was establishing a centralized preadmission unit that provides initial nursing history and assessment, coordinates completion of ordered tests, consults, initiates care, and performs preliminary discharge planning. The CHCS was employed to generate patient instructions, improve the results reporting for tests, increase the third party reimbursements due to timely completion of preadmit requirements, improve the accuracy of the medical record information, and to create a template that allows scheduling of "appointments" for preadmission services. In addition to decreasing the [length of stay] for patients admitted to the facility, additional benefits were realized: increased patient, physician, and nurse satisfaction; improved quality of care; improved patient accountability; decreased waiting time for non-emergent patients; and decreased patient complaints.

3.2 Scheduling of Patients for the Operating Room

At another facility, a multidisciplinary team of physicians, nurses, and administrative staff elected to establish a more efficient operating room scheduling process which would meet the needs of physicians and operating room, recovery room, and ancillary staff while improving the timeliness of, and access to, care for the patient population. In analyzing the current process, it was determined that lack of planning and communication were the two primary "breakdowns" in the process. Automating and centralizing the scheduling process in the operating room was the solution overwhelmingly recommended by the PAT. The PAT thought that a centralized scheduling process would elicit a "one-stop shopping" concept for scheduling, retrieval of information for pre-certification, and better utilization of facilities, supplies, and equipment. The team also recommended development of a preference card system resulting in efficient preparation and readiness of surgical suites, implementation of a patient tracking system to address communication breakdowns, and establishment of a pre-admission nurse position to enhance the timeliness of information retrieval for pre-certification and third party reimbursements. The outcomes of this business practice redesign effort were an increase in operating room procedures performed, a decrease in the number of surgical cancellations, an increase in both staff and patient satisfaction, a decrease in patient waiting time, improved inventory management, cost containment of supplies and equipment, and improved communication among the staff.

3.3 Notification of Patients Concerning Pap Smear Results

One process that is a common problem at facilities is the way in which providers and patients are notified of Pap Smear results. A PAT at one facility embarked on improving this process in the Family Practice Clinic. The recommendations for improvement fell into four key areas: Patient and specimen intake, specimen screening, resulting of the specimen, and reporting of the results. The solutions for improving this process rely heavily on the use of the CHCS to create an automated bulletin for reporting of abnormal results, automated generation of a negative results report, and use of a daily CHCS ad hoc report to monitor the number of exams performed. Re-engineering this process resulted in improved quality of care and patient outcomes, a reduction in the number of patient related complaints, and increased patient, physician, and nurse satisfaction.

3.4 Communication Between Nursing and Other Hospital Staff

One of the most unanticipated benefits derived from the system and fostered through the Benefits Realization Improvement Program has been the nursing time saved due to improved communication. Recent studies indicate that the use of the CHCS electronic mail (E-Mail) function has resulted in a time savings from 15 minutes to more than three hours per day with an average of 37 minutes saved per staff member. Nurses are the greatest beneficiaries of time savings when using E-Mail for patient care activities such as communicating with other nurses concerning patient care plans, interdepartmental communication regarding test results and patient status, clarifying physician orders, etc. Nurses were the second rank beneficiaries of time savings when using E-Mail for administrative purposes such as in lieu of conducting meetings, scheduling and assigning duties, training/inservices, coordinating services, etc.

4. Summary

In conclusion, planning, organizing, and implementing a BPI program requires dedication and a concentrated focus on one goal: maximizing the effective use of a new technology and capitalizing on automation capabilities to the fullest extent possible for improving business practices. The CHCS Benefits Realization Improvement Program is a proactive process for documenting the anticipated benefits, assisting the facilities to attain those benefits, and evaluating/documenting the changes that occur. The nursing staff who implement the innovations enjoy several improvement outcomes: a greater control of their own resources; improved efficiencies; overall improvement in nursing operations; improved quality of care and patient outcomes; and increased staff satisfaction. In the words of James Carville, a political strategist for the Clinton administration, the most noteworthy outcome is a shift from "Why we can't people" to "How we can people."

5. References

[1]   Glaser J, Drazen E and Cohen L. Maximizing the Benefits of Health Care Information Systems. *J Med Syst* 1986, 10:51-56.

[2]   Mackie, P L: Realizing Benefits from Health Information Systems in Australia. In: Proceedings of the 1993 Annual Health Care Information and Management Systems Society (HIMSS) Conference. San Diego, CA: 1993: Volume Four, 81-93.

[3]   Carville, J. A speech presented during a General Session at the 1993 Annual HIMSS Conference. March, 1993. San Diego, CA.

[4]   Minard, B; *Health Care Computer Systems for the 1990's; Critical Executive Decisions*. Ann Arbor: American College of Healthcare Executives, 1991.

[5]   Page, J; The Paradigm Has Shifted: A Quality Vision For Healthcare; *Healthcare Information Management Journal;* Health Care Information and Management Systems Society of the American Hospital Association, Summer 1990, Volume 4, Number 3, 11-13.

Nursing Informatics: An International Overview for Nursing in a Technological Era
S.J. Grobe and E.S.P. Pluyter-Wenting, eds.

A Benefits Realisation "Rescue" Plan for a Nursing Information System

Strachan H [a] Cogan M [a] Kelly K [a] Webber A [a]

[a] *Riverside Health, Department of Computing and Information, Charing Cross Hospital, Fulham Palace Road, London W6 8RF.*

This paper describes the project stages of a nursing information system implemented at Riverside Health in London. The main features of the nursing information system which include: nurse scheduling; care planning; and workload assessment; are described. Expected benefits of the project are outlined and the final evaluation methodology and results are reported. A description is given of the benefits realisation "rescue" plan which resulted from issues identified during the project evaluation and as a consequence of concerns raised during the change management experience.

1. Introduction

Riverside Health is situated in the heart of London on the banks of the River Thames. It consists of two large medical and nursing teaching hospitals. Charing Cross Hospital which has 600 beds, provides acute services and regional specialities including neuroscience, renal medicine, oncology and plastic surgery. The Chelsea and Westminster Hospital provides acute, obstetric and children's services and has 650 beds. There are 1110 full time nursing posts.

Following the implementation of a computerised nurse scheduling and workload assessment system in Riverside, an evaluation of benefits was undertaken. Although benefits had been achieved following the previous pilot study of the system, few benefits were realised following full hospital implementation. As a result of this evaluation a plan was formulated which attempted to identify the obstacles that prevented the realisation of benefits and recommended actions to remove these obstacles.

2. Project Phases

The nursing information system project began in January 1988. It was divided into four phases: the *scoping phase*, which sought to identify nursing information requirements and analysed the existing manual information systems; the *exploratory phase* defined user requirements and examined existing commercial packages; the *development phase* included piloting the applications, evaluating benefits and recommending software enhancements. These three phases took approximately two years. Once the enhanced versions had been fully tested, the final *start-up phase* was undertaken. [1] This included implementing the solution and evaluating the success of the project. Full implementation of the nurse scheduling and workload assessment system into 50 wards took approximately one year. Although a care planning system was piloted it was not implemented as no benefits were attained during the pilot stage. The final evaluation was undertaken in August 1992.

3. System Features

The nurse scheduling system had the ability to maintain an 8 week standard roster which could be used as a basis for planning actual duty rosters. Facilities were also available to assist in the generation of entirely new duty rosters. These included the automatic calculation of nurses' hours and daily skill mix. Information regarding; past off duty; shift and off duty requests; annual leave and study leave entitlement; and student nurses ward allocations; were available online. The roster could be updated easily to record changes to shifts, absences, overtime and the use of agency nurses. Updated rosters could be printed at any time and a variety of manpower, payroll and personnel reports could be generated automatically.

The workload assessment system allowed the entry of patients' dependencies and other ward activities. A comparison of required and available nursing hours were calculated automatically and available online or as monthly and daily reports.

The care planning system allowed the recording of a nursing admission assessment. A standard care plan could be retrieved from a library of standard care plans by entering key words. These stndard care plans could be individualised for each patient as required. An evaluation of whether outcomes had been met could be recorded.

4. Benefits Realisation

In order to realise benefits fully, they must be defined at the beginning of the project. Both managerial and clinical commitment is required to consciously plan and obtain these benefits during implementation. [2]

At the beginning of the project, potential benefits were identified for each system. The anticipated benefits of the nurse scheduling system included: saving time formulating duty rosters and producing manpower/personnel/ payroll reports; and improved monitoring and control of nursing resources by improved collection, retrieval and accuracy of appropriate data. [3] Monitoring workload was expected to: assist with daily staff scheduling; and improve roster planning, establishment setting and work organisation, by identifying trends and working patterns in relation to patients needs. [4] The care planning system was expected to: save time planning and recording nursing care; improve legibility and conciseness of nursing records; and assist in quality assurance and nursing audit activities. [5]

During implementation activities were directed towards securing these benefits. This included: general awareness training on computers in nursing; "hands on" training and follow up support; meetings with staff to examine reports and discuss their usage; the establishment of a user group to agree operational procedures; and meetings with the various departments to plan the replacement of manual reports with the computerised reports.

5. Computerised Care Planning System Pilot

Although the care planning system met the majority of user requirements, no benefits were achieved. No nursing time was saved and, since the hand written care plans on the pilot ward were excellent, an improvement here was not relevant. Our evaluation concluded that considerable attention was required to the screen and report designs, and the menu structure. The wealth of information stored in the system was not organised or retrieved in any meaningful way, and output was limited to printed care plans.

6. Method of Evaluation

Following implementation of the nurse scheduling and workload assessment system a survey technique was used to evaluate the benefits of the project. The target population was defined as the ward managers because they were the main users of both the system and the information. A random sample of 20 ward managers was selected from a total population of 50. A questionnaire was designed and structured interviews were undertaken by the nursing system managers. Some of the ward managers asked if they could complete the questionnaire in their own time. They stated that this would allow them to be more critical of the system because some degree of anonymity would be maintained. There were a mixture of open and closed questions which were directed at ascertaining: what benefits had been achieved in relation to time saved and the use made of information produced by the system; information required in nurses roles; other benefits or detrimental effects of the system; and what improvements the users would like to see.

7. Results

7.1 Workload Assessment and Roster Criteria

Of the ward managers questioned, 32% were collecting workload information on a daily basis. 58% of these found it useful for daily scheduling, roster planning or examining work organisation. Where information was not used it was generally found to be as a result of an inability to change previously planned rosters.

Thirty four percent stated they would like to collect workload information. Those who did not wish to collect workload information also agreed it was difficult to change the roster once it was planned. They also believed financial constraints meant increasing staffing establishments would be unlikely. Other reasons included: too time consuming to collect; unsure of benefits; and poor inter-rater reliability.

Ward managers were asked to identify their criteria or priorities for planning the roster. 100% stated that meeting nurses' requests for particular off duty or shifts was a criterion. 75% stated minimum number of trained staff, pre-defined skill mix/numbers per shift, and team or primary nursing. Other criteria mentioned included 24 hour workload patterns and weekly trends.

7.2 Formulating Rosters

Various facilities are provided to reduce time formulating a roster if it is entered directly onto the computer. However, 68% of users did not use the computer to enter their roster directly. Reasons given included: inconvenient location and limited availability of the terminal; insufficient time; frequent interruptions; lack of confidence with the computer; not easy to use; staff details not up to date; and no facilities to produce team rosters.

Those staff who did use the computer to enter their rosters directly, 33% stated it was between 50 - 66% quicker than the paper and pen method. The remainder said that it took a similar amount of time. The facilities that helped save time included, easy correction of shifts, and automatic totalling of staff numbers and hours.

7.3 Information Use

Seventy five percent of the ward managers found the manpower information obtained from the system saved them time and was useful to monitor additional resource usage, vacancies and time out. Those who did not find this information useful stated that they did not require or understand it. Only 25% of ward managers obtained further information themselves. The reasons given for not extracting information included a lack of awareness of, what information was available, and how to obtain or use it.

When asked what information they would like the system to produce the following items were identified: student nurse absences; payroll; training; and staff costs. These reports are required by either payroll or personnel and are being formulated manually at present. All however, were available from the system in a limited form.

7.4 Other Benefits, Effects and Suggested Improvements

Other benefits identified by staff included: improved communication for night duty managers, improved retrieval of information; more accurate information; and the provision of information not previously available. Disbenefits of the system were identified as: time consuming; slow responses; lack of confidence that the information was up to date. Suggested improvements included: auto rostering; improving ease of use and lay out of reports; providing on line access to past rosters; more flexible agency and team rostering; up to date staff information; and more training.

7.5 Technical Issues

A number of technical problems, which prevented benefits from being realised, were identified by the system managers. These included: reliance on central processing prior to obtaining reports; reliance on all users being up to date before undertaking central processing; frequent failure and protracted duration of central processing; inaccurate staff cost calculations; ridged report formats; and no links to the manpower/payroll system.

8. Change Management

Implementing technology into Riverside was a considerable change for the majority of ward managers who had little or no experience with computers. Although some benefits had been achieved, they were sporadic and inconsistent. Apart from some of the obvious technical and educational issues, it is not easy to be certain why the change was not fully successful. Moss Kanter identifies five blocks for productive change which provide a guide to how change should be managed, and can assist in the evaluation of the success of change. [6]

The first block, *departure from tradition*, relates to the reason for changing a method. The second block, *a crisis or galvanised event*, is also concerned with the reason the change was initiated. Was it forced upon staff or was it a need that was identified because of a particular event? In many ways Riverside was ahead in its thinking. It was recognised by the Directors of Nursing that these tools would be required with the forthcoming introduction of Resource Management and the resulting devolution of accountability for resources. However, it did appear to be a top down approach and we were offering ward managers the tools, prior to the need being recognised by them. Role change did not take place in conjunction with the implementation.

The third block involves *strategic decisions* which need to be taken. It requires strong leadership, mission statements and an overall plan. In Riverside, the aims and objectives of the project were defined in line with the goals of nursing. Project management principles were followed and a dedicated project manager was employed.

The need for leadership is highlighted in block four, *prime movers*. During the project in Riverside this element was not stable. The Directors of Nursing who initiated the project, left Riverside during the project. It was also a time of considerable change elsewhere in the organisation. The introduction of a new management structure meant considerable changes in senior nursing personnel. The introduction of new technology was not seen as a priority at this time.

The final block includes *action vehicles*. The change must impinge on other structures within the organisation to ensure its success. It must become the new way of working. It must produce the right results early enough to produce success. Unfortunately, the system had some technical and design problems that prevented the complete replacement of the manual rostering and reporting system. These problems prevented major benefits being achieved early in the project.

9. Recommendations

In order to rectify this situation a *benefits realisation "rescue" plan* was drawn up. This plan identified the expected benefits, how they should be achieved, the beneficiary, what the obstacles to achieving the benefits were, the actions required to remove these obstacles, including a named person responsible for the action and a date by when it should be achieved.

Recommendations included:
- provide further support and education regarding information needs, use and availability;
- reconsider accountability of the ward manager in relation to staff budgets;
- provide additional terminals and printers and relocate other terminals;
- agree enhancements with the company or find an alternative system that meets users needs regarding, ease of use, team rostering, auto rostering, flexible report formats;
- develop links with manpower/payroll system to ensure staff details are up to date;
- re-assess available workload assessment system and link to scheduling.

The Nursing Project Board, which consisted of the Director and Assistant Director of Nursing, the Nursing Project Manager and the Director of Computing and Information, were responsible for implementing the recommendations. A number of actions were agreed. An educational programme was established to promote awareness of the relationship between nurses roles, objectives and information needs. A new senior nurse advisor post was created with a specific responsibility for information. The new clinical directorate structure meant the responsibility for managing staff budgets was devolved to ward level. No agreement with the software company could be reached regarding improvements to the system and it was decided to decommission the system. The search for a more suitable nursing system that would more closely meet the needs of nurses, address the technical short comings of the previous system, and ensure links with other hospital systems, was incorporated as part of the Hospital Information Support System (HISS) project. More terminals would be made available as part of the HISS project. An Information Forum, with representatives from all Clinical Directorates, was set up to look at nursing information issues, in particular workload assessment.

10. Conclusion

Management of the change process, and ensuring implementation is directed towards appropriately identified benefits, is essential to the success of any project of this nature. The introduction of new technology requires changes to tasks, roles and organisational structures if the change from manual processes to computerisation is going to be successful. Providing leadership and support for staff, as well as involving them at all stages of the project and in the ongoing development of the system, should gain ownership of the system. Operational benefits should be provided to the nurses who collected and entered the data, and management information must be a by-product. In Riverside, the most significant areas that required attention were: the education of nurses in the use of information; their roles and responsibilities; full integration of the nursing system with other hospital systems, and the need for both suppliers and the system to be flexible to ensure continuing development of the system to meet the evolving needs of the users. Although few tangible benefits were achieved, there has been an increased awareness of the need for information by many staff, less fear of computers, and more knowledge about the sort of nursing information systems required by nurses. If at first you don't succeed...................

11. References

[1] Strachan H. The Development of a Nursing Information System Strategy for the Acute Hospital Setting. In: *MEDINFO '89*. Barber B, Cao D, Qin D, Wagner G (eds). Amsterdam: North Holland, 1989: 675-678.

[2] Peterson H, Gerdin Jelger U. Evaluation: A Means to Better Results. In: *Nursing Informatics: Where Caring and Technology Meet*. Ball M, Hannah K, Gerdin Jelger U, Peterson H (eds). New York: Springer-Verlag, 1988: 64-77.

[3] Halligan M, McCormack R, Thompson J. Nursing Information Management Systems. In: *Nursing and Computers: Third International Symposium on Nursing Use of Computers and Information Science*. St Louis: Mosby, 1988: 406-411.

[4] Seppala A. The Use of Information Technology for Monitoring Patient Dependency and Needs for Resources in the Helsinki University Central Hospital. In: *Nursing Informatics '91*. Hovenga E, Hannah K, McCormick K, Ronald J (eds). Berlin: Springer-Verlag, 1991: 261-265.

[5] Woods K. The Development of a Clinical Nursing Computer System. In: *MEDINFO '89*. Barber B, Cao D, Qin D, Wagner G (eds). Amsterdam: North Holland, 1989: 658-662.

[6] Moss Kanter R. *The Change Masters*. London: Routlidge, 1983.

Nursing Informatics: An International Overview for Nursing in a Technological Era
S.J. Grobe and E.S.P. Pluyter-Wenting, eds.

Multidisciplinary Order Entry System: Its Benefits

Goodman J[a] Assang W[b] and Clement H[c]

[a]*Department of M.I.S., Children's Hospital of Eastern Ontario, Ottawa, Ontario, Canada.*

[b]*Department of Nursing, Children's Hospital of Eastern Ontario, Ottawa, Ontario, Canada.*

[c]*Client Services, HealthVISION™ Corporation, Mississauga, Ontario, Canada*

The implementation of a multidisciplinary order entry system was identified as a strategy to maintain/improve quality of care and gain efficiencies in human and material resources. The results of a comparative analysis of the manual to the automated order entry/result reporting systems, in selected clinical care areas, will be reviewed. The analysis will outline the identified issues, and the impact of the implementation of the multidisciplinary order entry system, *CareVISION*™. The benefits realized in the delivery of patient care, and the impact on clinical practice, administrative activities, staff, quality assurance, and the overall organization will be summarized. In conclusion, issues and challenges requiring further review will be discussed.

1. Introduction

The Children's Hospital of Eastern Ontario (CHEO), Ottawa, Canada is a 168 bed, pediatric teaching facility associated with the University of Ottawa. It serves the pediatric population of Eastern Ontario and Western Quebec. CHEO has on average 10,000 inpatient admissions and 160,000 outpatient visits per year. The current cost constraints within the health care sector necessitated the development of alternatives to facilitate the delivery of quality patient care. To achieve this goal, an automated patient care system, *CareVISION*, was implemented. The objectives of this project were to maintain/improve quality of care while at the same time to gain efficiencies in human and material resources. The first modules to be implemented were the order entry and results reporting modules. The concept of PROVIDER order entry (i.e.physician order entry) provided the framework for the implementation of the order entry component.

2. Descriptive Study

A descriptive study was conducted to determine the degree to which the objectives of the project were met. [1] Quality and efficiency indicators were identified and used to compare the manual against the automated order entry and result reporting system on the two pilot units and on two control units.

3. Quality Indicators

3.1 Transcriptions and Interpretation Errors

These errors are expected to be eliminated using automated order entry due to one time data entry and improved legibility. Incident reports were compared during the pre and post study periods. [2, 3]

3.2 Completeness of Orders

The information required for order entry was defined in the automated system to eliminate incomplete order errors. Requisitions (laboratory, pharmacy, radiology, etc.) were examined during the pre and post study period to determine how many tests were ordered without required or with inappropriate information. Incident reports were compared to determine how many incomplete orders such as laboratory, pharmacy, radiology were submitted. [3]

3.3 Timeliness of Treatment

Orders are transmitted immediately to the appropriate departments to facilitate initiation of treatment. Patient information is readily available (e.g.lab results) enabling diagnosis and/or treatment decisions to be made in a timely fashion. [4] The average length of time when orders (pharmacy, laboratory, radiology, etc.) were written or entered into the system and when the order was processed, were compared pre and post study periods. [3] The time treatment was initiated (such as first medication dose, laboratory specimen collection time, scheduling of radiology exam) were compared. [5, 6]

3.4 Consistency of Orders

Hospital policies and procedures can be built into the automated system during implementation to ensure consistency of ordering practice, such as the legal requirements for ordering medications like digoxin; pharmacy stop order dates; and other general ordering practices. [3]

3.5 Quality Management

The software provides an audit trail facilitating the review of order entry / result review transactions that occur. Quality assurance procedures can be established that were not possible prior to implementation. [7]

4. Efficiency Indicators

4.1 Appropriate Use of Human Resources

The implementation of a multidisciplinary system eliminates the need for repetitive and redundant manipulation of order processing and results receiving. [4] The time spent transcribing orders was measured pre and post implementation. The number of phone calls and need for portering reports and requisitions to and from various departments was documented.

4.2 Reduction of Paper Costs

Automation eliminates the need for paper requisitions. Multi-part requisitions are expensive. These forms have been replaced by specimen labels and/or on-line messages. On-line result reporting has substantially reduced the need to print daily interim laboratory results. [2]

5. Issues Surrounding Provider Order Entry

The results from this study will outline the implications for nursing with the implementation of a multidisciplinary order entry / result review system.

5.1 Change in Roles and Practice

Provider order entry, specifically physician order entry, changes the traditional roles of all health care providers. The change process must be managed so that users understand the need for and are involved in defining the changes. This will help to ensure that the new roles are accepted. [4, 8, 2]

The committee structure that was put in place at CHEO involved all levels of users. Terms of reference mandated communication to and from constituents. The new roles must be clearly defined and communicated to all users. [3] With the implementation of order entry, the providers who were involved, the types of orders and the conditions under which they would be entered were clearly defined so that all health care providers (allied health, nurses, physicians, etc.) were aware of the scope of the project and the roles of those involved. [8, 9]

5.2 Training

The training is a very expensive but essential component for the successful implementation of any system. [8] Therefore, it is critical to ensure that the time invested in training is used effectively and efficiently. Excellent documentation and training material tailored to the hospital must be developed. The software must be "user friendly" and "intuitive" to decrease training requirements. [3]

The hospital must identify "Expert Users" that will be used as resources on an on-going basis. These expert users have an extra task since they may be called on to do training, data entry, etc. [10] Reward mechanism must be put in place to recognize the effort of the "expert users" throughout the hospital.

An ongoing training program must be put in place to ensure that all users received adequate training. [7]

5.3 Legal, Security and Confidentiality Issues

The electronic signature must be approved by the hospital as the legal authorization of physician orders. Confidentiality of patient information must be addressed when implementing an automated multidisciplinary system. Security procedures must be explicit and followed by users and system managers alike. [11, 12]

5.4 Paper Generation

The information required on hard copy must be identified to determine when and how orders are printed as the legal chart copy. In the early phases of implementation, users rely on paper. After developing confidence in the system, the printed copies may be eliminated. [2]

5.5 Job Satisfaction

At this time it is difficult to evaluate the impact of job satisfaction on quality of care issues. However, with changes such as provider order entry, it is important to be aware of the impact that change has on job satisfaction. [4, 7]

6. Conclusion

Automation has been identified as a mechanism for the management of clinical data to facilitate the delivery of quality care. Implementing a multi-disciplinary order entry system should not interfere with and must accommodate the practice of all health care providers.

7. References

[1] Malec BT. The Benefit-cost Justification of Executive Information Ssytems: A Model and Case Study. In: Proceedings of the 1992 Annual Healthcare Information and Management System Society (HIMSS) of the American Hospital Association. Glasser JP et al (eds). Chicago: American Hospital Association, 1992: 133-138.

[2] Carrol T. The Costs and Benefits of a Hospital Information System. In: Proceedings of the Seventh World Congress on Medical Informatics. Lun KC, Degoulet P, Piemme ET, Rienhoff O (eds). North-Holland: Amsterdam, 1992:1212-1220.

[3] Teich JM, Hurley JF, Beckley RF, Aranow M. Design of an Easy-to-Use Physician Order Entry System with Support for Nursing and Ancillary Departments. In: Symposium on Computer Applications in Medical Care (SCAMC) 1993. Clayton PD (ed) New York: McGraw Hill Inc, 1993: 99-103.

[4] Mackie PL. Realizing Benefits From Health Information Systems in Australia. In: Proceedings of the 1993 Annual Health Care Information and Management Systems Society (HIMSS) of the American Hospital Association. HIMSS, AHA (ed). Chicago: American Hospital Association, 1993: Volume 4, 81-93

[5] Palmer B. How to Harness the Power of Information Technology to Benefit Patient Care. In: Nursing Informatics'91, Proceedings of the Fourth International Conference on Nursing Use of Computers and Information Science. Hovenga EJS, Hannah KJ, Jelger UG, Peterson H. (eds). Berlin: Springer-Verlag, 1991: 151-157.

[6] Alvarez, RC and al. A Provincial Health Information Processing Strategy: A Case Study. In: Proceedings of the Seventh World Congress on Medical Informatics. Lun KC, Degoulet P, Piemme ET, Rienhoff O (eds). North-Holland: Amsterdam, 1992: 1180-1185.

[7] Cho S, Clement H, Gillis R, Matthews S, Salois-Swallow D, Tamaki C. Framework for the Planning - Nursing Information Systems. Edmonton: HealthCare & Computing, 1993.

[8] Fredericksen L. Benefits from Automation: A Myth or Realty? In: Proceedings of the 1993 Annual Health Care Information and Management Systems Society (HIMSS) of the American Hospital Association. HIMSS, AHA (ed). Chicago: American Hospital Association, 1993: Volume 4, 105-113.

[9] Shamian J, Nagle LM, Hannah KJ. Optimizing Outcomes of Nursing Informatization. In: Proceedings of the Seventh World Congress on Medical Informatics. Lun KC, Degoulet P, Piemme ET, Rienhoff O (eds). North-Holland: Amsterdam, 1992: 976-980.

[10] Abendroth, TW. End-user Participation in the Needs Assessment for a Clinical Information System. In: Symposium on Computer Applications in Medical Care (SCAMC) 1993. Clayton PD (ed) New York: McGraw Hill Inc, 1993: 233-237.

[11] Robinson D. A Legal Examination of Format, Signature and Confidentiality Aspects of Computerized Health Information. In: Proceedings of the Seventh World Congress on Medical Informatics. Lun KC, Degoulet P, Piemme ET, Rienhoff O (eds). North-Holland: Amsterdam, 1992: 1554-1560.

[12] COACH. Guidelines to Promote the Confidentiality and Security of Automated Health Related Information. Edmonton: COACH, 1989.

Nursing Informatics: An International Overview for Nursing in a Technological Era
S.J. Grobe and E.S.P. Pluyter-Wenting, eds.

Benefits Of Hospital Information Systems As Seen By Front-line Staff: Implications For System Evaluation, Design, And Marketing

Nauright, L P[a] and Simpson, R L[b]

[a]*Nell Hodgson Woodruff School of Nursing, Emory University, Atlanta, GA, 30322*

[b]*HBO and Company, Inc., 301 Perimeter Center North, Atlanta, GA 30346, USA*

The purpose of these descriptive, correlational studies was to identify benefits realized from computerized hospital information systems (HIS) and the value of those benefits as perceived by front line system users. A total of 697 respondents from six hospitals describe benefits related to quality of care as being realized to a greater extent, and more important, than those related to cost-savings/productivity or professionalism/recruitment/retention. Perceptions of nurses were not significantly different than those of general hospital staff. Scattered significant correlations were revealed between demographic and organizational variables and instrument scale and subscale scores. Findings appear useful to researchers studying HIS benefits and to system designers and vendors endeavoring to make HIS more user-friendly, functional, and marketable.

1. Research Questions

1.1 What are the perceptions of nurses and general hospital staff regarding the extent to which potential benefits of implementing an HIS are realized in their institution and the relative importance of those benefits?

1.2 How do selected demographic characteristics and organizational variables influence perceptions of benefits realized and benefit importance?

1.3 Do nurses and general hospital staff differ with regard to their perceptions of benefits realized and benefit importance?

2. Review of Literature

A review of related literature revealed two broad areas of emphasis--identification of benefits and attitudes of staff, usually nursing staff, about computerization. Major studies of benefits realized included studies by Romano and others [1], Norwood, Hawkins & Gall [2], Schmitz, Ellerbrake & Williams [3] and comprehensive reviews of studies by Hendrickson & Kovner [4] and Staggers [5]. Literature examining attitudes of nurses included reviews of literature by Ihde [6] and Bongartz [7], philosophical and theoretical issues presented by Ford [8] and McLaughlin, et. al. [9], and research findings of Happ [10], Krampf and Robinson [11], Stonge & Brodt [12], Jacobson, et. al .[13], Schwirian, Malone, Stone, Nunley, and Francisco [14], Burkes [15], and Scarpa, Smeltzer and Jaisin [16]. Generally the review of the literature revealed benefits related to efficiency, productivity and cost effectiveness of computerization with some concern over its dehumanizing effects on either patients or nurses. Attitudes of nurses were reported as mostly positive and not linked consistently to demographic characteristics. Emerging discussion was noted by Cocoran-Perry and Graves [17] and Swenson-Feldman, et al [18] of potential benefits for nursing research, quality of care, and professionalism. Little was written concerning the potential of HIS for recruitment, retention, or professional development.

3. Questionnaire

The questionnaire was developed from review of vendor materials, literature review, focus groups, and consultation with content and design experts. Two Likert-type scales were developed, one for the extent to which potential benefits were realized in the institution and a second for the importance of benefits to the respondent. Both the extent and importance scales had three subscales related to cost-savings/productivity, quality of care, and professionalism/recruitment/retention. Because of slight differences in terminology, two versions of the questionnaire were administered--one for nurses and one for general hospital staff.

4. Methodology

Data were collected from eleven sample populations at six hospitals in Georgia, using intermediaries employed by the participating hospitals. Data were analyzed using descriptive statistics, Pearson's r and t-test. Chronbach's alpha was used to test for internal consistency and reliability coefficients were above .94. Factor analysis was conducted to analyze subscales for internal consistency.

The sample consists of 324 nurses and 373 general hospital staff (GHS). Response rates averaged 39%. The respondents were predominantly female (nurses 93%, GHS 83%) with mean ages of 39 for nurses and 36 for GHS. Mean years employed was nine and mean years in position was six for both groups. Highest levels of education ranged from high school to doctorate with baccalaureate the most frequent response. A majority of respondents reported little or no prior experience with computers before the HIS; less than half of each group used a computer at home. Order entry and patient classification were the predominant applications of computer use reported.

5. Findings

5.1 Perceptions regarding extent benefits are realized.

For each instrument, the extent scale was analyzed by determining means for each item and for the entire scale and each of its subscales. To compare relative ratings of the extent to which potential benefits are realized, scale and subscale average item scores were calculated by dividing the subscale mean by the number of items on the scale or subscale. The responses of the extent scale available to the sample were: 1=not realized; 2=somewhat; 3=moderate; and 4=great. As indicated in Table 1, the average item scores on the extent scale were 2.33 for nurses and 2.48 for GHS with ranges among the respondent subgroups from 2.04 to 2.76. Benefits related to quality of care received the highest extent ratings from all populations.

Table 1
Average Item Scores for Extent Realized

| | ALL RESPONDENTS | | RANGE AMONG SUBSAMPLES | |
	Nses	GHS	Nses	GHS
Extent Scale	2.33	2.48	2.28 - 2.65	2.17 - 2.76
Subscale Quality of Care	2.46	2.46	2.29 - 2.69	2.28 - 2.87
Subscale Cost-Savings/Productivity	2.26	2.26	2.09 - 2.65	2.04 - 2.75
Subscale Professionalism/ Recruitment/Retention	2.21	2.21	2.08 - 2.59	2.13 - 2.59

5.2 Perceptions regarding importance of benefits.

Responses to importance data were analyzed in the same fashion. Average item scores for importance are reflected in Table 2. Average item scores on the importance scale were 3.06 for nurses and 2.82 for GHS, with ranges among subgroups from 2.64 to 3.43. Quality subscale items were ranked highest by all subgroups, followed by cost-savings/productivity subscale items and items related to professionalism/recruitment/retention.

Table 2
Average Item Scores for Importance

| | ALL RESPONDENTS | | RANGE AMONG SUBSAMPLES | |
	Nses	GHS	Nses	GHS
Importance Scale	3.06	2.82	3.12 - 3.33	2.64 - 3.33
Subscale Quality of Care	3.21	2.96	3.11 - 3.43	2.82 - 3.39
Subscale Cost-Savings/Productivity	3.04	2.78	2.83 - 3.40	2.48 - 3.35
Subscale Professionalism/ Recruitment/Retention	2.92	2.71	2.88 - 3.33	2.65 - 3.12

5.3 Influence of selected demographic characteristics and organizational variables.

Correlations between scale and subscale scores and the demographic variables are reported below for the total population of nurses and the total population of general hospital staff. Significant correlations are indicated in Table 3. Correlations were also performed for these variables for the eleven subsamples from the six hospitals and reported to those institutions.

Table 3
Significant Correlations Between Scale and Subscale Scores and Demographic Variables

N=Nses; G=GHS VARIABLE	EXTENT SCALE	SUBSCALES Qual	Cost	Prof	IMPORTANCE SCALE	SUBSCALES Qual	Cost	Prof
Age								
Years of Employment	N+							
Years in Position		N+		G-				G-
Education	G-	G-	G-	G-			N+	
Extent of Computerization in Department	N+	N+G+			G+	G+	G+	G+
Prior Experience with Computers	N-G+	N-G+	G+	G+	G+	G+	G+	G+
Gender								
Use of Computer at Home								

Response means for each subscale were compared with *age, years of employment, and years in position* and tested for significance using Pearson's r. For the total populations of nurses and general hospital staff, no significant differences were found between scale and subscale scores and the variable of *age*.

For nurses, *years of employment* correlated positively with the extent subscale quality. For general hospital staff, no significant correlation was found between *years of employment* and scale or subscale scores. For the total population of nurses, *years in position* correlated positively with the extent subscale quality. For the total population of general hospital staff, *years in position* was negatively correlated with the extent and importance subscales of professionalism/recruitment/retention.

Nurses and general hospital staff were grouped into less than baccalaureate degree and baccalaureate and above and their responses tested for significance using Spearman's rho. For the total population of nurses, *education* was positively correlated with the importance subscale cost-savings. For the total population of general hospital staff, *education* was negatively correlated with the extent scale and all of its subscales.

Extent of computerization in the department was calculated by giving one point for each computer application indicated. For the total population of nurses, *extent of computerization in the department* was positively correlated with the extent scale and its subscale quality. For general hospital staff, this variable was positively correlated with the importance scale and all of its subscales as well as with the extent subscale quality.

Correlation coefficients were calculated for *prior experience with computers* and tested for significance using Spearman's rho. For the total population of nurses *prior experience with computers* was negatively correlated with the extent subscale quality. T-test confirmed this correlation and also indicated a negative correlation with the entire extent scale. For the total population of general hospital staff, *prior experience with computers* was positively correlated with the extent scale, the importance scale and all subscales.

Demographic variables of *gender* and *utilization of a computer in the home* were compared to scale and subscale means and tested for significance using the t-test. For the total population of nurses and general hospital staff, no significant differences were found between the variables of *gender* and *use of a computer at home* and scale or subscale scores.

5.4 Differences in perceptions of nurses and general hospital staff.

Scale and subscale means for nurses and general hospital staff in each sample were compared and tested for significance using t-test. There were no significant differences in the perceptions of nurses and general hospital staff regarding benefits realized or benefit importance. Similarly, within individual hospitals, no significant differences were found between the scores of nurses and general hospital staff.

6. Conclusions

Generally, the data reveal that nurses and general hospital staff feel benefits are being realized from the HIS, at least to a modest extent. They believe that potential benefits are of moderate to considerable importance. The benefits seen as most realized and most important to staff tended to be those related to quality of care, followed closely by those related to cost-savings/productivity and those related to professionalism/ recruitment/retention. These consistent ratings of quality of care benefits as the predominant by front line caregivers is important, particularly in light of the current interest in total quality management and patient outcomes. The strong showing of benefits related to professionalism/recruitment/retention indicates an area of benefits not currently described in the literature or in vendor materials. There may be untapped resources within the HIS for marketing the institution and for recruitment and retention.

Correlations between demographic and organization data and scale and subscale scores revealed no impact on perceptions of nurses or general hospital staff by the variables of age, gender, or use of a computer in the home. For nurses, isolated positive correlations were noted between some subscale scores and years of employment, years in position, education, and extent of computerization in the department. Prior experience with computers was negatively correlated with one subscale.

For general hospital staff, isolated positive correlations were found between scale and subscale scores and extent of computerization in the department and prior experience with computers. Isolated negative correlations were found between subscale scores and the variables of years in position and education.

It is important to note that there were no significant differences between nurses and general hospital staff totally or in any institution surveyed with regard to their perceptions of benefits realized or benefit importance. If indeed, nurses and general hospital staff do not see the system differently, there may be no need to market systems differently to these populations or to conduct separate staff development/orientation programs.

7. References

[1] Romano C, Ryan L, Harris J, Boykin P & Power M. A Decade of Decisions. *Comput in Nurs*, 1985, 3(2): 65 -67.

[2] Norwood D, Hawkins R & Gall J. Information System Benefits Hospital, Improves Care. *Hospitals*, 1976, 50(18): 79-83.

[3] Schmitz H, Ellerbrake R & Williams T. Study Evaluates Effects of New Communication System. *Hospitals*, 1976, 50(21): 129-134.

[4] Hendrickson G & Kovner C. Effects of Computers on Nursing Resource Use: Do Computers Save Nurses Time? *Comput in Nurs*, 1990, 8(1): 16-22.

[5] Staggers N. Using Computers in Nursing: Documented Benefits and Needed Studies. *Comput in Nurs*, 1988, 6(4): 164-169.

[6] Ihde D. A Phenomenology of Man-Machine Relations. In *Work Technology and Education*, Feinberg W & Rosemont H (eds.) Urbana: University of Illinois Press, 1975: 186-203.

[7] Bongartz C. Computer-oriented Patient Care: A Comparison of Nurses' Attitudes and Perceptions. *Comput in Nurs*, 1988, 4(2): 82-86.

[8] Ford J. Computers and Nursing: Possibilities for Transforming Nursing. *Comput in Nurs*, 1990, 8(4): 160-164.

[9] McLaughlin K, Taylor S, Bliss-Holty J & Sayers P. Shaping the Future: The Marriage of Nursing Theory and Informatics. *Comput in Nurs*, 1990, 8(4): 174-178.

[10] Happ B. Should Computers be Used in the Nursing Care of Patients? *Nurs Manage*, 1983, 14(7): 31-35.

[11] Krampf S & Robinson S. Managing Nurses' Attitudes Toward Computers. *Nurs Manage*, 1984, 215(7): 29-34.

[12] Stronge J & Brodt A. Assessment of Nurses' Attitudes Toward Computerization. *Comput in Nurs*, 1985, 3(4): 154-158.

[13] Jacobson S, Holder M & Dearner J. Computer Anxiety Among Nursing Students, Educators, Staff and Administrators. *Comput in Nurs*, 1989, 7(6): 266-272.

[14] Schwirian P, Malone J, Stone V, Nunley B & Francisco T. Computers in Nursing Practice: A Comparison of the Attitudes of Nurses and Nursing Students. *Comput in Nurs*, 1989, 7(4): 168-176.

[15] Burkes M. Identifying and Relating Nurses' Attitudes Toward Computer Use. *Comput in Nurs*, 1991, 9,(5): 190-201.

[16] Scarpa R, Smeltzer S & Jaisin B. Attitudes of Nurses Toward Computerization: A Replication. *Comput in Nurs*, 1992, 10(2): 72-79.

[17] Cocoran-Perry & Graves J. Supplemental-Information-Seeking Behavior of Cardiovascular Nurses. *Res in Nurs and Health*, 1990, 13: 119-127.

[18] Swenson-Feldman E & Brugge-Wiger P. Promotion of interdisciplinary practice through an automated information system. *Adv Nurs Sci*, 1985, 7(4): 39-47.

© 1994 Elsevier Science B.V. All rights reserved.
Nursing Informatics: An International Overview for Nursing in a Technological Era
S.J. Grobe and E.S.P. Pluyter-Wenting. eds.

Benefits Assessment

Roberts R[a] and Melvin B[b]

[a]Welsh Health Common Services Authority, Information Group, Crickhowell House, Pierhead St, Capital Waterside, Cardiff, CF1 5XT, Wales, United Kingdom

[b]Nursing Division, Welsh Office, Crown Building, Cathays Park, Cardiff, CF1 3NQ, Wales, United Kingdom

Nursing is one of the key strategic systems identified in the Information and Information Technology Strategy for Wales. Benefits of systems implementation are not automatic, the process of achieving a successful system implementation and realising benefits requires a structured and well planned approach. A practical guide to measure the attainment of benefits which result from implementation of nursing information systems has been developed by the Welsh Project Nurses Forum. A field trial tested its appropriateness. The material provided can be used as it stands or adapted to local requirements. The benefits assessment tools are being used by the first implementation site to quantify the benefits of the procured nursing information system. The NHS in Wales, as a learning organisation, is committed to disseminating information on the progress of the project and highlighting the achievements, benefits and potential problems for other sites considering purchase of the nursing information system.

1. Introduction

The Information and Information Technology Strategy for the National Health Service in Wales was introduced in advance of the National Health Service and Community Care Act 1990 which heralded a new approach to the commissioning and provision of health care throughout the U.K. The Information and Information Technology programme consists of 22 projects all of which are project managed and are at various stages of development. Some are concerned with systems procurement; others look at system requirements; a number aim to improve National Health Service information and its use; and supporting projects address organisational development and training, data quality and standards, and telecommunications. All are geared to the effective use of resources and improvements in services to patients. Nursing is one of the key strategic systems identified in the Strategy.

The Nursing Project has been organised in three stages and has concentrated as much on awareness training, dissemination of good practice, education and training in the use of information in managing the nursing resource as system development.

Stage 1 surveyed systems already in use and defined the education and training needs.

Stage 2 identified the upgrades necessary for systems already implemented, provided guidance on good practice and produced a Benefits Assessment Tool.

Stage 3 is the procurement and implementation of a Nursing Information System for eleven hospital sites.

2. Development of the Guide

The core specification for a Nursing Information System in Wales [1] includes the following functionality: Patient/Nursing Administration, Care Planning, Pre-Discharge Planning, Workload, Rostering, Costing, Quality Assurance and Decision Support.

The Nursing Information Systems Project Board recognised the need for a Benefits Assessment guide which would provide a set of studies that would be practical and inexpensive relative to the cost of the system being implemented. The types of benefits expected from implementation of a Nursing Information System are not all of the same nature and some will be easier to quantify than others. Benefits assessment studies should be integral to the whole process of system implementation. American studies have tended to examine the use of Hospital Information Systems rather than just the nursing elements of the system [2]. In the UK the Audit Commission's Report on Nursing Management and Information Systems [3] identified that none of the hospitals studied had conducted a full evaluation of the costs and benefits of continuing to operate a nursing management system. Some hospitals had made changes in nursing shift patterns following activity analysis undertaken during the implementation of workload assessment systems; but "broad evaluations of the effects on delivery of patient care appear to be rare" [4].

The basis for the "Benefits Assessment Studies - A Practical Guide" [5] was a study undertaken during 1990/1991, to measure changes in the working practices of staff which results from the introduction of the All Wales Clinical Nursing Information System [6]. The Guide has two sections:

Section 1. provides a discussion of the types of benefits that could be expected as a result of implementing a nursing information system; the ways in which benefits might be categorised and an approach to prioritising the benefits that will be most worthwhile and practical to assess.

Section 2. takes the reader through each of the phases:

Figure 1

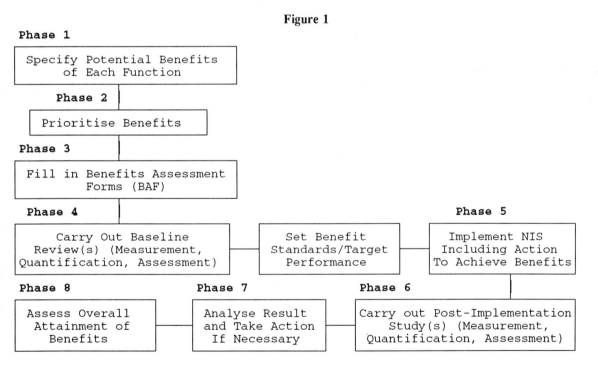

Benefits Assessment Studies (Phases 1-8)

It includes practical advice on how to carry out the study, examples of the types of documentation that will be necessary and sample Benefits Assessment Studies for workload, care planning and rostering functionality. The Guide stresses that hospitals should adjust the details to fit local circumstances.

A field trial was undertaken to ensure that the Guide was workable and easily understood by those not involved with its development. Amendments were then incorporated. The Guide is not viewed as a final product but the starting point for benefits assessment studies.

The Guide was launched at a seminar which highlighted the purpose and content of the Guide as well as providing an update on the Welsh Information Strategy and the Nursing Information Project. To inform other Nurses and Information Managers within the UK, publicity information appeared in several health service and nursing computer journals.

3. Benefits Realisation Study

Ceredigion and Mid Wales NHS Trust is the first site to implement the procured Nursing Information System (NIS). The Trust has established a NIS Project Board, Project Manager, Project Assurance Team plus Task Teams and is using PRINCE [7] as the project management methodology. A formal methodology is essential to ensure that clear lines of responsibility are established, the scope of the project is agreed and that project plans are prepared and agreed. The NHS has adopted PRINCE as the standard for managing IT projects.

One of the task teams is responsible for ensuring that the potential benefits of the NIS are identified, in particular those benefits which contribute towards tangible improvements in patient care, and to facilitate the way in which those benefits can be realised, in partnership with nurses, other directorate staff and managers in the Trust. One key support tool in this process will be the use of the "Benefits Assessment Studies - A Practical Guide". The team has produced an outline plan defining timescales, resources, assumptions and constraints plus main responsibilities. The timetable of this plan has been influenced by the timetable of the stages of implementation of the system. As the project progresses the actual resources and time are recorded. The team is being led by the Project Manager with the support of the All Wales Project Manager for Benefits Realisation. The team is accountable, through the Project Manager, to the Project Board and is responsible for providing up to date reports to the Project Board.

In realising benefits some effort, such as staff training or changes in working practices and organisation, will be required often necessitating management action. The team will clarify the policy, with the Project Board, on the management of the realised benefits. The Benefits Analysis and Realisation Team has also identified the need to note and follow up those areas of perceived disadvantage from implementation of the NIS.

A balance needs to be maintained when identifying which benefits will be monitored in detail, otherwise the level of effort and money invested in the process will outweigh the benefit likely to be realised. "Benefits realisation planning encourages commitment to an information systems investment by focusing the efforts of staff on areas which bring tangible and desirable benefits. Furthermore, it ensures expectations remain realistic, avoiding future disappointment or unmet demands by budget holders." [8]

Care planning will be the first functionality of the NIS to be implemented. Potential benefits for this functionality are listed in the Benefits Assessment Guide, one is that care plans will be more accurate, complete and consistent. The Director of Nursing Services for the Trust had previously identified this as an area for improvement and some work has been undertaken to improve nurses record keeping. The Benefits Assessment Form (see figure 2) identifies that the Standard or Target Performance is x% of care plans will be accurate, complete and consistent. It is unrealistic to expect this to be 100% so the Senior Nurse for each unit in the hospital has to determine the realistic percentage. Even though the hardware and software have not yet been installed at the hospital, the baseline review for this benefit is being carried out using Evaluation of Care Planning documentation and a staff questionnaire from the Benefits Assessment Studies. The staff questionnaire includes staff perceptions as to the usefulness of computerised care planning. These tools will be used again for the Post Implementation study at 6 months and 12 months.

Figure 2

Function: Care Planning		Ward:	
Key Benefit: Data more accurate/accessible		Code: C2	
	Date	Result	
Baseline Review			
Post-Implementation Study (1)			
Post-Implementation Study (2)			

Benefit:

Care Plans will be more accurate, complete and consistent.

Standard or Target Performance:

x% Care Plans will be accurate, complete and consistent.

Implementation:

Implementation of Care Planning function as agreed.

Benefits Assessment Tool:

Carry out Baseline Review immediately prior to implementing the care planning functionality and the Post-Implementation Study 6 and/or 12 months later.

Care Plan Audit using "Evaluation of Care Planning Documentation (Benefits Assessment Tool 5 - instructions on how to sample and sample size with BAT 5).

Staff Questionnaire (Benefits Assessment Tool 2) Questions 7 & 15 (Sample as C1).

Results Analysis and Action:

Assess against Target Performance Indicators agreed - see Standards above.

Compare accuracy before and after Implementation.

Take action as agreed eg. undertake further staff training.

BENEFITS ASSESSMENT FORM

Cost benefits analysis is briefly discussed in an appendix of the Benefits Assessment Studies. The All Wales NIS Project Board will be expecting a five year life cycle cost as part of the evaluation of implementation. This analysis will need to provide the initial capital cost, implementation costs and on going running costs, off set against the organisational benefits. "Investment Appraisal and Benefits Realisation for IM&T"[9] provides more specific information about costs identification and quantification and will be used to ensure that all cost issues are covered and information collected.

The costs of undertaking benefits realisation will need to be included in the cost analysis. The benefits realisation plan will be used to record actual resources (time and money) against planned resources. The All Wales Project Manager for Benefits Realisation is currently looking at software packages to find ways of reducing the work of documentation of the benefits realisation process, produce the calculations required and to see if there is a way of facilitating staff in Trusts to brainstorm the benefits expected from implementation of systems.

Cost benefits analysis is briefly discussed in an appendix of the Benefits Assessment Studies. The All Wales NIS Project Board will be expecting a five year life cycle cost as part of the evaluation of implementation. This analysis will need to provide the initial capital cost, implementation costs and on going running costs, off set against the organisational benefits. "Investment Appraisal and Benefits Realisation for IM&T"[9] provides more specific information about costs identification and quantification and will be used to ensure that all cost issues are covered and information collected.

The costs of undertaking benefits realisation will need to be included in the cost analysis, the benefits realisation plan will be used to record actual resources (time and money) against planned resources. The All Wales Project Manager for Benefits Realisation is currently looking at software packages to find ways of reducing the work of documentation of the benefits realisation process, produce the calculations required and to see if there is a way of facilitating staff in Trusts to brainstorm the benefits expected from implementation of systems.

The need for achieving value for money in the NHS is becoming paramount as the pressure on limited healthcare resources increases, there is a need to ensure that the investment placed in NIS results in demonstrable benefits to patient care and the organisation. The NHS in Wales, as a learning organisation, is committed to disseminating information on the progress of the project and highlighting the achievements, benefits and any potential problems for other sites considering the purchase of the nursing information system.

4. References

[1] *Resource Management Core Specification Nursing.* Welsh Health Common Services Authority. Cardiff: 1990.

[2] Kjerulff K H. The Integration of Hospital Information Systems into Nursing Practice: A Literature Review. In: *Nursing Informatics Where Caring and Technology Meet.* Ball MJ, Hannah KJ, Jelger UG, Peterson H (eds). New York: Springer-Verlag, 1988: 243-249.

[3] Audit Commission. *Caring Systems: A Handbook for Managers of Nursing and Project Managers.* London: HMSO, 1992: 56.

[4] Peel V. Money is the Root of All Systems. *Health Services Journal*, 31 October 1991, Volume 101: No 5276: 19.

[5] Information and Information Technology Project Nurses Forum. *Benefits Assessment Studies - A Practical Guide.* Welsh Health Common Services Authority. Cardiff: 1992.

[6] Lewis B, Carver N and Roberts R. Getting into the System. *Nursing Times,* August 5, 1992, Volume 88: No 32: 62-64.

[7] The National Computing Centre Ltd. *PRINCE: structured project support.* NCC Blackwell, Oxford: 1990

[8] Information Management Group, NHS Management Executive *Investment Appraisal and Benefits Realisation for IM&T Volume II: The Approach* Department of Health, Leeds: April 1993: 82

[9] Information Management Group, NHS Management Executive *Investment Appraisal and Benefits Realisation for IM&T Volume II: The Approach* Department of Health, Leeds: April 1993: 54-66

ADMINISTRATION

D. Nursing minimum dataset

Nursing Informatics: An International Overview for Nursing in a Technological Era
S.J. Grobe and E.S.P. Pluyter-Wenting, eds.

Using NMDS-Information for the Allocation of Budgets to Nursing Units

Vandewal D [a] and Vanden Boer G [b]

[a] *Nursing Logistics Officer, University Hospitals of Leuven, Belgium.*

[b] *Research assistant, Centre of Health Services Research & Nursing, Catholic University of Leuven , Belgium.*

The demand for better Health Care increases. Consequently, new technologies and treatments are being introduced, mostly bringing along increased costs. The patient emancipates and the contribution to the system also increases. For this reason he rightly demands the best possible treatment and care. The days of plenty, however, seem to be over and finally there is a general acknowledgement that resources are finite and have to be used and allocated carefully. Within the Nursing Department of the University Hospitals of Leuven (4 acute care hospitals - 2055 beds -130 nursing units) a project was started in 1986, to develop instruments that would make possible a justified allocation of manpower and resources. We report upon instruments as the Cost Control- report, Fingerprints, NMDS-profiles and a Weighted Patient Day.

1. What preceded

In 1986 a multidisciplinary committee was set up with the principal aim to study the cost of the utilisation of material resources and to make propositions for a more efficient use of them. From the past 8 years we can report that
- as for the *material resources*, we focused on distribution systems, stock management with bar-coding [1] and standardisation.
- as for the *personnel*, the San Joaquin classification system had already been introduced in 1978.
Time sampling studies enabled us to make better use of manpower. A huge step forward was made with the study and introduction of the Nursing Minimum Data Set (NMDS) as a tool for measuring nursing activities on nursing units. The combination of a patient classification system and the registration of a NMDS 4 times a fortnight a year open new horizons for a more efficient use of human resources [2].
- Fairly soon, we were in need of an instrument that would regularly gather some essential management data. The *Cost Control-report for nursing units (CC- report)* was published for the first time in 1987. It presented the actual situation of the use of material resources and the input of manpower in relation to a patient day. It also gave us the possibility to bring together all data of all nursing units in one report. From that moment on, the study could start with the following goals :

finding   - a basis to compare nursing units with one another,
               - a method to detect over- or underconsumption of resources,
               - a way to budget resources for direct patient care, taking into account the evolution of patient acuity on the specific nursing unit.

2. Looking for a basis to compare nursing units

Despite of the fact that the Cost Control-Report primarily focuses on the use of material resources and manpower, there is still a need for a sound basis to compare the use of resources on nursing units.
We strongly believe the Nursing Minimum Data Set bears this information.
What does a Nursing Minimum Data Set (NMDS) in Belgium mean ?
In September 1985, a research project was started at the Catholic University of Leuven, to develop one national nursing care registration instrument. For two months, data were collected in 13 Flemish hospitals, 92 nursing units and about 12000 patients [3].
At the same time, a similar research project was conducted in the French speaking part of Belgium by a research team of the Faculté Notre Dame de Paix, Namur. Both studies converged in one national nursing care registration instrument consisting of a list of 23 minimal nursing activities (Figure 1) which were approved by the General Association of Belgian Nurses.

1. Hygiene care
2. Mobility care
3. Elimination care
4. Feeding care
5. Gavage feeding
6. Complete care on mouth, nose, eyes
7. Decubitus preventive care
8. Assisting in getting dressed
9. Attending on tracheostomy or ventilation
10. Interviewing patient or relatives
11. Teaching indiv. patients or relatives
12. Supporting patient / highly emotionally disturbed
13. Supervision to mentally disturbed patient
14. Isolation
15. Monitoring of vital signs
16. Monitoring of clinical signs
17. Attending on continuos traction or cast
18. Drawing of blood specimen
19. Medication I.M., S.C.
20. Medication I.V.
21. I.V. therapy
22. Surgical wound care
23a. Surface of the traumatic wound
23b. Traumatic wound care

Figure 1 List of 23 minimal nursing activities.

This NMDS has to be collected in every Belgian hospital 4 times a year during a 15-day sampling period pointed out by the Minister of Public Health. These NMDS have to be collected daily for every patient hospitalised during this 15-day period.

Vandewal a.o. 1991 [4] demonstrate that a correlation exists on the nursing unit level, between a selected set of MNDS-items and their specific material consumption. In a first study a set of nursing activities and sterile materials that were indicative for the overall sterile material consumption, were selected. A correlation study between these costs and the specific NMDS-items allowed us to discover a mutual coherence. The use of bandages, syringes, needles, infusion material, aspiration material and patient care materials is strongly linked to the NMDS-items hygiene, elimination, tube-nutrition, medication, IV-infusion, attending on tracheostomy and wound care. In function of sterile material consumption only, the nursing units are compared on the basis of 7 NMDS-items, namely Medication I.M., Surgical Wound Care, Blood Drawing, Attending on Tracheostomy, Permanent Infusion, Gavage Feed and Medication IV.

This instrument is further refined in a second study. A new analysis, restricted to 23 surgical nursing units (644 beds), was made of annual returns between 1990 and 1992.

The Pearson Correlation Coefficients[(*)](Figure 2 and 3) clearly indicated a correlation between the following NMDS-items and their specific material consumption:

NMDS-item	Material	Coef.	Cost Category
-Medication IV	Material IV-medication	$(0,82)^{(*)}$	Steril Material
-Medication IV	Syringes/Needles	$(0,82)^{(*)}$	Steril Material
-IV Therapy	Material IV Therapy	$(0,71)^{(*)}$	Steril Material
-Surg.Wound	Surg.Wound Sets	$(0,78)^{(*)}$	Steril Material
-Ment.Disturbance	Linen	$(0,60)^{(*)}$	Linen
-Isolation	Pat.Care Material	$(0,68)^{(*)}$	Non Steril Material
-Dressing	Non-woven dispos.	$(0,61)^{(*)}$	Non Steril Material

Figure 2

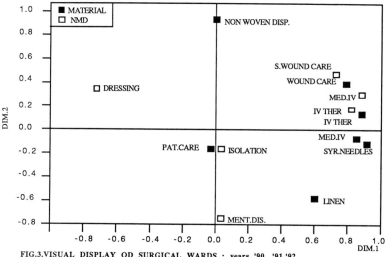

FIG.3.VISUAL DISPLAY OD SURGICAL WARDS : years '90, '91,'92
COST INDICATORS + SELECTED NURSING ACTIVITIES

The selection of these items (IV-material, syringes and needles and wound care materials) represents between 67 and 73% of the total sterile material consumption of a nursing unit, and 47 to 71% of the non-sterile materials.
These data reflect a correlation, but they do not say anything about the quantity or quality of the consumed materials with regard to the provided nursing care.

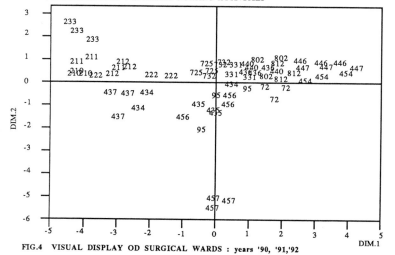

FIG.4 VISUAL DISPLAY OD SURGICAL WARDS : years '90, '91,'92

Mapping the correlation's by means of a multidimensional scaling technique (Figure 4) gives a better display of the relations between the different nursing units.

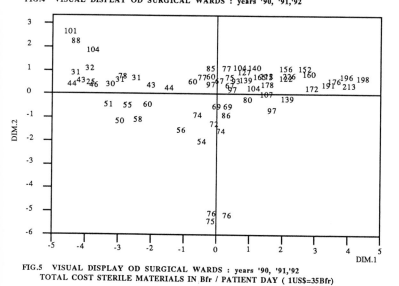

FIG.5 VISUAL DISPLAY OD SURGICAL WARDS : years '90, '91,'92
TOTAL COST STERILE MATERIALS IN Bfr / PATIENT DAY (1US$=35Bfr)

If we project the prime cost of consumed sterile materials on these units we can detect a number of prime cost quadrants (Figure 5). These quadrants give us an idea of the quantity of their use.
To find out more about the quality of the use of their resources, we relate them to the corresponding NMDS-items.

132

2.1. The search for a method to detect over- or underconsumption:

Here we made use of "Fingerprints"(Figure 6). The study is limited to the same 23 nursing units over a period from 1989 until 1992. All data are processed in SAS®, and *"interactively"* put on the screen by means of Excel 4.0®. The average of each consumption figure per sort of cost is separately calculated. The positive or negative deviations for each nursing unit are represented on the fingerprint.

This means that a specific nursing unit can score significantly higher or lower than the average of all nursing units taken together (i.e. the group of reference / peers)[5]. A similar reasoning is used for the NMDS-items, on the understanding that the averages are replaced by the average riditscores.

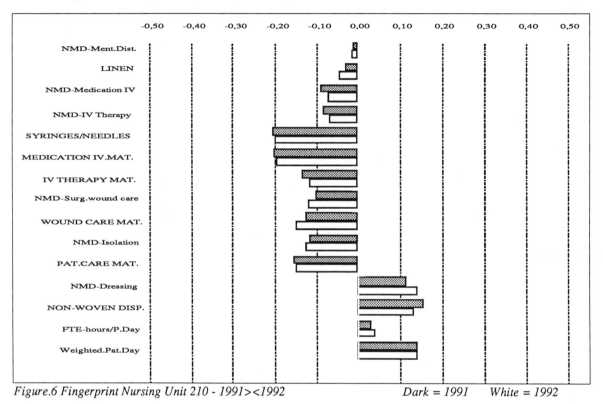

Figure.6 Fingerprint Nursing Unit 210 - 1991><1992   *Dark = 1991   White = 1992*

A fingerprint is a vertical "Bar-chart", showing a specific NMDS-score or use of materials in relation to a point of reference.(the point "0"). The point of reference in this study is each time the average of the 23 surgical units over a period of 3 years.

A fingerprint enables us to compare the consumption behaviour of a specific unit with its NMDS-profile. The reference point is the average of all nursing units. Alternative comparisons for a nursing unit are its own evolution in time and/or the comparison to any other nursing ward in the study group over any period of time.

We answered the quality question in so far that we are able to determine the under or overconsumption with regard to the related NMDS. The head nurse of the nursing unit concerned will be consulted for further information. Meanwhile, in order to build up a frame of reference, standard protocols are being developed per medical discipline. The protocols are qualitatively checked and the prices per protocol mapped in co-operation with the department of Hospital Infection Control.

2.2. The search for a way to budget resources in function of direct patient care:

After what precedes the question remains how to allocate the budget, taking into account the evolution of the NMDS-profile of the nursing unit. In order to represent the evolution of the NMDS-profile, the location of the nursing units on the first dimension of the Belgian NMDS-map is used as an indicator in the CC-report. The overall patient acuity is represented as a figure between 0 and 1000. This figure is a global measure that principally shows the continuum "nursing intensity" and is based on the 23 NMDS-items. This means more specifically that "the more intensive the care a patient receives is (e.g. IV-medication, infusion, monitoring, ...), the closer to 1000 the figure will be; or the more a patient is able to take care of him- or herself or is stimulated to do so, the closer it will be to 0 ". The average figure in our study was 156,8.

		Reference Per.(R.F.)	Actual Per.(A.P.)	DEV.1	
PROFITS	PATIENT DAYS (PD)	7177	7453	3,85	
	BED OCCUPANCY	73,7	75,5	2,4	
	AVERAGE STAY.	8,5	9,0	5,8	DEV.2
	NMDS-PROFILE	165,6	172,8	4,3	8,36
	FTE hours/PATIENT DAY	3,7	3,5	-3,95	-4,1
	Salary	3128,0	3009,0	900	
COSTS	STER.MAT./PATIENT DAY	297,5	318,5	7,1	6,5
	N.STER.MAT/PATIENT DAY	63,8	68,7	7,8	7,1
	LINEN/PATIENT DAY	128,0	129,9	1,5	1,3
	TOTAL / PATIENT DAY	3626,8	3543,3	-2,3	-2,5

Figure 7   DEV.1 = Deviation per Patient Day   DEV.2 = Deviation per Weighted Patient Day

With regard to the budgeting of a nursing unit, a *"weighted patient day"* is estimated, based on the patient acuity figures represented in the NMDS-profile. Due to this, the evolution of the use of recourses is not only corrected regarding the number of patient days, but also with regard to a change in the NMDS-profile.
On the one hand, the increase or decrease is represented with regard to the number of actual patient days (mass). This is done for the resource consumption figures, as well as for the NMDS-profile. (Dev. 1)
This increase or decrease of the costs per patient day is, on the other hand, further adjusted using the evolution of the NMDS-profile. We obtain this evolution by measuring the relation between two "weighted" periods. It gives us insight in the actual evolution of the nursing workload. (Dev. 2).We call the difference in weight between two periods in relation to their NMDS-profile " *the weighted patient day* ". To this end we multiply the number of patient days (PD) with the measured NMDS-profile. The calculation is done as follows (see also Figure 7):
Weighted Patient Day Deviation in % =
(((PD A.P. x NMDS-Profile A.P.) / (PD R.P. x NMDS-Profile R.P.)-1)x100)

Nursing units whose weighted patient day increases, have to obtain more resources, nursing units whose weighted patient day decreases however, have to give in. These data are currently being processed in the Cost-Control-report and are presented to the heads of our nursing departments, who must evaluate them.
Finally it is our intention to further develop a costs matrix on which we will calculate the expenditure (manpower, sterile and non-sterile materials and linen) per weighted patient day for each medical discipline. This would enable us to account the expenditures, and later on we might be able to draw up a budget that could be continually evaluated and refined, using these data. Refining this instrument will be our basic concern for the following years and should lead to a justified allocation of budgets in order to make qualitatively high-ranking patient care possible.

3. References

[1] Vandewal D. Nursing Portable Unit and barcodes : a useful technology on a nursing ward?
Nursing and Computers ,Proceedings Dublin, Mosby, St.Louis USA, 1988, pp.498-505.

[2] Vanden Boer G and Sermeus W. Operational linkage of NMDS and Patient Classification Systems. Paper to be presented during "Nursing Informatics '94", San Antonio, USA, June 1994.

[3] Sermeus W and Delesie L. Registration of the NMDS in Belgium: 8 years experience. Paper to be presented during "Nursing Informatics '94", San Antonio, USA, June 1994.

[4] Vandewal D,Vanden boer G, Dombrecht P and Sermeus W. Material utilisation efficiency in patient care: a case study. *"Nursing Informatics '91"* , Melbourne, Australia, Springer-Verlag pp.272-278

[5] Fleiss J.L : *Statistical Methods for Rates and Proportions*, J.Whiley & Sons, New-York, 1981, p.102-108.

Nursing Informatics: An International Overview for Nursing in a Technological Era
S.J. Grobe and E.S.P. Pluyter-Wenting, eds.

Spinal Cord Injury Nursing: Database Analysis
A Pilot Study

Kraft M R[a] and Lang B J[b]

[a]Associate Chief, Nursing Service, VA Edward Hines Jr Hospital, Hines, Il., 60141

[b]Project Manager, Information Systems Center, Department of Veterans Affairs, Hines, Il., 60141

The contributions of nursing to cost-effective spinal cord injury (SCI) care and positive patient outcomes must be demonstrated with objective data. The computerization of nursing data permits documentation, retrieval and analysis of nursing practice information that can be used to describe and evaluate nursing care, to investigate the quality and outcomes of care, to support resource allocation, and to stimulate nursing practice research. Participation of a VA SCI Nursing Service as an ALPHA site in the development of the VA Decentralized Hospital Computer Program (DHCP) Nursing Package resulted in a SCI nursing data base that offered the opportunity to study actual practice within a SCI population. Since the VA computerized information system includes all elements of the Nursing Minimum Data Set (NMDS) proposed by Werley and others (1990), the utility of the NMDS is tested as a framework for data collection. Existing SCI care phenomena gathered from a real life/real time perspective defines demographic characteristics of the SCI population, nursing diagnosis identified and nursing care provided.   Further statistical analysis explores possible relationships between nursing diagnoses, interventions, patient acuity, length of stay and patient outcomes. It is expected that exploration of this descriptive data will improve current care delivery, support resource management decisions, and encourage standards and guideline development.

1. Introduction

The advancement of Spinal Cord Injury Nursing as a research-based specialty area of the discipline of Nursing presents an exciting challenge. In this era of diminished resources, the profession must produce objective data that demonstrates nursing's contribution to patient outcomes and cost-effective care delivery. Subjective and anecdotal information cannot continue to be used as a basis for practice or resource allocation.

Research is needed to identify what is cost-effective care as well as to obtain objective facts to support and refute cost-containment measures. Generation and exploration of descriptive data can improve current care delivery; direct resource management, policy and standards development; guide the definition of the content and process dimensions of nursing practice; and promote further research in nursing practice. Research related to SCI nursing diagnoses and SCI nursing interventions can demonstrate under which particular circumstances specific interventions promote the most effective outcomes for SCI patients.

The initial purpose of this study is to test a methodology useful for analysis and descriptions of SCI nursing from the practice perspective of an existing database. Sixty-five episodes of care representing 10% of the database in November, 1992, are used to determine the ability to retrieve and manipulate data, and create files for purposes of analysis. The ultimate goal of the project is a full database analysis to describe SCI nursing practice at this site. Knowledge obtained from descriptive studies of SCI nursing may generate perspective knowledge.

Data Collection and documentation are costly aspects of nursing care. A retrospective application study of the NMDS done by Grier, Grier, Grainer and Stanhope (1991) indicates that the NMDS could be useful in decreasing the collection of redundant and non-essential data. In addition, reduced data collection could lead to greater consistency in data collected. The value of standardized data cannot be over-estimated and the use of the NMDS can lead to cost-effective improvements in the documentation of nursing care. The inclusion of the NMDS elements in the DHCP software provides an opportunity to use the NMDS as a framework for data review. The SCI nursing data base in this study exists in the DHCP system.

2. DHCP

The Department of Veterans Affairs(VA) development of a Decentralized Hospital Computer Program (DHCP) includes a nursing package within its enhanced core system. The VA nursing package is complementary and supplementary to other on-line packages and interfaces with the entire integrated hospital information system.

DHCP at the study site runs on a Digital Equipment Corporation VAC computer system. Software for DHCP is written in MUMPS (Massachusetts General Utility Multi-Programming System) which is an ANSI (American National Standards Institute) programming language now referred to as "M". The nursing software includes patient acuity data and care plan data. Since the inception of this study, functionality of the DHCP nursing software has been increased to allow frequency ranking of nursing diagnoses; nursing diagnoses with frequency ranking of associated interventions, and frequency ranking of nursing interventions. This functionality is used in the study.

3. Nursing Diagnosis and Intervention

The VA nursing care plan package and the NMDS both utilize North American Nursing Diagnosis Association (NANDA) diagnostic language which facilitates analysis of care plans. Nursing is defined as "the diagnosis and treatment of human responses to actual or potential health problems" (ANA, 1980). Creeson (1988) indicates that agreement must be reached on what it means to diagnose and treat human responses if this definition of nursing is to have meaning. NANDA formulated an official definition of nursing diagnosis at the 1990 General Assembly:

> "A nursing diagnosis is a clinical judgment about an individual, family, or community response to actual or potential health problems/life processes which provides the basis for definitive therapy toward achievement of outcomes for which the nurse is accountable." (Carroll-Johnson, 1991, p65)

Nursing diagnosis is the responsibility of the professional nurse and requires objectivity, critical thinking, and decision-making which in turn requires deliberation, judgment, and choice. Nursing diagnosis is both a process and an outcome. The diagnostic process involves collection of data by observation and assessment as well as interpretation of data based on the nurse's experience and knowledge base which culminates in a diagnostic statement. The focus of the nursing process elements has now expanded to include interventions and outcomes as well as diagnoses.

"Nursing intervention" is defined by Bulechek and McCloskey (1985) as " an autonomous action based on scientific rationale that is executed to benefit the client in a predicted way related to nursing diagnosis and stated goals" (p8). Nursing intervention was further defined as:

"...any direct care treatment that a nurse performs on behalf of a patient. These treatments include nurse-initiated treatments resulting from medical diagnoses, and performance of the daily essential functions for the client who cannot do ..." (Bulechek and McCloskey, 1989)

4. Methodology of Analysis

The SCI computerized data base at the study site accumulated 650 nursing care plans from July, 1989 to November, 1992. For purposes of the pilot study the first 60 care plans were dropped to eliminate early learning problems. The 65 episodes of care included in the study were chosen randomly using the SYSTAT random table of numbers. Sixty-five records in the pilot represented 10% of the entire database. A prevalence study conducted the study site on October 1, 1992, resulted in a list of 54 diagnoses and 624 associated interventions in a population of 51 in-patients. Frequency ranking of the nursing diagnoses in the entire data base revealed 90 nursing diagnoses. The rank and frequency of the top ten diagnoses are listed:

4.1 Table 1

SCI Nursing Diagnoses N= 650 episodes of care	
Rank	Frequency
1. Skin integrity, Impairment (actual)	205
2. Self-Care Deficit (Specify)	178
3. Skin Integrity, Impairment (potential)	110
4. Mobility, Impaired Physical	100
5. Urinary Elimination, Alteration in	85
6. Infection Potential (Specific to Elimination)	68
7. Health Maintenance, Alteration in	65
8. Infection Potential (Specific to Integument)	64
9. Skin Ulcer	58
10. Incontinence, Urine	57

Data abstracted from DHCP according the elements of the NMDS has been moved via Pro-Comm, a transportation software, to Word Perfect 5.1 files for purposes of graph production and to SYSTAT files for purposes of statistical analysis. This has proved to be a laborious process. Data analysis currently in process is seeking evidence of relationships between age, length of stay, specific nursing and medical diagnoses, numbers of diagnoses, and patient acuity as determined in the on-line VA SCI classification system. Daily classification is required and inter-rater reliability of the classification system is maintained at least 95%.

Interventions most frequently chosen for a specific diagnosis are being analyzed and since a chosen intervention may relate to several diagnoses, attention is being given to determination of the "usual" patterns of nursing care. This data is being reduced to conceptual clusters that could have potential significance for standards of nursing care. For instance, as a result of identification of alteration in skin integrity as the highest ranked diagnosis, interventions were reviewed and an assessment standard related to skin was built into the SCI assessment tool, and a care map was developed for the stages of pressure ulcers. This care map has become the standard of care and is also used as a documentation tool.

Analysis of nursing interventions will seek to determine those unique to the practice domain of SCI nursing. Nursing interventions in the study episodes of care will be classified with taxonomy suggested by Bulechek and McCloskey. (1989, ob cit) Documented description of nursing activities will be systematically organized in the language of practicing nurses.

5. Nurses as Diagnosticians

Since the study database represents actual practice, not value judgments have been made about whether diagnoses are accurate and interventions are appropriate. They are simply being described. A survey of nursing staff involved in the development of the database was done to determine SCI nursing experience as well as familiarity and comfort with the concept of nursing diagnosis. A semantic differential instrument "positions on Nursing Diagnosis" developed by Lunney and Krenz (1992) was administered to staff. This is a bipolar tool that scores 20 items from a negative score (40) to a positive score (120). As a group nurses in the study scored between 80-120. Fifty-two percent of the group reported either formal coursework or continuing education in Nursing Diagnosis. The self-reported comfort level with the use of Nursing Diagnosis on a scale of low/average/high was low 18%, average 56% and high 28%. This same group reported a comfort level with SCI nursing as average 44% and high 54%.

6. Summary

Few studies have been published on nursing diagnoses in general or specialty practice areas. None of the studies published address SCI nursing or a computerized data base. Rehabilitation Nursing (Swain and Heard, 1992) reported on a study of 346 nurses who responded to a list of nursing diagnoses to indicate those most commonly used in their practice. Twelve of the top 20 diagnoses in the rehabilitation data are in the top 25 diagnoses of this SCI study. Hardy, Maas, and Akins (1988) published on the prevalence of nursing diagnoses in long term care (LTC). Their study showed some closely related frequency rankings.

6.1 Table 2

Nursing Diagnosis	SCI	LTC	REHAB
Skin Integrity, Impairment	1	7	5
Self-Care Deficit	2	1	2
Mobility, Impaired Physical	4	2	1
Health Maintenance, Alteration in	7	8	

The opportunity to analyze current SCI nursing practice has presented a challenge in determining a methodology to retrieve and review data. The study described is a project in process and will be completed in March, 1994. Results of data analysis will be available at that time.

138

7. References

[1] Werley H. Devine E. and Zorn, *C. Nursing Minimum Data Set Collection Manual*. University of Wisconsin-Milwaukee, 1990.

[2] Grier M. Grier J. Greiner P and Stanhope M. Savings from use of the nursing minimum data set in Hovega E., Hannah K. McCormack K and Ronald J (Eds) *Proceedings of the Fourth International Conference on Nursing Use of Computers and Information Science*. Berlin: Springer-Verlag, 105-109, 1991.

[3] American Nurses Association. *Social Policy Statement*, 1980.

[4] Creeson N. Need for precision in the definition of elements for the nursing minimum data set in Werley H and Lang,N (Eds) *Identification of the Nursing Minimum Data Set*. New York: Spring Publishing Company, 289- 299, 1988.

[5] Carroll-Johnson R. (Ed) *Classification of Nursing Diagnoses, Proceedings of the Ninth Conference*. Philadelphia, Lippincott, 65, 1991.

[6] Bulechek G and McCloskey J. *Nursing Interventions: Treatments for Nursing Diagnosis*. Philadelphia: W B Saunders, 1985.

[7] Bulechek G and McCloskey J. Nursing intervention taxonomy development in McCloskey J and Grace H (Eds) *Current Issues in Nursing*. 3rd edition, St. Louis: Mosby, 23-28, 1985.

[8] Lunney M and Krenz M. An instrument to measure attitude toward nursing diagnosis .Referenced in *Nursing Diagnosis* (letter) Jan-Mr 3(1):44,1992. .

[9] Sawin K and Heard L. Nursing diagnoses used most frequently in rehabilitation nursing practice. *Rehabilitation Nursing*, 17: 5: 256-267, 1992.

[10] Hardy M A. Maas M and Akins J. The prevalence of nursing diagnoses among elderly and long term care residents: a descriptive comparison. *Recent Advances in Nursing*, 21: 144-158, 1988.

Nursing Informatics: An International Overview for Nursing in a Technological Era
S.J. Grobe and E.S.P. Pluyter-Wenting, eds.

139

The Use of the Nursing Minimum Data Set in
Several Clinical Populations

Sheil E P[a] and Wierenga M E[b]

[a]Health Maintenance Department, School of Nursing, University of Wisconsin-Milwaukee, Box 413, Milwaukee, Wisconsin, 53201.

[b]Health Restoration Department, School of Nursing, University of Wisconsin-Milwaukee, Box 413, Milwaukee, Wisconsin, 53201.

The overall purpose of this descriptive study was to demonstrate the effectiveness of the Nursing Minimum Data Set (NMDS) in two clinical populations. Populations under investigation included hospitalized patients with DRGs related to diabetes as primary or secondary diagnosis and women with normal vaginal delivery.

Description of the frequencies of, and relationships among, nursing diagnoses, nursing interventions, and nursing outcomes were explored as little information exists about the nursing diagnoses used for patients with specific DRGs. Even less data are available concerning nursing interventions used for specific nursing diagnoses.

The research questions were: (a) what nursing diagnoses were made for patients with the selected DRGs? (b) what nursing interventions were used with these diagnoses? (c) what were the outcomes of the identified nursing interventions?

Data are in electronic form obtained from a large medical complex. Descriptive and inferential statistics are used to investigate the research questions. Differences among age groups, racial/ethnic groups, residence, and type of insurance were investigated. Analysis of these data will provide information regarding the useability of the NMDS for standardizing essential nursing data. Results from this study will provide information on the effectiveness of the specified nursing interventions with the nursing diagnoses. The relationship between DRGs and nursing diagnoses for this sample can be assessed. Patient outcomes of nursing interventions are examined.

1. Study Purpose

The overall purpose of this project was to determine the effectiveness of the Nursing Minimum Data Set (NMDS) to establish comparability across clinical populations. The specific purpose of this study was to describe the nursing diagnoses, nursing interventions, and outcomes of nursing care for three Diagnostic Related Groups (DRGs); diabetes as primary diagnosis, diabetes as secondary diagnosis and normal delivery of mother. The effort to develop international [1] as well as national standards and guidelines would be enhanced by a minimum set of data which met the needs of multiple users [2]. Currently, the data set most used in the United States is the Uniform Hospital Data Set (UHDDS). However, the UHDDS does not include data regarding nursing care and outcomes, a costly component of health care. The NMDS represents the first attempt to quantify essential nursing data; information which is used on a regular basis by the majority of nurses across settings [3]. Simpson [4] supports the use of the NMDS and recommends that demonstration projects be undertaken to validate it.

Before data can be compared across sites, data from at least one system needs to be analyzed, it is important to learn the most efficient and cost effective means of accessing it, and to identify problems related to access and interpretation of the data. In this study, two broad populations were selected to begin the testing of the NMDS in one hospital. Exploration of the frequencies of, and relationships among, nursing diagnoses, nursing intervention, nursing outcomes, and intensity of nursing care for hospitalized persons is necessary because little information exists about this. Therefore, using the NMDS as it exists in one agency, the research questions are (a) what are the nursing diagnoses used for patients with these DRGs, (b) what are the nursing interventions used with these diagnoses, and (c) what are the outcomes of these nursing actions.

2. Method

The research design was secondary analysis of existing computerized service data. Adherence to agency guidelines for access to records of discharged patients and use of code numbers insured confidentiality. The project was approved by the IRBs of both the University and of the clinical agency.

The sample consisted of data for persons with nursing diagnoses who were patients during 1991 of a 350 bed county hospital and who had a medical diagnosis of diabetes, uncomplicated adult (DRG 250); diabetes, complicated adult (DRG 250.90); or normal vaginal delivery (DRG 650). All discharges from the hospital in 1991 made up the data set including multiple discharges for the same patient. Persons who utilize the hospital from which the sample was drawn are primarily from the urban community. A majority are economically disadvantaged, many are from ethnic groups other than Caucasian, and most have a low educational background. Specific information on the sociodemographic characteristics of the sample including gender, race, and age will be presented.

The NMDS was the measure used to gather data. A conference of experts in nursing, information systems, health policy, health care organizations, and health records developed the NMDS consensually during the three day conference in 1985 [5,6,7]. According to Werley and colleagues [3], the purposes of the NMDS are to: (a) establish comparability of nursing data across populations, settings, geographic areas, and time; (b) describe the nursing care of patients and their families; (c) demonstrate or project trends for nursing care and allocation of resources; and (d) stimulate nursing research through links to the data existing in health care information systems (HCISs). The four nursing care elements of the NMDS are nursing diagnosis, nursing diagnoses, nursing intervention, nursing outcome and intensity of nursing care. Patient or client demographic elements and service elements (except for the unique health record number of the patient or client and of the principal registered nurse provider) are already included in the UHDDS. The nursing diagnosis labels used in this data set were from the eighth national NANDA conference [8].

3. Process

Data were accessed through the previously identified DRG classifications. Multiple minor problems were experienced in transferring the data to our files, in assuring the very large amount of computer space for data management and manipulation, and subsequently in interpreting the data. Once data were received from hospital personnel, the time needed to organize and analyze the data set became a function of computer space at the University. Limitations were size of the data set and the need for very large amounts of computer space to organize, manipulate and sort the data. It was necessary to manipulate the data in segments as well as to take advantage of slower usage times on the mainframe, such as in the middle of the night.

Although the elements of the NMDS were already available within the hospital records, each episode of recording patient care appeared as a separate report in the file. In order to evaluate the presence of a nursing diagnosis for each admission, the records first needed to be aggregated by person. The number of times a nursing diagnosis was used could have been confounded by length of stay. Since we were interested in the presence or absence of a nursing diagnosis more time was needed to aggregate the records than was envisioned in the research plan. This work could not have been achieved without the dedication and skill of computer and statistic literate support persons. Nursing diagnosis, nursing interventions, and outcomes of nursing care will be presented.

4. Results

There were a total of 580 admissions for complicated and uncomplicated diabetes during the year studied, although only 9 patients were admitted with a primary diagnosis of diabetes. The uncomplicated diabetes admissions ($\underline{n}$ = 502) were composed of 282 (56%) females and 189 (38%) African American. The mean age of this group was 59.51 years (s.d. = 15.25), the mean length of stay was 7.99 days (s.d. = 11.61). The number of nursing diagnoses for persons with diabetes ranged from 1 to 9. Those with uncomplicated diabetes ($\underline{n}$ = 502) had slightly fewer nursing diagnoses (M = 1.88, s.d. = 1.05) than did the ($\underline{n}$ = 78) patients with complicated diabetes (M = 1.97, s.d. = 1.27). The ten most frequently occurring nursing diagnoses identified are listed in Table 1.

Table 1
Ten most frequent nursing diagnoses of persons with diabetes

Nursing Diagnosis	n	%
Pain	213	36
Potential Injury	180	31
Decreased Cardiac Output	124	21
Anxiety	73	13
Knowledge Deficit	47	8
Health Maintenance Alteration	43	7
Potential Infection	35	6
Impaired Mobility	34	6
Ineffective Breathing Pattern	34	6
Self-care Deficit	28	5

Data for 641 admissions of women who delivered babies without Cesarian section are reported. The nursing care plan for this group begins upon admission, follows the mother through labor and to the post partum unit. Ages ranged from 12 years to 43 years (M = 23.3 years; s.d. = 6.35), 621 women had single live births, 20 delivered twins. The minimum length of stay was less than one day, the maximum was 37 days (M = 3.15; s.d. = 2.5). African Americans accounted for 49% of the sample, Caucasians for 40%. The remaining 11% included American Indians, Hispanics, Asians and others. At this hospital, a separate nursing care plan for the baby was begun only in those instances where the neonate remained in the hospital following the mother's discharge. Therefore, no separate information is available related to nursing care of the normal neonate in this data set. For this population, 1022 nursing diagnosis labels were identified (mean = 1.59). The ten most frequently identified nursing diagnoses for mothers are found in Table 2.

Table 2
Ten most frequent nursing diagnoses of mothers

Nursing Diagnosis	n	%
Altered Parenting, Potential	226	35
Pain	174	27
Family Coping, Growth	153	24
Anxiety	114	18
Individual Coping, Ineffective	99	15
Breastfeeding	92	14
Fear	86	13
Communication, Impaired	17	3
Spiritual Distress	16	2
Self-care Deficit	5	1

Among the ten most frequently identified nursing diagnoses in both populations, there were two nursing diagnoses that were similar across aggregates. The number and percentage of the total number nursing diagnoses for the respective groups are compared in Table 3.

Table 3
Common nursing diagnoses across aggregates

Nursing Diagnosis	Diabetes		Mothers	
	n	%	n	%
Pain	213	36	174	27
Anxiety	73	13	114	18

To understand the relationship in this data set of nursing diagnosis category, defining characteristics, nursing interventions and outcomes, information related to the population of mothers follows. In the 641 mothers for the 1022 nursing diagnosis categories which were used 20 or more times, 5911 modifiers (or "related to" statements) were used. One intervention was identified for each of the 5911 nursing diagnosis with modifiers. Thus 5911 interventions were identified

In defining the NMDS elements, outcome was described as being measured by the resolution states of each nursing diagnosis as "resolved" or "not resolved" (Werley, Devine, & Zorn, 1990, p. 33). In this data set, in addition to this information, outcome was identified by a specific narrative statement including a action verb. In this data set, outcomes of the interventions were identified but were not linked to the individual interventions, therefore only 3826 specific outcomes were identified. These will not be discussed in this paper.

A comparison of interventions used in both populations for the nursing diagnosis "anxiety" and "pain" are presented in Table 4. Interventions that were noted 50 or more times in each population were categorized into groupings falling out of the data.

Table 4
Comparison of commonly used interventions for persons reported for both populations with nursing diagnoses of Anxiety and Pain

Intervention	Diabetes	Mothers	Diabetes	Mothers
	Anxiety		Pain	
Assess	109 (21%)	60 (10%)	344 (28%)	109 (12%)
Teach	141 (28%)	117 (19%)	260 (22%)	224 (25%)
Explain	47 (9%)	137 (22%)		
Encourage	102 (20%)	159 (25%)		
Comfort/Support			22 (2%)	363 (42%)
Give Medications			83 (7%)	106 (12%)
Others	114 (22%)	145 (24%)	493 (41%)	108 (9%)
Total	513 (100%)	615 (100%)	1202	910 (100%)

For the maternity population, 96% of the outcomes identified the nursing diagnosis, for Anxiety, were achieved; 93% of the outcomes identified for Pain were achieved. For the diabetic population, 68% of the outcomes for Anxiety were achieved; 82% of the outcomes for Pain.

5. Discussion

Following agreement to share the NMDS and approval of the research to protect human subjects, the process of actually obtaining the data and preparing it for analysis was more time and labor intensive than was originally visualized. Personnel at both the hospital and the university worked cooperatively over many months and continue to do so in order to achieve the purposes of this study. When planning similar studies, attention needs to be given to the cost of such support which may be greater than anticipated.

Similarities and differences in relation to nursing diagnosis exist between the two aggregates. Notably, nursing diagnoses of pain and anxiety are important to both groups. If commonly used interventions to treat nursing diagnoses can be identified with other nursing diagnoses and other populations as they have been in these five populations, we should have a much clearer picture of what actions nurses actually employ in caring for their patients. This has implications for nursing education and continuing nursing research. Future research will involve comparisons of the nursing interventions from this work with those of Bulechek & McCloskey [9].

Before data from the NMDS can be compared across sites, analysis of the remaining data from this one system needs to be completed. Some problems which were encountered included the need for more computer space and support than initially envisioned, the fact that this was the first time these data had been accessed for research purposes and the need to identify the most efficient ways of interpreting the large amount of information.

We also learned that it is important to involve clinical and administrative persons in the hospital on any research team involving the NMDS. They are essential sources of information to explain confusing or unexpected findings as well as for their specific expertise with the populations and nursing personnel at the agency.

6. References

[1] Clark J and Lang N. Nursing's Next Advance: An Internal Classification for Nursing Practice. *Int Nurs Rev* 1992, 39:109-111, 128.

[2] Health Information Policy Council: Background Paper: Uniform Minimum Health Data Sets (unpublished). Washington, D.C., U.S. Department of Health and Human Services, 1983:3.

[3] Werley H, Devine E and Zorn C. *Nursing Minimum Data Set Data Collection Manual.* Milwaukee, WI: University of Wisconsin-Milwaukee, School of Nursing, 1990.

[4] Simpson R. Adopting a Nursing Minimum Data Set. *Nurs Manage* 1991, 22:20-21.

[5] Werley H and Lang N. *Identification of the Nursing Minimum Data Set.* New York: Springer, 1988.

[6] Werley H, Lang N and Westlake S. Brief Summary of the Nursing Minimum Data Set Conference. *Nurs Manage* 1986, 17:42-45.

[7] Werley H, Lang N and Westlake S. The Nursing Minimum Data Set Conference: Executive Summary. *J Prof Nurs* 1986, 2:217-224.

[8] Carroll-Johnson M. *Classification of Nursing Diagnosis: Proceedings of the Eighth National Conference.* Philadelphia: J.B. Lippincott, 1989.

[9] Bulecheck GM and McCloskey JC. *Nursing Interventions: Essential Nursing Treatments, 2nd ed.* Philadelphia, PA: W.B. Saunders Co., 1992.

Nursing Informatics: An International Overview for Nursing in a Technological Era
S.J. Grobe and E.S.P. Pluyter-Wenting, eds.

144

The registration of a Nursing Minimum Data Set in Belgium: Six years of experience

Sermeus W[a] and Delesie L[a]

[a] *School of Public Health, Catholic University of Leuven, Kapucijnenvoer 35, 3000 Leuven, Belgium*

Since January 1st, 1988, all Belgian general hospitals are required by law to collect 4 times a year a Nursing Minimum Data Set. This article reports on how this Minimum Data Set is developed. This process consists in 3 steps: transformation of nursing practice to data which implies the construction of a uniform nursing language. The second step consists in the transformation of data to information. Most effort is put in this step. Eight conditions need to be fulfilled: sampling, multivariate approach, systematic, graphical presentation, feedback, unit of analysis, uniform frame of reference. The third step is the transformation of information to decision making. The use of this data set is shown by few examples.

1. Introduction

On April 18, 1986, Belgium got its new hospital law which gave the legal basis for the registration of patient data in the broadest sense. Since then, some royal decrees have been implemented the law. A Royal Decree of August 14, 1987 started to monitor as of January 1, 1988 a minimum number of variables, called the Nursing Minimum Data Set (NMDS).

The construction and implementation of such a Nursing Minimum Data Set nation-wide , goes slowly. In this process, each step is a challenge. The first step is the translation of nursing practice to nursing data. The second step is the translation of these nursing data into information. The third step is the use of this information for communication and decision making. The last step is the transformation of nursing practice based on decision making. The process will be illustrated by the use of the Nursing Minimum Data Set in Belgium which is collected in all general Belgian hospitals since 1988.

2. From nursing practice to nursing data

To transform nursing practice in nursing data, a 'uniform nursing language' is necessary. In a lot of countries, nurse researchers are developing nursing languages to describe patient problems from a nursing perspective. Examples are the Nursing Diagnosis list from the NANDA[1], the development of a nursing taxonomy in the Netherlands, in Scotland, in Denmark and in the UK. Similar research work is done in the field of nursing interventions. Examples are the research work of Bulechek & Mc Closkey[2], Grobe[3], Saba[4] in the USA, Ehnfors[5] in Sweden. The International Council of Nurses (ICN) is developing a overall framework for a international Classification of Nursing Practice. These languages are necessary to communicate among nurses all over the world.

Most countries put a lot of scientific effort in this first step. In Belgium this step was handled in a very pragmatic way. In 1985, the Belgian Nurses Association[6] developed a list of 111 nursing interventions. This list has been used as the nursing language to describe nursing practice in Belgium.

3. From nursing data to information

While most countries concentrate on the first step, in Belgium most effort has been put in this second step. Eight conditions have to be fulfilled to transform data into information.

The first condition is the use of samples instead of populations. The idea of sampling is integrated in the concept "Minimum" data set. Minimum means that not all aspects of nursing care have to be described but that a selection of the most relevant aspects has to be made. This has been done by the reduction of the whole list of 111 nursing interventions to a selected list of 23. These 23 nursing interventions are selected on statistical and professional grounds and contains 80% of the statistical information of the whole list of 111.
Secondly, samples have been introduced in delineating the registration frequency. The nursing minimum data set doesn't have to be collected each day but only 4 times a year during a 15 days sampling period. Out of this series of 15 days , 5 random days are selected and are sent the Ministry of Public Health.

A second condition is the multivariate approach. All attempts so simplify the complex process of patient care into an overall measure have failed. The length of stay, the medical diagnosis, the medical activities, the severity, the nursing interventions, the total cost of care, the intensity of the care, the drug consumption, the nursing workload, etc. all tell something on the patient and the care he receives. No one variable though is capable to give a full answer. How tempting this search for the holy grail may be to some, it is of no avail.
Some of these measures deal with the patient himself - his demand for care -, some measures deal with the care that the patient receives - the care provided: hence, the diversity of the patient population on the one hand and the variability in the practice patterns on the other hand. In Belgium, data about the diversity of the patient population (medical diagnosis, age, degree of dependency on daily activities) and the variability of the practice variations (23 nursing interventions, length of stay, number of nursing staff, level of qualification of the nursing staff) are registered.

A third condition is the systematic approach of the data collection. All the data are collected on a similar way in all Belgian general hospitals. Each year about 1,2 million data records are collected by the Ministry of Public Health.
The interrater-reliability of the Nursing Minimum Data Set was controlled in 70 Belgian Hospitals for 4000 records[7]. The global reliability of the data collection is 79%. The basic care and technical interventions are very reliably collected (more than 80%). Interventions such as emotional support, patient teaching are only weakly reliable. Their impact on the global reliability figure is however limited.

A fourth condition is the way these samples are taken: cross-sectional or longitudinal. Belgium has chosen for a cross-sectional approach. The argument is that nursing is not characterised by an individual interaction between an individual patient and an individual nurse but consists in many-to-many interactions[8]. The time that nurse X spend on patient Y, depends on the demands of the other patients assigned to nurse X and the presence and competence of the other nurses on a nursing unit. The care for an individual patient can only be discussed if you know something about the nursing care on all other patients.

A fifth condition is a micro/macro- design. It means that the data set must hold the necessary detail to describe a nursing speciality (oncology, intensive care, geriatric care) but is not too specific so that it also can be discussed on a more general level. A micro/macro design enforces both local and global comparison and at the same time, avoids the disruption of context switching[9].
This micro/macro design is built in the Belgian NMDS on a twofold way. Firstly, the number of combinations based on this 23 nursing interventions far exceeds 1.7 million billion of possible combinations. It means that 23 nursing interventions are enough sensitive to describe very specific care combinations. Secondly, in the presentation of the information, two presentation techniques have been used: the fingerprint and the national map. The fingerprint gives all detailed information within a general frame of reference and is meant for the inside world of the nursing unit. The national map presents a summary of this information for all nursing units and is meant for the outside world.

The fingerprint consists technically in horizontal bar charts for each of the 23 nursing interventions. The fingerprint of the nursing unit's practice compares the interventions of every nursing unit with the same interventions of some reference nursing unit: the sum-nursing unit in Belgium in 1988 or the theoretical nursing unit which we obtain by lumping together all data for all nursing units in Belgium. Figure 1 gives a example of such a fingerprint. A deflection to the left means that the intervention grades lower in the nursing unit than in the sum-nursing unit. A deflection to the right means that this interventions grades higher than in the sum-nursing unit. More-over, these deflections are standardised for the whole country. Utmost to the left and to the right, we find the most extreme deflections which are observed in Belgium in 1988. If a particular nursing unit would not differentiate itself whatsoever from the sum-nursing unit, no deflections would be visible. The fingerprint puts equal emphasis on nursing interventions that are present as on nursing interventions that are absent in each nursing unit. Although most people accentuate the positive, often one learns as much from the things one does observe as from the things that do not occur.

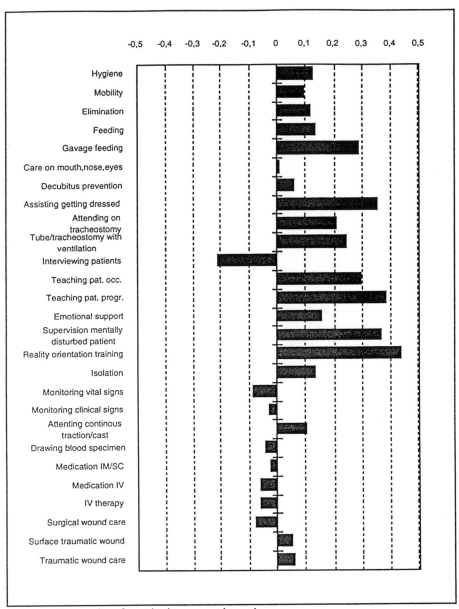

Figure 1: Fingerprint of a geriatric care nursing unit

The national map (figure 2) uses a specific graphic projection technique to show the position of all 2757 nursing units in Belgium with respect to all other nursing units on the basis of their fingerprint of nursing practice. Each nursing unit has its location on the map. Symbol I (right down) stands for intensive care nursing units. Symbols V and G (at the top) stand for geriatric care nursing units). Symbols C and D (in the middle) stand for surgical nursing units and internal medicine nursing units respectively.

The national map also indicates to what extent the NMDS allow to group nursing units with a similar nursing practice. Figure 2 shows that intensive care nursing units are not very homogeneous.

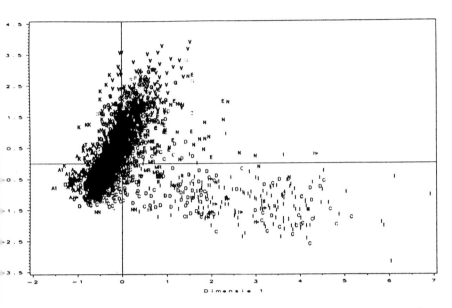

Figure 2: National statistics - national map: localisation of all Belgian nursing units 1988

Defining the 2 dimensions, helps in understanding the national map (figure 3). The first dimension (from the east to the west) is related to the conceptual framework of Orem[10]. A deflection to the east means that nursing interventions are characterised by "doing for". A deflection to the west means that nursing interventions are characterised by "doing with or self care". The second dimension (south to the north) indicates a balance between care and cure activities. More to the north means that the nursing care profile is dominated by care activities. More to the south, means that the nursing care profile is dominated by the cure activities supporting medical diagnosis and treatment. A strong relationship (68%) has been found between the first dimension and nursing intensity, based on the traditional patient classification systems such as the San Joaquin system. Moving in an eastern direction is associated with an increasing intensity of the nursing care.

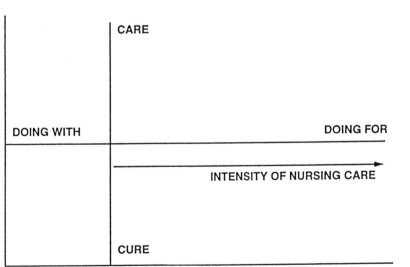

Figure 3: Frame of reference national statistics

A sixth condition is the feedback. People can only be motivated to collect data if they have timely results. This feedback is realised on different ways. First of all, a booklet "National Statistics"[11] is published by the Ministry of Public Health, which gives the general framework of nursing practice in Belgium. Secondly a computer diskette is developed which makes it possible for each hospital and nursing unit in Belgium to produce their own fingerprints right after the data collection in comparison with the stable reference point of 1988. Thirdly, education programs have been developed in co-operation with the 7 Belgian universities to teach nursing directors, head nurses to work with the program and to learn to read the fingerprints and national map.

A seventh condition is the degree of aggregation. In the "National Statistics" nursing data are aggregated at the level of the nursing unit. By lumping together all the units, we do obtain the location of hospital. Figure 2 points out that this "point of gravity" is just theoretical. A hospital is not very homogeneous concerning nursing care. It is however a

148

fallacy to believe that a nursing unit is more homogeneous with respect to nursing care. The nursing care also varies from patient to patient and even from day to day. That's why ways have been sought to zoom in the world of the nursing unit and to describe individual patients and patient days within the general framework set-up on the level of nursing units[12]. Again on all different levels of aggregation, fingerprints and national maps can be derived. Figure 4 shows the location of 207 inpatient days for a coronary care nursing unit. The black cross indicates the "point of gravity" which corresponds with one of the symbols in the "National Statistics". The figure makes clear that the variability of care in this nursing unit is very high. Some patient are intensive care patients, while other patients are self care patients.

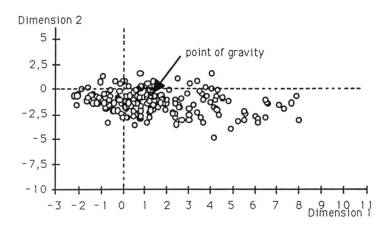

Figure 4: Projection of the nursing profile on the national map of 207 inpatient days from a coronary care nursing unit.

A eighth condition is the common denominator used to present the information. In the National statistics, the common denominator is the nursing unit. All patients hospitalised on the same nursing unit are taken together. But patients have other characteristics in common: their medical diagnosis, age, day of admission. Again it is possible to change the perspective to choose another common denominator e.g. medical diagnosis. Even more interesting are Diagnosis Related Groups (DRG's). Since 1982 a lot of research has been done all over the world to show the homo(hetero)geneity of DRG's in relation to nursing care. Several research studies reveal that DRG's explain only about 20-30% of the variation in nursing intensity[13][14][15]. Based on the NMDS the homogeneity of DRG's in relation to nursing care can be shown. Figure 5 shows the location of 182 inpatient days for the DRG014 "specific cerebrovascular disorders except TIA". The figure makes clear in a spot that this DRG is not homogeneous in relation to nursing care. Some patients are intensive care patients, some patients have high emphasis on basic care, some patients are self care patients. For a selection of DRG's in one Belgian hospital, the variability in nursing care has been calculated. DRG's explained about 25% of the variability in the intensity of nursing care (first dimension NMDS-framework).

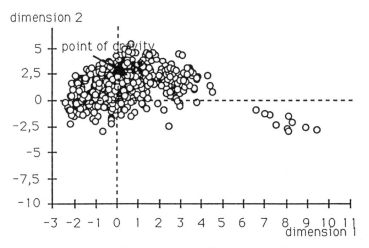

Figure 5: Projection of the nursing profile on the national map of 182 inpatient days for patients in DRG014: Specific disorders except TIA

4. From information to decision making

Despite the fact that the introduction of the NMDS was situated in a new hospital financing scheme in Belgium, the process goes very slowly. Data have to be collected. Then policy makers have to "trust" these data. Confidence is more than just reliability. In the national statistics of 1989 and 1990, the national map of Belgium has hardly changed for 0.2%. It means that the frame of reference is stable. It means that in 2 years time Belgium hasn't become sicker. At micro level, at the level of hospitals and nursing units, changes are more outspoken. A study investigating the dynamics over the period 1988-1991 has started. The stable frame of reference has strengthened the confidence in the information. At this moment a governmental work group is preparing a proposal to use the NMDS-information to determine the hospital's budget.

Besides this use by the government, these data are used within the hospital for management purposes. A first purpose is budgeting. Once the hospital's budget is determined, the budget has to be divided to departments, nursing units and finally to how many nurse you need to care for how many patients. This process is mainly a process of communication. The nursing director uses by preference a top-down approach to calculate fair budgets for each nursing unit. The head nurses use predominantly some bottom-up approaches in showing how many patients they are admitting, how long they stay, with what problems they are dealing, what they are doing with these patients, what they want to do next year, their workload etc. All these expectations mosly far exceed the budget what means that priorities have to be made. NMDS-information can be very helpful to support this communication process. Information is also needed to monitor the budget the top management and the head nurses have agreed upon. We call them dashboard instruments, because you need them while driving your nursing unit in the good direction. Several dashboard instruments have been developed based upon this NMDS: controlling nurses' workload by comparing this NMDS with patient classification systems[16] ; controlling material consumption [17].

The development of Minimum Data Sets has just begun. More and more, othet processes are monitored such as social processes, drug administration etc. All these process data finally will lead to patient outcomes and quality of life indicators. Finally that is what's all about: Delivering good patient care to a reasonable cost.

5. Reference list:

[1]   NANDA, *Taxonomy I - revised 1990 - with official nursing diagnoses*, NANDA, St. Louis, 1990
[2]   McCloskey JC & Bulechek GM (Eds). *Nursing Intervention Classification*, St. Louis, Mosby, 1992
[3]   Grobe SJ. Nursing intervention lexicon and taxonomy study: language and classification methods, *ANS Adv Nurs Sci*, 13 (2), 1990, p.22-34.
[4]   Saba V.et al, A nursing intervention taxonomy for home health care, *Nurs Health Care*, 12(6), 1991, P.296-299.
[5]   Ehnfors M. et al, Towards basic nursing information in patient records, *Var i norden*, 21(11), 1991, p.12-31
[6]   AUVB-UGIB, *Profiel van de verpleegkundige zorgverlening en de minimale verpleegkundige gegevens, cahiers 1 en 2*, AUVB-UGIB, 1985
[7]   Sermeus W, Delesie L. Betrouwbaarheid van de registratie van minimale verpleegkundige gegevens, *Acta Hospitalia*, 32(2), 1992, p.39-54.
[8]   Halloran EJ, Conceptual considerations, decision criteria, and guidelines for the nursing minimum data set from a administrative perspective in Werley HH & Lang NM (Eds), Identification of the nursing minimum data set, Springer Publ. Co, New York, 1988, p.48-66.
[9]   Tufte ER. *The visual display of quantitative information*, Graphic Press, Cheshire, 1983
[10]   Orem DE. *Nursing: concepts of practice 3th ed.*, Mc Graw Hill, New York, 1985
[11]   Ministerie van Volksgezondheid en Leefmilieu & Centrum voor Ziekenhuiswetenschap. *Medische Activiteiten in algemene ziekenhuizen:Nationale Statistieken 1988*, Brussel-Leuven, 1991
[12]   Sermeus W. *Variabiliteit van verpleegkundige verzorging*, Ph.D. thesis, Leuven, 1992
[13]   Atwood JR et al, Relationships among nursing care requirements, nursing resources and charges, in Shaffer FA (ed.), Patients & purse strings: patient classification and cost management, NLN, New York, 1986, p. 99-120
[14]   Green J et al. Severity of illness and nursing intensity: going beyond DRGs, in Scherubel JC & Shaffer FA (eds). Patients & purse strings II, NLN, 1988, p.207-230.
[15]   Halloran EJ. Nursing workload, medical diagnosis related groups and nursing diagnoses, *Res Nurs Health*, 8(4), 1985,p.421-433.
[16]   Vanden Boer G & Sermeus W. Linkage of NMDS and patient classification systems, Nursing Informatics San Antonio, USA, 1994, (submitted).
[17]   Vandewal D & Vanden Boer G., Using NMDS-information for the allocation of budgets to nursing units, Nursing Informatics San Antonio, USA, 1994, (submitted).

Nursing Informatics: An International Overview for Nursing in a Technological Era
S.J. Grobe and E.S.P. Pluyter-Wenting, eds.

Nursing Minimum Data Sets: Historical Perspective and Australian Development

Foster J[a] and Conrick M[b]

[a]*School of Nursing, Queensland University of Technology, Locked Bag No 2, Red Hill, QLD, 4059, Australia.*

[b]*School of Nursing, Griffith University, Nathan, QLD, 4111, Australia.*

Florence Nightingale began gathering minimum health data over a century ago, yet nursing has been very slow to realise the uniqueness of its data and position in the health care system. With the drive for computerisation of health care information nurses must become zealous about gathering, ordering and using nursing data. Nurses must design a minimum set of data elements essential to nursing practice, which will ensure quality, cost effective and equitable health care. This paper will discuss and compare developments in Nursing Minimum Data Sets and the plans for an Australian Nursing Minimum data Set.

1. Introduction

Patient level data for medical care has been available through the International Classification of Diseases for many years. The International Council of Nurses and other groups worldwide are attempting to develop internationally agreed nursing classification systems and nursing minimum data sets which are critical to support the processes of nursing practice and to advance nursing knowledge necessary for quality cost effective and equitable health care [1] & [2]. There are a number of countries currently undertaking developments in the area of Nursing Minimum Data Sets. These developments are all at differing stages and take differing stances, with only one country, Belgium, having a Nursing Minimum Data Set accepted and information collected by the Government.

The majority of Australian Hospital Information Systems are using ICD9–CM and perhaps ICD10, DRG's and Casemix as the standard for understanding and controlling the production process of health care delivery. These standards will probably be used for future funding and resource allocation but nursing data are not adequately represented in any of these systems and cannot receive appropriate funding or resource allocation because standardised nursing data has never been collected. –

2. International History of Minimum Data Sets

The pioneering development of the Data Set for nursing was undertaken by Professor Harriet Werley in the USA in the mid seventies. Professor Werley defines a Nursing Minimum Data Set (NMDS) as "a minimum set of items of information with uniform definitions and categories concerning the specific dimension of professional nursing, which meets the information needs of multiple users in the health care system" [3]. This is also the definition applied to the uniform minimum health data sets written by United States Health Information Policy Council. Werley & Zorn [4] emphasise strongly the need for multiple data users across all nursing practice settings to be considered in the definition of data elements. Also, central to the development of a NMDS is the development of standard uniform definitions and terminology for the data elements included [5].

The minimum data set concept was formulated in 1969 at a working conference in the USA. The aim was to collect the records of patients discharged from all hospitals and to develop a minimum set of core elements. The organisers of this conference recognised a need to order information, to contain rising health care costs, equitable distribution of services, and accountable resource use. These needs and the rapid developments in computer technology made it possible to design programs to manage large amounts of data [6].

The embryonic stage of the US Minimum Data Set was the Uniform Hospital Discharge Data Set (UHDDS) which originated from a conference attended by key health care providers and health data users. Unfortunately, a precedent was set, the UHDDS contained no nursing data. Around the same time in England, the budget shortfall for health was escalating and the National Health Service was under intense pressure, forcing Government intervention. The resultant investigation revealed problems in areas of data collection, processing, timeliness, accuracy and comparability. From this investigation the Steering Group on Health Services Information was born. This steering group identified, defined and tested those data elements to be included in a National Health Services Data Set and developed strategies for the collection of this data and this led to the 'Korner Report'. This report outlined the collection of data and use of information about hospital clinical activity, ambulance services, manpower, activity in hospitals and the community, services for and in the community and finance [7]. Once again no nursing data was collected. However, Wheeler [8] indicated that the 'Korner Data Set' has evolved to include nursing elements, reflecting the changing role of nurses in the United Kingdom. But, once again these nursing data elements focus only on facilities and not on nursing activities. In Canada in 1990 a National Task Force on Health Information (NTFHI) was begun to develop a plan for a National System for Health Information, NTFHI, 1990. The elements were defined but again there is no clinical nursing data.

In response to the inequity in nursing data collection, the nurses in the USA have developed a NMDS, which is currently undergoing testing and evaluation. It has received a positive review by the Health Information Policy Council of the US and the National Committee on Vital and Health Statistics. In Canada the information revolution has prompted initiatives to develop automated information systems focused on utilisation of data for the purpose of resource allocation, and to facilitate the evolution of a national system for health information built on essential and comparable data [9]. According to Hannah [10], the significance of the development of the NMDS is best understood through an examination of the context within which it was developed.

In the United Kingdom the National Health Service Centre for Coding and Classification (NHS CCC) was established in 1990 and it forms part of the Information Management Group (IMG) of the NHS Management Executive (NHS ME), but has a Supervisory Board drawn from the professions. Its main functions are to maintain and develop further the Read Codes, to collaborate with the professions in the development of specialty data sets to satisfy the detailed requirements of the professions, by expanding the Read Codes (which have been the recommended standard in UK General Practice since 1990) to from a comprehensive Clinical Thesaurus by 1994. Nursing in the UK has recently completed a Scoping Project to explore nursing terminology and assess the Read Codes for their appropriateness to the nursing profession, and to liaise with the various nursing professional bodies, groups and members to establish current known work and experience in this field. The task of identifying and coding all terms required is being assessed to determine the resources needed to develop the nursing terminology in the Read Codes to be suitable across all services and sectors of the NHS [11].

Belgium has had a National Minimum Data Set of Nursing Interventions since 1987, under Royal Decree, and this allows national availability of all health information on medical and nursing activities in hospitals. The Nursing Minimum Data Set consists of a selected list of twenty three (23) nursing activities. These activities monitor basic care activities, technical activities and some very typical activities and are collected four times per year [12].

Australia has National Minimum data Set for Community Nursing (Australian – Community Nursing Minimum Data Set, CNMDSA) and this is currently in the pilot stage and results are being formulated. As there are only three NMDS available a comparison of these displays the similarities and differences in identified data elements. The USA have sixteen elements covering three main areas which are nursing care elements, patient or client demographic elements and service elements. In contrast the Belgium NMDS has twenty seven elements based on the Activities of Daily Living and the Australian CNMDS has eighteen elements. The differences between these data sets are exemplified in Table 1 below.

2.1 Comparison of Nursing Minimum Data Sets

Table 1
Comparison of three Nursing Minimum Data Sets

AUSTRALIA CNMDSA	UNITED STATES of AMERICA	BELGIUM
1. Admission date	**Nursing Care Elements:**	1. Hygiene
2. Agency Identifier	1. Nursing Diagnosis	2. Mobility
3. Carer Availability	2. Nursing Intervention	3. Elimination
4. Client dependency	3. Nursing Outcome	4. Feeding
5. Date of Birth	4. Intensity of Nursing Care	5. Gavage Feeding
6. Discharge date	**Patient or Client Demographic Elements:**	6. Care on mouth, nose, eyes
7. Discharge destination	5. Personal Identification	7. Decubitus Prevention
8. Ethnicity	6. Date of Birth	8. Assisting in getting dressed
9. Sex of client	7. Sex	9. Attending to Tracheostomy
10. Location of client	8. Race and Ethnicity	10. Tracheostomy with ventilation
11. Medical diagnosis	9. Residence	11. Interviewing patients
12. Nursing intervention	**Service Elements:**	12. Teaching patient occasionally
13. Nursing diagnosis	10. Unique Facility or Service Agency Number	13. Teaching patient fixed program
14. Nursing goal	11. Unique Health Record Number of Patient or Client	14. Emotional support
15. Resource utilisation		15. Supervision to mentally disturbed patient
16. Source of referral	12. Unique Number of Principal Registered Nurse Provider	16. Reality Orientation Training
17. Unique client identifier		17. Isolation
18. Other support services	13. Episode Admission or Encounter Date	18. Monitoring of Vital Signs
	14. Discharge or Termination Date	19. Monitoring of Clinical Signs
	15. Disposition of Patient or Client	20. Attending on continuous traction or cast
	16. Expected Payer for Most of This Bill (Anticipated Financial Guarantor for Services).	21. Drawing of blood specimen
		22. Medication IM/SC
		23. Medication IV
		24. IV Therapy
		25. Surgical wound care
		26. Surface traumatic wound
		27. Traumatic wound care

Adapted from Werley H et al, 1991 and National Statistics, Belgium, 1988, and The Community Nursing Minimum Data Set Australia Project, Gliddon T and Weaver C, 1993 [13].

Clark & Lang [14], state there is an urgent need for an international classification for nursing practice that will provide nursing with a nomenclature, language and classification system that can be used to describe and organise nursing data. A model which clarifies the process of this development has been identified and is encompassed on a continuum with nursing practice. This is exemplified below in Figure 1.

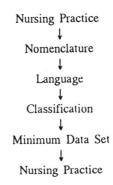

Nursing Practice
↓
Nomenclature
↓
Language
↓
Classification
↓
Minimum Data Set
↓
Nursing Practice

Figure 1. Model of a Nursing Classification System Modified from Clark & Lang, 1992, p111.

3. Australian Data Set Development

Ensuring quality cost effective, equitable health care in Australia is a national priority and an appropriate information base is required for monitoring and evaluation. The development of the National Health Minimum Data Set for Institutional Care and the Australian Health Care Data Dictionary under the auspices of the Australian Health Ministers Advisory Council (AHMAC), are crucial moves in the information systems area. Nursing, a vital component of health care, is responding, by developing a National Nursing Minimum Data Set (NNMDS) for incorporation into these data sets.

The NNMDS not only offers nursing the opportunity to order its data but has profound implications for all areas of nursing. With the advent of data collection for Casemix and DRG's means that large quantities of nursing data are being collected and standards formulated by individual institutions. This will be an important complementary activity with the initial steps of the NNMDS – the development of a National Nursing Thesaurus which will collect and standardise this data.

An NMDS must standardise data both nationally and internationally and the fragmentation of data collection must be contained, but in reality we cannot set nursing apart and regard it as a separate entity from health care. It is ludicrous to suggest that we can, given that nurses are the biggest group of care givers within the Health Care System.

On several occasions we have corresponded and discussed our national and international notion and thoughts on future directions with Professor Werley. Since beginning this project some two(2) years ago, we have had many letters and corresponded with nursing groups and other interested people worldwide. The message is loud and clear – there must be integration of all health data and there must be standardised data for all health care. Not nursing in isolation – not medicine in isolation – not administration in isolation as we are all health care givers. But, the development of the Australian Health Minimum Data Set, true to early development in other countries contains no nursing data. The revision of this project began in 1991–1992 and once more the omission was repeated! The Government has now made a priority on the development of the National Health Care Data dictionary as it became aware that standard definitions are necessary before one can develop a minium data set [15].

At this stage we have support from many sectors of health care for this development as it is seen to be critical for health care information systems and are awaiting funding to commence development of the NNMDS. Because of the enormity of the task we have broken the project into attainable segments:
1) development of an Australian Thesaurus,
2) development of an Australian Taxonomy
3) definition of data definitions and classification,
4) data base format development
5) assembly of the NNMDS [16].

The authors see data being collected by nursing, medicine and the paramedical areas and being integrated into a National Health Minimum Data Set (NHMDS). The collection of nursing data is too important to be kept institution specific and isolated from the nursing community. We need to work together in this important area to accomplish the most efficient usage of scarce resources.

4. Conclusion

This project has the potential to be valuable in many areas yet being separate in identity and scope from all. The identification of an Australian Taxonomy and the National Minimum Data Set would be invaluable to the automation of Nursing Information and Management Systems while the Classification of nursing data would be invaluable to the Casemix project. The introduction of a NNMDS and standardised nursing data would break down one of the greatest barriers presently hindering nursing research on a national and international basis and it would support the process of nursing practice and advance the knowledge necessary for the cost-effective delivery of quality nursing care.

5. References

[1] Clark J and Lang N. Nursing's next advance: An international classification for nursing practice. *Int Nurs Rev* 1992, 39 (4): 109-112, 128.

[2] Wheeler M. What do we have in common. *Information Technology in Nursing* 1991, 4 (3): 12-15.

[3] Werley H, Devine E, Zorn C, Ryan P and Westra B. The Nursing Minimum Data Set: Abstraction Tool for Standardised, Comparable, Essential Data. *Am Jnl of Pub Hlth* 1991, 18 (4): 421-426.

[4] Werley H and Zorn C. The Nursing Minimum Data Set and its Relationship to Classifications for Describing Nursing Practice. *Classification Systems for Describing Nursing Practice.* Kansas City: American Nurses Association, 1989: 50-54.

[5] Werley H, Devine E, Zorn C, Ryan P and Westra B. The Nursing Minimum Data Set: Abstraction Tool for Standardised, Comparable, Essential Data. *Am Jnl of Pub Hlth* 1991, 18(4): 421-426.

[6] Murnaghan J and White K. Hospital Discharge Data: Report of the Conference on Hospital Discharge Abstracts systems. *Medical Care* 1970, 8:1-215.

[7] Hanna K and Anderson J. Background Paper: Nursing Minimum Data Set. *Unpublished paper* 1992.

[8] Wheeler M. Nurses do count. *Nursing Times* 1991, 87 (16): 64-65.

[9] Hanna K and Anderson J. Background Paper: Nursing Minimum Data Set. *Unpublished paper* 1992.

[10] Hanna K and Anderson J. Background Paper: Nursing Minimum Data Set. *Unpublished paper* 1992.

[11] NHS Management Executive. Nursing terms (scoping) project workshops. *NHS Centre for Coding and Classification - General Information* 1993.

[12] Sermeus W. Hospital care financing and drg's: How Belgium takes nursing care into account. *Inforum* 1991, 12: 31-37.

[13] Werley H, Devine E, Zorn C, Ryan P and Westra B. The Nursing Minimum Data Set: Abstraction Tool for Standardised, Comparable, Essential Data. *Am Jnl of Pub Hlth* 1991, 18(4): 421-426.
Belgium Government. *National Statistics.* Leuven: Belgium, 1988
Gliddon T and Weaver C. The community Nursing Minimum Data Set Australia: Project: Real life issues of operationalising a common data set in diverse community nursing environments. In: *HIC'93.* Hovenga E, Whymark G (eds). Melbourne: Australia, 1993: 81-90.

[14] Clark J and Lang N. Nursing's next advance: An international classification for nursing practice. *Int Nurs Rev* 1992, 39 (4): 109-112, 128.

[15] Foster J and Conrick M. A national nursing minimum data set: Challenge to alter inequity. *Health Informatics: Now and tomorrow.* Nursing Informatics Australia (Inc) (eds). Melbourne: Australia. 1992.

[16] Conrick M and Foster J. Submission to the Health Minister: National Nursing Minimum Data Set. *Unpublished submission.* 1992.

1994 Elsevier Science B.V. All rights reserved.
rsing Informatics: An International Overview for Nursing in a Technological Era
J. Grobe and E.S.P. Pluyter-Wenting, eds.

A Nursing Management Minimum Data Set

Delaney C[a] Gardner Huber D[a] Mehmert M[b] Crossley J[c] and Ellerbe S[b]

College of Nursing, The University of Iowa, Iowa City, Iowa

University of Iowa Hospitals and Clinics, Iowa City, Iowa

Mercy Hospital, Davenport, Iowa

Complexity, rapid change, the high technology health care environment, and increasing economic pressures demand access to nursing data and information for decision making. Specifically, no common data set exists to facilitate nursing management and administrative decision making. Work is underway to establish a nursing minimum data set, a collection of core data elements needed by nurse administrators to make decisions and compare effectiveness of nursing care among institutions. Built to complement the Nursing Minimum Data Set, the NMMDS will facilitate decision making and policy development in such areas as costs of nursing services, allocation of nursing personnel, and comparison of nursing care delivery methods, and will foster data collection, retrieval, analysis, and comparison of nursing management outcomes across settings, populations, time, and geographic regions. The purpose of this research was to identify a universal set of variable for evaluating nursing administration effectiveness. Following a one-state pilot study from which 25 core variables and their definitions were derived, a national Delphi study was conducted. A stratified random sample (N=1199) was selected from the membership of the American Organization of Nurse Executives. Through rating necessity, collectibility, and measurability, consensus was sought on the core variables, their definitions, and measures. The proposed NMMDS elements and corresponding definitions are reported. Implications for testing the NMMDS in clinical sites are addressed.

Background and Significance

Every aspect of health care delivery in the United States has come under scrutiny. The industry-wide revolution requires the identification of creative solutions to deliver care more efficiently while improving quality. In large part, his survival is dependent upon developing effective quality management practices. Kratz [1] emphasizes the need for nursing to attend to those priorities which have the greatest impact on results: the high risk, high volume, problem prone, and high costs aspects of nursing service.

Moreover, nursing as a service must have a mechanism for monitoring and evaluating activities. Kratz and Green have advanced the "Blueprint for Quality Management" model, unique because it defines the clinical, professional, and administrative aspects of nursing within a quality assurance model. In serving our constituents, data must be available o support decision making that ensures patient satisfaction, quality results, and cost effectiveness. Data needs related to he patient are being addressed through the identified Nursing Minimum Data Set; data needs related to staff are being addressed by personnel database initiatives as well as personnel databases maintained within individual institutions and agencies; the nursing management minimum data set is proposed to meet the data needs reflecting the system within which health care is delivered.

The NMMDS is defined as an identified minimum collection of core variables, with their definitions and measures, needed by nurse managers and administrators to make decisions and deliver nursing care at lowest cost and highest level of patient outcomes achievement. That is, access to an NMMDS would support efficient accomplishment of NSA outcomes related to resource allocation, effective personnel management, and quality of care.

The NMDS as identified by Werley and colleagues and the Iowa Model of Nursing Administration formed th conceptual framework for this research. A descriptive survey approach was used for identifying the elements, relate definitions, and measures. The Development Phase consisted of three stages: pilot test, national Delphi, and consensu conference. This paper reports the results of the national Delphi.

2. Method

A single state pilot survey generated a questionnaire containing 25 data elements. This questionnaire served as th instrument for the three round national Delphi. The questionnaire was sent to a stratified random sample of 30% (N=1199) of the mailing list of the American Organization of Nursing Executives. Stratification occurred in relation t geographic region and bed size. Respondents were asked to rate the necessity, clarity, and collectibility of each item and to provide feedback on deletions and additions needed. Necessity was described as that data element that is clearl basic and important for nurse administrators to have to evaluate and manage nursing services. The highest rating v given to those items consider so important as to be essential. How clearly the definition was stated constituted the clarity rating. Collectibility was defined as the degree to which the element was available and easy to collect in th respondent's setting.

The response rate was 66% (N=791) for round 1; 69% (N=539) for round 2; and 62% (N=333) for round three Descriptive statistics were calculated. The level of inclusion of data elements was both a necessity mean and mod greater than 3.5 on a 1-5, low to high scale.

3. Results

The results of the three round national Delphi yielded 18 elements to be collected annually at the unit or institutiona levels. Nine unit level data elements were identified: type of nursing unit; method of care delivery; nurse manager/administrator demographic characteristics; unit of service/workload unit; size of nursing unit; costs; nursing resources; average intensity of nursing care.

Nine institutional level variables were identified: medicare case mix; occupancy; staff mix; budget; revenues satisfaction; achievement of accrediting body standards; nursing administration complexity; and nursing demographics Sixteen of the 18 elements exhibited necessity means greater than 4.00, with the exception of "Years of service o nursing staff" (3.81) and "Certification of nursing staff" (3.71).

Means for the clarity rating ranged from a low of 4.01 for nurse manager demographics to 4.82 for occupancy, tota admissions. Respondents ratings of the collectibility of the elements ranged from a mean of 2.81 to 4.94. Element receiving collectibility ratings less than 3.5 were satisfaction, physician (2.81); satisfaction, nurse (3.19); and costs indirect (3.39).

Although results indicate consensus on identification of the elements, qualitative data analysis revealed numerou definitional and measurement issues. For example, type of nursing unit was defined as the unique name (cost cente number, geographic location, or other identifier) and a description of the primary patient population or service unit Issues arose as to when type was determined by most common DRG grouping served, age of patient population, nursing diagnosis, and designation of unit when multiple populations are served. Costs per nursing unit were defined a. including a) direct costs, that is costs attributed to direct patient care, and b) indirect costs, costs of supporting activitie of the unit. Questions arose as to how ancillary services should be calculated and the need to separate direct personne costs from direct material/supply costs. Nursing resources were defined to be the actual full time equivalents (FTE) by classification, the total number of productive nurses, and the total number of nonproductive nurses. Questions arose a: to specific definition of productive and nonproductive and the placement of nurse practitioners and clinical nurse specialists. The nursing unit budget was defined as including components of direct labor, indirect labor, non-labor, and nursing unit revenue. Respondents questioned the inclusion of "revenue", some asserting that only expenses are relevant. Concerns arose as to how to report variance between budgeted and actual FTE's; how to report revenue when salaried physicians are paid from nursing unit revenue; and how charges are adjusted for contractual agreements.

At the institutional level numerous issues were also identified. For example, nursing demographics included turnover, vacancy rate, educational profile of nursing staff, years of professional experience and certification Respondents raised questions as to: consistent measurement of internal transfers; persons who leave nursing but remain within the institution or agency; reporting of educational preparation as highest preparation or all preparation;and eporting of certification data. Satisfaction encompassed patients, nursing staff, and physicians. Issues arose as to the availability of tools/scales to measure this variable in all populations.

4. Discussion

It is clear that a national consensus conference is needed to promote clarification and consistency of measurement of the NMMDS elements. In addition, adaptation of the proposed NMMDS to long term care, community and home health care is essential. Moreover, clinical testing must ensue.

The NMMDS has the potential to facilitate data collection, retrieval, and analysis that reflects the contextual variables in nursing practice. It will promote comparison of nursing management interventions across unit, site, and setting. As proposed, the NMMDS will interface with other data bases to enhance decision making. Finally, nursing's position to participate in policy development to reform the health care delivery system will be enhanced.

5. References

[1] Kratz, J. and Green, E. *Managing quality: A guide to monitoring and evaluating nursing services.* St. Louis: The C.V.Mosby Company, 1992.

Nursing Informatics: An International Overview for Nursing in a Technological Era
S.J. Grobe and E.S.P. Pluyter-Wenting, eds.

Linkage of NMDS -information and Patient Classification Systems

Vanden Boer G [a] and Sermeus W [b]

[a] Research assistant, School of Public Health, Catholic University of Leuven, Leuven, Belgium

[b] Assistant Professor, School of Public Health, Catholic University of Leuven, Leuven, Belgium

Since 1980 the University Hospitals of Leuven use the San Joaquin PCS [1] to monitor patient acuity on nursing units. This system, using 4 classes of patients (no help, average, more than average, intensive care), is based on traditional timesampling studies for calibration. Through a pair-wise comparison of time study-results of 1980 and 1990 for the same nursing units, we discovered that on the average the same amount of minutes direct patient care were measured for the same class of patients over the two periods. This was quite surprising because over those 10 years the length of stay decreased from 13 to 9 days and the complexity of the population on the nursing units increased (minor surgery went to short stay). This raised the question of the validity of the time-values per class. Therefore the traditional path was left and the classes were linked to the national NMDS-information: the proces is documented with NMDS data and PCS data as well as NRG's for the burncenter.

1. The PCS-system linked to the NMDS.

The on-line registration of the San Joaquin class is done on a daily basis for every nursing unit. In fact the 4 classes are used as a "global language" to describe the activity per nursing unit in the whole hospital (except for ICU and Pediatrics). Besides this registration we collect a Nursing Minimum Data Set (NMDS) 4 times a year during a 15-day sampling period. This nursing minimum data set, which contains 23 selected nursing interventions, is registered for every patient hospitalised during the 15 days [2]. It is possible to link the San Joaquin class to the NMDS for every patient in this 15-day period. In the Belgian NMDS all information is available to generate the San Joaquin classes. Sermeus W. [3] used this property to check on the validity of the Belgian NMDS in relation to intensity of nursing care. In addition to these indicators 17 other selected nursing interventions are part of the "minimal national nursing language". This gives this NMDS-language a broader and more detailed spectrum. A *national frame of reference* with regard to content of nursing care in Belgium [4], is used in the analysis and presentation of the NMDS-information.

1.1. Association of the clinical and algorithmic use of the SJ instrument

Table 1 shows a comparison between the San Joaquin class registered by the nurses on the unit and the San Joaquin class generated by an algorithm using NMDS-information for a surgical nursing unit and for the burncenter.

Table 1
Association between Class scored by nurses and Class score based on NMDS

		\multicolumn{5}{c}{Class scored by nurses on}					
		\multicolumn{4}{c}{A=Burncenter}		\multicolumn{4}{c}{B=Surgical ward}	
		1	2	3	4		1	2	3	4	
Class	1	1	5	0	0	6	123	15	14	0	152
generated	2	1	45	0	1	47	55	86	23	0	164
using	3	2	42	2	41	87	10	34	51	15	110
NMDS	4	1	20	23	96	140	0	10	52	33	95
		5	112	25	138	280	188	145	140	48	521
		\multicolumn{5}{c}{Kendall's tau-b = 0,50}		\multicolumn{5}{c}{Kendall's tau-b = 0,65}

The correspondence between the two scores is moderate on nursing unit B and weak for nursing unit A. This is to be expected since the PCS doesn't fit so well for the burncenter's population as it does for a common medical or surgical ward. The moderate association of 0,65 on unit B has several reasons. First, the possibility in the San Joaquin system to place a patient one category higher on the basis of clinical insight. Second the fact that the scoring of the categories is done implicitly. In the beginning the nurses use a scoring-tool but after a while they drop it and the scoring then is much more based on global clinical insight (the 4 classes are 'locally adopted/calibrated'). To monitor this normal process there is a need for regular reliability check (cfr. table 1) and content analysis by means of the NMDS.

1.2. Content analysis of the PCS

The 4 categories can be analysed using the much richer vocabulary of the NMDS (i.e. 23 nursing activities - see figure 1). Let us compare the class 3 patients for the surgical ward and the burncenter. Figure 1 presents the fingerprints for class 3 patients for both wards (black bars indicating the surgical ward, white bars the burncenter), and the location of all classes on the national NMDS-map. On the fingerprint the 0,0 value indicates the national median value for the corresponding nursing activity (the national frame of reference): a deflection to the left means that the activity, measured by patient and by day, grades lower in the nursing unit than in the "sum-nursing unit" of Belgium; a deflection to the right means a higher grading. So we see that the nursing care for class 3 patients on the surgical ward is oriented to basic care (hygiene, mobility, elimination & feeding), vital signs, attending on traction, IV therapy and of course surgical wound care. less monitoring ... On the burncenter the nursing care for class 3 patients is characterised by basic care (notice the lower grade for feeding), special care on nose, mouth, eyes; prevention of decubitus, giving emotional support, monitoring vital signs, less IV's and the combination of surgical and traumatic wound care... This way we get a fairly global picture of the two groups of patients. The right part of figure 1 shows the location of the 'median' class 1, 2, 3 and 4 patient for both units on the map : east-west means from total dependency to self-care - south-north means from technical, diagnostic care to basic care. Notice the diversion of classes 3 and 4 (more care oriented for the surgical ward, more cure oriented for the burncenter).

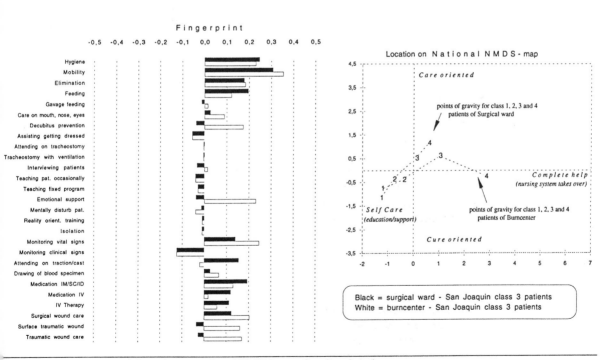

Figure 1. *Fingerprint* and *Location* on national NMDS-map for class 3 patients.

The global nursing profile is supported with a detailed picture of the variability within the specified class of patients (micro-macro phenomenon in the population [2]): this is done through projection of each individual patient per day on the national NMDS-map. Figure 2 and 3 illustrate this for the two nursing units: although the point of gravity gives us

160

the central tendency of the class 3 patients we see that within each group there is some variability, which we can take into account.

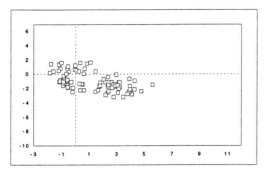

Figure 2. *Visual display* of patient days on national
NMDS-map, class 3 patients, burncenter.

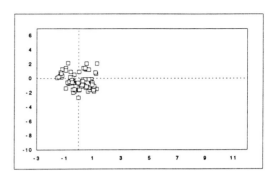

Figure 3. *Visual display* of patient days on national
NMDS-map, class 3 patients, surgical ward.

2. Using the system

The on-line registration of the 4 classes is rather simple and low cost - the collection of the NMDS has a higher cost as of today. For this reason the PCS is used on a daily basis and the NMDS, which is used for calibration, is collected 4 times a year. The presentation of the PCS-information is done as follows:

1. For each nursing unit a reference frequency distribution for the San Joaquin classes is generated using NMDS data of the 2 recent years (i.e. samples of ± 2000-2500 patient days per nursing unit)
2. This frequency distribution is used as a point of reference for the nursing unit by means of ridit-analysis [5] (the reference distribution can be updated on a yearly or two-yearly basis)
3. The frequency distribution of a particular day or week or period is compared with this point of reference: the result is expressed in a mean ridit for the period of interest and can be interpreted as a chance (table 2 gives an example). The mean ridit of 0,50 means that the chance that a randomly chosen patient from the reference group has a more intense nursing profile than again, another random patient from the reference group is one out of two. The mean ridit of 0,56 is 12% above 'the reference level of nursing unit activity'. This patient profile information is combined with actual staffing figures and bed occupancy rates.
4. The point of reference can be altered e.g. it can be the global frequency distribution over all the surgical wards - this way a comparison is made of the actual nursing unit with 'the reference level of global surgical activity'.
5. Four times a year the fingerprints for the 4 classes and for the whole nursing unit, as well as the location on the national map, including the variability in patient days, are generated. This information gives insight in the nursing profile of nursing unit and the 4 classes. A combination with 'local coding systems' is underway (see 3.).

Table 2
Calculation of mean ridit for a period of interest

San Joaquin class	Reference distribution	Riditscores (rescaled classes)	Period of interest 1 weekday
1	392	0,093	4
2	623	0,336	6
3	777	0,671	16
4	301	0,928	4
Total:	2093		30
Mean ridit		0,50 [6]	0,56 [7]

3. Mapping relevant clinical patient groups on the unit-level to the NMDS

On the level of a nursing unit the population is often divided in 'relevant clinical groups' (NRG) based on global clinical insight (a mixture of nursing and medical knowledge). This local, often implicitly used, system of communication or classification based on some or more relevant patient groups, can be mapped to the *NMDS frame of reference*: i.e. producing fingerprints per group and making the projection of the groups on the national NMDS map (point of gravity as well as individual patient days). Through this mapping the groups or the local coding system are brought into the open and can be validated. The linkage of the relevant patient groups often means the first practical clinical use of the NMDS information for the nurses on the ward. Let's illustrate the method using the burncenter's local coding system, introduced by the headnurse for day to day use instead of the San Joaquin classes (the system was introduced in september 1992). This center of 8 beds also functions as a small 'intensive care' unit (4 beds) for critical recovery patients. Nine classes are used:

	n
1: no burns - often breast correction or surgical decubitus therapy	58
2: burns < 20% of body - no special bath therapy - no ventilation	59
3: burns < 20% of body + special bath therapy - no ventilation	28
4: burns > 20% of body - no ventilation	24
5: burns < 20% of body + ventilation	0
6: burns > 20% of body + ventilation	2
7: recovery patient - no ventilation	73
8: recovery patient + ventilation - patient is not critical	20
9: recovery patient + ventilation - patient is critical	16
Total	280

To show the difference in the clinical relevance of the three systems, we compare, for the burncenter, the variability in patient days (through projection on the national NMDS map) for the following groupings:
1 = the grouping on the basis of San Joaquin classes (SJ-classes) generated by the algorithm (figure 4)
2 = the grouping on the basis of San Joaquin classes generated by the nurses global clinical insight (figure 5)
3 = the 9 groups used by the head nurse: of which 1, 2, 3, 4, 7 and 8 & 9 combined are de facto used (figure 6)

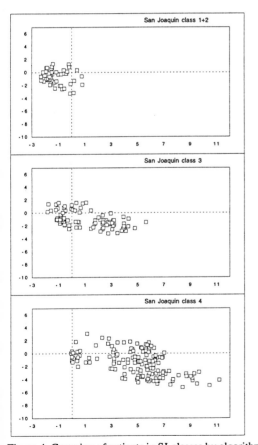

Figure 4. Grouping of patients in SJ-classes by algorithm

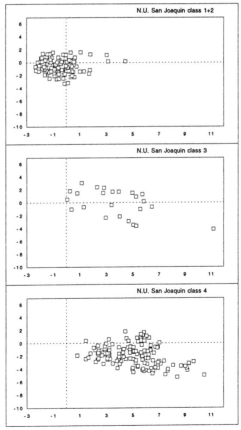

Figure 5. Grouping of patients in SJ-classes by nurses

Altough the comparison is based on one NMDS registration period, we see that the whole cloud of patient days (figure 6) is broken up into relevant groups on various levels of details. Of course the full detail of every single patient day can not be used for local management purposes - neither can a grouping into one single group. What the head nurse is

162

looking for is a system that is fine tuned for her unit and based on the variability shown in figure 4-6 her own system gives 'the most information', the spread over the four SJ-classes based on the algorithm is the lowest, then come the adopted SJ-classes, followed by the local coding system. This illustrates the micro-macro phenomenon in the language used.

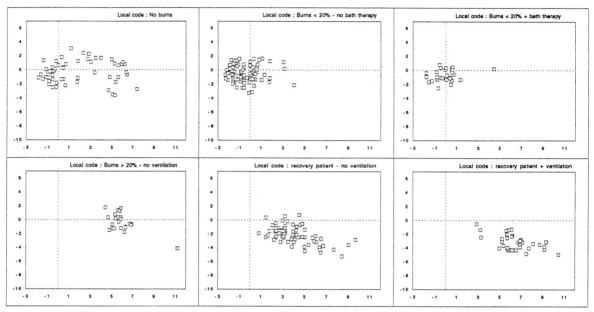

Figure 6. Grouping of patients by classification system of burncenter

4. Conclusion

The Belgian national NMDS functions as a worthwhile micro-macro frame of reference, by bypassing the context switching which often makes communication so difficult, and putting forward a sound methodolgy for information handling. Local coding systems linked to a common communication platform (NMDS) seem to have strong potentials with regard to resource and clinical management on a unit. [8] [9]

5. References

[1] Murphy LN, et. al., *Methods for studying nurse staffing in a patient unit, a manual to aid hospitals in making use of personnel*, DHEW publication HRA 78-3, Hyattsville, 1978, pp. 226.

[2] Delesie L. et.al., Identifying the hospitals' practice variations. micro/macro readings. In Delesie L. (ed)., *New Trends in Hospital Management*, Centre for Health Services Research, Catholic University Leuven, Leuven, june 1992, p. 41-71.

[3] Sermeus W. *Variabiliteit van Verpleegkundige verzorging in Algemene Ziekenhuizen*, doctoraatsthesis, Centrum voor Ziekenhuiswetenschap, K.U.Leuven, Leuven, 1992, p. 65-95.

[4] Ministerie van Volksgezondheid en Leefmilieu, Bestuur der Verzorgingsinstellingen en Centrum voor Ziekenhuiswetenschap, Katholieke Universiteit Leuven, *Medische Activiteiten in de Algemene Ziekenhuizen - Activités Médicales dans les Hôpitaux Généraux - Medical Activities in the General Hospitals*, Nationale statistieken - Statistiques nationales 1988, 1991 (in Dutch, French and English), pp. 88.

[5] Fleiss JL. *Statistical methods for rates and proportions*, John Wiley & Sons, New York, 1981, pp. 223.

[6] $0{,}50 = (392*0{,}093 + 623*0{,}336 + 777*0{,}671 + 301*0{,}928) / 2093$

[7] $0{,}56 = (4*0{,}093 + 6*0{,}336 + 16*0{,}671 + 4*0{,}928) / 30$

[8] Vandewal D and Vanden Boer G. Using NMDS-Information for the Allocation of Budgets to Nursing Units, Paper to be presented during "Nursing Informatics '94", San Antonio, USA, june 1994.

[9] Finnigan SA, et. al. Automated Patient Acuity, Linking Nursing Systems and Quality Measurement with Patient Outcomes, J *Nurs Adm.* 1993, vol. 23, No. 5, 62-71

Nursing Informatics: An International Overview for Nursing in a Technological Era
S.J. Grobe and E.S.P. Pluyter-Wenting, eds.

The Community Nursing Minimum Data Set Australia - From Definition to the Real World

Gliddon T [a] and Weaver C [b]

[a]Community Nursing Minimum Data Set Australia Pilot Implementation Project, c/- 45 Victoria Pde, Collingwood VIC 3066 Australia

[b]Fleming Associates (Australia) P/L, PO Box 1014 Chatswood, NSW 2057, Australia

The Community Nursing Minimum Data Set Australia (CNMDSA), was developed in 1990-1991. The CNMDSA Pilot Implementation Project commenced in June 1992 and aims over an eighteen month period to test the eighteen CNMDSA data items in context. This has involved intensive examination of the ability of the existing information systems in ten selected Community Nursing Services to provide the data items, followed by a three-month pilot data collection in eight of these. The database of approximately 6,500 discharges will undergo extensive analysis to determine whether its information and reporting capabilities meet the needs of all stakeholders; it will include some exploration of the potential of the data to develop a Casemix Classification for the domiciliary nursing environment. This paper reports on implementation and methodological issues mid-way through the project. A final version of the data set and results of the analysis will be available early in 1994.

1. Project Background

Community nursing in Australia has been working on developing a minimum data set under the auspices of the Australian Council of Community Nursing Services (ACCNS) since 1987. The initiative began as an attempt to develop a common patient record for domiciliary nursing services [1]. The project demonstrated that it was not feasible to develop a record which would fit the diverse environments within which domiciliary nursing services are delivered. It became clear that the focus needed to be on identifying and standardising the *information*, rather than the means of collecting it.

The impetus for pursuing the aim of a standardised information set was strengthened by rapid and major changes occurring in health services and health care funding. Many community nursing services faced these without the means to demonstrate demand, manage resources or reflect the dependency levels, needs, resource utilisation and outcomes of the clients they served. With this background of change and sometimes chaos across the health services, ACCNS members decided at a National forum to seek support for the development of a minimum data set which would describe community nursing practice and help to address these problems. Conceptualisation for the undertaking took direction from the significant inroads made by Werley and colleagues into the development of a Nursing Minimum Data Set (NMDS) in the USA [2]. Note was also taken of Werley's powerful case for the extension of the NMDS' principles to nursing in other contexts and countries [3].

The objective of the CNMDSA proposal which ensued was to introduce standardisation and comparability into the data collections which described the area of community nursing. The proposal aimed to identify and gain consensus on an agreed set of data items and definitions which would constitute a minimum set of data for community nursing. This concept was submitted as a proposal by ACCNS and the National Community Health Program funded the proposal in 1989. Dr James Turley was appointed as Project Director and commenced work in June, 1990, successfully identifying the Community Nursing Minimum Data Set Australia (CNMDSA) by May, 1991. The data items were derived through a Delphi technique, with major input from domiciliary nurses across Australia. This process was guided by a Steering Committee to which fell the task of finalising and further defining the seventeen identified items [4].

2. Community Nursing Minimum Data Set Australia Pilot Implementation Project

Before the newly defined CNMDSA data items could be operationalised as a minimum data set, a number of questions needed to be answered. The data set needed to be trialed to answer how easily this information could be obtained and how much of it was already a part of existing information systems. ACCNS thus sought funding for a pilot implementation of the CNMDSA and received this from the Home and Community Care Program (HACC) early in 1992. The time period for this project is eighteen months, concluding in January, 1994. The pilot implementation is guided by a Steering Committee with representatives from the ACCNS, HACC, the Australian Institute of Health and Welfare, and the National Casemix Unit. The Steering Committee has significant decision-making input into any development which affects the data items and also oversights the project. Based on ongoing developments, one further item has been added and definitions substantially modified via this process. (See Fig 1 for full list of items)

3. Study Design

The Pilot Implementation encompasses two distinct phases. The first phase involved conducting a national audit of ten community nursing services to determine the extent to which the CNMDSA defined data items were already collected. The second phase involves actually trialing the CNMDSA data set in a three-month data collection by eight of the ten agencies which participated in the Phase 1 Audit. At the time of this writing, the Phase 1 Audit has been completed, and eight sites are in the process of doing the three-month data collection.

The ten Community Nursing Services participating in the audit were selected by the Project Steering Committee to be broadly representative of the different structures, size and contexts of domiciliary nursing services across Australia. Each Australian State and Territory was represented in the sampling. The study's scope did not make it possible to include the full range of Community Nursing, although two of the participating agencies had generalist services including Infant-Maternal, Child and School Health and Primary Care Clinics.

The audit was preceded by a two day meeting/workshop of Project Coordinators (one from each of the selected sites), at which the Data-Set was discussed and methodology of the project and details of the audit were outlined. Each agency participating in the audit completed a 10 percent sampling of their client records. A standardised audit form was provided to each Project Coordinator to use in recording the audit results. At completion, the Project Coordinators sent their audit forms to the Project Director for analysis. The Project Director visited each site while the audits were in process and reviewed the preliminary results of each site's audit with the Project Coordinator. These discussions focused on identifying discrepancies between definitions, missing CNMDSA data items and possible source/s for deriving the data, and processes or practices which could complicate their collection for the CNMDSA. Based on the findings from the site visit and the audit results, the Project Director prepared a summary report on each site. The site visit reports served as the basis for proceeding to the preparatory tasks needed to initiate Phase 2. Using the site reports as a baseline description, The Project Consultant worked with each site to develop site-specific methodologies for the CNMDSA three-month data collection. These methodologies were then completed in collaboration with the Site Coordinators over the ensuing weeks.

Even though six of the eight agencies who proceeded on to Phase 2 had information systems, it became evident from the first site visits, that the agencies would not be able to modify their systems in time to accommodate the CNMDSA data collection. Three of the eight sites actually committed to developing systems with the CNMDSA data items incorporated. To avoid the prospect of manual data collection in five of the eight sites, the project developed a CNMDSA data collection software system. The developed software supported data collection, storage, retrieval and transfer at the site level, and supported data aggregation, reporting and data analysis at the Central site level. The three-month data collection period is to be undertaken in each Site during the period May through August, 1993.

4. Focus for Project Findings and Data Analysis

During and following the data collection, some reliability and validity testing of the data items will take place and the feasibility of implementation on a wide scale will be examined. In addition, aggregation and analysis of the resulting database will address the question of whether the information adequately reflects community nursing practice, including nursing problems and interventions and the associated resource consumption and patient outcomes, and whether it meets the needs of service providers and Government. The major concern of this project is the quality and integrity of the data content, and the value of the data set. However, the technical aspects of data collection and transfer will also be addressed, as will the issue of standards, including structure of data items, and privacy and security of information. In addition the question of when, how and to what extent the CNMDSA could or should be collected from individual service providers and "stored", in a central "repository" will be examined.

There are many factors and issues which have been considered during the development of the CNMDSA which are receiving further attention during this implementation project. The inevitable and ongoing tension between maintaining the integrity of the CNMDSA, (in particular those items which reflect nursing practice), and ensuring consistency with other data collections and compliance with national and international standards for health care information systems, is a challenging aspect. So too are the coding schemes and definitions of the included items. The data-set as it stands has undergone and withstood some rigorous development and testing up to this time and has satisfied the Steering Committees involved in its development. Nevertheless some issues have always been present, and indeed were identified as requiring further attention in the proposal which secured the funding for this project. The remainder of this paper will address the key issues currently facing the project.

5. Outcomes

The only outcome variable in the data set at this time is *Discharge Destination*. Its fourteen-odd codes describe the final outcome of a care episode, in terms of resolution of the client problem, or need for and source of ongoing care, or death. While this summary information is critical, there is and always has been an interest in obtaining resolution status of the specific problems which prompt admission for care and/or which develop during the course of an episode. Clearly it would be advantageous to link outcomes to nursing problems, (care-plan) goals, nursing interventions and nursing resource utilisation, but the often long-term nature of community care introduces a level of complexity into this problem which makes it a difficult one to address in a minimum data set. Nevertheless it is being further examined during the project.

6. Impact on Practice

By definition the CNMDSA is a standard set of items, with standard definitions, codes and instructions for its implementation and use. On the surface it seems that this would not be difficult to achieve. However the apparent simplicity of the items is deceptive, especially those which are embedded in the traditional practice of the individual services. One such example is DISCHARGE DATE, and the variable which by definition must accompany this, DISCHARGE DESTINATION. Some agencies have a practice of placing "on-hold" those clients who are admitted to acute or respite care, or even who go on holiday, when this is both planned and for a known and limited period of time. This practice avoids (for the practitioner and the client) the "hassle" of readmission, and in some agencies also avoids the "loss" of patients requiring their follow-up care, when hospital referral practices are not well developed or community-oriented. Changing this practice to ensure compliance with the CNMDSA will result in major change at the clinical level, in agency information processing and in the throughput statistics which ensue. For example, some agencies have in the vicinity of 10% of their current client population "on-hold" at any one time. Their length-of-stay and turnover statistics will differ substantially from equivalent agencies which by their rules would discharge the same patients.

For some agencies participating in this trial, and many more community nursing services as this data set is more widely implemented, there will be major implications of standardising to the CNMDSA in relation to DISCHARGE DATE. For example CNMDSA data would need to be provided for the hundreds of "on-hold" patients as the system is purged at the outset. It will also be more resource-intensive and unpopular at the clinical level unless admission and information processing are substantially streamlined to compensate for the added demands. Though only one example of the ramifications of standardisation, this is also an excellent illustration of the need to pilot-test a data set such as this one, in order to lay open and reach agreement regarding the underlying problems and practices which have dictated the need for it in the first place.

7. Medical Diagnosis

There are several items in the CNMDSA which have been seen as essential components of the data set, which are nevertheless difficult in terms of the effort required to obtain them or indeed their value, given this. A major example of this is MEDICAL DIAGNOSIS. Saba demonstrated in the USA that medical diagnosis is a much weaker predictor of the need for care than nursing diagnosis in a home health care setting [5]. For community nursing services in Australia which typically have up to half of their admissions from the acute hospitals and a large proportion of the remainder from general practitioners, the provision and often relevance of a medical diagnosis may be of dubious and certainly differing quality and timeliness. Many clients admitted for home care may not have a "medical diagnosis" per sé. Nevertheless until this information is routinely obtained in a structured format its presence, nature, relevance to, and capacity to predict the need for community nursing services in Australia can not be examined. Furthermore, while there is some doubt that medical diagnosis is a major consideration in terms of the required nursing care and interventions, it is often argued that it must be taken into account as nursing care is planned. Finally, until epidemiological analyses of health services and their recipients, including some description of medical diagnosis, are applied across the spectrum of care settings, the full impact and importance of community services will not be recognised or realised.

By definition the inclusion of this item in a minimum data set carries with it the requirement that it also be coded in a recognised and standardised way, including the selection of the correct diagnoses and then the identification of a correct code. The ICD-9-CM classification is the taxonomy which "drives" the DRG system and as such is used across this country and has been included in the National Health Data Dictionary [6]. This influenced its selection for the CNMDSA. However the implications of this are significant as it is operationalised. Given the unwieldy nature of the three-volume classification, the fact that morbidity coding is a specialised skill for which nurses do not receive training, the unsuitability of many of the "diagnoses" of community-nursed clients for classification in this way (or at this level), and the likelihood of highly compromised data given all of the above, the inclusion of medical diagnosis and the use of the ICD-9-CM classification must be, and is being, carefully examined during this project.

8. Resource Utilisation

The definition of Admission and Discharge Dates and the current requirement that only the resources utilised between these are "eligible" for inclusion in the CNMDSA, has caused some concern for those Services which undertake a considerable amount of activity prior to or after these events. For example, pre-admission assessment and work-ups, hospital liaison, bereavement counselling. Added to this, no further definition of what goes into the resource utilisation has been attempted at this stage. The definition of "Direct Care" (which will be measured) and the other "Indirect" activities which must take place to facilitate it (which will only be measured if taking place in the home), can only be addressed by a more detailed breakdown of nursing activities. Descriptions of the type and level of staffing involved in the resource expenditure will also become more critical as deregulation of the health care industry continues. Again the CNMDSA has not attempted to address this, given the difficulty which would be engendered obtaining this sort of information over long episodes of care with ever-changing care plans, and needs for different types and levels of care.

9. Scope of the CNMDSA

The development of the original set of items of the CNMDSA through a Delphi technique, and the largely but not exclusively domiciliary nursing membership of the ACCNS has resulted in a data set which is heavily biased toward this area of Community Nursing practice. This project is examining the extent to which the data set can be used in all community nursing settings and will make recommendations concerning those items which could be considered to be generic, and those which may need to be "modularised" to incorporate the different aspects of community nursing. For example, screening programs, infant and child health, school health, homeless persons programs and many others. Outside community nursing, the scope and interface of the data set across other areas of nursing practice within Australia and across nursing in other countries, and across other care settings and disciplines, are being considered as the project proceeds.

In conclusion, the eighteen data items are presented as they are, in the mid-stage of this pilot implementation [Fig 1]. Final specification and definitions will be an output of the project in early 1994. The table below enables comparison with other known minimum data sets. (See also, Wheeler, [7] for a useful comparison of the CNMDSA with three other NMDS's).

COMPARISON OF COMMUNITY NURSING MINIMUM DATA SET AUSTRALIA (CNMDSA) WITH OTHER KNOWN MINIMUM DATA SETS

CNMDSA ITEM	ACAT MDS [1]	NHDD [2]	NMDS-USA [3]
DEMOGRAPHIC ELEMENTS			
Birth Date of Client	*	*	*
Sex of Client	*	*	*
Ethnicity - Country of Birth	*	*	*
Ethnicity - Language Spoken at Home		*	
Location of Client	*		*
SERVICE ELEMENTS			
Agency Identifier		*	*
Client Identifier	*	*	*
Admission Date	Assessment	*	*
Referral Source		*	
Discharge Date	Not Applicable	*	*
Discharge Destination (Also a Nursing element)	Referral Recommendations	*	*
Other Support Services	*		
NURSING ELEMENTS			
Client Dependency	Minimal Detail		Nursing Intensity
Nursing Diagnosis			*
Nursing Goal			
Nursing Intervention	Action Plan		*
Nursing Resource Utilisation			*
OTHER			
Medical Diagnosis	Broad category	*	
Carer Availability			

1. Aged Care Assessment Program National Minimum Data Set. [8].
2. National Health Data Dictionary - Institutional Health Care. [6].
3. Nursing Minimum Data Set - USA [2].

Fig. 1

10. References

[1] Gliddon T, *for* Australian Council of Community Nursing Services, Victorian Branch. *Standardised Patient Record Evaluation.* Melbourne: Royal District Nursing Service, *1988.*

[2] Werley H, and Lang N (eds). *Identification of the Nursing Minimum Data Set.* New York: Springer Publishing Company, 1988.

[3] Werley H. Use and Implementation of the Nursing Minimum Data Set. *4th International Conference on Nursing Use of Computers, Melbourne, 1991.*

[4] Turley J, *for* Australian Council of Community Nursing Services. *Community Nursing Minimum Data Set Australia. Final Report.* Melbourne: Australian Council of Community Nursing Services, 1991.

[5] Saba V, and Coopey M. *Develop and Demonstrate a Method for Classifying Home Health Patients to Predict Resource Requirements and to Measure Outcomes.* Home Health Care Classification Project, Georgetown University, School of Nursing. Georgetown: February, 1991.

[6] Australian Institute of Health and Welfare. *National Health Data Dictionary - Institutional Health Care.* Canberra: Australian Institute of Health and Welfare, 1993.

[7] Wheeler, M. What Do We Have In Common? A Review of Patient-related Data in Nursing and Health Care Minimum Data Sets in Four Countries. *Information Technology in Nursing, 1992: Vol 4.3.*

[8] Aged Care Research Group. *Aged Care Assessment Program National Minimum Data Set.* Melbourne: Latrobe University, 1993.

1994 Elsevier Science B.V. All rights reserved.
ursing Informatics: An International Overview for Nursing in a Technological Era
J. Grobe and E.S.P. Pluyter-Wenting, eds.

Establishment of the Research Value of Nursing Minimum Data Sets

C Delaney[a] M Mehmert[b] C Prophet[c] and J Crossley[d]

College of Nursing, The University of Iowa, Iowa City, Iowa

Mercy Hospital, Davenport, Iowa

University of Iowa Hospitals and Clinics, Iowa City, Iowa

University Hospitals of Cleveland, Cleveland, Ohio

The purpose of this research was to begin to establish the research value, of the computerized Nursing Minimum Data Set (NMDS). This work is essential if the NMDS is to be used in large patient-linked, standardized datasets and facilitate use of these data sets in nursing research within and beyond the United States. This work is part of a program of research which focuses on core indicators of quality - quality of nurse clinical decision making, quality of information technology, and quality of nursing care data elements in large patient-linked databases The study focuses on their potential to assist professional nursing to support nursing practice and outcomes research efforts through information systems. This paper presents a summary of findings from seven studies conducted to establish the research value of the NMDS. Grant support includes a NIH Biomedical Research Grant, an American Nurses Foundation/HBO & Company Grant, and a Sigma Theta Tau, Gamma Chapter Grant.

1. Background and Significance

Ready access to and use of nursing data are critical to implementing wise stewardship of health care resources. The US health care system faces increased costs, increased numbers of uninsured, cost-shifting, and lack of accountability for cost and outcomes. Standardized data sets provide an essential means of communication among the multiple units of this complex system. They allow comparisons across systems, sites, and settings, helping to identify areas of over utilization and underuse of resources, as well as services that are cost effective.

The development and implementation of standardized, uniform data sets in health care have been prolific. In the US multiple federal medical and health services standardized data bases exist, including administrative, clinical, disease registries, and death registries. Other data bases have been developed.[1] Additionally, over 30 of the states in the US maintain hospital discharge data systems or collect financial data. These data systems rely at least in part on the collection of minimum data sets, including: Uniform Hospital Discharge Data Set (UHDDS), the Long-Term Health Care (LTC) Client Uniform Data Set (UDS), and the Uniform Ambulatory Medical Care Data Set (UACDS). [2,3,4] Because nursing data is absence from these data sets, critical data related to nursing's decision making and interventions are not available to monitor quality, reimbursement, and outcomes.

The development of the Nursing Minimum Data Set (NMDS) was initiated in the 1970's by Harriet Werley.[5] The NMDS, by definition, includes the essential nursing data used on a regular basis by the majority of nurses across all settings in the delivery of care. Sixteen NMDS elements are organized within three categories of patient demographics, . service and nursing care. Patient demographic elements include personal identification, date of birth, sex, race and ethnicity, and residence. The service category includes the unique facility number, unique health record number, unique number of principal registered nurse provider, episode admission and discharge dates, disposition of patient, and expected payor of the bill. Four data elements comprise the nursing care category: nursing diagnosis, nursing intervention, nursing outcome, and nursing intensity. All elementsof the patient demographic and service categories of the NMDS, with the exception of the "unique number of registered nurse provider" are contained in the UHDDS and have been collected since 1975 on all Medicare patients.

Although the four nursing care elements present validity, reliability, utility, and standardization problems, the International Council for Nurses Board did approve a year of planning for the International Classification of Nursing Practice (ICN-ICNP) which includes three of the four nursing care elements of the NMDS, nursing diagnosis, intervention, and outcome. This paper addresses nursing's efforts to test the NMDS.

2. Methods

A non-experimental ex-post facto design was used to begin to investigate the research value of the computerized NMDS. Research value was defined as utility, the condition of providing usefulness within the context of a specific investigation and to the discipline of nursing.[6] Utility of the NMDS was operationally defined as the ability to a) be a cost effective data abstraction tool for nursing, b) produce patient profiles for each nursing diagnosis group, c) establish retrospective validation of the defining characteristics for nursing diagnoses, d) determine costs of direct nursing care, and d) forecast/trend nursing diagnoses.

Two clinical sites were used for the work reported here. Site A is a 265-bed, private, midwestern, secondary acute health care center. Site B is a 1000-bed, public, midwestern, tertiary health care center. Sites A and B are nationally recognized sites which use computerized nursing care planning systems based on the NANDA approved nursing diagnosis taxonomy. Both sites have extensive ongoing educational programs and quality monitoring activities to maintain data quality.

Seven data sets containing the elements of the NMDS with the addition of defining characteristics and etiologies for each nursing diagnosis were collected from the computerized information systems of each facility. Two of the data sets (one from each site) were manually retrieved (N=200, N=26 respectively); five data sets were electronically retrieved (4 from Site A and 1 from Site B). The number of patient records in each electronically retrieved data set was: #1 = 704; #2 = 4,248; and #3 = 1,066. The fourth electronically retrieved data set was comprised of 69,427 nursing diagnoses documented from 1987-1990 in Site A. The fifth electronically retrieved data set consisted of a stratified random sample of all patients with Diagnostic Related Group #209 (N=211).

3. Results

Analysis of five data sets was completed to establish the availability of each NMDS element and related cost of using the NMDS as a data abstraction tool. The availability of the NMDS elements, with the exception of unique registered nurse provider number which is not available in the US, ranged from 95.5-100%. Cost analysis was completed. Cost for manual retrieval of one data set from each site ranged from $20.20-82.50 per patient record. Cost analysis related to three electronically retrieved data sets, two from Site A and one from Site B, ranged from $0.05-$.50 per patient record. Three electronically retrieved datasets have realized a cost savings of approximately $187,000.

Demographic profiles were established for all nursing diagnostic categories in all data sets. The patient demographic profile consisted of sex, age, race and ethnicity, disposition, and length of stay (determined from date of admission and discharge elements). Table 1 illustrates the patient profiles for three nursing diagnoses based on data from one data set extracted from Site A. This showed that diagnostic groups were not significantly different in sex, race, or discharge disposition. However, significant differences ($p < .05$) in age and length of stay were noted among the three diagnostic categories. Patients who exhibited fluid volume excess were significantly older and had significantly longer lengths of stay than patient in other categories. Patients 0-14 years old had more fluid volume deficit related to active loss compared to other fluid volume diagnoses. For patients 15-65 years old, fluid volume deficit related to active loss was significantly more prevalent, whereas fluid volume excess was significantly less prevalent than other diagnosis.

Table 1

Patient Demographic Profile by NDX (Percent/Mean)

		Fluid Volume Deficit-Regulatory Mechanism	Fluid Volume Deficit-Active Loss	Fluid Volume Excess
Number		28	78	28
Sex	Male	44%	52%	37%
	Female	56%	48%	63%
Age		54.7	40.7	68.3
Race	White	89%	97%	100%
	Non-white	11%	3%	0%
Discharge	Home	89%	94%	82%
	Other	11%	6%	18%
LOS		6.2	6.5	16.3

Retrospective validation of defining characteristics for nursing diagnoses was completed within and across datasets from within and between sites. Sensitivity was used to determine validation; levels were evaluated consistent with the North American Nursing Diagnosis Association Guidelines for major (present in 80-100% of the population) and minor (present in 50-79% of the population) characteristics. Table 2 illustrates the sensitivity measures for the defining characteristics of fluid volume deficit related to regulatory mechanism for patients selected from two different datasets extracted from Site A. Two characteristics qualified as minor in the first dataset, one of the two again qualified as minor in a second dataset from the same site. Likewise, a comparison of sensitivities for fluid volume deficit related to active loss from two datasets within the same site demonstrated that five of the six characteristics exhibited similar sensitivities. Table 3 illustrates sensitivity of one defining characteristic, dependent edema, for the nursing diagnosis fluid volume excess across two data sets from Site A and one dataset from Site B.

Table 2

Sensitivity of Defining Characteristics of Fluid Volume Deficit Related to Regulatory Mechanism Across Datasets Within Site

Defining Characteristics	Sensitivity	
	Dataset 1	Dataset 2
Dry skin, mucous membrane	57.0	58.3
Weakness	57.0	33.3
Increased skin turgor	39.0	33.3
Increased body temperature	32.0	16.7
Thirst	21.0	8.3

The utility of the NMDS for determining direct nursing care costs within a specific Diagnostic Related Group (DRG) was determined by obtaining a stratified random sample of all patients in the DRG category #209: major joint and limb reattachment procedures within a four year period (N=211). Length of stay, average and total acuities, an frequency of nursing diagnoses were quantified. The average length of stay (8.57 days) was significantly (p<.05 shorter for 1990 compared to 1988 (11.2) and 1989 (11.02). The average acuity for 1990 was significantly highe (73.24 pints) compared to 1987 (62.37) and 1988 (65.24). This sample represented a total of 826 nursing diagnoses Two diagnoses occurred in greater than 50% of the patients in this DRG category: pain (91.9%) and impaire mobility (82%). Other diagnoses represented were self care deficit, bathing and hygiene (38.4%), knowledge defici regarding orthopedic status (36.5%), impaired shin integrity (23.7%), and potential for infection (10%). Nursin interventions documented in the NMDS represented actual care delivered. Hours of direct nursing care per patier were consequently determined. The mean total nursing time per patient hospital stay was 68.38 hours. Using th staff mix component of the intensity element of the NMDS the mean costs for direct nursing care were calculated t be $1641.20 based on an average $24/hour pay rate. Given a Medicare DRG charge of $12,765 and a reimbursemen of $8,944 per patient, 21.3% of the reimbursement was consumed for direct nursing care.[7]

Table 3 Validation of Defining Characteristic Dependent Edema for Fluid Volume Excess Across Sites

Defining Characteristic	Sensitivity	
	Site A	Site B
Dependent edema	68.0	57.2
	66.7	

The research utility of the NMDS for forecasting frequency and trends in nursing diagnoses was analyzed. The frequency of occurrence of each nursing diagnosis was compiled from 1987-1990 in Site A. Profiles of the frequency of each diagnosis for each year were established. Data analysis using multiple linear regression techniques yielded R values ranging from 0.920-0.929. It appeared that it is possible to predict the frequency of occurrence of nursing diagnoses. If coupled with the cost analysis data related to direct nursing care, this approach may provide a quantifiable method for more precisely predicting consumption of nursing resources.

4. Summary

Seven studies have begun to establish the usefulness of the NMDS. The NMDS elements were available in two acute care sites. A cost efficient method for electronic data retrieval has been established. The NMDS has been used to develop patient demographic profiles within nursing diagnostic categories. Retrospective nurse validation of nursing diagnoses has occurred within and between sites. One method for demonstrating the forecasting capability of the NMDS has been demonstrated. Moreover, a method for using the *intensity* element of the NMDS to determine costs of direct nursing care has been developed.

Although the NMDS has the potential to provide the data necessary to measure patient outcomes, increased standardization of the nursing taxonomies for nursing diagnoses, interventions, and outcomes must occur. Lastly, studies to determine costs of nursing care and consumption of resources rely on the availability of the *intensity of nursing care* element as well as the other nursing care elements of the NMDS

References

1] Agency for Health Care Policy and Research. *Report to Congress: The feasibility of linking research-related data bases to federal and non-federal medical administrative data bases.* (AHCPR Pub. No. 91-0003), 1991. Washington, DC: U.S. Government Printing Office.

2] National Committee on Vital and Health Statistics. *Long-term health care: Minimum data set* (DHHS Pub. No., PHS 80-1158). Hyattsville, MD: National Center for Health Statistics, 1980.

3] National Committee on Vital and Health Statistics. *Uniform hospital discharge data: Minimum data set* (DHHS Pub. No., PHS 80-1157). Hyattsville, MD: National Center for Health Statistics. 1980.

4] National Committee on Vital and Health Statistics. *Uniform ambulatory medical care: Minimum data set* (DHHS Pub. No., PHS 81-1161). Hyattsville, MD: National Center for Health Statistics, 1981.

5] Werley H, Lang N and Westlake S. (1986). Brief summary of the nursing minimum data set. *Nursing Management*, 17(7), 42-45.

6] Waltz C, Strickland C, and Lenz E. *Measurement in research.* Philadelphia: F.A. Davis Company, 1984.

7] *Hospital Technology Scanner.* November, 1992.

Nursing Informatics: An International Overview for Nursing in a Technological Era
S.J. Grobe and E.S.P. Pluyter-Wenting, eds.

174

Prevalence and Relationships Among Elements
of the Nursing Minimum Data Set

Ryan P[a] Coenen A[b] Devine E C[c] Werley H H[c]
Sutton J[a] and Kelber S[c]

[a] *Dept. of Nursing, Milwaukee County Medical Complex, 8700 W. Wisconsin Ave., Milwaukee, WI 53226*

[b] *College of Nursing, Marquette University, 530 N. 16th, Milwaukee, WI 53233*

[c] *School of Nursing, University of Wisconsin-Milwaukee, Box 413, Milwaukee, WI 53201*

The purpose of this study was to describe the prevalence and relationships among elements of the Nursing Minimum Data Set for select patients in an acute care hospital during one year. Among the results of this study it was noted that nursing diagnoses are similar within and across medical diagnostic categories; Related Factors clearly influenced the selection of nursing interventions; there was large range of nursing time for all Related Factors and a small range of skill mix; and approximately 75% of outcomes were achieved by the time patients were discharged from the hospital. It was concluded that the NMDS provided a valuable framework for the examination of clinical nursing data.

The Nursing Minimum Data Set (NMDS) was derived from the concept of the Uniform Minimum Health Data Sets, and it is a standardized set of elements that facilitates the abstraction of minimum, essential, core, nursing data from health records. The NMDS elements have been documented in patient records from hospitals, nursing homes, home health care agencies, community nursing centers, and ambulatory clinics [1-5]. At this time data-based descriptions of nursing practice are not widespread. The purpose of this study was to describe the prevalence and relationships among elements of the NMDS for select patients in an acute care hospital during the year 1991.

Research Questions

1. What are the nursing diagnoses (NsgD) for patients with five of the most frequently occurring primary medical diagnoses (MedD) and five of the most frequently occurring primary surgical procedures (SurgP)?
2. What are the nursing interventions, patient outcomes, and intensity of nursing care in patients with each of the six most frequently occurring NsgD?

Method

The setting was a public hospital that shared services with six other facilities comprising a Regional Health Care Center in the Midwest. The number of patients admitted to the hospital during 1991 was 13,135. The hospital had a computerized nursing information system (NIS) that linked the elements of the NMDS and used the North American Diagnosis Association (NANDA) classification system [6]. On-line care planning provided the professional nurse with the framework for selecting aspects of standardized care plans, while individualizing the plan to meet the needs of each patient. Records of patients with selected MedD, SurgP, and NsgD were sampled. The primary MedD and SurgP were abstracted by medical record's personnel following discharge during 1991.

Elements of the NMDS were downloaded from the computerized NIS, placed in a fixed American Standard Code for Information Interchange (ASCII) file, and transferred to a University computer center for analysis. Approval by the appropriate Committees for the Protection of Human Subjects was obtained.

Question One. The most frequently occurring primary MedD included: maintenance chemotherapy (n = 322), chest pain (n = 292), congestive heart failure (n = 269), intermediate coronary syndrome (n = 219), and acute pancreatitis (n = 191). The most frequently occurring primary SurgP included: open reduction fixation tibia/fibula (n = 142), wound debridement (n = 107), vitrectomy (n = 60), total cholecystectomy (n = 59), and appendectomy (n = 51). The diagnostic categories in this setting reflected the distribution of services shared across the medical center. The mean age for the MedD and SurgP groups were 53 and 41 years respectively. In general, there was an even distribution of men and women across MedD categories, with the exception of more male patients with acute pancreatitis (78%). More men had SurgP except for total cholestectomies (61% women). Of the total sample for question one, 52% Caucasians, 41% African Americans, and 7% Others. Diagnoses that did not reflect this trend included vitrectomy (91.7% Caucasians) and acute pancreatitis (63.3% African Americans). Payer source was primarily governmental, reflecting the case mix of the patients served by this public facility.

Identification of the five most frequent NursD for each MedD and SurgP suggests that select NursD were used for each diagnosis or procedure (Table 1). Two NursD (Pain and Injury Potential) were among the NursD used most frequently for patients with all of the MedD and SurgP. However there was a wide range in the frequency that the diagnoses were used. Pain was the most prevalent diagnosis for seven of the MedD procedures. The second most prevalent NursD differed for each of the other MedD and SurgP.

Clusters of NursD were apparent within each MedD and SurgP. Some NursD (e.g., Cardiac Output/Decreased) were more common with the selected MedD and others (e.g., infection potential) more common with selected SurgP. The mean number of NursD for patients with either MedD or SurgP was identical (mean = 1.74). However a greater number of the diagnostic labels from the 1988 (NANDA) Approved Nursing Diagnostic Categories [6] were used in the primary MedD group (M = 29, range 24 - 33) than the SurgP group (M = 21, range 8 - 34) (t [8] = 3.54, p < 0.05).

Question Two. The most frequently occurring NursD for patients hospitalized during 1991 included: pain (n = 4397), potential for injury (n = 2942), anxiety (n = 2474), decreased cardiac output (n = 1796), potential for infection (n = 1038), and knowledge deficit (n = 996). The mean age was 47 years. In general, there was an even distribution of men and women across selected NsgD categories. In the sample for question two, 60% were Caucasians, 34% African Americans, and 6% Others. Payer source was similar to the sample for question one. There was a wide range in length of stay for all NsgD categories, with a mean of 8.6 days and a median of 4.0 days for the total sample.

The prevalence of Related Factors for each diagnostic label was examined. A Related Factor was defined as condition/circumstance that contributes to the development/maintenance of a NsgD [7]. Although each diagnostic label may have many multiple Related Factors, only two or three of these Related Factors were used frequently. For example, for patients with the diagnosis of anxiety the five Related Factor occurred 49%, 28%, 4%, 2%, and 2% of the time (Table 2). This pattern was the same for all six NsgD.

The prevalence of nursing interventions were examined according to the 16 category classification system proposed by the Task Force of the NMDS Conference Group [8]. Intervention categories associated with two of the six diagnostic labels are displayed on Table 2. The intervention categories differed across Related Factors of the NsgD suggesting that in addition to the diagnostic label, the Related Factors clearly influenced the selection of interventions. For example, in patients with anxiety, the intervention of "emotional support" was used most frequently (48%) for the Related Factor of unfamiliar surroundings, tests, or procedures (hereforth called unfamiliar procedure); "teaching" was used most frequently (75%) with patients having surgery; and, "coordination and collaboration" was most common (63%) with patients with uncertain discharge plans.

Multiple outcomes were identified for each Related Factor, with a mean of 2.6 to 3.7 outcomes per factor. Outcomes reflected the acute nature of the patient condition or status. Two examples of outcomes linked to the diagnostic label of decreased cardiac output were "demonstrated adequate system perfusion" and "demonstrated improved cardiac output within base line range." The NsgD and outcomes were re-evaluated at regular intervals during the hospital stay and at discharge. Approximately 75% of the outcomes were achieved and the NsgD were discontinued. Approximately 3% of the outcomes were not achieved. Of the remaining outcomes it was not possible to determine whether (a) the diagnosis remained active, or (b) if the diagnosis and outcomes were not re-

Table 1.
Number (%) of the Five Most Frequent Nursing Diagnoses for Select Medical Diagnoses and Surgical Procedures

	Primary Medical Diagnoses					Primary Surgical Procedures				
Nursing Diagnosis	Mchem $n=322$	CPain $n=292$	CHF $n=269$	ICS $n=219$	APanc $n=191$	ORFT/F $n=142$	WDebri $n=107$	Vitrec $n=60$	TChole $n=59$	Append $n=51$
Nutrition/ Impaired	126 (39)									
Knowledge Deficit	119 (37)					15 (11)		26 (43.3)		
Injury/ Potential	56 (17)	21 (7)	71 (26)	29 (13)	75 (39)	17 (12)	21 (20)	9 (15.0)	28 (47)	11 (22)
Anxiety	47 (14)	43 (14)		29 (13)			18 (17)	29 (48.3)	15 (25)	14 (27)
Pain	37 (12)	166 (57)	35 (13)	142 (65)	160 (84)	79 (56)	60 (56)	15 (25.0)	53 (90)	44 (86)
CO/ Decreased		109 (37)	141 (52)	123 (56)						
Coping Ineffect		20 (7)			39 (20)					
Fluid Vol. Alter			80 (30)						5 (9)	
Breathing Pattern			40 (15)	13 (1)						
Health Maint.					98 (51)	7 (5)			3 (5)	
Infect. Pot.					17 (4)		26 (24)			6 (12)
Mobil. Impaired						39 (27)		3 (5.0)		
Skin Integ. Impaired							19 (18)			
Commun. Impaired										5 (10)

Note: Column % totals may exceed 100 as patients frequently have multiple nursing diagnoses. Empty cells do not equal 0, as only the five most frequent nursing diagnoses were reported for each primary medical diagnoses/surgical procedure.

Key: Abbreviation, Diagnosis, and ICD9 Code
MChem - Maintenance Chemotherapy, V581
Cpain - Chest Pain, 78650
CHF - Congestive Heart Failure, 4280
ICS - Intermediate Coronary Syndrome, 4111
Apanc - Acute Pancreatitis, 5770
ORFT/F - Open Reduction Fixation Tibia/Fibia, 7936
Wdebri - Wound Debridement, 8622
Vitrec - Vitrectomy, 1474
Tchole - Total Cholecystectomy, 5122
Append - Incidental Appendectomy, 471

Table 2

Prevalence and Percent of Intervention Categories for Select Nursing Diagnoses and Related Factors

Nursing Diagnoses / Related Factors n (%)	INTERVENTION CATEGORIES*										Total n (%)
	1	2	3	6	8	9	10	11	12	13	
PAIN n = 4397 (100)	4422 (19)	1879 (8)	4548 (19)	2571 (11)	687 (3)	7685 (33)		1328 (6)	1 (<1)	38 (<1)	23646 (100)
Altered comfort n = 1928 (44)	2479 (18)	1497 (11)	3043 (22)	1756 (13)		3911 (28)		1145 (8)			13834 (59)
Surgical incision n = 638 (15)	869 (16)		1361 (26)	869 (16)	662 (12)	1684 (32)					5338 (23)
Chest pain n = 393 (8)	1036 (37)	359 (13)				1441 (50)					2838 (12)
Immobility, Limb n = 43 (<1)						59 (65)			29 (32)		88 (<1)
ANXIETY n = 2474 (100)	443 (3)	23 (<1)		23 (<1)	5304 (34)	7911 (51)	1143 (7)	81 (<1)	23 (<1)		15472 (100)
Unfamiliar surrounding n = 1233 (49)		58 (<1)			3494 (48)	2918 (40)	14 (<1)				7245 (46)
Surgical procedure n = 701 (28)	267 (7)				332 (8)	2922 (75)	371 (10)				3888 (25)
Uncertain discharge plans n = 122 (4)	15 (3)	60 (11)			98 (18)	11 (2)	348 (63)				549 (35)
Transfer to unfam. hospital n = 54 (2)					110 (41)	23 (9)	31 (12)		15 (6)		266 (2)
Hickman catheter n = 51 (2)	7 (2)				49 (15)	220 (69)	21 (7)		8 (3)		320 (2)

*Key Intervention Categories

1 Monitoring/surveillance
2 Activities of daily living
3 Comfort
4 Airway maintenance+
5 Applications/treatments+ +
6 Medications
7 Invasive insertions+ +
8 Emotions support/counseling

9 Teaching
10 Coordination/collaboration
11 Protection
12 Assisting others providers
13 Preventative services+ +
14 Providing a therapeutic environment+ +
15 Nutrition and fluid balance+ +
16 Therapeutic activities+

+ Not used.
+ + Less than 1%

evaluated. Each outcome also was achieved approximately 75% of the time.

Within the NMDS nursing intensity was defined by the two subelements of total time of nursing care and staff mix [8]. The NIS contained time (predetermined for each nursing intervention) and staff mix for all direct and indirect patient care. The total time and staff mix were determined for the most frequent Related Factors within each NsgD. There was great variation in time for each Related Factor. For example, the total time for "anxiety related to unfamiliar surroundings/ procedures/test" ranged from 0 to 492 hours of nursing care, with a mean of 10.0 hours and a median of 2.9 hours. Consistently more time was required of the professional (registered nurse) than the skilled (license practical nurse) and unskilled (nursing assistant) care provider.

Discussion and Conclusions

NsgD for the most frequent MedD and SurgP were identified. A greater number of distinct categories from the NANDA Accepted Nursing Diagnosis List [6] were selected for the MedD group than for the SurgP group. Persons in the surgical group, with the exception of wound debridement, had similar NsgD. Given the variability of NsgD within MedD groups, this finding has implications for the development of critical paths.

Nursing interventions were associated with Related Factors for each diagnostic label. Although it has been suggested that Related Factor, as well as the diagnostic label, are determinates of the intervention, the results of this study support this conclusion empirically. Further development of the NANDA classification system to include Related Factors is recommended. In addition, future efforts to link any classification system of nursing interventions with NsgD requires further exploration of these relationships.

The nursing care element of intensity currently includes measures of both time and skill mix [8]. It would be helpful in describing practice across settings to aggregate intensity by patient encounter (e.g., hospital shift/day, clinic visit) rather than length of stay.

It was proposed originally that the variables contributing to the difference in outcome achievement could be examined with these data. However, the majority of outcomes were resolved by the time patients were discharged from the hospital. It was apparent that these outcome indicators were short term, acute care focused, and should be resolved prior to discharge. This finding has implications for the development of a classification of outcome measures and the need to consider the multiple settings across a continuum of care.

The use of the NMDS, a computerized NIS, and a consistent language (e.g., NANDA) provided data that were aggregated and elements of the NMDS that were linked in order to describe nursing practice. It is recommended that data from this one setting be compared with data from other acute care settings.

References

[1] Devine EC and Werley HH. Test of the Nursing Minimum Data Set: Availability of data and reliability. *Research in Nursing and Health* 1988, 11: 97-104.

[2] Tillman HJ. Test of the Nursing Minimum Data Set in a Nursing Center. Unpublished Master's Thesis: Marquette University, Milwaukee WI, 1990.

[3] Hays BJ. Nursing Care Requirements and Resource Consumption in Home Health Care. Nursing Research 1992, 41: 138-143.

[4] Marek KD. Analysis of the Relationships Among Nursing Diagnosis and Other Selected Patient Factors. Unpublished Doctoral Dissertation, University of Wisconsin-Milwaukee, Milwaukee, WI, 1992.

[5] Martin K, Scheet N and Stegman MR. Home Health Clients: A Descriptive Analysis of their Problems, Outcomes of Care, and Nursing Interventions. *American Journal of Public Health*, in press.

[6] Approved Nursing Diagnostic Categories. In *Classification of Nursing Diagnoses: Proceedings of the Eight Conference.* Carroll-Johnson RM (ed). Philadelphia: JB Lippincott, 1989:515-516.

[7] Nursing Diagnosis Submission Guidelines and Diagnostic Review Cycle. In *Classification of Nursing Diagnoses: Proceedings of the Ninth Conference.* Carroll-Johnson RM (ed). Philadelphia: JB Lippincott, 1991: 373-377.

[8] Werley HH and Lang NM. *Identification of the Nursing Minimum Data Set.* New York: Springer Publishing, 1988.

NURSING HEALTH INFORMATION SYSTEMS

A. Development, implementation and evaluation

Nursing Informatics: An International Overview for Nursing in a Technological Era
S.J. Grobe and E.S.P. Pluyter-Wenting, eds.

The whole patient: I T connects the pieces

Marr P B

Hospital Information System, New York University Medical Center, 550 First Avenue, New York, NY 10016

The age of information is here and healthcare is playing an active role in its evolutionary process. The Institute of Medicine has recommended that by the year 2001 healthcare will have in place a computerized comprehensive patient record. The impact of large, longitudinal, relational databases on healthcare will be positive, but its total impact will be left for others in the future to assess. This new approach to patient records will provide a base of knowledge for clinical practice, research, education and administration to enhance our ability to effectively and efficiently deliver quality patient care. The ethical issues of privacy, confidentiality, compliance and cultural beliefs will present challenges to all of us as we progress along the continuum of this new frontier.

1. Introduction

The Institute of Medicine has recommended that by the year 2001 healthcare delivery systems will use a computerized comprehensive, longitudinal patient record to provide all clinical, financial and research data. The significant word in "Computerized Patient Record" is the word patient. To date, efforts have been directed toward the computerization of the medical record which serves as the documentation for care delivered to a patient by an inpatient facility and remains the property of that facility. The computerization of a patient record implies the intent for the information to transcend institutional boundaries and the patient becomes the center of focus, not the service or care provider.[1] The traditional practice of providing care based on clinical data collected during a single episode in one care setting is no longer acceptable; care decisions and expected outcomes need to be based on information gathered over the lifetime of the patient, regardless of the provider or clinical setting.[2]

2. Impact on Healthcare

Lifetime, individual health records will allow us to trend diseases by decade of life, environmental impact, cultural differences, genetic mapping and the interrelationship of two or more variables. Information that results from pooled data will enable researchers to solve many of the disease mysteries facing us today. The "not so common" occurrences will form populations large enough for relationships to provide ready answers. And, because we will be able to more quickly determine what does and does not work, our ability to deliver quality healthcare should greatly improve. This new approach to patient records will provide a base of knowledge for clinical practice, research, education and administration that currently is beyond our comprehension.

For example, individuals will become more active participants in their healthcare. Each will have a current, up-to-date health record starting at birth, continuing through childhood immunizations to puberty, early adulthood, child bearing years and then on to late-life health episodes. As a result of this increased participation in one's healthcare, it is expected that the current trend of wellness and disease prevention will be enhanced. But as we develop the new patient record, we must tend to the delicate balance between maintaining patient confidentiality and the need to address the healthcare issues of the larger population.

3. Computer-Based Patient Record Institute, Inc.

Achieving a computerized patient record will be an evolutionary, not a revolutionary process. Both national and international healthcare providers are starting at various points along the continuum of information technology (IT), developing from their own institutional foundations. The goal of a total computerized record thus requires us to coordinate multiple activities, in a way that has not been previously necessary. In January, 1992, the Computer-Based Patient Record Institute, Inc. (CPRI) was formed to provide this coordination. Representation in CPRI is broad-based, since organizations which traditionally have divergent views must be involved. Membership from the major healthcare organizations include the American Nurses Association, American Hospital Association, American Medical Informatics Association, American College of Physicians, American Medical Association, and the American Health Information Management Association. Additionally, there are representatives from vendors, insurers, healthcare facilities, consumer and patient advocacy groups, employers and the business community.

Five major work groups have been formed within the CPRI to address the major issues in greater depth.[3] The Codes and Structure Group is responsible for developing standard messages and identifiers. This will enable the data elements to be combined - as well as define a communication vehicle - from which the large databases will be created. As the Agency for Health Care Policy and Research (AHCPR) continues developing clinical practice guidelines, outcomes can be evaluated for their effectiveness and efficiency. The CPRI Justification Group will attempt to demonstrate how various concepts and approaches can be used for optimal results. Demonstration projects will be designed to measure various approaches to determine the attributes most beneficial to the individual as well as the larger population. Patient and provider confidentiality issues will be addressed by the Confidentiality, Privacy and Legislation Group. Patient confidentiality is perhaps the area of greatest concern for those individuals initially exposed to computerization. After further consideration, one often realizes that the present manual system is far from secure. It is highly likely that well-designed computerized patient databases will provide a level of security that is impossible in the manual system. Barry Barber from the United Kingdom has stated that the widespread availability of micro-computers, computer networks and powerful multi-access centralized systems increase both the risks to confidentiality and the opportunities for securing effective security at the same time.[4] The Professional Dialogue Group will enhance CPRI work by stimulating interest and developing knowledgeable users and consumers. Their task is to articulate the possibilities and benefits to be gained from this massive endeavor. Visionaries are required to inspire and motivate the numerous healthcare disciplines for the long, tedious task ahead. The fifth work group and arguably the most important is Finance. They are responsible for obtaining funding sources through contributions, grants, and endowments.

4. Issues

We assume that progress will occur rapidly in some areas while others will be delayed by major obstacles. It is too early to know when or where this will occur. We only know that for the creation of the computerized patient record all the major issues must be addressed and resolved. When protocols are developed,
guidelines are agreed upon, and data transmission standards attain universal acceptance, we will be well down the road toward universal healthcare.

A multitude of issues needs to be addressed along the way. Who is responsible for maintaining the accuracy and completeness of the individual record - the provider of the care or the individual client? Is the individual compelled to document socially aberrant behavior? Is the termination of an unwanted pregnancy to be available in the life time record? As knowledge is gained in treatment protocols resulting in disease prevention or cure, what is the relationship to compliance? Will society carry the costs of those individuals who willingly choose not to comply to known health maintenance standards? Further, not all societies or cultures share the same definitions for health and sickness; but as national databases mature, these differences will become more obvious. A means must be found for maintaining cultural uniqueness and diversity while promoting international healthcare.[5]

5. Approach of One Healthcare Provider

Following are examples of how one healthcare provider is starting to connect the pieces of information technology. This institution's nursing documentation committee, meeting over a number of years, has imbedded standards of care and practice guidelines in the computerized documentation process. Patient assessment requirements by clinical specialty and/or disease process have been computerized, thereby enabling the practitioner to move from the general to the specific as is appropriate for an individual patient. This has enhanced the accuracy and completeness of the documentation and presents it in a logical, thorough manner. In the rehabilitation division the initial Functional Independence Measure (FIM) data are entered into the computer as well as functionality at time of discharge. This information is used to compare various treatment modalities within the institution and is then transferred to a national database for inter-institutional outcome comparisons.

Quality assurance activities are supported in numerous ways via the computer. Medication alerts are automatically generated on the patient care worksheet when the patient is receiving one of these drugs: they inform the nurse of untoward interactions, administration, dosage or side effects. Reminders are provided automatically to the nurse if medications have not been documented within a specific time frame. Informational screens guide the practitioner in preparing a patient for various invasive procedures. They also provide laboratory test collection guidelines. The practitioner is alerted if a service is available only during certain hours or if specific pre-procedure protocols are mandatory. Data are collected on individual patient activities and then aggregated with other patient data, helping thereby to determine trends and/or the effectiveness of a specific quality assurance program.

Regulatory compliance is met in various ways. For example, recertification of cardio-pulmonary resuscitation (CPR) skills are required at defined intervals depending on the clinical specialty. The didactic portion of this review is on the computer, followed by a multiple choice questionnaire, to be completed at the nurse's convenience during working hours. At the end of the tour of duty, the nurse delivers the answer sheet to the nursing practice laboratory where the manual CPR can be performed quickly, completing the certification process. Female patients were not routinely being questioned when they last had a pap smear. This question was placed in the initial admission assessment pathway and follow-up audits revealed near total compliance.

When patients are awaiting transfer from the acute care setting to a less acute setting they are placed on an alternate level of care (ALOC) status. Regulations in this instance require that these patients be followed by a nutritionist and a recreational therapist and when appropriate, by a rehabilitation therapist. When a physician orders that the patient be sent to a less acute setting, the nutritionist, recreational therapist and appropriate others are automatically notified.

6. Summary

In some clinical settings the pieces of the puzzle are already being put together. These early efforts have provided major advances in the effectiveness and efficiency in the delivery of healthcare at these institutions. So this is not a dream but a reality, which makes it all the more exciting. Much needs to be done before we reach the goal of a computerized, longitudinal patient record but if we combine our intellect, creativity, energy and resourcefulness it will happen.

7. References

[1]   Hanson RL. Message from the chair of the 1992 HIMSS publications committee. In: *Healthcare Information Management* 1993:7-1.

[2]   Boyer AG and Levine HS. Clinical information needs in ambulatory care: Building a longitudinal patient record. In: *Healthcare Information Management* 1993:7-1.

[3]   Computer-based Patient Record Institute, Inc. 1992.

[4]   Barber B. Data protection and a secure environment for nursing: Information technology security. In: *Lecture Notes in Medical Informatics '91*. Marr PB, Axford RL, Newbold SK (eds). Heidelberg: Springer-Verlag 1991:157-159.

[5]   Mandil SH. On the interaction between health informatics, the individual and society. In: *Lecture Notes in Medical Informatics '91*. Marr PB, Axford RL, Newbold SK (eds). Heidelberg: Springer-Verlag, 1991:3-8.

Nursing Informatics: An International Overview for Nursing in a Technological Era
S.J. Grobe and E.S.P. Pluyter-Wenting, eds.

184

Planning, Implementation and Evaluation of System Downtime Procedures

Wierz C

Nursing Information Systems, Fairfax Hospital, 3300 Gallows Road, Falls Church, Virginia 22046, USA

Clinicians agree that the benefits of computerizing the medical record certainly outweigh those of the current manual systems found in most health care institutions. The list of benefits has been well documented over the years, with little argument over its effects.

What has not been discussed or documented as thoroughly is the issue of documentation backup procedures to help process orders and administer medicines in the event (and it does happen) that computer systems fail or "crash." Consistent, manageable, and easily initiated backup documentation procedures are as important as the computer system itself. The health care industry's growing dependency on computer systems should be tempered with uptodate downtime procedures that will support current nursing practice in the event of system downtime and that will sustain clinicians until systems are again online.

Our institution recently developed and implemented downtime procedural policies specific to the order entry, report retrieval and medication administration documentation processes. These new policies not only will support our clinicians during system downtime but also will provide the backup procedures essential to possible future system upgrades.

1. Identification of Need

Our clinical staff found that our current downtime procedures do not adequately support our daily clinical operations, specifically order communications and medication administration documentation. Instead, these current procedures created confusion, stress, and chaos. For example, ordering of lab tests were done by telephone on some units, and by manual requisitions on other units. Theses differences made recovery of orders into the computer system quite difficult once the system was again online.

To correct this situation, the Nursing Information Systems Downtime Task Force, a subcommittee of the Nursing Information Systems Council, was developed, consisting of staff RNs, unit secretarial support, and nursing management. This task force was assigned the responsibility of developing system downtime procedures that would support both manual order communication practices and manual medication administration documentation.

2. Policy Objectives Stage

In order to successfully plan and implement manual downtime procedures, the task force developed four policy objectives to ensure that desired outcomes would be achieved. These objectives were as follows:

1. Downtime order entry procedures must be easy to initiate and follow.
2. Procedures must follow current practices, with minimal changes in process.
3. All departments must share the responsibility of developing the policies, with subsequent responsibility in actual order processing during downtime.
4. Procedures must be developed that are standard, regardless of the computer system being used in the institution.

3. Data Gathering Stage

The task force began gathering data on current procedures used during scheduled and unscheduled system downtimes. This information was necessary to identify those outdated practices that would need to be corrected in the development of new procedures. In addition, this data would provide the task force with information on "underground" or unitspecific procedures that have been developed to cope with system downtimes in the absence of standardized procedures.

The major issues identified in the datagathering stage included the following:

1. Clinical departments, for example, radiology and laboratory had different ideas about the exact procedures that were to be followed by clinicians during a system downtime. For example, radiology expected the nursing staff to recover orders into the computer system once it was again online whereas laboratory wanted to perform the task of recovery themselves.

2. These informal procedures were not documented and, therefore were difficult to adhere to.

3. Timeframes for initiating downtime procedures were inconsistent from department to department. Some departments expected downtime procedures to begin immediately following the beginning of the downtime whereas some departments wanted the procedures to begin after a specific period of time into the downtime.

4. Manual requisitions and forms, if available, were not in a standard format or in a central location. Those departments lacking manual requisitions relied too heavily on the telephone to process orders, often slowing up order processing. This slowdown was due to duplicate communications, once by telephone and then by manual requisition.

5. Units had developed their own internal mechanisms for tracking active orders. Examples of these mechanisms included carbon-copied notepads, handwritten kardexes, and perpetual reuse of the last systemgenerated worksheets.

6. Units had assumed responsibility for recovery of all orders once the system was again available. This created general confusion for ancillary departments and additional workload for nursing units. This confusion came because of the different ideas about procedures that were to be followed, (as explained in #1).

7. Medication administration documentation was done in the progress notes during system downtime, creating fragmented medication records and information that was generally unavailable for other clinicians.

4. Policy Development Stage

Using the four criteria formulated in the policy objectives stage and the seven major issues identified in the datagathering stage, the task force began drafting a proposed policy. The structure of the policy would be general in scope, with subsequent addendum addressing each of the major ancillary departments and their specific procedures.

Formulating the general policy proved to be extremely challenging for the task force because major rules and timelines had to be developed that would affect all clinical areas. Three major policy statements were adopted:

1. All ancillary departments are responsible for recovering their own manual downtime orders. By adding this responsibility in the context of greater control over ordering statistics, workload, and charging, the departments readily accepted this new function.

2. The timeframe for recovery of downtime orders will occur according to the following criteria:
    a. If downtime lasts less than 8 hours, orders will be recovered within 2 hours.
    b. If downtime lasts more than 8 hours, orders will be recovered within 24 hours of the time the system came back online.

3. Downtime procedures would begin once the system was unavailable for more than 1 hour, allowing for flexibility in the event the downtime is short.

This second policy statement was adopted to provide timely information for all clinicians. Given the increased acuity and shorter lengths of stay for hospitalized patients, it is important that information be recovered as soon as possible once systems are again available. Once the major policy statements were identified and written, manual forms and downtime requisitions were developed to provide a clear and concise paper audit trail regarding orders communications and medication administration.

In total, nine requisitions and two manual forms were created in collaboration with the appropriate ancillary departments. The two manual forms developed were the Downtime Plan of Care and the Downtime Medication Record. Once completed, the policy included nine addendum addressing specific ancillary requirements and three addendum addressing specific issues or needs, listed below:

1. Procedures for Scheduled System Downtimes--Addresses the specific needs of each department during a scheduled downtime, when predetermined activities and tasks can be done in advance of the downtime.

2. Procedures for Filling Out the Downtime Plan of Care During Systems Downtimes--Describes the uses of the Downtime Plan of Care (manual kardex), which provides a paper audit trail of active orders during system downtime.

3. List of Departmental Downtime Requisitions--Provides a quick reference for the type and location of requisitions available for use during system downtime.

During this policy development stage, the task force worked closely with various departments and individuals to ensure the development of mutually agreedupon procedures. Those consulted included Corporate Information Systems, Volunteer Services, Nursing Education and Research, the Nursing Documentation Task Force, the Nursing Quality Improvement Council, and members of the nursing management team. Each contact provided valuable information and suggestions that were incorporated into the policy.

5. Testing and Approval Process Stage

To ensure that the primary objectives would be met, the draft policy needed to be tested. During the lengthy policy development stage, a number of scheduled and unscheduled system downtimes occurred that provided us with "live" test experiences. The task force seized these testing opportunities and conducted postdowntime meetings with key individuals to obtain feedback on the policy. These meetings proved valuable with regard to finetuning the draft.

Within one year of task startup, the task force sought final approval for its recommended system downtime procedures. From the Nursing Practice Congress, a shared governance model, the task force turned for final input and approval to 70 delegates (staff nurses representing all specialties and clinical areas). These 70 professionals actively participated in discussions involving downtime policy that affected their respective areas of clinical practice. The Nursing Practice Congress serves as the body to which structures supporting practice are accountable, as well as serves a primary role in integrating the activities of nursing committees that support nursing practice. The Nursing Practice Congress granted final approval of the recommended procedures after two sessions, allowing the task force to begin policy implementation.

In addition to approval from the Nursing Practice Congress, the task force obtained signoff and approval from all departments affected by the policy as well as from the other individuals and departments whose input and feedback was requested. Signoff criteria were developed to ensure that all parties were clear as to their new roles and responsibilities.

6. Implementation Stage

Recognizing that conscientious efforts had gone into developing this policy, the task force determined that similar efforts should go into the implementation of this work.

Continuing its collaboration, the task force solicited the input of unit clerical staff (unit secretaries) who have long been known to be key innovators of operational activities. The task force's purpose in doing so was to brainstorm for ideas on how to best implement the new policy and forms. This process generated the following ideas:

1. Distributing "Code Green" boxes, similar in idea to a crash cart, which would contain all information, forms, requisitions, manuals, and so forth necessary to efficiently continue orders communications and medication administration documentation during a system downtime. ("Code Green" in our institution was the definition of a system downtime.)

2. Developing posters to be used during unit inservices of these new policies and procedures. These posters showed sample completed forms and requisitions, addressing specific unit needs if necessary.

3. Creating a System Downtime Manual that includes all vital policy information.

Additional measures were taken to ensure successful policy implementation:

1. The task force provided system order communication and medication administration documentation recovery inservices. These inservices lasted approximately 1/2 hour each and gave both the task force and the participants (those who would recover orders) an opportunity to discuss outstanding issues and refamiliarize themselves with system functions.

2. Each member of the task force provided inservices to their assigned units/departments, using the posters discussed above. During these inservices, the "Code Green" boxes were also distributed, each containing a "starter set" of requisitions and forms, as well as the new System Downtime Manual.

3. The new system downtime policy was incorporated into the bimonthly nursing orientation program to ensure that all new staff are familiar with the process.

7. Evaluation Stage

Since the implementation of the policies and procedures, there have been no unscheduled computer system downtimes, therefore there is limited experience with which to evaluate the new process. The task force will continue to assemble focus groups to evaluate the effectiveness of the policy after scheduled and unscheduled system downtimes. Under the institution's continuous quality improvement philosophy, the policy document remains subject to changes and revisions.

Developing system downtime procedures has given the task force the opportunity to improve the operations of the clinical departments and units during system downtimes. Nursing's objectives have been met and will continue to be evaluated to ensure that, in the event of a system downtime, backup procedures remain consistent, manageable, and easy to carry out.

Nursing Informatics: An International Overview for Nursing in a Technological Era
S.J. Grobe and E.S.P. Pluyter-Wenting, eds.

Rapid Prototyping in the development of Nursing Information Systems: creating and using databases to improve patient care

Hoy JD, Hyslop A and Wojcik E

Management Executive of the National Health Service in Scotland, Directorate of Information Services, Health Systems Division, Keith House, 2 Redheughs Rigg, Edinburgh EH12 9DQ, Scotland.

Interest is growing in using the *output* from clinical systems, and particularly in exploiting the power of new technology in aggregating and widening access to clinical information for audit and research. The creation of such databases is now a matter of high priority and will influence the future use of information systems by nurses.

Development of effective information systems depends on three things: the satisfactory definition of user information requirements; the availability of affordable systems which support these requirements; and the implementation of these systems in the context of practice.

Experience with Nursing Information systems (NIS) has shown that system development has relied on the use of methodologies that have required users to have clear and readily specifiable statements of information requirements before development can begin. Inadequate specification produces systems that require revision following delivery as inadequacies are exposed, and users get a clearer idea of requirements through experience. This ongoing revision may delay delivery, add considerably to costs, and dent user confidence.

The continuing controversy over, for example, care planning, workload estimation, patient costing, and nursing classification, demonstrates the difficulty nurses have in defining exactly how a NIS will behave. Rapid Prototyping (RP) can be of use in situations where clients cannot initially define their requirements to the extent of producing a hard specification. Its use has grown recently as software engineering techniques have delivered rapid development platforms which can result in production-quality software. RP offers iterative development of a system specification with users guiding it along the way as they gain insight into what is achievable. This effectively brings the processes of information requirements analysis and system design much closer together.

A project using RP techniques to assist the development of commercial and centrally-funded NIS is described.

1. Development of NIS

1.1. The traditional approach

To date, Nursing Information Systems in Scotland have been either developed and funded by the national Health Service (NHS), or developed commercially. Whilst the first option offers advantages in control over development, and greater scope for participation of users, it has brought home the difficulties of involving users in system design and specification.

Most of our users have little or no experience of information systems. Present systems are uncertain in their methodology, and are being introduced in a climate of change which is resulting in uncertain practice and organisational structure. Uncertain users have problems with the hard specifications we have required for system development to date.

The result has tended towards the automation of existing practices, for example, in patient documentation, with tentative new development. This is a well-documented early phase in the adoption of technology to support new information systems [1].

1.2. Emerging standards

Emerging standards in information systems include a strong focus on data, with standard definitions and coding systems, and standard ways of accessing, protecting, exchanging and sharing data [2].

Of equal importance is a system's ability to respond to the rapidly changing context of health care, and achieve consistency across application.

With this goal in mind, the current trend is toward the use of business process modelling, using software to develop and maintain the resultant models, and then automate the production of software. Where these techniques are used effectively, the model can be updated and new software generated to reflect these changes [3].

1.3. Rapid Prototyping

Prototyping is an integral part of this process, allowing speedy development of partially-functioning systems, realistic enough to allow user interaction and reassessment of requirements. This is then used to amend the model, and a cycle of develop, test, and redevelop is maintained until an agreed level of functionality is reached [4].

NHS experience with the use of RP in large-scale projects is limited, but is being gained through projects such as the Directorate of Information Services' CARDEX project, which has developed a hospital-based medication ordering and administration system.

However, new PC-based applications are making small-scale projects more feasible. These projects may be useful in developing new methodologies, 'process' modelling, or working on information requirement's analysis.

Technology has made available new, more powerful, and more user-friendly PC packages able to access 'open' data over computer networks. These tools offer the flexibility and accessibility required for projects which bring together skilled users with clinical nurses to allow exploration of potential in systems and data. Such small-scale prototyping projects can guide the development of methods, e.g. new forms of care planning, or multidisciplinary records.

Results can be achieved quicker, using few resources, and should be closer to requirements because of early user involvement.

1.4. Advantages in development of NIS

From our experience, it is clear that even experienced users have difficulty in dealing with formal specifications of operational requirements. Prototyping is attractive in allowing early iterative development with users, analysts and system designers working together to define requirements. This addresses the old problem of users not knowing the full potential of a system until they have it.

While this inevitably extends the time required for this part of system development, there are reported gains in coding time, and more particularly in 'maintenance', which is often a euphemism for the correction of mistakes in the original specification, and can be very expensive [4].

2. Expectations from Ward Nursing Information Systems

Nurses in Scotland have over 20 years experience with Ward Nursing Information Systems (WNIS) as the CANIS system was first developed in Dundee in 1973. Based on this experience, a formal policy and strategy for nursing information systems was agreed with all interested parties in 1989. The key to this strategy was that a WNIS should support the following integrated functions:

- *care planning*
- *staffing and rostering*
- *workload estimation*
- *patient costing*
- *clinical audit*

While the first three functions are now in daily use in our hospitals, the last two are not, though for different reasons. Data to support costing, and the agreed methodologies to process it, are not available, while the early focus on care planning, which includes data on actual outcomes, has provided a large database of patient-related clinical information which is largely unused beyond the production of documentation.

2.1. Information for audit and research

Our systems therefore present us with a rich source of nursing information for clinical audit and research, but without the means to access it. The use of proprietary file formats precluded the use of third party database reporting software, while the complexity of the care planning data made ad hoc reporting facilities within the systems ineffective.

2.2. Audit and system evolution

These systems to date have simply swallowed up clinical data offering only labour-saving production of paper care plans as a benefit. Clinical data is therefore not structured and stored with retrieval in mind.

The current flurry of audit activity offers a means of tackling this. The use of care plans to support clinical audit will allow refinement of these care plans with an increased emphasis on information retrieval.

In short, given the tools to access aggregated clinical data, users will quickly discover how useful their documentation practices are.

3. Experience with Rapid Prototyping

3.1. The Ninewells' project

Sites with a computer based ward nursing information system have generally put a high value on innovation, and regarded their system as evidence of this. Paradoxically, these sites may become difficult test-beds for further innovation. Changes in methodology are likely to involve alterations to software and data structures, which may be costly and time-consuming, even assuming co-operation from suppliers.

However, work at Ninewells Hospital, in Dundee General Unit, has suggested ways of getting round this problem. Ninewells is an exceptional site, as a computer assisted WNIS has been in use there since 1973. Directorate of Information Services (DIS) nurses have been working with a small group of nurses making use of PC tools to develop the audit potential in the nursing record.

At Ninewells, the system produces a report of the nursing episode, made up of some demographic data, a record of patient movements within the hospital episode, and then a list of all items from the nursing care plan, including free text entries, all with the date of adding to, or deletion from, the care plan, and the identity of the user making the change. These records contain identified problems, expected and actual outcomes, and the associated interventions.

Nurses then have a history of all the nursing care given to a patient during the hospital stay, as far as it is present in the care plan. This has proved a useful concise document for filing in the patient's record, with the proviso that nurses must be satisfied that the care plan is an accurate account of the care actually delivered.

The potential for audit of this episode care plan was apparent. A simple modification of the system software allowed these records to be captured as text files whenever they were printed out as part of the discharge routine. These text files were transferred to a PC and data access and reporting software used to analyse them.

Simple statistics such as distribution of patients by age, sex, speciality and length of stay were readily produced. By querying the care plan data, reports on the incidence of particular problems could be generated, along with their associated outcomes.

The care plan libraries used on the system contained keywords for each library item, allowing reports to aggregate problems, for example, by keyword. Using this feature, one report allowed nurses to view actual outcomes by problem group, such as pain, wound care, etc.

3.2. Expected benefits

Using such information, we might expect two questions to arise:
- *does this information inform us about patient care?*
- *if so, what aspects of our practice do we need to address?*

The first question would look at care planning and documentation skills, and the extent to which the record tells nurses about what they are doing. If data are found to be missing or inadequate, then care planning libraries or documentation practices can be reviewed. This process will be easier if it is guided by system output aimed at a specific use.

As the record evolves to an acceptable form, the implications for practice can be considered. If, for example, pain is seen as being the most frequently occurring patient problem, and recorded outcomes show standards are not being achieved, then perhaps more specific outcomes are required to provide more accurate information. The care plan libraries can be amended with new outcome measures, and reports monitored following this to allow changes in pain management to be evaluated for clinical effect.

As a consequence, further benefits related to NIS development are expected. A frequent criticism of efforts aimed at improving documentation, or charting, is that resultant improvements in care are often claimed but seldom demonstrated [5, 6]. The development and use of a nursing database as described can allow the information in the nursing record to influence patient care.

This work has clarified the information requirements of clinical nurses and suggested ideas for developing care planning into a more useful and effective activity. Suppliers have shown a keen interest, and modification of existing systems is already in progress to make clinical data more accessible to the use of third party data access and reporting software.

4. Conclusions

Many of the information requirements for management and research functions hinge on the success of clinical systems in capturing patient or client-related data. Unless users perceive the effort of using these systems as worthwhile, the systems will fail [7].

By deriving new outputs from systems which up till now have asked clinical users simply to input data, these users will have a greater stake in the success of these systems, and find it easier to articulate, or even demonstrate, their future requirements to suppliers. Prototyping offers a means to facilitate this process and speed the evolution of more effective information systems.

Much of the work on standards, for example in clinical language and data definitions, will require the use of prototyping to demonstrate and win the hears and minds of users. By focussing on the demonstrable benefits of nursing databases based on patient or client records we are shifting the emphasis from clinical use feeding the system, to system feeding the user.

5. References

[1] Edwards C, Ward J, Bytheway A. *The Essence of Information Systems*. London: Prentice Hall, 1991.

[2] Directorate of Information Services of the National Health Service in Scotland. *National Technical Standards for Information Systems*. Unpublished, 1993.

[3] Rock-Evans R. *Data Modelling and Process Modelling*. Oxford, England: Butterworth-Heinemann Ltd, 1992.

[4] Maude T, Willis G. *Rapid prototyping: The management of software risk*. London: Pitman Publishing, 1991.

[5] Aidroos, N. Use and effectiveness of psychiatric nursing care plans. *Advanced Nursing* 1991, 16: 177-81.

[6] Holzemer WL, Henry SB, Klemm V. Comparison of computerized and manually generated nursing care plans. In: *Nursing Informatics* 1991. Hovenga EJS, Hannah KJ, McCormick KA, Ronald JS (eds). Berlin: Springer-Verlag, 1991: 447-51.

[7] Audit Commission. *Caring Systems: Effective Implementation of Ward Nursing Management Systems*. London: HMSO, 1992.

Nursing Informatics: An International Overview for Nursing in a Technological Era
S.J. Grobe and E.S.P. Pluyter-Wenting, eds.

Software Quality Assurance: A Critical Part of the Software Development Life Cycle

Zimmet J A

Nursing Administration, Good Samaritan Regional Medical Center, 1111 E. McDowell Rd., Phoenix, AZ 85006, U.S.A.

As Clinical Information Systems are developed to re-engineer the health care system, they are more complex in structure and design, and hence more prone to defects. Software used in health care is critical in scope and requires the utmost integrity. Knowledge about software quality assurance is important for the nurse involved in software development as well as for the nurse involved in the selection, purchase and installation of a clinical information system. This paper will provide a foundation for understanding software testing and validation as part of the software development cycle by defining and describing: the phases of the software development cycle, the stages of testing within each test phase and the testing techniques which can be employed during each phase. Examples of software applications and the testing techniques which should be employed are given.

1. Introduction

Clinical Information Systems (CIS) are now being developed to re-engineer the health care system. From structure and design perspectives, the clinical information system is comprised of code written in various languages, system and application programs, multiple databases, graphical user interfaces (GUIs), and interfaces among other information systems and monitoring devices. This increasingly complex software provides more opportunities for software defects or "bugs" to develop, and often more likely that fixing the bugs will result in new ones as a side effect. In both cases, these defects become increasingly difficult to detect. Unfortunately, in software quality assurance there is no perfect or complete test. A testing technique which may work on one project may not work on another. In order to meet the high integrity requirements of health care software which is life critical in scope, software quality assurance must uncover as many errors as possible earlier in the software life cycle with the least number of resources.

2. The Software Development Cycle

Numerous methods for software development exist. Some of the more common models include the waterfall model, testing with parallel development (the V model), the spiral model, object-oriented development, rapid prototyping model, clean room software engineering, and formal verification. The project scope of the software drives the testing goals which in turn drive the selection of a test methodology. For health care software, parallel development with comparison tests of the V Model (Figure 1) is recommended.

The V Model shows test development being conducted in parallel with software development. The left side represents development activities with requirements analysis, preliminary design, detailed design and code phases while the right side represents the corresponding test stages contained in the test phases. The dotted lines show control flow while the solid lines show information flow. The entire model demonstrates overlap and sequential dependence between both sides. For example, system tests are developed while software requirements are being analyzed, integration tests are designed while structure charts are being developed, and unit tests are designed and implemented while pseudocode is being written. Reviews are held for all phases.

During the Unit Test phase each developed software module is tested as an individual entity. Incremental testing of groups of software modules or subsystems while building larger software entities occurs during the Integration Test Phases. System testing tests the completed, integrated system. Alpha, Beta and Acceptance testing may occur on site depending on the number of sites which will receive the software.

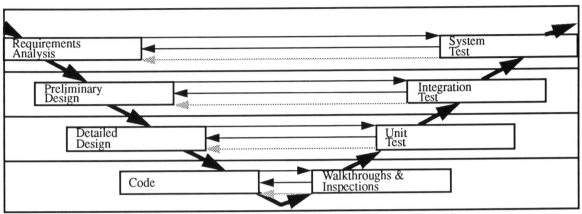

Figure 1. The V Model (Cartwright, 1989, p.III-6).

3. Stages of the Test Phase

Five stages comprise each test phase of the development life cycle. During the test plan and design stage the test plan and test design are generated based on the defined test phase objectives and the selected test strategy. Test cases and test procedures are developed during the test creation stages. Test code (e.g. test drivers, stubs, responders, test scripts, etc.) which is used for testing purposes only is also developed. In the test execution and result reporting stage tests are run according to the documentation generated in the previous two stages. Any failures detected are reported to a failure tracking system for defect isolation and fixing as well as metrics data collection. Status reports are created throughout this stage to report the progress of testing. The defect isolation and fixing (debugging) stage is composed of two substages. Change requests which have been evaluated by the change control board are implemented by the software developers. Defect fixes are then regression tested by the testers. The last stage consists of a postmortem meeting where problems that occurred during the test phases are identified and determination of what should have been done differently is made. Important feedback is provided to the developers and testers of this project and to the other projects within the organization

4. Unit Testing: Functional Testing

Unit testing employs functional testing and structural testing techniques. Functional testing is a dynamic testing technique that uses information about the inputs, outputs and the actions which must take place. Six basic functional testing methods can be used. These include: equivalence partitioning, boundary value analysis, cause and effect, syntax-directed, transition-flow and state-transition. In equivalence class partitioning the domain is partitioned into valid and invalid inputs. The assumption is made that if one value in an equivalence class is tested, then all the values in the equivalence class are tested thereby performing a limited amount of tests, but decreasing the possibility that errors exist. Boundary value analysis is a special case of equivalence class partitioning which focuses both on the input and output equivalence class. Conditions that are directly on, above, and beneath the edges of the input/output equivalence classes are explored. The cause and effect technique transforms functional specifications into a graph and then into a cause-effect decision matrix. By mapping inputs to outputs, the incompleteness and ambiguities are pointed out and the developer can select only those test cases which return the highest yield of errors. The syntax-directed method validates the system's tolerance for bad stream data through data parsing and handling input. Inputs and delimiters can be divided into valid and invalid cases. The transition flow technique verifies the flow of data through processes or computer programs. By the use of transition flow graphs, test cases are derived to meet path and loop coverages including extreme and peculiar cases. The state transition technique uses the finite state graph or table to verify the sequence of events in which the order of inputs is important. After a state-transition graph is created, the same path testing approach used with the transition flow testing technique is employed.

5. Unit Testing: Structural testing

Structural testing techniques look at the implementation details e.g. programming style, control method, source language, database design and coding details, and select test data based on the logic of the implementation to satisfy specified code coverage criteria. Common structural testing techniques include statement coverage, branch coverage, path coverage and data flow coverage. Statement coverage tests every executable and reachable statement in the program. While this method is easy it does not test the structure of the program. Branch coverages exercise every branch out of each decision node and every entry point to a block of code. Generally, all the statements are covered, but not all the conditions are exercised in each node. Condition coverage testing forces the true and false outcomes for each logical condition in a decision node, but not all the branches of each decision node are traversed. Path coverage is the strongest structural testing technique. All possible control paths are executed. Data flow analysis looks at both control flow and data flow. The path from where a data element is defined to where it is used is examined. By stringing the segments together, paths to test and the data that will force these paths to be followed are derived.

6. Integration testing

Integration testing demonstrates that even though components operated satisfactorily as individual units from unit testing, when the components are combined into larger entities new defects can be introduced. Integration testing can be divided into the areas of hierarchical and network integration

Hierarchical testing consists of top-down, bottom-up and sandwich testing techniques. Top-down testing starts with testing the topmost element over simplified programs which simulate the response provided by the real function called stubs. As testing is completed on the top-level component, the stubs of the next level are replaced with the real element and retesting is done to confirm that the real element is working correctly. Bottom-up testing starts with testing at the bottommost part. The next layer of functions are integrated and retesting occurs until the topmost level has been successfully integrated and tested. Sandwich testing is a hybrid technique which involves top-down and bottom-up testing simultaneously.

Network integration testing tests intertask communication, intertask synchronization, resource utilization among the components and hardware device interfacing.

7. System Testing

System Testing tests the complete product from the user's perspective. The following common testing categories should be exercised during the system test interval. Functional or system level testing demonstrates whether the system meets system specification objectives. Testing whether existing features continue to work occurs during regressions testing. Performance testing determines if the system's performance objectives are met. Attempts to "break" the system by stressing all its resources occurs during stress testing. Background testing subjects the system to real loads instead of no load. Configuration testing assures that the system operates under the logical/physical device assignment combination. Recovery testing verifies whether the system can recover from hardware/software failures and data errors. Usability, compatibility/conversion, reliability, security and volume are other testing categories which are also desirable to be performed during the system test interval.

8. Examples

8.1 Equivalence Partitioning and Boundary Value Analysis

Equivalence partitioning and boundary value analysis techniques can be used to test fields that comprise non-invasive blood pressure. In a clinical information system where the systolic and diastolic non-invasive blood pressure values are defined as XXX where X is an integer, and the systolic value must be greater than the diastolic value, and configurable ranges of unacceptable values are 300 and 0 for systolic, and 200 and 0 for diastolic, and the ranges for the limits for maximum warning are 299-200 for systolic and 199-120 for diastolic, and the limits for minimum warning are 70-1 for systolic and 20-1 for diastolic, the following values should be used:

Testing the limits of unacceptable values: 301/60,300/60, 299/60,1/0, 2/1, 0/-1, -1/-2, 220/201, 220/200, 220/199, 120/1, 120/0, and 120/-1

Testing the limits of warning: 300/60, 299/60, 298/60, 201/60, 200/60, 199/60, 71/60, 70/60, 69/60, 2/1, 1/0, 0/-1, 201/200, 200/199, 199/198, 180/121, 180/120, 180/119, 180/21, 180/20, 180/19, 180/2, 180/1 and 180/0

Testing systolic greater than diastolic: 80/90

Testing systolic and diastolic field properties: 9999/60, 120/9999, -9999/60, 120/-9999, 999/60, 120/999, -999/60, 120/-999, a/60, and 120/a where a equals any character.

Order of data input: test systolic then diastolic, test diastolic then systolic, test systolic alone, test diastolic alone.

The data above contains values which are one above, one below, borders as well as special cases.

8.2 Top-Down Testing

A top-down testing approach can be used to test the graphical display of non-invasive blood pressure values. In a clinical information system where data entered in a field can be displayed in user configurable graphs, the following values and approaches should be taken:

The fields should be tested as described in example 8.1 to verify that the functionality works correctly.

Different test cases which test the configuration capabilities of the graphs e.g. mix graph properties, mix the data types which can be displayed on the graph, should be set up.

Test cases which will test the limits of the graphs should be loaded through the non-invasive blood pressure field -- two non-invasive blood pressure values at the same time, non-invasive blood pressure values at the different limits (300/0, 300/200, 0/0, 201/200 and 100/60) at varying frequencies and durations over minutes, hours, days, weeks and months.

The following items should be verified -- data appears only where it should appear, the data displayed on the graph is the same as the data entered in the field in value and in any attached detailed information, the graphed data has full functionality as designed, the data entered in the fields is displayed on the graph as specified in the graph configuration and that the applications do not "crash".

8.3 System Testing

Functional and regression system testing techniques can be used to test system wide changes such as the impact of rollover to and from Daylight Savings Time. In a clinical information system all flowsheets, graphical display of data, reports, interfaces to other systems and system processes triggered by a specific time should be tested to ensure that none of the components malfunctioned and to ensure that the components functioned according to design for the Daylight Savings Time changeover.

8.4 Interfaces

Interfaces between systems range from non-standard proprietary to well-defined standards such as Health Level 7 (HL7). The lowest level of an interface consists of the physical line and hardware connections which allow data transmission. The hardware connections should be validated before proceeding. The next interface level consists of low level communication protocols. This level is the level where system "B" receives data from system "A" in the format that system "A" transmitted the data. The following sample state graph (Figure 2) represents a particular low-level protocol; state transmission testing should be performed using the delineated paths:

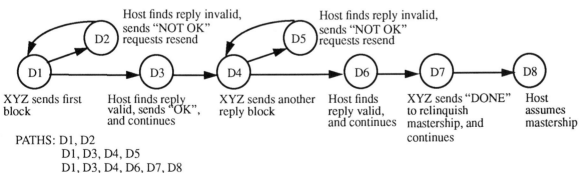

PATHS: D1, D2
D1, D3, D4, D5
D1, D3, D4, D6, D7, D8

Figure 2. Sample State Graph

Interpretation of the message occurs at the next highest interface level. A message is composed of positionally identified fields with reserved characters called delimiters separating one field from the next. Syntax directed testing will determine if the messages are correct and whether the application on the host side is functioning as designed. Given the fields and delimiter(e.g. |) of the expected message MSH|^~\&|LAB|222222|ADT|222222<CR>, different combinations and permutations of the message such as wrong or missing fields, etc. and/or delimiters should be created and passed.

The testing of the highest interface level concerns whether the application functions in the manner it was designed to. Similar to low level communication testing, the following state table would be tested according to state transition testing techniques through the creation of a state graph and then through the identification of different path combinations:

Table 1
State Table

EVENT	CONDITION FROM BED STATE	TO BED STATE	RESULTS
Transfer	Empty bed	A Unit which doesn't exist	An error message is logged
Transfer	Empty bed	Empty bed	Patient admitted, State=3
Transfer	Bed occupied by a different patient	Bed doesn't exist, unit does	Patient is admitted to a holding bed in unit, State=1

9. Conclusion: Implications for Nursing

The nurse who is a project manager on a software development project must incorporate testability into the software design, and must utilize the proper testing techniques at the appropriate phases and stages within the software life cycle to minimize costs, resources and time, and to maximize quality. The nurse who is involved in the selection of a CIS should evaluate metrics obtained from software testing during development, the testing process employed by the developer, the role that testing will take in the implementation process as outlined by the developer, and the implications of being an alpha or beta test site. Similar to the nurse involved in software development, the nurse who is involved in implementing a CIS must incorporate software quality assurance techniques in all phases of implementation--especially in any configuration tasks--and should work with the developer in creating and executing test plans.

10. Acknowledgment

The author wishes to express thanks to her husband for his professional, technical and emotional support during this endeavor.

11. References

[1] Cartwright, Jeff. *Software Testing Course Notes.* Schaumberg, IL: Motorola University, July 10, 1989.

[2] *Unit and Integration Testing Participant Guide.* Schaumberg, IL: Motorola University, November 24, 1991.

[3] *Software System Testing Workshop.* Chicago, IL: AT&T, December 2, 1987.

[4] Health Level Seven. *An Application Protocol for Electronic Data Exchange in Healthcare Environments.* Ann Arbor, MI: Health Level Seven, Inc., June 30, 1990.

[5] *Operation/Technical Manual SpaceGate Serial Interface.* Redmond, WA: SpaceLabs, Inc., April, 1988.

Nursing Informatics: An International Overview for Nursing in a Technological Era
S.J. Grobe and E.S.P. Pluyter-Wenting, eds.

Interfacing and Linking Nursing Information Systems to Optimize Patient Care

McDermott S

Nursing Service, Department of Veterans Affairs Medical Center, 50 Irving Street NW, Washington D.C. 20422

Living in an age of information and technology explosion, nurses are expected to process clinical information quickly, intervene and document care. On large nursing units or with acutely ill patients the quantity of information a nurse is expected to assimilate in providing care for one shift is difficult to effectively manage. Nurses need patient information at the point of care, i.e. where patients are treated, for timely clinical decision making. Nursing and hospital information systems (NIS and HIS) exist on a wide variety of multi-vendor personal computers, minicomputers, and mainframes that may not share clinical information. Linking and interfacing systems provides communication between two or more computer systems now, the future holds the expectation of "seamless" data base management information systems (DBMS) that may provide optimal access to patient information and decision support.

1. Introduction

Nurses spend a great deal of time gathering and assimilating information to provide patient care. Lange [1] notes that nurses spend the first part of their shift in information seeking behavior related to planning interventions and other patient activities. In addition, Lange notes that medication schedules and other information related to medications are the most frequently sought type of information yet assessments and nursing summaries require more time for retrieval. With computerized nursing documentation systems interfaced to other hospital systems more information would be available for nursing computer displays and reports. Many hospitals have or plan NIS based entirely upon a network of microcomputers not interfaced to HIS. Local area networks (LANS) are increasingly being utilized in hospitals because personal computers are becoming more powerful and capable of handling textual and graphic information which is a major requirement of nursing information systems.[2]

HIS and ancillary department systems, e.g. nursing, laboratory, radiology, and pharmacy, may run on different computers. Stand-alone systems or LAN based systems are often more advanced and provide more detailed information than HIS however both departmental and HIS applications need to share data.[3] HIS developers have a significant task to try and keep every application current whereas the specialized systems may more effectively create and update applications for a specific group of users, i.e., nurses. HIS vendors may purchase and interface nursing and ancillary department systems and market the entire package as an HIS.

Significant benefits exist from integrating healthcare data collected by all of the computerized information systems in the hospital setting.[3] Valuable nursing outputs in the form of computer displays and reports should save nurses some of the data collection time. Transformation of data to information is also possible with computerized information systems. Patient assignment reports or intervention lists for an individual or groups of patients can put individual patient information in the nurses hand without copying the kardex and making notes from other documentation. With these tools, nursing care should be more organized, efficient, and effectively provided.

Change of shift reports may include the following data: medications, critical lab results, nursing interventions/orders, physician orders, e.g. IVs, catheters, previous V.S. and amount left hanging in Ivs, patients' schedules for PT, OT, radiology and surgery. Integrated clinical databases can bring nursing, lab, radiology, pharmacy, medicine, surgery, dietetics, and other information together for informed clinical decision making. Nursing data is more useful when entered real time at the point of care and made immediately available to all of the patients' healthcare providers throughout the hospital.

2. Current Trends

The value of computerized information systems for nursing and hospitals is widely accepted therefore many institutions are hastening to purchase systems to meet information needs. Nursing and other hospital departments may purchase systems as an answer to their current local information needs without considering the long term need to share clinical data across departments. Currently, networks and interfaces are employed to transmit data between systems and applications.[4] Many computer interfaces are one-of-a-kind which make them costly to build and maintain therefore minimal essential data is transmitted between systems. With stand-alone departmental systems the clinical data base is usually not completely interfaced with the HIS. For systems not interfaced, two terminals may exist in clinical areas, e.g., a HIS terminal and a lab terminal with their databases remaining separate and distinct. Linking systems for terminal emulation using windows provides a view onto one system from another system without data transmission between the systems. Interfaces actually transmit data between systems.

Data base management systems and telecommunications are two building blocks for trends in developing information systems. Databases make data integration possible and telecommunications brings information closer to the end users.[4] A hospital database consists of the collection of data within the hospital and its departments. If there are stand-alone departmental systems, the data may not be transmitted across systems unless data requirements have been well defined and appropriate programs have been implemented. An interface capable of transparently passing any requested set of data from one system to the second system is necessary to support integrating processes.[3] Local area networks allow the sharing of programs, data and peripherals by providing common access to local and remote resources. There is immense pressure to link resources to increase productivity. Technological innovation and commercial offerings for LANs is increasing because of users' demand for greater data transmission speed and capacity.[5]

Telecommunications and network terminology is quite complex to the nontechnical consumer and includes but is not limited to the following components. Several common types of networks are star, ring and bus/tree connections. Types of LAN servers include file, mail, print and gateway servers. To select a LAN one must understand its growth limits, available number of nodes, and data rate limits. The media used to connect LANs may be shielded and unshielded twisted pair, coaxial cable, or fiberoptic cable. Each of these have performance, cost and installation issues. Hardware components include transceivers, multi-station access units, repeaters, and network interface cards. To interconnect LANs one must understand the physical layer relays, e.g., repeaters, amplifiers, and token ring stations as well as the logical link layer bridges, e.g. source routing bridges, transparent bridges, inter-operability, filter rate, and copy rate.[4]

Interface software may be written for one way communication of data, e.g., lab data transmitted to a nursing information system, or bidirectional, e.g., NIS sending data to and receiving data from the HIS. Technical knowledge and experience is needed to understand what a computer department is recommending or a particular vendor is offering when a LAN is being discussed. Since telecommunications is a rapidly evolving field, the hospital computer department may not have the technical expertise needed for decision making, or to create and troubleshoot networks and interfaces. Vendors and consultants often offer services to install and maintain networks and interfaces. Although network terminology may be foreign to nurses, a diagram that labels each device in the LAN by function may assist in understanding networks. Technical advice is recommended before contract negotiations begin involving networks or interfaces.

"When a network is considered, the nursing informatician and nurse administrator may want to consider these types of questions. How many workstations may be added to the network? How many days of an active patient record can be maintained on-line? Are patients records archived or purged after x number of days? How much time will it take nurses to log onto the NIS? What is the average response time for other users who have the same or similar network?, How reliable will the link or interface to other systems be, i.e. percentage of time available? What, if any, data will be transmitted to and from the HIS? Interfaces may add costs to an already itemized bill. Are the data stored in a data base and can ad hoc reports be generated? Are the system and reports site configurable by non-programming staff? The answers to these questions are important in assuring desired benefits are realized from a NIS.

Networking to hospital information systems is becoming easier with interface standards development. Use of standards will facilitate technical progress toward the "plug and play" environment where all types of computers will easily and transparently transmit data between each other. Interface standards make it possible to build complex systems from simple standard parts.[5] Standards committees for facilitating patient data exchange include ASTM (American Society for Testing and Materials), HL7 (Health Level 7), MIB (Medical Information Bus), and MEDIX. HL7 does not require special software or specific network protocols. MEDIX is an application level protocol and is built on the IOS (International Organization for Standardization) protocol. The MIB committee has developed interchange standards for critical care devices such as physiologic monitors, automatic intravenous infusion pumps, etc.[5] ASTM standards deal mainly with the exchange of laboratory data. All three specify messages, record types and data elements. The focus has been on transfer of coded data, which provides definite advantages for database retrieval and decision making.[6]

3. Data Capture and Output

Completely stand-alone networks without an interface to a HIS eliminate benefits from the automated NIS data. Data on integrated systems may be readily accessed and utilized from a cathode ray tube (CRT) without combing through a chart that is usually less meticulously organized and complete. Various input screens and devices can be utilized to capture data for different disciplines. Similarly separate outputs can be designed for nurses, physicians, and the different clinical departments without duplication of data on separate information systems. Nursing, like other disciplines, utilizes specialized knowledge and skills throughout the nursing process therefore the information desired and how to display it on screens and reports may be unique.

4. The Decentralized Hospital Computer Program (DHCP)

The Decentralized Hospital Computer Program (DHCP) consists of approximately 20 separate clinical and administrative software applications that reside on a dual VAX mainframe system at the Washington, D.C. Veterans Affairs Medical Center (VAMC). Applications include: admission, discharge and transfer; medical record tracking; lab; radiology; nursing; allergies; vital signs; medicine; surgery; pharmacy; order entry; health summaries; dietetics; oncology; progress notes; consults; mental health; social work; and, quality management. The data entered through these multiple applications reside in an integrated data base. All programs and data may be accessed from every hospital CRT. With access to these databases, data from multiple applications may be displayed or generate a report. The data may also be sorted and manipulated from the database.

The recent implementation of physician order entry utilizing the DHCP applications at the Washington, D.C. VAMC allows physicians to enter all orders on patients. The orders are entered through the "Order Entry/Result Retrieval" application. The orders are transmitted to the ancillary services applications, e.g. lab, radiology, and pharmacy. The nurses and physicians utilize the orders data base to review current orders on patients without searching through order sheets on the chart. Orders for a specific department may be displayed, e.g., all active pharmacy orders or all orders including discontinued and expired orders. All orders for all services may also be displayed in reverse chronological order.

From pharmacy orders nurses print automated medication administration records and pharmacy prints profiles without transcribing orders or later recopying the record. Nurses can also print current physician or nursing orders and utilize these as kardexes. Included in the nursing orders printout are the responsible physician(s), diagnosis, condition, V.S. frequency, activity level, I&O, etc. With an integrated database many providers can utilize the same information in a context most meaningful to their discipline.

In another application physicians, nurses, pharmacists, radiologists, and dietitians can enter and display allergies, i.e., in an allergies application, which then print on nurses' medication administration records, display on the CRT when physicians enter orders, and display and print on pharmacists' and dietitians' profiles. All of this occurs with the simple entry of allergies by any user.

The "Health Summaries" application retrieves information from all clinical applications mentioned previously plus a clinic scheduler. A health summary displays real-time data and may be interacted with on-line or printed. Specific data may be displayed or printed as requested, e.g., the amount of data may be altered or the format of the data may be changed. Health summaries have been created for the diabetic nurse practitioner, cardiac rehabilitation nurses, nursing home clinicians, pharmacists review of antibiotics and microbiology reports, dietetic profiles, cardiac clinic, inpatient medicine, surgery, et.al. Each user may create a health summary to meet their needs. Without an integrated database, this type of data retrieval and output would not be available.

5. The Future

Open Systems Interconnection (OSI) represents the goal of the "seamless" DBMS when all data is available across platforms and applications. OSI is an architectural framework defining standards for linking heterogeneous computer networks. The term "open" denotes the ability of a computer of one design to connect with any other computer conforming to a reference model and the associated standard protocols. The goal is to have applications on one computer communicate with applications on another computer through the OSI environment[4]. This "plug and play" environment would eliminate the need for programming interfaces to exchange data between systems and applications. MEDIX is the standard intended to bring all clinical data interchanges within the ISO scope.

Two technology centers for healthcare information systems that now exist are the Hospital of the Future for Andersen Consulting is in Dallas and the Healthcare Information Technology Center for Coopers & Lybrand is in Parsippany, N.J. New technologies that enable disparate systems to communicate and share information are demonstrated.[7]

Although decision support and expert systems technologies are relatively rare in healthcare institutions today, they will clearly be a standard in future systems. Integrated clinical DBMS are the foundation of these advanced tools. Automation of simple alerts are among the first application of expert systems in hospitals. Many current systems provide clinical alerts. In DHCP, alerts are generated for duplicate orders, critical lab results, abnormal radiology reports, unsigned orders, and for order clarification.

6. Benefits to Patients

With the DHCP order entry/result retrieval system, orders are entered through one application and received instantaneously in all ancillary services. Patients' receive and are started on medications sooner, are having laboratory tests and radiology exams completed more quickly, and diagnostic results available sooner. Duplicate order checking also avoids the inconvenience of duplicate testing of the patient and its associated costs. To the patient these may mean earlier effective treatment and a shorter length of stay.

One of the challenges to each department is the implementation of effective quality improvement programs. Measuring and attempting to improve the quality of healthcare are becoming increasingly important and expensive. Outcomes from nursing interventions and their impact on the patients' outcomes and course of illness may be more easily tracked in an automated nursing data base. Nursing quality improvement (QI) and research are facilitated by information systems that are designed to meet these needs. QI and clinical nursing research provide objective feedback about the quality of clinical practices which should lead to better patient care.

7. Summary

Nurses' needs for information processing are in the early stages of identification and development. Who was it that said, "how do you know what to ask for unless you know (or can dream) of what's possible." NIS can so clearly assist in processing the volume of data in patient care, education, administration and research. Increased attention must be paid to providing universal access to the clinical content of each department's data base.[3] Networking and integration strategy should build upon the existing technology base[9]. Ideally all information in the future will be available in an apparently "seamless" DBMS so that relevant data may be accessed for clinical decision support. Clinical warning or alert systems are available to bring prompt attention to critical clinical events. Nurses participating in system selections and strategic information system planning may benefit from understanding the value of linking and interfacing NIS and HIS using the current telecommunications standards as a method of achieving the "seamless" clinical DBMS and "plug compatible programming."

Connectivity of future NIS and HIS should be evaluated during selection processes to achieve the greatest access to clinical data for nurses. Hardware and software contracts must include the cost and time frame for systems integration. Standards utilized for systems must also be considered. Design, implementation, and evaluation proceed more readily when hardware and software integration is planned. Also, current and future software functionality are understood. When comprehensive nursing computer applications are accessible at the bedside including documentation, retrieving previous multi-disciplinary documentation, all clinical results, entering and retrieving orders, obtaining operating room and on-call schedules, using electronic mail, and accessing staffing schedules, nurses remain at the patient's bedside rather than calling for results, signing on to different terminals, or walking up the hall looking for patients charts and other information.

References:

[1] Lange L. Information Seeking by Nurses During Beginning-of-Shift Activities. *Proceedings Sixteenth Annual Symposium on Computer Applications in Medical Care*. Frisse ME(ed). McGraw-Hill,1993,317-321.

[2] Poggio F. Little Packages with big power. A Micro-Network to Meet Nursing Information Needs. *Comput Nurs*. 1990 8(6) 256-260.

[3] Haug P,Pryor T and Frederick P. Integrating Radiology and Hospital Information Systems: the Advantage of Shared Data. *Proceedings Sixteenth Annual Symposium on Computer Applications in Medical Care*. Frisse M E(ed). McGraw-Hill, 1993, 187-191.

[4] Held G and Sarch R. *Data Communications: A Comprehensive Approach* Edition II. New York: McGraw-Hill. 1989,396-426 and 495-500.

[5] Ahituv N and Neuman S. *Principles of Information Systems for Management* Third Edition. Dubuque: William C. Brown. 1990,587-622.

[6] McDonald C. Standards for the Electronic Transfer of Clinical Data: Progress, Promises, and the Conductor's Wand. *Fourteenth Annual Symposium on Computer Applications in Medical Care: Standards in Medical Informatics*. Miller R(ed). Los Alamitos: IEEE Computer Society Press.1990,9-14.

[7] Sideli R, Johnson S et.al. Adopting HL7 as a Standard for the Exchange of Clinical Test Reports. *Proceedings Fourteenth Annual Symposium on Computer Applications in Medical Care: Standards in Medical Informatics*.Miller R(ed). Los Alamitos: IEEE Society Press.1990,226-229.

[8] Dunbar C. Technology Centers Showcase. *Comput Nurs*. 1991,12(1),24-25.

[9] Panko W and Wilson M. A Path to Integration in an Academic Health Science Center. *Proceedings Sixteenth Annual Symposium on Computer Application in Medical Care*. Frisse M E(ed). McGraw-Hill,1993,278-282.

[10]Greenes R. Promoting Productivity by Propagating the Practice of "Plug-Compatible" Programming. *Proceedings Fourteenth Annual Symposium on Computer Applications in Medical Care: Standards in Medical Informatics*. Miller R(ed). Los Alamitos: IEEE Computer Society Press, 1990,22-26.

© 1994 Elsevier Science B.V. All rights reserved
Nursing Informatics: An International Overview for Nursing in a Technological Er
S.J. Grobe and E.S.P. Pluyter-Wenting, eds

Use of Total Quality Management Techniques to Facilitate
Determination of System Requirements

Blessing B B

Headquarters, Air Force Medical Support Agency, Office of the Surgeon General, Brooks Air Force Base Texas

The process of defining system requirements can be a very time consuming and tedious task, and certainly accounts for the reason many institutions are purchasing systems after looking at just a few. This article discusses the use of various Total Quality Management tools to facilitate analysis of systems requirements for automating nursing documentation. The outcome was a document which not only was comprehensive but had nurses "buy-in" from all levels of nursing in the Army, Air Force, and Navy.

1. Introduction

Total Quality Management (TQM) is more than a 1990's buzz word. It offers the potential to positively affect every major healthcare constituency. Within the military, medical facilities are beginning to use TQM techniques to empower people to work together to analyze and improve work processes. When nurses were challenged to write the specific detailed requirements for the next major version of the Department of Defense's Composite Healthcare System software, it was decided that several of the TQM techniques might prove beneficial in facilitating a thorough discussion of the issues. The challenge for this group of nurses was to design a system to meet the needs of Army, Air Force and Navy nurses assigned to different types of facilities, ranging from the small clinic to the very large medical center. This paper focuses on the activities that led not only to the development of those detailed requirements, but also a "buying in to the solution" by this diversified group. Nurse representatives from the three military services met as a group and used brainstorming, cause and effect diagrams, and small group tasking to analyze how care is provided and documented. From these procedures, the nurses were able to clearly specify the requirements for a system which would support not only current practice, but one which would have the flexibility to adapt to future changes. Additionally, the processes used to facilitate discussions allowed the group to discuss the specific details of input screens, output products, rules, process, styles, etc. At the end of the session, a document was written that clearly represented a consensus of the desired capability of the next major software version. At a time when nurses are being challenged to define nursing needs, this technique allowed an opportunity to analyze how nurses practice, and what capabilities a computer must have to support that practice.

2. Literature Review

Defining system requirements is a process that few people look forward to performing. In these days of fast foods, and high tech solutions to problems, many hospitals are procuring expensive medical information systems based on demonstrations of only two or three products. Often decisions are made on the best looking screens or the slickest "tools". However, once users begin to use the system, they often find that it doesn't meet the needs or is not consistent with the work flow, or patterns of logic. The step of analyzing work processes to define user needs is viewed by many as an unnecessary exercise. However, it is an important first step in determining what the system must do to meet user needs. Crowther [1] recommends establishing a steering committee to develop an information systems plan that will meet the organization's needs in the future and will support the organization's business plan. Berg [2] a pioneer in obtaining nursing involvement in system procurement, stated that nurses need to first understand the manual system, and then analyze what parts would benefit from automation. Happ [3] recommends that the expected benefits be clearly established, and that the system be designed to achieve those benefits. Mills [4] provides a checklist which can be used to guide the process of developing requirements. It is apparent that many authors advocate analyzing needs to support the definition of requirements. Few authors, however, provide guidance on how to expedite this very tedious, time-consuming process. The method being proposed by this author is to use various Total Quality Management (TQM) techniques to facilitate defining requirements of the system. TQM is indeed rapidly changing the way we do business in our medical facilities. The literature is replete with articles on the definition and use of TQM to improve business practices. Many authors describe general tips to assist CEOs with introducing this concept into the organization [5-8]. However, there is limited documentation on the successful application of TQM within medical treatment facilities, and much less with system design to support those facilities. This is probably due in part to the relative newness of the concept of TQM. This portion of the literature review will focus on a general overview of TQM, with a specific focus on the use of "tools" to assist in the analysis of problems or issues.

Labovitz [9] describes TQM as a top down process, driven by senior managers who shape and communicate a unifying vision of quality, set clear quality improvement goals, and serve as the organization's most avid champions. At lower levels in the organization, people use TQM to analyze and modify processes, with a goal of continuous improvement. One good example of effective use of some of the TQM tools was presented by Stratton [10], a quality manager at AT&T. He facilitated problem analysis, using Ishikawa's Cause and Effect analysis (Fishbone Diagram). The group found that the effects could be better understood when the causes of them were reviewed in detail. Stratton use Force Field analysis to identify the forces on the situation, both the driving forces and the restraining ones. He helped his group to analyze the problem, using the Cause and Effect analysis and then used Force Field analysis to map the solution.

The application of TQM principles to improve practice in health care in undergoing testing at Rush-Presbyterian, St. Luke's Medical Center, Chicago. To date they are pleased with the program and are beginning to see "real" return on investments in areas such as Radiology, Laboratory, and Billing [11]. Melum [12] remains skeptical, and has reported that it is too soon to evaluate TQM's impact on health care. However the author offered some strategies to promote its success. One of the strategies presented includes integrating TQM with efforts to improve clinical outcomes. This focus has been effective in getting health care professionals interested because it answers the question "what is in it for me?"

3. Discussion

The Composite Health Care System (CHCS), integrated hospital information system, is undergoing testing by the Department of Defense in 14 Tri-Service Medical Facilities. In July of 1991, approximately 50 Tri-Service Nurses and Physicians representing each of those facilities met to discuss the requirements of the next major software version. The intent of the group was to ensure that CHCS would better meet the needs of the clinical user. The Tri-Service Nursing representative at that meeting identified three specific functions that were required. These were Patient History, Patient Assessment, and Nurses Notes. The system currently has documentation capability, but does not support the detailed descriptions of the patient assessment or the care provided. These would need to be designed. The original functional description included these capabilities, but did not provide specific details. It was decided at the meeting that the nurse would need to provide an exact description of both the required capabilities and output products of the nursing documentation portion of CHCS.

The challenge put before the group was clear. Unequivocally articulate the specifications for the new areas to be designed, using the approved functional description. With this challenge came two constraints. The first was the need to consider the original functional description. This meant that each specification had to be a clarification of a line in the requirement. This did not pose much of a problem, because the requirements were generally vague and allowed considerable room for creativity. The second constraint was the time limitation. The document has to be completed within the next 60 days, and would require a consensus by all three services. Although 60 days may sound like a long time for some, within DOD, this equates to nanoseconds. The challenge was then to identify a methodology that would allow the group to complete the tasking in a very short period of time.

The Air Force took the lead on this tasking. One of the goals for the Air Force Medical Service, established by the Air Force Surgeon General, is to "capitalize on the opportunity to improve processes at all levels." The accepted Air Force methodology for accomplishing this is Total Quality Management. Since a new process was needed, it was felt that TQM would provide an excellent framework for analyzing needs and defining requirements. The three techniques chosen to support the analysis were brainstorming, cause and effect analysis, and small group tasking.

Brainstorming is a technique to encourage expansion of ideas and promote the opportunity to include all dimensions of a problem or solution [13]. The DOD group used brainstorming to clarify how the three functions of nursing documentation would be addressed to identify the critical issues that needed to be discussed within each function to define the specific requirements. The group agreed that each of the three functional areas (Assessment, History, and Nursing Notes) should be defined separately. Although it is apparent that they are intertwined in thought processes, addressing them separately would allow the group to focus on the specific details of each portion of the process. Their next step would be to identify the issues. The brainstorming technique proved to be invaluable in this area because helped the group identify the various dimensions of the topic. many ideas were proposed and discussed. Howeve under the guidance of a skilled facilitator, the group was able to define the absolutely critical issues.

The process of identifying critical issues is used to provide the focus for the next step which is to "sketch" th requirements needed to support the identified issues. Therefore it was imperative all participants agreed that the list o requirements was complete and clearly understood the definition of each of the issues. Getting group consensus for the list was the last step in the brainstorming process. The diagram shows the tool used to define the critical issues.

In essence, the group identified seven critical issues that would need to be addressed in order to achieve the goal of developing a comprehensive set of requirements. These were as follows:

Figure 1. Diagram to facilitate discussion/analysis of critical issues

1. Each new function would need to be integrated with other portions of the system.
2. Input should be consistent with thought processes and be user friendly
3. Throughput rules must be defined to establish how data would be moved within the system
4. Output screens should provide information in a logical format.
5. All new functions must meet the documentation requirements for the various regulatory bodies.
6. Information should be easily retrievable and meet user needs for flexibility.
7. System must support he various documentation styles being used in facilities.

Once the issues were defined, the group was ready to move to a more complex level of analysis: definition of the specifications that pertained to each issue. It was determined that the "Cause and Effect Diagram" would help the group identify the relationship between the issue and the achievement of the goal. For example, when analyzing Input Screens, the group would define requirements needed to make the input screen acceptable to the user. These migh include what information needs to be on the screen, when the user could use that screen, or how the user would ente the information (i.e. pick lists). On the other hand, when Style was discussed the group analyzed the differen documentation and practice styles. They had to understand how a difference in style impacted the system success o this phase of the analysis. The group wanted to analyze each issue to the greatest degree of detail possible. However, i was not the purpose of this large group to analyze at the micro level. The purpose of this phase was to identify the general requirements related to the critical issue. Once this was accomplished, the group was ready to move to the third phase.

The next phase is the actual writing of the detailed specification. The methodology use for this phase was 'small group work" or "process actions teams." The advantage of small groups is the ability to get to detailed levels, analyze the absolute requirements, and produce a document that incorporates the general requirements for ONLY the critical issue that they were assigned. The benefit of this was the ability to focus on only one aspect and not the whole piece. A potential problem with this type of methodology is the small groups could write requirements in one section that might conflict with those written by other groups. To a certain degree, this was resolved in the large group discussion of the issue. However, this type of approach requires the group to have the opportunity to reconcile conflicts that may develop.

The final phase was designed for this reconciliation. Each group explained their document and reviewed the proposed specifications line by line. Discussion centered around how the specifications could complement each other. Conflicts were resolved during these discussions. Once the specifications were agreed upon, they were adopted.

The reader is reminded that the group decided that the three pieces of nursing documentation should be written separately. Therefore, this process was completed for History, Assessment, and Nursing Notes. Once all documented were written, the group had to combine them to insure that they would work together. This process also provided the opportunity to determine if something was included in one section and inadvertently left out of another. It became obvious that the group had learned a great deal from the earlier efforts, because they were more efficient at identifying what needed to be included, and less discussion was required as the process was repeated.

At the end of this session the group reviewed all documents and came to the consensus that they had defined requirements that would be compatible with their specific work flow patterns. They were proud of the work that they had accomplished and were eager to have the document presented to the Nurse Corps Chiefs from each of the services. It was presented to the Corps Chiefs and wholeheartedly approved.

4. Keys to Success

The process used for this tasking was complex and really required a great deal of support to bring it to fruition. There are some issues that should be considered if this is to be replicated successfully.

1. The undivided attention of individual is required. The process of determining complex system requirements was complex and required a great deal of thought and work by the participants. If the participants are subject to being pulled out of the session to work other issues, group dynamics change and the goal may not be able to be achieved. The participants in this project were taken to a remote location.

2. Clearly establish the rules, roles, and goals of the session. Prior to beginning the session, participants were told of the rules for successful group process, their role as representative of all the nurses from their facility, and the goals for the session.

3. Provide users with reference material to better prepare them for the tasking. If there are references or information that needs to be reviewed prior to the meeting, this should be sent to the participants well ahead of time. It is critical that each individual is prepared to discuss the topics from the outset. For example, the participants were provided copies of regulations, JCAHO requirements, and ANA standards.

4. Determine how much authority the group will have to change current practice. Since this group was defining how to best automate a task being performed manually, it was important to know how much leeway the group had to improve practice at the same time. The Chiefs of the nurse Corps from each service were asked to define any constraints on changing the Service defined documentation practices.

5. Finally, the key to success is the support of facilitators, scribes, and typists, as well as the need for technological support with computers, copy machines, and PAPER, PAPER, PAPER.

5. Summary

The process of defining system requirements is not easy. However, it is one that nurses need to be involved in to insure that the system being procured for their use will in fact meet their needs. The use of this methodology for facilitating analysis is one that worked very well for this diversified group. The use of brainstorming to initiate the process provided a framework that the group could build upon to achieve the level of detail required. The cause and effect analysis allowed users the opportunity to clarify what was needed in the different phases of documentation, as well as the impact of styles and regulatory concerns. And finally the small group work allowed the users the opportunity to clarify the specific details that would be required. Because clear guidance had been provided by the large groups and they were given only small areas to deal with, participants were not frustrated by getting taskings that were too large to accomplish or in which they had inadequate guidance.

6. References

[1] Crowther B. High ground: The administrator's role in system's procurement. *Computers in Healthcare*, December 1991.

[2]   Berg CM. The importance of nurses' input for the selection of computerized systems. In: *The Impact of Computers on Nursing.* M Scholes, Y Bryant and B Barber (eds) Elsevier Science Publishers, BV (North Holland), IFIP-IMIA, 1983.

[3]   Happ B. Defining information system requirements. Presented at the *Nursing Informatics Summer Institute* Jul. 10, 1991.

[4]   Mills ME. Nursing input to the selection of Hospital Information Systems. In: *Nursing Informatics.* MJ Ball, NJ Hannah, UG Jelger, and H Peterson (eds). New York: Springer-Verlag, 1988; 353-365.

[5]   Harrington HJ. *Excellence -- The IBM way.* American Society for Quality Control: Milwaukee, WI 1988.

[6]   Thompson RE. The six faces of quality. *Healthcare Executive,* 1991 6(2), 26-27.

[7]   Berger S and Sudman SK. Making TQM work. *Healthcare Executive.* 1991 6(2), 22-25.

[8]   Merry MD. Illusion vs. reality. *Healthcare Executive,* 1991 6(2), 18-21.

[9]   Labovitz GH. Beyond the total quality management mystique. *Healthcare Executive,* 1991 6(2), 15-17.

[10]   Stratton DA. *An Approach to Quality Improvement that Works.* American Society for Quality Control: Milwaukee, WI, 1988.

[11]   Koska MT. Case study: Quality improvement in a diversified health center. *Hospitals,* 1990, 38-39.

[12]   Melum MM. Total quality management: Steps to success. *Hospitals,* 1990, 42-44.

[13]   Caspary R, et al. The Memory Jogger: *A pocket guide for the tools for continuous quality improvement.* Methuen, MA: GOAL/QPC, 1988.

Nursing Informatics: An International Overview for Nursing in a Technological Era
S.J. Grobe and E.S.P. Pluyter-Wenting, eds.

The Collaborative Approach to the Development of a Nursing Information System Environment in a Medical Center Setting

Sweeny M E[a] and Post H D[b]

[a] Nursing Education, Nursing Service, Veterans Affairs Medical Center, Wilmington, Delaware, 19805

[b] Information Resources Management Service, Veterans Affairs Medical Center, Wilmington, Delaware, 19805

This paper will describe the development of a functional Nursing Information system within a Medical Center. Both mainframe and personal computer hardware and software make up the operational environment. The primary focus will be on the joint efforts of the ADP Application Coordinator from the Nursing Service and the Computer Specialist from the Center's Information Resources Management Service. The work of the two individuals in identifying and resolving computer related issues will be reviewed. The availability and acceptance of computerization by the Center's nursing staff has evolved rapidly. Online patient classification, care plans and electronic mail have allowed the inexperienced computer user to become proficient quickly. The process that allowed this to happen will be reviewed and evaluated. Identifying individual unit-based needs; planning, implementing and evaluating hardware and software solutions; implementing nursing software packages; examining various teaching methods; developing user training; marketing computer resources to nursing staff; networking; consulting; and mentoring will be addressed. The strengths and weaknesses of the collaboration can serve as guidelines for nursing departments who are in the early stages of computerization.

1. INTRODUCTION

According to Catellier [1] successful ADP Coordinators possess expertise in three areas, which are listed in order of priority: *Knowledge of the Service Itself; Interpersonal and Managerial Skills; and Knowledge of Automated Data Processing*. The authors professional relationship was formed from their experiences, educational backgrounds, knowledge of information systems technology, and an understanding of organizational culture. These factors provided a solid foundation for their collaboration to implement nursing informatics. Their strengths and pitfalls of this collaboration are described throughout this paper and summarized in a table as part of the conclusion.

2. RESOURCES

The information system environment evolved and continues through the availability of internal resources that includes management support, funding, hardware and software, adequate staffing, and staff willingness to learn and use computers. Nursing staff not having access to terminals, plus lack of training on software that could be used in their practice were concerns that were identified by the authors. As resources became available and with management's support these short comings gradually disappeared. Externally, access to special interest user groups, professional organizations, literature and vendors contributed to the authors' growth and development. In retrospect, our greatest asset has been the support from both Nursing Service and Center management. The authors' self-motivation was encouraged by their collaboration and exchange of knowledge. This sharing of information took the place of formal classroom training, which was limited because of insufficient resources.

208

3. IMPLEMENTATION

In July, 1989, three goals were set for the Nursing ADP Coordinator: implement the patient classification section of the Nursing package, design databases to track unit based medication errors and falls, and analyze the service's use of overtime. At that time, the hardware resources only included one terminal connected to the DHCP (Decentralized Hospital Computer Program) and one printer on each of the thirteen nursing units. The nursing administrative offices had one personal computer; and one DHCP terminal which was located in the Chief Nurse's office, and shared by the ADP Coordinator. Sharing the Chief Nurse's terminal and office gave the ADP Coordinator the benefit of communicating the progress of implementation on a daily basis. The authors identified lack of access to computer terminals hampered package implementation and led them to request additional terminals being placed on the nursing units and one in every head nurse office. Figure 1 displays the growth in related areas.

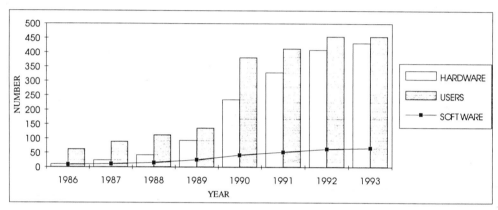

Figure 1. Center 's DHCP hardware, and software packages in use, and the number of nursing staff users from 1986-1993

4. PATIENT CLASSIFICATION

Implementation of the patient classification module occurred on a unit by unit basis. Head nurses were taught to use the module first, and they were then responsible for instructing their staffs. Head nurses and the ADP Coordinator identified nurses on each unit who could serve as resource person(s). This allowed the ADP Coordinator to focus on other issues while delegating teaching responsibilities to the unit level, since staff shortage did not allow for formal classroom training This plan of action has been paralleled by Scarpa, et al in 1992 [2]. The Computer Specialist monitored the software to identify and correct any programming problems, and also alerted the ADP Coordinator to any user entry problems. This collaboration allowed the ADP Coordinator to follow-up on unit problems and to provide staff with information to better implement the nursing informatics system. The ADP Coordinator receiving daily communication and training by the Computer Specialist were principal factors responsible for the successful implementation.

5. OTHER SECTIONS OF THE NURSING PACKAGE

Along with the online classification system, the nursing software package also contained an education tracking module. Use of this module was determined to be an efficient means of recording training activities by the education department. Individual staff members were able to view and print their educational records. This feature worked as an incentive to motivate staff to learn and to use the computer, and specifically use the patient classification system online. Within two months, all units were using the computer to classify their patients, and obtain their educational records. The administrative module of the package was utilized to track employees' personnel records. After being in use for eighteen months, computerized nursing care plans were suspended until editing functionality has been refined. Nursing staff continues to enter their direct care hours along with their daily classification. This information provides online reports that Nursing management use in their daily operations to staff units.

5. DATABASES: FALLS, MEDICATION ERRORS, AND OVERTIME DATA

The second goal was to establish tracking systems for medication errors and patient falls. A database was created on a personal computer to record medication errors and another database was created on the DHCP mainframe to track the occurrence of falls. Both databases failed due to insufficient input time, lack of user training, and staff resistance to change. From this experience, the authors concluded that having only one person responsible for all entry of data is doomed for failure. When an updated release of incident tracking software became available for the DHCP, the authors and the Center's Quality Management Specialist met to coordinate its implementation. The software allowed the staff of each nursing unit to enter incidents as they occurred. With that feature, one person was no longer responsible for the collection and entry of all incident data. Decentralizing the recording of data allowed more timely reporting by distributing the task of data entry. Management support, along with adequate training, decreased the resistance of the staff.

The third goal was to analyze the overtime used by Nursing Service. For five years, the ADP Coordinator had been using a personal computer relational database to analyze this overtime data. The authors collaboration led to Fiscal service providing the ADP Coordinator with a disk of the previous pay period's data. Unfortunately, the data was not consistently provided in a timely manner, so a manual system was implemented. Head nurses were required to keep track of their overtime dollars spent. This manually collected data became the basis for computer generated graphic presentations used for annual management reviews and JCAHO visits. In 1992, Fiscal began to provide Nursing with the payroll data in hard copy format. In the near future, this data will be available as part of the Nursing package, allowing downloading into personal computer spreadsheets and graphs for analysis.

6. NETWORKING

In September 1989, the ADP Coordinator began communicating with colleagues at other VA facilities, the project manager for the Nursing software package, and computer users in other health care facilities. Interactions provided information regarding conferences such as the Symposium on Computer Applications in Medical Care (SCAMC), and the existence of nursing networking groups. Coincidentally, a local nursing network was in its developmental stages. Participation in that group led to the identification of local resource persons and a broader awareness of nursing informatics applications. The authors continually attend local, regional and national conferences to exchange ideas and to keep challenged by this ever changing field.

7. ELECTRONIC MAIL

Within the Veterans Health Administration, a national electronic mail system (FORUM) exists. This system provides 172 Medical Centers, 53 outpatient clinics and the VA Central Office with instant online communications. Currently, there are over 30,000 users registered in the FORUM System[3]. This exchange is an effective mechanism which provides information in a timely fashion. The system is used to resolve problems, provide training, issue corrections/patches to existing software, and allows users a platform for idea exchange.

A similar electronic mail system is used locally at each medical center. This electronic mail system (MailMan) had the greatest impact on communications, not only within the Nursing Service, but among other services throughout the Center. The Nursing Education department has used electronic mail to schedule classes, distribute quizzes, and conduct surveys. The Computer Specialist and ADP Coordinator continuously provide formal and informal training to all nursing staff on the utilization of MailMan. New staff computer orientation mainly focuses on teaching MailMan. This provides the staff the means to communicate with each other, as a unit, as a service, and as a facility.

8. MARKETING

Some people are resistant to change; some people are resistant to computers; some are resistant to both. Faced with individuals in all three categories, implementation of computers may be a frustrating experience [4]. The authors found through their experiences that showing people how to use computers in their practice was more successful than telling them. The most effective method to market nursing informatics was management's use of electronic mail as a communication tool. Equally effective was providing key individuals with reports and graphs of the data they previously entered in the computer. Having key individuals demonstrate their accomplishments in using the computer was the most effective tool for acceptance of computers in this nursing service.

9. MENTORING

In 1991, the authors became mentors for an undergraduate nursing student. The ADP Coordinator and Computer Specialist obtained and alpha tested a quality assurance statistical package for this project. The student's course work was to computerize the Nursing Service quality assurance monitor for documentation of the nursing process. This experience was the student's first exposure to computerized analysis of patient data. Working with a novice computer user required the basic research and computer skills to be taught [5].

10. CONSULTING

The authors have served as resource persons to other institutions. Other facility's ADP coordinators have visited our Center to see first hand how the software is utilized. Sharing information with others has been beneficial to them as well as to the authors. In the Center, assistance has been provided in the selection and use of personal computer software and hardware for staff. Forms, graphs and charts have been created for staff to assist them in their preparation of reports. Databases were created to monitor hemodialysis acuity levels, track compliance in the tuberculin testing program, and automate employee health records. Instructional pamphlets on computer security, DHCP software guides, and clinical nursing guides were developed. Training has been provided and encouraged so individuals can become self-sufficient in creating their own computer generated output. ADP Coordinator and the Computer Specialist are not members of the Center's strategic planning committees. However, they provide committee members with current computer technology information insuring appropriate future planning and decision making.

11. CONCLUSIONS

The authors collaborative approach in implementing nursing informatics was solidified by their feedback to each other, their willingness to make changes, their ability to stay focused on goals, their complementary knowledge base/expertise, their determination, and continual evaluation of their activities. An effective collaboration can be aided by a set of guidelines to assist implementors meet their goals [6]. Table 1 shows what assisted and blocked the authors progress during the past five years.

Table 1
Collaboration strengths and pitfalls

COLLABORATORS STRENGTHS	COLLABORATORS PITFALLS
Communication skills	Insufficient resources
Knowledge of organizational culture	Not being involved in organizational planning
Awareness of resources	Lack of training
Managerial skills	Insufficient time
Knowledge of computer technology	Inadequate staffing levels
Self-motivation	Staff resistance to change
Teaching skills	Staff perception of computers
Ability to recognize failure	User lack of understanding/acceptance of informatists

12. REFERENCES

[1] Catellier J. ADP Coordinator: An Essential Service Level Position for Effective Integration of Automation into a Hospital System. (Unpublished paper)

[2] Scarpa R, Smeltzer S and Jasion B. Attitudes of Nurses Toward Computerization: A Replication. *Comput Nurs* 1992, 10:72-80.

[3] Morris, C. *Forum New User's Guide.* Washington: US Department of Veterans Affairs, 1992.

[4] Summers S. Attitudes of Nurses Toward Hospital Computerization: Brain Dominance Model For Learning. In *Symposium on Computer Application in Medical Care. '90.* Miller R A. (ed) . Los Alamitos: IEEE Computer Society Press, 1990: 902-905.

[5] Fochtman M and Kavanaugh S. A Nursing Service-Education Model for Introducing Baccalaureate Nursing Students to Research and Computer Concepts. *Comput Nurs* 1991, 9:152-158.

[6] Pluyter-Wenting E. Experiences with Selection and Implementation of an Integrated Hospital Information System. In: *Nursing Informatics '91: Proceedings of the Post Conference of Health Care Information Technology.* Marr P, Aaxford R and Newbold S (eds). Berlin: Springer-Verlag, 1991:125-130.

Nursing Informatics: An International Overview for Nursing in a Technological Era
S.J. Grobe and E.S.P. Pluyter-Wenting, eds.

212

Construction and Utilization of a Nurse Database

Murakami T[a], Miura K[a], Moriya Y[a], Ito Y[a], Andou K[a], Shimoda H[a].Takemoto Y[a], Narita Y[b], Sato M[b] and Tamamoto H[b]

[a]Akita Red Cross Hospital, 1-4-36 Nakadori, Akita City, Japan.

[b]Department of Information Engineering, Mining College, Akita University, 1-1 Gakuenmachi Tegata, Akita City, Japan

A nursing personnel database system utilizing a personal computer was designed by systems engineers and nurses at the Akita Red Cross Hospital. To facilitate the maintenance and utilization of the system by nurses with minimal help from experts in computer technology, the data structure of the database was formed in a fixed-length format for multiple entry data (e.g. employment history, training qualification, researching history) in addition to single entry data such as name and address. With the completion of a retrieval system that is easily used by nurses at all levels, administrators have been freed from providing their section members with information such as nurses' education, training projects, and personal placement plans. Furthermore, since they are now able to retrieve information previously unavailable, they can make high level decisions related to the information available.

1. Introduction

Nursing work has been computerized at Akita Red Cross Hospital using distributed processing with personal computers since 1989 [1]~[3]. Since 1990, each nurse employed by the hospital has been provided with yearly training in information technology so that he/she can interact with the nursing personnel database. Systems for various labor saving projects using personal computers (PCs) have been developed and implemented by those nurses who participated in the educational program. [4]~[6]. In 1992, a database to monitor nurses' technological level and facilitate adequate manpower placement was developed. Several reports are available from the database [7]~[11]. Developing a networked, PC based database with a simplified data structure has made it possible for nurses to work with the system effectively. There are few database systems for which this is true. Nurses have learned how to use the data obtained from the databases as the basis for intelligent judgments and informed decision making.

2. Nurse Database

2.1 An outline of the system

The nurse database was placed on the UNIX work station (hereafter called EWS). The EWS is connected to a sub-network that is linked by Ethernet to the medical system which has an in-hospital mini-computer as a host computer. Furthermore the database management system is on multiple PCs linked with EWS via an Ethernet connection. Any MS-DOS PC can be connected to the network. [2]

2.2 Specifications of the database

To enable nurses who are provided with information technology training to perform database maintenance and management, specifications that are easy to comprehend and simple in structure have been adopted as shown below:

1)   The main data file will be 1 set, and 1 record will be used for each nurse. The total number of records will be permitted to exceed 319, the number of the nurses currently employed in the hospital.

2)   The data for one person will be expressed in ASCII characters, in fixed-length records of 4096 bytes.

3)   Specification files on which the ASCII characters of the database are described will always be available.

4)   Items for which multiple entries are required such as career, educational background, training history will be

retrieved using a method of first-in/first-out. The information exceeding the maximum recording times will be added to a permanent record with ID codes and dates attached to it. For example, the maximum number of recordings for personal training history is limited to 50.

5) Careful protection of privacy should be provided with the personal database which may be accessed by many and unspecified users [12]. To protect personal information , information protection codes will be defined on specification description files. Items that can be accessed will be restricted by individual security codes assigned to each user. When a user tries to access data not permitted by his security code, only the allowable data will be provided.

2.3 A database management system

A database management system is broadly classified into a data entry system and a retrieval system. The data entry system can change the database specifications by reading in the specification description file referred to above at the time of execution without changing execution programs. To enable everyone to enter and retrieve data without training, almost all the work was designed to be performed with ten function keys and cursor keys. The retrieval system allows retrieval of multiple items to be made simultaneously by describing retrieval items and/or conditions. The retrieval condition permits a single set of conditions by applying the "AND" operator to items. (See Example 1) In most cases, the retrieval result meets the nurse's informations needs and is helpful in making decisions. However, when higher level judgments are required, it is advisable to use a simplified judgment system developed by us for a clinical survey [13]. (See Example 2) This system conducts a 4-step analysis of as many as 20 items by applying judgment rules in an if/then style of 3-AND/3-OR using a forward reasoning chain. All the programs were written in C-language to facilitate their use on different computers [2]. A schematic diagram of the management system is illustrated in Figure 1.

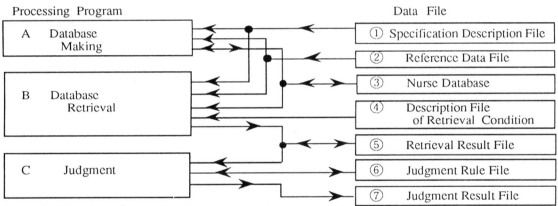

Figure 1. The view of nurse database

3.   Examples of Simple and Complex Database Queries

3.1   Example 1

Simple Query   Select a nurse for Training Program C, who has been working at the hospital for more than Y years and has had neither Training A nor Training B.

The first step in answering this query would be to build a retrieval condition to obtain the occurrence of Training A and Training B on a retrieval condition description file. Following this, it would be necessary to register the rule, "if there is a person who has been working for the hospital for more than Y years and whose grades in both Training A and B equal 0, then record 'true' in the judgment system. The retrieval result file, obtained by executing the retrieval system, will then be processed by the judgment system to produce a response to the query.

3.1   Example 2

Complex Query   Choose many items such as work career, training qualification, and study history for a specific nurse, and let the data be judged from a general viewpoint.

Judgment from a general viewpoint requires simultaneous analysis of many items. The first step is to build a retrieval condition description file to provide retrieval results required by the judgment system. The second step is to register the rules required for the individual query in the judgment system. The judgment system can combine many criteria for the retrieval results. The judgment results are exhibited using the four numerical values of 0 (sufficient), 1 (rather sufficient), 2 (close to sufficient) and 3 (insufficient). Table 1 shows an application of the 4-step judgment rules with results showing the sufficiency of nurses participation in training by number of years worked.

Table 1
Four step judgment rules and results corresponding to the "Training Estimate"

Times of Paticipation in the Training	Nursing Carrier (years)		
	0~4	5~9	10~
20~	0	0	0
10~19	0	0	1
5~ 9	0	1	2
3~ 4	1	2	3
1~ 2	2	3	3
0	3	3	3

Result 0: sufficient , 1: rather sufficient , 2: close to sufficient , 3: insufficient

The sufficiency is based on the number of times a nurse participated in training programs. Figure 2 shows the registered screen of "sufficient" case according to the rule in the judgment system.

```
Judgment item [Training ] Judgment class  Sufficient

   Nurs   Carrier    from 10   to  99        and
   NoOfTraining      from 20   to  99        or
                     from      to
   Nurs   Carrier    from 5    to  9         and
   NoOfTraining      from 10   to  19        or
                     from      to
   Nurs   Carrier    from 0    to  4         and
   NoOfTraining      from 5    to  9         or
                     from      to

   Do you modify judgment of this class?
            Yes->'RETURN'   No->'0'
```

Figure 2. A judgment of this class "Sufficient"
estimation of rules shown in Table 1

The registration of the judgment rules can be done easily on the screen, even by an inexperienced PC user. A user can modify his query with little difficulty by changing the rule as needed. However, if the user registers an improper or contradictory rule, the result tells her/him that the judgment is not possible because of improper rules.

Table 2 shows the sufficiency of training for four nurses with different careers based on an application of the judgment rules described above.

The administrators are willing to use the results obtained in this way to assist them in making decisions about promotion, education, and training plans.

By carrying out the retrieval and judgment separately, utilization of the system is simple and straight forward. Although the method is not entirely trouble-free, most nurses with minimal knowledge of information technology are able to utilize the database without difficulty.

Table 2
Judgment result by applying rules shown in Table 1

Nurse	Nursing Carrier	Times of participation in the Training	Results
1	23	14	1
2	25	36	0
3	19	7	2
4	16	6	2

4. Conclusions

Collaboration between nurses and systems engineers at Akita Red Cross Hospital resulted in the successful development and implementation of a nurse database management system that can be utilized by nurses having no previous knowledge of information-processing technology. The database resides on PC network. In-house development was chosen because many commercially available database management systems for PCs are relational databases and have many functions so that they can be used for a wide range of applications. Such systems are not user-oriented, and their use is complicated for nurses with no background in information-processing technology.

The success of the system developed can be attributed to effective communication between the nursing division staff and the in-hospital system engineers. This was facilitated by training nurses in information-processing technology. The system has replaced recording various kinds of data about nurses in multiple hand-written notebooks with subsequent difficult and time-consuming retrieval of data needed for decision making. In contrast, the new system allows nurses to retrieve any data or simple judgments that they need, rapidly and easily. In addition, administrators are able to obtain information that forms the basis for judgments required to make decisions about nurse placement, education, and training plan.

5. References

[1] Andou K, Takemoto Y, Narita Y, Tamamoto H, Tateoka M and Ohba H. *A Trial to Structure a Medical Information System by Means of LAN*. 9th Joint Conference on Medical Informatics (JCMI) 1990: 421-424.

[2] Narita Y, Tamamoto H, Takemoto Y, Miyasita M and Ohba Hi. Unification of Program Execution under a Multi-Vendor Environment for Personal Computers. *Japan Journal of Medical Informatics* (JJMI) 1991.11(1):43-52.

[3] Narita Y, Tamamoto H, Andou K, Shimoda H, Takemoto Y and Ohba H. *Aiming at Building up Hospital Information System by Midget Computers*. The 1st Report. 12th JCMI 1992: 223-226.

[4] Miura K, Murakami T, Miyasita M, Ito Y, Andou K, Takemoto Y and Narita Y. *Improvement of Hand Writing Works Using Tagform Design System*. 10th JCMI 1990: 415-418.

[5] Miura K, Konno R, Karasu T, Moriya Y, Andou K, Takemoto Y and Narita Y. *Development and Evaluation of a Nursing Service Schedule System Giving Importance to Operability and Versatility*. 12th JCMI 1992: 745-748.

[6] Handa I, Karasu T, Ito Y, Andou K, Takemoto Y and Narita Y. *A Trial for an Electronic Manual Drawing System for an MS-DOS Personal Computer*. 12th JCMI 1992: 439-442.

[7] Tamarisk NK. Personal Computer Databases for Middle Managers. *Nurs Management* 1990,21(7): 49-51.

[8] Kanamori Y, Taoka K, Yamamoto C, Iwata K, Nosaka S and Noguchi H. *The Development of Computer-Assisted Central Administration System of Personal Affairs of Nurses in Our Hospital*. 11th JCMI 1991: 567-570.

[9] Thede LQ. Databases Demystified. *Nurs Management* 1991,22(7): 38-42.

[10] Anderson RA, Dobal MT and Blessing BB. Theory-Based Approach to Computer Skill Development in Nursing Administration. *Comput in Nurs* 1992,10(4): 152-157.

[11] McClean S, Reid N, Devine C, Gribbin O and Thompson K. Using a Manpower Database to Analyse the Nurse Limbo Stock. *Journal of Advanced Nursing* 1992,17:992-1001.

[12] Rittman MR and Gorman RH. Computerized Databases: Privacy Issues in the Development of the Nursing Minimum Data Set. *Comp in Nurs* 1992,10(1):14-18.

[13] Narita Y, Fukushima S, Takemoto Y, Miyashita M, Takahashi K, Murakami T and Andou K. *Simplified Expert System for the Human Dry Dock Diagnosis*. 9th JCMI 1990:847-850.

© 1994 Elsevier Science B.V. All rights reserved.
Nursing Informatics: An International Overview for Nursing in a Technological Era
S.J. Grobe and E.S.P. Pluyter-Wenting, eds.

Nursing experiences from a PC-based monitoring and information system resulting in a paperless ICU

Palmkvist Berg M

Dept of Cardiology, Medical Intensive Care Unit, Söder Hospital, S-118 83 Stockholm, Sweden.

Experience is reported from a Medical Intensive Care Unit with 21 beds in a university affiliated county hospital (1000 beds) with a yearly admission rate of 3000 patients. During the period 1979-1991 the unit was equipped with a mini computer based central central information and monitoring system which reduced the paper work by some 50%. The system helped to reduce staff number and cost by some 8%. From 1992 the mini computer system has been replaced by a PC-based system. A database is up-dated on-line from bedside monitoring modules, the chemical and other laboratories. Doctors records and orders and nursing care documentation are entered through PC's. All information is available all over the ward in PC's. Therefore, no paper records or sheets are needed or produced during the care. When a patient is discharged, a hard-copy is produced for further care of the patient.

1. Background

The Medical Intensive Care unit at Söder Hospital in Stockholm is a 21 bed university affiliated hospital. The unit has a long tradition and vast experience from automatic monitoring systems. During the period 1979 to 1991 the unit was equipped with a minicomputer based arrhythmia-monitoring and information system previously described by us [1, 2]. The system resulted in an approximately eight percent cut in cost for staffing. The hallmarks of our philosophy has been:
  -automatic non-invasive monitoring of cardio-pulmonary vital parameters
  -all pertinent patient information included
  -wireless paging system at alarms
  -decentralized access to all information
  -user friendly interface
  -high degree of safety by extensive back-up systems
The number of data generated in an ICU is enormous and the computer-ripeness of the ICU-staff is over the last decade highly enhanced. Therefore we have decided to go the full way and to introduce the paper-less ward.

2. The Patient Care Manager

In 1992 the minicomputer-based system was replaced by a personal-computer based information system, the *Patient Care Manager* (Siemens-Elema). There is one PC for each bed and the system is connected in a local area network with fileservers. PC's are also located in nurses-stations, doctors offices, the local dispensary and conference rooms. A total of 50 PC's are distributed throughout the ward.

3. Bedside monitoring

By an interface the *Patient Care Manager* is normally on-line fed with all non-invasively monitored parameters, i.e. cardiac rhythm, blood-pressure, temperature, oximetry from a Sirecust (Siemens-Elema) and, if in use, respiratory mechanics from the ventilator. Invasive parameters from the central circulation are also automatically entered to the *Patient Care Manager* when a Swan-Ganz-catheter is in position.

4. Laboratory information

Blood chemical and other laboratory data are recovered directly from the laboratory computer to the *Patient Care Manager*-system but has to be accepted (or rejected) and electronically signed by the physician. Laboratory data can be presented in a variety of manners and in optional combinations and trends.

5. Documentation and doctors orders

Case records and nursing care notes are entered directly by the keyboard by physicians, staff nurses or by secretary after dictation. Doctors orders are entered directly to the system by the physician. Default doses for drugs and routes for administration are predefined in the system. Tests for incompatibility are automatically performed. Proposals for medication timetable and iv-nutrition schedule are automatically generated. All documentation is readily accessible in standardized and structured forms in the computers and hard-copy is normally not generated until the patient is discharged from the ICU.

6. User-friendly interface and security

Emphasis has been put on the construction of a user-friendly graphical interface. The system is easy-to-handle and after a few hours of introduction a new staff-member can start to use the *Patient Care Manager*. The software is working in an OS-2 environment and all information can be acquired by the use of a roller-mouse. All users are given security-ID-codes with different accessibility to the system. All data in the system either accepted after being fed on line, or manually entered by keyboard can be derived to the staff-members ID. Comprehensive back-up is automatically undertaken and after discharge data-reduction is performed whereafter data is stored on optical disk for future use. The function of the highest priority is the arrhythmia monitoring system which is detached to a devoted terminal (cardiac work station).

7. Intelligent alarms

Alert signals and alarms are generated by the Sirecust-system. Three levels of seriousness are defined, from the lowest (informative) priority, i.e. "point of time for administration of ..... is overdue" to the most malignant (life-threatening), i.e. "ventricular fibrillation" or "disconnected ventilator-tubing". Alarms are displayed on the Sirecusts but also thorough a wire-less paging system. Every nurse on duty carries a pocket-receiver which gives off different characteristic sounds according to seriousness. It also displays bed-number and cause of alarm.

8. Experience

The compliance of the staff has, as expected, been good. The reason for this is most certainly found in the heritage from the "old" system but also in the managements decision to introduce the new system feature-by-feature.

The experience from a good year use of the system is that the staff-nurses to an increasing part of working hours are engaged with bedside tasks in direct contact with their patients and to a less degree in administrative functions. The on-line sampling of vital-parameters (i.e. blood-pressure, heart rate, temperature, etc.) and the automatic construction of flow-sheets and diagrams of the variables has released nurses from the former manual registration and drawing of charts.

The quality of care has increased thanks to uncomplicated and distinct care plans and nurses diagnosis implemented in computer. A consequence of these features is that a good part of information which previously was passed over only verbally now is perpetuate on disk. All steps taken by nurses are related to a "problem" (i.e. pain, insomnia, malaise) and are also "evaluated". The chain "*problem-step taken-evaluation*" which is visualized on the PC-screen has reduced duplication of work since a nurse easily can see what has been the result of actions taken by her predecessor. The electronically filed material also guarantees that all staff-nurses have access to the same information regarding the patient. The previously verbal reporting between shifts, three times daily, has largely been replaced by mutual scrutiny of care plans and nurses diagnosis in the *Patient Care Manager*. The wireless paging-system has led to that nurses no longer are tied to monitors for to supervise cardiac rhythm. Thanks to the pocket receivers the sound level can be kept low and is as good as noiseless in the patients room which creates a peaceful atmosphere for the critically ill patient and his relatives.

9. Conclusions and summary

-a completely paperless ICU has been realized with success
-staff acceptance of the system is good, and
-nursing quality and medical security have increased.

10. References

[1] Matell G, Hulting J et al. Computerized monitoring and information processing in the ICU. Attempts at an evaluation. In Medinfo 1983, pp 84-87.

[2] Baehrendtz S, Hulting J et al. Clinical evaluation of automated arrhythmia monitoring and its integration with respiratory monitoring in a general computerized information system. In *Proceedings of the first International Symposium on Computers in Critical Care and Pulmonary Medicine*, 1980, ISBN 0-306-40449-4, pp 269.

[3] Hulting J, Baehrendtz S et al. Non-invasive continuous or frequent computer-based monitoring of vital parameters in a medical intensive care unit. In *Proceedings of the 5th Nordic Meeting on Medical and Biological Engineering*, 1981, ISBN 91-7260-531-6, pp 319.

Nursing Informatics: An International Overview for Nursing in a Technological Era
S.J. Grobe and E.S.P. Pluyter-Wenting, eds.

Implementation of an Administration and Clinical Information System for Nurses

Carr R L

Implementation Project Leader, Management Information Systems, Auckland Healthcare.
Greenlane/National Womens' Hospital New Zealand.

This paper describes how 5000 Nursing staff of a large area health board are introduced into a total administration and clinical information system.   The author is a member of the Implementation Team comprised of computer analysts, and health care workers , both clerical staff and nurses, who had previously worked in the clinical field.

The team's role is to ensure that a full understanding is achieved for the requirements of the ultimate users of the system - nurses, doctors, data managers and hospital administrative staff. Thus leaving more time for *quality patient care - the ultimate goal of the nurse.*

1. INTRODUCTION

New Zealand is not alone in experiencing the struggle between political expediency and traditional medical service values.

Presently nurses in New Zealand experience much pressure within a high workload, in part due to insufficient budget, which frustrates the employment of quality staff in sufficient numbers. This has resulted in burnout, nurses leaving the field of nursing, increased absenteeism from work and consequently increased workload for the remaining nurses

Recognising this situation the Government, through the Area Health Boards, have been initiating the development and implementation of information and communication technology, including integrated hospital information systems. In Auckland we commenced with our development in the latter part of 1991.

This paper summarises the key points of the Implementation of a Patient Administration System (PAS) together with Service Request & Reporting (SRR). The latter is directly driven, and serviced, by clinicians. The information needs analysis had previously been done and the system chosen. The scope of the implementation only covers those activities required for the successful completion up to "Go-live". The first phase of the implementation was conducted as a pilot, initially involving a single site. On satisfactory completion of this initial site the system was rolled out to other sites in the Auckland Area Health Board (AAHB).

The Board's customer market is spread over 2,800 square kilometres and supports the health needs of one million people. There are four major base sites and fourteen satellite units. These eighteen sites encompass over 4,000 beds while employing 5,000 nurses. Annual nurse turnover is very high at 20 percent.

Middlemore Hospital is a large, stand alone unit encompassing mainly general, orthopaedic, plastic and gynaecology surgery plus a good mix of medical wards. This hospital was identified as the most suitable site for the pilot, both with PAS and SRR. Also it was not bound by any perceived speciality restrictions. In addition, of all the major hospital units in Auckland, the staff at Middlemore had the vision and will to encompass the gains to be made by the introduction of computer systems into other than purely administrative areas.

2. PLANNING

A considerable amount of background work was done before the implementation was due to commence. The AAHB provided early involvement of the project by arranging a core group of health professionals, together with administration staff from its' major hospitals, to assist in the assessment of the presentation given by the final three vendors for supply of the administration system. The initial investment being US$ 10 million.

Resource requirements are of vital importance. It was seen as essential that qualified staff were available to execute the implementation. The initial implementation team consisted of computer business analysts and health care workers (some seconded from the hospitals). These were drawn from both clerical and nursing areas. A Medical Adviser was available to the team to advise on the more complex or technical medical issues. This adviser was actively involved as part of the implementation team during the approach to the clinical module (SRR).

The initial structure of each team varied depending on the availability of personnel - which in the early stages was an unknown and untried commodity. At this stage it was necessary to draw on help from the systems contractor.

As time passed team structures were amended to zero into the skills that emerged, not only in the technical area but also recognising the use of people who would be "acceptable" to end users. Inherent in this was the need for a system of reporting lines that could work to and from a number of task force groups invariably scattered across the hospital sites. All concerned lived and worked with the concept of control change management.

3. WHAT WERE OUR AIMS ?

* Reduce manual processes
* Increase productivity
* Optimise scarce or expensive resources
* Improve quality control
* Encourage clinical ownership of the information process thereby ensuring data integrity
* Examine requirements in the light of new information possibilities
* Improve production processes through better access to information
* Improve allocation of resources and reduction of paper work
* Improved flexibility, management information and decision making
* Control costs including duplication and waste

All these things aim to give health care professionals a better opportunity to provide quality of service. This to increase time physically with the patient, observing and treating, to ensure total quality care.

4. IMPLEMENTATION

The implementation team commenced in the pilot area by undertaking a thorough review of the current procedures, proposed new procedures, identifying hardware requirements, training etc.

4.1 The Pre-Implementation Review
The review was essential both in meeting the end user requirements and identifying exactly how they carried out the daily procedures within their department. It was of vital importance that the system being implemented would at least meet the standard already present but should offer better!

4.2 Hardware Requirements
Hardware needed to be of a quality and quantity that ensured the health care workers' daily tasks were fully enhanced and in no way perceived to cause extra work in the long term. The Occupational Health Officer on site was required to check the area to be used in regards to ergonomics. Additional resources were identified as stationery, labels, printer ribbons etc.

An un-planned bonus during the placing of computer cabling was the realisation by end users that their, hitherto, inefficient office spaces could be re-shaped. This not purely to place the work station in an optimum position but to bring the use of total space into the 90's.

4.3 Communication

Interaction both within the Team and especially with the hospital workers, was essential. This was assisted by the part time secondment of clerical and nursing staff from target departments. Demonstrations of the system were shown to all staff in the hospital/department, both administration and clinical, to familiarise them with the system and its facilities. These seminars were used to brief the staff on tasks to be undertaken, what goals were expected to be achieved and when, what part individuals and groups were expected to play in the project, how it impacted on various staff groups' working practices, and what benefits were expected.

Setting up a steering group, which met regularly, was essential in bringing the Information Systems team and hospital staff together to plan and iron out any issues which arose, throughout the implementation. To assist the continuity of the project it was essential that implementation teams lived " on site " becoming de facto local staff members, sharing staff facilities etc. This was found to greatly enhance the speed of implementation and also ensured swift and believable responses to the myriad of "what if" questions.

Regular use was made of newsletters, strictly defined for particular sites, in which the concepts and gains of computerisation were "sold" to prospective users. In addition the senior management of each site was always included in the planning and decision making to ensure that enthusiasm and ideas emanating from the workforce level were not stifled or frustrated.

4.4 Reports

The aim of investing in Health Information Systems is usually to gain benefits in productivity, management control , strategic placement, effectiveness and efficiency. Reports required by the hospitals were identified to ensure the system met the majority of the statistical needs. During the project work has constantly been carried out upgrading the system to meet the changing demands of the business.

4.5 New Procedures

Procedures needed to be planned by all involved with the implementation, with emphasis on a standard equal or better than was presently in place within the department. This gave further opportunity to review all procedures and, if necessary, overhaul them if they were not applicable to the new system.

4.6 Training

Training was an integral part of the implementation and we found it had to be taken at the speed necessary for the end user to feel both comfortable and ready to accept the system. Clear " user " manuals for the student to follow were prepared and we targeted tutors who understood the working conditions of the users being taught. In this way the teaching, and eventually the use of the system, were blended in with their daily tasks. Both clerical and nursing staff were trained initially in a quiet, computer equipped room away from the work area, to enable total concentration without interruptions. Two 2 hour sessions were given initially and a further 2 hours offered for those requesting or requiring more. The fifth and sixth hour were rarely needed.

4.7 Go-Live

An exciting and apprehensive time for all. Full support at the workface was given for 1 -2 weeks depending on the size and need of the particular area. A phone - in Help Desk was also available on a 24 hours basis. Each hospital had a site liaison person who met fortnightly with the Account Manager of IS to discuss any necessities arising with the system. These meetings were still being held eighteen months down track, not only to target individual site problems, but also to facilitate the pan-hospital sharing of ideas and experiences.

4.8 Post Implementation Review

The Review was undertaken 2-3 months post go-live to ensure a quality job had been done and the area was running as planned. This was achieved in two ways . Initially the end user maintained manual statistics for a period of three months as a check against computer generated information. A further safeguard was achieved, in conjunction with hospitals Quality of Service Departments, by the use of a "customer" questionnaire seeking commentary and a critique of achievements versus expectations. This process is still ongoing therefore, at the time of writing, a total achievement measurement is not available. We can advise that we are not totally satisfying the last of our aims (Section 3) as users have yet to break away from a reliance on paper generated reports. It was, and still is, important that the users should never feel that they were cut adrift five minutes after Go Live.

4.9 Ongoing Training

Site liaison personnel took on this responsibility. These people had to be regularly updated in order that they were aware of changes and additions within the system. Thus they were charged with passing on these amendments to the end users. Some difficulty was experienced in ensuring that stand alone sites followed up with training and re-training of staff.

Each main site is equipped with a suitably supported training room yet we are not achieving the continuity that is desirable. This, in part, is due to the very high nursing staff turnover highlighted earlier in the paper. A further complication is the irregular use of bureau (part time hired in) nurses which disrupts continuity.

4.10 Issues Perceived by Health Workers as End Users:

These have been found to fall within three categories. The system, information and personal issues.

System problems emerging saw staff realising that there will always be a wider picture. While, invariably, there is frustration with system down time (luckily minimal) there is a constant thirst for upgrades, system support and a desire to be informed on " what is coming in the future?"

Information - ever a "buzz" word - has become more meaningful in that there has been a realisation that the ownership of the information is regularly challenged. How is it to be used, patient and employee confidentiality, the ownership of the data and does the information have a downside use outside of the immediate hospital system? Indeed, is it a tradeable commercial commodity? This last point could evoke a number of in depth debates!

Personal matters were allied to training and perhaps a lack of staff confidence. This should reduce as time passes but in the early stages covered the fear of mistakes, "loss" of information, a concern with destruction/deleting of data and the awareness that these issues proved the requirement for on-going training and support.

5. SUMMARY

5.1 Delivering a Health Information System

It is necessary for hospitals to have sophisticated though achievable information systems to operate effectively. The aim of investing in Health Information Systems is to gain benefits in productivity, management control and strategic placement.

" Nurses must become involved in the decision making concerning the installation of computerised systems in their hospitals" [1]. In order to be able to respond to this demand, a solid knowledge background of data processing in the hospital is required. Proper education in this field is imperative. Often ideologies, attitudes and workload are hindering nurses to undertake the necessary steps to acquire computer literacy. It is necessary to integrate the technology with nurses' work, taking into account their interests, knowledge and experience.

The successful implementation of PAS was due to a collaborative approach by Health Care workers (management, administration and clinical) and Information Services through the implementation team, working together within the constraints of time and resources. It is important that any major systems set-up in hospitals identifies and acknowledges the need for Health Care professionals to be part of the planning and implementing of systems to be used in the hospital. All parties involved have to realise and accept the **need for change.**

References:

[1]BERG CM (1983). The importance of nurses input for the selection of Computerised Systems. In: Scholes M, Bryant Y, Barber B(eds). *The impact of computers on Nursing*-an international review North Holland Amsterdam. pp 42-58

Nursing Informatics: An International Overview for Nursing in a Technological Era
S.J. Grobe and E.S.P. Pluyter-Wenting, eds.

Adapting the Nursing Informatics Pyramid to Implementation Monitoring

Spranzo L G

School of Nursing, University of Maryland, 655 West Lombard Street, Baltimore, Maryland 21201, U.S.A.

As a colleague and in the interest of advancing the field of nursing informatics this work is presented posthumously. This paper was edited by C A Gassert, School of Nursing, University of Maryland, 655 West Lombard Street, Baltimore, Maryland 21201, U.S.A

The process of system implementation poses a multi-faceted challenge for the conduct of evaluation research in Nursing Informatics (NI). Paradigms and frameworks that guide such inquiry are required. Schwirian's Pyramid Model for NI research offers a cogent and flexible example of the necessary elements to include for relevant investigations in this field. This paper presents an adaptation of the Pyramid Model which was used as a conceptual framework for the monitoring of activities and responses surrounding the implementation of a computerized nurse care planning system. Major topics include a description of the elements, features and their relationships, suggested refinements to the framework and recommendations for its future use. An illustration of the conceptual framework is also provided.

1. Introduction

Advances in nursing informatics (NI) research will require the development and testing of conceptual models and frameworks that incorporate the unique attributes of this field. Attributes that reflect the combination of nursing science, information science, information technology and associated data-information-knowledge transformations are important model components [1]. Models depicting direction, interaction and purpose among components provide focus and guidance to research. Such models foster replication, refinement through comparative analyses and cumulative knowledge development in nursing informatics. The purpose of this paper is to describe and illustrate an example of adapting an existing research model into a framework for a systematic study of the process of implementation in NI. As a result of the development and application of this framework, several refinements and uses are recommended in the spirit of stimulating further study in the area of system implementation.

2. Background

Implementation monitoring is a tool used in evaluation studies involving a complex intervention such as the implementation of a computerized system. Its purpose is to assess the manner and extent of activities associated with an intervention in order to ascertain its construct validity, that is, to determine the relative strength of the intervention as an independent variable [2]. Implementation monitoring is often used to assess variations of an intervention that may alter achievement of outcomes among experimental groups. This was the basis for its use in an evaluation study measuring the effects of a computerized nurse careplanning system (CNCP) on nursing practice, patient outcomes and nursing staff [3].

Recommended study methods for an implementation assessment include qualitative approaches, such as interviews with personnel, observation checklists, surveys and content analyses techniques. A categorical scheme or conceptual framework that illustrates the relevant aspects of the intervention facilitates a systematic approach to data collection and analysis. Such a scheme needs to reflect comprehensiveness, dynamic interaction between users and technology, and characteristics associated with implementation that influence the actual use of the system.

Research based literature addressing implementation in nursing or health care is scant and usually focused on selected aspects of implementation such as training, user involvement or user satisfaction [4]. Implementation monitoring applied to computerized systems generally only addresses system performance and not the implementation process itself [5]. Conceptualizing the process of implementation required expanding a more general, yet, flexible model.

3. Conceptual Framework for Implementation Monitoring

Schwirian's Pyramid Model for NI research was selected because of its relevance to nursing informatics and its applicability to a variety of research purposes [6]. Schwirian's triangular model depicts the three base elements of information, user context, and technology which interact to create nursing informatics activity. The apex of the model is considered as the goal toward which the three base elements are directed. This model displays bi-directional arrows to illustrate the interaction among the base elements and their relationship to the goal.

Adapting this model as a framework required expanding each of the base elements to include features reflecting the process of implementing CNCP within hospital nursing units. For example, the user context was the staff nurses on the nursing units where CNCP was implemented. Features selected to represent this element were training, implementation stress and user perceptions. The features within each element were conceptualized to be modified by certain characteristics. For example, training could be modified by the characteristic of how much time was available for training. The feature of implementation stress could be modified by the workload characteristics on the nursing units during implementation. And finally, the feature of user perceptions could be modified by nurse characteristics.

The goal toward which the base elements and features were directed was the production and actual use of the careplan by the nurse users of the system. This goal was selected to reflect the purpose of the framework as a guide to data collection and analysis on the nursing units receiving CNCP as a treatment variable. For this reason, the relationship of the elements, features and modifiers were depicted as an influence diagram. Bi-directional and straight arrows are used to indicate the interaction and direction among features of the elements and their relationship to the goal. Bent arrows are used to indicate the influence of modifiers.

Figure 1 illustrates the conceptual model applied to implementation monitoring. This adapted model differs from the Pyramid model in that it is more linear and temporal, a depiction that is consistent with implementation activities. However, the base elements are still considered interactive as illustrated by the dotted connecting lines. Following is a brief description of each element which includes suggested refinements based on findings from the application of this framework.

3.1 Information Element

The nurse care planning information, care planning data elements and the standards of care upon which care planning was based are considered as the information element. The feature of modification of CNCP was included to indicate its policy implications, in that, the information contained in the CNCP must be a reflection of the standards of care consistent with nursing as practiced in this setting. The amount of flexibility available to the users in modifying, adding and building the system to match their needs was considered essential to the successful use of the system. The data were analyzed to reflect themes related to the importance of information modification to match end users' needs, flexibility in modification and user involvement in this process.

Inclusion of these features proved appropriate given that, in actuality, significant modification of the CNCP had to take place in order for user involvement to take place. However, a recommended refinement is to include the modifier to user involvement that reflects the *value of the information* as a resource in patient care. In this case, nurses did not demonstrate a strong value of care planning information beyond the requirements of documentation. This finding tended to modify both the user involvement feature and user perceptions and consequently limit full use of the CNCP.

3.2 User Context Element

The user context element includes training, implementation stress and user perceptions. Training is modified by methods, frequency, personnel and time for preparing the nurses for use of the system. Kjerulff's conceptualization of the environmental factors to consider when studying the adoption of innovations contributed the characteristics for the user context element [7]. Workload characteristics such as staffing to patient ratios, patient intensity for nursing care time and census can increase the amount of implementation stress when incorporating a new technology. User perceptions can also relate to benefits to practice, changes in role expectations and expectations of continued use. Communication from management in support of technology incorporation influences the user's perceptions of the benefits of the technology to their practice.

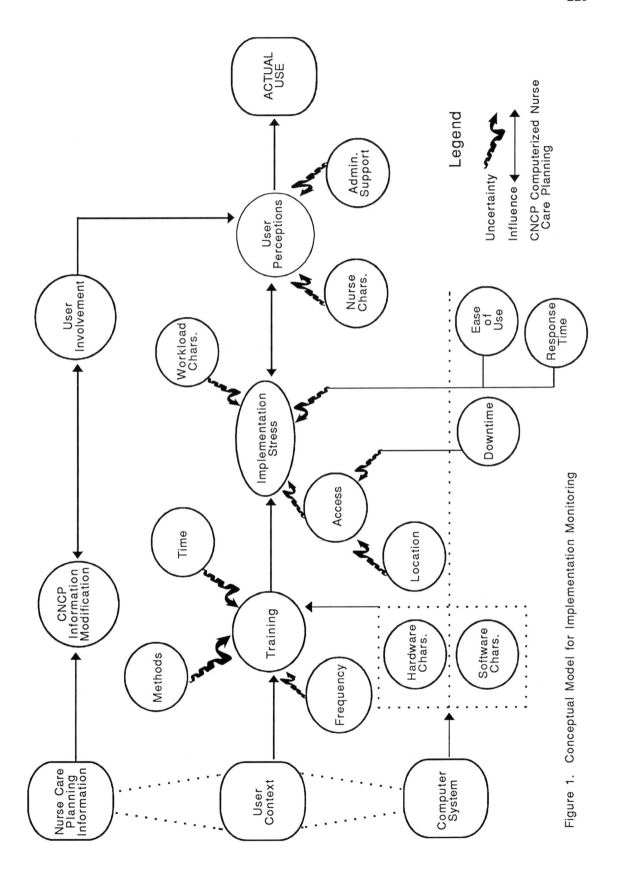

Figure 1. Conceptual Model for Implementation Monitoring

A modifier that warrants inclusion and refinement is *leadership*. Characteristics of leadership in promoting the incorporation of a system into practice can be demonstrated by administration or staff. The relationship of leadership to successful implementations of systems is relatively under-investigated.

3.3 Technology Element

The element of technology or computer system included a description of the hardware and software and methods of input and output. Additionally, the location and accessibility of terminals and printers to the user group was assessed to determine variations in access. The characteristics of downtime, response time and ease of use were considered to influence the implementation and consequently user perceptions of the system. These features reflected the system's quality in terms of the service it provides.

A modifier which was not included in the framework but found to be influential was the *flexibility of the software (configurability)* in terms of its capacity to be modified to match the information needs of the user. A low level of software flexibility was found to limit the degree of user involvement and consequently alter user perceptions of the system.

4. Recommendations

The conceptual framework warrants further investigation and refinement. Future research could improve operationalization and measurement of the modifiers and examine their relationships to the goals of implementation. With this refinement the conceptual framework would become a tool with several uses. It can continue to be used to monitor the implementation process and provide ongoing feedback on the strengths and weaknesses of each element. It can also be used as a guide to retrospective analysis of implementation and offer predictions of elements and features that require additional resources to improve the effectiveness of implementation.

With further refinement, the conceptual model can provide the framework for studying the implementation process as an intervention in itself. Methods designed to strengthen selected aspects of the implementation could be developed and compared with conventional implementation methods. The results from such comparisons could provide feedback on the cost effectiveness of implementation methods in achieving successful use of computerized systems.

5. Conclusion

The application of the framework and use of qualitative methods for implementation monitoring provided several advantages to the evaluation of the effects of CNCP. First, the findings from the implementation monitoring were shared with the nursing information systems specialist who could then bolster the implementation and training as necessary. Second, the framework used as a guide to data collection was sufficiently comprehensive to assure that relevant aspects of the implementation process were addressed and provided insight to future areas of study. And finally, Schwirian's Pyramid model proved a valuable aid in conceptualizing the process of implementation as a dynamic interaction of user, information and technology.

6. References

[1]   Graves J and Corcoran S. The Study of Nursing Informatics. *Image* 1989, 21: 227-231.

[2]   Mark M and Cook T. Design of randomized experiments and quasi-experiments. In Rutman L (ed). *Evaluation Research Methods*. Beverly Hills: Sage, 1984: 65-119.

[3]   Keller-Spranzo L, McDermott S and Alt-White A. Effects of computerized nurse careplanning on selected health care effectiveness measures. In: SCAMC. Clayton P(ed). New York: McGraw-Hill, 1991: 38-42.

[4]   Bailey J and Rollier D. An empirical study of the factors which affect user satisfaction in hospitals. In: SCAMC. Greenes R A (ed). New York: IEEE Computer Society, 1988: 843-846

[5]   Drazen E and Seidel J. Implementation monitoring: A critical step towards realizing benefits from hospital information systems. In: SCAMC. Cohen G (ed). Los Angeles:IEEE Computer Society, 1984: 148-151.

[6]   Schwirian P. The NI Pyramid: A Model for Research in Nursing Informatics. *Comput Nurs* 1986, 4: 134-136.

[7]   Kjerulff K. A theoretical framework for the study of nursing information systems. In: SCAMC. New York: IEEE Computer Society, 1988: 796-800.

Nursing Informatics: An International Overview for Nursing in a Technological Era
S.J. Grobe and E.S.P. Pluyter-Wenting, eds.

228

Impact Evaluation of Automated Bedside Documentation in ICUs and on a Medical-Surgical Unit

Bergersen M P[a] Falco S M[b] and Murphy J[c]

[a]*St. Luke's Medical Center, Information Services, 2900 W. Oklahoma Avenue, P.O.Box 2901, Milwaukee, WI. 53201-2901.*

[b]*University of Wisconsin-Milwaukee School of Nursing, P.O. Box 201, Milwaukee, WI. 53201.*

[c]*Aurora Health Care, Information Services, 3031 W. Montana Street, P.O.Box 343910, Milwaukee, WI. 53234-3910.*

Increasingly, automation is having its effect on nursing and patient care activities, with resulting changes occurring almost on a daily basis. The older, more limited, first generation systems are being replaced by second and even third generation systems that have greater complexity, sophistication, and potential. How these new systems can best be implemented within the hospital is a much explored subject. Consequently, this project was designed to evaluate the method of implementation for a second generation computer system. Impact evaluation surveys were conducted at ten and twenty month intervals. Staff nurse attitudes re: training, support, workstation ergonomics, system response time, and application efficiency were assessed. Nurses voiced opinions on the advantages/disadvantages of automated documentation and bedside accessibility, as well as their impression of the impact on planning and delivery of patient care. Each of these factors plays a major role in continued use of the system.

1. The System

Automated bedside documentation had it's advent at St. Luke's Medical Center in Milwaukee, Wisconsin in 1979. St. Luke's Medical Center is a 711 bed nonprofit, private, teaching hospital which serves as a regional, national and international referral center for it's Centers of Excellence in Cardiac Care, Cancer Treatment, Rehabilitation, Women's Health and Emergency Medicine.

The first Clinical Information Management System was installed in 63 critical care beds. Although limited in scope primarily to vital sign documentation, hemodynamic calculations, drug infusion calculations and an on-line reference library, this system was successfully implemented and served the Intensive Care Units (ICUs) well for over ten years. Moving into the 90's, its capabilities fell short of rising nursing expectations and new technologies offering open architecture workstations. It also became apparent that there were obvious bedside information management needs in the medical-surgical environment, as well as the ICU. Although there was a good amount of Hospital Information System (HIS) functionality in place (order entry, result reporting, acuity entry, charge capture, etc.), terminals were all located centrally in the nursing station and there was no automation supporting nursing documentation at the point of care delivery. In 1990, an extensive evaluation looked at replacement of the ICU system, as well as assessing the efficacy of expanding use of automated bedside documentation to the general hospital units. The goal was to focus on improvements in care through implementation of technologies to facilitate enhanced availability of data and information management, as well as to create a foundation for the growth of an integrated environment for clinical information.

The current system was implemented in May of 1991 on two pilot units, a ten bed Medical Respiratory Intensive Care Unit (MRICU) and a thirty-six bed General Medical Unit (GMU). An additional nine bed Cardiovascular Intensive Care Unit (CVICU) was added to the pilot in February of 1992, and the MRICU increased its beds to sixteen in September of 1992 bringing the network to 70 workstations and 4 printers. Bedside workstations were placed in all MRICU and CVICU rooms and in eight GMU rooms (one of four wings of the medical unit). In addition, there were GMU decentralized workstations located in the nursing station, conference room and one centered down each of the three remaining wings.

Initial functionality focused on matching applications with those from the first generation system. Added functions included interfaces to Laboratory and Admission/Discharge/Transfer (ADT) systems, as well as terminal emulation for HIS applications. Physical Assessment applications were added the first year.

2. The Evaluation

In order to assess the impact of this second generation system, the staff of each pilot nursing unit was surveyed. A multi-item questionnaire was developed to collect information on the staff's perception of the benefits and problems of the computerized documentation system, as well as demographic information about the responding sample. Of particular interest were the areas of system training, support, workstation ergonomics, workstation location, system response time, ease of documentation/retrieval, and application efficiency for this second generation system.

The questionnaire consisted of 14 demographic items, 21 5-interval Likert-type questions for attitudes about specific elements of the system, 25 5-interval Likert-type questions related to the placement of the equipment on a general medical unit (at time 1 only), and 7 comment items. Data were calculated by using a Likert-type attitude scale questionnaire as this is the one most referenced in literature and most commonly used. [1] Example of Likert-type instructions and format used:

Directions - Read each statement carefully, then circle one of the 5 responses. Give your first reaction and response. 1= Strongly Agree, 2= Agree, 3= Uncertain, 4= Disagree, 5= Strongly Disagree.
   1. Charting has been made easier......... 1 2 3 4 5.

Through these common items, nurses voiced opinions on the advantages and disadvantages of automated documentation and bedside accessibility, as well as their impressions of the impact on planning and delivery of patient care.

Following receipt of Human Subjects Approval of the Nursing Research Committee, questionnaires were sent to all professional nursing staff members working on the pilot units at ten month and twenty month intervals following installation of the system. *(NOTE: The CVICU data was only collected for the ten month interval and not the twenty month interval as this was installed eight months after the original pilot units.)* These intervals were selected in order to allow ample time for adjustment to the new system. The ICU and GMU sample sizes and identification of factors were not discreet individually, so they were combined. The data was analyzed using descriptive statistics.

The number of questionnaires returned totaled 118 (52 at 10 months and 66 at 20 months). Regardless of the study time or the nursing unit, the typical respondent was female, between 24 and 44 years of age, who worked three to five days a week. She had a baccalaureate degree in nursing and was at step 3 in the 4 step career ladder. Although she had not taken a computer class, she had experience using the computer for lab results inquiry and patient acuity entry. Approximately half the sample also used the computer for order entry of physician orders.

As was expected, the respondents felt very positive about many aspects of the system. For example, at the ten month interval they felt they had adequate training for the system (73.4%), felt comfortable using the system (82.7%), and liked having computers on the unit (76.9%). After 20 months, each of these percentages increased to 92.4%, 93.9%, and 84.9% respectively. Many comments were consistent with this viewpoint. For example, the drug dosage calculator, vital sign trending, and hemodynamic calculation functions were viewed as great time savers. Other aspects, however, did not fare as well, as Table 1 indicates.

Table 1
Positive Responses (Combined Scores of 1 or 2) to Selected Items at 10 and 20 months

SELECTED ITEM	10 MONTH	20 MONTH	% DIFFERENCE
Training was Adequate	79.2%	96.8%	+ 17.6%
Comfortable using system	91.6%	95.3%	+ 3.7%
Efficient using system	80.8%	95.1%	+ 14.3%
Know who to call with questions	95.9%	96.7%	+ 0.8%
Resource person Available as needed	86.3%	74.5%	- 11.8%
Know how to call HELP DESK	74.3%	90.0%	+ 15.7%
Problem resolution/communication Okay	80.0%	39.5%	- 40.5%
Change Requests handled Okay	77.4%	34.1%	- 43.3%
Using computer saves time	63.4%	66.7%	+ 3.3%
Charting is easier	39.8%	66.0%	+ 27.0%
Data retrieval is easier	47.4%	55.6%	+ 8.2%
Like computer reports	61.9%	78.6%	+ 16.7%
Shift Report is Easier	37.1%	64.7%	+ 27.6%
Response time is acceptable	13.9%	16.9%	+ 3.0%
Prefer return to manual/old system	33.3%	46.0%	- 12.7%
Want more charting in computer	70.0%	54.9%	- 15.1%
Like computers on the unit	88.9%	91.8%	+ 2.9%
Like computers in Patient Room	85.1%	90.6%	+ 5.5%
Like computer for charting	73.8%	80.0%	+ 6.2%
Like computer for data retrieval	73.3%	79.7%	+ 6.4%
Enough Workstations, no waiting	73.9%	95.0%	+ 21.1%

Although most of these percentages improved with time, they clearly indicate there were problems with the new system. Specific comments supported these results. The pivotal factor seemed to be response time. Comments included: screen-to-screen movement needs to be quicker, speed of retrieval is way too long, too many keystrokes, and too much down time. With unacceptable response time, respondents found it difficult to feel positive about doing more with the system, or finding it easier or faster to use. A further explanation for these results can be found in other comments related to computer use. For example, keyboard covers were felt to contribute to making key entry errors. "Help Desk" personnel were not able to troubleshoot the system well. Newly admitted clients were not in the system when the staff was ready to retrieve and/or chart information. Clearly, the system was viewed as not living up to expectations.

3. Response Time

Response time, as noted, had been poor. Initial patient and user volume tests run on the system did not demonstrate any problems. The system went live without flowsheet review capability for several weeks and no significant problems with response time were seen. However, once the system was in full use (flowsheet inquiry, system archiving and purging of unverified data) significant response time issues became apparent. The vendor exchanged hard disks, installed silicon drives on the files servers and tuned application and system software, without appreciable improvement in response time. System performance standards related to seconds of response time were specifically stated in the contract, which resulted in final acceptance criteria for the original pilot units never being met. Multiple response time testings throughout the many system changes revealed that response time is affected more by system wide activity (archiving, purging, report printing than it was by the volume of users. Addition of workstations in the remaining rooms on the GMU did not significantly change the response time, although this could not be clearly evaluated due to the multiple system changes noted above.

4. Workstation Location

The location of the workstations was evaluated at the ten month post-implementation time period for the GMU, as justification for completing system expansion to all bedsides on the GMU as needed. As Table 2 indicates, the placement of the computer at the bedside facilitated both charting and patient care. Documentation had been in the Charting By Exception format with documentation forms located at the bedside [2]. Moving to decentralized workstations resulted in 69.6% of the respondents needing to document data on an intermediary form which in turn impacted directly on how current the on-line patient chart was at any one point in time. In addition, without a workstation in the patient room, staff often had to leave the room to search elsewhere for information or to complete documentation. Respondents estimated the average time from assessment to documentation as 4.7 minutes for the bedside workstation and 47.5 minutes for the decentralized workstation. Comments, however, indicated some problems with bedside computers ranging from the physical (room too small, safety hazard due to location, too many cords) to the psychological. For example, respondents had concerns about turning their backs on the patient to enter data, feeling it might be rude.

The survey showed overwhelmingly, that 70.0% of the staff preferred access to bedside computers for documentation. Results reported in Table 2 support their request. Consequently, all rooms on the GMU now contain a workstation. The decentralized workstations were also left in place.

Table 2
Positive Responses (scores of 1 or 2) to Selected Items Related to Workstation Location at Ten Months

SELECTED ITEM	BEDSIDE	HALLWAY/ALCOVE/ CONFERENCE ROOM
Easy access to computer and keyboard	100.0%	52.2%
Efficient and thorough documentation entry	100.0%	69.6%
Comfortable charting (patient only in room)	68.8%	----
Comfortable charting (patient & family in room)	41.2%	----
Comfortable charting Nursing Station,hallway/alcove	----	70.2%
Comfortable charting in conference room	----	75.0%
Convenient patient data retrieval	83.3%	40.0%
Immediate Data entry after collection	81.8%	38.1%
Data entry without Intermediate Form	75.0%	30.4%
Increased time with patient	61.9%	21.1%
Decreased time in hall	64.7%	31.3%
Decreased interruptions to care	35.3%	11.8%
Decreased time charting	41.2%	20.0%
Preferred Charting Location	70.0%	30.0%

5. Conclusions

The results of the study indicate that the second generation computer system has met some expectations and not others. Because it impacts on so many other areas, the element of response time is critical for meeting expectations. With the perception of the system as being down all the time or being too slow executing its functions, the system is viewed as more of a hindrance than a help. In an effort to stabilize the system, requests for new development and enhancements were placed on hold. This contributed to dissatisfaction with problem resolution and change requests. To help address concerns, silicon disks were added to the fileservers by the vendor. Software was reviewed and more efficient code and search patterns were invoked. In addition, system archiving was moved to non-peak use times.

Given that so few of the respondents have any computer or word-processing experience, the abilities of the "Help Desk" personnel is critical. Therefore, additional training classes have been given to these personnel on the hardware and the software, as well as classes on communication skills. To make data entry easier and more accurate, the keyboard covers were removed from all keyboards located outside patient rooms.

The study showed that even with unacceptable response time, respondents believed the system increased their time with patients. This differs from results reported in other studies, Hendrickson [3] and Sultana [4], and is supported by Kahl [5] and Staggers [6].

Perhaps the biggest impact is what was learned from the entire process. The experiences throughout implementation gave nursing insight into methods to increase functionality to support patient care and hospital management. This system was purchased looking towards a future of *one* CIMS system for the entire hospital. Is this the right direction? With the burgeoning of technology, we remain uncertain and continue to analyze the marketplace for solutions. Experienced and wiser, we embrace other projects with excitement and an emphasis on "what is" melded with a cautious anticipation for "what can be".

6. References

[1] Polit DF and Hungler BP. 1987 *Nursing Research. Principles and Methods.* Philadelphia: J B Lippincott,1987.

[2] Burke L and Murphy J. *Charting by Exception: A Cost-Effective, Quality Approach.* New York: Delmar,1988.

[3] Hendrickson G and Kovner CT. Effects of Computers on Nursing Resource Use: Do computers Save Nurses Time? *Comput Nurs* 1990, (8)1:16-22.

[4] Sultana N. Nurses' attitudes towards computerization in clinical practice. *J Adv Nurs* 1990,15:698-702.

[5] Kahl K, Ivancin L and Fuhrmann M. Automated Nursing Documentation System Permits a Favorable Return on Investment. *J Nurs Adm* 1991,21(11): 44-51.

[6] Staggers N. Using Computers in Nursing: Documented Benefits and Needed Studies. *Comput Nurs* 1988,6(4):164-170.

Nursing Informatics: An International Overview for Nursing in a Technological Era
S.J. Grobe and E.S.P. Pluyter-Wenting, eds.

A Computer Blueprint For Nursing Care Planning: How Effective Was It?

Dominiak T [a] and Falco S [b]

[a]*Aurora Health Care, Information Services, 3031 W. Montana Ave., P.O. Box 343910, Milwaukee, WI. 53234-3910*

[b]*University of Wisconsin-Milwaukee School of Nursing, P.O. Box 401, Milwaukee, WI. 53201*

Nursing care planning is a highly complex, multi-faceted, individualized process that uses an extensive amount of information. Because a computer is designed to store, sort, and retrieve vast amounts of information rapidly, the potential impact on nursing care planning is tremendous. Exactly what information will be managed by nurses for their care planning activities, and how that data will be stored and retrieved forms the basis for a computer blueprint. The various components of this computer blueprint and the impact of its implementation are discussed. The effectiveness is measured by the nurses' perceptions of the use of computers for nursing care planning. A quasi-experimental approach was used to study nurses' attitudes toward, and factors facilitating or impeding, the use of the computer for nursing care planning. Over a two year period, data was collected before, during, and following computer implementation from the staff on three units using the Stronge & Brodt's "Nurses' Attitudes Toward Computerization" Questionnaire and Allen's Semantic Differential Scale. Opened-ended questions collected data on factors that facilitated or impeded use. Demographic data were collected in order to adequately describe the sample. Data were analyzed using content analysis and analysis of variance.

1. Introduction

St. Luke's Medical Center is a 711-bed, nonprofit, private, teaching hospital which receives regional, national, and international referrals for its Centers of Excellence in heart, cancer, rehabilitation, women's health, and emergency medicine. This study was part of a pilot project to replace an aging clinical information system, and at the same time to extend the new clinical information system into a Medical-Surgical environment. The vision of the pilot was an integrated clinical information environment which would ultimately encompass our care planning process and incorporate the ability to document against the plan of care, retaining the current charting by exception format.

Nursing is a data-intense profession. Since computers have the ability to store, sort and retrieve vast amounts of data quickly and efficiently, these machines have the potential to impact nursing in many valuable ways. How best to tap this potential requires the development of blueprints that blend nursing's needs with the computer's abilities.

2. The Blueprint

A major data-based nursing activity is the care planning process. Although the process consists of many components, the pivotal one was determined to be the assessment. The assessment is the basis for initiating the plan, selecting interventions, and evaluating goal achievement. Thus, the first blueprint developed dealt with assessment data needed for care planning.

Given the mass of assessment data available, creating a manageable blueprint loomed as an enormous task. Consequently, two major areas were developed. Essential data were defined as information needed for all clients regardless of reason for admission. This data included vital signs and hemodynamic values, along with their derived calculated values, height, weight, and in critical care areas, continuous vasoactive intravenous infusion monitoring.

Physical assessment data were defined as information related to reason for admission and was divided into categories. These categories included body systems, such as neurological, cardiovascular, integumentary, respiratory, gastrointestinal, genitourinary, and musculoskeletal; and manifestations such as pain, dressings, and incisional care.

How the blueprint was computerized, particularly in a charting by exception environment, was a major challenge. In the manual system, a check indicated that the data for that parameter were within normal limits as defined by institution standards. If findings were outside normal limits, an asterisk denotes the existance of a detailed note on the abnormal findings. If findings were unchanged from the previous assessment, the nurse only needed to draw an arrow horizontally through the box for that assessment [1]. With staff involvement the computerization challenge was met through screen design. For example, the first time a screen was accessed, normal assessment values were provided. The nurse documenting the initial assessment needed only to change the parameters which were outside normal limits. The system was designed so this could be done by accessing pop-up windows and choosing the appropriate descriptor. Once the screen was stored, the next time that screen was accessed, the most recently stored data appeared, and the nurse needed only to document further changes. A note screen could be accessed for any parameter that required more detailed documentation or explanation. The system allowed logical progression through a head-to-toe assessment without having to back out to the main menu after each body system. The capability also existed to pick and choose from the main menu the systems being assessed on an individual basis.

Since the computer allows information retrieval in multiple formats, there existed a wide range of choices for information display and paper documentation. This flexibility allowed graphical display of vital signs for one unit, while another chose to display the vital signs in a list form, with vasoactive support drugs and dosages displayed opposite the vital signs for that time period. This flexibility also allowed the creation of a printed flowsheet form which recreated the handwritten forms in a more legible manner. In addition, it allowed the construction of report sheets based on unique unit needs, where data about predetermined patient parameters were printed on the report sheet, thus shortening the amount of time spent in shift-to-shift report.

Throughout this development process, there was much staff involvement. There were committees for assessment of needs, determination of wishes, construction of screens and reports, and evaluation of prototypes. There were reports of progress at staff meetings, and educational offerings for computer use. As a result, interest and enthusiasm was high as implementation of the blueprint began to be phased in on three nursing units--two critical care units, and one general unit.

3. Its Effectiveness

The effectiveness of this blueprint was measured by the nurses' perceptions of the use of computers for nursing care planning. Because true experimental control was not possible, a quasi-experimental design was used to study nurses' attitudes toward, and factors facilitating or impeding, the use of the computer for nursing care planning. A simple interrupted time series approach [2] was chosen to collect data over a two year period, before, during, and following computer implementation from the staff on the three units using Stronge and Brodt's Nurses' Attitudes Toward Computerization Questionnaire [3], and Allen's Semantic Differential Scale [4]. Open-ended questions collected data on factors that facilitated or impeded computer use. Demographic data were collected in order to adequately describe the sample.

Following receipt of Human Subjects Approval from the Nursing Research Committee, questionnaires were sent to all professional staff members working on the three selected units. The number of questionnaires returned totaled 178 (60 for initial data collection before the computer system was implemented; 52 at 10 months post implementation and 66 at 20 months following implementation). Regardless of the study time or nursing unit, the typical respondent was female, between 24 and 44 years of age, who worked three to five days a week. She had a baccalaureate degree in nursing and was at step 3 in the 4-step career ladder. Although she had not taken a computer class, she had experience using the computer for laboratory result inquiry and patient acuity entry. Approximately half the sample also used the computer for entry of physician orders.

The Stronge and Brodt's Nurses' Attitudes Toward Computerization Questionnaire consisted of 20 Likert-type items with a 5-point scale. The possible score range was 20 to 100 with 20 being the ideal score and 60 the midpoint. Allen's Semantic Differential Scale consisted of 14 pairs of adjectives which were rated along a 7-point scale. The possible score range was 14 to 98 with 98 the ideal score and 56 the midpoint. Table 1 provides total mean scores for both instruments at each testing period. Using a one-way analysis of variance, no significant difference was found for either instrument.

Table 1
Total mean scores

	(Ideal score)	Initial	10 months	20 months
Stronge & Brodt Questionnaire	(20)	45.8	50.9	47.6
Allen's Semantic Differential	(98)	65.3	62.6	64.3

Inspection of these mean scores revealed scores closest to the ideal were those collected before computer implementation; those obtained following implementation moved initially away, then marginally back toward the ideal. Although movement was not great, this trend suggested that reality was not consistent with expectations. In other words, clinical staff's attitudes about computerization were slightly more positive before they worked with them, than after. This conclusion was supported by the comments received.

The subjects were asked to identify factors that facilitated or impeded computer use. Factors facilitating computer use were identified as time-saving and appropriate data entry, easier and quicker record access, ability to complete and enter the assessment all at once, elimination of duplicate documentation, and the positive feelings and excitement about the new system. Most of these were responses from the initial data collection questionnaires and consequently, can be viewed as expectations

Factors impeding computer use were found predominantly on the 10-month and 20-month questionnaires. Overwhelmingly, the most frequently cited impeding factors were that the system was too slow, particularly in data retrieval, log-in acceptance, and screen-to-screen moves; and that the system was "down" too much. Other factors included physician resistance to learning the system, which required the nurse to take time to retrieve information for the physician; unfamiliarity with the content of various available reports; the difficulty in correcting erroneous data; excessive steps to access the multiple screens; and excessive keystrokes throughout the system.

Based on the content and volume of the comments, it was clear that the implementation of the blueprint for assessment was not meeting expectations. The subjects were not able to efficiently and effectively carry out their tasks using the computer. Sultana [5] reported similar results, finding that nurses perceived no reduction in paperwork, no increased efficiency or time saved, and that nurses' jobs were not made easier by computerization. Without consistent positive experiences, it would be unlikely that positive attitudes towards the computer would be further developed. This is borne out by the results of the study reported by Burkes [6] wherein nurses' computer-use satisfaction and beliefs were related to each other and to nurses' motivation to further use the computer. The results obtained in this study demonstrated an absence of significant differences in the attitude scores over time.

4. Summary

In conclusion, no matter how well developed the computer blueprint for nursing care planning, nor how extensive the involvement of the clinical staff in development of the system, it will be the quality of the system that implements the blueprint that determines its effectiveness. Of paramount importance to the user is the time involved in using the computer. Items perceived as time consuming are:
- lengthy screen to screen response time
- frequency of log-in/log-out procedures during the course of the day
- degree of effort required to correct errors
- frequency of system nonavailability or computer downtime
- the amount of time required by nurses to assist other users.

Thus, recommendations for improving the effectiveness and acceptance of a system would address these and other related points. If the system does not have the ability to meet basic performance criteria, clinical staff will not have very positive attitudes about computer use.

5. Reference List

[1] Burke L and Murphy J. *Charting By Exception: A Cost-Effective, Quality Approach*. New York: Delmar Publishers, 1988.

[2] Burns N and Grove SK. *The Practice of Nursing Research: Conduct, Critique and Utilization, 2nd Edition*. Philadelphia: WB Saunders, 1993.

[3] Stronge JH and Brodt A. Assessment of Nurses' Attitudes Toward Computerization. *Comput Nurs* 1985, 3(4):154-158.

[4] Allen L. Measuring Attitude Toward Computer Assisted Instruction: The Development of a Semantic Differential Tool. *Comput Nurs* 1986, 4(4):144-151.

[5] Sultana N. Nurses' Attitudes Towards Computerization in Clinical Practice. *J Adv Nurs* 1990, 15:696-702.

[6] Burkes M. Identifying and Relating Nurses' Attitudes Toward Computer Use. *Comput Nurs* 1991, 9(5):190-201.

Nursing Informatics: An International Overview for Nursing in a Technological Era
S.J. Grobe and E.S.P. Pluyter-Wenting, eds.

Measuring the Effectiveness of Critical Care Systems

Milholland D K[a]

[a]Senior Policy Fellow, Research and Databases, American Nurses Association, 600 Maryland Ave, SW, Suite 100 W, Washington, DC

Patient data management systems (PDMS) are designed to help critical care nurses cope with large volumes of multi-variate, multi-source data. This research focused on developing and testing a generic, non-vendor-specific effectiveness measure for PDMS. Eight literature-based PDMS goals were identified and operationalized as the 79 item PDMS Effectiveness Measure. Instrument testing addressed internal consistency reliability (.9098), test-retest reliability (Pearson's r = .8941) and content validity (content validity index = 0.66). Construct validity was assessed through contrasted groups analysis with higher scores (p<.05) for nursing units with PDMS. The PDMS Effectiveness Measure is a reliable, valid measure of the effectiveness of PDMS for critical care nurses. PDMS effectively assist critical care nurses in information management.

1. Introduction

The PDMS Effectiveness Measure (PEM) is designed to evaluate the effectiveness of generic, non-vendor-specific patient data management systems (PDMS) from a clinical nursing perspective. The research described here focused on the development and testing of this measure.

PDMS are hardware/software systems which support collection, integration, retrieval and interpretation of large volumes of multi-variate, multi-source critical care data. PDMS are designed to improve clinical data collection and care provider decision making by organizing, manipulating and displaying information in meaningful ways [1]. Nurses are primary patient information managers and primary users of PDMS. Given the time and capital expenses associated with installation, implementation, and maintenance of PDMS, their effectiveness for critical care nurses is important in the current cost conscious, resource limited healthcare environment.

2. Background

The literature on evaluation of PDMS has been dominated by anecdotal, personal reports of staff and organizational responses to an institution's clinical computer system [2,3,4]. Even in formal evaluations the tendency has been to focus on the systems' impact on discrete nursing tasks or patient outcomes of mortality and morbidity [5,6,7,8]. Instruments and methods employed in these studies have had limited or no assessment of reliability and validity. Thus, the applicability of the results to other systems and environments is questionable. Further, research does not examine how PDMS impact clinical nursing practice. When the focus is on nursing, nursing is viewed as a collection of tasks amenable to efficiency techniques and requiring automation to enforce their execution. Certainly, nursing practice encompasses more then the execution of serial tasks.

Because of this lack, this research was conducted to develop a reliable, valid measure that adequately addresses information management from a clinical nursing practice perspective. The measure was designed to assess the effectiveness of computer systems in facilitating nurses information management activities and processes in critical care.

Interaction between nurses and a PDMS is conceptualized as two open systems connected to each other via the device-human interface. There is a shared, overlap area in each system's functions resulting from intersystem connections. The patient care unit environment is shared, but otherwise, each system operates independently of the other. However, because of the shared area, functions of one system may influence functions of the other.

Evaluation research is the utilization of scientific methods to study how effectively knowledge has been applied; that is, identify how well a program works or compare different programs [9]. Effectiveness is the key term and can be the achievement of progress, rather than 100% fulfillment of goals [10].

For this research, critical attributes of system effectiveness were identified as goals, degree, and achievement. System goals progress along a continuum of achievement and degree is the extent of goal progression at any point in time.

3. Instrument Development

Using the techniques described by Waltz, Strickland and Lenz [11], a norm-referenced approach was employed for measurement development. Aspects of PDMS effectiveness were derived from PDMS design goals and system user goals via examination and analysis of research and descriptive literature on PDMS. The PDMS literature was analyzed to identify explicit and implied system goals as perceived by the authors. From these statements, 8 PDMS goals were identified: improve data management (MANAGE), improve data analysis (ANALYZE), help the staff (HELP), improve data quality (QUALITY), improve access to data (ACCESS), provide savings (SAVINGS), improve the quality of patient care (CARE), and totally computerize the patient chart (COMPUTERIZE).

A theoretical definition was developed: the degree to which the system has achieved these goals in terms of the experiences and perceptions of the nurses who interact with the system. A highly effective PDMS has a high degree of achievement for all goals. There may be full achievement of some goals and lower achievement for others.

Operational definition of PDMS effectiveness involved development of definitions and observable indicators for each goal, specification of the criteria for goal achievement, and establishment of the objective for the measure. Using the observable indicators as guides, items were developed, along with directions for administration and scoring. Items were oriented general principles of data management. The intent was that the cumulative score would determine system effectiveness, rather than items explicitly asking about computer systems. The result: a 79 item instrument, the PDMS Effectiveness Measure.

4. Instrument Testing (Methods and Results)

A non-random sample of 71 nurses was obtained from two critical care units with functioning PDMS (Unit 1 and Unit 2) and from two medical-surgical units with no computer system (Unit 3 and Unit 4.) The two critical care units were in different hospitals. The PDMS in the two critical care units had been in active, regular use for ten years. Unit 3 was in the same hospital as Unit 2. Unit 4 was in a different hospital. The hospitals ranged from a university medical center to a rural, community hospital. The sites were chosen to provide contrasts between units with PDMS and those without PDMS. Two rounds of questionnaires were distributed and retrieved by on-site staff with a six week interval between each round.

There were approximately equal numbers of respondents from each type of unit. The respondents did not differ significantly in demographic characteristics. Respondents from the critical care units were significantly more comfortable with computers and had more computer experiences than their counterparts from the medical-surgical units.

The possible range of scores for the PDMS Effectiveness Measure 79 - 395 if all items were answered. The sample's range of scores was 210 to 339 with a mean of 272.24. The first critical care unit (Unit 1) had a mean score of 283.95 and a range from 217 to 339. A mean of 295.53 and a range of 264 to 329 was achieved by Unit 2. The mean score for Unit 3 was 260.35 with a range of 233 to 298. Unit 4 had a mean score of 224.33 and the range was 210 to 260.

Most of the scores from Unit 1 and all of the scores from Unit 2 were in the upper half of the possible range of scores. Most of the scores of Unit 3 were also in the upper half of possible scores, with a smaller range. Most of Unit 4 scores are at or below the halfway point for the range of possible scores. The data management systems in all of these units are at least moderately effective and, in the units with PDMS they are very moderately effective.

Instrument testing addressed: internal consistency reliability through calculation of alpha coefficients; test-retest reliability using the Pearson Product Moment Correlation Coefficient; content validity through use of the content validity index; and construct validity via contrasted groups analysis. An acceptance level of 0.62 was set a priori for the internal consistency, test-retest, and content validity assessments. A significance level of .05 was set a priori for the analysis of contrasted groups.

Internal consistency reliability of .9098 was estimated for the instrument as a whole. Alpha coefficients were calculated for each PDMS goal sub-scale. These were as follows: ACCESS (.4215), CARE (.5048), DATA QUALITY (.5359), SAVINGS (.7337), ANALYZE (.6525), MANAGE (.7578), HELP (.7400), and COMPUTERIZE (.7263). The range of alpha coefficients in the face of the very acceptable alpha value for the measure as a whole may indicate that the subscales are not independent factors within the measure; that is, the set of items comprising the measure assesses PDMS effectiveness, but the individual goals which were to be assessed by the subscales cannot be measured separately.

For test-retest reliability, a Pearson's r of .8941 ($p<.05$) was calculated, indicating 79.9% agreement. This is a very good coefficient for a new measure and can be interpreted to mean the measure as a whole is stable over time. All of the subscales had significant correlation coefficients ($p<.05$) and ranged in value from .6087 to .8527.

Two expert judges, external to all of the research sites, familiar with PDMS assessed content validity. The judges were asked to evaluate the relevancy of the measure's items to the content domain. This resulted in a content validity index (CVI) of 0.65. This means there was 65% agreement among the judges. While not a robust finding, this is an acceptable value.

One way analysis of variance (ANOVA) assessed the differences in mean scores of the respondents from different units. This contrasted groups analysis revealed significant differences among the units ($F=13.0760$, $p<.05$). Post-hoc analysis with Tukeys HSD range test identified the two units with functioning PDMS as having significantly higher PDMS Effectiveness scores.

5. Conclusions

The PDMS Effectiveness Measure has demonstrated acceptable reliability and validity characteristics. The measure is able to discriminate differences in the effectiveness of data management systems among nursing units. In addition, the PDMS functioning in the participating critical care units can be considered as nearly fully effective in achieving their design goals. The PDMS Effectiveness Measure has demonstrated its potential for use in research aimed at understanding the impact of critical care systems on clinical nurses and clinical nursing practice.

6. References

[1] Milholland K. Patient Data Management Systems (PDMS) Computer Technology for Critical Care Nurses. *CIN* 1988, 6:237 - 243.

[2] Cook M and McDowell W. Changing to An Automated Information System. *AJN* 1975, 75:46-51.

[3] Beckman E, Cammack B and Harris B. Observation on Computers in An Intensive Care Unit. *H&L* 1981, 10:1055-1057.

[4] Diaz O and Haudenschild C. Implementation of An Integrated Critical Care Computer. In: *Computers in Critical Care and Pulmonary Medicine*. Nair, I. (ed). New York: Plenum Press, 1983.

[5] Hilberman M, Kamm B, Tarter M and Osborn J. An Evaluation of Computer-based Patient Monitoring at Pacific Medical Center. *Computers and Biomedical Research* 1975, 8:447-460.

[6] Tolbert S and Partuz A. Study Shows How Computerization Affects Nursing Activities in ICU. *Hospitals, J.A.H.A.* 1977, 51:79-84.

[7] Miller J, Preston T, Dann P, Bailey J and Tobin, G. Charting vs Computers in A Postoperative Cardiothoracic ITU. *Nursing Times* 1978, August 24:1423-1425.

[8] Bradshaw KE, Setting DF, Gardner RM, Pryor TA, and Budd M. Improving Efficiency and Quality in A Computerized ICU. In: *Proceedings of the Twelfth Annual Symposium on Computer Applications in Medical Care*. Greenes RA (ed). Los Angeles, Ca: IEEE Computer Society, 1988:763-767.

[9] Suchman E. *Evaluative Research*. New York: Russel Sage Foundation, 1967.

[10] Rutman L. *Evaluation Research Methods: A Basic Guide*. Beverly Hills: Sage Publications, 1977.

[11] Waltz C, Strickland O and Lenz E. *Measurement in Nursing Research*. Philadelphia: FA Davis Company, 1984.

NURSING HEALTH INFORMATION SYSTEMS

B. Bedside systems; point-of-care systems

Nursing Informatics: An International Overview for Nursing in a Technological Era
S.J. Grobe and E.S.P. Pluyter-Wenting, eds.

Building Computer Interfaces With a Human Touch

Bartos CE[a] Mascara CM[a] Nelson R[b] and Rafferty D[c]

[a]Nursing Informatics Department, University of Pittsburgh Medical Center, DeSoto at O'Hara Street, Pittsburgh, Pennsylvania

[b]Nursing Informatics Department, University of Pittsburgh Medical Center, and University of Pittsburgh School of Nursing, DeSoto at O'Hara Street, Pittsburgh, Pennsylvania

[c]Clinical Administration, University of Pittsburgh Medical Center, DeSoto at O'Hara Street, Pittsburgh, Pennsylvania

As health care facilities interface clinical computer systems, the process used to accomplish this task is critical. Most health care facilities have all of the appropriate people to accomplish this interface process effectively. Unfortunately, the right people may be utilized in the wrong sequence. Clinical personnel involved at the onset of the project, insure a patient care oriented approach. The resulting interface of the systems improves patient care, is efficient for the users, and is ultimately a more cost effective method for the facility.

Patient data are the key resources that nurses use in identifying and meeting patient needs. In acute care settings these data are split across departmental computer systems. Building an interface between computer systems can expedite and augment patient care, *if* the process is established and guided by the clinical users. Most health care facilities have all of the appropriate people to accomplish this interface process effectively. Unfortunately, the right people may be utilized in the wrong sequence.

1. Who decides it's time to interface?

The decision to interface systems may be initiated from many sources within a health care institution. For example, the decision to interface two clinical department computer systems may be made by fiscal management to expedite and enhance patient billing procedures. Interfacing allows automated charge capturing. Once the decision is made, the task of building the interface is assigned to the computer programmers. Unfortunately if the request for the interface is initiated from a non-clinical source, improved patient care may become a secondary goal. The interface design is based on the goals of the fiscal department and the technical constraints of each system. After the technical interface is created, it is delivered to the clinical users. Their task is to create the human interface between the systems. The clinical users establish goals, procedures and lines of communication based on the developed interface. In effect, the computer system dictates clinical practice.

This type of situation is riddled with hidden costs to the institution. Excessive "meeting time" is required as clinical users search for common goals and lines of communication within the constraints of the interfaced systems. Complex procedures are established to deal with system constraints. Each new procedure requires training time, documentation and an expectation of error until the complex procedures are learned. Often, redesign of the system is necessary if the interfaced systems produce too much of a handicap to patient care.

This approach fails to build upon existing relationships and communication between the clinical departments. It leaves the clinical users believing that they have no ownership in the development process. They feel the interface has been forced upon them. Once the system is implemented, clinical users on either side of the interface find fault with the "other system." The frustration spills over and begins to destroy inter-departmental communication. In the end the clinical users in the other department become the villains.

NURSING PROCESS	SYSTEMS DEVELOPMENT LIFE CYCLE
1. ASSESSING	1. Identifying problems, opportunities and objectives.
	2. Determining information requirements.
	3. Analyzing system needs.
2. PLANNING	4. Designing the recommended system.
	5. Developing and documenting software.
3. IMPLEMENTING	6. Testing and maintaining the system.
4. EVALUATING	7. Implementing and evaluating the system.

Figure 1. Nursing Process and SDLC.

2. Get the sequence right

To prevent this outcome, the process must begin with the clinical users in the departments to be interfaced. They must establish common goals, recognize information needs and identify points of conflict before programming is done. The interfaced system can then be designed to support those goals, provide the information and eliminate the points of conflict. Administrative support, including fiscal management, is critical to the success of this approach.

Just as nursing has identified the four phases of the nursing process as a method for identifying and resolving a patient's health care needs[1], a similar process exists for computer system development. This process is called the systems development life cycle (SDLC) and consists of seven phases[2]. However, the seven phases of the SDLC can be easily translated into the nursing process (See Figure 1). By integrating these two processes, you have the foundation for the Interface Development Process for clinical systems.

Beginning this clinically oriented interface requires a core group of practicing nursing and ancillary personnel, a "steering committee" (See Figure 2). The committee is co-chaired by a representative from nursing and the ancillary area. Ownership of the system and the goals begins with this committee. This committee should also have representation from the staff nurses, unit secretaries, and ancillary personnel that will be using the system to provide patient care. Clinical personnel already interact routinely. Their input into automated, inter-departmental communication is realistic. Representation from the programming areas allows the programmers the opportunity to understand the rationale and ask questions as decisions are made. It may also be necessary to include representation from administration and fiscal management on an as needed basis. Their input can assist in major policy or charging decisions. A systems analyst or clinical informatics specialist is necessary to this committee to bring together the patient care and technical aspects.

The systems analyst is helpful to guide the information sharing and goal setting process. Ideally, the individual has a clinical background and a functional understanding of both systems. The systems analyst encourages that ideal goals be stated in realistic, achievable terms. Building an interface between two systems requires some compromises. When compromise is necessary, the goal should be better patient care.

STEERING COMMITTEE MEMBERSHIP	INTERFACE DEVELOPMENT PROCESS
Co-Chairs: Nursing Manager Ancillary Manager Staff Nurses / Unit Secretaries Ancillary Personnel Systems Analyst Programmer from Nursing System Programmer from Ancillary System As needed: Fiscal Representative Administrator	1. Form Steering Committee 2. Establish joint, patient oriented goals Determine mutual information needs Define any existing points of conflict 3. Determine what the interface can do to accomplish these goals and needs. 4. Program the interface. 5. Jointly create procedures to address what the interface cannot resolve. 6. Pilot the interfaced systems. 7. Evaluate the pilot. 8. Extend the pilot, if necessary. 9. Implement the interfaced systems.

Figure 2. Summary of Interface Development.

Once the clinical focus is established, the programmers become actively involved. They attempt to make the system accomplish the established goals. The programmers work as closely to what the users want as possible. The systems analyst assists with screen design and wording to insure that the system remains "clinically user friendly." If programming is unable to achieve the desired results, procedures, established jointly, are used to overcome system limitations.

Once a usable system and realistic procedures are developed, the system is piloted. The steering committee determines the criteria for success or failure of the pilot project. This requires establishing baseline criteria before implementing the pilot and a method for gathering data. Data are also collected from the employees working in the pilot area. New ideas or problems are often identified by that group.

At the end of the pilot, the steering committee compares the results to the established criteria. They determine if changes to the system or procedures will improve those results. If the needed changes are significant, a continuation of the pilot is necessary.

3. Conclusion

System interface is achieved unless a detriment to patient care results from the process. If the clinical users feel an ownership of the system and responsibility for its success or failure, they will work to achieve its success. No system can run without people making it run, so the most important element to any system interface is the human interface.

4. References

[1] Kelly LY. *Dimensions of Professional Nursing Sixth Edition.* New York: Pergamon Press, 1991.

[2] Kendall KE and Kendall JE. *Systems Analysis and Design.* Englewood Cliffs, NJ: Prentice-Hall, Inc., 1992.

Nursing Informatics: An International Overview for Nursing in a Technological Era
S.J. Grobe and E.S.P. Pluyter-Wenting, eds.

The Patient-Oriented Bedside Terminal

Meehan N K

Department of Nursing Science, College of Nursing, Clemson University, Clemson, South Carolina, 29634-1703, USA

Bedside terminals are fast becoming as important to hospitals as billing systems. In 1987, C. L. Packer [1] reported that two out of every three hospitals in the United States were interested in information systems that collect and retrieve data at the bedside. Yet the bedside terminal is currently not affordable for most hospitals. And the most common reason given for not buying bedside terminals is cost. As prices decline more hospitals will purchase them. Therefore, patient contact with a bedside terminal is an inevitability.

Since the bedside terminal inhabits valuable space in an already crowded patient room, the terminal is difficult for patients to ignore. Patients' natural curiosity, increased computer skills and illness-specific concerns may prompt them to interact with the terminal.

This paper will investigate a new approach to nursing care by discussing the possibility of a patient-oriented interface for the bedside terminal. The paper is organized in three sections. The first section covers the nurse's role in designing this patient-oriented interface. The second section discusses what defines a 'patient-oriented' interface for the bedside terminal. The third section addresses the question, "Would patients utilize a patient-oriented interface?" This paper concludes by providing suggestions for the development of a patient-oriented interface for the bedside terminal.

1. Nurse's role in design of a patient-oriented interface

Nurses have been patients' advocates for decades. Nurses act as patients' representatives to hospital administration and ties to the health care team. Presently, nurses function as patients' communication link with the bedside terminal. Nurses also fulfill many other roles. Nurses are educators who assess patients' needs for information about their disease and supply necessary information. Nurses also provide direct care to patients. Patients generally choose to share their fears and anxieties with nurse members of the health care team.

Basically, nurses are "information managers," managing data pertinent for patients' return to health. Nurses interact with patients in many ways and are familiar with their information needs. Therefore, nurses should be involved in the design of a patient-oriented interface.

Nurses should also encourage patients to have input into the design of a patient-oriented interface. Nurses can include patients by asking them to assist with information system committee duties. Yet patient representatives seldom have the commitment necessary to remain with the committee until completion. Therefore, nurses should be the primary patient representative when designing and selecting a patient-oriented interface for the bedside terminal.

2. Definition of a 'Patient-Oriented' Interface for the Bedside System

The question, "What defines a 'patient-oriented' interface for the bedside system?" is an interesting one. The single most important component of a patient-oriented interface is the ability of patients to interact with the computer. First, consider the information patients desire. Patients want to learn about their disease or condition and the possibility of future illness. They want to know if their test results are normal. Patients have questions concerning their level of activity or pain medication. They want to understand medical procedures and to obtain a daily schedule of meals, diagnostic tests, and treatments. The type of information frequently requested by patients falls into three categories: 1) information patients can access directly from their computer record, 2) information in patients' records that necessitates interpretation, and 3) information not available from the computer record.

2.1 Data Directly Available from Record

Patients frequently request information they could obtain directly from their medical record. Many patients want access to information in their medical record. Patients have a right to this information. Putting a medical record on a computer system should not affect that right. With a patient-oriented interface, patients can directly access parts of their medical record. However, allowing patients direct access to information from the medical record introduces new problems.

The first problem that arises is safeguarding the privacy of patients' records. Nurses have always been concerned with patient privacy. Traditional methods for insuring privacy do not work with the computerized record. Faaoso [2] states that an increase in the number of terminal locations has multiplied the possibilities for access. If patients are allowed access to their records, the sheer number of individuals having access to patient data increases the chances of a breech of privacy.

The next problem is identifying parts of the record that patients can be allowed direct access. Certain parts of the medical record are self-explanatory. Patients could access their demographic information with the ability to mark errors for correction. Patients could access charges and give the medical facility input about these charges. Allowing patients direct access introduces the issue of accuracy. If patients are given direct access to their medical records, who should be responsible for the accuracy of the record? Should the patient, the medical facility or the nurse assume this responsibility? These are just a few of the problems introduced when patients have direct access to their data.

2.2 Data Indirectly Available from Record

A second type of information the patient frequently requests is information that necessitates interpretation. Certain information obtained from patients' records requires interpretation by a medical professional. The legal ramifications of patients directly accessing this information without some form of interpretation are staggering. Patients want information about their medication. Listing the medication, dosage, and administration times does not provide patients enough information. Patients want to understand their test results. Lab results alone mean nothing to patients. Most lab results need some explanation of the findings. A patient might misunderstand that a negative finding on a biopsy means cancer was not found.

A patient-oriented interface for the bedside terminal could access patients' medical records and then present this data in a way to educate patients about their diseases. Patients could be given an interpretation of the data. For instance, patients could request information about blood tests for hemoglobin. A patient-oriented interface could give patients their hemoglobin results, explain the normal range for their particular gender and age, and then explain problems associated with a high or low hemoglobin. The patient-oriented interface could incorporate the results of tests with a "lay" explanation of the findings.

2.3 Data Not Available from Record

The last category of information that patients desire is data that is not available from their medical record. Patients want information about their diagnosis. They want to understand their illness and the treatment options available to them. Patients want to know any special diet or exercise limitations. One method of providing this data is similar to that suggested by Blue Cross / Blue Shield [3]. The company developed a "Shared Decision Making" system composed of a laser disk system which gives patients information about the treatment options available to them. The system gives information about patients' illness and pros and cons available for those treatments. In this way, patients are able to make better decisions about their own care.

3. Patients' utilization of a patient-oriented interface

Another area of discussion is the utilization of a patient-oriented interface. Today almost all individuals have interacted at some time with a computer. ATMs (automated teller machines) and grocery store bar code readers are just a few examples of how computers are incorporated into our everyday life. Most people do not realize that they deal with computers daily. These interactions seem too commonplace to be considered computer interactions.

For patients to get medical data from their bedside terminals, systems must be user-friendly. A patient-oriented interface should encourage patient interaction with the bedside terminal. If a computer interface is appealing and easy-to-use, patients are more likely to use the system to participate in their health care.

One suggested method of providing information meaningful to patients while allowing a user-friendly interface is to have a question / answer component. Richards et al. [4] developed a computer system that contained a section called "Personalised Dialogue." The dialogue section allowed patients to enter into a conversation with the computer in the same way they would talk with a nurse or doctor. However, answers would be available 24 hours a day and patients would not have to wait for physicians to make rounds before they could get answers.

Sometimes patients have questions they find too embarrassing to ask nurses or physicians. A dialogue section could enable patients to ask questions they feel uncomfortable asking a health care professional. A study by Van Cura et al. [5] found some interesting results concerning information patients consider personal. The study found that the majority of patients would rather give personal information to a computer than share it directly with nurses or physicians.

The way the system presents data to patients is a second component important in defining a patient-oriented interface. For years, health educators have been using visual images to teach patients about their illnesses. Patients learn more when they visualize an abnormality or disease. One research study by Hinohara et al. [6] used the computer's color graphic capability to educate patients about their cardiovascular risk factors. Color graphics were used to plot an individual's risk factors within a circle. The further the plotted points fell from the center of the circle the fewer the significant risk factors.

Another major area of consideration is that some features of a patient-oriented interface might discourage patient utilization. One study by Robinson and Walters [7] looked at a computer network called Health-Net. The network was made available to graduate and undergraduate students at Stanford University.

Health-Net provided an electronic mail system, an electronic bulletin board, an information and referral listing, and a self-help / health information library. However only students with computer experience used the system often. Other students said Health-Net was intimidating and too difficult to learn to use. They also said they did not have convenient access to a computer terminal, they did not know how to use computers, and did not trust computers.

Computers are still too complex and frightening for average patients. And, until using bedside terminals becomes as easy as using the ATM, most patients will probably avoid using a patient-oriented interface for the bedside terminal. To encourage all patients to interact with their bedside terminals, voice recognition abilities are essential. The patient-oriented interface should provide language options and multiple data entry methods to accommodate handicaps. In this way, the patient-oriented bedside terminal could meet the needs of most patients.

4. Suggestions for Development of a Patient-Oriented Interface

In summary, suggestions for development of a patient-oriented interface for the bedside terminal must address three areas. First, the nurse must identify information important to patients. Nurses are the likely health care professionals to be involved with the design of a patient-oriented interface.

The second suggestion for development concerns operationally defining a 'patient-oriented' interface for the bedside system. This category must consider two types of data: data available from medical records and data not available from medical records. Data from patients' records are necessary to educate patients about their particular disease, medication, etc. Patients need to understand their lab results in relationship to their disease process. Patients also want other educational tools to guarantee the understanding of their illness.

The third area for development targets the use of the patient-oriented interface. This interface should be so inviting that patients would choose to utilize the system to participate in their health care. The patient-oriented interface should allow patients 24 hour access, the ability to share in decision-making, and easy-to-understand graphic capabilities.

In summary, the bedside terminal is coming. In the future, patients *will* have some interaction with bedside terminals. The type and quality of that interaction is the responsibility of nursing. Representing patients on a information system committee, nurses can provide input on the best methods to encourage patients' utilization of their bedside terminals.

5. References

[1] Packer CL. Point-of-Care Terminals: Interest Abounds. *Hospitals* 1987, 61: 72.

[2] Faaoso N. Automated Patient Care Systems: The Ethical Impact. *Nurs Management* 1992, 23: 46-48.

[3] Patients Hit Computer Age. *The Greenville News*. Friday, March 05, 1993.

[4] Richards B, Cadman J, Farmiloe H, Leong F and Wong K. The Value of Computer-Aided Patient Education For Nurses In General Practice. In: *Proceedings of the Fourth International Conference on Nursing Use of Computers and Information Science*. Hovenga EJS, Hannah KJ, McCormick KA and Ronald JS (eds). New York: Springer-Verlag, 1991: 545-549.

[5] Van Cura LJ, Jensen NM, Greist JH, Lewis WR and Frey SR. Venereal Disease. Interviewing and Teaching by Computer. *Am J Public Health* 1975, 65: 1159-1164.

[6] Hinohara S, Takahashi T, Uemura H, Robinson D and Stehle G. The Use of Computerized Risk Assessment for Personal Instruction in the Primary Prevention of Ischaemic Heart Disease in a Japanese Automated Multiphasic Health Testing and Services Center. *Med Inf* 1990, 15: 1-9.

[7] Robinson TN and Walters PA. Changing Community Health Behaviors with a Health Promotion Computer Network: Preliminary Findings from Stanford Health-Net. In: *SCAMC '87*. November 1987: 514-520.

A nursing interface

Thom JB[a] Chu SC[b] McCrann L[c] Chandler G[c] Rogers S[d] Edgecumbe J[e]

[a]*Clinical Consultant (Nursing Information Systems) and Systems Analyst, Nursing Information Systems, Melbourne, Australia*

[b]*Coordinator, Computer Studies & Nursing Informatics, School of Nursing Deakin University, Victoria, Australia*

[c]*Systems Designer, Nursing Information Systems, Melbourne, Australia*

[d]*Systems Coordinator, Nursing Information Systems, Melbourne, Australia*

[e]*President, Nursing Informatics Australia, 431 St. Kilda Road, Melbourne, Australia*

A glaring problem with healthcare software design is the aessumption that healthcare professionals operate in the same way as any other desk-bound office worker and the focus had, in the past, always been placed on the technology instead of the users. The rapid development in information technology, new knowledge in software engineering and a shifting focus onto the users demand a total re-think of healthcare software design. New conceptual and design approaches have been adopted for the development of a new generation Clinical Information Systems. The new design focuses on useability, user tailorability, expansibility and portability as the fundamental features. To ensure these features, we choose an object oriented approach in our design and integrate interface design closely with system functionality. The central object-library and data store are well shielded from users to protect system integrity but users are encouraged to define and develop their own children "action objects." The system is designed to be delivered on the state-of-the-art technology like pen-computers and is fully capable of being run on conventional desktops.

1. Introduction

The man-machine interface remains one of the most crucial areas of software design and along with the programs functionality logic forms the basis of any system from the user perspective. When be began to look at the various interfaces available for systems in the early 90s, one thing that became clear was that the office orientation of these interfaces was not particularly relevant to our task of designing a high end Clinical Information System as a research prototype.

The reasons for this perceived inadequacy were basically that these systems were designed to be used by a desk bound office worker, and thus were designed as a generic work environment that mirrored the established office. Our aim was to develop a system specifically for care providers in particular, in this early form, nurses in the acute care hospital environment. So our system was seen as a very specific tool that is used in what marketing people would call a vertical application.

2. The Interface Features

We believe the interface must reflect the reality of the clinical environment and the functionality of the system must be closely embedded in and related to the interface to make the system as intuitive as possible. By embedded functionality we mean the actual "doing" parts of the application which we feel in such a system are indivisible from the interface in the users perception of the system. These embedded functions must be user tailorable to enable the best fit to the practise standards of the institution and its constituent members. Yet the concept of a single reliable and predictable interface standard was seen as imperative to prevent a hodge podge of interface types and technologies that would destroy consistency in the system, and lift the duration and slope of the learning curve to the point where the system was without value. Thus functionality and interface for our purposes became indivisible in an overall conceptual context although they remain separate but closely related in the physical design. So our intent came to be, the design of a system that provided the functionality required by the bedside clinician with an interface that was as simple as possible within the demands of the functionality. The interface therefore needed to be a natural and intuitive reflection of the work environment [1], and this is conceptually the most difficult part of the system to design, and our major interface and system design parameters are as follows:

1. To be intuitive and incorporate natural human information processing parameters. Human dialogue relies on speech, images, touch, and gestures. Handwriting and speech are two intuitive skills that we have acquired and developed since childhood. Such data input methods are believed by many researchers as the ultimate interfaces to the computerized medical records [2] and should be incorporated into the user interface design whenever technologies permit.

2. Easy to learn and use, as our common household electronic devices like the telephone, the television sets or the fully automatic 35mm camera. They should make all technical encumbrance such as the input/output devices, operating systems, networks, and applications transparent from the users.

3. Consistent, simple, reliable, convenient and highly portable.

4. Based on user needs not analyst perceptions.

5. The system should conform to the concept of "What You Want is What You Get [WYWWYG], that is the user should be able to individualize displayed information sets.

To achieve these aims we entered into a long period of analysis with ideas constantly being brought into the system developed, dissected, used or, if necessary, discarded. This process of constant analysis continues and allows the system to be extremely flexible and evolutionary. Early in this process we found that our knowledge of information technology and the capability of current and future pieces of hardware became critical. It is possible to design today a system that would be totally dependent on voice control and holographic output, it is not however possible to build it in even a prototype stage as the technology is not yet well enough advanced. Yet a system needs to use the best available technology that will most enable the users to perform their jobs in the most effective and efficient manner. So the challenge becomes one of designing a conceptual model that is adaptable and open to change, yet can make use of the speed and capability of changing system architectures, and it is our firm contention that without solid knowledge of the state of technological innovation that such design is simply not possible. You must have a vision of future possibilities to design for the future.

3. The object oriented paradigm

The design uses a object orientated theoretical basis [3][4][5] which allows for the design of "doing" objects which perform some designated functionality but also are uniquely responsible for their interaction with the user through an association with a communication object. An example would be the best way to explain what we mean here.

If the end user wishes to create a way to store say blood pressure she would call up a data store object and here would tell it what sort of information it was to store.

- Three numeric values [Systolic, Diastolic, and a calculated mean]
- The unit of measure [mm Hg]
- Alert ranges [institution, unit, ward, practitioner, patient, age range, diagnosis]
- Priority of alert ranges

The data store object would automatically create its needed data store files in the central data base which initially would be a RDBMS such as Sybase. The user would then call a communication object to define a suitable set of data entry and egress routines which would handle the display and interface needs of the data type and these routines can be defined by user or group. Object orientated DBMS are, in our opinion, not yet sufficiently developed for the complexity of the task of managing a Clinical Information System [CIS] at the time this paper is written. However, we are keeping a close watch in the development of object-oriented DBMS in healthcare systems. Active development of such systems for use in Europe as part of the EEC Ward Information System has recently been reported [6]. When the object-orient DBMS technology is ready we will incorporate its use in our system.

The data store and communication objects so defined become "children" of the original "parent" objects through inheritance with specific attributes as a result of their polymorphic changes. These two objects are then combined into a single object that becomes the BP action object for that group of users. This action object can then be combined with other specific vital sign action objects and a specialized trend display communication object to form a larger total vital signs action object. Figure 1 illustrates this concept.

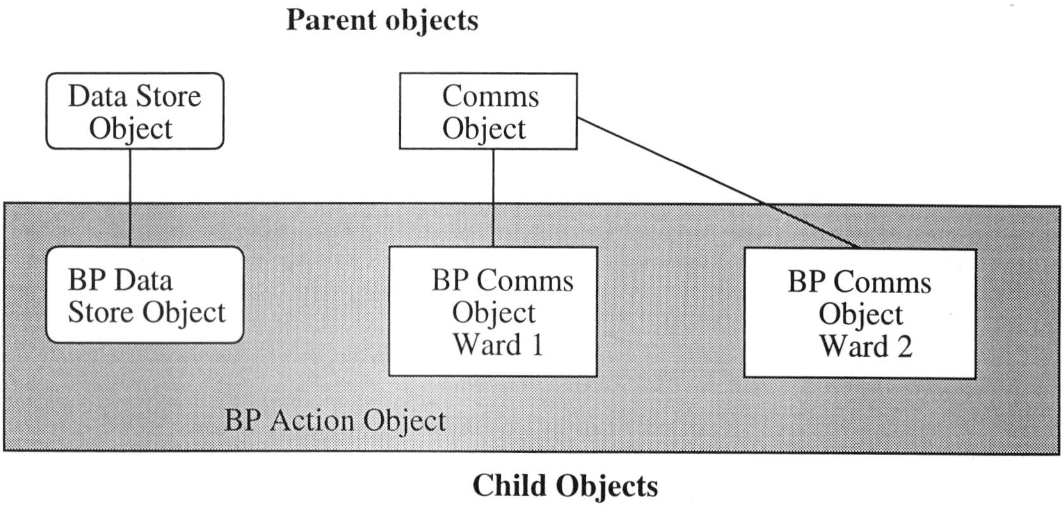

Parent objects

Child Objects

Fig. 1 A simple hierarchy of objects, in this example two wards prefer to have slightly different interfaces for collection and displaying patients' blood pressure so there are two different communication objects, one used in each ward, yet only one data store object.

These objects would be allowed to be remarkably freeform due to the fact that the data storage part of the system is firmer in that the system deals with all the RDBMS data store functionality and to the users this functionality is largely a black box that they need not be aware of at all [7]. We make a firm distinction between the input and output of data from and to the user and the entry and egress of data to the RDBMS. Data input and output is a function of communication objects whilst entry and egress is far more rigorous and definite in its methodology to enable speed of RDBMS access and reliability. Thus we can allow the institutions to develop their own objects from a set of pre-defined functionality in "parent" objects and we take this one step further by allowing suitably qualified users to write their own communication objects and so extend the functionality of their system in ways that the system analysts never initially envisioned.

It is through this separation of "church and state" in the form of data and user interface functionality that is core to our systems ability to be many things to many users yet still maintain the patient data in a patient centric manner that is reliable and most importantly easy to support. This allows for the richness of a working environment that will mirror the variety that is intrinsic in the medical record, and patient charts even in its current limited paper form. It is the primary responsibility of the data objects to provide safe and reliable data entry and egress from the central data engines in the system, they would be by their nature and design guardians of the data provided to them and would be responsible for the final integrity of data that has offered for use by communication objects. The communication object is the way users interact with the CIS, together forming the systems interface and the interface can be extended to suit the needs of particular institutions.

Currently we would anticipate that such new objects would need to be tested and certified at the original development centre to ensure that they are safe, but once that was done they would remain the property of the author and they could be swapped liked any other collectable between institutions. This would enable other vendors to come into the market as well to write add on functionality for the system and the basic specifications would be placed in the public domain to encourage this. Licensing and copyright of these new objects could be commercial or public domain depending on the developers aims, although distribution would have to be tightly controlled to ensure that objects were the original certified ones and not altered or infected. The fact that they were certified however would mean that they could be used with confidence.

Data store objects would be more difficult to develop generally as they would need access to the DBMS routines and data dictionary definitions. It would be anticipated that third parties and users could create "child" objects with enhanced functionality but that they would still have the same data elements, storage routines and audit trails. It would be possible to give out new data dictionary elements but obviously this would need to be centrally controlled and the process of certification of this sort of object would be complex and probably expensive. However if the core system provides an adequate data dictionary there should be little need for extensions and those that are required due to changing practise methods and new treatment modalities, will be required by many users and thus cost justifiable.

Thus the entire system from user interface to central RDBMS store will be user definable to a level that is unknown in current systems. This means that the system will be tailorable to the needs of the institution and the practitioners within it, thus the users perceptions will be of a set of functionality that matches their needs and is consistent with their work practises, this brings us to the issue of what the system would actually look like to the user, and in particular the bedside clinicians.

4. Cutting edge technologies

As we noted originally the idea of a office metaphor is appropriate for people who work in offices but bedside clinicians do not work in offices, they work with patients in wards, and clinical departments. Therefore the system must reflect this reality and must use perception aids that reflect that reality to enable the user to"use" the knowledge of their environment in their navigation through "their" CIS. So we would anticipate that the system would be navigated through a series of layouts or maps of the work environment, so that the user could locate the environment they were working in the the patients in that environment.

The system would for the most part organise data around the patient so that we would represent the patient graphically with the various devices around the patient also represented. Highlighting one of these devices would bring up all of the information known on that area. For instance if the patient was being treated with intravenous fluid therapy, the data behind its icon would include the orders, fluid balance chart, dates of cannula insertion, line changes, dressings, and a hypermedia help on how to care for this patient in relation to this therapy and the sort of therapeutic agents being used. The data set for this therapy could also include digital still and motion video images of the IV site and written and verbal anecdotal notes about the management of the therapy. Finally trended data could also be displayed.

The system would be based in Pen Computing technology as this allows for what we consider to be the most natural interface currently available [8]. Whilst also providing minimal distraction in patient clinician interaction allowing the system to be used naturally during patient care, without the social disruption and limitations of conventional keyboard and mouse interfaces. Also this system has the obvious benefits of portability, scalability to large displays in suitable areas such as critical care and central stations. It is envisaged that the concept of scalability would lead to differing devices being used from Apple Newton, NCR 3130 and Toshiba Dynapad T100X type devices right up to A3/A2 sized displays in critical care at the patients bed or at the Triage Desk in the emergency department. Also the ability of such systems to use radio transmission based LANs means that the user with a portable device becomes truly mobile, and all patients records are always available. Currently our development work is based in using Microsoft Windows for Pen as it has the benefit of market presence and a well established technical community. Object oriented operating systems are definitely going to have an impact in the area of CISs but we feel that at the moment these technologies are not stable enough, although a pen capable version of NEXT would be wonderful.

We would see voice data input and output and system controls as a near term aim along with cursive handwriting recognition. In the longer term there will be great benefit in three dimensional and virtual reality interface, these would obviously be of use in medical imaging but also in the area of data manipulation such as the new tools being developed by Xerox at PARC in Palo Alto [8] (it appears that once again that Xerox will be central to the development of a new critical information technology). How such interfaces could be applied at the bedside is unclear due to their very antisocial nature with goggles and data gloves. Not to mention the issue of combining a virtual reality with the "real reality". Also of importance will be the emergence of high end object oriented data bases and finally artificial intelligence and in particular the concepts of agents and expert systems will be important to long term development.

5. Conclusion

In conclusion we have now gone a fair way into the process of suitable design methodologies for complex Clinical Information Systems and are now at the stage of prototyping some of the concepts involved. We perceive that should such a system be brought to commercial development that it would need to be seen as a relatively open environment, and developments encouraged by many software vendors.

6. References

[1] Lindgaard G. Human Factors in Professional Computing. *Professional Computing*. 1992, 79: 24-28.

[2] Gabriel, ER. Electronic Healthcare Records: A Discourse. *Journal of Clinical Computing*. 1990, 18(5/6): 130-142.

[3] Yourdon E and Coad P *Object Oriented Analysis*. Prentice Hall. 1991.

[4] Booch G. *Object Oriented Design with Applications*. The Benjamin/Cummings Pub. Co. Inc. 1991.

[5] Meyer B. *Objected-oriented Software Construction*. Englewoods Cliffs, Prentice Hall. 1988.

[6] Rasmus DW. Object Databases Find Their Niche. *Byte*. 1992, 17(14): 164-165.

[7] Kim Wand and Lochovsky FH. *Objected Oriented Concepts, Databases & Applications*. Addison-Wesley. 1989.

[8] Rees MJ. New Directions in Graphic User Interfaces. *Professional Computing*. 1992, 80: 20-24.

Nursing Informatics: An International Overview for Nursing in a Technological Era
S.J. Grobe and E.S.P. Pluyter-Wenting, eds.

The Nursing Process Meets Technology:
The Evolution of Care Elements for a Point of Care System

Dzugan R

Nursing Information Services, Chedoke McMaster Hospitals, 1200 Main Street West, Hamilton, Ontario, Canada

A strategic partnership between Ubitrex Corporation and Chedoke McMaster Hospitals was formed to collaborate in the design, development, and testing of a Point of Care system which supports the delivery of direct patient care. The initial step was to conceptualize a means to lend structure to the system and to maximize clinical orientation in a manner useful to nursing. This design concept focused on defining patient care needs within the context of the nursing process. The building block of the Point of Care system became the "Care Element." A Care Element is a symbolic representation of discipline specific information in a technologically meaningful format. Care Elements are flexible and can be structured to reflect any patient care delivery system, professional practice model, or patient population. This flexibility guarantees that Care Elements will continue to serve in developmental models for protocols, care planning based on nursing diagnosis, case management, critical paths, care maps, outcome based care, and patient focused care.

1. Introduction

The Chedoke McMaster/Ubitrex initiative unlocks the potential value of point of care technology and provides a tool that transforms the documentation aspects of nursing care into a technologically advanced milieu. The Point of Care system consists of a computerized nursing workstation linked to hand held portable units that record and retrieve clinical information wherever patient care is delivered. At the workstation, nurses use "Care Elements" to create an electronic patient Kardex which is based on physician orders and nursing diagnoses. Kardex information is downloaded to the portable device where the nurse accesses the documentation system by scanning user and patient identification numbers and entering in a four digit password.[1] Patient specific information is captured immediately following delivery of care and is available for viewing on the main computer system by any member of the health care team. This paper will describe the conceptual and technical process of Care Element development and the ways in which Care Elements are used. Links will be made in relation to Care Elements, Point of Care technology, and contemporary issues of current nursing practice.

2. Development

Nursing has recognized the need to standardize and formalize health related information. There is increased focus on the quality of care and the potential of information technology to gather data indicators contributing to the advance of patient care management and nursing knowledge. To support these concepts the Care Element was developed as the heart of the Point of Care system. The Care Element is a nursing data element which defines and characterizes patient care.

Clinical experts from all levels of nursing contributed to Care Element development. In order to maximize usefulness to nursing and to demonstrate value to practice, education, research, and administration, Care Elements were developed in the presence of a clearly defined view of how care planning activities could be automated. The concept of Care Elements was tightly focused on a patient centred design and built with and to nursing requirements. At the onset of development, it was necessary to come to terms with the concept and structure of the Care Element and to define the infrastructure of the Point of Care application. As the Care Element would be the building block of the system, determination needed to be made about: what a Care Element should be; what it should do; what ideas it should capture; what was the taxonomy and nomenclature; and what were its rules.[2] Care Elements needed to respond to nursing intervention language that formed the nursing lexicon and to represent labels that provided clinical meaning.[3] Consequently, the Care Element became an innovative combination of preexisting knowledge that could be structured for automation.[4]

From a systems perspective, the Care Element was a distinct and mutually exclusive data element. The initial phase of Care Element prototyping was done with a Supercard software development package on a MacIntosh. Supercard software flexibility allowed rapid modification to accommodate the structural evolution of Care Elements.

Intensive hardware and software testing consistently underscored all Point of Care developmental activities. The major challenge to the system was to convert patient care information on the manual Kardex into Care Elements which were accurately displayed on the electronic Kardex. The associated challenge was to document all patient care activities using the Point of Care device without any loss or corruption of data. Constant modification of Care Elements occurred during all testing phases.

3. Description of Care Elements

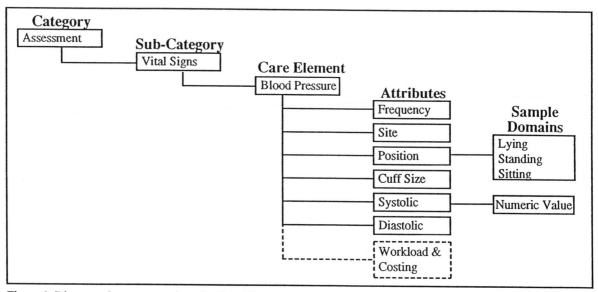

Figure 1. Diagramatic representation of a Care Element.

Care Elements are the smallest unit of nursing activity and reflect the functional component of nursing actions. Care Elements are symbolic representations of discipline specific information and the phenomena which concerns nursing practice.[5] By design, Care Elements are action oriented, event specific, dynamic, and user definable. Care Elements describe relevant nursing actions and interventions complete with all the diversity and complexity present within the nursing environment. Their characteristics are flexible and useful in customizing care planning according to patient needs. Care Elements are structured in three main sections: the Care Element itself, associated attributes, and associated domains or values. The composition of Care Elements are further described as follows:

3.1 Care Elements
- are a descriptor of clinical activity that is clinically meaningful
- are the building block of the electronic Kardex and the source of all documentation
- can be grouped and electronically linked to nursing diagnostic care plans, protocols, or documents
- have associated groups of attributes

3.2 Attributes

- describe the characteristics of a Care Element
- may be optional or required
- have an associated domain

3.3 Domains

- describe all possible values for an attribute
- may be: single choice from a pick list
  multiple choice from a pick list
  number within a range
  free text

To lend order to the system, Care Elements were grouped into distinguished units or categories. Categories were classified into sub-categories of related Care Elements. The electronic Kardex and the portable Point of Care device were designed to match categories. Care Elements were assigned to one of six categories as outlined in Figure 2.

Assessment	Activities of Daily Living	Medications	Tests	Treatments	Education/Communication
•vital signs •specific assessments	•activity •comfort •elimination •hygiene •nutrition •safety	•I.V. •blood products •routine meds •prn meds •1x meds	•specimen collection •diagnostic tests	•wound care •tube care •supportive devices •respiratory therapy	•ward orientation •teach-condition •teach-procedure •teach-health promotion •communication - supportive •communication - therapeutic

Figure 2. Categories and related subcategories.

All Care Elements are clustered in their subject categories on the electronic Kardex and are available to view, create, modify, or discontinue. The electronic Kardex, provides a comprehensive overview of current planned care similar in nature to the manually generated Kardex. Point of Care and the supporting structure of Care Elements provides a means to facilitate evidence of patient care by care planning, Kardex creation, documentation, report generation, historical recall, and immediate output of data on a real time basis.

4. Care Elements and the Nursing Process

The nursing process is an integral component of nursing care. It is an efficient method of organizing thought processes for clinical decision making and problem solving.[6] Care Elements support the nursing process through the use of nursing diagnoses by forming the basis of data building and data collection. Care Elements are clinically oriented and therefore support the steps in the nursing process model. An individualized care plan for the patient is built by selecting Care Elements from the six categories of care. The Care Elements are customized in response to a specific patient need or problem. Care Elements enable on line modification of standard documents for patient care which are derived from dependent, interdependent, and independent orders.[7] The scope of Care Elements encompass clinical orders related to nursing, laboratory, pharmacy, nutrition, and diagnostics. Point of Care provides the link between patient care information on the Kardex or care plan and the information technology which enables electronic documentation of care.

The following process describes the continuum of care beginning with the Doctor's order to documentation of care by the nurse. The Physician writes an order for "occlusive dressing to sacral ulcer." The nurse selects a Care Element from the treatment category. The Kardex entry is electronically displayed on the workstation as "Wound Care: impaired skin integrity: duoderm to sacral ulcer, change Q5 days." When the nurse has completed the wound care on the patient and is ready to document the activity at the bedside, the treatment category button on the Point of Care device is pressed. The prompt on the Point of Care device is displayed as "Wound Care: impaired skin integrity: duoderm to sacral ulcer, change Q5 days. Dressing status? Wound appearance? Patient response?" The nurse responds to the prompts by selecting values from choice lists. The documentation note is displayed on the Point of Care device with date, time, and the electronic signature of the nurse providing care and appears as "Wound Care: impaired skin integrity: duoderm to sacral ulcer, change Q5 days. Dressing status: changed. Appearance: moderate exudate, open, reddened. Patient response: mild discomfort."

Table 1 illustrates the way in which the Care Element "wound care" facilitates the nursing process.

Table 1
Nursing process supported by a Care Element

NURSING PROCESS	DEFINED IN	SYSTEM ENTRY POINT	SPECIFICATIONS	DOMAINS/VALUES
ASSESSMENT	Care Element	Kardex	wound assessment/care	
NURSING DIAGNOSIS	Care Element	Kardex	impaired skin integrity related to immobility	
PLANNING and INTERVENTION	Attribute	Kardex	site	sacral ulcer
	Attribute	Kardex	dressing	Duoderm
	Attribute	Kardex	frequency	q. 5 days
EVALUATION	Attribute	Point of Care device	dressing status	changed
	Attribute	Point of Care device	appearance	moderate exudate, open, reddened
	Attribute	Point of Care device	patient response	mild discomfort

5. Scope

Care Elements accommodate a wide parameter of application and may be utilized to:

5.1 Support Nursing Functions

Care Elements support patient care management through the ability to: create nursing care plans based on nursing diagnoses; maintain current nursing care plans and nursing care records; facilitate individualized patient care planning process; and document planned care according to nursing diagnoses, goal statements, milestones, and patient outcomes. Delegated Tasks are supported by the use of Care Elements to: transcribe and document physician driven protocols, treatments, diagnostic tests, medications, and parenteral fluids; and tailor physican orders to meet individual patient care needs. Finally Care Elements support nursing therapies by the ability to: document patient teaching, supportive and therapeutic communications; modify care plan based on nursing judgement; and customize nursing orders to enable a unique care approach for each patient.

5.2 Facilitate Quality Assurance

Care Elements facilitate Quality Assurance activities as they are built: using standard nursing terminology according to quality assurance standards and documentation guidelines; to match care codes in the GRASP workload measurement system; and to provide a database for planned versus actual care or prospective versus retrospective care.

5.3 Provide a Tool for Nursing Research

The use of standardized patient care terminology can generate a clinical database for nursing research.

5.4 Support Professional Practice

Care Elements are adaptable to any: professional practice model; theoretical base; care delivery system; and philosophy of care.

5.5 Determine Per Patient Costing/Workload Measurement

Dollars and workload measurement units can be assigned to the care element, attribute, or domain. The system has the ability to generate costing and workload measurement reports. The Point of Care system can interface with other applications such as a staff scheduling system.

6. Conclusion

Care Elements, which are the building blocks of the Point of Care system, enable nurses to plan and document patient care activities. With the use of Care Elements nurses conceptualize the communication and documentation of care in a technologically structured manner and shift to a new paradigm of practice. Written in common nursing language and comprehensively structured, Care Elements reflect the direction and continuity of care by facilitating the planning process among care givers. Care Elements span the scope of nursing and physician driven orders and are the written coordination of care. Clinical nursing care data collected and retained by Point of Care operational procedures provides timely and reliable information. The ability of the Point of Care system to collect, retain, and retrieve data expedites clinical decision making by the nurse. Clinical information and specific aspects of nursing minimum datasets such as patient outcomes related to planned care are accessible from powerful datasets extracted from the use of Care Elements. Nursing care activities can be described in a variety of settings for comparability across clinical populations.[8] Care Elements are a significant contribution to nursing efforts in the fields of practice, administration, research, and education.

6. References

[1] McKenna J, Blight Dr.W, Dietiker W, McLachlan L, Webster M. *COACH: Guidelines to Promote the Confidentiality and Security of Automated Health Related Information, 1989.*

[2] Clark J, Lang N. Nursing's Next Advance: An International Classification for Nursing Practice. *Int Nurs Rev* 1992, 39(4) 109-128.

[3] Grobe SJ. Nursing Intervention Lexicon And Taxonomy: Methodological Aspects. In: *Proceedings, The Fourth International Conference on Nursing Use of Computers.* Berlin, Springer-Verlag, 1991: 126-131.

[4] Romano CA. Innovation, The Promise and Perils for Nursing and Information Technology. *Comput Nurs* 1990, 8(3) 99-103.

[5] Graves JR, Corcoran S. The Study of Nursing Informatics. *IMAGE:* 1989, 21(4) 227-231.

[6] Doenges M, Moorhouse M. Nursing Process. In: *Nursing Diagnoses With Interventions.* Philadelphia: F.A. Davis 1988: 5-8.

[7] Zielstorff RD, McHugh ML, Clinton J. *Computer Design Criteria, For Systems That Support The Nursing Process.* Kansas City: American Nurses' Association, 1988.

[8] Werley HH. Use And Implementation of the Nursing Minimum Data Set. In, *Proceedings, The Fourth International Conference on Nursing Use of Computers.* Australia, 1991.

Nursing Informatics: An International Overview for Nursing in a Technological Era
S.J. Grobe and E.S.P. Pluyter-Wenting, eds.

What is the Impact of Bedside Technology on Nursing Care?

Happ B A

The Analytic Sciences Corporation (TASC), Arlington, VA, USA

Dramatic changes are taking place in the technologies used by health care providers. Many acute care facilities are implementing bedside computers or point of care devices to improve patient care documentation and nursing productivity. Research on the actual effectiveness and consequences of bedside computers is lacking. A descriptive and quasi-experimental study was conducted in three hospitals to describe the effect of bedside computers on the patient and to examine changes in quality of care. Patient interviews indicated positive perception about the bedside technology in their room, although overall quality of care measurements were lower on units with bedside computers. The social impact of the technology on patients and the recommendations for bedside implementation and use are described.

1. Problem

Bedside computer systems are being selected and installed in many hospitals because it is thought that they assist the nurse with documentation and delivery of patient care. There are few studies in the literature which describe improvements in patient satisfaction and patient care documentation. Thus, the effectiveness of this technology is untested. In addition, patients' personal preferences, perceptions of self, locus of control, coping styles, patient-provider relationship and belief systems in relationship to bedside computers have not been described. The cost and safety of new information systems technologies at a patients bedside must be considered. With a range from $1200-$35,000 per bed, health care administrators need to be aware of the return on investment and documented benefits of bedside systems.

2. Conceptual Framework

The Health Care Technology Assessment (HCTA) framework was used for this study to examine the impact of bedside computers on patient care. This included the examination of the cost, safety, effectiveness and social impact of the technology. The HCTA framework was developed by the Office of Technology Assessment [1] to assist in ensuring that technologies which have potential benefits and acceptable risks are made available. Table 1 illustrates the use of the framework for this study.

3. Literature Review

Technologies are drugs, devices, procedures or systems used by health care providers. Computers in nursing are categorized as systems and procedures. While critical care nursing has dramatically changed because of technologies, there have been only a few studies which document changes in acute nursing care delivery with the introduction of computers in nursing. The effectiveness of information systems in health care is not well documented and only three empirical studies actually describe the impact of bedside computers on the patient and quality of care. Kahl, Ivancin and Fuhrmann [2], describe a significant financial savings with bedside computers and Marr [3] reports positive patient perceptions. Knickman, Kovner, Hendrickson and Finkler [4] found no changes in patient satisfaction, increase costs and a positive impact on nurse recruitment and retention when studying the impact of two types of information systems in acute care settings (bedside and hospital information systems).

Bedside computers are still an emerging technology with few empirical studies on the consequences of the patient and quality of care.

Table 1
The Health Care Technology Assessment Framework (HCTA) For Evaluating Bedside Computers

Effectiveness (Quality)	Social Impact	Cost/ Safety
Chart Audit Patient Satisfaction Questionnaires	Patient Interviews	Literature Review

4. Study Design

Two patient satisfaction questionnaires were administered and a chart audit was conducted. A convenience sample of 90 patients on five units in three hospitals participated in the study. A sub-sample of the same patients were interviewed to assess the social impact of bedside computers. The units included a pretest and posttest and two comparison experimental units. A time block (Time 1, Time 2) was used to analyze the effects of bedside over time. Table 2 illustrates the study design.

Table 2
Study Design

Hospital Units No Bedside/ Bedside Computers	Time 1	Time 2
	Hospital A pre Bedside	Hospital A post Bedside
Bedside	Hospital B Bedside	Hospital C Bedside
No Bedside	Hospital B No Bedside	Hospital C No Bedside

The independent variable was the bedside computer and the dependent variables was the quality of patient care as measured by patient satisfaction and patient care documentation. The covariates were gender, race, age and computer experience. Hinshaw and Atwoods's [5] Patient Satisfaction Instrument (PSI) and an author developed Patient Perception of Computer Related/Technology Related Care Instrument (PPCI) were used to measure patient satisfaction (PSI) (as one measure of quality of care) and to relate patient satisfaction to the independent variable (PPCI).

The Joint Commission on Accreditation of Health Care Organization (JCAHO) Nursing Care Standard, NC.1, 1991 was used as the chart audit instrument. This consisted of 27, yes/no questions used by a trained auditor to assess the patient's chart. ("Admission completed by RN" etc). An author developed Patient Interview Guide was used to gather descriptive data on the social impact of technology on the patient. One way and two way analysis of variance and multiple regression were used to analyze the data.

5. Study Findings

Although patients were generally very satisfied with patient care and the presence of the computer in their room, this study found that the quality of patient care as measured by patient satisfaction and chart compliance to standards, was better on units without bedside computers. The literature indicated that the costs of the technology do not out weigh the benefits. There were no studies on the safety of bedside computers.

6. Discussion and Recommendations

The implications of computer technology in a patient's room are many. First, patients who were interviewed had positive perceptions of the machines. However, overall quality indicators found that the technology did not improve patient care. Nursing administrators must review the goals of increasing the technology surrounding the patient area. In this case, computers were installed because patient documentation and nursing care delivery were thought to be improved by automation at the point of patient encounter. Examination of the placement (these were fixed terminal at the foot of the bed), the computer system implementation process and nursing attitudes must be considered. The most important issue may be to ask what processes are being used to deliver nursing care delivery before computerization. Automation of the present paper process may not bring improvements in quality. Computerization must include changes the nursing care delivery system to include movement toward patient focused care. Patient care redesign along with considerations for non-fixed or mobile technology may assist in quality of care improvements through automation for nursing. More study is needed on bedside computers to justify continued acquisition and implementation of this technology.

7. References

[1] Office of Technology Assessment. *Assessing the efficacy and safety of medical technology.* 1978 (NTIS No. PB 286 929).

[2] Kahl K, Ivancin L and Fuhrmann, M. Automated nursing documentation system provides a favorable return on investment. *J of Nurs Adm* 1991,11:44-51.

[3] Marr PB. NYU study supports community general's stance. *Healthcare Informatics.* 1992 May:72.

[4] Knickman J, Kovner C, Hendrickson G, and Finkler S, *An evaluation of the New Jersey nursing incentive reimbursement awards program: Final report and Appendix.* NYU, The Health Research Program. 1992, June.

[5] Hinshaw, AS and Atwood JR A patient satisfaction instrument: Precision by replication, *Nurs Res* 1992,3:170-175, 191.

Nursing Informatics: An International Overview for Nursing in a Technological Era
S.J. Grobe and E.S.P. Pluyter-Wenting, eds.

263

Point of Care: A Move Toward a Paperless Process

Lang B J[a] Gallien-Patterson Q[b] Chou J Y[a]

[a]Department of Veterans Affairs, Hines Information Systems, P.O.Box 7008, Hines, IL, USA, 60141-7008

[b]Department of Veterans Affairs, Chicago-Westside Medical Center, Damen Avenue, Chicago, IL

This paper discusses the implementation of a bedside terminal project and its impact on the Nursing personnel in a Veterans Affairs Medical Center as part of the point of care (POC) plan of the Department of Veterans Affairs, Decentralized Hospital Computer Program. Other POC projects are also mentioned.

1. Introduction

Point of Care is defined according to Andrews [1] as a clinical information system (CIS) which is designed to support the patient care delivery process and automate the nursing and other caregiver documentation process at the patient bedside, treatment area, or point of care. Some characteristics of a point of care system are:

- Computerized terminals/devices, either fixed or portable, located at the bedside, or available to, the patient bedside or (any) point of care.
- Information processing capabilities (input & output) are provided by various technologies.
- Assistance or automation of routine, repetitive clinical tasks and activities performed by nursing staff and other caregivers.
- Supports quality assurance and audit processes to ensure delivery of quality patient care.
- Provides for need-to-know access to other pertinent data at the point of care via integration or interface with other information systems; also allows for the transmission of patient data to other need-to-know information systems in the organization.

The approach and technology used in choosing and implementing a point of care (POC) system within a patient care setting is based on the type of care provided to the patient, the structural environment, and the complexity of the tasks or activities of the care giver. In general, a categorization of the types of POC including hardware preferences would differ in acute care medical/surgical areas, long term care settings, psychiatric units, ambulatory care areas, and critical care units. Devices used in the POC approach might be fixed terminals in intensive care units and ambulatory care settings, and portable and fixed devices in acute care, long term care, and psychiatric settings. Device types can be summarized as monitoring equipment, workstations, regular data terminals (Keyboard, Touch Screen, Light Pen, Bar Code Reader, etc.) and voice technology. The number of device types associated with a specific point of care system would vary based on the type of patient and complexity of care provided.

2. Bedside Terminal Project

2.1 Purpose of Study

This study is designed to examine the benefits of implementing a bedside clinical information or monitoring system on a typical acute care medical unit. In recent years bedside monitoring has generated much interest in the private sector; however, very little diffusion has occurred. In general, bedside monitoring is a concept which expands centralized patient care systems with bedside terminals placed at the "point of care", i.e., the patient's bedside. The terminal at the bed-side reflects a difference in the way caregivers document and communicate care. Care documented at the bedside is immediately available for access by other caregivers. Currently, there is little data to document the benefits of a bedside monitoring system in the public sector. A decision to automate must include careful analysis of benefits.

2.2 Objectives of the Study
- Describe the nurses' perceptions of implementation of a bedside monitoring system.
- Identify quantitative and qualitative benefits attributable to installation of a bedside monitoring system.
- Examine the variation of nursing hours during selected nursing care prior to and after implementation of the bedside terminal system.
- Identify hardware and software requirements for point-of-care.
- Identify installation considerations for hardware installation.

2.3 Background /Literature Review
Bedside terminals were introduced into the market primarily to capture immediately observed patient data [2,3,4]. Facilitating timely monitoring of patient data assures more informed clinical decision-making by nurses, according to Herring [6]. After almost a decade of talk about terminals at the bedside, 99 of 100 bedsides remain terminal-free. Of hospitals with more than 100 beds about 5% plan to buy bedside terminal systems, according to information from industry consultants of Dorenfest and Associates [7,8].

Gardner [5] suggests that one reason customers hesitate to implement an automated bedside system is that many do not have a good underlying patient care information system, without which a stand-alone bedside terminal system has limited usefulness. When information system budgets are virtually flat, bedside terminals are difficult to justify in hospitals that lack those basic systems.

Herring [6] also reports many benefits of bedside monitoring: fewer errors of omission, greater accuracy and completeness of documentation, improved standardization of charting quality, increased accountability for charting, more timely response to patient's needs, more accurate and up-to-date care plans, greater timeliness of tests and procedures, and more time available to provide patient education.

2.4 Relevance to the Veterans Health Administration
Is bedside computing needed to achieve high-quality care? Will it really save nursing time? The purchase of a bedside terminal implementation will be a major financial investment for the Veterans Health Administration. The current perceptions are that such systems will increase the quality of patient care and increase productivity. Other perceived benefits include reduced nurse overtime, retaining/attracting nursing staff, better accounting of clinical costs, reducing patient length of stay, liability reduction, and standardization of patient care according to Denger et al [2]. Unfortunately, few quantitative benefit studies are available to substantiate these claims. Providing a benefit analysis would, therefore, be extremely valuable.

Hospitals using bedside systems have also shown that they contribute to nursing satisfaction. Although this has not yet been translated into dollars, most nursing directors and hospital administrators certainly value highly any impact improved satisfaction will have on retention of nursing staff especially in the VA where recruitment and retention shows some evidence of decline.

The results of this study provide data which will help VA hospital administrators make a more informed decision relative to the advantages and disadvantages of implementing bedside monitoring systems. In addition, this study identifies the nursing staff's response to utilizing a bedside monitoring system.

2.5 Methodology
This study was conducted at the VA Chicago-West Side Medical Center with medical center management approval and support for approximately 1 year (July, 1991-July, 1992). Most of the hardware installation was completed on a twenty-eight bed medical unit in July, 1991. Two tools were developed; one to assess staffs' perceptions and another to measure time required by nurses to perform and document care for the following procedures:
- Admission Assessment
- Vital Signs
- Intake and Output
- Nursing Care Plan Development & Revisions
- End-of-Shift Reporting

An activity definition of each of the selected nursing care events was identified and used as a yardstick for measuring time required to complete activity pre and post bedside terminal installation. A time and motion study associated with the previous procedural listing was performed prior to (Sept.-Nov., 1991) and six months after the bedside terminal installation (May-June, 1992). This provided time for the staff to be trained and adjust to the software and the new documentation system.

The tool to assess the staffs' perceptions is a pen and pencil test that was administered to all of the nursing staff on the POC unit. The pre assessment of the nursing staffs' perceptions was administered January, 1991 and the post assessment was administered in June, 1992. The following is a list of questions asked the nursing staff in the pen and pencil perception survey:

1. Do you feel the POC bedside monitoring system will increase productivity?
2. Do you feel POC will decrease the amount of overtime and compensatory time used?
3. Will POC improve the accuracy/legibility and quality of documentation?
4. Will POC increase accessibility/availability of data?
5. Will POC improve information gathering/retrieval?
6. Are you optimistic of the concept of POC bedside monitoring?
7. Do you feel that the patients will feel intruded upon with the installation of the hardware?
8. Do you feel that you will adjust quickly to the POC bedside monitoring system?
9. Do you feel that POC will eventually be a time saving measure?
10. Do you feel there will be cost benefits with POC?
11. What type of hardware do you prefer?
    a. Portable
    b. Stationary

2.6 Hardware

Stationary, wall-mounted VT320 terminals with standard keyboards (42 inches from the floor) were selected. There was a 1:1 terminal to bed ratio. All terminals were connected to a 386 processor speed personal computer through an Arnet board. The 386 processor ran all clinical Decentralized Hospital Computer Program (DHCP) applications and was used as a file server transferring data to a Digital Corporation VAX computer where the patient data was permanently stored. Response time was almost instantaneous, i.e., there appeared to be no perceptible delays. Three laser printers supported the project.

2.7 Unit Profile

This is a typical medical unit in this medical center with regards to staffing ratio and clinical practice. It is somewhat unique in its physical layout for it is situated around an intensive care unit and each room is structurally different with a bed complement of 1, 2, or 3 beds.

The unit has one head nurse, nine staff nurses and three staff licensed practical nurses and a bed capacity of 28 patients. The daily patient-nurse ratio is approximately 7:1. The educational preparation of the staff is summarized:

Bachelor of Nursing Science = 5
Associate Degree in Nursing = 1
Nursing Diploma = 4
License Practical Nurse Diploma = 3.

The average daily census pre-POC equaled 22; average daily census post-POC was 25.

2.8 Staff Perceptions

Thirteen surveys pre-POC and twelve surveys post-POC were administered and returned. The nursing staff was optimistic about the concept; 69% pre-installation and 100% post-installation. It was felt both pre and post installation that bedside terminals would increase nurse productivity, improve accuracy/legibility and quality of documentation, increase accessibility of patient data, and improve information gathering/retrieval (100%).

Seventy-seven percent of staff felt a quick adjustment to POC pre-installation as compared to 100% post-installation indicating that the POC system is user-friendly. Stationary terminals were preferred 53% pre-installation and 100% post-installation.

While the staff was not as convinced of the time savings and cost benefits of POC monitoring it is significant to note that perceptions relative to time savings increased by 25% and cost benefits increased by 47% when the Pre-POC and Post-POC are compared. Also, it is well to note that 63% of the staff felt that the terminals would intrude upon the patients pre-installation and 0% of the staff saw terminals as intrusive to patients post-installation.

7B Nursing Staff's Perceptions

Pre-POC
N=13

Post POC
N=12

Questions	Yes	No	NR		Yes	No	NR
Increase Productivity	13	0	0		12	0	0
Decrease OT	11	0	0		12	0	0
Improve Quality of Documentation	13	0	0		12	0	0
Increase Access	13	0	0		12	0	0
Improve Retrieval	13	0	0		12	0	0
Optimistic	9	3	1		12	0	0
Pt Intruded Upon	7	4	2		0	12	0
Quick Adjustment	7	5	1		12	0	0
Time Saving	5	4	3		9	3	0
Cost Beneficial	4	7	2		10	2	0
Stationary Terminal	7	3	1		12	0	0

2.9 Overtime/Compensatory Use

Data was collected to monitor overtime and compensatory time use for Ward 7B for the first and second quarters of fiscal year 1991 and fiscal year 1992. The 1st and 2nd quarters of fiscal year 1991 represents Pre-POC; 1st and 2nd quarters of fiscal year 1992 represents Post-POC. While use of overtime and compensatory time decreased during FY'92, it is difficult to credit this occurrence to the presence of the POC bedside monitoring system. Reasons noted for request of overtime and compensatory time were varied, i.e., to augment staffing, complete documentation, replace staffing, etc. A closer monitoring of the reasons for overtime and compensatory time is needed to make this measure statistically significant.

2.10 Time and Motion Studies

A total of ten (10) measures for each of five events (vitals, intake & output, patient admission, new care plan development, and care plan revisions) were collected on all three shifts. It is worth noting that nurses rarely performed these activities independently of other tasks. Every attempt was made to isolate and exclude all interruptions, even if it was well within that which is considered nursing care. Some activities noted were patient teaching, engaging of side rails, suctioning the patient, preparing the patient and his tray during mealtimes, etc.

A comparison of Pre-POC and Post-POC data showed that each time an activity was performed, there was a decrease in the amount of time required to take and record vital signs (one minute), measure and record intake and output (1.5 minutes), admit a patient (five minutes), develop a patient care plan (1.5 minutes) and updating a care plan (3.5 minutes). Overall a potential time savings of 13.5 minutes/patient was realized on a single tour of duty when all activities were performed with a patient with the POC system.

On this 28 bed unit, if all patients have vital signs taken on a single tour of duty, there is a potential savings of forty-two minutes. If five patients on this unit (on one tour of duty) are on intake and output (I&O), a potential saving of a minimum of 7.5 minutes is identified. Overall, there is almost fifty minutes of time saved which could be applied to performing patient education, staff training, and other patient care related duties.

3.0 Findings

The implementation of POC at the Chicago-Westside VA Medical Center have indicated the following benefits:
1. Patient information is readily available and easily retrievable by all health care providers, e.g., nurses, physicians, pharmacists, dietitians,
2. Point of care is labor saving and reduces the time required to document patient care.
3. Data entry of patient information into a computer database contributes towards the enhancement of a nursing knowledge base which could be used in developing decision supports tools to enhance patient care.
4. There is improved timeliness in the accessing of patient data throughout all hospitals areas; no waiting for the paper medical record to either record or retrieve information.
5. Clinical record documentation is improved; documentation contains less omissions.
6. There is improved patient care due to the accessibility of patient information.
7. Improved unit efficiency has resulted.
8. POC supports reduced paper filing and reduction in clerical functions and errors.

9. The installation of bedside terminals does not interfere with the delivery of patient care nor is it considered an environmental safety hazard.

4. 0 Other POC Implementation Projects

The following is a summary of several additional POC projects implemented in the DVA medical centers. Preliminary information regarding the outcome of the implementation is being accumulated. This data will be available by April 30,1994.

- Topeka, Kansas VA Medical Center is using a radio frequency hand-held device in the acute care area for the purpose of documenting patient information such as vital signs, intake and output, and the administration of medications.
- Baltimore, Maryland VA Medical Center is implementing a fixed bedside "terminal" approach by using Apple Powerbooks mounted on pull down arms. Several specialty care units and an acute care unit are testing this hardware. In the ICU, data will be transferred from the Marquette monitors to the DHCP environment.
- Atlanta, Georgia; Temple, Texas; Mountain Home, Tennessee, and Philadelphia, Pennsylvania VA Medical Centers are implementing fixed bedside terminals similar to that outlined in the Chicago-Westside project.
- Marlin, Texas VA Medical Center is investigating the feasibility of implementing a moveable PC based system using a wireless LAN to capture and display patient information.

5.0 Conclusions

The implementation of a point of care care system at the Chicago-Westside Veterans Affairs Medical Center has provided the Veterans Health Administration with a prototype point of care module. Future implementations of point of care systems should have a positive impact on the quality of care provided to the veteran patient. Finally, POC systems will have a significant impact on the cost savings related to clinical FTEE and the associated operating costs of multiple hospital services.

References
[1] Andrews, William F., '92 Bedside Systems Report, *Healthcare Informatics. May, 1992.*

[2] Denger, S. and et al, Implementing an Integrated Clinical Information System. *Journal of Nursing Administration, 18 28-34.*

[3] Edmunds, L., Computers For Inpatient Nursing Care. *Computers in Nursing, 1986, 4 102-204.*

[4] Evans-Paganelli B., Criteria for Selection of a Bedside Information System for Acute Care Units, *Computers in Nursing, 1989 Sept/Oct 7(5) 214-221.*

[5] Gardner,Elizabeth, Hospitals Not in a Hurry to Plug in Computers by the Bedside. *Modern Healthcare, 1990 July 31-55.*

[6] Herring, Donette, A Closer Look At Bedside Terminals. *Nursing Management 1990 July 21(7) 54-61.*

[7] Kahl, Ken, Identifying the Savings Potential from Use of Bedside Terminals. Case Presentation at Hospital Information Management System Conference held in New Orleans, 1990 February 1-10.

[8] Johnson, Joyce, Psychological Impact. Case Presentation at Bedside Computer Terminals, Future Technology Emerging Conference held in Washington, DC, 1988 February, 31-70.

NURSING HEALTH INFORMATION SYSTEMS

C. Order management; care plans; computerized care record

Nursing Informatics: An International Overview for Nursing in a Technological Era
S.J. Grobe and E.S.P. Pluyter-Wenting, eds.

Bedside Charting by Exception
in a Computerized Patient Care Plan System

Murphy J [a] and Hoffmann M [b]

[a]*Aurora Health Care, Information Services, 3031 W Montana Ave, PO Box 343910, Milwaukee, WI, 53234-3910.*

[b]*St. Luke's Medical Center, Nursing Education, 2900 W Oklahoma Ave, PO Box 2901, Milwaukee, WI, 53201-2901.*

Professional staff nurses in acute care settings have been struggling with care planning and documentation models for decades. This paper explores the innovative approach taken by St. Luke's Medical Center in Milwaukee, Wisconsin to facilitate a comprehensive and efficient patient record. Charting By Exception (CBE), which has been used in a manual mode for over 10 years, is now integrated into an automated bedside documentation system. Once the Plan of Care is established, whether by Nursing Diagnosis, Protocol, Critical Pathway, or other Care Plan framework, documentation against the plan takes place in the exception format. This facilitates ease of documentation and clear identification of significant findings and variance data. It also expedites data retrieval for trend analysis. Completion of orders from the Plan of Care are documented directly from an automated "Task List". CBE creates a mechanism for quick and easy documentation, which works well at the bedside while the nurse is delivering patient care. It eliminates writing information on an intermediary form for later computer entry. Nurses document immediately, which removes lag time from collection of information to accessibility in the computer system. Although CBE has proved effective and efficient in a manual mode, bedside automation has synergistically impacted on the cost and quality effects seen.

1. Project Scope and Objectives

When St. Luke's Medical Center investigated automated bedside nursing documentation systems, one functional requirement was the ability to maintain the principles of Charting By Exception. The nurses at St. Luke's were very used to the ease of significant data entry and retrieval at the bedside, using unique Nursing/Physician Order Flowsheets [1, 2, 3, 4]. Although at the writing of this paper, the automation of documentation has not been accomplished throughout the medical center, the principles of CBE have simplified the design and development of an automated documentation system on a pilot nursing unit.

St. Luke's Medical Center is a 711-bed, nonprofit, private, teaching hospital which receives regional, national and international referrals for its Centers of Excellence in heart, cancer, rehabilitation, women's health and emergency medicine. Clinical Systems had their advent at St. Luke's Medical Center in the early 1980's, with the installation of a Patient Data Management System (PDMS) for 63 critical care beds. Moving toward the 1990's, however, its capabilities began to fall short of rising expectations and technologies offering open architecture workstations. It also became apparent that there were obvious bedside information management needs in the Med-Surg environment, as well as the ICU. Although there was a good amount of hospital information system (HIS) functionality in place (order entry, result reporting, acuity entry, charge capture, etc.), terminals were all located centrally in the nursing station and there was no automation supporting nursing documentation at the point of care delivery.

A second phase began in 1990 with an extensive clinical system vendor evaluation. The major goal was to find a product that could meet the requirements for both an ICU and Med-Surg environment: support the nursing process components common to both, and focus on improvements in care through implementation of technologies to enhance data availability and information management, as well as create a foundation for the growth of an integrated environment for clinical information. An extensive list of functional and technical specifications was created.

However, there were no products on the market at that time that were capable of providing CBE to the extent of the manual CBE system already in place. Investigation turned to finding a vendor that would provide the greatest capability for software flexibility and was eager be a developmental partner in this endeavor. The development process began in fall of 1990 and the pilot system went live in May of 1991.

The pilot unit is a 36-bed general medical unit, with workstations at several locations around the nursing station and in every patient room. Although the need for bedside data entry with automated documentation systems continues to be controversial from a cost/benefits standpoint [5, 6, 7, 8], it is an essential element for the CBE system in order to facilitate immediate data trending and identify if a change or significant finding (i.e., "exception" data) has occurred. Documenting current data in the context of all previous data also eliminates the need to transfer volumes of information from one nurse to another at shift report and avoids transcription of data onto intermediary forms prior to computer entry. Information is immediately accessible in the system and is not subject to availability of the chart or the nurse [9, 10].

2. Pilot Unit Functions Incorporating CBE Features

Initial functionality included documentation of vital signs, intake and output, bedside glucose monitor results, height/weight, and physical assessments. The pilot proved that the concepts of CBE can be adapted to an automated system, as long as the software has flexible, robust software configuration tools. Interestingly, use of CBE also supported the pilot use of computers by nursing, as entry of only significant or changed data kept the time spent at terminals to a minimum, thereby reducing the fear of any nurses intimidated by computers.

2.1. Standard Assessments

The standard assessments that had already been established as part of the CBE philosophy made data entry screen design an easier process than anticipated. Since parameters were already established for 10 assessments [11], much of the initial analysis was eliminated. The assessments and their associated parameters are shown in Table 1.

Table 1
Standard assessment parameters

Category	Parameters
Respiratory	Rate, characteristics, nailbeds, CRT, mucous menbranes, cough, sputum, breath sounds
Cardiovascular	Apical pulse, edema, neck veins, CRT, calf tenderness, peripheral pulses
Neurological	Orientation, movement, sensation, pupils, memory, quality of speech/swallowing
Integumentary	Skin color, temperature, integrity, condition of mucous membranes
Gastrointestinal	Abdominal appearance, bowel sounds, palpation, diet tolerance, stools
Urinary	Urine characteristics, bladder distension, voiding patterns
Musculoskeletal	Muscle strength, joint swelling/tenderness, ROM limitations, condition of surrounding tissue
Pain	Location, description, intensity, duration, radiation, precipitating factors, alleviating factors
Neurovascular	Color, temperature, movement, peripheral pulses, CRT, sensation to affected extremity
Surgical site	Dressing/incision characteristics; color, temperature, tenderness of surrounding tissue; condition of sutures/staples/steri-strips; approximation of wound edges; drainage

The screens were designed by arranging the already defined parameters for each system so the entry fields flowed logically. Each parameter then had the following identified: definition of normal findings, list of predictable choices for abnormal/significant findings, field length, whether the field entry would be mandatory or not, and whether free text was to be allowed. The list of predictable choices was drawn from the same textbook [11] from which the standard assessments were developed and was made available from a pop-up window attached to each field.

2.2. Initial Assessments

Entry screens supported CBE by initially displaying the findings defined as a "negative/normal" system assessment. Required fields were used to force appropriate baseline parameters to be addressed. When documenting an assessment, the nurse had only to review the screen and change any parameters to "abnormal/significant" findings using the pop-up window.

Another feature was added to the entry screens to further minimize data entry and make use of the established negative system assessments. When a parameter had numerous possibilities for entry and the norm could not be limited to one entry, the use of the phrase "WNL (within normal limits) except" became a useful addition to the field title as a support for CBE. For example, when documenting perfusion on the cardiovascular screen, it was obvious that there is no one pulse grade or skin color that is the norm for all patients. The field titled "Perfusion WNL except" allows the nurse to use an empty field to indicate insignificant findings, and requires only significant data entry. In these cases, the normal system assessment parameters do not display, instead the fields are blank.

2.3. Ongoing Assessments

After the initial assessment entry, successive screens display with the previously entered data "carried forward", whether normal or significant data. If no assessment change is noted, it requires only two keystrokes to document the same data for the current time. If assessment changes are noted, the appropriate parameters are changed using the pop-up window selections or free text. If the assessment was significant and now all parameters are returned to normal, one keystroke allows the retrieval of normal findings. Again, only one more keystroke allows this to be documented for the current time.

2.4. Highlighting of Significant Information

All screens were designed so that significant data entered was immediately flagged via inverse video display, so that it drew the immediate attention of the user. This flagging made it possible for any clinician entering, retrieving or reviewing information to identify significant data at a glance. It was also important to build into this flagging feature the ability to unflag an otherwise significant entry. This allowed the nurse to indicate that data typically thought of as significant for most patients was insignificant for a particular patient. For example, the absence of right pedal pulses is typically significant, but would be insignificant for a patient with a history of right lower leg amputation. This aids all clinicians, as only *patient-specific* pertinent data is highlighted for quick review.

2.5. Assessment Report

The Assessment Report generated by automated documentation of assessment data was most helpful and acceptable as it took on the appearance of the Nurse/Physician Order Flow Sheet already familiar to the staff. The report prints daily and summarizes assessment data so that review of the information takes minimal time and easily identifies the significant pieces. The detailed assessment data only prints when there are significant findings.

There was much discussion about what to print when designing the Assessment Report. With automation, it would have taken no additional staff effort to detail both normal and significant assessment findings on the report, as the normals could have been pulled out of the system data base. However, staff felt they would have lost the ease of *quick significant* data review on the report if these findings were buried in voluminous detailed text notes. Thus, staff chose to maintain the policy of only printing detail information for significant findings.

Another advantage of automation is used when creating and printing the Assessment Report. With the manual process, a new flow sheet is started every 24 hours. This requires detailed charting of significant findings for the first entry of each day even if the assessment remains unchanged, as policy states that an arrow (CBE symbol) cannot be used to reference back to notes on previous flow sheets from previous days. The automated record does not have that requirement; the two keystrokes used to "carry forward" the unchanged detail from the last documented significant finding can elicit a detail print for the first entry on the report.

2.6. Shift Worksheet Report

The Shift Worksheet is printed by each nurse at shift start and is designed to print all significant data from the most recent physical assessment documented. Since the nurses at St. Luke's also report by exception, the automation of CBE reduced shift report time. Time is saved by the nurse giving report, who does not have to verbally repeat the information already printed on the Shift Worksheet. Time is also saved by the nurse receiving report, who does not have to write down information already available in printed form.

3. Future Directions for Expanding Use of CBE Features

The computer design team continues to work to define the direction for completing the automation of CBE documentation. Their vision will be incorporated into new software that will be used on the pilot unit, and eventually expanded throughout the hospital. Below are some examples of areas of development.

3.1. Documentation Against a Pre-Established Plan of Care

CBE incorporates documentation against an established plan of care. Once the Plan of Care is established, whether organized by Critical Pathway, Problem, Focus, Nursing Diagnosis, Protocol, or any other framework, documentation against the plan of care can take place in an exception format. This includes both nursing assessments, and all other nursing intervention and physician order completion. A patient-specific "task list" can be derived from the plan of care and provide the linkage to the documentation screens [12, 13, 14].

Completion of any intervention/order from the plan of care should be able to be documented using the exception format directly from an automated "task list", organized by outcome and orders for the shift or day. Options from the "task list" should include: (1) Done/no exceptions, documentation complete, (2) Done/with exceptions, branch to detail documentation screen for significant data entry, (3) Not Done/reschedule, branch to scheduling screen for new time entry, (4) Not Done, branch to order cancellation screen for reason entry. When the order is completed without significant findings and the expected result is obtained (option 1), documentation should be as simple as one keystroke. When the order is completed and significant findings are noted or the expected result is not obtained (option 2), one keystroke from the "task list" should branch to a detail entry screen to document the exception. When the order is not done and needs to be re-scheduled (option 3), one keystroke from the "task list" should branch to a screen for re-scheduling the order. When the order is not done and needs to be cancelled (option 4), one keystroke from the "task list" should branch to a screen for cancelling the order and documenting why. This functionality would promote efficient data entry and provide a robust data base for quality monitoring [15, 16].

3.2. Using CBE to Identify Variance Data for Case Management

Within a computer system, the benefits of CBE can be expanded beyond those seen when documenting for any one patient. By incorporating CBE concepts with an integrated information system, historical data across patient populations can be captured and turned into information that directly guides patient care management. The system can assist the nurse in: identifying achievement of expected or standardized outcomes of care; determination of causes for variances from expected outcomes; promotion of collaborative practice, coordinated care and continuity of care; promotion of appropriate/reduced utilization of resources; and, facilitation of early discharge or discharge within an appropriate length of stay. The use of critical pathways within a case management model helps define "best practice" pattern for a specific patient population. The database of information collected about every patient is used to help identify the most appropriate expected outcomes and the most effective interventions for each defined patient group.

Once a critical pathway is established, documentation of outcome achievement and intervention completion can easily take place in the exception format as described in the previous sections. CBE can be used to help document variances: expected outcomes that are not achieved as planned; interventions that are not completed as planned; and, interventions that are completed as planned, but have an unexpected or significant response. Additional entry may be required to categorize the cause of any variance, such as: patient, caregiver, ancillary department, etc. As long as the exceptions are clearly tagged in the computer system database, variance analysis can take place to facilitate re-evaluation/revision of the critical pathway or identify corrective action to eliminate causes for variance.

3.3. Patient Care Management By Exception

One of the most difficult tasks for patient care providers is assuring that all relevant patient information is reviewed and acted on in a timely manner. Clinicians spend a tremendous amount of time pouring over the paper record, attempting to separate new information from old and important from unimportant. CBE eliminates this critical and time-intensive task by automatically highlighting new and significant information. Computer systems can be programmed to automatically route new and significant information to the appropriate clinician(s). The information can sit in the clinician's "review queue" until the next time they sign on, at which time they are notified of the significant data. Furthermore, through the use of audit trail capabilities, computer systems can document when the clinician has reviewed the new and significant information. This design feature provides a tremendous cost containment and quality improvement advantage to the organization.

4. Summary

The exception format facilitates ease of documentation as well as clear identification of significant findings and variance data. This, in turn, supports data retrieval and analysis by all health care professionals and promotes quality of care. Although this type of system is effective and efficient in a manual mode, bedside automation synergistically impacts on the cost and quality effects seen.

5. References

[1]   Burke L and Murphy J. *Charting By Exception: Cost-Effective, Quality Documentation Approaches*. New York: Delmar Publishers, 1993.

[2]   Burke L and Murphy J. *Charting By Exception: A Cost-Effective, Quality Approach*. New York: Delmar Publishers, 1988.

[3]   Murphy J, Beglinger J and Johnson B. Charting By Exception: Meeting the Challenge of Cost Containment. *Nurs Manage* 1988, 19(2):56-72.

[4]   Murphy J and Burke L. Charting By Exception: An Efficient Way to Document. *Nursing* 1990, 20(5):65-69.

[5]   Barry C and Gibbons L. Information Systems Technology: Barriers and Challenges to Implementation. *J Nurs Adm* 1990, 20(2):40-42.

[6]   Herring D and Rochman R. A Closer Look at Bedside Terminals. *Nurs Manage* 1990, 21(7):54-61.

[7]   Nieman H and Bakker A. Vision on Bedside Nursing Information Systems. In: *Nursing Informatics '91*. Turley J, Newbold S (eds). Berlin: Springer-Verlag, 1991:15-23.

[8]   Shamian J, Hagen B, Brenner R and Lohman P. Point of Care Terminals: A Blessing or a Curse? In: *Nursing Informatics '91*. Turley J, Newbold S (eds). Berlin: Springer-Verlag, 1991:26-30.

[9]   Cline A. Streamlined Documentation Through Exceptional Charting. *Nurs Manage* 1989, 20(2):62-64.

[10] Volden C. Decentralization of Patient Charts: What Does It Accomplish? *Appl Nurs Res* 1988, 1(3):132-139.

[11] Bates B. *A Guide to Physical Examination, 5th Edition*. Philadelphia: J B Lippincott, 1991.

[12] Brider P. Who Killed the Nursing Care Plan? *Am J Nurs* 1991, 91(5):35-38.

[13] Fiesta J. If It Wasn't Charted, It Was Done - Law for the Nurse Manager. *Nurs Manage* 1991, 22(8):17.

[14] Worthy M and Siegrist-Mueller L. Integrating a "Plan of Care" Into Documentation Systems. *Nurs Manage* 1992, 23(10):68-72.

[15] Wake M. Nursing Care Delivery Systems Status and Vision. *J Nurs Adm* 1990, 20(5):47-51.

[16] Zielstorff R, McHugh M and Clinton J. *Computer Design Criteria That Support the Nursing Process*. Kansas City: American Nurses' Association, 1988.

Nursing Informatics: An International Overview for Nursing in a Technological Era
S.J. Grobe and E.S.P. Pluyter-Wenting, eds.

Order Management in a Nursing Perspective

Nieman H B J Bakker A R and Duffhauss J H

BAZIS Central Development and Support Group Hospital Information Systems, Schipholweg 97, 2316 XA Leiden, The Netherlands

Order management systems support order entry activities and the communication of data between the nursing unit and ancillary services. This paper first describes the functions of the early order communication applications in the U.S.A. The characteristics of these systems and the new clinical-oriented systems, are then compared. The requirements for clinical order management systems that support patient care activities of nurses and doctors, are explored. As an example, the order management features of an integrated nursing information system (VISION), are presented.

1. Introduction

Patient care in hospitals is an order-driven process :
In the paper based system health care providers generate orders for medication, tests, treatments and examinations. The original doctor's orders are translated by nurses and ward secretaries into request forms that are sent to ancillary departments e.g., the pharmacy, laboratories and radiology. The orders are processed there. Results are then reported back to the ward and documented in patient records. The order management process consists of 4 major components: order entry, order communication, order processing and results reporting.

Manual management of orders requires a considerable amount of paperwork and manhours. Research on data handling by nurses in a 18 bed unit at the Leiden University Hospital indicated the following number of procedures per year [1]:

Lab. Tests	33,857	IV Medication	4,692
Consults	772	ECG	678
Radiology examinations	558	Miscellaneous	2,257

In total between 2 and 5 orders per day per patient are being written, each to be translated into 50-70 data items on requisition forms. These figures illustrate the order related workload for the ancillaries as well as the clerical efforts for the nursing units.
Computer systems can provide support for more efficient and effective management of orders.

2. History

Applications for order handling by computer and especially order entry in the ward, became available in U.S. hospitals already in the early seventies [2]. These systems were aiming at more complete patient charges, cost reduction and improved order/result communication.
Main incentives for the introduction were:
- Fast and complete billing.
  In the pre-DRG (diagnosis related group) era, the costs of tests and procedures were reimbursed to the hospital.
- Order information.
  Information on orders to be retrievable online e.g., an overview of outstanding orders for a patient with status-information, indicating the progress of order handling, in summary or full detail.
- Results reporting and inquiry.
  Reports of results of tests ordered, to be available online for wards and outpatient departments.

The early order management applications can be characterized as 'message routing' systems that replaced order forms and result reports by electronic documents. Data for billing was captured from the orders entered into these administrative systems.
New developments in the U.S.A address clinical and nursing aspects of order management [3].

In a survey of one of the AIM projects of the European Commission it was found that most European hospital information systems offer, even today, only limited functionality with respect to order entry at the source and the communication of computerized orders [4]. The development efforts were concentrated on the realization of an integrated HIS, while data for billing and results reporting is captured from a central database, filled by the HIS-subsystems that support the ancillary departments. Request forms are still sent to the ancillary services, where the order data is being entered into the computer.
However, there is a growing interest in more efficient order entry and communication facilities as machine-readable order forms are being introduced and developments take place to prepare for order entry in the nursing unit.

3.   Administrative vs. clinical order management systems

3.1   The adminstrative system

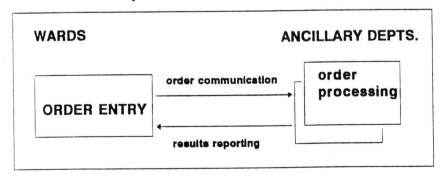

Figure 1. Functional components of an administrative order management system.

The dataflow in an administrative system is a rather simple one. Orders are being entered in the ward, authorized and sent to the ancillary service. The orders are verified and processed there and the results are reported to the nursing unit. Order status information (e.g. order: entered, cancelled, modified, processed) can be reviewed online with these systems.

An administrative order management system is suited for speeding up the communication between the ward and the ancillaries. By using such systems the number of order forms in the hospital will be reduced as well as the turn around time of the order handling process. The system might provide for automatic billing, easy access to readable order/result information on multiple locations. Errors from transcribing orders might be eliminated. A reduction of clerical staff in the central service departments is achieved by spreading the order entry workload over the hospital units.

3.2 The clinical system

The impact of an administrative order entry system on the quality and efficiency of direct patient care is rather limited. Administrative systems were not designed in a patient oriented way. Seperate and manual nurse charting is still required. When order information is not automatically stored in computerized nursing documentation, order entry requires additional clerical effort of nurses.

However, billing based on order entry data has become less important because financial practices have changed. New developments focus on clinical and nursing aspects of order entry and results reporting , as ever more health care professionals recognize the potential benefits of integrated order management facilities.

A clinical order management system should provide for [5]:
-       Screens and menus that are customized to the needs and the terminology of the nursing unit. [6]
-       Checks on conflicting orders, duplication of orders, contra indications and allergies.
-       Efficient and 'smart' order entry facilities, like ward specific and personal order sets as well as protocols, that reduce the time spent for order entry. Protocols allow users to order a series of tests and treatments, 'with one keystroke'.
-       Screens that list the most common orders of the ward and that make information available on the patient's past and current orders.
-       Automatic generation of sub orders related to a primary order. A request for refilling the drug stock on the nursing unit should be produced as a by-product of a medication order. Patient transport might be organized as a result of an order for a radiology examination.
-       Automatic updating of the computerized nusing documentation as a new order is being entered.
-       Presentation of information on past and active orders, per patient, ward, physician, order category.
-       Integrated graphical presentation of results of various order categories, e.g. an automated chart-print showing vital signs, fluid balance data, diagnoses, allergies, medication and (lab.) test results.
-       Scheduling of resources of ancillary services, taking into account the care program of the patient.
   A clinical order management system should be integrated with other systems in the nursing unit.

In a recent study, 46 main functions of an integrated ward information system were identified [7]. Over 50% of these functions are related to order management processes.

A study in the Wishard Memorial Hospital, Indianapolis, demonstrated the feasability of a clinical order management system where physicians enter orders on workstations [11].

The study showed potential savings of more than $ 3 million in charges annually. However, the system equired an increase of time for order entry of 5 minutes per patient per day.

4. The VISION case

In 1987 the BAZIS foundation started the VISION project: the development and implementation of an integrated nursing information system (NIS), based on the use of bedside, patient room, or nursing desk terminals [8,9]. The VISION system is an integrated part of the BAZIS Hospital Information System (HIS). Modules for vital signs, care planning, nursing notes and a nursing work plan have been developed and are implemented now in 5 Dutch hospitals. Apart from functions for support of nursing activities regarding admission and discharge of patients, the developments are concentrating now on the order management process. Figure 2 shows the major functional components of VISION:

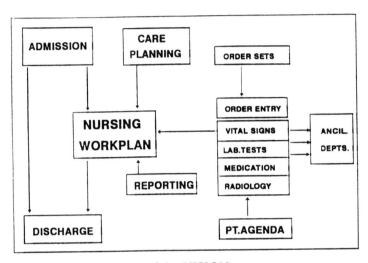

Figure 2. Functional components of the VISION system.

The major functional components of VISION are the care plan, the work plan and order entry facilities. The care plan contains all problems identified for an individual patient, together with the corresponding nursing interventions and goals. The work plan shows all nursing activities for a single patient to be performed in a shift. It contains nursing interventions from the care plan as well as nursing activities based on orders from physicians as well as nurses. The patient agenda reflects the work plan in a patient-oriented way, in terms that can be understood by the patient. Order entry functions document nursing activities in the work plan, using both the patient agenda and information stored in protocols and personal order sets.

The relation between VISION, HIS functions and the order management process, is illustrated by the following example.
When an appointment for a colon X-ray is made, the order 'explodes behind the screen' into a series of separate registrations and communications:
First the system checks if there are possible contra-indications for the x-ray or conflicts with other appointments for this patient. Then the resources of the radiology department are checked to find out if facilities are available at the desired date and time.
When the appointment is made all nursing activities related to the colon X-ray are identified and recorded in the nursing workplan, e.g. preps, patient education, vital signs and enema. Medication orders to prepare the patient for the examination, are activated automatically. Sub-orders are generated and communicated to the corresponding services: for transport of the patient to radiology, refilling the drug stock at the nursing unit and to inform the kitchen about the patient's diet.

In order to investigate and demonstrate the feasibility of this approach, a VISION maquette was developed [10]. This 'motion picture model' shows the functions of the (bedside) nursing information system as well as the HIS and order management features. The maquette has been presented to hundreds of nurses in BAZIS hospitals. We found that the nurses recognize and appreciate our approach of an integrated NIS, HIS and Order Management System.

In June 1992 a two-year study in three hospitals in the Netherlands started [12]. Together with the BAZIS foundation, the hospitals assess the effects of VISION. This technology assessment project is financially supported by the Dutch Ministry of Welfare, Health and Education.
The aim of the project is to provide, where possible in quantitative measures, data on effects of integrated information systems in nursing wards of a university, a general and a psychiatric hospital.

5. Conclusion

Order management systems provide powerful tools for speeding up the communication between the nursing unit and the ancillary departments. Administrative systems have been introduced mainly to support the processes in the service departments and to enable automatic charge capture.
New clinical order management systems focus on the support of the patient-oriented activities of nurses and doctors. Bringing in this 'clinical perspective', opportunities are provided for improvement of both the quality and efficiency of patient care.

6. References

[1]   Heemskerk-van Holtz P R B. Data handling in a nursing unit. *Proceedings third symposium on nursing use of computers and information science*. Daly N, Hannah K (eds), St.Louis: Mosby, 1988: 796-803.

[2]   Duffhauss J, Nieman H B J, Bijl K. Verslag studiereis ordercommunicatie. *BAZIS-report*, 1991.

[3]   Brady M. Bedside nursing/HIS integration must include productivity gains for nursing. *Computers in nursing*. 9(4), 1991: 134-138.

[4]   Heemskerk-van Holtz, Nieman H B J, Kraamer K. The use of computer applications by nurses at clinical wards in European hospitals; An exploratory survey. *PRECISE project no. A.1043: prospects for an extra-mural and clinical information system environment*. 1990.

[5]   Mills M E. Order communications/nursing system requirements questionnaire. *Nursing informatics, where caring and technology meet*. Ball M. Hannah K, Jelger U G, Peterson H (eds), New York: Springer-Verlag, 1988: 353-364.

[6]   Rubino A. Installing order entry using a loaned staff concept. *Healthcare Informatics*. 1990: 22-24

[7]   Baud R, Scherrer J-R, Coignard J, Lucas L. The concept of a ward information system. *Proceedings MIE Conference*. Adlassnig K, Grabner G, Bengtson S, Hansen R (eds), 1991: 81-85.

[8]   Bakker A R. An integrated hospital information system in the Netherlands. *Clinical computing*. 7(2), 1990: 91-97.

[9]   Nieman H B J, Bakker A R. Bedside nursing information systems: the missing link. *Proceedings Nursing Informatics '91*. Hovenga E, Hannah K, Mc Cormick K, Ronald J (eds), Berlin: Springer-Verlag,1991: 424-429.

[10]   Gondelach J, Bik S. Prototype developments for a nursing information system. *Proceedings MIE Conference*. Hansen R, Solheim B, O'Moore R, Rogiers F (eds), 1988: 147-151.

[11]   Tierney W M, Miller M E, Overhage J M, McDonald C J. Physician inpatient order writing on microcomputer workstations. *Journal of the American Medical Association,* January 20, 269(3), 1993: 379-383.

[12]   Van Gennip E M S J, Klaassen-Leil C C, Stokman R A M, Van Valkenburg R K J, Technology Assessment of an Integrated Nursing Information System in three Dutch Hospitals, *This volume,* 1994.

Nursing Informatics: An International Overview for Nursing in a Technological Era
S.J. Grobe and E.S.P. Pluyter-Wenting, eds

Delivering the payoff from clinician order entry: addressing the organisational issues

Soar JN[a] and Ayres D[b]

[a] Senior Consultant (Clinical Applications), Information Management Division, Health Department, New South Wales, Locked Bag 961, North Sydney, NSW, Australia, 2059

[b] Assistant Director of Nursing (Information Systems), Concord Hospital, Concord, New South Wales, Australia, 2039

Realisation of many of the benefits of a HIS (Hospital Information System) is dependent upon direct clinician use for enter of their own orders. These benefits include accuracy, efficiency and elimination of duplication. A goal of recent HIS implementations in Australia has been to achieve order entry by clinicians, and by physicians in particular. Success in encouraging clinicians to use order entry systems requires a strategy for marketing, education and for organisational issues to be identified and addressed.

This paper reports on a case of successful implementation of clinician order entry into an Australian hospital. Planning and training were key features of the strategy. Well planned strategies will deliver benefits in quality of patient care and throughout the hospital from improved communications.

Direct use of order communications (order entry and result reporting) by clinicians, and by physicians in particular, is central to the anticipated benefits from the large investment in information systems that is underway in the New South Wales (Australia) public health system. There has been very little research on the use of these systems by physicians, on factors for successful adoption of this technology by physicians, on factors critical for realisation of the anticipated benefits, and on what the challenges and risks are.

As physician utilisation of a HIS (Hospital Information System) is uncommon, this paper will focus on the successful adoption of order communications by physicians in Concord Hospital, Sydney, New South Wales, Australia. Nurses also use this system for a range of patient administration and communication functions. An empirical case-study based research was undertaken which focussed on factors related to the use of order communications by physicians. Physicians directly use the HIS to access patient information, place orders for diagnostic services and retrieve results.

1. Order Communication Systems

Order communications is the functional core of a HIS. It is the communications channel between wards, physicians' offices, outpatient clinics and all other hospital departments. Orders are placed, enquiries can be made on the status of an order and results are available to all authorised clinicians with access to a computer terminal.

This communication functionality and the inherent information dissemination capability is the basis for many of the tangible and intangible benefits from the implementation of a HIS. Physicians are the principal originators of orders for diagnostic tests and the main consumers of clinical information. Such systems can assist the physician to enter complete orders that will not be questioned or misinterpreted and can create a forced review of orders to reduce duplication and inappropriate orders.

Other benefits include more timely and accurate communication of information. Information concerning a patient will be available at a single point to assist in timely decision making. The legibility of computer-based orders eliminates errors of transcription and reduces time wastage. Work-load information will be immediately available to managers to assist in decision-making, utilisation review and research. Information on ordering activity will benefit of clinicians, hospital management and health authorities. These benefits are expected to lead to a reduction in the average inpatient length of stay.

The results of the research by Finn et al [1] vividly demonstrate a benefit of computer-based order communications. Their research indicated that alteration of physicians' hand-written orders by clerical and laboratory staff was a common occurrence. Order communications can assist clinicians in planning and delivery of patient care. If physicians still handwrite or dictate orders to other staff after the implementation of order communication systems, some of the benefits, such as greater accuracy and efficiency, will not be realised.

2. Literature Review

Physicians are keen to exploit information technology and can identify the advantages. In a survey of attitudes towards the potential use of bedside computer terminals[2], physicians identified a range of potential benefits including improved legibility, accuracy, accountability, charting consistency, access to patient information, and the ability to enter orders or retrieve information at any computer terminal location. There are, however, only a very small number of reports of direct physician utilisation of HIS.

Schreier [3] describes a case of direct physician use of order communications in a Chicago hospital. Physicians were involved in this implementation from the beginning of the project. Lapierre [4] describes physician utilisation of a HIS. This includes remote links to physicians offices for test results, care procedures, vital signs and reports. Copeland [5] reports on physician order communications at a US Army Medical Centre. There, all physician orders are entered into the system by the physicians themselves. The success described in this case study is linked to the military nature of the hospital. Peterson [6] reports on significant cost savings and other benefits from a hospital which encouraged physicians to directly use the HIS.

There is a lack of academic research about physician utilisation of HIS. Anderson et al [7] note that the development of policies regarding computer-based medical technology is hampered by a lack of knowledge about the process by which such applications are adopted and utilised by physicians.

3. Physician Order Communications at Concord Hospital

Concord Hospital, a 725 bed teaching hospital of the University of Sydney, is in the forefront of HIS utilisation in the Australasian region. Three modules of an integrated Hospital Information System have been installed using the PCS (Patient Care System) system provided by IBM and Baxter Healthcare. These modules are for patient management, clinic appointment scheduling, and order communications [8]. The Concord Hospital physician order communications system was the first implementation in an Australian Hospital.

Physicians are key producers and consumers of patient information. Because of their time constraints and work-loads, encouraging physicians to directly use systems can be a challenge. At Concord Hospital this required strong executive support, adequate training, firm policies that departments would only accept electronic orders and not hand-written or telephone requests, and that other staff will not use systems on behalf of physicians. Medical administration at Concord Hospital insisted that physicians would directly use systems and nursing administration required nurses not to undertake the physicians computing for them.

4. Methods and Findings

Research was undertaken at Concord Hospital with the objective of evaluating the utilisation, benefits and other aspects of the direct use of computer systems by physicians for patient administration and order communication systems. Physicians were surveyed on their use of the computer system as part of a PIR (Post-Implementation Review)[9] of the implementation. The order communications system was implemented in July 1990 for Diagnostic Imaging orders. Diagnostic Imaging orders are only placed by physicians and it is a hospital requirement that physicians use the computer system to place any orders that are available on the computer system. Later that year Microbiology orders were also available on-line. The implementation of the system for order communications with other laboratories and other hospital departments is continuing and now covers most diagnostic services.

The PIR was completed in early 1991. It found that physicians accepted the system but with many reservations. Major concerns were the slow response time of the computer system and a perceived insufficient number of computer terminals on the wards. Frustrations included the need to use both the hand-written and computer systems as not all orders were available on-line. Physicians reported that the system was less efficient than the hand-written one for placing orders however this was offset by significant benefits. Benefits included accountability, legibility, accuracy, access to patient data, the ability to remote order from any computer terminal located in the hospital, improved quality of results which could be viewed on-line and printed at ward level, duplicate order checking and the ability to order tests in advance.

The survey questionnaire was distributed to 64 randomly selected physicians from those who were recorded as having received training in the use of the order communications system. Physicians reported an increase in time spent generating requests and commented on the inability to order at the patient bed-side while on ward rounds. There were benefits in the ability to remote order, retrieve results at all hours and the improved legibility of data. 60% reported that the system had assisted in doing their job more efficiently. 66% agreed that there had been a decrease in time spent in finding results. 66% reported a decrease in time spent telephoning departments. Over 70% agreed that the system provided easier review of patient data and that it provided efficient ordering of tests and procedures.

71% doubted that the system allowed more time for patient care. Interestingly the responses to whether the system increased their workload were mixed: 29% believed their workload had increased, 24% that it had decreased and 42% reported no change to their workload. 60% responded that the system had assisted them in doing their job more effectively while 36% responded that it had not. Detailed comments of the benefits included speedier results, remote ordering ability, legibility, out-of-hours ordering and advance ordering. A comparative survey is currently underway to replicate some of the questions in the PIR to determine changes in experiences and perceptions of physicians. When other hospitals in NSW install similar technology it is intended to conduct comparative studies.

5. Strategies for Physician Utilisation of HIS

Copeland [5] suggests that to be successful, the computer system needs to save time or at least provide benefits to offset any additional time taken. It is almost impossible for a computer system to accept orders faster than they can be written on a form, consequently attention must be paid to maximise and advertise the conveniences and time savers in other functions to offset the block of time that the physician must spend on order entry.

The factors for success identified by the survey of the Concord Hospital implementation were similar to those mentioned by Copeland. These include rapid screen change response times; sufficient computer terminals in convenient locations; complete on-line services so as to avoid having to jump back and forth between the computer and hand-written forms; integrity of physical infrastructure such as a reliable power supply; sufficient training to avoid frustration and inefficient use; the involvement of physicians in the design of the screens that they were to use; efficient screen design; ease of use of the system; streamlining of work-practices and procedures; flexibility and rapid response to change to keep pace with changing medical practices and organisational change.

The research by Anderson et al [7] indicate that physicians rely heavily upon their colleagues for advice and evaluative information when considering changes in their practices. Attempts to influence physicians to adopt new technology must directly involve the physicians. At Concord Hospital the benefits of the computer system were promoted including the financial savings that could be directed towards medical equipment.

A strategy for physician utilisation of a HIS must begin with early involvement of physicians. This should begin with marketing and education. Influential physicians should be invited to be on steering committees and working parties. It may be prudent to establish a physician user committee. The computer system must be as user-friendly as possible. Computer terminals should be located in convenient locations. Consideration should be given to locating computer terminals in physician lounges, resident quarters, physician offices and even their homes. Concord Hospital is currently planning to locate a computer terminal in the medical library for the convenience of physicians.

Strassman claims that many of the reported productivity gains from research studies have resulted from changing procedures based upon the employee's suggestions [10]. In both Copeland's case-study and the Concord Hospital implementation, the physicians were able to suggest organisational and procedural changes to make the system work effectively.

6. Training

The strategy for encouraging physicians to use the HIS at Concord Hospital began by reaching the younger and newer medical staff. Training in the use of the systems is part of orientation for new staff. Logon names and passwords are only provided to staff who undertake training courses. While the more junior physicians are the main users of the systems, every effort has been made to provide training to suit the work demands on specialists. Frequent invitations have been issued offering training to suit their times and locations.

Training must be on physicians' own terms. The training should be task oriented, well enough for physicians to perform their functions, not become system experts. Success depends upon the availability of training staff, training content, strategy, personal attention and perserverence. Schreier suggests hiring a physician to conduct the training and to train the most influential physicians first as leadership and example within the medical staff are critical to success [3]. At Concord Hospital it was found that by training the interns first, senior physicians were keen to enrol in training. Anecdotal evidence is that the more senior staff did not want the interns to have more skills and access to greater knowledge than they had.

At Concord Hospital the on-line bulletin is an effective means of keeping clinicians up-to-date with developments with the computer systems. Short courses or seminars provide a second opportunity to introduce the new computer-based practice.

7. Conclusion

At Concord Hospital physicians are responsible for direct use of the HIS to enter their own patient orders and to retrieve results. This system has been used for several years by physicians. Where physicians have access to the system they will only use the system to place orders and only computer-based orders will be accepted by service departments. There is much to learn from this success.

9. References

[1]   Finn A Jr, Valenstein P and Burke M. Alteration of physicians' orders by non-physicians. *JAMA, 1988, May 6; 259(17): 2549-52.*

[2]   Ayres D. A US developed nursing system - will it work in Australia? In: *Nursing Informatics '91, Pre-Conference Proceedings VII. Turley J P and Newbold S K (eds). Heidelberg: Springer-Verlag, 1991: 6-14.*

[3]   Schreier J. Physicians who use the system help hospitals gain advantage. *Comput Healthcare, August 1991: 30-33.*

[4]   Lapierre D. Installing a patient care system physicians will use. *Comput Healthcare. January, 1990: 22-24*

[5]   Copeland R L. A physicians' perspective on the implementation of a patient care system. In: ECHO (IBM Healthcare User Group) Phoenix Meeting, Proceedings, September, 1990: 14 -26.

[6]   Peterson P. Computerised HIS as a tool in quality medicine. *Comput Healthcare.October 1990; 37-38.*

[7]   Anderson J, Jay S, Schweer H and Anderson M. Physician utilisation of computers in medical practice: policy implications based on a structural model. *Soc Sci Med 1986, 23(3): 259-267.*

[8]   Soar, J. Health Information Systems - strategies for success. In: ACC'91 MOSAIC - Fitting the IT pieces together, Australian Computer Conference, Adelaide, 1991.

[9]   Soar J Ayres D and Van der Weegen L. Achieving change and altering behaviour through direct doctor utilisation of a Hospital Information System for order communications, *Aust Health Review*, 1994;16(4)

[10]   Strassman P A. *The business value of computers, an executives guide, New Canaan, Connecticut: The Information Economics Press, 1990: 397.*

© 1994 Elsevier Science B.V. All rights reserved.
Nursing Informatics: An International Overview for Nursing in a Technological Era
S.J. Grobe and E.S.P. Pluyter-Wenting, eds.

Nurses' Orders in Manual and Computerized Systems

Prophet CM

Department of Nursing, University of Iowa Hospitals and Clinics, 200 Hawkins Drive, Iowa City, Iowa, USA

In order to retrieve and report nursing data locally, nationally, and internationally in the advancement of nursing care and the profession of nursing, automated Nursing Information Systems (NISs) are required. This research study examined the impact of computerized order entry via NIS on nurses' orders for selected patient populations in a tertiary care hospital. The research questions addressed the relationships among the order entry mode (manual versus computerized) and the number and type (assessments versus interventions) of nurses' orders in terms of the patient variables of age, sex, marital status, medical diagnosis, order categories, and nursing diagnosis. Additionally, the relationships of order entry mode and nurses' orders to the patient care unit variables of average daily census, care delivery method, staff mix, and educational preparation of nurse managers were investigated. Data were collected during three periods (one month before, and one month and 6 months after system installation) from 238 patient records on five patient care units.

A significant relationship was found between the order entry mode and nurses' orders in that the number of nurses' orders increased significantly with computerized order entry. Moreover, all computerized patient records had some nurses' orders whereas the majority of manual patient records had none. With minor exceptions, there were no significant relationships between nurses' orders and both the patient and patient care unit variables. In summary, this study demonstrated that the implementation of a NIS enhanced the capture, retrieval, and comparison of nursing data required for the purposes of research, administration, education, and clinical practice.

1. Purpose of the Study

The purpose of this study was to examine the impact of computerized order entry on the number and type of nurses' orders for selected patient populations in a tertiary-care facility.

2. Research Questions

The following research questions were addressed:

(1) What is the relationship between the mode of order entry (manual versus computerized) and the number of nurses' orders?

(2) What is the relationship between the mode of order entry (manual versus computerized) and the type of nurses' orders (assessments versus interventions)?

(3) What is the difference/relationship between the number and type of nurses' orders in manual and computerized systems, and the patient variables of age, sex, marital status, medical diagnosis, order categories, and nursing diagnosis?

(4) What is the difference between the number and type of nurses' orders in manual and computerized systems and patient care unit variables of average daily census, care delivery method, staff mix, and educational preparation of assistant and head nurses?

3. Definitions

The following definitions for nurses' orders and order types were used in this study.

(1) *Nurses' orders* are care prescriptions of the Registered Nurse in response to the patient's needs and nursing diagnoses, as obtained on a written or computer-generated care plan.

(2) Each nurses' order is delineated by *order type* which specifies the intent of the order in terms of the patient, either an assessment or an intervention.

(3) An *assessment* is intended to determine the patient's physical and psychosocial status whereas an *intervention* is intended to maintain or improve the patient's physical or psychosocial status.

4. Methods

Data were collected at three different times: (1) manual (one month prior to the system implementation), (2) computerized-1 month, and (3) computerized-6 months after system installation. The duration of each data collection period was one month to six weeks, depending upon the availability of patient records to obtain or match the sample.

5. Sample

For this study, a total of 238 patient records were selected from five patient care units: (1) gynecological--60 records; (2) neurosurgical--39 records; (3) obstetrical--66 records; (4) pediatric newborn--52 records; (5) medical--21 records.

The number of patient records examined for each data collection period were 90 for manual, 67 for 1 month post-computerization, and 81 at 6 months post-computerization. These patient records were sorted by two, three, or four diagnostic-related groups (DRGs) appropriate to each unit for a total of fourteen DRGs. Depending upon the DRG, data were collected either on hospital day three or post-op day two.

6. Data Items

For each patient record, four patient demographic variables were collected: (1) age, (2) sex, (3) marital status, and (4) medical diagnosis (DRG). For each nurses' order, the order type (assessment versus intervention), order category, (for example, comfort), and any associated nursing diagnoses were obtained. Additionally, the total number of nurses' orders and the sub-totals of assessments and interventions were tallied. To establish baseline and note alterations, five patient care unit variables were noted on each patient care unit at each data collection period: (1) average daily census, (2) care delivery method, (3) staff mix, (4) educational preparation of the assistant head nurse, and (5) educational preparation of the head nurse.

7. Data Analysis

Data were analyzed using descriptive statistics, frequency and percentage tabulations, Chi-square test statistic, Pearson correlation coefficients, and General Linear Models (GLM) procedures. To control type 1 errors, Tukey's studentized range test was used for the comparisons of means of nurses' orders.

8. Summary of Findings

Following data analysis, significant relationships were found between order entry mode and the number and type of nurses' orders. With certain exceptions, there were no significant differences between the number and type of nurses' orders and patient and care unit variables.

The first research question was: "What is the relationship between the mode of order entry and the number of nurses' orders?" Utilizing GLM procedures, Tukey's, and 95% confidence intervals, a significant relationship between order entry mode and the number of nurses' orders was found. The mean number of nurses' orders was 1.77 for manual, 9.93 and 11.32 for one month and six months after system installation.

Comparing manual to one month after computerization, there was a large and significant increase in the number of nurses' orders. At six months post-implementation, nurses' orders continued to increase, and, on some patient care units, to a significant degree. In the manual data collection period, the majority of patient records contained 0 to 5 nurses' orders whereas after computerization, the majority contained 6-34 nurses' orders.

The second research question was "What is the relationship between the mode of order entry and the type of nurses' orders?" Utilizing Chi-square tests, the type of nurses' orders was found significantly related to the mode of order entry only between the computerized data collection periods. Between computer-1 month and computer-6 months, the number of assessments decreased and the number of interventions increased significantly.

The third research question was "What is the difference/relationship between the number and type of nurses' orders in manual and computerized systems, and the patient variables of age, sex, marital status, medical diagnosis, order categories, and nursing diagnosis?" With specific exceptions for age on one patient care unit, and for age and sex on another unit, there were no significant differences/relationships between the number of nurses' orders and age, sex, marital status, and medical diagnosis (DRG). For order type of all orders, the number of assessments exceeded the number of interventions. Moreover, significantly more assessments and, correspondingly, fewer interventions were recorded for males versus females and for patients under one year, specifically 3 day-old newborns, versus patients over one year.

Additionally, there were no significant differences/relationships between the number and type of nurses' orders and order categories, and nursing diagnosis. The majority of nurses' orders in every data collection period were captured by eight of the 24 possible order categories. The categories with the most orders were: reproductive/sexual, knowledge, fluid/electrolytes, skin/wound, comfort, psychosocial, bowel elimination, and respiration. Moreover, with computerization, nurses' orders were more likely to be classified into one of these eight categories.

Differences in the number of nurses' orders in particular categories appeared more related to the patient care unit specialty rather than mode of order entry; for example, 161 or 32% of the orders on the obstetrical unit were categorized "reproductive/sexual."

The relationship between nurses' orders and associated nursing diagnoses were analyzed for the manual and computer-6 months data collection periods only. Of the sum of 1,077 nurses' orders in these two data collections, the majority 856 or 80% were not associated with a nursing diagnosis. Moreover, the majority (153 or 90%) of the total number of 171 patient records had no nurses' orders associated with a nursing diagnosis.

The fourth research question was: "What is the difference between the number and type of nurses' orders in manual and computerized systems and the patient care unit variables of average daily census, care delivery method, staff mix, and the educational preparation of the assistant and head nurses?"

For all units in this study, there were no changes between data collection periods for care delivery method and educational levels, and minor changes in average daily census and staff mix. With only five patient care units, there were insufficient data to determine if the number and type of nurses' orders changed based upon differences in patient care unit variables.

The nursing research literature did not offer any explanation of the relationship between nurses' orders and the mode of order entry [1]. With the advent of a new system, expectations and anxieties heighten, and users are given a great deal of attention whereby their suggestions and participation are solicited by administration. Therefore, it is not altogether surprising that the number of nurses' orders increased significantly immediately following system installation. However, the number of nurses' orders did not decrease in six months, although the attention had diminished.

9. Implications for Nursing

Automated NISs are required for the capture, storage, retrieval and reporting of nursing data locally, nationally, and internationally in the advancement of nursing care and of the profession of nursing. This study demonstrated that the number of nurses' orders increased significantly with computerized order entry. Moreover, all patient records in computerized order entry had some nurse' orders whereas in the manual system, the majority of patient records (51%) had no nurses' orders. As stated by many authors, nursing seems invisible, and evidence of nursing's contribution to patient care, in the form of nursing data, is lacking [2]. The capture, presentation, comparison, and research of nursing data via NISs increases the visibility of nursing.

In efforts to define nursing, investigators often endeavor to state what it is by what it does. Attempts to capture these data -- "what it does" -- are facilitated by automated NISs. The availability and retrievability of nursing data, especially nurses' orders, will enhance efforts to refine nursing data base classifications. Moreover, NISs provide powerful mechanisms for the implementation of professional guidelines and standards.

Furthermore, with the inherent clinical focus of NISs, the clinical implications are of paramount importance. As information systems develop, nurses will be provided expert systems to improve their decision making. By means of NISs, research studies can be conducted to examine the clinical effectiveness of particular nursing interventions in the achievement of nurse-sensitive patient outcomes. Given the efficiency of many NISs, time spent by nurses in laborious manual recording procedures will be available for patient care. Computerized NISs facilitate the capture and communication of nursing data, including nurses' orders, while enhancing data retrieval for many other objectives for the profession of nursing.

10. References

[1] Prophet C. *Nurses' Orders in Systems.* Master's Thesis, University of Iowa College of Nursing, Iowa City, 1991.

[2] Zielstorff R. Why Aren't There More Significant Automated Nursing Information Systems? *J Nurs Adm* 1984, 14:7-10.

Nursing Informatics: An International Overview for Nursing in a Technological Era
S.J. Grobe and E.S.P. Pluyter-Wenting, eds.

290

Temporal data management: A model for nursing home resident care plans

Hassett C M [a] Hassett M R [b] and Rupp S [c]

[a]Dept of Computer Information Systems & Quantitative Methods, Fort Hays State University, 600 Park St, MC 311, Hays, KS 67601-4099 USA

[b]Dept of Nursing, Fort Hays State University, 600 Park St, STH 137, Hays, KS 67601-4099 USA

[c]Director of Nursing, Good Samaritan Center of Hays, 27th & Canal, Hays, KS 67601 USA

A temporal database model represents the progression of *states* of nursing home residents' care plans over intervals of time. A *no re-write* policy is adhered to; all changes in the database are viewed as additions. This affords access to historical data; that is, past *states* of the database: points in time and durations. Findings from an on-going three-year study in one nursing home in the Midwest are presented (analysis of preliminary data and model will be completed: March 1994). Nurse managers in nursing home settings need access to residents' care plan data, over time. Since information is dynamic rather than static, a temporal database is needed to provide for management decisions. The goal for the model is to provide and maintain valuable nursing care plan information (such as nursing diagnoses) in relation to Standards of Care, throughout the resident's stay in the nursing home. The Nursing Minimum Data Set is used with the Nursing Interventions Classification of the Iowa Project.

1. Introduction

This ongoing descriptive exploratory investigation examines the progression of *states* of nursing home residents' care plans over intervals of time. An extension to the relational database model [1] that will represent this progression is under development. A language such as the temporal query language (TQuel) [2] will be used or a new language specific to healthcare temporal databases will be developed. The language will query temporal databases.

Medical information systems have a growing need for temporal information (*i.e.*, over intervals of time) [3] as does nursing information systems. A diagnosis is often strongly affected by temporal relationships between/among client symptoms or problems. Bloom examined a time-oriented clinical database in which plotting of patient data could be done either by visit or by time [4]. Nursing home intervals could be plotted, for example, by shift or by transaction date.

The Nursing Minimum Data Set (NMDS) was developed for clinical nursing data [5] and is used in this study along with the nursing process. Further, the Nursing Interventions Classification (NIC) of the Iowa Intervention Project provides intervention labels [6].

Uses for the temporal data management model are discussed. Segments of actual nursing home resident care plans will illustrate temporal data management.

2. Present Status of Databases in Healthcare Industry

When computerizing manual data processing systems, healthcare providers have used *traditional file management systems*. These are systems in which data and computer programs are *dependent*. The program defines the format for the data and the functionality for accessing the data. Only that program has access to the data, and if the data format needs changing, the program must be rewritten. This results in high maintenance costs and uncontrolled data redundancy (multiple copies of data without cross referencing) because data cannot be shared. There is presently a trend toward the *database approach* in which data are *independent* of any specific program.

A database is a repository for stored data; it is both integrated and shared [7]. The database approach provides developers with a *data dictionary* describing the data formats, access routes to data elements, and levels of access authority. Data, in this approach, belongs to the organization and may be shared by many applications. Where redundancy exists, it is controlled. The software that allows for use and/or modification of data is a database management system (DBMS). The database approach also provides a number of formal database models. The most popular of these is the relational model. The relational database model is a logical structure in which all data are viewed as tables (two-dimensional), with each row having the same format [8].

The move from traditional file processing to a database approach requires a *paradigm shift*. The database approach requires viewing information as any other asset of the organization is viewed. This implies that information can be managed in much the same way as other assets are managed. The task of this management must be assigned to persons high on the organization chart. This approach requires long-range planning for information needs.

A paradigm shift to the database approach has taken place in some healthcare organizations. A second paradigm shift is needed: information viewed in the context of time rather than currency. Databases that include the context of time are called *temporal databases*.

3. Overview of Temporal Database

There is a major body of research on temporal databases [7] dating from 1956. Different approaches include extending the relational model. Most healthcare databases represent the state of organizational data at a single moment of time. As the data change the contents of the database continues to change. These changes are represented as modifications to the state, with old data being deleted from the database. The current state (contents) of the database can be viewed as a snapshot of the organization. The out-of-date data (past states) being deleted from the database, if preserved, could provide valuable information. Figure 1 is an example of a query on a traditional (snapshot) database and reveals that JANE and MARY have Mobility Impaired Physical. Figure 2 is an example of a query on a temporal database for the same nursing home residents. The temporal database query not only reveals that JANE and MARY presently have Mobility Impaired Physical but also that MARY has had it in the past. Additionally, the temporal database query reveals that JOE has had Mobility Impaired Physical in the past but presently does not. This information was lost in the traditional database query. Further, the durations shown in the temporal database query of Mobility Impaired Physical were never recorded in the traditional database.

Process (Resident, Diagnosis)

RESIDENT	DIAGNOSIS
JOHN	NONCOMPLIANCE
JANE	MOBILITY IMPAIRED PHYSICAL
MARY	MOBILITY IMPAIRED PHYSICAL
TOM	POTENTIAL FOR INFECTION
MARK	NONCOMPLIANCE

Query: Mobility Impaired Physical (Name)

RESIDENT
JANE
MARY

Figure 1. Traditional Database and Query

4. Research Questions

Many time-oriented databases have been developed within the healthcare industry during the past decade [4]. Such databases should be widely used by healthcare providers such as nursing homes. Current databases in use are instantaneous or *snapshot* databases. However, time is a multifaceted and subtle component of data. Presently, most nursing home personnel that think they are using a database are actually using a file manager. Often, the output *believed* to be from a database is items programmed to be printed on a care plan, such as a set of nursing interventions commonly used for a particular nursing diagnosis. Questions for this ongoing study are:
  (a) How do present nursing home databases handle time?
  (b) Why is time is important for nursing home databases?
  (c) How can time be added to nursing home databases?

(d) What method, *e.g.*, query language, is appropriate to access nursing home temporal database?

Process (Resident, Diagnosis)

		Valid time		Transaction time	
RESIDENT	**DIAGNOSIS**	**(from)**	**(to)**	**(from)**	**(to)**
MARY	MOBILITY IMPAIRED PHYSICAL	01-20-92	04-21-92	03-01-92	07-1-92
JOHN	NONCOMPLIANCE	01-04-92	∞	03-01-92	∞
JANE	MOBILITY IMPAIRED PHYSICAL	06-22-92	∞	07-01-92	∞
MARY	MOBILITY IMPAIRED PHYSICAL	01-01-93	∞	04-01-93	∞
TOM	POTENTIAL FOR INFECTION	01-02-93	∞	04-01-93	∞
MARK	NONCOMPLIANCE	02-06-93	∞	04-01-93	∞
JOE	MOBILITY IMPAIRED PHYSICAL	02-23-93	04-24-93	04-01-93	∞

Query: Mobility Impaired Physical (Name)

	Valid time		Transaction time	
RESIDENT	**(from)**	**(to)**	**(from)**	**(to)**
MARY	01-20-92	04-21-92	03-01-92	07-1-92
JANE	06-22-92	∞	07-01-92	∞
MARY	01-01-93	∞	04-01-93	∞
JOE	02-23-93	04-24-93	04-01-93	∞

Figure 2. Temporal Database and Query

5. Study Timeline

The study timeline includes:
(a) analyze present system; define data structures (completion: September 1993);
(b) build a traditional relational prototype database; analyze and further extend traditional relational prototype database (completion: January 1994);
(c) implement traditional relational prototype database (estimated completion: March 1994); and
(d) extend traditional relational model to include temporal data; implement query language for accessing the temporal database (estimated completion: June 1994).
Research-based tools include: the NMDS Form B (Inpatient Long-Term Care) and NIC's 366 intervention labels.

6. Conclusions

If nurses can review and select historical care plan information and incorporate it with the resident's new problem savings will be realized in terms of (a) time going through old charts, and (b) re-entries. Using the information gleaned from historical data also allows for more informed choices regarding present and future decision making Further, effectiveness of nursing interventions for various diagnoses may be compared across nursing home resident Those who are developing taxonomies such as outcomes for interventions need to address temporal data issues. T proposed model will assist in addressing these issues. The new language developed to query temporal databases w also benefit the database approach in nursing homes.

7. References

[1]   Lorentzos NA and Johnson RG. Requirements Specification for a Temporal Extension to the Relational Mod *Database Engin* 1988, 7:26-33.

[2]   Snodgrass R. The Temporal Query Language TQuel. *ACM Trans Database Sys* 1987, 12:247-298.

[3]   Ariav G and Clifford J. Temporal data management: Models and systems. In: *New Directions for Databa Systems.* Ariav G, Clifford J (eds). Norwood, NJ: Ablex, 1986: 169.

[4]   Bloom RL. Displaying Clinical Data from a Time-Oriented Database. *Comput Biol Med* 1981, 4:197-210.

[5] Werley HH, Devin EC and Zorn CR. *The Nursing Minimum Data Set (NMDS) Data Collection Manual.* Milwaukee, WI: University of Wisconsin-Milwaukee School of Nursing, (1992).

[6] McCloskey JC and Bulechek GM (eds.). *Nursing Interventions Classification (NIC).* St. Louis: Mosby-Year, 1992.

[7] Date CJ. *An Introduction to Database Systems* (3rd ed.). Reading, MA: Addison-Wesley, 1981.

[8] O'Brien JA. *Management Information Systems: A Managerial End User Perspective.* Homewood, IL: Richard D. Irwin, 1990.

[9] Snodgrass R. Temporal Databases--Status and Research Directions. *SIGMOD Record* 1987, 17: 83-89.

Nursing Informatics: An International Overview for Nursing in a Technological Era
S.J. Grobe and E.S.P. Pluyter-Wenting, eds.

A knowledge based system for nursing care planning.

Goossen WTF[a] and Smulders J[b]

[a] School of Nursing, Leeuwarden Polytechnic, PO Box 1080, 8900 CB, Leeuwarden, The Netherlands, E-mail: Goossen@F2.NHL.NL

[b] Bolesian BV, Steenovenweg 19, 5708 HN, Helmond, The Netherlands.

Abstract. A prototype Knowledge Based System (KBS) for nursing diagnosis and care planning is developed by means of the Structured Knowledge Engineering (SKE) Methodology. The study involved a multi method approach for the knowledge analysis. Documented knowledge about nursing diagnosis and care planning and practical knowledge about nursing care for patients with leukemia is used. This is supplemented with a case study of diagnosing and planning of one expert nurse clinician. The aggregated knowledge is categorized into a four layer knowledge model which served as the foundation of the system design. The system design included a forward as well as a backward driven approach for nursing diagnosis and care planning. Only the forward driven approach is implemented in the prototype KBS. After refinement the prototype may serve as a basis for the development of a "second generation" Intelligent Tutoring System for nursing education.

1. Introduction

This paper discusses a pilot study involved in the development of a Knowledge Based System (KBS) for nursing diagnosis and care planning, and the background theoretical concepts, design, implementation and implications issues of the study.

The study was initiated and carried out as a joint project of the school of nursing of Leeuwarden Polytechnic and Bolesian. Bolesian is a Dutch company specialized in building knowledge based systems. This project was partly funded by the Dutch Board of Professional Education (HBO Raad) program to keep professional education up to date with developments in society and industry.

The short term goal of this study was to investigate the possibilities to build a KBS by means of the Structured Knowledge Engineering (SKE) methodology, which supports nursing diagnosis and care planning in a well defined area. The area of leukemia for the development of the KBS was chosen only for practical reasons. The long term goal is to investigate the possibilities of the SKE method to develop an Intelligent Tutoring System (ITS) with interactive video for (Dutch) student nurses.

2. Structured Knowledge Engineering

Bolesian's Structured Knowledge Engineering is a useful methodology for the realization and control of projects for the development of Knowledge Based Systems [1]. The SKE methodology has previously proven to be of use in building an experimental KBS and ITS in the field of Health Care (The FysioDisk [R]).

An attractive feature of SKE is that it allows a multi-method approach for knowledge acquisition. Within SKE the real world, as envisioned by the expert, is taken as the base to build a conceptual knowledge model. This model serves as the guide for the realisation of the KBS. SKE consists of seven phases: 1) Project proposal, 2) Feasibility study, 3) Analysis, 4) Design, 5) Realization, 6) Testing and 7) Maintenance [1]. It is not within the scope of this paper to present all of these phases in detail. Only the analysis and design stage will be presented, but first attention will be given to ITS and KBS in nursing.

3. Intelligent Tutoring Systems

An ITS analyses the students learning behaviour in problem solving before the system gives feedback. ITS is considered a more adequate learning tool because the feedback is intelligent and individualized instead of the more standard yes/no of several Computer Assisted Instruction tools. A traditional ITS consists of a number of experts. These experts are: 1) A Domain expert, 2) The Student expert, 3) The Teaching or Didactic expert [2]. If one looks at the knowledge the experts use, there is a huge overlap. Another problem in this traditional ITS is the confusion of functions [2]. Winkels is a major researcher in the field of ITS. He suggests a new metaphor for ITS: coaching as process control. This "second generation" ITS consists of two components. The proposed components include: 1) The problem solving task, represented in a knowledge based system, 2) A computer coach that follows the learning process. The problem solving tasks are performed both by the student and the coach. These tasks are: 1) Selecting the learning actions, 2) Monitoring of the students learning behaviour, 3) Diagnosing the learning problems. Feedback is given when the student asks questions or when the performance of the student indicates that feedback is necessary or desirable. This implicates that the student himself can establish what knowledge is missing for successful completion of the problem solving tasks. In cases where this is difficult for the student, the coach is expected to take the initiative. The initial step in developing such an ITS lays in the construction of the KBS. After the KBS is realized the system can be enhanced with patient cases on interactive video or CD-I. Finally the the teaching coach can be produced. For this reason the project started with the investigation of the knowledge based system.

4. Knowledge based systems in nursing

A review of the literature concerning KBS in nursing shows a growing trend towards constraining the domain [3, 4, 5, 6, 7, 8, 9, 20]. All described systems have in common the subject of nursing care planning. Criteria for the construction and use of KBS are cited in two of the articles [10, 11,]. One essential criteria is to limit the nursing domain to a specific, well-defined sphere of involvement [11]. No detailed criteria for this limitation of scope are given. It is further suggested to use a multi-method approach for knowledge acquisition [10]. Although several KBS have a teaching component, a report in the literature about the use of a KBS as base for an ITS in nursing could not be found by time of writing [14, 15, 16, 20]. This may be because it is not done before, or the literature search was not thorough enough, especially for developments in 1992 and later.

5. Feasibility

A working example from the actual study illustrates the study's feasibility. The project envolved the cooperation of a clinical nurse expert and the heamatology ward of the Groningen University Hospital. The domain was constrained to the nursing diagnosis and care planning for patients with Acute Myeloid Leukemia (AML). A list of Orem's categories of self care requisites was used for scoring during the knowledge acquisition [19]. Several patient cases were constructed by other ward nurses based on prototype patients. The care planning was devided into the tasks within the nursing process. Documented knowledge about the nursing process and the care of patients with AML was available. Practical knowledge was available in a core careplan for patients with chemotherapy which encompassed knowledge of the heamatology ward.

6. Analysis stage

Within the analysis phase several studies took place; the first of which was the "knowledge analysis". The existing aggregation of knowledge was supplemented with a concurrent case study of one nurse expert. The nurse clinician scored areas of care in order of priority using a constructed scoring scale of Orem's selfcare requisites [19]. The initial scoring was considered the base score. In the 6 following sessions the nurse clinician was required to score priorities for individual cases of prototype patients. The results revealed that the individual circumstances of the case patients influenced the priority scoring of the clinician. Findings based on the scoring included: essential patient data, crucial decision making, actions towards more information gathering, as well as a confirmation of hypothesis testing. In later sessions the expert arranged priorities for 6 new cases. These new cases had profiles similar to the first 6 cases. The results of the scores were comparable to the first sessions.

The four layer knowledge model derived from the aggregated knowledge is shown in figure 1. A user-computer interaction analysis and technical requirement analysis took place, but it is beyond the scope of this article to give complete results. Just a few features will be discussed. The computer-nurse interaction has the following possibility. The computer presents questions on the screen about nursing assessment, signs and symptoms. Possible answering options differ from; yes/no options, single choice options, values, multiple choice options. The questions sometimes go 7 levels deep, depending on the knowledge available. If a broad category of signs and symptoms is selected at a higher level and the nurse selects a certain answer, questions at a detailed level are skipped or presented, depending on the relations. E.g. The question: "Does the patient have problems with heartrate?" can be answered by yes or no and with a value for the heartrate. If the value is below or above a certain standard and/or if the nurse gives yes as answer more detailed questions are presented to gain in depth information. Otherwise the next category of questions is presented.

Strategic knowledge.
Deciding which task to do.

Tasks.
    1) Initial care planning.
    2) Modifying the careplan.
    3) Discharge.

Inferences.
    1) For initial diagnosing and care planning.
    2) For modification of the careplan.
    3) For discharging the patient.

Domain knowledge.
  1) Declarative: categories, entities, atributes, values.
  2) Procedural: relations between data, categories, solutions.
  3) Solutions: nursing diagnosis, goals and interventions.

Figure 1. Four layer knowledge model.

7. Design and realization stages

The system design includes a data driven approach (first input of all data, then conclusions, or 'forward chaining') and a diagnosis driven approach (after initial data are known, potential nursing diagnoses are ruled in or out, or 'backward chaining'). The system consists of: 1) Patient identification database, 2) Patient assessment database, 3) Knowledge base (combines data by use of 175 If-Then rules into nursing diagnosis), 4) A list of detected diagnoses (nurse problems) and careplans, 5) A listing of the result of every rule. (Firing of rules gives more data about the individual patient), 6) Modification tool to: delete, tailor or create a nursing diagnosis and careplan, 7) List of all available nursing diagnosis, careplans and rules. The final careplans consists of a statement of the problem (nursing diagnosis), expected outcomes and nursing interventions. It is possible to have five types of careplans in the system:

- derived from the rules and accepted.
- derived from the rules and modified by the nurse for the individual patient.
- derived from the rules and deleted by the nurse for the individual patient.
- picked from the list of diagnoses by the nurse.
- completely written by the nurse in a free-text careplan screen.

Not all the design features could be programmed due of time limitations for the study. The system uses only the forward chaining approach. The KBS is realized in the Prolog language because this is very flexible.

8. Discussion and conclusions

The purpose of this pilot study was to investigate the possibilities of building a KBS for nursing care planning by means of the SKE methodology. The use of the SKE methodology lead to a working prototype in a relatively short period of time. It is feasible to build KBS for nursing with this method. This means that the short term goal of the project is met. It seems to be possible to enhance this prototype for assisting in care planning. Nonetheless several problems should be mentioned. Orem's self care requisites do not cover all the possible problem areas in nursing [5]. The scoring list may prove to be incomplete. The reliability and the validity of subsequent research, especially the interpretation of the inferences and the knowledge model, can be enhanced by using a panel of experts from the domain.

At present only the forward chaining data driven approach is in use; while the literature suggests that the backward chaining or combined approaches would be more appropriate [17, 18]. More research is needed with respect to the most suitable approach for mimicking the diagnostic process of nurses.

The rules in the system may be inappropriate or incomplete and need careful refinement.

The instability of Prolog as a programming language does not hinder its use in a prototype, but renders it unsuitable for a working system. Prolog uses the systems memory in a very inefficient way. Currently, adequate and stable expertshells are available which can combine a patient database, a knowledge base and a teaching coach.

It is clear that for the future development of the ITS additional research regarding the KBS is necessary. Also the development of "second generation" ITS is still in an experimental stage.

The prototype KBS was intended to develop complete careplans for patients with leukemia. Even this narrow scope of the domain can be too much to cover in one system. It is advised to limit the domain to one nursing diagnosis or a few interrelated nursing diagnoses. This point of approach will be taken if and when the complete ITS is to be developed. Currently we are looking for partners and funding to continue the development of an ITS. The results of the present study; the prototype KBS and the theoretical background is being used as examples in the nursing informatics courses of Leeuwarden School of Nursing.

9. References

[1] Smulders J. Structured Knowledge Engineering. *Informatie* 1990; 32 (5):425-512.

[2] Winkels R. *Explorations in Intelligent Tutoring and Help*. Amsterdam: IOS Press, 1992.

[3] Ryan, S.A. An expert system for nursing practice. *Comput Nurs* 1985, 3, (2):77-84.

[4] Bloom KC, Leitner JE, Solano JL. Development of an expert system prototype to generate nursing care plans based on nursing diagnoses. *Comput Nurs* 1987; 5 (4):140 - 145.

[5] Ozbolt, J.G. Knowledge-Based Systems for Supporting Clinical Nursing Decisions. In: Ball MJ, Hannah KJ, Gerdin-Jelger U, Peterson H. *Nursing Informatics: were caring and technology meet*. New York, Springer Verlag, 1988.

[6] Chang BL, Roth K, Gonzales E, Caswell D, DiStefano J. CANDI. A knowledge-based system for nursing diagnoses. *Comput Nurs* 1988; 6 (1): 13-21.

[7] Heriot C, Graves J, Bouhaddou O, Armstrong M, Wigertz G, Ben Said M. (1988). A pain management decision support system for nurses. In: Greenes RA (Ed.). *Proceedings of the Twelfth Annual Symposium on Computer Applications in Medical Care*. Washington DC, IEEE Computer Society Press, pp. 63-68.

[8] Probst CL, Rush J. The Careplan Knowledge Base. A prototype expert system for postpartum nursing care. *Comput Nurs* 1990; 8(5): 206-213.

[9] Woolley N. A computerised assessment for clinical care. *Professional Nurse* 1990; 632-638.

[10] Woolery L. Expert Nurses and Expert Systems. Research and development issues. *Comput Nurs* 1990; 8 (1): 23-28.

[11] Hannah KJ, Warnock-Matheron A. Application and Implication of expert systems for clinical nursing practice: a meta analysis. IN: *MEDINFO '89*. Barber B, Cao D, Qin D, Wagner, G (eds). Amsterdam: North Holland, 1989: 34 - 39.

[14] Bolwell C. *Directory of educational software for nursing*. 4th Ed. New York, NLN; Athens, Fuld Institute 1991.

[15] Ullmer EJ. *Interactive Technology*. Bethesda, National Library of Medicine 1990.

[16] Sparks SM. *Computer based education in nursing*. Bethesda, National Library of Medicine 1990.

[17] Benner P. From novice to expert. *Am J Nurs* 1982, 82: 402-407.

[18] Tanner CA, Padrick KP, Westfall UE, Putzier DJ. Diagnostic Reasoning Strategies of Nurses and Nursing Students. *Nurs Res* 1987, 36,(6):358-363.

[19] Orem DE. *Nursing, concepts of practice* (3rd ed.). New York, McGraw-Hill 1985.

[20] Grobe S, et al. Decision Support Systems in Nursing Education. In: Ozbolt JG, Vandewal D, Hannah KJ (eds.) *Decision Support Systems in Nursing*. St. Louis, The CV Mosby Company 1990.

Nursing Informatics: An International Overview for Nursing in a Technological Era
S.J. Grobe and E.S.P. Pluyter-Wenting, eds.

Computerized nursing care plan

Ryhanen S M[a] and Eronen M I[b]

[a]*School of Nursing, Käkelänkatu 3, 53100 Lappeenranta, Finland.*

[b]*Home for Mentally Retarded, Kanavakoti, 53300 Lappeenranta, Finland.*

This paper presents a project for computerizing written nursing care plans. We wanted to increase the use of computers in nursing. Our purpose was to improve nursing care plans through computer programming. This computer program of nursing is based on the nursing process utilizing a lexicon which was created for nursing diagnoses and interventions. By analyzing written nursing care plans (105 plans) we got the first version of the lexicon which was then expanded by using nursing literature.

1. Introduction

In the health care center of Lappeenranta, Finland, the computerized health care data system called "Finstar" has been used since 1983. Health care units are widely spread throughout the county, which is why computers are convenient when exchanging information among practitioners.

Our computer system has grown from consisting only of statistical data to include data from clinical charts. The documentation of nursing care was scant because at this point, the computer system was not completely operative. That is why the project for computerizing nursing care plans was started.

A well-written nursing care plan provides a central source of information about the client with a description of his problems and a plan of action to solve them.

2. Aims of the project

Our intention is to computerize nursing care planning based on the nursing process model, which is used in our manual nursing care plans. The documentation/charting in nursing records is a combination of problem oriented and process oriented documentation. The idea of our computerized nursing care plan is as follows: Only essential data from the admission interview is documented by computer. Goals, data of implementation and evaluation are documented in freehand. Developing the lexicon of nursing diagnoses and nursing interventions was the most time-consuming phase of our project.

3. The lexicon of nursing diagnoses and nursing interventions

Two approaches were used to develop the lexicon for nursing diagnoses and nursing interventions. The first approach was to take a random sample of 105 manually written nursing care plans. Nursing care plans were from the surgical, medical and long-term wards, outpatient clinics, home health care department and day-hospital. The documentation of nursing care plans was analyzed and from them we devised our first version of practical nursing diagnoses and interventions.

The second approach was to search through nursing literature for terms/concepts, which would be comprehensive for our purpose. After reviewing the nursing literature which was available to us [1-8], we made a synthesis of natural language and concepts of nursing theories. This was the first version of the lexicon of nursing diagnoses and interventions. The list of terms for nursing diagnoses and nursing interventions are on two levels. The primary level contains the main categories, with sub-categories being found on the second level.

4. The taxonomy of the lexicon

The next phase was to find a taxonomy for a list of nursing diagnoses and nursing interventions. The taxonomy should be logical and suitable for practice. Nursing practice encompasses care provided by one human being for another. Both people come to the situation with various life experiences. Each person for whom the nurse has responsibility is unique and individual. All people must meet their own needs differently. Having examined the client and his situation, the nurse will have collected certain data that are analyzed.

The review of nursing theories didn't give us a taxonomy suitable for our purpose, then we selected the view of man by Rauhala as a taxonomy for our lexicon [9]. Rauhala's holistic view of man divides human existence into three dimensions of being: situation, psychological and physiological. According to Rauhala situational existence means the situation and circumstances of human's life. He says: "We are always a member of some society." The importance of situational existence is clearly seen when the human's self-image is formed. Psychological existence means a wholeness of human experience and physiological existence includes physical being and needs.

5. The computer program

This computer program of nursing care is based on the nursing process model, in which the lexicon was created for nursing diagnoses and nursing interventions. The lexicon of nursing diagnoses and nursing interventions makes it possible to computerize a data base and to create different kinds of files and statistics. Simultaneously, the conceptual framework will be more clear and accurate. The data from the admission interview is documented in freehand, likewise the data of nursing goals and evaluation. The correspondence between the concepts of the nursing process model and the nursing data in our program is shown in the following figure:

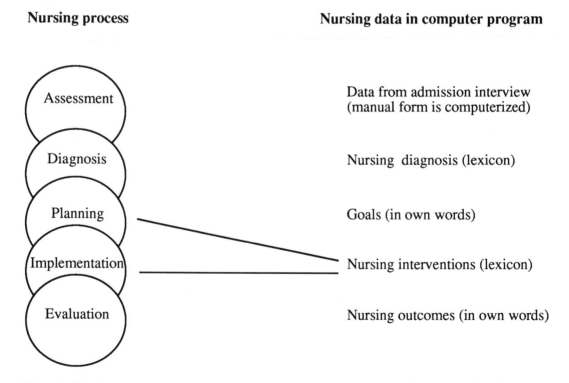

Nursing process

Nursing data in computer program

Assessment — Data from admission interview (manual form is computerized)

Diagnosis — Nursing diagnosis (lexicon)

Planning — Goals (in own words)

Implementation — Nursing interventions (lexicon)

Evaluation — Nursing outcomes (in own words)

Figure 1: Nursing process and data in the computer

This computer program of nursing follows the nursing process model. The data of admission interview/nursing assessment is documented in freehand according to these codes: housing, social environment, state of mind, functioning and capacities of life and living, selfcare, domestic and supporting services, orders of treatment. The nursing diagnoses are chosen from the lexicon and nursing goals are set for each one of the diagnoses in freehand.

Nursing interventions are planned from the lexicon. The data of implementation and evaluation is also documented in freehand.

Nursing diagnoses and interventions can be recorded as follows: The lexicon of nursing diagnoses and interventions are grouped into three dimensions; situation, psychological and physiological existence; as mentioned before. If an exact and appropriate concept is not found, the nearest suitable concept can be chosen and tailored to the patient's situation. For example: One can computerize from the situational group of codes, "social environment" and the exact code, "lack of privacy". In this case one can chose from the lexicon of nursing interventions the code "to provide privacy" and the exact code "individual territory". Each code can also be clarified in freehand.

6. The experiences of users

This computer program is used in the day-hospital, home health care department, and in some long-term wards. The first experiences are promising, although it takes plenty of time to learn the program and its possibilities. The lack of terminals makes it difficult nowadays to use this program.

Computerized nursing care plans are suitable for teaching the nursing process model and improving the contents of nursing care plans. In the autumn 1993, the nursing school of Lappeenranta implemented this computer program for teaching the nursing process model and concepts of nursing theories.

7. Summary

The ultimate purpose of this project was to develop the lexicon of the nursing diagnoses and interventions and to computerize the nursing care plans based on the nursing process model. We are convinced that the computer system will be helpful in nursing practice and education.

8. References

[1] Stevens BJ. *Nursing theory. Analysis, application, evaluation.* Boston: Little Brown, 1979.

[2] Riehl JP and Roy C. *Conseptual models for nursing practice.* New York: Appleton-Century-Crofts, 1980.

[3] Carpenito LJ. *Nursing diagnosis. Application to clinical practice.* Philadelphia: J.B. Lippincott Company, 1983.

[4] Fawcett J. *A framework for analysis and evaluation of coceptual models of nursing.* Philadelphia: F.A. Davis Company, 1984.

[5] Ziegler SM, Vaughan-Wrobel BC and Erlen JA. *Nursing process, nursing diagnosis, nursing knowledge. Avenues to autonomy.* Norwalk, Connecticut: Appleton-Century-Crofts, 1985.

[6] Ehnfors M, Thorell-Ekstrand I and Ehrenberg A. Towards Basic Nursing Information in Patient Records. *Vard i Norden* 1991, 3:12-31.

[7] Meleis AI. *Theoretical nursing: Development & progress.* Philadelphia: J.B. Lippincott Company, 1991.

[8] Nicoll LH. *Perspectives on nursing theory.* Philadelphia: J.B. Lippincott Company, 1992.

[9] Rauhala L. Ihmiskäsitys ihmistyössä. Helsinki: Gaudeamus, 1983. (in Finnish)

Nursing Informatics: An International Overview for Nursing in a Technological Era
S.J. Grobe and E.S.P. Pluyter-Wenting, eds.

302

STRUCTURING NURSING DATA
FOR THE COMPUTER-BASED PATIENT RECORD (CPR)

McHugh ML

The Wichita State University School of Nursing, 1845 N. Fairmount, Wichita, Kansas, 67260-0041, U.S.A.

If the promise of the CPR is to be realized, a paradigm shift in patient care documentation is required. The CPR can provide important benefits to patients, the health care system and to nurses. Recently, the CPR has also become recognized as an important tool for continuous quality improvement in health care. However, these advantages cannot be achieved with narrative documentation models. Data selection, mapping, coding schemes, logical and physical storage structures, and retrieval and analysis processes and technology must be changed. At St. Francis Regional Medical Center in Wichita, Kansas, the theory and practice of clinical documentation is being shifted from a paper-based standard to an electronic record paradigm. The old charting paradigm focused on documenting care. It was organized around clinical services. It promoted department specific and poorly structured forms, narrative reporting, and a weak focus on outcomes. Data retrieval was often difficult and time consuming. The new paradigm focuses on the patient's problems, care requirements and changes in health and functional status. As such, it is derived from the Problem Oriented Medical Record (POMR) model described by Weed [1]. It employs highly structured forms composed almost entirely of coded data elements. The new system is designed to *guide* as well as to document care, to reduce the incidence of clinical errors, to streamline documentation, and to improve the quality of information in the chart. Thus, the entire system is designed to support care quality.

1. Components of Successful Design

Properly designed, the Computer-based Patient Record (CPR) has great potential. It can be used to facilitate continual improvement of quality patient care. At the same time, it can help with cost control. The CPR can produce these advantages by improving accessibility and utility of data related to patient care. Ultimately, it should enable clinicians to better understand the effects of clinical decisions on patient care outcomes. Clinicians can use that new knowledge to change practice in a way that improves the success of clinical protocols. The key to achievement of these benefits lies in the design of the system. The purpose of this paper is to describe one facet of the design of the CPR; design of the structure for the clinical content of the CPR.

Design of the CPR has four main components. They are, design of the hardware configuration, database management system (DBMS) design, applications software design, and design of the structure of the content data to be placed in the CPR. Details of the hardware design are usually a function of the requirements of the software. Users specify the requisite functionality of the applications software. Vendors design the internal structure of their software packages to meet the customer's requirements. Sometimes, customers and their consultants collaborate with vendors on software design. When the system involves a database, the specific DBMS software must be purchased or developed. Once the DBMS is selected, the file structures and the internal linkages among the various databases, files and tables or records must be addressed. These layers provide the foundation for a powerful computer based clinical record. With a clinical database, an additional layer of structure needs to be developed. That layer consists of the structure of the clinical information that is to be placed in the CPR. Structuring of the content data to be accessed and stored by the system is as important to the success of a CPR as is the computer-based medium itself.

History has demonstrated the problems with simply "computerizing" existing paper system. The benefits of the CPR were not achieved when vendors transferred existing documentation models designed for paper record systems to a computer record system. The primary problems with that approach were inefficiency and the inability of users to aggregate data across groups of patients for the purposes of analysis of clinical and financial performance. If the promise of the CPR is to be realized, a paradigm shift in the structuring of patient care documentation is required. Data selection, mapping, coding schemes, data item interrelationships, and data retrieval and analysis processes and technology must be changed so that they provide a better fit with a computer information system paradigm [2].

At St. Francis Regional Medical Center in Wichita, Kansas, the theory and practice of clinical documentation is being shifted from a paper-based standard to an electronic record paradigm. The old charting paradigm focused on documenting patient assessments and clinicians' actions. It was organized around clinical services. It promoted department specific forms, which were unstructured or minimally structured. Narrative descriptions were common, as was a weak focus on outcomes. Data retrieval was often difficult and time consuming. The new paradigm focuses on the patient's problems and care requirements, and changes in health and functional status as the focus of the documentation system. It employs highly structured forms composed almost entirely of coded data elements. Many of the concepts and ideas used in this redesign were derived from the writings of Dr. Lawrence L. Weed. Further clarification was obtained when Dr. Weed came to St. Francis in 1991 to discuss his ideas with members of the hospital staff involved in documentation system redesign.

2. System Functionality and Design Processes

As suggested by Weed [1], the new system has been designed to *guide* as well as document care. Design focused on ways to reduce the incidence of clinical errors, to streamline documentation, and to improve the quality of information in the chart. Thus, the entire system is designed to support care quality. It guides practice by using flow sheets rather than narrative charting formats. Flow sheets list as many of the clinical assessment, intervention and evaluation activities performed by nurses as possible. Clinical errors of omission are reduced by a format that inherently reminds the nurse of care that needs to be performed. The new format is expected to facilitate quality improvement efforts by making available in a timely manner, data required to track care processes, and to monitor and evaluate the outcomes of patient care. It is also expected to help support many of the financial analysis, clinical, research, and education needs that are now so poorly supported by the manual systems.

The St. Francis task force began by identifying the purposes to be served by the new system. The task force recognized that the first and most important purpose for the patient record was communication of clinical events. The patient record or "chart" is to be used to help the care givers to record their observations and their actions. These recordings are used by all care givers involved with the patient to communicate care directions, patient health and knowledge deficits, and other information that will help to ensure that optimal care is delivered by all staff who come into contact with the patient. In addition to clinical communication, the chart needs to be used by utilization review personnel, by representatives of third party payers who check for correct billing and quality of care provided. The chart is also the legal record of care and must sometimes be made available to attorneys and to the patients. Regulatory agencies, such as public health departments, nuclear regulatory agencies, and environmental protection agencies, among others, may require certain patient records to evaluate compliance with various regulations. Finally, it was recognized that a tool that made explicit the logic of clinical decision processes [3] would serve our mission as a teaching hospital better than the existing model.

The Task Force recommended a charting methodology focused on the patient rather than the caregiver, location of care or procedures as the center of the documentation effort. That is, the clinical record designed around the need to identify patient problems, record clinical actions taken to deal with those problems, and document the effects on patient health status or functional status of those clinical services. (It is understood that a "problem" may be either an actual or potential problem). Intrinsically, the new approach will meet Joint Commission on Accreditation of Health Care Organizations requirement that the linkage between caregiver actions and patient problems be explicit. It will also enable clinical managers to begin the process of linking costs of care to patient outcomes.

3. Documentation System Redesign Principles.

There are two basic drivers for the new system. The first driver is focused on diagnoses. The diagnoses made by each of the clinical subspecialty practitioners are logged onto the *Patient Problem List*. The Patient Problem List is envisioned as becoming the "driving force" for clinical action planning. All other documents are being designed to support problem identification, to document plans and interventions designed to resolve or ameliorate those problems, or to document outcomes of care. In this way, the system will make clear the thinking of clinicians, and the logic of clinical decisions. The system is designed to replace the nursing care plan and other clinical care planning documents. An important goal of the new system will be parsimony. That is, the least amount of paper (or file space) needed will be used to capture the maximum amount of clinical information.

The nurses on the task force identified an issue important to nurses that was not addressed by our consultants or by the POMR literature. Nurses must repeatedly document some of the same assessment/monitoring and care items over the length of stay. Some of these items are not associated with a problem but rather with unit routines and basic hygienic care. The system had to support documentation of *both* problem-derived and other nursing care documentation needs. This was accomplished with the second type of forms. The second driver of the system is the set of *Flow Sheets*, composed of highly structured screens or paper forms. The flow sheets are used to document assessment data, interventions and patient outcomes in the form of changes in functional or health status. These structured forms are similar to the flow sheets that have long been in use in most critical care units. The entire documentation system is being redesigned around these two drivers. Once the drivers were selected, design principles were elaborated to guide the redesign process.

The principles of chart redesign are:

1. The organization of the chart forms and data elements selected for inclusion are designed to represent the structure of care.
2. All possible information is recorded coded data elements rather than a narrative format.
3. The documentation format is designed with as many items of assessment, diagnosis, interventions and patient care outcomes specifically named in lists. The clinician chooses words from the list to enter into the clinical record. The choice made by the clinician is represented by a code in the computer's memory.
4. The record is integrated around patient problems, rather than fragmented into forms that reflect the hospital's departmental and service structure. Thus, the patient problem list becomes the organizing focus of clinical documentation.
5. The structure of the flow sheets is specifically designed to help maintain minimum standards of care. This principle is actualized through flow sheets that guide assessment and care. The words used in the flow sheets, and the sequencing of the interrogatory structure of assessment and care documentation are designed to prevent errors of omission by supporting memory and clinical pattern recognition.

4. Goals and Anticipated Outcomes of the Redesigned Documentation System

Use of these principles produces a document that offers many memory supports to the nurse. Blanks in a document serve to remind the nurse to perform an assessment, or to provide a treatment. The Medication Administration Record (MAR) in use by most hospitals is a document that exemplifies many of the desired characteristics. Each of the patient's ordered medications is listed, along with the correct dose, time of administration, route, and if appropriate, concentration in admixture. These items serve to help nurses maintain a high degree of accuracy in medication administration. The new forms are designed to garner these benefits for the majority of patient care work of the nurse.

The main objective of the redesign is to develop a more effective and efficient clinical documentation system. The system will be used for the following purposes: improve quality of care through improved clinical communication, maximize reimbursement, support accreditation of the medical center and service units within the center, meet the requirements of regulatory agencies, and when necessary, provide legal evidence of care.

The anticipated outcomes of the redesigned documentation system are:

1. The system will increase overall efficiency by reducing the amount of time and effort staff spend entering or retrieving data from the clinical record
2. The system will make recording and retrieving clinical information substantially easier for physicians.
3. The redesigned documentation system will facilitate and document care integration across and among the departments.
4. The system will lower clinical errors of omission as well as errors related to incomplete or missing documentation.
5. The system will improve clinical communication by increasing the ease with which important information can be retrieved as well as by decreasing problems of incomplete or missing documentation, and by increasing the

legibility of the record.
6. The system will make clear the linkages among patient problems, care delivered and the effect of that care on patient outcomes.
7. The system will reduce the volume of the clinical record.

5. Goals of the Redesign Process

The task force also delineated a variety of goals for the documentation system redesign process itself. It was recognized that a healthy, inclusive process would increase the probability that the main objectives would be achieved. The process goals were:
1. Representatives of all patient record user groups would be included in the redesign effort. Where feasible, legitimate external users were to be consulted about redesign concepts or products.
2. To the extent possible, the system would encourage house-wide, common forms rather than area or specialty specific forms.
3. To the extent possible, the system is to avoid the use of narrative notes. This was to be accomplished through the use of codifiable data formats, such as numeric entry, checklists, graphic representations of information, etc.
4. The system was to be designed to serve as a memory support system for clinicians.
5. Data entry simplification was to be an important goal for both the manual and computer-based implementations of the new documentation system.
6. The system was to be designed to provide a method by which the outcomes of patient care could be clearly and concisely documented.
7. The system design process was to focus on ways to reduce data redundancy in the clinical record.

6. General Approach to Documentation, and Rationale

The new documentation system is a Patient Centered, Problem Oriented charting system. The patient centered chart will be achieved through a focus on the list of patient problems. (Depending upon the preference of each hospital's medical staff, the list of medical diagnoses may head up the problem list, or physician documentation may be kept entirely separate.) Nursing at St. Francis uses the NANDA words and coding scheme for nursing diagnoses in the design of the nursing component of the documentation system. Other nomenclatures and coding schemes such as those developed at Iowa [4] are under review.

The new documentation system is designed to be parsimonious. That is, it must be concise, yet extremely complete. The quality of succinctness will be achieved by limiting redundancy and the amount of narrative charting as much as possible. Forms and procedures are being redesigned to avoid repetitive entry of the same data. For example, if nursing has recorded information about the patient's family and living situation, social service will need only to ask information that is not already collected. The patient's age and gender are standard items stamped or printed onto every form. The nursing assessment has this information. There is no reason for any other form to have a place for the clinician to re-enter the patient's age and gender. Parsimony is also encouraged through checklists, numeric representations of information, and other forms of entry that can be coded. Narrative charting is not parsimonious.

Reduction of narrative charting carries a variety of benefits to the institution. First, it takes more time to write a paragraph than to make two or three check marks on a list. Second, personal script is often illegible. Numeric or check list formats are far more likely to be understandable to the user. Third, this approach helps to reduce the amount of extraneous and unnecessary notation often found in narrative notes. Superfluous items increase the volume of the chart without a concurrent increase in communication. Even more serious, such notations may be prejudicial to the hospital, its staff or physicians in litigation. Fourth, narrative charting makes the job of those who must perform quality studies, abstract the chart, or otherwise search out and summarize information across multiple patients, very time consuming and difficult. Fifth, the design of flow sheets (which is the basis of the codifiable charting format) intrinsically serves to support the memory of the caregiver. Sixth, narrative charting formats offer no supports to the memories of clinicians. Seventh, the specific structure chosen by St. Francis uses the initial nursing assessment to lead directly into identification of the nursing diagnoses, which then -- along with the medical diagnoses -- form the patient problem list. Thus, the system serves to focus and guide care as well as to document care.

The St. Francis clinical record system is being reengineered to provide many memory supports in aid of complete documentation. Common care-related items are listed for check-off to help remind staff of important items that are easily forgotten. Insofar as possible, care information was represented numerically, or through checklists and codifiable formats. The new Nursing Admission Assessment is designed to guide the nurse through a complete assessment, and to extract information from that assessment to use in building the problem list. The reason for these new approaches is futuristic, and at the same time pragmatically focused on the current need for efficiency and a very high degree of completeness (effectiveness) in the St. Francis clinical documentation system. Existing research demonstrates that a minimum of 35% to 40% of nursing time is spent handling information. Given the cost and cyclical scarcity of nursing resources in the United States, and the very high complexity of St. Francis patients, the need to achieve the most efficient use of nursing staff time is critical.

Incomplete or inaccurate charting is most serious. It is ineffective for the purpose of clinical communication. It can therefore have deleterious effects on the quality of patient care. Insufficient documentation can have very serious financial and perhaps even public image consequences for the institution. HCFA publishes information about mortality rates in hospitals, and has a stringent quality review system that can provide very severe punishments for quality problems in hospitals. Since those quality reviews are based on review of the clinical record, a complete, concise clinical record is an important tool for demonstrating quality care to third party payers and other reviewers.

The proposed system will eliminate the Nursing Care Plan (NCP). Information in the NCP should be in the clinical record. Nurses complain that NCPs are very difficult and time consuming to generate, yet have contributed little to quality patient care. Using a Problem Centered system creates a mindset in which actions are deliberate, and explicitly related to recognized patient problems and needs. The NCP was a device to encourage such deliberate action. The new system is focused on impelling the caregiver to consciously act in an organized manner that is directed toward solution of the patient's problems and needs that the NCP becomes unnecessary as a separate document. With a more structured format, the work of coders, abstracters and reviewers should be greatly streamlined. A variety of approaches could be used. Many of the items these staff need could be easily located on the problem or intervention lists, or placed on a flowsheet type of form. In an automated system, these items could be retrieved with the help of a   Third, the volume of the chart may be reduced, thus saving costs associated with paper purchases, record storage costs and people time in searching form information on the chart.

7. Conclusion

The proposed changes are a significant departure from typical paper-based, manual documentation systems. The paper systems can best be described as care giver, service center or department focused or procedure focus. The new paradigm is focused on the patient and his/her problems and needs. It also is designed to take account of the need to provide a system to support human memory in a complex, rapidly changing work environment. The paper-based model depended far too much on human short and long term memory. As a result, human limitations too often resulted in clinical errors. The redesign of the structure of the documentation system will serve as a support system as well as a documentation system to clinicians. As a result, patients will receive better care; and the best justification for an automated system is that it improves patient care.

8. References

[1] Weed LL. *Medical Records, Medical Education, and Patient Care: The Problem-Oriented Record as a Basic Tool.* Cleveland: Press of Case Western Reserve University, 1969.

[2] McHugh ML. Increasing Productivity Through Computer Communications. *Dim Critical Care Nsg* 1986 5(5):294-302.

[3] Weed LL, and Zimny NJ. The Problem-Oriented System, Problem-Knowledge Coupling and Clinical Decision Making. *Phys Ther* 1989, Jul;69(7):565-8.

[4] Bulecheck GM and McCloskey JC. Nursing Intervention Taxonomy Development. In: *Current Issues in NUrsing* 3rd ed. McCloskey JC, Grace HK (eds). St. Louis: CV Mosby Company, 1990.

Nursing Informatics: An International Overview for Nursing in a Technological Era
S.J. Grobe and E.S.P. Pluyter-Wenting, eds.

Nursing Information in Patient Records: The use of the VIPS-model in Clinical Nursing Education

Thorell-Ekstrand I [a, b], Björvell H [b]

[a] *Stockholm University College of Health Sciences, Box 17913, S-118 95 Stockholm , Sweden.*

[b] *R & D Unit for Nursing, the Center of Caring Scienes North, Borgmästarvillan, plan 1, Karolinska Hospital S-171 76 Stockholm, Sweden.*

Nursing students have shown to have been poorly clinically educated about writing patient care plans. It was hoped that the VIPS model for nursing documentation , consisting of a list of key words and guidelines [1], might be used as a teaching tool and affect their learning of individualized patient care, including the writing of care plans. The model was used by nursing students as a charting strategy while they learned about documentation during their clinical allocations.

Hypotheses formulated were that documenting nursing care by using the VIPS model may:
1) enhance learning of patient care planning, 2) facilitate structure and readability of the documentation, and 3) reinforce students' attention to patient participation. In a descriptive evaluative approach, a group students (n=87) used the key words when writing care plans during their final clinical training. In addition to the students' assignments, copies of the real patient records were analyzed. After the care plans and copies were delivered, a questionnaire was answered by the students. The data collection took place in June 1993.

1. Introduction

This paper is a description of the use of a model for nursing documentation as a teaching model for the integration of theory and practice in a final stage of nursing education. Deficiencies and difficulties have been reported in earlier studies that described a group of students' theoretical preparation of how to write care plans [2], the knowledge and experience among a group of students' preceptors [3] and an evaluation of the perceived amount of clinical training of care planning activities [4]. In a parallell project the VIPS model for nursing information in patient records was developed [1]. This model was used by a group of nursing students (n=87) for a care planning assignment during their last clinical placements at medical and long term care units.

1.1. The writing of patient care plans in Sweden

The long history of the development of case studies as care plans as was described by Hege dus [5] has not been seen in Sweden. The writing of nursing care plans was introduced not more than a decade ago as a mean to systematize and individualize patient care. As in most of the world, it was most quickly and widely adopted by the nursing education as a method of teaching the nursing process. However, its implementation in nursing practice has been slow, a fact that has had implications upon the clinical parts of the nursing education. The writing of care plans seems to have been conserved as an educational task that has little in common with Swedish health care reality.

Instead there is a strong oral tradition, shown at the repeated, regular "report meetings" when there is talk about observations, medical orders, and changes of patient conditions. Nurses often express pride over the substantial oral reports given on their unit. Swedish authorities have recently emphasized the importance of systematically noted nursing information in patient records as a tool for patient security and a basis for quality care [6]. This has resulted in a growing awareness of the necessity to develop proper nursing records and patient care plans. However, resistance to documentation still exists and as late as January 1993 only minor improvements were shown to have affected the training of nursing students during their clinical education, compared to 1990, as shown among a group of nursing students [4].

2. Critique of the care planning model

Problems and resistance to document has not only been seen in Sweden, although the reasons may be different. A growing concern has been described about the deficiencies inherent in the way care planning has developed . A "slavishly" use of formal analytical tools are believed to limit the development of more flexible ways to collect and describe information about the patient and the situation [7]. A complain over standardized, comprehensive care plans, described as being of a "wide-spread unpopularity" was described by Brider in 1991 [8]. It was concluded that there is a need to fundamentally reform the nursing documentation system using a "critical pathway" of a day-by-day summary of the patient's stay, highlighting only deviations from projected daily outcomes. It was also suggested that nursing care plans must be part of the permanent patient record and as such constructed in collaboration with physicians. These comments also mirror the common Swedish concern of finding a documentation system that will function as being primarily practical to use.

The faculty's emphasis on teaching the nursing process in theory vis-á-vis the problems of applying it in clinical practice has been discussed by Moss [9] and Daws [10]. Although the writing of care plans has a history as an educational tool, little empirical evidence supports that the written nursing care plan provides a reliable instructional method [11].

3. Theoretical framework

The clinical nursing education is in Sweden organized in blocks of 7-8 weeks, using a preceptorship model where the student is assigned to work along with a specific staff nurse, called a preceptor or supervisor. Each student has a preceptor at each clinical placement and the staff nurses are assigned to be preceptors in turn. Preceptor training courses are optional and of different length and content. Educational situations in a preceptor system assume that students learn from their experience in work situations in which teaching-learning not is the main focus. The preceptor's major responsibility is to give good patient care, not to teach. The students' learning in the preceptor system may be explained by the theory of experiential learning [12]. According to experiential learning reflection is a necessary assumption for high quality of learning. It is further assumed that reflection does not happen by itself, it must be observed and practiced, a form of cognitive training [13, 14]. Perhaps the most obvious educational effect in this situation is that reflection is developed by formulating written words. Ong [15] states that writing sharpens the analytic skills as the single words are given a more demanding task when written than when spoken. Reflection is thought to be forced because writing is slower than oral description. Therefore nursing documentation and writing of care plans training is seen as a vital teaching and learning issue; and, the use of the VIPS model should be carefully followed to explore its potential effects on learning.

4. Study purpose

The purpose of the present study was twofold: to involve the students in the evaluation of the usefulness of the model, and, to gain experience in observing the educational effects of the model.

The study should be considered as explorative. Its aim was to reveal any difficulties that could be avoided in a later planned randomized trial. A special interest was focused on the students' use of intervention key words and their descriptions.The questions were:
1. Which key words did students use?
2. How relevant was the students' use of chosen keywords, especially the interventions?
3. How was patient participation worded?
4. How well were the students' care plans correlated with the patient problems noted in the copied original record?

4.1 A pilot study

The development of the VIPS model has quickly gained great attention among both clinical practitioners and nurse educators throughout Sweden. It was therefore natural to present it to students as a way of teaching documentation of nursing care. However, the teaching of new ideas in the classroom is completely different from its application in practice. Well aware of this fact, the project leaders asked for ten interested students to volonteer to try and use the VIPS model with the keywords during their clinical education as they were completing their care plans.
The trial was considered a failure since the students used only some of the keywords. They did not use any key words for interventions, and none used the complete VIPS model. Therefore, it could not be concluded that the model was the problem; however it was more likely that this failure was due to insufficient preparation of the students, teachers and preceptors.
The next attempt to introduce the Vips model in students' clinical training was preceded by intensive discussion with the involved educators. A major problem that became obvious was the educators' lack of experience in writing care plans. Their experience consisted only of the teaching of care planning that was done only in classroom exercises and in correcting students' care plan assignments.

5. Study methods

All students (n=93) attending the last course of the General Nursing Program at one of three units of Stockholm College of Health and Caring Sciences during the spring term of 1993 agreed to participate in the study.

5. 1 Procedures

The study was designed using a descriptive evaluation approach. Students agreed to practice using the model during their clinical training at medical and long term care units, and, agreed to have their last assigned care plan examined by the research team. The examination of the care plan included a comparison of it with the ordinary nursing documentation in patient records. A copy of the original patient care plan, temperture list and progress notes, all unidentified, were enclosed as material for the researcher's examination. Letters of request to all chief clinical managers, head nurses and the students' preceptors preceded the study. Extra personal information about the the model or/and the project was offered upon request to all participants. Participating students were encouraged to contact the project team regarding any difficulty or uncertainty. Confidentiality was assured and the students agreed not to be anonymous and were in return promised personal comments upon the care plan to be sent by mail at a later date.
The care plans were reviewed by a research team and analysed according to three instruments, two developed by Ehnfors [16] and one developed for this study: 1) Components of the nursing process and key words, 2) Protocol for review of comprehensiveness of recorded nursing problems, and 3) template for educational review of relevance and nursing knowledge. The third intrument was developed in cooperation with two experienced educators with the intention that it be tested as a review instrument, and later possibly introduced as a teaching/learning tool. It was thought that it might be a useful tool for helping students develop their care plans continuously. This latter instrument used a 4 point scale based on 9 criteria.

In addition a questionnaire was answered by the students, once their care plans were delivered. Questions concerned perceived amount of education and conditions of importance for the application of the model.. Each key word in the model was evaluated as to usefulness and difficulty to use on two four-point scales with the extremes "1=always useful" and "1= very easy to use" to "4=never useful" and "4=very difficult to use".

5.2 Preliminary results

The project was successfully accomplished in the sense that the students implemented the task and delivered their own nicely typed care plans together with the ordinary hand written records with enthusiasm. Two students had experienced computerized recording with the VIPS model at their placement unit.

Although only 53% of the participating students expressed satisfaction with the education about the model, the key words were evaluated as both useful and easy to use. The two exceptions were the assessment of "sexuality" and "spritual needs". The key words for interventions were considered more difficult to use than those for assessment.

The students' care plans were due to the key words easier to read than the authentic nursing notes. However, many identified problems were not satisfactually recorded through the nursing process; the recorded key words for interventions were few and outcome was seldom recorded.

5.3 Implications for nursing

It is important that nurses in the future learn to use a common language in order to communicate and identify the essence in the delivery of quality health care. Thus, these students' evaluation of their education and experience of the VIPS model may useful in the further development of nursing information in patient records.

6. References

[1]   Ehnfors M, Thorell-Ekstrand I, & Ehrenberg A. Towards Basic Nursing Information in Patient Records. *Vård i Norden*, 1991, 21:3/4, 12-31.

[2]   Thorell-Ekstrand I. & Björevell H. Preparedness for Clinical Nursing Education. Accepted 1993. *Scand J Car Sci.*.

[3]   Thorell-Ekstrand I., Björvell H. & Blanchard- Ceasar L. Preceptorship in Clinical Nursing Education in Sweden: Aspects of Quality Assurance. *Quality Assurance in Health Care. 1993. Vol 5* In press.

[4]   Thorell-Ekstrand I & Björvell H. The teaching and learning of writing care plans in clinical nursing education. Submitted.

[5]   Hegedus KS. From case study to plans for caring. *West J Nurs Res*, 1991, Oct; 13(5): 653-7.

[6]   Socialstyrelsen. *Socialstyrelsens allmänna råd (SOSFS 1990:15) i omvårdnad inom sluten somatisk vård och primärvård*, Stockholm:Socialstyrelsen.1990. (In Swedish).

[7]   Benner P. & Tanner C. From beginner to expert. *ANS Adv Nurs Sci*. 1992, Mar 14(3) 13-28.

[8]   Brider, P. Who killed the nursing care plan? *Am J Nurs* 1991, May 35-39.

[9]   Moss AR. Determinants of patient care: nursing process or nursing attitudes? *J Adv Nurs* , 1988, 13, 615-620.

[10]   Daws J. An inquiry into the attitudes of qualified nursing staff towards tjhe use of individualized nursing care plans as a teaching tool. *J Adv Nurs,* 1988, 13, 139-146.

[11]   Tanner C. The Nursing Care Plan As a Teaching Method: Reason or Ritual? *Nurse Educator,* 1986. Vol 11, No 4. 8-10.

[12]   Kolb D. 1984. *Experiential learning.* Prentice-Hall Inc., London.

[13]   Burnard P. 1992. Learning from expererience: nurse tutors' and student nurses' perceptions of experiential learning in nurse education: some initial findings. *Int. J Nurs Stud.* Vol 29, No2, pp. 151-161.

[14]   Bandura A. 1977. *Social Learning Theory.* Prentice-Hall, Englewood Cliffs, New Jersey.

[15]   Ong W.J. (1982) *Orality and Literay. The Technology of the Word.* Methuen & Co. (1990 Swedish ed., Anthropos, Göteborg.)

[16]   Ehnfors M. *Quality of Care form a Nursing Perspective. Methodological Considerations and Development of a Model for Nursing Documentation.* Acta Universitatis Upsaliensis. Comprehensive Summaries of Uppsala Dissertations from Faculty of Medicine 415, Uppsala: Uppsala University, 1993. (Dissertation)

Computerised Nursing Care Record
- A Case Study -

Cheminat C. and Elsig Y.

Department of Nursing, Geneva Canton University Hospital (HCUG), Geneva, Switzerland

The computerisation of the "nursing process" is a dream that nursing care personnel, coming from different professional horizons, have succeeded in achieving by creating GEPSI (Groupe d'étude pour un processus de soins informatisé) which is a study group for a computerised nursing care record. The following describes an experiment made within a nursing unit at the Geneva Canton University Hospital (HCUG). The training of the nursing personnel, the integration of computer tools into the work environment and the organisational changes which this form of communication entails, are the steps experienced by a team of nurses having, initially, no particular computer training. The test was set up within a research framework with the aim of proposing its use to different hospitals in the Canton of Geneva. A model of the nursing process can be reintegrated into all future Ward Information Systems (WIS) and should also include the medical and administrative record as a whole.

1.   Introduction

GEPSI, which was set up in 1988, brings together care personnel who have very different professional diplomas or nursing qualifications. The participants conducted their research centering themselves on the best methods of problem solving, bearing in mind that the basic concept of the computerised nursing record is the possibility of its use by either general care or psychiatric nurses. The computer tools proposed had also to interface with the different information systems already installed [1].

1.1. The prototype tested comprised of:
a) the nursing process: a personalised care plan manager for each patient based on a four column layout, objectives, nursing activities and completion of follow-up notes or evaluation.

b) the patient care daily charting tool: testing the originality of the application, its ability to link a problem to the objectives, nursing activities, follow-up notes and evaluation.

The setting up of the process was made easier by the use of a nomenclature, or vocabulary, based on the "Fourteen Patient Needs" as defined in the philosophy of Virginia Henderson [2].

1.2. The prototype was tested in four care units:
1 psychiatric unit; 2 geriatric units and 1 orthopaedic reeducation unit. The four care units have two points in common: first, they belong to EPMG (Etablissements Publics Médicaux Genevois) and second, they are either medium or longterm nursing units.

2. Choice of location for case study at HCUG (Hôpital Cantonal Universitaire de Genève)

The 2 AK unit was considered suitable for this case study as it is one of the 120 nursing care units at HCUG and receives patients undergoing orthopaedic reeducation.

As well as this, one of the nurses in the care team regularly attended the GEPSI nomenclature group meetings. The chief nurse for the unit followed a training course for nursing quality assurance and belongs to the special Nursing Informatics Group of the Department of Nursing (Informatique et Soins Infirmiers - ISIS) at HCUG. The nursing staff worked with the same care record common to all units and voluntarily complied with the demands of the test.

3. Preparation for the case study: training

The 12 nursing staff comprised: 8 nurses and 4 hospital assistants. Even though they were familiar with the hospital information system - DIOGENE (Division Informatique hOpital GENEve), they had never before used a personal computer (PC), a keyboard, nor a mouse. To demystify these computer tools the first task was to train the personnel to use the PC. A PC (MACintosh) with a large screen was installed outside the nursing unit in an office accessible 24 hours per day. In this location 5 hours of training and support were offered to each person to enable them to learn how to use the PC, its keyboard and mouse, the diskettes, and how to set up a programme and use the printer, etc.

The objective of the first phase of training - adaptation to the computer tools - was thus accomplished. A word-processor, printer and relevant software were then put at the disposal of the personnel being trained to allow them to practice. This enabled the introduction of the second phase of training - learning to use the software developed by the nursing computer scientist. It took just 10 hours to train each person to use this prototype and then they continued by practicing on their own. Throughout this period of training the PC remained outside the care unit.

4. Integration of the tool in the working place

An area was then prepared, in the already limited space of the care unit, to accommodate the material necessary to make the test. By modifying a cupboard and adding a small table, an agreeable working space was created. The PC MACintosh and DIOGENE system could then be used in the care unit.

5. Test of the GEPSI prototype in the 2 AK unit

At the end of May 1992, the PC was installed in the 2 AK nursing unit. After a running-in period, the proper testing began on June 3, 1992 and terminated on December 31, 1992. By common agreement, the nursing team decided to treat the care records of 4 patients hospitalised in rooms with 1 or 2 beds.

Each nurse was asked to introduce into the computer the data of the patients she was responsible for and evaluations were foreseen at 1 month, 2 months, 4 months and 6 months, with the participation of the person responsible for the test and the head nurse.

The software offered three principal menus:

Menu I - Nursing Process

This sets out: problems, objectives, nursing interventions and follow-up notes.

These four elements are shown on the screen *in summary form* (with key words for rapid reading of the nursing procedure) or *in detailed form* (description of the problem's nature, cause, care and priorities).

It is possible to access and link together the two above formats. The collection of nursing data or anamnese is accomplished using the hard copy (paper) support of the usual nursing record (Fig. 1).

Menu II - Patient care plan manager

The daily tasks which the nurse must complete for each patient. This plan is determined by the activities undertaken in the initial nursing care process (Fig. 2).

Menu III - The nursing nomenclature

The nursing nomenclature is based on the Virginia Henderson philosophy of nursing theory and has two functions. Firstly, assistance in setting up the nursing process, giving directions as the appropriate request is entered by way of the keyboard (or mouse). Secondly, direct validation of the contents of the nursing nomenclature at the set up of the nursing process.

During the course of the first month of use, much time was spent developing the care process, as well as learning the subtleties of the software and the temperament of the computer hardware. The nursing record was made in duplicate: a backup copy stored in the computer and a traditional "hard copy" on paper. When trying to eliminate the need for the duplicate hard copy paper support, out of the 17 nursing records in the test, it was possible to eliminate only two of them. The reason was that, in the orthopaedic reeducation unit, not all the team members looking after the patients were trained to use the computerised nursing record (physiotherapists, occupational theraphists, dieticians etc.). After the initial minor equipment problems were resolved the time needed to enter and process the nursing record diminished. During the whole of the test, the program developer and the person in charge of the test for HCUG, responded to all requests for assistance and fully supported the set up and follow up of the test.

6. The experience and the benefits

Introduction of the nursing care record prompted an interest from the medical profession as a whole. It served as a means of communication on the methods used by nurses in establishing the process of nursing care and the patient care plan, following Virginia Henderson's philosophy for the care of patients. The following positive points were noted: 1) Access to information concerning the patients was rapid and gave a good global view of the problems and their priorities. 2) The test permitted the nursing team to apply the nursing care process more thoroughly. 3) The nursing nomenclature permitted a better knowledge of nursing diagnostics. Furthermore, it was used for compiling a nursing care process and also used didactically for teaching students and new nursing staff. 4) The printed characters were easy to read and errors easily corrected, leaving no trace. 5) The computer was also used as a word-processor for compiling the Minutes of the unit's meetings.

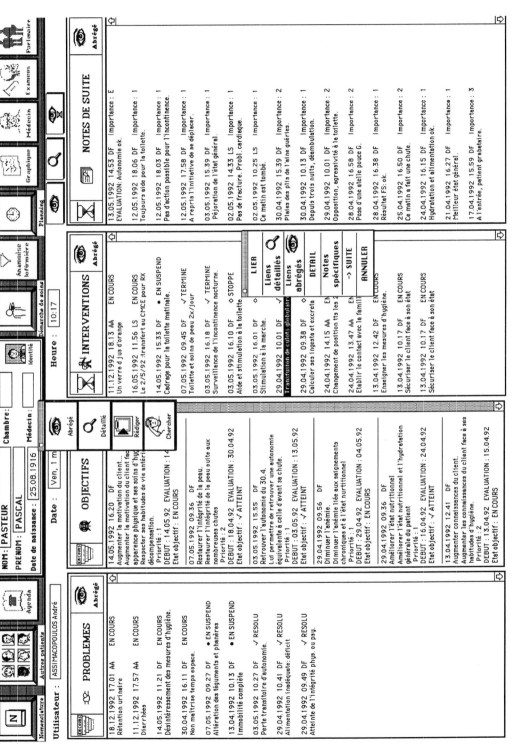

Fig. 1

315

316

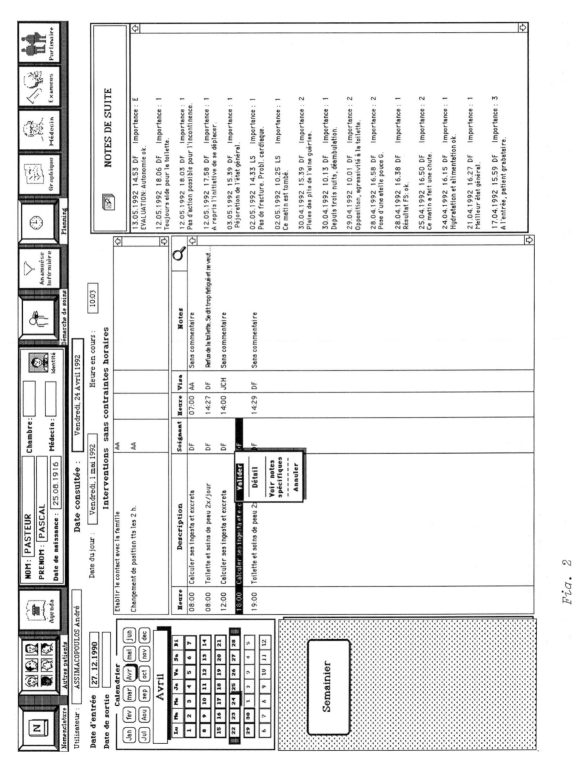

Fig. 2

7. Conclusion

Apart from brief teething problems inherent to this prototype, we felt that the experience gained by the nursing staff on the use of the computer, now an important part of the modern nurse's equipment, allowed them to develop an up-to-date nursing procedure. A report concerning the four test locations has been given to the Directors of the Nursing Department of EPMG, and we await news of the decisions taken.

The conditions for success:
-       To succeed in the introduction of a computerised nursing process in a care unit, it is essential that the computer tool be user-friendly so it can be used by staff who do not have any particular computer training. To facilitate this we must integrate all the medical and nursing teams in the computerisation process of patient care.
-       The software for the nursing record should interface with HIS and integrate the anamnese and the patient's daily chart. This means the computer equipment should be placed near enough to the patient to enable easy retrieval of this information. The computer tool must be flexible and adaptable to the usual working practices of different care units.

There is a particular approach given to the setting up of a computerised nursing care record for which *standard nursing terminology* is obligatory. The process of care being the data continually updated 24-hours a day by the nurses can, therefore, be considered as an autonomous document as well as a medical or administrative record.

8. References

[1] Wagenknecht A, Arnet PA, Borgazzi A, Butel J, Elsig Y, Rougé A, Assimacopoulos A. Tomorrow's Nursing; No Paperwork. Lecture Notes in Medical Informatics : *Proceedings of Nursing Informatics '91,* Melbourne, Australia. April 1991: p.54.

[2] Assimacopoulos A, Borgazzi A. An electronic patient record combining free text and coded nomenclature: Application to nursing process. Lecture Notes in Medical Informatics : *Proceedings of Nursing Informatics '91,* Melbourne, Australia. April 1991 p.746.

NURSING HEALTH INFORMATION SYSTEMS

D. Expertise/expert systems; decision support systems

Nursing Informatics: An International Overview for Nursing in a Technological Era
S.J. Grobe and E.S.P. Pluyter-Wenting, eds.

A Computer-based Approach to Knowledge Acquisition For Expert System Development

Henry SB[a] Holzemer WL[a] and Gennari J[b]

[a]*Department of Mental Health, Community, and Administrative Nursing, University of California, San Francisco, CA 94143*

[b]*Section on Medical Informatics, Stanford School of Medicine, Stanford, CA 94130*

Knowledge acquisition, which consists of knowledge elicitation and knowledge representation, is often considered the weakest link in the design of expert systems. Systems are frequently built on the knowledge of one expert and require extensive use of knowledge engineering techniques to elicit the knowledge from the expert. Machine learning algorithms are a potential alternative method of knowledge acquisition for expert system development. The aim of this pilot study was to examine the feasibility of applying machine learning techniques (inductive algorithms) to an existing research database as a method for knowledge elicitation and knowledge representation for expert system development. The data are from NIH-NR02215, "Quality of Nursing Care of People with AIDS" (WL Holzemer, Principal Investigator). The output of the inductive algorithms will be judged on two criteria, reliability and comprehensibility.

1. Background

Persons with HIV are now living longer and increasing numbers are receiving medical and nursing care in community-based primary care settings rather than in the high census areas.[1,2] Research has demonstrated that HIV care is often superior in settings caring for a high volume of HIV patients. Holzemer and Henry [3] described a wide variation in the nursing care plans for patients with HIV within four geographically close medical centers. An expert system focused on HIV nursing care has the potential to improve the quality of nursing care for patients by providing computer-based clinical practice The task of knowledge acquisition for such an expert system is formidable.

Knowledge acquisition, which consists of knowledge elicitation and knowledge representation, is often considered the weakest link in the design of expert systems. Systems are frequently built on the knowledge of one expert and require extensive use of knowledge engineering techniques to elicit the knowledge from the expert.[4] Critics of this method of knowledge elicitation state that experts often tell more than they can know.[5] In other words, the "how" of decision making (procedural knowledge) may not be accessible to the conscious mind for recall and verbalization. This lack of accessibility to procedural knowledge is a characteristic of expertise well-described in nursing by Benner.[6]

Machine learning algorithms are a potential alternative method of knowledge acquisition for expert system development. Abraham et al. [7] described the potential for inductive algorithms to discover the nursing knowledge embedded in databases. This point was recently reiterated and expanded by Jones [8] in an excellent review article.

The essence of induction is to construct a formalism that correctly classifies not only objects from the training set, but other unseen objects as well.[9] Spackman [10] identified the context for the appropriate use of machine learning or inductive algorithms: 1) the goal of the learning is to produce a decision formalism that is

Funding: This project was supported by grants from the University of California, San Francisco, School of Nursing Annual Fund (SB Henry, PI) and from the National Institutes of Health NR02215 (WL Holzemer, PI).

readable by humans (i.e.. decision tree, criteria table, production rules); 2) a classification or decision is the main outcome of the derived knowledge and the assignment of a probability estimate for the certainty of the decision is only a secondary goal; and 3) a relatively large set of training examples exists. He further states that "if a human-consumable knowledge representation is not important, then one should consider the numerous alternatives available as pattern recognition, statistical, probabilistic, and/or connectionist learning models" (p.641). Logistic regression and neural networks are examples of approaches in which the knowledge representation is not readily human-consumable.

Michalski and colleagues [11] in their classic work categorized machine learning techniques according to the amount of inference required and according to the type of knowledge acquired. If a computer is programmed directly it requires no inference while computer-based discovery learning requires extensive inference. A number of investigators have studied the capabilities of various inductive algorithms to classify healthcare data or to predict healthcare outcomes. Krusinska et al. [12] described an integrated approach for designing medical decision support systems with knowledge extracted from clinical databases by statistical methods. Their approach comprises data quality and semantic analyses as well as statistical data structure analysis which may include neural networks, inductive algorithms, and probabilistic methods. Spackman [10] compared C4 and CRLS algorithms for the prediction of breast cancer recurrence and the medical diagnosis of hyperthyroidism.

Jones [8] described the use of automated rule induction (SuperExpert) as a method of knowledge acquisition for four nursing expert systems in the domains of pressure sore risk assessment, priority nursing actions during ICU admissions, manpower deployment, and care plan generation. His findings indicated that automated rule induction compared favorably with cognitive modeling and statistical approaches to knowledge acquisition when careful attention was paid to the choice of training set attributes.

Grobe [13] examined the reliability of the ID3 algorithm for the classification of nursing interventions expressed in natural language into one of ten intervention categories. Agreement between the algorithm and human experts was greater than 79% for all but one category.

The questions to be addressed in this experiment meet the criteria proposed by Spackman [10] for the appropriate use of inductive algorithms. Additionally, a number of investigations have demonstrated the feasibility and reliability of using inductive algorithms to classify healthcare data and to predict healthcare outcomes. No investigations that focused on the application of inductive algorithms in the HIV disease domain were located. The complexity of the domain presents both great challenge and potential for contribution to methods for knowledge elicitation and knowledge representation.

2. Study Questions

The aim of this pilot study is to examine the feasibility of applying machine learning techniques (inductive algorithms) to an existing research database as a method for knowledge elicitation and knowledge representation for expert system development. The specific questions to be addressed in the feasibility study are: 1) Can machine learning algorithms accurately predict patient outcomes six months post-hospitalization for persons living with AIDS (PLWAs) hospitalized for Pneumocystis carinii pneumonia? and 2) Is the knowledge representation inducted from the machine learning algorithms comprehensible and adequate?

3. Methods

3.1 Design

The method for this experiment was a secondary analysis of an existing research database. The data are from "Quality of Nursing Care of Persons with AIDS" (NIH-NR02215, WL Holzemer, Principal Investigator). The data were collected from patient interviews, nurse interviews, and chart audits of 201 patients hospitalized for Pneumocystis carinii pneumonia during the years 1989-1991. The sample for this study was the 179 patients for whom six month outcome data were available. The initial set of variables submitted to the inductive algorithms are listed in Table 1.

3.2 Preparation of the Data

The data related to patient problems, nursing interventions, and patient medications are stored in a relational database. Patient demographics, laboratory findings, and patient outcomes including quality of life

(HIV-Quality Audit Marker [HIV-QAM]) [14], length of hospital stay, health services utilization for six months post-hospitalization, and mortality are stored as statistical files. Data were first merged into a single computer-readable file and then exported as an ascii file.

3.3 Selection of the Algorithms

The prognostic task in this study falls into the Michalski category of learning by examples which requires a moderate amount of inference. In this method the algorithm learns from a training set of data. The subsequent algorithm is then tested with a second set of data (test set). The resultant knowledge will be represented in human-consumable form as a decision tree and/or as a series of production rules (if-then statements). The selection of the algorithms for testing is in progress.

Several inductive algorithms including ID3, C4, CART, and SuperExpert are under consideration for the analysis. The final selection of at least two inductive algorithms for testing will occur after the existing data structures are examined Criteria to be considered in the selection of the inductive algorithms include type of knowledge representation produced, size of training set required, ability of the algorithm to be implemented with the data structures present in the research database, method for dealing with noise (inaccuracy inherent in real-world data), and method for dealing with missing data.[9,10]

Table 1
Variables in data set for machine learning algorithms

Laboratory	HIV-QAM Scales	Clinical
White blood count	(At admission)	Temperature
Absolute lymphocyte count	Self-care	Heart rate
CD4 count	Ambulation	Respiratory rate
T4/T8 ratio	Psychological distress	Blood pressure
		Breath sounds
Patient Problems	Demographics	O2 rate
Shortness of breath	Age	
Fatigue	Transmission category	Outcome Variables
Poor appetite	Payor	(At six months)
Anxiety	Clinical site	Mortality
Nausea		Number of hospitalizations
Elimination	Physical Condition	Number of hospitalized days
	Patient rating	HIV-QAM self-care
	Nurse rating	HIV-QAM ambulation
Chest Radiograph		HIV-QAM psych distress
Infiltrates	Psychological Support	
	Patient rating	
	Nurse rating	

4. Results

The selection and testing of the algorithms is in progress. The output of the inductive algorithms will be judged on two criteria, reliability and comprehensibility. Cohen's kappa statistic will be used to calculate the agreement between the predicted outcomes and actual patient outcomes (reliability) for both the training and testing sets. Percent error rates will also be reported.[10] The comprehensibility of the knowledge representation will be independently judged by five nurses expert in the nursing care of PLWAs. The adequacy of the knowledge representation will be judged by a panel of three healthcare informaticists.

5. Discussion

The research described in this paper is one arm of three-pronged approach to knowledge acquisition for expert system development for HIV nursing care. The inductive algorithm approach has been preceded by traditional statistical processing methods (i.e. correlational techniques, cluster analysis) and will be succeeded and supplemented by a computer-based knowledge engineering approach such as Protege II or KADS.[15] The significance of research on machine learning techniques was recently addressed in a report by the National Center for Nursing Research' priority expert panel on nursing informatics [16] which states that "...algorithms or structured methods for transforming clinical information from the databases in clinical nursing information systems into new knowledge, that is, new and interesting relationships between variables of interest to nursing, is a fruitful direction for research..." (p.51). A recurring theme throughout the priority panel report is the need to link the structure, process, and outcomes of nursing care through the use of information technology. This research study focuses on the linkage of structure (patient problems and patient characteristics) and outcomes of care (mortality, health services utilization, and quality of life). Subsequent experiments will focus on the relationships between nursing interventions and patient outcomes.

6. Literature Cited

[1]   Moore RD, Hidalgo J, Sugland BW and Chaisson RE. Zidovudine and the natural history of theAcquired Immunodeficiency Syndrome. *NEJM* 1991, 324:1412-1416.

[2]   Lemp GF, Hirozawa AM, Araneta MR, Young K and Nieri G. Improved survival for persons with AIDS in San Francisco. In:*Proceedings of the VII International Conference on AIDS* 1991:66.

[3]   Holzemer WL and Henry SB. Nursing care plans for people with HIV/AIDS: Confusion or consensus? *J Adv Nurs* 1991, 16:257-261.

[4]   Musen MA. In:*Second general expert systems*. David JM, Krivine,JP, Simmons R(eds), in press.

[5]   Nisbett RE and Wilson TD. Telling more than we can know: Verbal reports on mental processes. *Psychological Review* 1977, 84:231-259.

[6]   Benner P. *From novice to expert: Excellence and power in clinical nursing practice*. Menlo Park, CA: Addison-Wesley, 1984.

[7]   Abraham IL, Fitzpatrick JJ and Jewell JA. The artificial intelligence in nursing project: Developing advanced technology for expert care. In:*Clinical judgment and and decision-making: The future with nursing diagnosis*. Hannah KJ, Reimer M, Mills WC and Letourneau (eds). NewYork: John Wiley & Sons 1986:468-470.

[8]   Jones BT. Building nursing expert systems using automated rule induction. *Comput Nurs* 1990, 9:52-60.

[9]   Quinlin, J.R. Induction of decision trees. *Machine Learning* 1986,1:81-106.

[10]   Spackman KA. A comparison of two methods of inductive knowledge acquisition for medical knowledge based systems. *Proceedings of the Fourteenth Annual Symposium on Computer Applications in Medical Care* 1990, 641-644.

[11]   Michalski RS, Carbonell JG and Mitchell TM. *Machine learning: An artificial intelligence approach*. New York: Morgan Kaufmann Publishers, Inc, 1983.

[12]   Krusinska E, Babic A, Chowdhury S, Wigertz O, Bodemar G and Mathiesen U. Integrated approach for designing medical decision support systems with knowledge extracted from clinical databases by statistical methods. *Proceedings of the Fifteenth Annual Symposium on Computer Applications in Medical Care* 1992, 353-357.

[13] Grobe S. Nursing intervention lexicon & taxonomy. *Proceedings of MedInfo92* . Amsterdam: North Holland, 1992: 981-986.

[14]   Holzemer WL, Henry SB, Stewart A and Janson-Bjerklie S. The HIVQAM: An outcome measure for HIV/AIDS. *Quality of Life Research* 1993, 2:99-107.

[15]   Musen MA. Dimensions of knowledge sharing and reuse. *Comp Biomedical Res* 1992, 25: 435-467.

[16]   Ozbolt J. *Nursing informatics: Enhancing patient care: A report of the NCNR priority expert panel on nursing informatics*. 1993, Bethesda, MD: US Department of Health and Human Services.

© 1994 Elsevier Science B.V. All rights reserved.
Nursing Informatics: An International Overview for Nursing in a Technological Era
S.J. Grobe and E.S.P. Pluyter-Wenting, eds.

Knowledge Solicitation from Expert Nurse Clinicians

Thompson CB[a] and Ryan SA[b]

[a]*Nursing Informatics Program, University of Utah College of Nursing, 25 South Medical Drive, Salt Lake City, UT 84112*

[b]*University of Rochester School of Nursing, 601 Elmwood, Rochester, NY 14642*

Clinical nurse experts have the ability to perform appropriate nursing actions, rapidly, after recognizing a minimal number of situational cues. Research supports the belief that it is not only the content of the nurse's knowledge, but its organization that is imperative for clinical expertise. Techniques now exist for eliciting the knowledge embedded in nursing practice directly from the expert. Pathfinder is a computer algorithm that has been used to create visual networks of the cognitive organization of clinical experts. Pathfinder uses ratings of the dissimilarity of concepts to create the networks. Examples of knowledge structures contained within the networks are presented.

1. Introduction

Clinical nurse experts have the ability to perform appropriate nursing actions, rapidly, after recognizing a minimal number of situational cues [1]. Knowledge, gained through experience and education, is often credited with being responsible for this ability. However, research supports the belief that it is not only the content of the nurses knowledge, but the organization of that knowledge that is imperative for clinical expertise.

Techniques now exist for eliciting the knowledge embedded in nursing practice directly from the expert. Pathfinder is a computer algorithm that has been used to create visual networks of an individual's cognitive organization of clinical concepts. Pathfinder uses ratings of the dissimilarity of concepts to create the networks.

This paper will discuss the usefulness of the Pathfinder technique as a method for the representation of clinical knowledge. Approaches to the use of the knowledge in expert systems also will be discussed.

2. Literature Review

Benner, Tanner, and Chesla [2] discuss the richness of nursing practice. They state that not all knowledge can be detailed in rationalistic propositions. Instead they use detailed personal accounts of clinical exemplars. These descriptions of nursing practice are eloquent and portray the resources available within specific clinical experts. Benner's accounts are based upon the assumption that clinicians learn through lived experiences. If knowledge must be gained through experience then this expertise is not available to add to clinical knowledge, to assist others in problem solving or to assist individuals to learn the practice of nursing. Nurses are in too great a shortage and patient needs too acute to allow the luxury of waiting for all nurses to learn the answers through experience. Methods must be found to document the clinical experience embedded within current clinical experts.

Newell and Simon [3] propose a theory of information processing as an explanation of how humans intake and process information to use in decision making. This theory states that sensory information (words, context, sensations) enter human short term memory. Additional relevant information is retrieved from long term memory and used in conjunction with the contents of short term memory in decision making.

The exact anatomical structures and physiological processes responsible for long term memory are unknown. The basic structures are assumed to be associative in nature, however[3]. This means that items are placed in memory not in isolation, but in reference to preexisting items. For example, the first time a student sees a patient become diaphoretic in response to hypotension this information is stored relative to the didactic information regarding hypotension.

If long term memory is associative, this might assist in explaining why experts cannot explicitly describe their reasoning processes. It may further contribute to understanding the difficulties encountered when attempting to demonstrate cognitive processing differences between novices and experts [4]. If knowledge is stored in associative networks, if-then rules might not exist and consequently require generation from stored associations. Novices and competent individuals might recall rules because rules have been taught and subsequently stored. Experts, however, no longer encounter rules on a daily basis, consequently they are no longer easily accessible within stored memory. Instead they have saved multiple actual examples.

A method for uncovering the structure of long term memory is needed. Similarity data analyzed by the Pathfinder algorithm is a proposed method for obtaining the knowledge embedded in experts' long term memory. Similarity data is obtained by asking individuals to rate the degree of similarity between concepts. For example, are the terms hypoxia and dyspnea related or unrelated. The response is given on a scale of from 0 to 9. A 0 indicates that the terms are exactly the same (no cognitive distance between them). A 9 indicates that the terms are not at all similar (their meanings are a great distance apart). Thus hypoxia and dyspnea may be rated a 0 or 1 and hypoxia and dobutamine may be rated much higher.

The advantage of similarity data is that it requires little cognitive processing. Subjects are asked to provide their first response to the questions of similarity in a given pair of concepts. Subjects can be requested to provide the response for a context free situation or within the framework of an actual clinical situation.

The raw similarity data is of little value without further analysis. An advantage of this fact is that individuals are unable to select a response set due to social desirability or other criteria. In addition, subjects are unable to predict and/or manipulate the networks that result from the raw data.

The Pathfinder algorithm used for data analysis was developed by Roger Schvaneveldt and colleagues at New Mexico State University [5]. It uses similarity data to derive visual representations of knowledge structures. It is based on graph theory and establishes interconcept connections by discarding all connections that do not represent the closest cognitive links within the data. This technique has been used by several researchers [6,7,8] who have demonstrated both construct and predictive validity. Reliability testing has been limited but suggests that ratings are stable across a two week time period.

3. Methods

Concepts to be included in the pairs rated for similarity were obtained during a pilot study. Potential concepts were obtained from the principal investigators personal clinical experience, clinical reference books, current literature, and written output from the Creighton On-line Multiple Modular Expert System. Potential concepts were given to an anonymous panel of nationally recognized experts for selection of those concepts most relevant to nursing care of a patient with congestive heart failure (CHF). Subjects for the pilot study were selected by Karen Sechrist R.N., Ph.D., the American Association of Critical Care Nurses Director for Research, based upon national recognition of their expertise. A total of 27 concepts (Table 1) were selected for inclusion within the study.

The study was conducted in two university-affiliated northeastern hospitals as part of the first author's dissertation research. Registered nurses employed on units admitting patients with a diagnosis of CHF, who could speak and understand English, were asked to participate. Subjects for this analysis were either novice or expert nurses. Novices were graduates from an program designed to prepare individuals for licensure as a registered nurse, who had less than six months nursing experience. Previous licensure as a practical nurse or previous employment to provide direct patient care prior to entering a nursing program were considered exclusionary criteria. Experts were nurses identified as expert by 75% of peers on their unit. A sample of 40 novices and 42 experts was obtained. For further detail see Thompson, Ryan, and Ingersoll [9].

Table 1
Concepts

air hunger	anxiety	arterial blood gases	capillary oncotic pressure
cough	crackles	diuretics	dobutamine
dyspnea	dysrhythmias	explanations	fatigue
fear of death	fluid overload	frothy sputum	furosemide (Lasix)
gallop rhythm	hypoxia	inotropic agents	left heart failure
morphine sulphate	myocardial contractility	oxygen	pulmonary edema
rales	right heart failure	stay with patient	

Approval for the study was obtained from Human Subjects Review committees and nursing administration at both institutions. Subjects volunteering to participate were given a cover letter explaining the nature of the study and informed written consent was obtained. Subjects completed a demographic form and provided similarity ratings for 356 pairs of concepts.

4. Analysis

A sample of 82 subjects was obtained, 40 novices and 42 experts. Fourteen potential subjects elected not to participate. Twelve subjects agreed to participate but were unable to schedule data collection appointments.

The quantitative analysis resulting from this study is presented elsewhere [9]. This analysis will focus on the specific knowledge embedded within the networks of novice and expert nurse clinicians.

Pathfinder networks were created for each subject. Subsequently, the similarity data from all novices and all experts were averaged and rounded to 3 digits (x.xx) A single Pathfinder network was created for the novices and for the experts from this averaged data (Figures 1 and 2).

The networks represent the cognitive relationships between concepts. Links between concepts indicate that the two joined concepts are more closely related to each other than to any other unlinked concept within the network. Concepts are positioned within the network to maximize clarity of the relationships. Relative position within the network is otherwise meaningless. Similarly, length of the link (in this representation) also is meaningless.

The overall pattern of links between the two averaged networks is similar. Pulmonary edema appears as a central point of both networks and each of the spokes contains similar concepts. Several differences are evident, however. Novices place class of drug further from the center (e.g. inotropic agents and diuretics), whereas experts place the class of drug closer to pulmonary edema and the specific drug (e.g. Dobutamine, Lasix) further from the center.

Interestingly, novices do not appear to connect several related concepts. The experts associate tachycardia with dysrhythmia. The novices, however, place the concepts widely apart and appear to conceptualize tachycardia as a heart rate phenomenon, not an electrophysiological concept. This difference may have its basis in undergraduate curriculums in which dysrhythmia interpretation is not included or is covered only briefly.

Another example of a difference in cognitive organization is between the terms fear of death and stay with patient. Experts have these two concepts connected directly. Experts appear to view staying with the patient as an appropriate nursing intervention when a patient is experiencing a fear of dying. Novices have not connected the two concepts. They may either have not connected staying as an indicated intervention or may not have overcome their own discomfort in dealing with a patient's fear of death.

5. Discussion

A qualitative difference in the cognitive organization of clinical knowledge was demonstrated within this sample of nurse clinicians. The technique of eliciting similarity data from nurse clinicians and using the Pathfinder algorithm to transform the data into visual networks was effective in capturing specific differences in cognitive organization of clinical knowledge of novices and experts. This technique has the potential for contributing to efforts to elicit the knowledge embedded in nursing practice directly from the expert.

Figure 1*
Expert Network

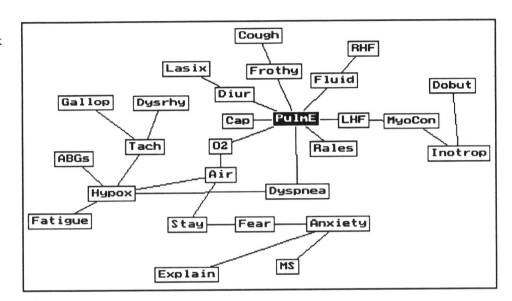

Figure 2*
Novice Network

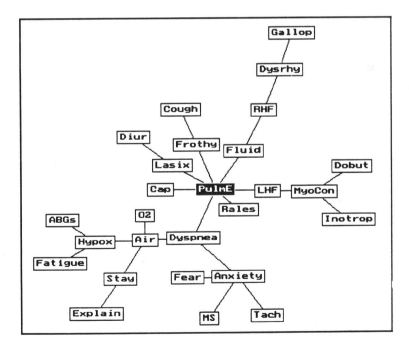

*Abbreviations frequently used for concepts. See Table 1 for list of concepts.

Although the relationship between the networks and actual clinical decision making was not investigated, the two derived networks (Figures 1 and 2) support the belief that experts reason from the abstract to the specific. Categories of medications are more closely related to central concepts than are the specific drugs. In contrast the novices connect first the specific drug and then the abstract drug category to the central concept of pulmonary edema. This is consistent with the work of Adelson [10] who state that experts are more abstract and novices more concrete in their reasoning processes.

Specific relationships demonstrated within the data reveal the knowledge used by expert clinicians in their practice. For example, the importance of staying with a patient is emphasized as a nursing intervention. This concept is connected to both air hunger and fear of dying, two specific patient responses to disease processes. Other links in the vicinity of stay with patient are hypoxia, anxiety and explanations. All concept linkages work at placing this intervention within a patient care situation creating relationships with both nursing and medical approaches. This visual representation is much richer than a statement of multiple if-then rules used to explain expert logic. In addition, this technique does not require the knowledge engineer to prompt the expert for the rules. If the relationships exist, it will be demonstrated. Further dialogue regarding the network(s) can then be used to elicit further expert knowledge.

Cooke and McDonald [7] indicate that Pathfinder networks also might provide an alternative method for directly representing knowledge within the knowledge base of a decision support system. Specific techniques remain to be developed, however. It is hypothesized that incoming data could be used to highlight specific concepts and that related links could be traversed to then highlight the indicated intervention. Graph theory and techniques from neural network development could be used to guide these efforts. Concept selection processes also would have to be modified so that the concepts would be specific enough to aid in decision making.

The Pathfinder algorithm has provided a new methodology for the examination of the cognitive organization of expert knowledge. Pathfinder networks have the ability to differentiate novice and expert thinking and may be useful for automating the process of clinical decision support.

[1] Thompson CB, Ryan SA, and Kitzman H. Expertise: The Basis for Expert System Development. *ANS Adv Nurs Sci* 1990, 12(2):1-10.

[2] Benner P, Tanner C, and Chesla C. From Beginner to Expert: Gaining a Differentiated Clinical World in Critical Care Nursing. *ANS Adv Nurs Sci* 1992, 14(3): 13-28.

[3] Newel A., and Simon H. *Human Problem Solving*. Englewood Cliffs, N. J.: Prentice-Hall, 1972.

[4] Corcoran SA. Planning by Expert and Novice Nurses in Cases of Varying Complexity, *Res Nurs Health* 1986, 9:155-162.

[5] Schvaneveldt RW, Durso F T, Goldsmith TE, Breen TJ, Cooke NM, Tucker RG, and De Maio JC. Measuring the Structure of Expertise. *Int J of Man-Mach Stud* 1985, 23: 699-728.

[6] Bradley JH. The Representation of Cognitive Structure in Expertise. (Doctoral dissertation, University of Texas at Arlington, 1990). Dissertation Abstracts International 1991.

[7] Cooke NM and McDonald JE. A Formal Methodology for Acquiring and Representing Expert Knowledge. *Proceedings of the Institute of Electrical and Electronics Engineers* 1986, 74:1422-1430.

[8] Goldsmith TE, Johnson PJ, and Acton WH. Assessing structural knowledge. *J Educ Psyc* 1991, 83:88-96.

[9] Thompson CB, Ryan SA, and Ingersoll G. Novice Expert Cognitive Differences (Under review).

[10] Adelson B. Problem Solving and the Development of Abstract Categories in Programming Languages. *Mem Cognit* 1981, 9:422-433.

Nursing Informatics: An International Overview for Nursing in a Technological Era
S.J. Grobe and E.S.P. Pluyter-Wenting, eds.

The Nature of Nursing Expertise

Fisher A A [a] and Fonteyn M E [b]

a, b School of Nursing, University of San Francisco, 2130 Fulton St., San Francisco, CA 94117-1080, USA.

Recent studies of nurse experts have begun to provide insights for the development of decision support systems. In this study, exploring the nature of nursing expertise using a triangulated method we identified four salient aspects of expert practice. These findings represent our analysis of a portion of the data collected from an on going study exploring expert critical care nurses' reasoning within and outside their domain knowledge and the patient outcomes associated with their reasoning strategies. We believe that an understanding of the nature of expert nurses' practice would be useful in the development of information systems that could assist administrators in decision making regarding staffing, patient assignments, and staff development needs.

1. Research Objectives

Interest in the practice of experts has a substantial history.[1-6] Studies of nurse experts have given us insight into how they reason to make judgments about patient care, and recently have begun to provide information useful in the development of decision support systems.[7-10] One potential use of these systems is to assist nurses' in their decision making with increasingly complex patient problems.

In addition to supporting the practice of nursing and the delivery of nursing care, decision support systems may be useful to administrators who have to balance such factors as cost effectiveness, job satisfaction, quality nursing care, and positive patient outcomes. Typically, systems utilized for administrative decision making include such indicators as census, budget, staff levels, patient acuity, and patient and physician service.[11] Jennings and Meleis[12] indicate that the generation of knowledge useful to nurse administrators requires a common ground between clinician and administrator, and that knowledge development which considers the patient, the nurse, the environment, and their interrelationship would assist in administrative decision making. Our study provides an initial understanding of the nature of nursing expertise with potential utility both for practitioners and administrators.

2. Setting and Sample

We conducted this study at a 600-bed tertiary care medical center in the Western United States on two intensive care units with distinctively different postoperative patient populations: a neurosurgical care unit and a cardiovascular care unit. The nursing staff on each of these individual units possess extensive (domain-specific) knowledge about the cases treated there and their clinical management.

Our sample consisted of three registered nurses who volunteered to be in our study after being identified by both the nurse manager and their peers as expert (in terms of their knowledge and experience) on their nursing unit. One subject had been identified as being able to function as expert on both the cardiovascular surgery and the neurosurgery

Acknowledgements

This study was partially funded by the Beta Gamma Chapter of Sigma Theta Tau International and the Faculty Development Fund of the University of San Francisco, School of Nursing.

unit (S1); a second subject was identified as expert on the neurosurgery unit (S2); and a third subject was identified as expert on the cardiovascular unit (S3). This sample size was adequate for our study, because our primary goal was to examine in detail the reasoning strategies and processes of individuals not to generalize across subjects.

3. Data Collection

We used a triangulated method, including think aloud technique, participant observation, and in-depth interviews that was tested in an earlier pilot study. Combining collection of verbal protocol data at the bedside while care was being given with a field research approach that sought to understand the complexity of the clinical environment and the routine and problematic aspects of clinical practice, provided a richer and more detailed understanding of expert nursing practice than could have been obtained using simulation outside the clinical setting.

After obtaining informed consent, we collected data from subjects during their nursing shifts when they were providing immediate post operative care for patients within their area of expertise and during shifts when they floated to the other intensive care unit, where they provided immediate post operative care for patients outside their area of expertise. S1, although currently working on the cardiovascular unit caring for open heart surgery patients, has had almost equal experience on both units and is considered by her peers and the nursing manager to be expert on both units. We studied her while caring for open heart surgery patients on the cardiovascular unit and then while caring for craniotomy patients on the neurosurgical unit. Her unique range of experience and domain knowledge allowed us to make comparisons in the nature of expert practice both within and across study subjects. We studied S2, who routinely works on the neurosurgical unit, first while caring for craniotomy patients on the neurosurgical unit, and then while caring for open heart surgery patients on the cardiovascular unit. Finally, we studied S3, who routinely works on the cardiovascular unit caring for open heart surgery patients, first while caring for these patients, and then when she floated to the neurosurgical unit, where she cared for craniotomy patients.

We conducted a pilot study to test the use of think aloud method in the practice setting and demonstrated that it was both logistically possible and safe to study nurses' clinical reasoning in the clinical setting while care was being given. Subsequent to our pilot study, we continued with our full investigation incorporating the three data collection techniques described below.

<u>Think aloud technique</u>. During data collection in the clinical setting, subjects carried a small portable tape recorder in their pocket, and wore a voice-activated microphone on their lapel. We prompted them to "think aloud" while they were reasoning and making decisions about their patient's care. These taped verbalizations were transcribed and subsequently analyzed, using a type of protocol analysis described by Fonteyn, Kuipers and Grobe.[14]

<u>Participant observation</u>. During data collection sessions, we took field notes regarding our subjects' patient care activities. At intervals, when subjects were not thinking aloud, we asked them questions that helped us clarify their reasoning strategies and to understand their actions. We asked subjects to identify their goals [expected outcomes] for patient care, and the data [outcome indicators] they were using to assess progress toward meeting these goals. These verbal interactions were also tape-recorded, transcribed, and later analyzed using dimensional analysis that has been described by Schatzman[15] and Fisher.[16]

<u>In-Depth interviews</u>. We conducted in-depth interviews with each subject at scheduled times outside the work environment. We asked questions designed to identify the dimensions and range of each subjects' expert nursing practice, to determine how they had acquired, enhanced, and maintained their knowledge and reasoning skills, and to substantiate and verify findings that we had obtained during the think aloud and participant observation data collection sessions. The guided interviews were tape recorded and subsequently transcribed and analyzed using dimensional analysis.

We used dimensional analysis, a variant of grounded theory methodology, to analyze the qualitative data from the in-depth interviews for the current investigation. It provides the analytic logic and plausibility to the interpretation of complex qualitative data. A brief account of the analytic operations follows. Data are coded using line-by-line analysis. This early analysis yields a list of codes as dimensions. Each code is further dimensionalized or subdimensionalized. Preliminary dimensions and considerations, initially identified without regard for their significance later become a complex framework of considerations. Ultimately, dimensional analysis allows the investigator to frame a narrative utilizing an explanatory matrix. The matrix lets the researcher check the data for plausibility and consistency in relation to context, conditions, and consequences.

The results that follow represent an early stage in this analytic process. Initial codes as dimensions have been identified through line by line analysis of the in-depth interview data. As these were subdimensionalized and speculative relationships among them identified, we reviewed them with our subjects to clarify, confirm, or correct the emerging scheme.

4. Results and Discussion

To date, four salient dimensions (aspects of expertise) related to the nature of nursing expertise have emerged from the analysis of our data: *knowing, familiarity, flexibility,* and *balancing*. Tentative definitions of each dimension with examples from the transcripts follow.

We defined *knowing* as: **the understanding of all the salient aspects of a particular clinical situation that is associated with expert reasoning and optimal patient outcomes.** *Knowing* seems to reflect both formal knowledge (resulting from educational programs) and informal knowledge (gained through experience with similar patient cases). From subjects' transcripts, we identified several types of *knowing*: the patient; the case type; the technology; the physiology; the setting; the medications and drips; and the resources. The following are three examples of *knowing the patient* from subject's transcripts:

It's good to know the patient...[because you are] trying to organize physical therapy,
occupational therapy, and trying to wean him and not tire him. S2
...it's telling when things are starting to go sour, like having a patient code...you can
see it coming, and you can start to intervene. S3
I just need to stay with my patient (versus running here and there) [when the patient's condition deteriorates] and push the drugs...I want to be there, I know what drugs the patient's getting and what I'm giving. I want to palpate their pulse, keep the air-way open. I know what's been happening with him all day. I'd want someone else to mix drugs for me, hand me drugs, do compressions, get the defibrillator. S3

These examples reinforce the centrality of knowledge to the practice of nurse experts. Our findings have significant implications for administrative decisions related to staff development and quality of care issues. They suggest that: nurses required to work outside their area of expertise and without adequate supervision (because of floating or per-diem assignments), may contribute to poor patient outcomes, unless these nurses are first provided with the necessary knowledge needed to function in the new clinical area.

We defined *familiarity* as: **the consequence of intimate knowledge of and comfort with the technology, setting, and case type within a specific clinical context.** In the following example, one of our nurse experts discussed *familiarity* with case types and associated treatment protocols:

I can look at the orders here in the cardiovascular unit and *you know, recognize automatically three things that might be omitted. Whereas, I wouldn't know over there [on the neurosurgery unit] with a new craniotomy.* S1

In the data that follows, S2 discussed how familiarity with the setting contributed to her ease in practice.

... The other thing that makes it easier for me [to practice], I know a lot of those
people, I've been here a long time.

In contrast, S2 discussed her lack of familiarity when she floated outside her area of expertise:

I just don't know where things are and my arms are outstretched when I go over there.
It seems to take longer for me to do things because I don't know where things are or I'm unfamiliar with the equipment.

These findings suggest the important role of familiarity in the practice of nurse experts, which has potential ramifications for administrative decisions regarding assigning nursing personnel to units with case types outside their range of expertise. Since it appears that familiarity with case type is a factor in expert practice, the variety of case types located within one intensive care unit may also have an impact on the ability of nurses to deliver consistently excellent care to patients. Administrators may need to consider the mix of nurses on those units where there is variability in case types, to ensure that an adequate number of experts with each type of case are available to both care for patients and to educate the other nurses about patient care outside their area of expertise.

The final two dimensions that we have identified are *flexibility* and *balancing*, both of which assist nurses in managing their multifaceted work. We defined *flexibility* as: **the ability to adapt and adjust to clinical circumstances.** One of our expert subjects indicated that, having *flexibility* allows her to take risks in her work and to define each clinical situation as manageable:

If you're flexible in your mind, I don't know any situation that has to be fearful. S1

Another subject indicated that unit work conditions created a need to be flexible:

...with the budget cuts, you just need to be more flexible. Sometimes you'll have four patients a day, and that's a lot. Some people are still trying to do everything. S3

We defined our final dimension, *balancing*, as **the capacity to manage competing demands and data in a complex, risky clinical situation.** An example of *balancing* competing demands follows:

He [the patient] just went to CT scan two days ago I don't understand why you two
[physicians] can't coordinate the care for this patient. You put him at risk every time
you move him with all his lines and traction. S2

Here our subject was trying to get the MD to balance the risk of moving the patient to a scan with the need [demand] for further diagnosis. She was aware that the patient was recently moved for a similar procedure, and thus she questions the need to do so again. The same subject provides us with an example of balancing data:

They [MDs] look at the flow sheet and everything looks good and I look at the patient
and he doesn't look good. He's kind of clammy; he's not real alert; and he seems real
fatigued; and I know what is going on. S2

In the above example our subject stresses the importance of balancing a variety of available competing data. Each of our experts suggest that while the technology reveals valuable data, it only serves to provide a slice of what must be looked at in light of all that is available. In this case, how the patient looked, felt, and responded told the nurse a different story than could be obtained from just a review of the flow sheet. Since nurses have the advantage of being with patients for longer stretches of time than the physicians, their input is invaluable in assisting physicians to balance clinical data with physical assessment data. Knowing this, administrators can take steps to promote this type of interdisciplinary sharing of patient information in order to ensure the best possible patient outcomes.

5. Summary and Conclusion

In this study, we used a triangulated method to identify and describe aspects of expertise. Our preliminary analysis yielded four salient features of expertise *knowledge, familiarity, flexibility, and balancing.*

Our findings would be useful in developing decision support systems to assist nursing administrators in decision making regarding staffing, patient assignment, and staff development needs. Additionally, an understanding of the nature of nursing expertise (generated from studies such as this one) has implications for administrative decisions at the organizational level. It is thus essential that investigators continue to examine expert nursing practice so as to describe the nature of nursing expertise with sufficient detail to allow both improvement in nursing practice and enhancement in the decisions nurse administrators must make regarding practice.

References

[1] Corcoran SA. Task complexity and nursing expertise as factors in decision making. *Nurs Res* 1986a, 35:107-112.

[2] Corcoran SA. Planning by expert and novice nurses in cases of varying complexity. *Res Nurs Health* 1986b, 9:155-162.

[3] Benner P. *From Novice to Expert.* Menlo Park: Addison-Wesley, 1984.

[4] Benner P, Tanner C and Chesla C. From beginner to expert: Gaining a differentiated clinical world in critical care nursing. *Adv Nurs Sci* 1992, 14:13-28.

[5] Fonteyn M. Clinical reasoning in critical care nursing. *Focus on Crit Care* 1991,18:322-327.

[6] Chi M, Glaser R and Farr M. *The nature of expertise.* New Jersey: Lawrence Erlbaum Associates, 1988.

[7] Thompson CB, Ryan SA and Kitzman H. Expertise: The basis for expert system development. *Adv Nurs Sci* 1990, 13:1-10.

[8] Fonteyn M, Grobe S. Expert nurses' clinical reasoning under uncertainty: Representation, structure, and process. *Proceedings of the sixteenth annual symposium on computer applications in medical care.* Los Alimitos, CA: IEEE, Computer Society Press, 1992.

[9] Graves J, Corcoran S. The study of nursing informatics. *Image: J Nurs Scholar* 1989, 4:227-231.

[10] Woolery L. Expert nurses and expert systems. *Computers in Nurs* 1990, 8:23-27.

[11] Simpson RL. The executive information system's basic eight. *Nurs Manage* 1993, 24:32-33.

[12] Jennings B, Meleis A. Nursing theory and administrative practice: Agenda for the 1990"s. *Adv Nurs Sci* 1988, 10:56-69.

[13] Fonteyn M, Grobe S and Kuipers B. A descriptive analysis of expert critical care nurses' clinical reasoning. In: *Nursing Informatics '91*. Hovenga E, Hannah K (eds). Holland: Springer-Verlag. 1991: 765-768.

[14] Fonteyn M, Kuipers B and Grobe S. A description of the use of think aloud method and protocol analysis. *Qual Health Res* 3(4), 430-441.

[15] Schatzman L. Dimensional analysis: Notes on an alternative approach to the grounding of theory. In: *Social organization and social process,* Maines D (ed). New York: Aldine de Gruyter, 1991: 303-314.

[16] Fisher A. Dimensional analysis as a vehicle for the study of dangerousness. Unpublished paper presented at the Western Society for Research in Nursing Annual Conference in Seattle, WA. April 20, 1993.

Nursing Informatics: An International Overview for Nursing in a Technological Era
S.J. Grobe and E.S.P. Pluyter-Wenting, eds.

336

Facing the Challenges of Nurse Expert Systems of the Future

Hendrickson MH and Paganelli B[a]

[a]Clinical Information Systems, Hewlett-Packard Company, 3000 Minuteman Road, Andover, MA 01810

Nurse Expert Systems can significantly impact nursing practice and potentially improve the quality of patient care [1]. However, these benefits cannot be realized until such systems are fully utilized. Remaining in the prototype state, many are highly specialized, stand-alone, and poorly adaptable, discouraging their full use. Developing an expert system that exceeds the prototype stage and expands into daily nursing practice is a challenge for the future. Such systems should be adaptable, easy-to-use, fast, and intuitive. In addition, they should electronically link their information source to their output consumer and provide override safety mechanisms. FLEXPERT is a prototype to demonstrate integration into a nursing documentation system and adaptability through configuration tools. Linking nursing diagnoses to symptoms, the expert system algorithm generates a list of suggested diagnoses. Evaluated by nurse experts, the system was found to be valid and easy-to-use, indicating readiness for the next step. Future plans includes additional clinical trails and possible incorporation of FLEXPERT concepts and algorithm into a currently available bedside information system.

1.0 Introduction

One of the most promising areas of nursing informatics is nurse expert systems. Many articles describe the application of expert system technology to a wide variety of clinical areas [2,3,4,5,6,7]. However, many nurse expert systems remain at the prototype stage, not yet reaching full integration into nursing practice. Although many obstacles face these systems, one main challenge for the future is incorporation into daily nursing practice.

An expert system uses procedures and techniques from artificial intelligence in combination with inference techniques and expert knowledge to analyze and potentially resolve problems [2]. Such systems in nursing promise many benefits. Clinical decision making can be enhanced in a wide variety of areas [1,5,7]. Expert systems can expand the abilities of inexperienced nurses or the nurses functioning outside of their area of expertise to assess, plan, implement, and evaluate patient care [1,5,7]. Identifying the unique needs and problems of patients, these systems assist the nurse to individualize care and prevent critical omissions [1]. Documentation resulting from such systems can be more complete and accurate, potentially improving communication amoung nurses. The time savings that such systems can potentially offer can be used for other critical tasks [1].

2.0 Examples of Current Expert Systems

The nursing literature describes many nurse expert systems. PACE, formerly known as COMMES (Creigton ON-Line Multiple Medical Expert System), addresses both the educational needs of nurses and the assessment and planning of nursing care [3]. Another system, CANDI (Computer Aided Nursing Diagnosis and Intervention), is written in LISP for use on a personal computer (PC) and generates nursing diagnoses from assessment data [4]. CAREPLAN, also PC based, is used for planning care for low-risk postpartum patients [5]. UNIS (Urological

Nursing Information System) is written using the expert system tool, NEXPERT OBJECT, to assist in planning the care of long-term patients with urinary incontinence [6].

These nurse expert systems have shown that nurse expertise can be collected and expressed in computer algorithms. However, system problems have impeded widespread use by nurses. Stand-alone expert systems cannot be integrated with nursing documentation systems and require redundant data entry. In addition, the cost of maintaining highly specialized expert systems may outweigh their benefits. Even maintaining more generalized systems can be difficult. Some systems necessitate programmer intervention for rule updates, costing time and money. The severe complexity and large number of rules of other systems also make impair maintenance. Some systems like PACE include literature references, requiring frequent updating as new literature is published [3]. These problems have impaired widespread use of nurse expert systems.

3.0 Expert System Requirements

To promote extensive use, nurse expert systems must meet at least seven key requirements: integration, adequate performance, ease of use, accessibility, promotion of safe use, accuracy, and adaptability. In addition, the system must meet the unique information processing needs of the nursing profession.

An expert system must be functionally and technologically integrated into a documentation system. Without functional integration, redundant data entry is required, costing time and money. Hospitals and nurses expect one point of entry for information [7]. They expect systems to easily lead them from one task to a related task. An integrated nurse expert system connects its information source to its output utilizer. For example, a system that generates nursing diagnoses should automatically use assessment information, generate results, and pass them to the care plan application. Integration should be transparent instead of intentional [7]. Intentional systems must be manually invoked while transparent systems are automatically invoked, thereby requiring less user-computer dialog [7].

For technological integration, an expert system must adapt to the documentation system's technological platform. Health care information systems function on a wide variety of platforms. Some are workstation based; others operate on PC's. Each may use different operating systems. For example, if the information system is an UNIX (tm) based system using Hewlett-Packard risc machines and a client-server model, then the expert system must also be able to function on that platform. The technological platform may dictate the tools available for expert system development. Likewise, the data definition must be consistent between the expert and documentation systems to allow communication. Consistent data dictionaries are becoming more of a reality as the standardization of nursing clinical data and development of the nursing minimum data set continues. Standardization of nursing diagnoses by North Atlantic Nursing Diagnosis Association and nursing interventions by the University of Iowa progresses [8]. In addition, both the American Nurses Association and the American Organization of Nurse Executives currently have committees developing minimum data sets [9]. In addition, any data used by the expert system must be coded. The documentation system must support the entry of coded information rather than nondescript text entry.

Nurses expect adequate system performance which is directly related to the power of the computer, the number of rules, and the complexity of the algorithms [7]. Fortunately, the stronger processing power of newly available computer hardware can potentially address the problem of performance. However, performance may still be inadequate for those systems plagued by numerous rules and extreme algorithm complexity. Although a system may have adequate performance, a poorly designed interface can simulate poor performance. Nurses do not have time for lengthy dialogs with the computer. Expert systems should be able to complete their task with minimal interaction, ideally, through a single pass of the patients data.

As with other systems, an expert system should be easy to use and accessible. Appropriate use of color and graphics, a well-designed intuitive user interface, and easy to use input devices such as trackballs, enhances a system's usability. To be accessible, expert systems may need to be available at the patient's bedside, and thus need to be integrated with bedside information systems. Other expert systems are needed at the nurses station and in the nurse manager's office.

An expert system must be sufficiently accurate to be useful. However, high system accuracy may be difficult to obtain. Although nursing knowledge is rapidly expanding, significant gaps remain, affecting accurate system development. In addition, complexity must be carefully balanced with accuracy. A highly accurate expert system may be plagued with numerous rules and a complex algorithm. Although accurate, such a system may not be used because it is difficult to maintain and slow. An expert system that is insufficiently accurate will not be useful. Between accuracy and complexity is the balance that will provide both usefulness and ease of maintenance.

An expert system can only advise; it is not and cannot always be correct [1]. Since high system accuracy cannot always be guaranteed, safety mechanisms must be included to promote appropriate use. One possible safety feature requires nurses to consciously approve the result of the nurse expert system. Another feature always permits the nurse to override the system's suggestions.

Perhaps, the most critical requirement is adaptability [7]. The rules must be easily updated to reflect changes in the nursing knowledge base. The ease of updating depends on the updating method and the complexity of the rules and algorithm. The ideal expert system provides easy to use configuration tools for nurses to add, change, and remove rules. An adaptable expert system also has minimal rules to maintain. The algorithm permits the rules to be expressed in an easy to understand format and does not require extensive rule interconnection. Although a system is adaptable, it does not guarantee validity. Significant effort through nursing research is often required to develop expert system rules.

The last requirement is meeting the unique informational processing needs of the nursing profession. An expert system designed for one profession cannot necessarily be used for another simply by changing rules. For example, a medical expert system generating medical diagnoses generally attempts to narrow down the output to one diagnosis. Whereas, nurses need an expert system which generates multiple nursing diagnoses. In addition, clinical reasoning can vary from profession to profession. An expert system must take into consideration the methods by which nurse experts reach their conclusions. The nursing profession has the responsibility of describing input and output requirements for a nursing expert system and providing the research describing nurses' clinical reasoning.

4.0 FLEXPERT

FLEXPERT is a prototype information system that meets some of the previously mentioned requirements. FLEXPERT address the key requirements of integration and adaptability through configuration tools. FLEXPERT also met other requirements such as easy to use and promoting safe use.

Written in DBase III, FLEXPERT was designed for use on a IBM personal computer. DBase III was selected for its relational database capabilities, programming abilities, user-interface features, and report capabilities. The relational database stores the expert system rules and clinical content. The forward chaining inference engine was written in the DBase III programming language using a quasi bayesiam approach. The bayesiam approach is an artificial intelligence method combining if-then rules and probabilities to reach conclusions [10]. The user-interface features support screen design for data entry and navigation. The author filled the roles of programmer, knowledge engineer, and nurse expert. Additional clinical content and nurse expertise was obtained from textbooks. The prototype focused on general medical-surgical patients, although any patient population type could have been selected. FLEXPERT contains three key components, the nurse care plan information system, the expert system algorithm, and the configuration tool.

4.1 Nurse Care Plan Information System

The nurse care plan information system permits the nurse to follow the nursing process from the collection of assessment data to the printing out of the initial nurse care plan. First, the nurse is asked to enter the patient's name, medical diagnosis, their name and title, and the current date. Next, the nurse is asked to select the patient's signs and symptoms from a list categorized by functional health patterns and body systems. After the nurse enters the assessment data, the system presents a prioritized list of suggested nursing diagnoses based upon the assessment data. The nurse then either selects one from the suggested list or can chose to override the expert system by selecting from the full list of nursing diagnoses. After the nurse makes a selection, the system asks for the etiologies. Next, the nurse enters outcomes for the problem, including target dates, and possible outcome criteria. After this, the nurse selects interventions from a list of anticipated interventions. For each intervention, the nurse enters frequency and possible additional instructions. After interventions are completed, the suggested list of diagnoses is displayed again. The nurse selects to add additional problems or to printout the completed care plan. Prior to printing, the nurse is asked to verify patient and own professional information. The care plan is then printed, providing a space for the nurse's legal signature.

4.2 Expert System Algorithm

The FLEXPERT algorithm contains three key parts. The first part assesses the priority value of the diagnosis. Each diagnosis has an associated priority value of 1 to 99. Diagnoses with a priority of 99 are the most critical to address for this population, diagnoses with a priority of 1 are the lowest priority for this population. For example, Lack of Knowledge may not be a priority diagnoses for the critical care patient, but has a high priority for the medical-surgical patient.

The second part of the algorithm contains the primary relationship rules. These rules match a diagnosis with specific signs and symptoms. An example of a primary relation rule is if the patient has this symptom, then they have a 99% chance of having this diagnosis. A diagnosis may have primary relationship to multiple symptoms, or a specific symptom may have a primary relationship to multiple diagnoses.

The third part of the FLEXPERT algorithm consists of secondary relationship rules. these rules also map a particular diagnosis with secondary signs and symptoms. Two other components of secondary relationship rules include the key number of signs and symptoms and the secondary relationship probability. These rules state that if the patient has at least this key number of secondary signs and symptoms, then they have the secondary relationship probability of having this diagnosis.

The algorithm passes over the assessment information twice. During the first pass, each diagnosis is assigned a running score starting with 0. The system examines each patient symptom and checks whether primary relationship rules exists. For each primary relationship rule, the diagnosis is found and the value of diagnosis priority value (multiplied by 99) is added to the diagnosis running score. Once a primary relationship rule is found for a particular diagnosis, the diagnosis is placed on the suggested list and is no longer included in the future searches.

In the second pass, the system searches for any secondary relationship rules that exist for a diagnosis. The system counts how many secondary rules addressed by the patient's symptoms match a specific diagnosis. If the number is equal to or more than the number required, then the value of secondary relationship probability multiplied by diagnosis priority value is added to the diagnosis running score. After all calculations, the list of diagnoses is prioritized by running scores and displayed in the care plan information system.

4.3 Configuration Tool

Nurses use the configuration tool to defined the expert system rules and the care plan content. Nursing diagnoses are added, deleted and revised. When the nurse adds a new diagnosis, the tool displays all other diagnoses and their priority values in sorted order and asks the nurse to assign a priority value for the new diagnosis. Then, the tool asks the nurse to select those symptoms that have a primary relationship with the diagnosis. The nurse cycles through the symptoms list, selecting those with a primary relationship. The tool asks the nurse to select those remaining symptoms that have a secondary relationship to the diagnosis. The nurse again cycles through the symptom list and selects appropriately. The nurse is asked how many of these symptoms must exist to indicate that this diagnosis has at least a 50% probability of being present. The nurse enters the key number and is asked for the exact probability. The configuration tool permits the nurse to change any of these values.

5.0 Evaluation

FLEXPERT was introduced as an initial trial to 5 clinical nurse experts. These experts had on an average of 25 years of nursing experience and were also experts in the area of nursing process and nursing diagnoses. All were nurse educators responsible for teaching nursing process either in the clinical environment and/or in the classroom. Each nurse tried out the system using a patient that they had cared for and completed a confidential questionnaire. The nurses were asked to rank accuracy and ease-of-use of the scale from 1 to 8. Accuracy average was 7.25 and ease-of-use was 6.8. The major complaint was performance, but poor performance was expected because the trial was conducted using a less powerful personal computer than normal.

The next goal is to expand the prototype stage by incorporating the concepts and algorithm demonstrated by FLEXPERT into a real information system. A well-known bedside information system company vision matches well with the concepts that FLEXPERT expresses, including integration and adaptability through configuration tools. FLEXPERT concepts and algorithm integrated with a real system can further meet the requirements of integration, adequate performance, ease of use, accessibility, and adaptability.

6.0 Conclusions

Although many nursing expert systems have been developed, most have not expanded beyond the prototype stage into daily use by nurses. Limitations such as poor performance, lack of integration into documentation systems, and difficult maintenance impair widespread acceptance of such systems. FLEXPERT was developed to address two key requirements of adaptability and integration. FLEXPERT was integrated with a care plan system. In addition, configuration tools were developed to allow nurses to define clinical content and expert system rules. Preliminary evaluations by nurse experts found FLEXPERT to be sufficiently accurate and easy to use. Future goals include additional tests, clinical trails, and possible integration into a currently available bedside information system.

7.0 References

[1] Sinclair V. Potential Effects of Decision Support Systems on the Role of the Nurse *Comput Nurs* March/April 1990: 60-65

[2] Chang B and Hirsch M. Knowledge Acquisition and Knowledge Representation in a Rule Based Expert System. *Comput Nurs* Sept/Oct 1991: 174-178

[3] Evans C. the COMMES Nursing Consultant System in *Decision Support Systems in Nursing*. Ozbolt J, Vandewal D, Hannah K (eds). St. Louis: CV Mosby 1990: 97-120

[4] Chang B, Roth K, Gonzales E, Caswell D, and DiStefano J. CANDI, A Knowledge Based System for Nursing Diagnosis. *Comput Nurs* Jan/Feb 1988: 13-21

[5] Probst C and Rush J. The CarePlan Knowledge Base, a Prototype Expert System for Postpartum Nursing Care. *Comput Nurs* Sept/Oct 1990: 206-213

[6] Petrucci K, Jacox A, McCormick K, Parks P, Kjerulff K, Baldwin B, Petrucci, P. Evaluating the Appropriateness of a Nurse Expert System's Patient Assessment. *Comput Nurs* Nov/Dec 1992: 243-249

[7] Brennan P. Decision Support Systems in Nursing, An Overview. In *Decision Support Systems in Nursing* Ozbolt J, Vandewal D, Hannah K (eds). St. Louis: CV Mosby 1990: 3-14

[8] McCloskey C and Bulecheck G. *Nursing Interventions Classification*. St. Louis: CV Mosby 1990

[9] Simpson R. Hospitals Redesign Demands Open Information Systems. *Nurs Manage* Aug 1993: 32-35

[10] Shapiro S. (ed) *Encyclopedia of Artificial Intelligence*. New York: John Wiley and Sons, 1992

© 1994 Elsevier Science B.V. All rights reserved.
Nursing Informatics: An International Overview for Nursing in a Technological Era
S.J. Grobe and E.S.P. Pluyter-Wenting, eds.

Ambulatory Care Clinician's Expert System: ACCESs

Brazile R.P.[a] and Hettinger B.J.[b]

[a] *Department of Computer Science, University of North Texas, Denton, Texas 76203*
[b] *Hettinger & Brazile, 221 Wellington, Denton, Texas 76201*

ACCESs, an ambulatory care clinician's expert system, was envisioned as a way to assist community health nurses in their daily practice. The facts for the expert system come from a database created by a clinical information system (CIS) designed by Brazile and Hettinger. The CIS, which features multiple problem schemes, group tracking, a longitudinal health care record, and the capability of creating individual portable electronic health care records, has been in use at a nurse-managed pediatric clinic since December, 1991. The database in July, 1993, contained data on several thousand children, primarily medicaid recipients, and about five hundred teen-age mothers. ACCESs features four modules, each designed to assist with a particular aspect of ambulatory care. The modules include 1) 'Well-Baby', health maintenance visit and immunization tracking; 2) Asthma, clinical management for asthma; 3) Case Management, referral tracking; and 4) appointment scheduling. Initial rules for the expert system were derived from published healthcare standards. Subsequent rules will be developed by consensus of the clinicians, thus capturing the unique expertise of the community health nurse.

1. Introduction

No data are currently available to summarize the number of persons who have received all appropriate health screening and immunization services [1]. The immunization of the population under age two is seen as a critical health need, and bills to establish a nationwide immunization tracking system were introduced into Congress in the spring of 1993 [2]. Health screening and immunizations are two services usually provided in ambulatory care settings by nurses, but nurses often lack the necessary computer services to assist them in their daily practice [3]. Lancaster [4] points out that "clinical information systems have not yet been able to effectively help clinicians absorb and interpret information so that they can make good clinical decisions" (p 3). If available, the use of an expert system in daily nursing practice would allow immediate feedback into practice of the knowledge gained by the use of the system, thus becoming a "springboard" to nursing science [5]. Clayton [6] identified the major challenge of building envisioned systems in the real world environment. "We can't easily show the benefit ... until our best visions are implemented."

An expert system, ACCESs, was created to assist community health nurses, and to focus in particular on pediatric aspects of ambulatory health care. Initially, a clinical information system (CIS) for data collection and storage had been developed based on a database design by Hettinger and Brazile [7]. The CIS features a longitudinal health care record, the use of multiple problem classification schemes, including NANDA, ICD-9, and the Omaha System [8], and facilitates retrieval of the Nursing Minimum Data Set [9]. The CIS has been in use at a nurse-managed pediatric clinic since December, 1991. The database in 1993 contained data on several thousand children, primarily medicaid recipients, and about five-hundred teen-age mothers. The pediatric nurse practitioners and clinic staff needed rapid access to information stored in the database, and a way transform the data into usable information to assist them in daily care management. In addition, the clinicians needed a system that could help monitor high risk clients.

An expert system that used the CIS database, and included rules concerning standard pediatric health maintenance and immunization routines was developed. However, standard rules have exceptions that may not be documented, and the expert practitioner has methods of handling those exceptions. These exception handling techniques will need to be added to the rulebase as they are identified and verified by clinicians. A modular design and implementation process that would allow the expert system to evolve in a busy clinic setting was chosen. The purpose of this paper is to describe the features desired in the expert system, and the first four modules, each designed to assist with a particular aspect of ambulatory care.

The modules include 1) 'Well-Baby', health maintenance visit and immunization tracking; 2) Asthma, a clinical module; 3) Case Management, for referral tracking; and 4) an appointment scheduler based on the recommended number and timing of pediatric health maintenance visits. Initial rules for the expert system were derived from published healthcare standards. Subsequent rules will be developed by consensus of the clinicians, thus capturing the unique expertise of the community health nurse.

2. Desirable features of an Expert System.

2.1 Incorporates existing classification systems

An expert system requires that nursing knowledge be organized and codified to allow accurate and efficient use of that knowledge. Much work has already been devoted to the development of classification systems, thus any new expert system should draw on that cumulative expertise [10]. Translating the information gathered by the nursing process into codes is the most precise and efficient way to represent that information, both for storage of the information and use of the information by the expert system. However, since there are many coding schemes, the system must be prepared to accept and make decisions based on any of the existing classification systems. A unique feature of the CIS that is used to enter data into the database is its ability to incorporate multiple classification systems. In this manner, the practicing nurse is not forced to choose from just one model.

2.2 Uses single concept input, multiple output documentation

A relational database allows one-time entry of data. To further assist the health care provider, a system should preform some of the required data entry for clinical visits with a single prompt.

2.3 Represents data in patterns for intellectual synthesis

Once data is stored at a detail level, it can be aggregated in many different ways; by looking at the same data organized and presented in new forms, new insights may begin to emerge. One of the most valuable capabilities of the computer is its ability to give feedback in a form entirely different from the data entry sheet.

2.4 Provides a means of analyzing practice

It is important for us to realize that at this stage of development of expert systems for community health, nurses may not be able to articulate the type of information processing that would assist them in achieving improved outcomes for their clients. It is sometimes difficult to imagine the potential of an expert system without seeing some concrete examples. The system under construction implements re-presentations of data, merged with practice 'rules', to elicit feedback. These examples are expected to stimulate ideas about other helpful features. In addition, the built-in coding will allow abstraction of data for comparison with other data sets.

2.5 Provides for growth

To allow the expert system the greatest flexibility for future enhancements, a modular approach to the design has been adopted. This technique allows the system to be implemented in steps, gathering feedback on each module and applying lessons learned to implement additional modules. This evolutionary technique to building the expert system has been proven to be a very effective technique for producing useful software systems [11].

2.6 Utilizes known techniques

There is recognition that common patterns of reasoning and knowledge representation transverse disciplines [12], and thus information regarding the structure and process of the knowledge is known. What is still needed is the specific unique knowledge possessed by practicing nurse experts. A description of the unique knowledge, both factual and heuristic, of community health nurses is especially needed. A modular approach to system design would capitalize on the phenomena of clinical expertise in specific selected conditions by allowing real-world nurses the opportunity to 'fine tune' a module representing their specialty.

2.7 Have a reality-based orientation

Grobe [13] proposes both classification and natural language methods be used to understand nursing practice. Language linked to classification allows subsequent retrieval for determination of equivalency between terms. A unique feature of the CIS allows inclusion of a user's own terminology to describe practice, paired with an expert system that allows the user to insert new 'rules' into the expert system's rulebase. Decisions made by the nurse, as represented retrospectively by the problem classification, interventions, and comments documented on the electronic healthcare record, will assist us in understanding the real world of nursing practice, and its relationship to formal nursing language.

3. The Expert System

3.1 ACCESs

'ACCESs', Ambulatory Care Clinician's Expert System, is an expert system incorporating the desired features. The prototype system was tailored to the needs of pediatric nurse practitioners in an ambulatory care clinic. The system design is modular, with implementation accomplished one module at a time. Three clinical modules were planned and a scheduling module was also included to support the clinical practice requirements.

3.2 Scheduling Module

An appointment scheduling module based on recommended number and timing of health maintenance visits was incorporated to assist in making appropriate appointments for well-child care. The expert scheduler uses the agency and provider files in the clinical database as the source of data regarding clinic hours and provider availability. These files can be updated by the system administrator. In addition, the user will be able to insert rules regarding a particular client into the rule base, for example, *IF CLIENT ID = n THEN SCHEDULE EVERY 30 DAYS* to override the standard health maintenance timing rules. The clinician can access the scheduler while remaining logged into the CIS. The scheduler can include visits to the social worker, nutritionist, or health educator as well as the nurse practitioner; all providers use the same longitudinal health care record. A family code links all family members and allows the practitioner to coordinate sibling visits and parent education time. Illness visits are also incorporated into the system, providing a comprehensive view of the clinical caseload at any one time.

Data that can be analyzed for the practitioner include the effect of appointment status (completed visits, cancellations) and illness episodes on the child's health maintenance program. By predicting events and comparing them to the actual database, the system will assist the practitioner to assess risk of non-completion of the health maintenance program, and to identify successful intervention strategies. The system can demonstrate the distribution of individual practitioner time if all children in the case load were to receive timely, comprehensive Well-Child care. The system can also provide managers with the number of staff required to give care to all the children registered at the clinic.

3.3 WELL-BABY Module

The term *WELL-BABY* was selected to indicate a health maintenance module with an initial focus on the population of healthy children age two years and under. The expert system WELL-BABY module was designed to assist the clinician to make decisions concerning:

1. do the children in my case load have all the recommended preventive health care?

2. if not, what are the steps necessary to remedy that situation?

To develop this section, it was necessary to define 'recommended preventive health care', determine what had already been done, what was still needed, decide when the uncompleted events were to be administered or accomplished, by whom, and if an exception to the basic rules existed. The critical pathway for children's health maintenance is based upon completion of all health maintenance visits at scheduled intervals. The system uses six expected health maintenance visits during the first year of life. These visits are timed to coincide with recommended immunization schedules, including requirements for Hepatitis B immunizations for infants [14]. The rules used to decide which actions are necessary were derived from the published standards, with each immunization requirement placed into the rulebase as one or more statements of the form *if condition then action.* For example, a typical rule would be *IF BABY IS AT LEAST 60 DAYS OLD AND BABY DOES NOT HAVE FIRST DPT, THEN BABY IS NOT IN COMPLIANCE WITH RECOMMENDED HEALTH CARE.* The baby's age and immunization records will be in the clinical data base. The expert system checks the database, and if all recommended preventive health care has been performed on time, no other activity is generated from this section. In the event that the client does not meet the criteria, the system sends a screen message to the clinician that the client does not meet all requirements for age, and identifies the missing data. The system will create a suggested next appointment with the client's primary provider, using a series of rules beginning with *IF BABY IS NOT IN COMPLIANCE WITH RECOMMENDED HEALTH CARE THEN SCHEDULE BABY FOR WELL-BABY VISIT.* If the client's primary provider is unavailable within an acceptable time frame, the system selects the first available appointment, and identifies the provider who would see the client. The clinician can then accept or reject the appointment, ask for a second choice of date or time, or type in a desired date and time and see if it is available. The 'Group' function of the system allows the practitioner to make queries about groups of clients, for example, a group of infants born in one time period. Managers can benefit by the systems ability to predict the number of clock hours needed to provide care for the registered clients.

3.4   Asthma Module

The second module will address the monitoring and treatment of problems identified either by the practitioner or by the system. The prototype exemplar selected is asthma, and asthma related conditions. The problem was selected to illustrate the usefulness of the system to practitioners managing children with a high risk condition. The CIS provides for clinical tracking of any group of clients. A 'group' is constructed by entering a client identification number, and the group name chosen. The expert system module can then access records of children in the 'ASTHMA' group, thus limiting the database search and shortening response time. The system uses Guidelines for the Diagnosis and Management of Asthma as a guide [16]. Again, rules were developed one at a time from the published guidelines by entering statements as facts. The practitioner will be able to ascertain which clients with asthma have had all the recommended asthma counseling/education activities, in addition to routine well-baby immunization and health maintenance activities. The return-to-clinic timeframe for a particular child, or medication 'alerts' are two examples of 'rules' that could be entered into the expert system rulebase by the clinician, if desired. When a clinician inserts 'asthma' or 'asthma-related problem' into any clinical record, the expert system checks to see if the client has been entered into the 'ASTHMA' group; if the client is not found in the 'ASTHMA' group, the system queries the user about adding this client to the ASTHMA group.

3.5   Case Management Module

Coordinating the care of the client in the community remains a challenge. The third module, termed 'Case Management', will focus on interactive aspects of care coordination, such as referrals to and from other providers and other agencies. It includes the use of an electronic patient care record carried by the client, for communication between providers. The use of a 3 1/2 " floppy disk to contain the record is currently being piloted [16].

3.6   The Expert System Platform

Software considerations for the expert system implementation were important. The selection criteria included reasonable cost, ability to access facts from the clinical database, and ease of constructing rules. For the prototype expert system the cost and database access criteria were critical. The first version of the prototype was written using the C programming language. This version satisfied the reasonable cost goal, but not the database access goal. A C language interface to the database is not supported by the vendor and thus would have required more development time to create that interface. The prototype was therefore re-constructed using CLARION, the language of the database system which holds the clinical database. This satisfied the cost and database access goals, but constructing rules for the expert system was not feasible for the user (health care provider) of the system. An expert system needs to have a rule base that can be modified, preferably by the user, as changes occur in clinical practice. Two possible solutions were studied; 1) rules embedded into the clinical database as data, and 2) converting to an expert system shell which had a user-friendly interface. Solution 1, which required no new software, was chosen, and the system design modified to its present form.

4. Conclusion and Future work.

The expert system prototype ACCESs is currently installed at a nurse-managed pediatric clinic, and development is continuing on the modules described in this paper. These initial modules are providing the nurse practitioners with a system that can provide daily assistance in monitoring health maintenance visits, immunizations, and selected health problems of groups of clients. Future work includes continuing knowledge acquisition from community health nurse experts. Verification of the system, that is, validating that the system comes to the same conclusion that a nurse expert would, will continue.

The long-term effect of technology and information sciences on clinical practice may have consequences currently unknown. When practitioners have the opportunity to study patterns of data retrieved from their daily caseload, it will increase their awareness of intervention effectiveness and may enable them to redirect their energy more productively. It is important that prototype systems be reality based and have this introspective capability built-in. Capturing daily practice is a necessary precursor to strengthen nursing science.

5. References

[1] Healthy Texans 2000. Austin, TX. TX Dept Health. stock no 4-156, 1991.

[2] deVries C. Update on Immunization Proposals in Congress. *The American Nurse.* May 93, 25:5, 22.

[3] Leske, JS and Werley HH. Use of the Nurs Minimum Data Set. *Comput Nurs.* Nov/Dec, 1992; 10:6, 259-263.

[4] Lancaster L. Nursing Information Systems in the Year 2000: Another Perspective. *Comput Nurs.* Jan/Feb 1993; 11:1, 3-5.

[5] Ozbolt JG, Schultz S, Swain MA, Abraham IL. A Proposed Expert System for Nurs Practice: A Springboard to Nurs Science. *J Med Syst.* 1985; 9:12, 57-68.

[6] Clayton PD (ed). Assessing Our Accomplishments. American Medical Informatics Assoc: *Proceedings of the 15th Annual Symposium on Comput Applications in Medical Care (SCAMC).* Washington, DC: Nov 17-20, 1991. McGraw-Hill, 1991: 173-176.

[7] Hettinger BJ and Brazile RP. A Database Design for Community Health Data. *Comput Nurs.* May/June, 1992; 10:3, 109-115.

[8] Martin KS and Scheet ND. *The Omaha System: Applications for Community Health Nursing.* Phil: WB Saunders Co, 1992.

[9] Werley HH and Lang NM, eds. *Identification of the Nursing Minimum Data Set.* NY: Springer, 1988.

[10] McCormick KA. A Unified Nursing Language System. In: *Nursing Informatics: Where Caring and Technology Meet.* Ball MJ, Hannah KJ , Jelger UG, and Peterson H (eds). NY: Springer-Verlag, 1988

[11] Rumbaugh, et al. *Object-Oriented Modeling and Design.* NJ: Prentice-Hall, 1991.

[12] Brachman RJ, Levesque HJ, and Reiter R. Introduction to the Special Volume on Knowledge Representation. *Artificial Intelligence.* 1991; 49, 1-3.

[13] Grobe S. Nursing Intervention Lexicon and Taxonomy Study: Language and Classification Methods. *Adv Nurs Sci.* 1990; 13:2, 22-33.

[14] Poon CY. Pediatric Pharmacology: Childhood Immunization (Part 1). *Journal of Pediatric Health Care.* 1992, 6:6, 370-376.

[15] Guidelines for the Diagnosis and Management of Asthma: National Heart, Lung, and Blood Institute, National Asthma Education Program, Expert Panel Report. *J Allergy Clin Immunol.* Sept 1991; 88:3. Supplement.

[16] Brazile RP and Hettinger BJ. Baby's Electronic Medical Record. Paper/demonstration given at the *11th Annual National Nurs Comput Conference.* Rutgers: NJ,Mar 25, 1993.

Nursing Informatics: An International Overview for Nursing in a Technological Era
S.J. Grobe and E.S.P. Pluyter-Wenting, eds.

Expert system in prenatal care: Validation and implementation

Marin HF[a], Ramos MP[b], Santos LA[b], Ançâo[b] and Sigulem D[b]

[a]Informatics Nursing Group, Escola Paulista de Medicina, São Paulo, Brasil

[b]Informatics Health Center, Escola Paulista de Medicina, São Paulo, Brasil

We developed a system in Prenatal Care field to identify potential obstetric complications and suggest appropriate interventions. The system's knowledge was acquired through interviews with experts in prenatal care and through the review of current literature. It was represented in backward chaining rules stored in seven different categorized files.

1. Introduction

Prenatal Care is currently considered to be the most efficient way to ensure a healthy pregnancy for its emphasis on prevention and early recognition of complications and its treatment [1]. Access to prenatal care must be fairly considered a woman's right, and although in many parts of Brazil this care is available, there are some areas where it is not found, resulting in a higher susceptibility to prenatal and obstetric complications. This failure is most prevalent on underprivileged rural areas, because health professionals are mainly found in the urban centers. Aiming to correct this inequity, we have designed an expert system to assist health care providers [2].

2. Objectives

This expert system performs the following tasks:

a) Identify potential obstetric complications
b) Recognize the risk's degree associated with these complications
c) Calculate patient-specific parameters during prenatal care
d) Suggest appropriate interventions
e) Permit independent access by consultants to the system's database

3. Material and Methods

The system was developed using the Clipper version 5.0 programming language to be run on MS-DOS platforms. The process was done in three steps: Knowledge acquisition; knowledge representation, and validation. The knowledge was acquired through open interviews with 5 (five) experts in prenatal care as well as through the review of current literature in the subject. The knowledge obtained was represented in 700 backward chaining rules stored in seven different categorized files.

The system collects the following data about each patient: Patient identification; personal and family history; obstetric follow-up; maternal weight; subsidiary examinations and procedure's information to calculate the predicted delivery date; current gestational age of the fetus and uterine development. These data are stored in database files.

After all the facts (data) have been entered into the database, backward chaining inference process produces the output regarding obstetric risk and, when appropriate, recommends referral to a specialized center. The system also contains a database that provides information regarding general purposes' services, such as: Immunizations, ultrasound, and nutritional counseling.

In the validation phase we will test the system using 200 prenatal cases of patients that were followed at the Ambulatory Prenatal Care Clinic, and have already gone through delivery. By using such cases, we will be able to compare the results produced by the system with the data about each case.

4. Discussion

In backward chaining inference, the expert system attempts to prove the hypothesis. It follows Harmon and Sawyer's [3] method used to produce the output diagnoses, mainly when there are more inputs than outputs. Those facts inferred by the inference process to prove the hypothesis, are assumed to be true and becomes the output recommendation [4]. Currently, we are on the knowledge base's validation process. The test of the system was initiated in August 1993 by graduate students in nursing who are providing prenatal care to patients at the Ambulatory Prenatal Care Center of the Hospital Amparo Maternal in Sao Paulo, Brazil.

5. Conclusion

There are many papers in the literature regarding prenatal care's importance. Expert systems such as this one, will improve the quality of prenatal care in poor and rural regions. They also will supply information's access to health care providers, allowing them to identify prenatal complications and choose appropriate interventions. By tracking statistics regarding prenatal complications, morbidity and mortality, the impact of the system use will be evaluated.

6. References

[1] Royston E and Armstrong S. *Preventing maternal deaths*. Geneva, World Health Organization, 1989.

[2] Marin HF. *Aquisiçao de Conhecimento e Desenvolvimento de protótipo de sistema Especialista em Assistencia Pré-Natal no atendimento de gestantes normais*. Dissertação de Mestrado. Escola Paulista de Medicina. São Paulo, 1991.

[3] Harmon P and Sawer B. *Creating Expert System for Business and Industry*. New York: John Wiley and Sons, 1990.

[4] Frenzel L. *Understanding expert systems*. Indianapolis, IN: Howard W. Sams, 1987.

Nursing Informatics: An International Overview for Nursing in a Technological Era
S.J. Grobe and E.S.P. Pluyter-Wenting, eds.

Decision Making in Nursing Care Process:
A Systematic Computerization

Zanotti R

International Institute of Nursing Research (ISIRI), Via Udine 6, Padua, Italy.

Expert systems could help nurses in practice settings by supporting decisions underlying nursing processes. A systematic computerization of such decision was implemented by ISIRI, based on matrix-algebra. Matrix-algebra makes possible the processing of amounts of data and it is can be easily used in many programming languages. Thus, matrix-algebra allows the continual upgrading of the internal knowledge with no changes in the shell The first part of the system supporting nursing diagnostic hypotheses is completed and in use in 7 Italian nursing schools. The second part regarding planning and control is in the advanced stage of development.

1. Nurses' decisions in the care process

Nursing practice is based on different and complex activities of caring. These activities are performed in order to help the patient to achieve better health and a higher quality of life. Caring for human beings requires technical knowledge, clinical expertise, and relational skills. Thus, many decisions are made under risk and uncertainty. In the nursing field, risk taking can be viewed as selecting an action, because the consequence of which could leave the patient worse off than if another action had been chosen [1]

A decision can be defined as an irrevocable commitment of resources that results from a deliberative process of examining the elements of a situation, relating the elements in a particular manner, determining the difference between what is and what is not desired, and selecting a strategy to remedy the discrepancy[2]. Decision means autonomy, that is, freedom to make choices that may affect the client's health, the cost of treatment, and amount of resources mobilized, within a legally defined and occupationally-regulated domain [3][4].

Expertise in complex human decision making makes possible the assessment of a patient's need for nursing care, a definition of goals and strategies of care, administering interventions, and monitoring results and quality of care. The use of a rational methodology of decision process in caring practice requires awareness about the area of nursing domain and an ability to process information. If the domain is unclear, then care plans will include medical-type diagnoses and interventions. On the medical-surgical units, patients with similar medical diagnoses often share similar nursing care plans based on medical interventions and instructions [5]. In a large number of articles in the nursing literature, a very high level of decision making in nursing practice is assumed. However, some studies report a very different reality, with much of a nurse's time used on mundane routine tasks, and the same formula being painstakingly written out in long hand on every occasion. The nursing care plan seems more like a legal document or an institutional requirement than as an aid to nursing care [6]. Often a nurse's decision process is within the typical set of instructions given by the physician. In this case the nurse processes a few simple information patterns because the decision concerns only a small segment of the patient's health problem. However, the use of computerized decision support systems could make sense when the following elements are present: (a) large amount of different kinds of data to process; (b) high complexity of internal relations among data, and (c) different values and weights of data in the complex set [7]. Computer-based modeling tools could help to analyze complex decision problem and determine the best course of action. Thus, a superior decision could result when nursing judgment is aided by an expert system [8]

2. Expert system shells

Basically, the structure of an expert system is quite simple. It has three essential parts, the triptych of data, the knowledge base and the shell [9]. The nursing knowledge necessary to build decision-support systems is found in nursing textbooks, specialized scientific magazines, experience acquired during clinical practice, at conferences, congresses, interdisciplinary panel of experts, and discussions with other professionals. In the system, the body of knowledge is commonly represented in the form of facts and rules. The shells use two main strategies to process the internal knowledge: (a) the "data-driven" method, where the available data are examined and all the applicable rules are operated, and (b) the "goal-driven" method, which identifies the conclusions it needs to establish its goals, and then examines the rules to see which ones contribute directly to these goals. These methods are both able to look repeatedly at the "if . . ." (part of the rules) in order to identify the data required to make the conclusion. The algorithms for providing this control are quite unsophisticated because the power of the system comes from the contents of the knowledge base rather than from sophisticated features of the shell. Rules and facts are the more ways of representing knowledge but other ways are possible as well. For example this knowledge can be implemented as networks of elementary relationships (semantic net) or more highly structured collections of interrelated materials (frames). A classic example of a semantic net implemented in a nursing computer application is COMMES [10] developed at Creighton University and able to process more than 20,000 terms linking their meaning.

The shell may use logical deduction to interpret the data, or it may use very different methods, such as fuzzy reasoning. This depends on the rules and facts in the knowledge base and the primitive functions which are available.

3. The ISIRI prototype

In 1988 an interdisciplinary team of the International Institute of Nursing Research (ISIRI) developed a mathematical model to represent the nursing process with the assumption that matrix algebra can be used to represent the relations among the variables involved in the nursing process. A characteristic of matrix-algebra is that one can manipulate and operate on large matrices of data with relative ease, when ordinary algebra will simply not do. A matrix can be conceived as a pattern of correlation between two vectors. Using matrix-algebra, the patterns of knowledge required for decision making in nursing practice have to be described in terms of vectors and matrices. Each cell of the matrices may or may not contain a numeric value depending on the degree of correlation between two items of the vectors. The information processed by the nurse during the caring process was categorized in terms of informative variables (e.g signs and symptoms, potential objectives, etc). The whole system of variables was analyzed as a three step information process: input, algorithm of calculus, and output. The knowledge used to implement the matrices was collected using interdisciplinary panels of experts, analysis of literature and surveys in clinical settings over several years. The theoretical framework was provided by the model "Nursing as stimulus of health and harmony" developed by Zanotti [11]. The model describes the patterns of signs, symptoms, and causes for each need, and provides criteria and

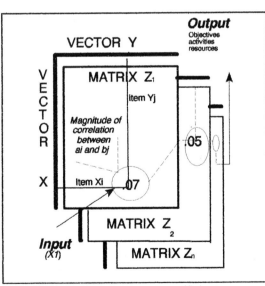

Figure 1 Vectors, matrices, and coefficients

extensive descriptions about the correlation between needs, objectives, and activities within the nursing domain [12]. The internal knowledge is stored in the vectors, then used as an interface with the nurse and the system's link matrices. The interface vectors provide an exhaustive array of items to choose from in correlation with the specific step of the nursing process. Once an item is chosen, a value from 1 through 10 has to be entered by the nurse, as indicating the item's importance about the current health status of the patient. The typed values are processed through the

350

coefficients of one or more link matrices and the output (results) are produced promptly as shown in Figure 1, 2, and 3. The function of the link matrices could be compared to the activity of correlating, comparing, and weighing information made by a nursing expert. One advantage of an expert system based on matrix-algebra is the independence of internal knowledge from the shell. This means that the upgrading of the system's knowledge is a very easy task that can be performed also by people with little or no competence in informatics. Each matrix is a file that is loaded when the program starts. Link matrices are easily updated through a particular subprogram that permits direct access to each matrix for editing or control. In order to validate the reliability of the outcomes, several pilot studies have been conducted in hospital and community settings in the last four years [13] [14] and others are still in process. Based on the studies' results, the matrices' knowledge has been revised and improved many times. The program is written in C++ for DOS, stand-alone computers. It uses a color, friendly graphics interface with pop-up menu bar and permits unlimited storage of patients' records in its own database. The database allows one to keep a record of several items about a patient's demography, style of life, past and current health, medical diagnoses and treatment. The database interacts with the link matrix of causes when something in the patient's story could be a cause of a health problem or a risk factor (e.g. daily abuse of alcohol, sedentariness, overweight, etc.) as shown in Figure 3. A different internal database records all the events regarding planning, activities carried out, and outcomes. Both databases are

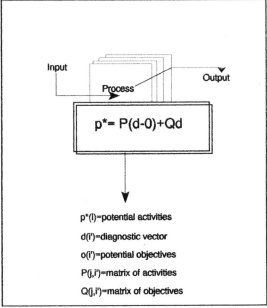

Figure 2   Output for activities

automatically updated each time new data about the patient are entered, and the outcomes are recalculated. All the database information as well as diagnosis, planning, and evaluation outcomes can be printed out as a complete or a

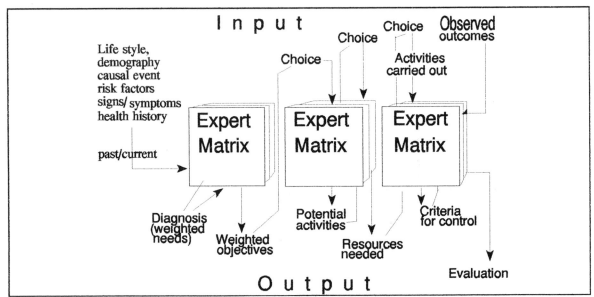

Figure 3 Overlook on the prototype

partial report in a form-like format. All the database files can be stored in secure sites because they are independent of the shell. In order to protect the privacy of the patients' data, a password has to be entered by the user.

The implementation of the computerized expert system is in an advanced stage. At the current time, the first part, called NIMMO (Nursing Information Matrix Model) is already used as an expert system for tutoring and training the students' diagnostic skills in some Italian nursing schools. The feature regarding objectives, activities, resources and evaluation are in the validation process through a multisite correlational study.

The major limitations of the ISIRI prototype are that (a) it does not consider nonlinear relationships between variables, and (b) some parameters, like the progression of the activities carried out, need more appropriate indicators and measurements.

4. Conclusions

The availability of computerized nursing expert knowledge for caring practice could improve reliability and quality of care if the system knowledge is actually wider than the average nurse's knowledge. Thus, the possibility to store large amounts of data, process a long array of information, and produce reports and many sophisticated analyses are tasks that a modern computer can perform with ease. Currently, many decision support systems for nursing are reported in scientific literature, but there is little evidence of the systematic use of these systems in caring settings [15]. Flexibility, easy upgradeability, interconnections among massive data bases, and the outcomes of a real professional expert are to be the goals when implementing a new decision support system. Because the use of matrix-algebra meets most of the above requirements, it could represent a different way to conceptualize and to implement such a system. The ISIRI prototype is the first to use matrix-algebra, and despite some important limits due to the nature of matrix-algebra, it can process more data and with greater flexibility then other rule-based systems. The ISIRI prototype requires the nurse to input weighted data and this means that the first step of the information process is completely controlled by the user. Sensibility, motivation, passion for the patient's health, and personal expertise are the required characteristics of the nurse for obtaining valid outcomes from this prototype. The use of a computer expert system like this one, despite its name of expert, requires nurses with a *high degree* of professional skills. This requisite highlights the complexity of the knowledge involved in decision making in nursing practice.

5. References

[1]	Grier MR & Schizler CP. Nurses' propensity to risk. *Nurs Res* 1979, 8:186-191.
[2]	Brennan PF. Computerized decision support beyond decision support. *Health Matrix* 1987, 5:31-34.
[3]	Goode WJ. The theoretical limits of professionalization. In: The professions and their Organizations. New York: Free Press 1969.
[4]	Friedson E. Profession & the occupational principle. In: The Professions and their Prospects. Friedson E (ed). Beverly Hills CA: Sage 1973
[5]	Larrabee JH. Rodgers VO Corsey R. Murff WE, Barnoud K and Knight M. Developing and Implementing computer-generated nursing care plans. *Journ of Nurs Care Qual* 1992, 6:56-62.
[6]	Porter S. A Participant Observation Study of power relations between nurses and doctors in a general hospital. *Journ of Adv Nurs* 1991, 16:728-735
[7]	Zanotti R and Fitzpatrick J J. Nursing Care and Decision Support Tools. *Inf Tech Nur* 1993, 5:5-7.
[8]	Brennan FP. Dcision support system in nursing. In: Proceedings from the third International Symposium on Nursing Use of Computers and Information Science. Ozbolt J and Vandewal D (eds). St. Louis: Mosby, 1990.
[9]	Fox J. Formal and Knowledge-based Methods in Decision Technology. *Acta Psychologica* 1984, 56:303-331.
[10]	Ryan AS. An Expert System for Nusing Practice. *Comp in Nurs* 1985, 3:76-84.
[11]	Zanotti R . Un modello teorico per la lettura dei bisogni della persona. In:Ricerca e Professione Infermieristica. Veneto Region (ed). Venezia Italy. 1988: 70-77.
[12]	Poletti P Vian F and Zanotti R. *Introduzione al Processo di Nursing*. Padova: Summa, 1989.
[13]	Fanton S and Zanotti R La rilevazione dei segnali di bisogno. In: Proceeding of the Third VRQ National Conference in Italy. : VRQ Ass (ed). Padova Italy 1992: 35-38

[14] Zanotti R. Sperimentazione del processo di nursing nell'assistenza domiciliare. In: Proceedings of the National Conference on Home Care. ULSS 19 (ed). Castelfranco, Treviso Italy, 1991:37-42.

[15] Jones TB. Expert System in Nursing: The wide chasm between promise and practice. *Inf Tech Nurs* 1991, 4:10-11

Nursing Informatics: An International Overview for Nursing in a Technological Era
S.J. Grobe and E.S.P. Pluyter-Wenting, eds.

Simulation as a Method to Plan Operating Room Schedules

O'Brien-Pallas LL[a] Carter M[b] McGillis L[a] and Blake J[b]

[a]Faculty of Nursing, University of Toronto, 50 St. George St., Toronto, Ontario, Canada M5S 1A1

[b]Department of Industrial Engineering, University of Toronto,, 4 Taddlecreek Rd., Toronto, Ontario, Canada, M5S 1A4

This paper describes the development of a portable desktop computer based simulation of hospital operating room schedules that can be used by hospital administrators to evaluate the impact of administrative decisions associated with operating room scheduling. The tool determines the systematic effects of modifying operating room schedules, restricting OR time to patients with particular age, sex or procedural characteristics, and adding and deleting ward bed space or nursing staff. This paper describes: a) the rationale for such a system, b) simulation methodology and the related literature, c) model considerations and development, d) model capabilities and outputs, and e) future directions for this research. Just as the surgical schedule drives the demand for hospital resources and influences the number and type of patients a hospital may treat, this model has great potential to assist with the resource utilization activities of many hospitals. An animal version of the model will be demonstrated as part of this presentation.

1. Scenario

"It's Thursday afternoon at 1415 hours and I've already had two patients return from the operating room. Orthopaedic patients need so much monitoring post-operatively. One of them is on constant nursing observation and the other one has q15-minute vital signs and pedal pulse checks. The other three patients on my assignment are only the second day post op and still need a great deal of care. Now my third OR patient of the day is coming back from the recovery room. Why is it that we always have ten patients going to the OR on Thursday when we have less staff on, and only three go on Mondays? It just doesn't make sense to me" Staff Nurse - Surgical Services, Anywhere Hospital.

2. Purpose

The above scenario repeats itself over in countless hospitals daily. Scenarios such as this prompted a team of researchers at the University of Toronto to ask the following research question: Is it possible to schedule operating room time to balance the impact of the operating room activities on the nursing units? Specifically, the study examined the development of a model capable of determining the overall impact of modifying: a) the number of surgical beds and the workload associated with patients in those bed; b)the number and availability of nursing staff on surgical wards; c) the operating room schedule; d) the age, sex and procedure characteristics of patients scheduled for surgery on any particular day; and e) patient arrival rates. The ultimate purpose of this study was to develop a decision aid for hospital administrators to examine the impact of trying different operating room schedules on various nursing and organizational outcomes. After an extensive review of the literature it was determined that simulation offered a feasible and practical solution of this question.

3. Simulation Methodology

Simulation is a technique for imitating the operation of a real world facility. The facility of interest is usually called a system. In order to study the system, we often have to make assumptions about how it works. These assumptions, which usually take the form of mathematical or logical relationships, constitute a model which is used to gain some understanding of how the corresponding system behaves.[1]

If the relationships that compose the model are simple, it may be possible to work out an exact answer to questions of interest using ordinary mathematics. This is called an analytic solution. However, since most real world systems are too complex to evaluate analytically, we use simulation. In a simulation we use a computer to evaluate a model numerically over a period of time. Data is then gathered from the model to estimate the true characteristics of the system.[2]

4. Literature

While a great deal of literature has been written about bed usage, admission procedures, demand analysis and operating room utilization, relatively few studies have explored comprehensive hospital planning models. Most models concerned with OR utilization do not consider a patient's use of resources (bed space and nursing care) outside of the surgical suite, nor do they attempt to determine the impact of a particular schedule on the entire hospital. Modelling health care facilities is generally regarded as a difficult task, due to the size and complexity of the systems involved. The unique characteristics of patients adds to the complexity of the health care system. As acute care centres become more technical, it is often difficult to develop profiles of typical patients, because many of these patients are gravely ill and present unique medical, nursing, social, and personal needs. Until recently the computational power required to model large systems was also a limiting factor: researchers were forced to either develop extremely simplified models or restrict their attention to small subsets of the overall problem.

Wright[3] describes a model developed for a health care district in Lancaster, England which was used to rationalize the number of urology and general surgery cases performed at two local hospitals. Wright used the operating room schedule to determine the admission patterns whose length of stay is correlated to service, sex, and type of operation. Wright does not make provisions for simulating the function of the surgical suite, the post-anaesthesia recovery room or the nursing unit on which the patient is housed.

In our study we expanded upon many of the basic principals established by Wright and developed the model using the surgical services of five Toronto hospitals. The scope of the model examines the exact flow of patients at each site from admission to discharge. Additionally, we include provisions for determining the utilization of beds on individual surgical units, the workload created by this, as well as the availability and use of nursing resources on these units. We asked nursing unit managers from each of the study hospitals to provide daily estimates of the time required to care for patients undergoing procedures that commonly occur on their units. These estimates were derived from their workload measurement systems. When the simulation model is run, the program uses these estimated to determine the daily amount of workload that will be consumed by patients on each of the surgical wards. As patients are admitted to, or transferred from, a ward, the estimate of nursing workload is updated.

As a result, the model is large and relatively complex. The availability of cheap, powerful desktop computers has overcome the traditional computational difficulties experienced during earlier attempts to model complex health care systems. We developed a custom interface to reduce the complexity of the model as experienced by the user.

5. Model Development and Validation

The model was developed by gathering data on patient flow through a series of interviews with surgical nurse managers and personnel from key hospital departments that interact with surgical patients. This data is then collated and converted into a flow chart which is validated at each site. Validation occurs through regularly scheduled meetings with a steering committee from the site, composed of nurses, administrators, and physicians who discuss the validity of the model as it is developed. Through an iterative process the model is refined until it is considered an accurate representation of surgical patient flow for that setting. The patient flow model is then converted into a computer simulation. Users from each hospital site review the software and comment on its face validity. Model validation is accomplished by comparing results from the simulation model to historical records from the site. These include both the number of admissions and the number of cases for each surgical service.

The model simulates all departments directly affecting the flow of surgical patients. These include: a) admitting and day surgery registration; b) surgical nursing wards (including day surgery); c) surgical operating rooms; d) post anaesthetic recovery rooms; e) surgical intensive care units; f) radiology units; and g) emergency rooms. Three substantive groups of patients emerged from the interview process that have come to constitute the key groups of patients in the flow model. These are elective surgical admissions, day surgical admissions, and emergency admissions requiring OR. Detailed admitting and block OR scheduling information is contained in the model, with ward preferences and priority systems for emergency patients also built in. Operating room time is assigned on a block booking basis where a period of time, or block is reserved for the exclusive use of a surgeon or service. A scheduling module assigns patients to defined blocks and develops an elective surgery admission list for each day of the simulated time period. When the model is run, any doctor's unused block time is made available for urgent and emergency surgery. Decision rules in the model allocate the time first to other surgeons within the scheduled doctor's service and then to any other surgeon with excess cases.

The model data base contains information describing patients, physicians, the operating room schedule, and physical entities in the hospital such as the number of beds, workload profiles of "usual" patients undergoing surgical procedures and the amount of nursing staff available on a ward. The model contains the rules and relationships which link the various departments and functional areas of a hospital. The model picks scheduled patients from the elective admission list and emergency patients from the database and admits them to the simulated hospital. These patients flow through the simulation in a manner analogous to that of patients in an actual hospital. Currently, the scope of the model has been limited to include only those areas of a hospital that directly impact the flow of surgical patients. Ancillary support services and diagnostic services are not currently included in the model.

6. Model Capability

The simulation model is able to predict the impact of changes to a number of key hospital parameters such as ward resources and non-scheduled patient arrival rates. Information about numbers of patients admitted and discharged, day surgery cases performed, scheduled cases deferred or cancelled, emergency and scheduled cases completed, and the amount of OR time use can be displayed for the entire hospital, surgical services, an individual doctor, or a specific operating room. Census and nursing workload information is also available for inpatient surgical wards, intensive care units, recovery rooms and day surgery wards.

Often the process of validation has constituted the initial use of the model at the hospital site. At one location during the validation process, it was found that the capacity of the OR schedule to not correspond to the caseload of a particular service. A number of surgical services routinely failed to fill their assigned blocks. This unused time was being used on an *ad hoc* basis by services with too little assigned time. Staff at the site were able, because of this information, to adjust their schedules to more accurately represent the practice at their hospital. Another site has used the model to trial various scenarios to alter the time allocated to the cardiovascular surgery service. The model determined that there was a potential to increase their OR case capability from 750 to 900 cases a year. The model is currently being installed at a third site where it is proposed to use to it to plan the expansion of the day surgery complement.

Blocking beds and closing whole wards or services for a specified period of time has been a technique used by Ontario hospitals to reduce the overall operating budgets for particular services. Ultimately, the impact of closing one unit may not reduce overall budgets if the flow of patients needs to be absorbed by other nursing units. The Operating Room Scheduling Simulation (ORSS) is uniquely able to assist hospital administrators to examine the impact of closing a ward or service on the overall resources used in the surgical services. Running a series of scenarios through the model allows managers to determine the critical threshold where overall cost savings are incurred in terms of resource use as opposed to simply passing costs on to another service. These permutations can be completed and outcomes determined before there is any interruption in the normal activity flow of the hospital's surgical services.

7. Model Outputs

The model is run on four simulated months of data (and takes approximately 4 hours on a 386-based PC), during which time statistics are collected on all aspects of the simulated hospital performance. At the end of the run users are presented with the summary statistics in both text and charts through the interface module.

8. Future Development

Currently the model provides utilization statistics around a number of procedures, hours of nursing care, and number of cases. While these data are useful for planning, the manager must convert them to cost estimates for practical applications. Given this, our immediate research activities will be directed at developing an overall cost module. Managers will then be able to weigh the overall cost implications of any proposed decisions they may entertain. We are also developing a module that will optimize the OR schedule given the parameters considered in the model. Providing an optimal schedule against which managers can compare current practice will greatly enhance the decision aid capabilities of the system.

The simulation is run on historical data reflecting the unique volumes and practices of the institution at this time. However these data bases reflect previous years' practices and may not reflect the rapid changes hospitals currently experience. We are now developing an interface that will allow the system to read current computerized perioperative data bases in those institutions where such resources exist.

While systems such as the OR simulation model may have intellectual and practical appeal to their developers and to senior administrators who wish to use these applications, middle managers and other end users may not share the same views. There are many factors which influence whether a new technology is integrated into day-to-day practice. Given that the five hospitals involved in this study have integrated the ORSS to varying degrees we are currently mounting a study to determine the extent to which this technology has been diffused through the organization. In order to find ways to help users maximize the potential application of technologies such as the ORSS we intend to study barriers and opportunities experienced during the implementation of the ORSS at each of the study hospitals.

References

[1,2]   Law A and Kelton W. *Simulation Modelling and Analysis.* New York: McGraw-Hill Series in Industrial Engineering and Systems Management, 1984.

[3]   Wright. The Application of a Surgical Bed Simulation Model. *European J Operational Res* 1987, 32:26-32.

Nursing Informatics: An International Overview for Nursing in a Technological Era
S.J. Grobe and E.S.P. Pluyter-Wenting, eds.

Machine Learning for Development of an Expert System to Support Nurses' Assessment of Preterm Birth Risk

Woolery L[a]   VanDyne M [b] Grzymala-Busse J [b] and Tsatsoulis C [b]

[a]S329 School of Nursing, University of Missouri, Columbia, MO, USA 65211

[b]University of Kansas Departments of Computer Science, Electrical Engineering, Lawrence, KS, USA 64055

Normal pregnancy involves a term of 40 weeks gestation. Problems associated with low birthweight and prematurity continue to plague childbearing families and the healthcare system because 8-12% of all newborns in the United States deliver prior to 37 weeks gestation. The purpose of this study was to develop a prototype expert system for assessment of preterm delivery risk in pregnant women. A knowledge base development methodology used machine learning, statistical analysis, and expert verification techniques with large datasets (n=18,890; 214 variables). The prototype expert system was more accurate in predicting preterm delivery than existing manual techniques.

1. The Problem

Early and accurate detection and treatment of preterm labor can prolong gestation with improved outcomes for both the infant and family. Review of the literature provided both theoretical and empirical support for research and development of an expert system to provide decision support for nurses' assessment of preterm labor risk. Determining preterm labor risk in pregnant women and making decisions about interventions remain problematic in the clinical setting [1]. The problems related to preterm labor risk assessment include a poorly-defined and complex knowledge base. The plethora of information about preterm labor risks remains disorganized and of little guidance to patients and providers of prenatal care. Review of the literature found no conceptual or theoretical models of preterm labor risk, which may account for poor reliability and validity of existing manual screening techniques [2]. Existing preterm labor risk screening instruments include factors that are not valid predictors of preterm labor and delivery risk, and fail to include factors reported in the literature that may be valid predictors of preterm labor [3,4,5] . Although existing instruments are only about 44% accurate, and are not adequately predictive of preterm delivery, current preterm labor prevention programs use these invalid, unreliable tools to intervene with pregnant women on a daily basis. This phenomenon has resulted in a trend that increasingly treats pregnant women as if they are 'high risk' for preterm labor. Alternative solutions to the problem may be achieved using machine learning and expert system technology to support nurses' assessments in this complex domain.

This research was supported by the National Center for Nursing Research (NCNR): Small Business Innovation Research (SBIR) funding 1 R43 NR02899-01A1.

2. Machine Learning

Machine learning is an emerging specialty in the field of artificial intelligence that developed during the 1980's [6]. Machine learning involves computer science techniques where mathematical algorithms are used to analyze patterns, frequencies, and sets within data. Using various algorithms and a variety of theoretical and mathematical approaches, machine learning offers powerful new tools for knowledge acquisition directly from nursing, and other, data.

3. Methodology

The methodology used in this study was refined from earlier knowledge base development methodology work [2, 7] by using multiple large datasets (n =18,890 subjects from three databases), multiple machine learning programs (ID3, LERS, CONCLUS, and a Bayesian classification program), and simplified classification schemes for machine learning analysis. The decision analyzed by machine learning programs was preterm or full term delivery, rather than weeks of gestation at delivery. The procedure included the following steps:

1. Acquire and load data into appropriate computers and formats. It is important to note that the data was split in half at this step. Half of the data was used for statistical and machine learning analysis. This is data that was used to generate the production rules for the prototype expert system. The other half of the data was used to test the prototype expert system with real patient cases.
2. Conduct exploratory factor analysis for data reduction purposes
3. Conduct multivariate regression analyses to determine predictors of preterm labor risk
4. Conduct machine learning knowledge acquisition to generate production rules directly from the data
5. Verify production rules using content validity techniques and nurse experts
6. Build and test the prototype expert system

4. Statistical Analysis Results   (Methodology Steps 2 and 3)

All statistical analyses were conducted with datasets that were used for production rule generation. Descriptive statistics, exploratory factor analyses, and multiple regression analyses were conducted for 9445 subjects and 214 variables. Descriptive statistics found the average age of women in all three databases was in their late twenties. Numbers of adolescent subjects were relatively small, so this data may not reflect risk factors of adolescent pregnancy. Only three of the subjects analyzed had received no prenatal care, thus this study was unable to address preterm labor risk in women who do not seek prenatal care. Dichotomous coding and small numbers of subjects with positive responses on numerous variables produced statistical results that contradict findings in the literature. Between 10.8% and 14.2% of the subjects were smokers, but smoking was recorded 'yes' or 'no', and multiple regression analyses did not detect a relationship between smoking and preterm delivery. This same phenomenon was true for substance abuse and a variety of medical diagnoses that complicate pregnancy. In general, conclusions drawn from descriptive data analysis were that the data was voluminous, sometimes erroneous, poorly organized, inconsistently recorded, frequently dichotomous, and data items needed were often not collected. Continued statistical analyses were conducted with caution to better understand the problems and to determine data needs for future studies.

Exploratory factor analyses that yielded the best results produced a four factor solution that accounted for 25.6% of the variance. There were no double loadings in the four factor solution, and factors were named with relative ease. Factor 1 was named 'Biophysical Markers' and included data items for blood pressure, pulse, weight, and mean arterial pressures. Factor 2 was named 'Age and Abortion History' and included data items for maternal age, number of pregnancies, first trimester bleeding, and several abortion variables. Factor 3 was named 'Reasons and Interventions' and included information about the average number of contractions, reasons given for patient contact, and patient interventions prescribed by the nurse. Although some of the interventions required physician collaboration and orders, they were initiated by the nurse. Factor 4 was named 'Preterm Labor Risk Factors' and included data items for previous preterm labor and delivery, cervical history, and pregnancy within one year of a previous pregnancy. In addition, Factor 4 included data items for years of maternal education and numbers of living children. Exploratory factor analyses partially confirmed construct validity of the data. Exploratory factor analyses was also conducted for purposes of data reduction to guide multiple regression analyses. Various factor solutions were used as models for multiple regression analyses.

Multiple regression analysis used weeks of gestation at delivery as the dependent variable and tested numerous regression models with varying configurations of the remaining 213 variables as predictors. Results found very low correlations between the dependent variable and most of the predictors tested. The inability to predict preterm delivery from the data was somewhat surprising, at first, but this finding can be clarified through several explanations. It is important to remember that the exact cause of labor, whether full term or preterm, remains unknown. The data in the perinatal database reflected risk factors [8] that are consistent with most preterm labor risk screening instruments currently in use. However, review of the literature found that preterm labor risk scoring indices have not been developed with attention to psychometric standards, and remain invalid and unreliable although they are used daily as a standard of practice in providing prenatal care [9]. The low correlations between predictor variables and the criterion variable are explained, in part, to a large volume of dichotomous data. The low correlations between predictor variables and the criterion variable may also be due, in part, to the possibility that healthcare providers continue to collect a great deal of data that has little to do with preterm labor risk. The multiple regression findings in this study may lend additional support to an earlier study [10] that found no statistically significant results for race, age, marital status, parity, or socioeconomic status and a study [11] that found no statistically significant differences in age, gravidity, parity or race. It is possible that current clinical practice operates with assumptions about risk factors for preterm labor that are invalid. Continued questions exist as to the relationship between demographic data and preterm labor risk. More work is needed to replicate and analyze preterm labor risk factors in relationship to age, race, and other items believed to predict or be strongly associated with preterm labor risk.

5. Machine Learning and Expert Verification Results (Methodology Steps 4 and 5)

Multiple approaches to machine learning were conducted using software programs named ID3, LERS, CONCLUS, and a Bayesian classification program. Examples with missing values and obvious errors, such as maternal 10 pound or 700 pound weights, systolic pressures of 14,000, and pulses of less than 40, were excluded from machine learning analysis. The details of this work are reported elsewhere [12]. LERS produced the only usable output, generating about 1600 production rules directly from the data. Expert verification of the rules was difficult due to the large volume and 'unfriendliness' of the rule output. Automated features built into LERS assisted with the rule verification process and programs were written to make the rule output easier for the experts to analyze. In general, the experts indicated that individual rules did not provide enough information and that important data were missing. Considering the prototype expert system results, described in the next section, limitations of expert verification in complex and disorganized domains need further study.

6. Prototype Expert System Results (Methodology Step 6)

The prototype expert system used 520 rules in an object oriented expert system shell named 'Kappa' that runs on a DOS platform in a Windows environment. Forward chaining techniques and priority encoding of the rules were used to develop the prototype. It is important to remember that none of the data used for testing was used in building the prototype. A computer program was written to 'feed' each of the 9445 test subjects through the prototype expert system to analyze the system's ability to accurately predict preterm delivery. Accuracy was tested by having the expert system analyze each test case's data and predict either preterm or full term delivery. The computer program then retrieved the actual preterm or full term outcome from the database, and the expert system prediction was compared with the actual patient outcome. Where the predicted outcome and the actual outcome matched, there was 100% accuracy. Accuracy rates are reported in Table 1.

While the ultimate goal of expert system development is to predict preterm *labor* risk, the definition of preterm labor and data needed to analyze preterm labor risk is less amenable to study at present. There were numerous confounding variables in the data that made prediction of preterm labor impossible. It was determined that accuracy of predicting preterm delivery was more viable, and that the purpose of this study was to determine the feasibility of using an expert system for prediction of preterm delivery. Future studies are planned to study the feasibility of using the expert system to predict preterm labor risk. Even so, the reader is reminded that existing manual systems are approximately 44% accurate in predicting preterm delivery. Each of the databases tested surpassed the manual accuracy rates. And the lower accuracy for Database 3 is still very encouraging because there were no rules used from this database. The 53.4% accuracy for Database 3 reflects data tested against rules from the other two databases.

Table 1
Expert System Prototype Accuracy Rates

	Database 1	Database 2	Database 3
Number of Test Cases	1593	1218	6608
Total Correctly Classified	1415 (88.8%)	722 (59.2%)	3533 (53.4%)
Total Misclassified	171 (10.7%)	456 (37.4%)	2796 (42.3%)
Total Unclassified	7 (.4%)	40 (3.2%)	279 (4.2%)

Considering the limitations with databases used, 'noisy' data, and difficulties encountered with expert verification, the accuracy rates reflected in Table 1 were both surprising and exciting. Future studies using prospective, carefully planned, and quality-controlled data collection methods should improve rule generation and accuracy predictions to very high levels in a fully implemented expert system that will provide valid and reliable decision support for nursing assessment of preterm labor risk. The statistical, machine learning, and prototype expert system findings from this study validated that preterm delivery risk assessment is a complex and disorganized knowledge domain. But even with this complexity, the research methodology and machine learning techniques used in this study were able to extract rules directly from data, and use these rules in a prototype expert system that was more accurate in predicting preterm delivery than existing manual systems. The knowledge base development methodology used in this study offers a mechanism to further develop linkages between technology, nursing science, and clinical nursing practice in a variety of settings.

Special thanks for data provided by St. Luke's Regional Perinatal Center (Kansas City, MO), Healthdyne Perinatal Services (Marietta, GA), and Tokos Corporation (Santa Ana, CA).

References
[1] Rosen M, Merkatz I, and Hill J. Caring for our future: a report of the expert panel on the content of prenatal care. *Ob Gyn*, 77 (5), 782-787, 1991.

[2] Woolery L *Knowledge Acquisition for Assessment of Preterm Labor Risk.* Unpublished doctoral dissertation. University of Kansas, 1992.

[3] Keirse M. An evaluation of formal risk scoring for preterm birth. *Am J Perinat*, 6 (2), 226-233, 1989.

[4] Alexander G, Weiss J, Hulsey T, and Papiernik E. Preterm birth prevention: an evaluation of programs in the United States. *Birth*, 18 (3), 160-169, 1991.

[5] VanDyne M and Woolery L. *An Expert System for Nurses' Preterm Labor Risk Assessment.* SBIR Phase I Summary Report, 1993.

[6] Forsyth R. *Machine Learning: Principles and Techniques.* New York: Chapman & Hall Publishers, 1989.

[7] Woolery L, Grzymala-Busse J, Summers S, and Budihardjo A. On the use of LERS-LB knowledge acquisition for expert system development in nursing. *Comput Nurs,* 9 (6), 227-234, 1991.

[8] Holbrook R, Laros R, and Creasy R. Evaluation of a risk-scoring system for prediction of preterm labor. *Am J Perinat*, 6 (1), 62-68, 1989.

[9] Keirse M. An evaluation of formal risk scoring for preterm birth. *Am J Perinat*, 6 (2), 226-233, 1989.

[10] Lockwood C, Senyei A, Dische M, Casal D, Shah K, Thung S, Jones L, Deligdisch L, and Garite, T. Fetal fibronectin in cervical and vaginal secretions as a predictor of preterm delivery. *New Engl J Med*, 315 (10). 669-674, 1991.

[11] McGregor J, French J, Richter R, Franco-Buff A, Johnson A, Hillier S, Judson F, and Todd, J. Antenatal microbiologic and maternal risk factors associated with prematurity. *Am J Ob Gyn* , 163 (5). 1465-1473, 1990.

[12] Grzymala-Busse J, Tsatsoulis C, VanDyne M, and Woolery L. multiple articles in progress.

© 1994 Elsevier Science B.V. All rights reserved
Nursing Informatics: An International Overview for Nursing in a Technological Er
S.J. Grobe and E.S.P. Pluyter-Wenting, eds

A decision support system for troubleshooting pulmonary artery catheter waveforms

Zielstorff R D   Barnett G O   Fitzmaurice J B   Oliver D E
Ford-Carleton P   Thompson B T   Estey G   Eccles R   Martin M

Massachusetts General Hospital, 32 Fruit Street, Boston, MA, USA 02114

On-line, real-time decision support for managing patient care problems is a rare commodity for clinicians. This paper describes a microcomputer system for providing computer-based access to synthesized expert knowledge, specifically in the area of troubleshooting pulmonary artery catheter waveforms. The system is used by both nurses and physicians in the intensive care setting. It uses state-of-the-art technology to quickly provide appropriate expert knowledge in a problem-solving context. It relies heavily on graphics, and was implemented with a popular commercial hypertext authoring tool. An evaluation protocol has been designed to examine the impact of the system on clinicians' knowledge, their decision-making skills, and their satisfaction with the system.

1. The Problem

The effectiveness of clinical decision making is receiving major attention from professional organizations, private health care groups, and federal agencies. Physicians and nurses are being called upon to provide care that is efficacious under ever-increasing time and resource constraints. Access to relevant information for making clinical decisions, as well as skill in clinical decision-making, are essential to efficacious care.

Technical solutions have been developed that attempt to provide access to information and knowledge (e.g., bibliographic retrieval systems, indexes to abstracts and to databases, on-line texts, etc.), but by and large these are not accessible to clinicians at the point of care. Even if they were, clinicians often have difficulty formulating searches that will answer a patient-specific question, and when relevant articles are found, they have difficulty evaluating the quality of the material. Failure to incorporate empirical knowledge into practice for these and other reasons is a well documented problem [1,2].

The technological solution to supporting clinical decision-making is the expert system. There are several reports of expert systems applied to nursing problems [3,4,5,6,7]. Several of these systems are in the prototype phase, and have not reached the stage of clinical implementation. Many have limited ability to teach or to provide rationales for their recommendations. In addition, there are indications that expert clinical judgment is founded on gestalt impressions and intuition, which bodes poorly for expert systems founded on mathematical models or production rules [8].

2. The Response

The solution we developed presents *synthesized* knowledge of domain experts in the context of *case-specific patient problems* selected by the clinician. It incorporates not only the empirical knowledge found in the accumulation of research about the specific problem, but also the expert's clinical knowledge that is gained only through experience. Instead of content experts having to dissect their knowledge into minute facts and associations, their knowledge is formalized in terms of "chunks" that are associated with a particular clinical context. Presenting knowledge in this way provides clinicians with easy access to expert knowledge that can be used both for case-specific consultation and for case-oriented education.

.1. Significance of the Clinical Topic

The pulmonary artery catheter has come into widespread clinical use during the past twenty years. However, use of the pulmonary artery catheter is not risk-free. Complications can occur, and the data may be misleading if appropriate attention is not given to technique and management of the PA catheter [9]. Evaluating whether a catheter is functioning properly and if not, finding and fixing the problem, becomes a basic requirement if use of this invasive technique is to be justified.

.2. System Design

The system runs under Microsoft Windows 3.0 or 3.1 on computers based on the Intel 80386 or 80486 microprocessors with 8 megabytes or more of memory and SuperVGA displays with resolution of 1024 x 768 and 256 colors. For reasons of performance, all systems installed on the intensive care units have been 80486-based computers with 16 megabytes of memory. Most programming for the system was done using the Toolbook authoring environment; some additional programming was done in C. Graphics used in the system came from several sources: many of the waveforms used in the system originated in the Massachusetts General Hospital /Marquette Foundation Database developed by other researchers at our institution; most of the illustrations in the system were drawn for use in the system using CorelDRAW or Micrografx Designer.

The content is organized hierarchically, first by waveform category (Right Atrium, Pulmonary Artery, or Pulmonary Capillary Wedge), then by specific types of waveform abnormalities (damping, respiratory variation, etc.) represented graphically on the screen. Having selected a waveform that looks similar to the problem, the user is then brought into the knowledge base. Knowledge about each waveform is "chunked" according to Characteristics, Causes, Management,

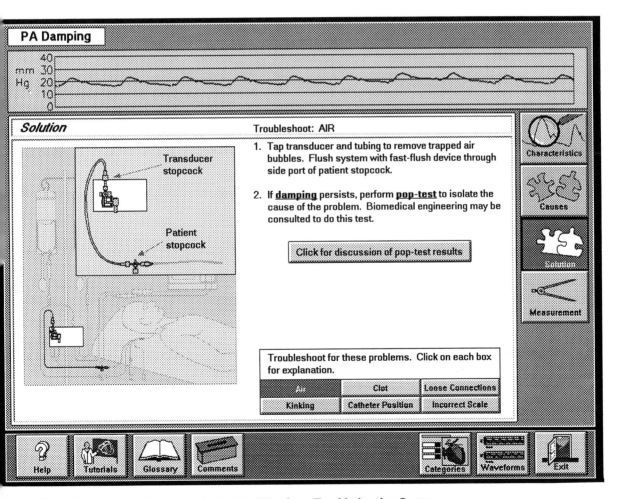

Figure 1. Representative screen in the PA Waveform Troubleshooting System

and obtaining the best Measurement. Graphics are used to illustrate the material as much as possible. Other media such as digitized X-rays and animation are utilized when that seems to be the most effective way to impart the knowledge. Within the text, terms that might need definition or further explication are designated as selectable "hot words." A consistent set of icons allows the user to navigate within the knowledge base. Some buttons allow the user to leave the waveform-specific knowledge and go into the glossary or into the tutorial section of the knowledge base. Of course, there are navigational buttons allowing the user to go back to the set of waveform choices, or to the waveform categories, or to exit the system entirely. Figure 1 shows a representative screen in the waveform knowledge base.

The final design of the system resulted from several years' experience with experimenting with hypertext methods of knowledge construction and presentation [10,11]. It was out of that experience, and out of an iterative process that included a formative evaluation and a three-month beta test in a volunteer intensive care unit that the current design evolved. In essence, the most pervasive lessons have been to keep the indexing methods problem-focused, to keep the knowledge constructs clinically meaningful, and to keep the text explanations as terse as possible [12].

2.3. Implementation of the System

In December 1992 the system was implemented on an 18-bed medical intensive care unit, where there are approximately 3-5 PA lines in place at any one time. As of the end of June, 1993, a total of 37 nurses, 24 physicians, 6 medical students, 6 graduate nursing students and 2 from other categories of personnel have registered to use the system. Of those who registered, 28 nurses, 18 physicians, 5 medical students and 3 nursing students have used the system at least once, for a total of 227 sessions, with a median session length of 3.9 minutes. In addition, we encourage group use of the system. In 43 sessions, those who logged into the system recorded that they were using it with at least one other person.

2.4 Use of the System

In 38 of the 227 sessions (17%), users indicated that the access was for "patient care." For example, a nurse or physician may see an unusual waveform on a patient monitor, and access the system to identify the waveform, its causes, and what to do about it, or if nothing can be done about it, how to at least obtain the best measurement in that circumstance. Half of the sessions (50%) were for "educational browsing." Many of these sessions are initiated by the unit clinical teacher. When a staff person comes to her with a question pertaining to waveform troubleshooting, she frequently brings the person to the computer, has them log on, and guides them to content in the system that answers the question, or that explicates her answer with illustrations, references, even animation when appropriate. The system is also used to supplement training and orientation of students and new personnel. Fifty sessions (22%) were used for this purpose. (See Figure 2.)

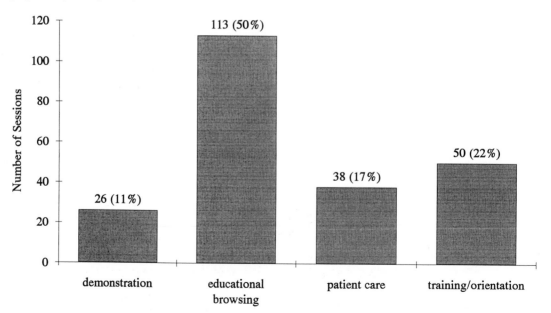

Figure 2. Reasons for use of PA Waveform Troubleshooting System

Evaluation of the System

An evaluation protocol has been designed to examine the system in several areas, including clinicians' knowledge, their decision-making skills, and their satisfaction with the system. The evaluation protocol is being carried out on the experimental unit, and also on a comparison medical intensive care unit whose personnel do not have access to the system. Clinicians' knowledge is assessed via a multiple-choice test developed for this project, which is administered prior to each person's use of the system, and after using it. Nurses' decision-making skills are assessed via case simulations developed for this project, administered before and after use of the system. Pre-tests have been completed, and after 6 months of use with the system, post-tests are in progress.

Satisfaction with the system is assessed in two ways. The first is by asking users at the end of each session to rate the usefulness of the information imparted to them, on a four-point scale ranging from "of little use" to "highly useful." We have ratings for 78 sessions. (The question is only asked if the user exits from the system, not if the system just times out. Most of the time, users leave without exiting, so the system just times out.) Of the 78 sessions rated, 61, or 78%, were rated as "quite useful" or "highly useful" (Figure 3).

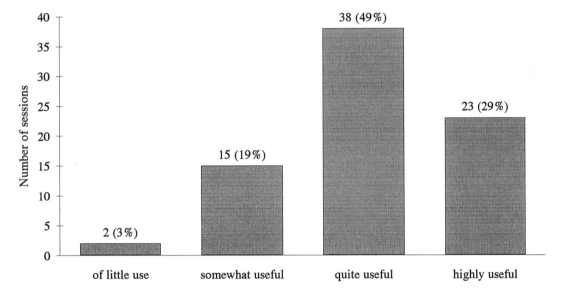

Figure 3. User evaluations of sessions

A second way of assessing user satisfaction is through a short written survey originally developed by Doll and Torkzadeh [13]. The survey was distributed to 30 users who met the following criteria: they had used the system more than one time, they used it for a total of at least 8 minutes, and they viewed at least 20 screens. Twenty-two (73%) have returned the survey at this writing. The twelve-item instrument uses a Likert-type scale to assess users' perceptions of five system dimensions. With 1 as lowest and 5 as highest, the summary scores for each of the dimensions were: Content, 3.4; Accuracy, 4.5; Format, 4.2; Ease of Use, 4.4; Timeliness, 4.1. Further results of the evaluation will be presented in future publications.

4. Conclusion

The system we described provides problem-focused access to expert knowledge for clinicians by emulating the successful qualities of other technologies while avoiding some of their limitations. Evaluation data will show whether using the system has positive effects on clinicians' knowledge and clinical decision-making skills, and on their satisfaction with use of the system. Experience with this topic will be applied to the design of similar systems to provide expert knowledge in the area of prevention and management of pressure ulcers, and in the management of patients on ventilators.

5. References

[1]   Bircumshaw D. The utilization of research findings in clinical nursing practice. *J Adv Nurs* 1990, 15(11):1272-1280.

[2]   Champion VL and Leach A. Variables related to research utilization in nursing: an empirical investigation. *Adv Nurs* 1989, 14(9):705-710.

[3]   Heriot C, Graves J, Bouhaddou O, et al (1988). A pain management decision support system for nurses. In *Proceedings of the Twelfth Annual Symposium on Computer Applications in Medical Care*. Greenes RA (ed) New York: IEEE Press, 1988:63-68.

[4]   Blaufuss JA and Tinker AK. Computerized falls alert: A new solution to an old problem. In: *Proceedings of the Twelfth Annual Symposium on Computer Applications in Medical Care*. Greenes RA (ed). New York: IEEE Press, 1988:69-72.

[5]   Chang BL, Roth K, Gonzales E, Caswell D and DiStefano J. CANDI: a knowledge based system for nursing diagnosis. *Comput Nurs* 1988, 6(1):13-21.

[6]   Bradburn C, Zeleznikow J and Adams A. FLORENCE: Synthesis of case-based and model-based reasoning in a nursing care planning system. *Comput Nurs* 1993, 11(1):20-24.

[7]   Ryan SA. An expert system for nursing practice. *Comput Nurs* 1985, 3(2):77-84.

[8]   Benner P and Tanner C. Clinical judgment: How expert nurses use intuition. *Am J Nurs* 1987,87:23-31

[9]   Civetta JM. Pulmonary artery catheter insertion. In: *The Pulmonary Artery Catheter, Methodology and Clinical Applications*. Sprung CL (ed). Baltimore: University Park Press, 1983:21-71.

[10]   Oliver DE, Estey G, Ford P, Burke S, Teplick R, Zielstorff RD, Barnett GO. Computer-based access to patient care guidelines. In: *Proceedings of the Fourteenth Annual Symposium on Computer Applications in Medical Care*. Miller, RA (ed). New York: IEEE Press, 1990: 398-402.

[11]   Estey G, Oliver DE, Chueh HC, Levinson JR, Zielstorff RD, Barnett GO. Problem-based knowledge access: useful design principles for clinical hypertexts. In: *Proceedings of the Fourteenth Annual Symposium on Computer Applications in Medical Care*. Miller RA (ed). New York: IEEE Press, 1990: 430-434.

[12]   Estey et al, ibid.

[13]   Doll WJ, and Torkzadeh G. The Measurement of End-User Computing Satisfaction. *MIS Quart* 1988, 12:259-274.

=========================

Toolbook is a registered trademark of Asymetrix Corporation. Microsoft and Windows are registered trademarks of Microsoft Corporation. CorelDRAW is a registered trademark of Corel Corporation. Micrografx and Micrografx Designer are trademarks of Micrografx Corporation.

Funded by Grant 5 R18 HS06575, Agency for Health Care Policy and Research, PHS, USDHHS; and by Grant 1 T15 LM07092 and Grant 5 R01 LM05200, National Library of Medicine, NIH, PHS, USDHHS; and by an educational grant from Hewlett Packard Corporation.

NURSING HEALTH INFORMATION SYSTEMS

E. Gerontology; community health; patient education

© 1994 Elsevier Science B.V. All rights reserved.
Nursing Informatics: An International Overview for Nursing in a Technological Era
S.J. Grobe and E.S.P. Pluyter-Wenting, eds.

Development of a Gerontological Nursing Information System

Arnold J M and Gristci K

College of Nursing - *Rutgers, The State University of New Jersey*

A review of the literature was conducted to determine the conceptual framework for a nursing information system(NIS) that links nursing diagnoses and nursing interventions. A relational database evolved from a paper database of 30 nursing diagnoses and related interventions based on six gerontological case studies. The NIS was designed using Paradox software and an IBM compatible microcomputer.

1. Purpose

There is a need to develop nursing information systems in order to computerize and document nursing practice. "A nursing information system is an automated system designed to manage information used by nurses to plan, give, manage, evaluate, document and improve patient care provided by nurses [1, p. 18] The classification of nursing diagnoses and interventions using a common framework within a database structures is presented. Database management stipulates the organization of information by categories in a logical manner for easy access and retrieval. The purpose of this report is to describe the process in developing a computerized gerontological nursing data base, which links nursing diagnoses and nursing interventions and nursing outcomes using a nursing model. The following review of the literature provided the foundation for the creation of a nursing framework for the design of the nursing information system.

2. Review of literature related to nursing diagnosis

The volume of literature and discussion generated by the use of the terms nursing diagnosis and nursing process resulted in attempts to develop a nursing diagnosis taxonomy. [2] The first national conference in 1973 set as its purpose to generate labels or names for nursing diagnosis and creation of a classification system [3]. At the fifth conference the group adopted Martha Rogers concept of Unitary Man [2] Kritek, questioned the utility of the patterns of unitary man for use in practice settings because of their abstract nature. [3] A classification system has been developed for the community health care setting. The Omaha Classification system has four domains: environmental, psychosocial, physiologic and health-related behaviors [4, p. 110] It has been validated through research with client records.

3. Review of literature related to nursing interventions

The review of the literature revealed the development of the term "nursing intervention." Early definitions of nursing included actions of nursing care such as caring for the sick. Florence Nightingale designed rules, which were to be followed for providing optimum care to patients thereby establishing written behaviors for nurses to use [5] As stated previously Harmer used the words nursing treatments in 1926 [6]. Kreuter in 1950s described the nurse as providing "ministrations" or nursing actions such as basic needs, ministering, observing, teaching, supervising, guiding, planning with and communicating with the patient [5, p.11].

At the Fifth NANDA conference mention was made of nursing interventions and it was concluded that "cues, interventions, and qualifiers were largely ignored during sorting of nursing diagnosis lists, but were viewed as germane to further classification tasks." Subsequent NANDA Conferences continue to focus solely on nursing diagnosis.

Work has been done on four proposals for describing nursing interventions which will be referred to as the Nursing Minimum Data Set (NMDS), Iowa Project, University of Texas Project and George Washington Home Health Project [7] [8], [9], [10]. The first task force related to nursing interventions was a part of the of the NMDS Conference in 1985. Nursing intervention was defined "as an action intended to benefit the patient or client and for which nurses are responsible" [7] Devine and Werley tested the 16 item nursing intervention classification scheme developed at the NMDS Conference resulting in a 87% inter-coder agreement [11]. Next this 16 item classification system was modified to a seven item classification scheme and tested yielding a 84% inter-coder agreement [11, p.104]. This testing was applied to patient records in four patient care delivery settings, hospital, nursing home, home health and two clinics. Respondents (46) in a study about usage of the Nursing Minimum Data set reported that "availability and use of nursing interventions and nursing outcomes appear to be the least consistently documented areas" [12, p.262]

In 1990 the Iowa Project distinguished three nursing intervention categories within seven groups of nursing activities. "Nursing interventions are primarily those treatments initiated by nurses in response to a nursing diagnosis [8]. In 1992, the Iowa Project reported the use of expert groups to define and validate nursing interventions which resulted in a list of interventions labels, "each with a conceptual definition and defining activities" [13, p.290]. Phase two of the Iowa Project was the placement of an intervention list into a taxonomy including domains and classes.

A preliminary nursing intervention lexicon and taxonomy reported by Grobe used language methodology with 94 masters prepared nurses to generate 1317 nursing intervention statements. Ten categories of nursing interventions were identified and 1,240 nursing interventions were assigned to one of these ten categories with 100% agreement by the three independent investigators. 81% (1006) of these interventions were assigned to the four categories; Care Environment Management, Care Need Determination, Care Information Provision and Therapeutic Care-General [9] These categories reflect coordination of care, assessment, teaching and provision of care. There was less inter-coder agreement regarding the remaining 77 items; 66% or less. This study described the structure of a nursing intervention statement as a verb phrase and one or more noun phrases.

A home care classification system based on 8,961 retrospective client records from 646 home care agencies has been developed. [10]. This system is used to predict resource requirements and measure outcomes. The twenty Home Health Care Components (HHCC) constitute the coding framework for the further classification of 147 nursing diagnosis and 166 nursing interventions. Two additional elements recorded are expected outcomes (improved, stabilized and deteriorated) and nursing intervention type (assess, direct care, teach and manage) [14]. Saba tested NANDA's nine human response patterns and Gordon's 11 functional health patterns, but found neither as relevant to the home health care setting as the 20 HHCC.

Teaching was identified as a nursing intervention in two recent empirically based classification studies [19] [9] A meta-analysis of nursing intervention research indication that 17 of 42 (40%) of these studies used instruction, teaching or information explanation as their type of intervention [15. p. 414].

A classification system has been developed that groups patients in to 11 functional health parameters based on prototypical descriptions of comprehensive nursing process needs on a four point scale [16]. Unlike other patient classification systems the Reitz intensity index uses the nursing process in its classification framework, including diagnosis, intervention and outcome and can be used in a variety of patient settings [16, p.30]. The index was pilot tested at John Hopkins Hospital retrospectively on patient records in surgery, medicine, pediatrics, ophthalmology, oncology, neurology psychiatry and gynecology/obstetrics for instrument validity and inter-rater agreement. This study yielded an average 90% inter-rater agreement across all clinical departments. A subsequent full scale study in the same institution yielded an average 84% inter-rater agreement across all clinical departments [16, p.32, 38].

4. Design of Nursing Information System

None of the studies discussed described a conceptual framework for designing a relational database of both nursing diagnoses and nursing interventions. The gerontological nursing information described is based on the data collection from six gerontological nursing case studies representing acute and community nursing care. Three acute and three community nursing care case studies were developed by the author with the assistance of gerontological master prepared nurses using the same model which was a scenario, listing of NANDA nursing diagnoses, objectives, criteria, nursing interventions and outcomes. Content validity and inter-rater reliability was established as described previously [17]. Thus an inductive approach was used to compile a database of thirty common nursing diagnoses and 283 related interventions.

The next phase of development for the gerontological NIS was the comprehensive review of the literature to compare the paper database with the existing classification schemes for nursing diagnoses and nursing interventions. A fundamental conceptual issue that related to the linking of nursing diagnoses and interventions is that nursing diagnosis reflect patient behavior and nursing interventions reflect nursing behavior. The majority of the literature reviewed failed to address this issue. The Reitz nursing intensity index was chosen for use as a nursing diagnosis classification scheme because (1) the patient is the unit of analysis rather then the discrete nursing intervention; (2) the nursing process serves as the fundamental framework [16] and (3) it is based on research. Concurrently existing databases developed for use with IBM compatible microcomputers were reviewed concluding with the choice of the Paradox relational database. Two NANDA problems were tested within gerontological NIS prototype incorporating Reitz classification systems. The decision to use the NMDS intervention categories was based on the following criteria; 1) availability of definitions for each category, 2) developed with nurse experts with a 78% inter-coder agreement, 3) further testing with consistent findings 40 likelihood that 7 categories would be more discriminating than four categories. 4) compatibility with Reitz classification system.

Design problems centered about the identification of requisite field, common fields, linkage schema, desired outputs of the system and overall conceptual framework. The design for the nursing information system is illustrated in Figure one. The fields for the diagnosis table include the diagnosis identification, functional health parameter and the NANDA problem. The diagnosis table is linked with the intervention table through Reitz's functional health parameters. The fields for the intervention table include the intervention identification, action category and specific intervention. There are four action categories; direct care, indirect care, monitor and teach. These categories evolved from terminology used by Werley, Saba, Bulechek and McCloskey [7,14,13]. The linkage flow chart will be used to provide examples of how the NIS can be used (see Figure 1).

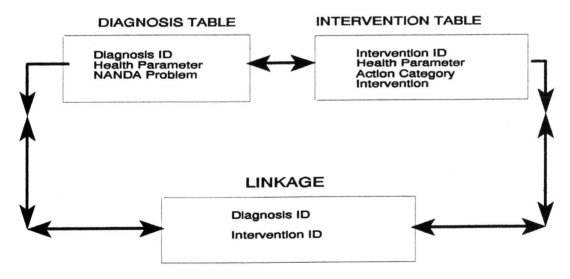

Figure 1. Linkage flow chart

The significance of this nursing information system is the creation of a conceptual framework to link nursing diagnoses and nursing interventions within a relational database. Once the NIS is established, anticipated benefits will include: 1) develop nursing care plans for gerontological clients, further define the domain of gerontological nursing practice, and teach database development. Future work involves the submission of the paper database to a gerontological expert panel to determine final placement of diagnoses within biophysical or behavioral health parameters. Validation of the gerontological database will occur through its use with gerontological nurses in a clinical setting.

372

5. References

[1] Poslusny S and McElmorry BJ. Developing Nursing Databases: Critical Considerations. *Vard I. Norden* 1990 2(3): 17-23.

[2] Aydelotte M and Peterson K. Keynote address: Nursing taxonomies - state of the art. In: *Classification of Nursing Diagnosis: Proceedings of the Seventh Conference.* McLane A (ed). Princeton: The C.V. Mosby Co., 1987: 1-15.

[3] Kritek PB. Development of a taxonomic structure for nursing diagnoses: A review and an update. In: *Classification of Nursing Diagnosis: Proceedings of the Sixth Conference.* Hurley, M. (ed). Princeton: The C.V. Mosby Co., 1986: 21-36.

[4] Hettinger BJ and Brazile RP. A Database Design for Community Health Data, *Comput Nurs* 1992, 10(3): 109-115.

[5] Yura H and Walsh MB. *The Nursing Process: Assessing, Planning, Implementing and Evaluating.* 3rd ed. New York: Appleton, Century & Crofts, 1978: 11.

[6] Harmer B. *Methods and Principles of Teaching the Practice of Nursing.* New York: Macmillan, 1926.

[7] Werley HH and Lang NM. *Identification of the Nursing Minimum Data Set.* New York: Springer Publishing Company, 1988.

[8] Bulechek GM and McCloskey JC. Nursing intervention taxonomy development. In: *Current Issues in Nursing.* McCloskey JC, Grace HR.(eds). 3rd ed. St. Louis: C.V. Mosby & Co., 1990: 23-28.

[9] Grobe SJ. Nursing intervention lexicon and taxonomy: preliminary categorization. In: *MEDINFO '92.* Lun KC, Degoulet P, Piemme TE, Reinhoff O. (eds). Holland: Elsevier Science Publishers, 1992: 981-986.

[10] Saba V. The Classification of Home Health Care Nursing: Diagnoses and Interventions. *Caring Magazine*, 1992, XI(3): 50-57.

[11] Devine EC and Werley HH. Test of the Nursing Minimum Data Set: Availability of Data and Reliability, *Res Nurs Health*, 1988, 11: 97-104.

[12] Leske JS and Werley HH. Use of the Nursing Minimum Data Set. *Comput Nurs*, 1992, 10(6): 259-63.

[13] Bulechek GM and McCloskey JC. Defining and Validating Nursing Interventions. *Nur Clin North*, 1992, 27(2): 289-299.

[14] Saba V and Zuckerman AE. A New Home Health Classification Method, *Caring Magazine*, 1992, X: 27-33.

[15] Holzemer WL. Quality and Cost of Nursing Care. *Nursing and Health Care*, 1991, 11(8): 412-415.

[16] Reitz JA. Toward a Comprehensive Nursing Intensity Index: Part I, Development. *Nursing Management,* 1985, 16(8): 21-30.

[17] Arnold JM. Development and testing of a diagnostic reasoning simulation In: *Measurement of Nursing Outcomes: Measuring Clinical Skills and Professional Development in Education and Practice.* Waltz, C. F., Strickland, O. L. (eds). New York: Springer. 1990, 3: 85-101.

© 1994 Elsevier Science B.V. All rights reserved.
Nursing Informatics: An International Overview for Nursing in a Technological Era
S.J. Grobe and E.S.P. Pluyter-Wenting, eds.

Where high-tech and high-touch meet:
A custom-designed database system for a
nursing outreach program to rural elderly

Currie L J and Abraham I L

Center on Aging and Health, University of Virginia, 170 Rugby Road, Charlottesville, Virginia 22903

The need to systematically and comprehensively manage data to support nursing services asserts itself in all areas and contexts where nursing services are delivered to patients and families. While most applications have targeted inpatient nursing services, several systems to sustain ambulatory nursing care have been proposed as well [1]. In this paper, we outline the purpose and general structure of a custom-designed computerized database management system to support the clinical, administrative, and research operations of a geriatric nursing outreach program in rural Virginia.

1. Introduction

Parallel to the need to continue developing systems to support clinical nursing operations in inpatient and outpatient environments, there is a need to extend the scope of clinical systems to all contexts of nursing care delivery, including nontraditional contexts where nursing is a leading discipline in the development and testing of new models of nursing and health care delivery. Furthermore, as this latter category may include innovative models of health care delivery in early experimental stages of development, there is an additional need to have access to data for program evaluation and related research efforts. In this paper, we outline the purpose and general structure of a custom-designed computerized database management system to support the clinical, administrative, and research operations of a geriatric nursing outreach program in rural Virginia.

2. Background

2.1. The Outreach Program

The Jefferson Area Rural Elder Health Consortium, a community partnership of the University of Virginia, the Jefferson Area Board for Aging (JABA), and the Region Ten Community Services Board, has developed an innovative outreach program that may serve as a model for other rural areas in the Southeast and South. The Rural Elder Outreach Program (REOP) aims to increase the accessibility of preventive, curative, and promotive health services to rural elderly and their families in the five county, 2,179 square mile area surrounding Charlottesville through in-home assessment, case management, and psychosocial support services. The Program's goal is to meet the health care needs of elderly residents in rural areas who do not have adequate access to health services and are at risk for institutionalization in nursing homes or psychiatric institutions, hospitalization in acute care facilities, or inappropriate use of emergency services. The major focus of the Program is to link formal community-based services, informal community resources, volunteer efforts, and academic resources in order to strengthen the self-reliance of rural communities to care for their elderly citizens.

The REOP provides outreach assessment, case management, and psychosocial support services by nurse case managers with masters preparation in psychogeriatric nursing. Potential clients are screened as to whether their needs are primarily of a health versus social service nature (with REOP assuming responsibility for the former). Initial telephone contact by the nurse clinicians is followed by an outreach visit. This visit includes a comprehensive psychogeriatric nursing assessment, caregiver assessment, collection of key medical data, and assessment of financial

374

and benefits information. Program services are explained and initial clinical action may be taken. Following initial intake, each case is presented at the weekly clinical staff meeting, which is attended by all disciplines involved in the program: nursing, social work, geriatrics, and geriatric psychiatry. Multidisciplinary care plans are developed and implementation strategies are discussed. This includes a discussion as to what the Program's involvement will be: (1) community referral; (2) referral to existing agency for care management, with the Program serving in a consultative capacity; or (3) care management by the Program. Procedures are also in place for follow-up, including re-assessments in the home and re-evaluation of service needs at specified later time points. For further description of services, see Abraham *et al* [2] and Buckwalter, Abraham, Smith, & Smullen [3].

2.2.Database Needs

The development of a computerized database system was a priority during REOP's start-up phase. The Program's clinical, research, and program management goals require a system capable of tracking clients and families throughout their association with the Program. Initial client data entry, as well as on-going data entry and tracking, requires the completion of numerous data collection forms and instruments; approximately 514 items per client and family (see Table 1). In addition, in order to accomplish both formative and summative evaluation of these goals, data need to be retrieved, analyzed, and reported every six months. Consequently, we required a database system which: (1) reflects the more than 514 unique variables of interest to REOP; (2) handles both numeric and character-type data; (3) possesses simple access and retrieval features; (4) allows migration of data to statistical software applications (in our case, SPSS/PC+); and (5) is capable of generating pre-programmed reports.

Furthermore, because most, if not all, of the data entry is performed by the nurse clinicians as part of their formal documentation procedures, the following features were also identified as requirements of the database system: (1) user-friendly menus and prompts commensurate with novice-user skill levels; (2) on-screen simulation of the forms and instruments to facilitate data entry ease and accuracy; and (3) print functions of on-screen simulated forms so that hard copies could be placed in patients' charts as official documentation.

Table 1
Data Collection Forms and Instruments

Title	Description*	Timetable
Initial Contact/REOP Referral Form	Basic demographics on patient, family, referral source; information on presenting problem. (24)	At intake
Financial Intake Form	Sources of monthly income for patient, spouse, other household members; insurance coverage; residence status; employment status; guardianship status. (63)	At intake
Intake Diagnosis Form	Clinical admission diagnosis based on DSM-III-R. (24)	At intake
Medical Assessment Form	Basic health status information: illness history, current problems, medications. (7)	At intake
Psychogeriatric Nursing Assessment Protocol (PNAP)	Physical and instrumental activities of daily living of patient and caregiver; cognitive status; depression scale; mood-dementia scale; geriatric behavioral scale; substance abuse; caregiver burden and coping; home environment. (250)	At intake, every 6 months, and at termination

Title	Description*	Timetable
Health Services Utilization Survey	Hospitalization; clinic visits; private doctors' office visits; emergency room visits; meal delivery or meal sites; nursing home; home health care; mental health services; transportation. (47)	At intake, every 6 months, and at termination
Multidisciplinary Progress Notes	Open-ended notes: telephone contact with patient or family; after home visits; after clinical staff meetings. (Text)	Ongoing
General Health Survey	Degree and type of physical limitations with particular activities; pain status; overall feeling of health. (20)	At intake and termination
Quality of Life Index	Level of physical activity, health, support, outlook. (6)	At intake and termination
Barriers & Facilitators Questionnaire	Specific aspects of REOP's services that positively or negatively influenced receipt of services. (27)	For patients and families: At termination
Satisfaction Questionnaire	Satisfaction with Program services. (16)	At termination
Termination Form	Summary of services provided, referrals, health status at termination. (6)	At termination
Termination Diagnosis Form	Clinical discharge diagnosis based on DSM-III-R. (24)	At termination

*Numbers in parentheses indicate the number of items associated with the form or instrument.

3. System Overview

The database management system is written in dBase IV to create a multi-relational, multi-module structure and is installed on a Novell network serving the offices of clinical, administrative, and research staff of the REOP. At this point in the system's development, the program is composed of 157 program files and uses slightly more than 2.9 Mb of disk space. When added to the 66 dBase IV program files, using approximately 3.4 Mb, the customized system requires almost 6.4 Mb. Therefore, since a typical patient record averages 8420 bytes, it is clear that this database system can be installed and used easily on a laptop PC with only a 20 MB hard disk.

The database program is invoked from the network's multi-user drive and thus can be accessed by multiple users simultaneously; however, individual client records can be opened by only one user at a time. This restriction prevents duplicate data entry.

Clients are automatically assigned an identification number based on the date and time of their initial entry into the system (e.g., John Doe: 1992-0106-11:53:32 was entered at 11:53:32 on January 6, 1992). System-assigned identification precludes the need for staff to check and maintain a list of identifying code numbers and prevents inadvertent duplication of identifiers. Client information and data can be retrieved and tracked according to either their first and/or last names, name initials, or all or part of their identifying number.

The program's opening screen lists the main menu selections: (1) Completion of the Forms and instruments listed in Table 1; (2) Printing Forms; (3) Producing Reports; and (4) Performing Database Maintenance. The Completion of Forms selection requires either entry of, or retrieval of, patients' basic demographic information so that their identifying number can be activated. Once this is done, pull-down menus for the specific forms and instruments are then invoked for data entry. At the top of each screen are user-activity selections (e.g., Zoom to invoke pull-down menus, Add a record, etc.). On the next line the individual's identifying number is displayed, as well as fields for entry of the date and the staff person's identifying initials. Actual data entry relies on both text and numeric characters. Numeric characters can either be typed in or the spacebar can be toggled to elicit the range of pre-programmed selections for the particular item. Since the on-screen form simulates the original hard copy form, the sequence of items for data entry is identical.

The Printing Forms feature can occur on either the network's laser printer for formal products or a dot matrix printer for rough drafts. The completed laser- printed forms are placed in the patient's chart as the Program's official clinical documentation.

The menu selection pertaining to Reports activates the retrieval of information concerning the Program's specific service delivery objectives, program evaluation procedures, and research questions. This process required the writing of additional customized program modules that identify the variables to be extracted from the database system at regular calendar intervals. At these times, the report-module programs perform listing, summarization, and basic tabulation activities on the pre-determined clusters of information. For more indepth analyses, data are migrated into SPSS/PC+ in order to conduct the necessary statistical tests.

The Database Maintenance menu item enables updating of demographic data on patients, families, referral sources, and staff. This feature expedites management of the database system since new or modified information entered in this feature is automatically distributed throughout the individual's record. Similarly, additions or changes regarding referral sources and REOP staff can be entered into the system at this one point and thereby activated throughout the database program.

Initial client and family data are entered into the program by the nurse clinicians from their laptop PCs following determination in the clinical staff meeting of the client's appropriateness for case management services. This can be done on-line by connecting laptop PCs to the network, or off-line on the laptops followed by downloading of data into the network at a later point in time. As clients continue to receive the Program's services, assessments are repeated on a regular basis by the nurse clinicians and entered into the database program (see Table 1).

3.1.System Security

System security is maintained by a number of methods. Since all database information is stored on the network server, manual and automatic tape back-ups are performed on a regular basis. In addition, the database program is also installed on one of the nine work station PCs, thus functioning as a back-up system upon which the data tapes can be downloaded. Data security, and thus client privacy and confidentiality, is protected by the limited number of total network users, restricting staff's knowledge of system access to a "need to know" basis, programming the network with automatic password expiration dates, and changing user's network passwords at random intervals. Furthermore, multiple attempts to enter an unrecognized password result in a lock-up of both the database program and the network, which can only be re-activated by the network supervisor.

At regular intervals the database system is momentarily inactivated so that all existing data can be transferred or downloaded to a duplicate, but separate, file. This second file is used for generating pre-programmed reports and facilitates the importing of data into SPSS/PC+ for statistical analyses. The temporary inactivation of the database program ensures that all patients' system files are closed during the moments of downloading, so that data complete the transfer process intact.

4. Applications

Although the emphasis of REOP's custom-designed data system is on data management rather than the formalized concept of decision support, it does have an important role in three primary areas of REOP's operations: clinical, administrative, and research. From a clinical perspective, the system facilitates the extensive clinical documentation that is required in case management when clients are followed on a long-term basis. Hand written and mental note-taking that occur in the field are more quickly and easily transferred into formal documentation via keyboard entry into the database program than with traditional hand written transcription. Similarly, information retrieval by the clinicians in order to update, or more importantly compare, a client's status from one visit to another is expedited by using the program since data can be located instantaneously. Furthermore, since data elements can be retrieved and analyzed according to almost any criteria, the nurse clinicians are able to obtain a description and analysis of their case load, by individual client or by groupings, in a matter of minutes.

The database program's clinical applications flow directly into its uses in administrative operations. REOP's program evaluation plan is anchored in the ongoing assessment of the information obtained from the instruments listed in Table 1. Formative and summative evaluations of REOP's goals and objectives are facilitated and expedited by staff administrators' and clinicians' ongoing current access to and utilization of the data obtained by the clinicians and entered in the database system. Data such as outreach penetration, client demographics, and clinical outcomes are regularly tabulated, analyzed, and summarized so that they can be used in administrative and clinical staff meetings to inform decision making regarding REOP's structure, organization, and service delivery activities.

Finally, the custom-designed system provides ready access to data needed to conduct and report research. Since the database system contains and manages only the variables of interest unique to REOP, research questions and findings can be readily identified and reported with regard to case management outreach to rural elderly.

5. Future Plans

We anticipate that our clinical, administrative, and research database management needs will continue to evolve, change, and expand. Consequently, we expect that the program will require further revisions and expansions. The advantage of the multi-modular design structure is that it readily lends itself to changes both within and across elements of the system. Furthermore, we hope to gain valuable feedback on the database program's design and features as it is tested in other settings that provide health care services similar to our Program's model. Based on our experience with the system, it is evident that it holds promise for being a convenient, useful, and cost-effective method of managing data in nontraditional health care delivery settings.

6. References

[1] Saba VK, Rieder KA and Pocklington DB. (Eds.). *Nursing and computers: An Anthology.* New York: Springer-Verlag, 1989.

[2] Abraham IL, Buckwalter KC, Snustad DG, Smullen DE, Thompson-Heisterman AA, Neese JB, and Smith M. Psychogeriatric outreach to rural families: The Iowa and Virginia models. *Int Psychogeriatr,* in press.

[3] Buckwalter KC, Abraham IL, Smith MA, and Smullen DE. Nursing outreach to the mentally ill rural elderly. *Hosp Community Psychiatry,* in press.

Nursing Informatics: An International Overview for Nursing in a Technological Era
S.J. Grobe and E.S.P. Pluyter-Wenting, eds.

378

Development of a Nursing-Diagnosis Based Integrated, Computerized Documentation and Care Planning System for Long-Term Care

Rantz M J

School of Nursing, University of Missouri-Columbia, Columbia, MO 65211

A committee consisting of Registered Nurses (three with advanced preparation in nursing) designed an overall plan for a computerized documentation system which has resulted in an integrated, computerized documentation and care planning sytem that is nursing diagnosis driven for a 328 bed county operated nursing home. This documentation system integrates with the federal regulations recently mandated for long term care. The system uses a nursing diagnosis framework including comprehensive assessment, nursing diagnoses, etiologies, defining characteristics, resident outcomes/goals, and interventions specific to long term care. Resident-specific nurse and nursing assistant care delivery directions and chart forms are generated from the system. The flexibility of the computer allows the user to expand the federally mandated assessment tool to meet internal needs of the facility while providing regulators with required assessment information. The documentation system facilitates nursing process and practice while satisfying regulatory documentation requirements. It analyszes specific documentation decisions made by the nursing staff related to regulations; additionally, the system generates required forms which indicate if care planning regulations have been met. The system facilitates the nursing process by allowing the nurse to focus on a complete assessment, make appropriate nursing diagnoses and develop an appropriate individualized care plan. It de-emphasizes the need to satisfy specific regulations which may or may not be germane to a specific resident's care. Audit trials were prepared to monitor user progress, compliance with documentation requirements, and reports for quality assurance evaluations.

1. Developing the Care Plan Data Base

A comprehensive system of preparing nursing care plans using a nursing diagnosis framework was implemented in a 328 - bed skilled nursing facility in 1982. Care plans developed throughout the years were the data source from which objectively validated care plan components were identified for the long-term care population. (The researcher for this project was hired as Nursing Administrator of this facility in 1981 and promoted to Administrator 1983-1992.)

The system of care planning that was implemented was carefully designed to provide valid data describing etiologies, defining characteristics, resident outcomes/goals, and interventions for North American Nursing Diagnosis Association (NANDA) accepted and commonly used nursing diagnosis labels. An additional intention in designing the system was to extend the work of the nursing diagnosis movement. A content analysis was undertaken from randomly selected care plans in our medical records system for the years 1984-1986.

Procedures for the content analysis included listing the identified etiologies, defining characteristics, resident outcomes/goals, and interventions in descending order of frequency of occurrence within the sample. The content analysis included multiple iterations completed by two masters-prepared nurses who evaluated items based on clinical practice relevancy and application to the population of elderly nursing home residents. An editing process included referencing material to NANDA, Gordon, and other relevant nursing diagnosis experts. The content analyses was completed in 1987 and provided an empirically sound data base to enter into a computerized documentation system. Previous efforts discussed in the literature have been directed toward group consensus of expert nurses or simple group consensus of staff in a particular agency. The scope of this content analysis is one of the broadest attempts to prepare a data base for use in a computerized charting system or any hard copy documentation for long-term care [1]. As computerization efforts began, other nurses participated in evaluating the applicability of the care plan content.

2. Developing a Nurse-Designed Computerized Charting and Care Planning System

The intent of the computerization effort was based on a professional practice model using organizational participation, active involvement in decision making and nursing diagnosis. The professional practice model was a driving force for the development of the nursing information system for our facility. A major complaint from our staff was the amount of time devoted to documentation. Time to handwrite care plans needed to be reduced, so that nurses had time to deal with increasing acuity of our residents. Additionally, we wanted to evaluate other options for documentation practices to comply with increasing volumes of regulations.

During 1987 and 1988 much time was devoted to reviewing existing software for care planning and charting relevant to long-term care. Staff opinion was that none of the commercially available systems they evaluated appropriately addressed the needs of the long-term care resident, nursing home regulations, and, most of all, the nursing process. Nursing staff consensus was that as an agency we should develop a system for long-term care based on a nursing diagnosis model that would support the nursing process and enhance strengths of our established care planning system. Additionally, the system had to support and enhance quality assurance/assessment activities [2] and incorporate the elements of the Nursing Minimum Data Set [3].

Efforts to fund a computerized charting system were begun in 1987. In the fall of 1988 funding was obtained to begin in 1989 for programming and hardware costs. Our agency had telephone line access to two main frame computers. One was handling billing, resident accounts, and payroll. A second provided computerized physicians' orders, pharmacy records, and a custom-designed dietary meal ticket system.

When funding was approved, many nurses volunteered to participate in a Computer Steering Committee to develop the system. As a group, the nurses were excited about the possibility of computerizing care plans and other charting. A solicitation memo was circulated to all licensed staff and all direct care departments asking volunteers to join the Computer Steering Committee. The committee was charged with designing the overall charting system, assisting with the specifics of development of chart forms, and critiquing work done by committee subgroups. This committee was projected to be the liaison with project programmers from the County Data Department.

Funds were available for a nursing computer consultant to assist our committee in the decision-making process. The doctorally prepared consultant attended a January 1989 meeting of the Computer Steering Committee. The consultant suggested that we select a subcommittee from the Computer Steering Committee to meet and reconceptualize the essential components of the projected computerized charting system.

3. Reconceptualizing the Documentation System

Volunteers were selected and a seven-member Computerization Subcommittee was formed. These members were two masters-prepared nurses from nursing administration, one masters-prepared clinical nurse specialist, two nurse managers, and two experienced registered nurses who had recently completed baccalaureate degrees in nursing. This subcommittee met for six hours without interruption and reconceptualized the charting system. Before the meeting, state and federal regulations, including OBRA '87 information, were circulated to each committee member with directions to carefully review code requirements related to documentation. The consultant suggested that we begin the meeting with directions to all committee members to attempt to "blank out any thoughts of the current charting system, to begin again by determining exactly what was necessary in the system, and to think about how we want to organize the necessary information."

Six hours in this small group reconceptualizing the system was time well spent in the development of the computerized charting system. By examining actual mandated requirements and then making decisions about what we really wanted the system to facilitate, the overall design became clear. Conceptualizing the documentation system as being driven by each resident-specific care plan was a key idea generated during this group effort. The group identified a cluster of four or five nursing diagnoses that contained information in etiologies, defining characteristics, outcomes/goals, and approaches that could be extracted by the computer and compiled for a nurse attendant worksheet and related documentation tool. Additionally, a licensed nurse worksheet and documentation tool could be extracted from the computer in the same way. These worksheets and documentation tools would then be specific to the care delivered to each resident. We anticipated retaining our current narrative documentation system that is problem-oriented, focusing on each nursing diagnosis and the current status of each resident's goal attainment. We thought the computer could enhance the narrative notation process by retrieving notations about a specific diagnosis to assist the nurse writing current status notes. Retrieval also would be important in retrospective auditing for quality assurance/assessment activities.

Having reconceptualized the overall nursing documentation system, the small group shifted attention to how this system would interface with other parts of the medical record used by other departments. To facilitate this effort, we used a hypothetical admission and brainstormed all documentation necessary for a new admission using the new system.

It must be noted that the people in this work group had limited computer backgrounds. The nurse computer consultant was not present during this Computerization Subcommittee meeting: her skills were used earlier and later in the development process. Explicit meeting minutes describing conceptualization of the documentation system were dictated and circulated to the entire Computer Steering Committee. The Computer Steering Committee then met, discussed, and concurred with the Computerization Subcommittee decisions made about the basic design of the system.

4. Refining Content and Information for the System

Subgroups were formed to refine key nursing diagnoses care plan content and to identify information that would automatically transfer to worksheets and other documentation forms. Other tasks included refining the current treatment card system, preparing information for computerized labels to be linked to physicians' orders and medication administration records, and redesigning assessment worksheets and reports. The enthusiasm of several staff members was contagious. Two staff registered nurses were especially enthusiastic. They informally shared their positive comments, and their enthusiasm for developing our own computerized charting system quickly spread throughout the nursing staff. The system was designed in a way that nurses would find useful, timesaving, and meets the individual needs of our residents. Most important, the system reinforces the nursing process, enhances nursing practice, and subsequently, the quality of care in our facility.

Concurrent with the development of these computerization efforts, the long-term care industry became aware of the federal OBRA '87 mandate that the minimum data set (MDS) be required for resident assessment by all nursing homes. As drafts became available, we evaluated the content of the assessment information and planned for enhancing the data required. From inception of the computer system, plans included computerization of the MDS and additional assessment tools.

Programming for the computerized documentation system began during 1989. The programmer met with the Computerization Subcommittee to develop a programming approach to meet our needs. Close relationships developed between the programming staff and nursing staff. Both were impressed with each others' respective expertise. The programmer attempted to learn as much as possible about what different nursing jobs entailed and how the computer system might be supportive. Testing of the computer programs by our nursing staff began in March of 1990. Subcommittee members were challenged to "break the system" to assist the programmer in "debugging" programs. Actual use of the system is an integral part of testing it.

5. Dealing with Regulations While Supporting Diagnostic Reasoning

The OBRA '87 mandated MDS was implemented nationwide in October 1990. Our MDS programming was in place and tested. The nurses believed strongly that the MDS required by OBRA was incomplete, and, while some individual questions were relevant, many components were missing. Also, we believed maintaining a nursing framework for the assessment tool was important. We had used Gordon's Functional Health Patterns for almost 10 years, and we believed it imperative to continue its use. Computerization Subcommittee members clustered the MDS questions into the appropriate sections of Gordon's framework. Using our prior assessment instruments, they brainstormed additional items and physical assessment questions to accompany the MDS items. Early in planning the assessment tool, the programmer accommodated our desire to use Gordon's framework in a more comprehensive assessment. We wanted to input the information from hard copy assessment worksheets into the computer and generate two reports: one report with the questions in the specific order and framework required by OBRA regulations for official level of care determinations by regulators and a second report with the complete assessment information organized in Gordon's Functional Health Patterns for our own internal clinical use.

In January 1991 the computer care plan module was thoroughly tested and initial testing was begun on the narrative note component of the system. Because we had not anticipated the regulations requiring the triggers and resident assessment protocols (RAPs), that particular programming was not completed until late 1990; we began testing those system components in 1991. The triggers and RAPs presented an interesting dilemma for nurses. Nationwide reports indicated that hours were being spent double checking RAPs and triggers when analysis of care plans was revealing that all items (or at least 98% of them) were already addressed in previously developed care plans. We decided our goal would be to design support for the triggers that would allow nurses to focus on the nursing process rather than focus on satisfying specific documentation requirements. The computer program was designed to check if specific care planning decisions were made by the nurse that would satisfy the triggers and generate the required RAPs Summary form that indicates which triggers have or have not been addressed in the care planning process. The computer allows the nurse to focus on the assessment, make appropriate nursing diagnoses, and develop an appropriate care plan, not simply focus on assuring compliance with regulations.

Many facilities have developed care planning systems generated from the MDS, triggers, and RAPs. The danger we envisioned in using the RAPs and trigger system as a foundation for care planning is that this approach conceptually interferes with diagnostic reasoning and the nursing process. According to Gordon [4], the word diagnosis has two meanings. It refers to the name for a health problem found in a classification system of nursing diagnosis, an it also means a process leading to a clinical judgment. By virtue of education and licensure, the professional nurse has the cognitive foundation necessary for acquiring and using clinical information. Gordon describes four areas of the diagnostic process: collecting the information, interpreting the information, clustering the information, and naming the cluster. This process is a cycle of perceptual and cognitive activities of the professional nurse that ultimately results in identifying a nursing diagnosis. The diagnostic reasoning process is influenced by the nurse's clinical knowledge and critical reasoning; ultimately, the diagnosis provides a focus for the nursing care planning and evaluation process.

The RAPs and triggers are limited to 18 problem-oriented assessment areas. We believe the nursing knowledge processing in each nurse's head is more extensive than the information within the 18 RAPs. Simply focusing on the triggered items from the MDS will not generate a comprehensive care plan and will severely limit the nursing assessment and diagnostic process. In our system, nurses consider and use the information from the RAPs and trigger system as required by regulators. We use this as supportive information to the entire comprehensive care planning process. Ultimately, a comprehensive care plan based on a more comprehensive assessment is generated by the nursing and interdisciplinary staffs.

6. Supporting On-going Implementation and Evaluation Activities

Consistent with the participative management model in place in our facility, a participative committee was formed in the spring of 1991 to assist in the final stages of implementation. This computer committee, the Bits and Bytes Committee, is a multidisciplinary group of users who are enthusiastic about the computer system. In a group process, they are making practical decisions about implementation and the policies related to care planning and documentation. They also are advising the data department when additional programming is needed to enhance specific features of the documentation system. They have participated in refining some content developed for use in the computer care plan system. They have made practical suggestions for changes in computer screens to make them user friendly. They are now an essential component to monitoring and evaluating the system.

During the summer of 1991, audit trails were programmed to monitor user compliance with the documentation requirements. We needed to have methods of identifying those nurses who were having difficulty learning how to use the computer system without examining the medical records of all our residents. Throughout 1991 other audits were made available by the data department to help us monitor and evaluate the system from a quality assurance/assessment perspective. We can identify frequencies from individual MDS items or care plan components that can function as quality indicators for analysis. With the capacity of the computer, analysis of defining characteristics, etiologies, resident outcomes/goals, and interventions as well as the myriad of other individual data can be accomplished from one point in time or from a longitudinal perspective. Diagnosis-specific evaluation of care plan components and outcomes can be conducted as well as evaluations across multiple diagnoses. Outcome evaluations linked to MDS assessment data can be undertaken. The limits of quality assurance/assessment activities are boundarized only by organizational commitment to support and encourage evaluation.

7. References

[1] Rantz MJ, and Miller TV. *Quality Documentation for Long-Term Care: A Nursing Diagnosis Approach.* Gaithersburg, MD: Aspen, 1993.

[2] Miller TV and Rantz MJ. *Quality Assurance for Long-Term Care: Guidelines and Procedures for Monitoring Practice.* Gaithersburg, MD: Aspen, 1992.

[3] Werley H. Nursing diagnosis and the nursing minimum data set. In: *Classification of Nursing Diagnosis - Proceedings of the Conferences of the North American Nursing Diagnosis Association.* McLane A (ed). St. Louis: Mosby, 1987: 21-36.

[4] Gordon M. *Nursing Diagnosis Process and Application.* New York: McGraw Hill, 1987.

Nursing Informatics: An International Overview for Nursing in a Technological Era
S.J. Grobe and E.S.P. Pluyter-Wenting, eds.

The reliability of summary descriptions of monitored nurse activities within a Care of the Elderly ward in a psychiatric hospital.

Rimmer P[a] Jones B T[b] Munro S[a] and Mc Mahon J[b]

[a]*Gartnavel Royal Hospital, Mental Health Unit, Greater Glasgow Health Board, Glasgow G12)XH, Scotland UK*

[b]*Department of Psychology (Nurse Information Processing Group), University of Glasgow G128QQ, Scotland UK*

To get good data from time-sampled activity monitoring exercises requires attention to be paid to two quite separate issues: the *validity* and *reliability* of the data recorded from the monitoring process. The former is a *professional* concern and is well-recognised. The latter is a *statistical* concern and is poorly-recognised by the profession - but, in practice, no less important. This paper describes one way of assessing the statistical reliability of, otherwise, valid data from a time-sampled activity monitoring exercise.

1. Background

There are many reasons for wanting to monitor the activity of nurses in hospital wards. Usually, these reasons relate to either costing, manpower planning, manpower management or care quality exercises [1].

Whatever is the nature of the exercise, activity monitoring sessions typically take 'snapshots' on a periodic basis of what the ward staff are doing and from this sample is derived an overall statement of ward work. Of course, there are difficulties. These difficulties relate to data *validity* and data *reliability*.

1.1. Data validity.

How well does the monitored record represent what is actually done?

(i). If the continuous process of nursing is to be represented in this way, it needs to be broken down to a finite list of well-define categories of activity that are exhaustive of what nurses do.

(ii). Once a particular activity has been identified as representing what a single nurse is doing at one point in time, it needs to be assumed that this single activity is the only activity that is immediately current.

(iii). Once regularly time-sampled representations of what a single nurse has been doing have been secured, extrapolations need to occur to turn the discrete and partial representation in to a continuous and whole one.

(iv). Once such a representation has been derived it needs to be 'aggregated-up' across nurses, shifts, days, wards, specialities, hospitals etc to serve whatever purpose the activity monitoring exercise was designed to address.

Those within nursing who put store by activity monitoring exercises such as this need to be careful to ensure that the data does, indeed, represent what they *think* it represents [2]. They need to be sure that the data is valid. Of course this problem is well-recognised and many procedures have been adopted to help *maximise* the data's validity (or quality). Indeed, many of the professional issues addressed in respect of this have to be also addressed when considering how valid is costing, planning and management information acquired from 'off the back of' careplans authored with ward-based nursing information systems [3] - because the discrete representation of continuous care to be subsequently aggregated-up for costing, planning and management is also a central feature of these machines (some would argue it is *the* central feature).

The procedures that help assure the quality or validity of monitored data are as interesting as they are important. They are not the focus of this paper, however. This paper focuses on an equally interesting and, perhaps, even *more* important issue than data validity - data reliability. We risk using the modifier 'more', here, because the issue appears to go unrecognised and for this reason it is potentially dangerous, potentially compromising apparently valid data.

1.2. Data reliability

How likely is it that the monitored record would be the same if it were collected again? Of course, if attention had not been properly paid to many of the points raised above in respect of validity, then the answer to this question might be "not very likely". Even if attention had been properly paid to these points, then it is no guarantee that the record would be a good one. There is compelling evidence that the reliability of data collected within the nursing workload management/planning framework, in general, is poor and misleading [4]. In our own case, for example, the nurse-monitor might not have been properly trained, might not have been sufficiently diligent or might have been honestly mistaken in judging what others were doing. It might even be that under some hitherto unidentified set of circumstances, valid monitoring is *simply not possible* (but this has not been realised). There is no magic solution to this, of course, but there *are* things that can be done to help ensure that even when there are good reasons for believing that the constituent data of a monitored record is professionally valid, it is also *statistically reliable*.

One procedure that we are routinely adopting to assess whether the monitored record is, indeed, statistically reliable is described below. (In practice, we find about one record in seven is not.)

2. The project

As one (but only one) of the inputs into a process for establishing a job-specification for different grades of nurse working in Care of the Elderly wards, an activity monitoring exercise was designed to discover what different grades of nurses *do* in a ward that had already been identified and assessed as delivering quality care [5]. In addition, since with the Project 2000 departure (nurse education's plan for a new future in the UK) student nurses were to become supernumerary as far as staffing wards is concerned, it was important to know what range of activities students had been carrying out *before* the P2000 implementation because these would have to be picked up by other current or additional ward staff.

Unfortunately, activity monitoring is cruelly labour-intensive [6,7] and what many forget is that transcribing the data for subsequent processing is even more so (let alone the transcription errors that regularly occur). Also, with traditional activity monitoring exercises, more cognitive effort is usually diverted towards recording what had been monitored (and this is something *anybody* can do) rather than towards the monitoring, itself, which we view as the intelligent application of nursing knowledge to decide what nursing is currently occurring (and this is definitely *not* something anybody can do). This describes a state of affairs that is exactly the wrong way round because *maximum* cognitive effort should be diverted towards the latter (monitoring) and *minimum* to the former (recording).

2.1. WAM and WIP

To help achieve this, Jones [8] has designed an easily-used computer-based recording program to relieve the nurse-monitor of as much cognitive effort as is conceivably possible. This *liberates* the nurse-monitor to direct more cognitive effort to classifying what is going on around her/him (monitoring). The program is called WAM (Ward Activity Monitor). It also by-passes the other labour-intensive part of activity monitoring exercises, namely, transcribing the data for subsequent analysis for once recorded (as a computer file) it is accessible to WIP (WAM Information Processor). This is now seen by those who consult in nurse manpower management/planning as having "developed the efficiency and effectiveness of recording nursing interventions" [7] and the approach has now been adopted by the largest health board in Scotland. What they have failed to appreciate, however, is that within this approach (within WIP) there is opportunity to *automatically* and *routinely* assess the data's statistical reliability.

Although WAM/WIP is being demonstrated at NI'94, a brief description follows to serve as an introduction to an account of the reliability assessment.

Original versions of WAM were written in HyperTalk (the scripting language of Apple's HyperCard) and implemented using a MacPlus. More recent versions have used PLUS2 instead of HyperCard for three reasons: (i) it has a better programmer's interface; (ii) it supports full colour more readily and (iii) it allows cross-platform access for there are versions of PLUS2 for both Apple and (IBM)-Compatible machines. Our current preferred machines are Apple LCs (cheap but bulky) and PowerBook 180cs (more expensive but conveniently small).

The WAM screen contains small, rectangular, colour-differentiated buttons that are activated by pressing them with the screen pointer under hand-mouse or hand-trackball control. Buttons represent and carry on their surface the different items from each of the following: (i) the names of nursing staff (grade information is hidden under the button); (ii) the list of nurse activities; (iii) the list of patients (dependency information is hidden under the button) and (iv) invisible buttons cover the important locations of a plan of the ward currently being monitored that is also held on the screen. Most importantly, nurse name/grade and patient name/dependency can be edited in momemts at any time during monitoring as nurses/patients arrive and leave the ward or their status changes. (WAM was developed, originally, for a fast-moving ENT ward that directly received accidents and emergencies and had a hefty day-surgery load and fast/easy editing of both nurse and patient information was an important prerequisite).

By pressing four buttons appropriately, the following information is recorded: *who* (and what grade) is doing *what*, to *whom* (and what dependency) and *where*. If the activity is not directly or indirectly patient-centered, then no patient need be selected. This process takes seconds. If monitoring is 10-minutely (the most frequently-used periodicity) and if there are a half dozen nurses to be monitored, then recording takes less than thirty seconds. A count-down clock is present on the screen to indicate what length of time away is the next sample to be taken. These time indications are for the nurse-monitor's guidance only because each button-press is automatically (real) time-logged to the nearest second and checks on periodicity can be subsequently carried out if required.

Subsequent shift-analyses can be by-nurse (individuals or grades), -locations, -activities, -patients (individuals or dependencies) or any of these can be aggregated-up to shift level. When shifts and wards are combined, subsequent analyses can be carried out by-shift and -ward. In addition, the forty or fifty individual nursing activities that are the basis of the monitoring can be combined. For example, in Care of the Elderly we are currently using the global categories: Direct care, Indirect care, Administration, Meetings, Housekeeping and Other (including personal time).

2.2. Rationale behind reliability testing

Consider the following: if time-sampled monitoring were to be carried out, then there is no real reason to believe that whatever profile the analyses produce for the first third of a shift should be the same as the middle third or the last third (take as a profile, the frequency of occurrence histogram of the nursing activities). Indeed, it would be a worrying surprise if the profiles *were* identical because different parts of any shift capture different patient needs and this would impact upon the frequency of occurrence of the different nursing activities (and this is particularly apparent in, but definitely not restricted to, Care of the Elderly).

However, if two independent monitoring processes were set up side-by-side then, whatever profiles were derived from them, *should* be identical no matter what part of the shift the analyses addressed. A useful reliabilty check could be carried out by *comparing the frequency of occurrence of activities* from each of the monitoring processes using a chi-square test. Parallel monitoring, however, is not only expensive but even more invasive than single monitoring and we rarely carry it out. *Virtual* parallel monitoring is how we have tried to solve this problem.

Virtual parallel monitoring allows us to derive two apparently-parallel monitoring processes from a single one (see Figure 1, over). If monitoring is *inconsistent*, so we have shown, then when the frequency of occurrence of the nursing activities from the two monitoring processes that come from virtual parallel monitoring are compared using chi-sq procedures, reliable differences are detected in the profiles. When monitoring is *consistent*, however, no reliable differences are found. We have usually used the six grouped nursing activities referred to above to do this because when the whole range of activities are individually employed (often as many as fifty), the test becomes too sensitive to the noise that is almost certainly a feature at this level of representation.

A word about inconsistent and consistent monitoring. We have *simulated* these two types of monitoring in a number of ways in order to explore the variability in reliability (using the chi-square test) that virtual parallel monitoring can potentially bring. We have examined the differences using WAM-untrained nurses, WAM-trained nurses, novices, WAM-trained nurses who were given (artificial) reasons for being *particularly* diligent in their efforts and WAM-trained nurses who were given (artificial) reasons for their efforts not *really* mattering. We have also, ourselves, monitored in an extremely slovenly fashion that bordered upon guessing!

2.3 Assessing reliability

What we have discovered is that in our simulations, no reliable differences are detected between the two virtual procedures when (i) monitoring is deliberately slovenly or when (ii) much effort goes into 'getting it right' by

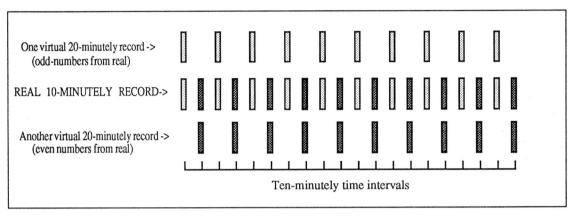

One virtual 20-minutely record -> (odd-numbers from real)

REAL 10-MINUTELY RECORD->

Another virtual 20-minutely record -> (even numbers from real)

Ten-minutely time intervals

Figure 1. Real 10-minutely activity sampling divided into two virtual 20-minutely parallel activity samplings

appropriately trained and motivated staff. Although the latter should not surprise, the former might. However, it does demonstrate when a reliable difference is *not* detected, it does not *always* mean that the monitoring is sound. Fortunately, such extreme circumstances will be very infrequent and they are easily detected by simply looking at the frequency profiles produced because they invariably will not make nursing sense.

On those occasions when monitoring was carried out by those (i) who were not necessarily motivated or (ii) who were not aware of the pitfalls of activity monitoring, in general, or WAM, in particular, reliable differences between the two virtual procedures were almost invariably detected. Table 1 illustrates this comparison for both a single unmotivated and a single motivated WAM-trained nurse monitor. The former was instructed that the WAM session was primarily designed to help accustom ward staff to the intrusion and the latter was instructed that the recorded information was to be the focus of a monthly ward management meeting that they would be invited to attend.

Table 1.
Comparing pairs of virtual records for a motivated and an unmotivated nurse monitor using grouped nurse activities

	Motivated		Unmotivated	
	virtual record		virtual record	
	odd	even	odd	even
Administration	15	16	6	15
Meetings	7	10	10	11
Housekeeping	14	12	19	10
Other	17	21	21	9
Direct care	56	49	36	55
Indirect care	12	14	20	12
χ^2	3.8		40.8	
df	5		5	
p	>0.5		<0.001	

. Conclusion

This encourages us to believe that it is possible to determine whether data produced by ward activity monitoring is reliable or not - and that it is an important assessment to be made *independently* of the validity question. Moreover, if ward activity monitoring is to be carried out in the least of labour-intensive ways (which in the days of limited resources is an important point) and if this observation is extended to included post-monitoring analysis, then computer-based recording is essential for the reasons discussed earlier. If the record of the monitoring is held as a computer file, then it is computationally trivial to automatically and routinely assess its statistical reliability along the lines indicated above. When the data is unreliable, of course, it should not be used. More to the point, though, when you don't *know* whether the data is reliable or not *it should not be used either!*

This paper has been designed to bring attention to this unrecognised problem. As a final note, any person who has taken part in an activity monitoring exercise (especially using stopwatches, clipboards, booklets of proforma and different coloured pencils to tick and cross appropriate boxes on appropriate pages every 10 minutes) knows that it is no straw man to suggest that due diligence might not *always* be securely in place. When individuals monitor for hours on end and even for whole shifts (which is routinely done with WAM), assuring the quality of the data goes *beyond* issues of professional validity.

Elsewhere, Jones [9] has argued for a working definition of informatics that embraces (among other things) the need to research the *use* to which data can be satisfactorilyput. The problem that this paper addresses and the attempt to find a solution are derived from this approach.

4. References

[1] Hurst K. Learning workforce planning from the school of hard knocks: Part 2 Nursing role, nursing grade mix and nursing quality. *International Journal of Health Informatics* 1992, 2/2:15-17.

[2] Jenkins-Clarke S. From lamps to laptops: Measuring nursing workload. *International Journal of Health Informatics* 1992, 2/1:11-14.

[3] Hoy D. Computer assisted nursing care planning in the UK *Information Technology in Nursing* 1990, 2/2):22-23

[4] Jenkins-Clarke S and Carr-Hill R. Nursing workload measures and case-mix: An investigation of the reliability and validity of nursing workload measures. Centre for Health Economics, University of York UK, 1991

[5] Ball J and Goldstone LA. 1984 Criteria for care - Manual. Newcastle-upon-Tyne Polytechnic Products Ltd, Newcastle-upon-Tyne UK, 1984.

[6] Jenkins-Clarke S. Measuring nursing workload: A cautionary tale. Health Economics Consortium Discussion Paper 96, University of York UK, 1992

[7] Hurst K. Learning workforce planning from the school of hard knocks: Part 1 Theory and practice of patient dependency measurement and nursing activity analysis. *International Journal of Health Informatics* 1992, 2/1:17-19.

[8] Jones BT and Buchanan M. Relieving the bottlenecks in Ward Activity Monitoring through I.T.: WAM and WIP, solutions using Apple's HyperCard. *Information Technology in Nursing*, 1989, 1/2: 27 - 31.

[9] Jones BT. Heeding, measuring,utilising, the informatics template: An explicit working definition for informatics. *International Journal of Health Informatics.* 1993, 2/2:in press.

Nursing Informatics: An International Overview for Nursing in a Technological Era
S.J. Grobe and E.S.P. Pluyter-Wenting, eds.

The Electronic Community:
An Alternative Health Care Approach

Skiba D J [a] and Mirque D T [b]

[a]*School of Nursing, University of Colorado Health Sciences Center, Campus Box C-288, 4200 E. Ninth Ave., Denver, CO 80262 USA.*

[b]*School of Nursing, University of Colorado Health Sciences Center, Campus Box C-288, 4200 E. Ninth Ave., Denver, CO 80262 USA.*

Electronic communities, not bound by distance or time barriers, will serve as an emerging technology for the delivery of health care in the 21st Century. The merger of information technology and telecommunications provide a fertile ground for the development of alternative health care delivery systems. National Health Care Reform and a renewed emphasis on health promotion and prevention are the building blocks for this development. Community computing systems and health-oriented telecommunications are being combined to foster the concept of "healthy communities" throughout the nation. The intent of this paper is to describe the implementation of the Denver Free-Net Project, an electronic community computing system, and its potential impact on the delivery of nursing care in the state of Colorado.

1. Background

Health care expenditures in the United States have reached staggering proportions, 761 billion dollars in 1990 representing 12.2% of the gross national product (GNP) [1]. There is consensus among the health care professions that much of the injuries and illnesses contributing to this cost can be prevented through widespread adoption of improved safety practices and healthier lifestyles [2]. The promotion of health and prevention of disease are the basis of the health care reform movement and of the government initiative, Healthy People 2000. Health promotion and disease prevention are considered methods to: dramatically cut health care costs, prevent premature onset of disease and disability, and help all Americans achieve healthier and more productive lives [3]. The National Agenda for Health Care is based upon three assumptions: personal responsibility is a key to good health, health care should be accessible and available to every citizen, and that prevention is described in its broadest perspective [3]. In Colorado, these initiatives are examined by a governor-appointed task force, the Colorado Health Care Reform Initiative [4].

To achieve the health goals, individuals must understand the relationship between lifestyle behaviors and their medical consequences. Individuals must have readily accessible health care information to promote this understanding. Further, the broad definition of health must extend beyond the notion of absence of disease. The World Health Organization defines a healthy community as "one that includes a clean, safe, high quality physical environment and a sustainable ecosystem; provision of basic needs; an optimum level of appropriate, high quality, accessible public health and sick care services; and a diverse, vital and innovative economy" [5]. To date, most printed information as well as computerized information systems remain accessible to only health care professionals [2]. Many [6, 2, 7] believe that taking self-care and health promotion into the home is of critical value in resolving the health care crisis. According to McDonald and Blum's [8]) report, 95% of all first-line health decisions are made at home or in the workplace by the person and family or friends. Additionally, most people (60%) wait too long to handle health care problems resulting in longer, more complex and costly care [8]. Certainly home health care and community based clinics are popular mechanisms advocating these notions of self-care and health promotion concepts [9].

An alternative for health care delivery advocates the use of computers and telecommunications. Information access and communication can be available on a 24 hour basis, 365 days a year. This approach is of particular importance for rural areas which traditionally have suffered from serious problems with health care access [10]. A recent report [8] states that a telecommunication infrastructure could provide health care to the neediest segments of our population. Health-oriented telecommunications "could save hundreds of billions of health care dollars over the next two decades" [8]. According to this report, this proposed interactive network could provide: access to patient electronic medical records, integration of clinical databases and preventive care, self-care medical advice and other health care information to consumers. The provision of distributed health information and health decision-making tools coupled with communication pathways to health care professionals will promote greater self-responsibility for one's health.

A review of the literature examining the use of electronic networks for the delivery of health care provided encouragement for the development of this project. The use of a computerized network to support persons living with AIDS/ARC [11] and support for caretakers of Alzheimer's patients [12] provided a solid foundation for the efficacy of health-oriented telecommunications. In both instances, patients and caretakers were receptive of the technology and used the network for information retrieval and communication. Hassett, Lowder and Rutan [13] studied the use of bulletin boards by the disabled population and found the technology could provide information, services and support for this population and their caretakers. Another study [14] also concurred that it is feasible to use interactive, computer-based systems to support people facing health-related crises such as breast cancer and AIDS/HIV infection. Brennan [11] summarized that a computer network provided the balance necessary to promote social support while providing information access and tools to foster self-care.

2. Denver Free-Net

2.1 Denver Free-Net Development

Since 1987, the School of Nursing at the University of Colorado Health Sciences Center has operated an electronic bulletin board called NurseLink. With initial funding from the regional telephone service entity (US WEST), NurseLink was designed as a communication vehicle to disseminate research findings to nurses in local clinical agencies. After an extensive evaluation [15], a decision was made to redesign NurseLink from an electronic bulletin board for health care professionals into a community computing system for consumer access to information and communication mechanisms. The evolution of NurseLink to the Denver Free-Net was facilitated by the receipt of a grant from The Colorado Trust, a philanthropic foundation dedicated to promoting the health and well-being of the citizens of Colorado.

The Denver Free-Net is modeled after the community computing system, the Cleveland Free-Net. Community computing, as described by the National Public Telecomputing Network (NPTN), establishes a community resource that is freely accessible by the citizens through a computerized network. By using a personal computer, telecommunications software and a modem, the community can access a Free-Net system on a 24 hour basis. The community itself defines the information resources and provides the necessary support to maintain the information resources as well as to sustain the concept of an electronic community. The Cleveland Free-Net originated at Case Western Reserve University in 1984. Presently, there are 10 free-net systems available worldwide and all are members of NPTN.

2.2 Denver Free-Net Description

The mission of the Denver Free-Net project is to promote the concept of community computing to citizens in the state of Colorado. Specific goals are: to provide citizens with free and open access to community information resources, particularly in health and human services and to foster the development of health-oriented telecommunications as a means of health care delivery within the state of Colorado. The Denver Free-Net system is available to anyone who has access to a computer, modem and telecommunication software. The system is available 24 hours per day and can be reached via six dial in phone lines (303-270-4936) or via Internet (telnet to 140.226.1.8). People may login as a guest or as a registered user. A guest can browse the system and register as a user via an online registration process. Register users have interactive privileges through electronic mail, chat functions and the ability to post questions, answers or messages. Presently, a total of 20 concurrent users are allowed online.

The Denver Free-Net is best conceptualized as an electronic city where a user enters buildings such as the Post Office, the School House and the Health Care Community Center. It is a menu-driven system that provides information in several formats: read only text information, databases, question and answer forums, and online conversation mode. The opening screen is the main menu and contains the numerous building a user can enter. As one can see, the buildings are similar to those in existence in many communities throughout the world.

2.2.1 Health Care Building

Let us take a tour of the Health Care Building and view a sample of the information and communication exchanges available. It is important to remember that the Denver Free-Net is a dynamic system in which new information can be added on a daily basis. The Health Care Building contains numerous menu selections categorized into several broad areas. One area focuses on health promotion and prevention materials categorized according to the Healthy People 2000 goals. For example, the Aurora Prevention Partnership, a federally funded resource center with educational materials, is listed under the goal--substance abuse. Another example is a list of "consumer tips" provided by sources such as University Hospital, Colorado Department of Health and the FDA. Also included in this broad category is the Consumer Health Question and Answer (Q & A) moderated by a consortium of medical librarians. The Q & A allows consumers to leave questions about health promotion and an experienced consumer health librarian provides an answer within a day or two. The Q & A sections are the most interactive component of the Free-Net system. The Q & A provides a comfortable, non-threatening environment for consumers to ask questions openly without fear of ignorance or embarrassment. This is a particular useful method for consumers to ask questions about sensitive topics. A similar Q & A is under construction for school health area. This Q & A is targeted for adolescents who will be able to leave anonymous questions to be answered by school nurses.

A special community area is the Support Group Center that houses a database of support groups available in the Denver metropolitan region. The Support Group Center, initiated by the Denver Free-Net staff, is continually updated by community information providers. The database contains over 600 support groups with specific information about the group, meeting times, address, phone numbers and contact person. All groups are classified by keywords to represent their focus areas such as grieving, cancer patients, eating disorders, etc. The database has a simple searching capabilities. There are plans to develop the searching capabilities.

Another room focuses on AIDS/HIV and contains a variety of information: online publications, database of support group and discussion groups. A highlight of this room is an AIDS discussion area that is part of a worldwide USENET newsgroup. This communication mechanism, delayed time discussion groups, allows users to participate in discussions with people from around the world.

Various organizations such as the Alzheimer's Group and the Parkinson's Disease Group maintain areas in the health care building. Information include items such as support group listing, newsletters, position papers (i.e. Directions in Alzheimer's research), and Frequently Asked Questions (FAQ) section that contains answers to consumers' most commonly asked questions.

The University of Colorado Health Sciences Center maintains a building which contains separate areas for the schools of nursing, medicine, dentistry and pharmacy. A variety of information and Q & A's are housed in this area. For example, the School of Nursing lists its courses, academic schedule, student and school newsletters, faculty phone numbers, faculty research interests and research announcements. The Colorado Nursing Task Force maintains information about the differentiated practice models and articulation programs available in Colorado and operates a Q & A to guide nurses about educational and career opportunities available statewide. The Health Sciences Library also maintains a room with a current list of available journals, available library courses, announcements and a newsletter. There is also a gateway for a connection to the Colorado Alliance of Research Library (CARL) system. The gateway provides a connection to a remote computer (telnet capability) that houses the CARL system. Computer conferencing classes are being planned by the School of Nursing with its outreach students using the discussion/newsgroup format available on the Denver Free-Net.

Online publications for health care professionals are also available in the Health Care Building. For example, the Center for Disease Control's biweekly publication of Federal Drug announcements and Weekly Mortality and Morbidity Reports are available via the Health InfoComm Newsletter. Health care professionals can read these documents within hours of their release rather than waiting for their arrival via the postal service.

These examples of the health care building are but a small fraction of what is available in this electronic city. The examples, though, represent a wide variety of information and communication formats. Information is available in various formats: text only (most of which can be downloaded) and searchable databases. Communication vehicles include Q & A formats, delayed time discussion and news groups, computer conferencing and the ability to connect to remote computers via the telnet function. Other capabilities of the Denver Free-Net system are described in the subsequent section.

2.2.2 Electronic Mail (email) and Chat

Registered users have two additional communication mechanisms available: email and chat. Each registered has full Internet mail access. In the Post Office, a user can check their mail, send mail, create a signature file, and use the directory services to find a user login name. Electronic mail includes messaging and the attachment of files to messages. The Communications Center Building allows one to communicate with others online. The chat function allows both a one-on-one chat or a multi-user chat. The one-on-one chat allows you to talk in real time to another registered user who is currently on the system. A multi-user chat allows several users to talk in real time. Both functions are quite popular and many of our Internet users partake in this function. This function will be particularly useful for our outreach students who can chat with each other the instructor.

2.2.3 Other Buildings

The Denver Free-Net boasts a wealth of consumer-based information in other buildings; the latest weather report for most North American cities can be found in the Science Building; the current performing arts schedules in the Arts Building; an electronic library in the Schoolhouse, the ability to explore other established Free-Nets in the Communications Building. As one can see a variety of essential consumer information exist to complement the Health Care Building and foster the healthy community concept.

3. Current Usage

The Denver Free-Net officially opened to the public on January 12, 1993. At the time of this writing (September, 1993), there are over seven thousand registered users. Most users are from the Denver metropolitan area and represent age groups from teenagers to senior citizens. Users from other Free-Nets throughout the United States and other Internet users in the United States and from various countries (France, England, China, Germany, Finland, Bulgaria and Italy) are also registered. Numerous health care projects have been initiated with the Denver Free-Net being used as a communication vehicle and as an information dissemination mechanism.

Besides the registered users, there are over 500 information providers who contribute information to the various buildings. In addition, a multitude of volunteers help to maintain the system by serving on committees, as technical back-up staff and moderators of special interest groups or discussion areas (Q & A's). Without the participation of the community, the Denver Free-Net would not exist.

Since the time period between the paper submission and presentation is lengthy, we know the health care applications of this system will increase dramatically over the next year. Therefore, the conference presentation will focus on the impact of this system as an alternative health care delivery system.

4. Summary

The Denver Free-Net project is achieving its mission to promote the concept of community computing in the state of Colorado. Health care and human services information is widely being distributed to all segments of the population. The uses of electronic community network is offering many opportunities as an alternative health care delivery system and is promoting the concepts of self-care, consumer-health care partnerships, and healthy communities. It is important to remember that "Telecommunications is not an end in itself but a means to an end which is to break down barriers... and ...that the highway of the 21st Century will transmit information, not people" [10].

5. References

[1]   Office of the Actuary, *Health Care Financing Administration*, Press Release, March, 1991.

[2]   Melmed A and Fisher FD. *Towards a National Information Infrastructure: Implications for Selected Social Sectors and Education*. New York University, 1991.

[3]   *Healthy People 2000: National Health Promotion and Disease Prevention Objectives.* Full report with commentary. Washington, D.C.: United States Department of Health and Human Services (PHS #91-50212).

[4]   *Colorado's Health Care Action Plan: From Concept to Proposal to Solution.* Denver: Governor Roy Romer's Office, 1992.

[5]   Colorado Trust Unveils Strategic Study. *The Colorado Trust Quarterly* 1992.

[6]   Grundner TM and Garrett R. Interactive Medical Telecomputing: An Alternative Approach to Community Health Education. *N Engl J Med* 1986, 15:982-985.

[7]   Olson R, Jones, MG, and Bezold C. *21st Century Learning and Health Care in the Home: Creating a National Telecommunications Network.* Washington, D.C.: Institute for Alternative Futures and The Consumer Interest Research Institute, 1992.

[8]   McDonald MD and Blum HL. *Health in the Information Age: The Emergence of Health Oriented Telecommunication Applications.* Berkeley, CA: University of California, 1992

[9]   Shugars D, O'Neil E and Bader J. *Healthy America: Practitioners for 2005, An Agenda for Action for U.S. Health Professional Schools.* Durham, NC: The Pew Health Profession Commission, 1991.

[10]   Puskin D. Telecommunications in Rural America: Opportunities and Challenges for the Health Care System. *Ann N Y Acad Sci* 1992, 670:67-75.

[11]   Brennan P, Ripich S, and Moore S. The Use of Home-Based Computers to Support Persons Living with AIDS/ARC. *J Community Health Nurs* 1991,8:3-14.

[12]   Brennan P, Moore S and Smyth K. ComputerLink: Electronic Support for the Home Giver. *ANS* 1991, 13:14-27.

[13]   Hassett M, Lowder C and Rutan D. Use of computer network bulletin board systems by disabled persons. In:SCAMC '92. Frisse M (ed). New York: McGraw-Hill, 1992: 151-155

[14]   Gustafson, D, Bosworth K, Hawkins R, Boberg E and Bricker E. CHESS: A computer-based system for providing information, referrals, decision support and social support to people facing medical and other health-related crisis. In:SCAMC '92. Frisse, M. (ed). New York: McGraw-Hill, 1992: 161-165

[15]   Skiba D, and Warren C. The impact of an electronic bulletin board to disseminate educational and research information to nursing colleagues. In: Nursing Informatics '91. Hovenga E, Hannah K, McCormick K and Ronald J (eds). Berlin: Springer-Verlag, 1991:704-709.

Nursing Informatics: An International Overview for Nursing in a Technological Era
S.J. Grobe and E.S.P. Pluyter-Wenting, eds.

The Automated Community Health Information System (ACHIS): A Relational Database Application of the Omaha System in a Community Nursing Center

Lundeen SP and Friedbacher BE

Nursing Center, School of Nursing, University of Wisconsin-Milwaukee, P.O. Box 413, Milwaukee, WI 53201

The need to systematically describe nursing practice has never been greater. The development of computerized clinical information systems is imperative if the clinical data collected in the process of delivering nursing care are to be effectively utilized by administrators, researchers, and policy makers. The Automated Community Health Information System is a relational clinical database application of the Omaha System. Developed for use in a community nursing center, the ACHIS is affordable, efficient, and effective. It provides community health nurses the opportunity to meet administrative and research agendas while simultaneously documenting the daily process and outcome of direct clinical service.

1. The Need for Community-Focused Health Information Systems

There is a critical need for professional nursing to describe, categorize, and test systematically the unique contributions that nurses make to the improvement and maintenance of the health status of various population groups. In order to provide data that will facilitate the integration of Nursing's Agenda for Health Policy Reform into the general health care public policy agenda, nurse researchers must investigate questions related to access, quality, and cost in the delivery of health care [1].

It is important that professional nurses address many of these questions related to policy issues such as: (a) What is the nature of the health problems (actual or potential) that nurses encounter in practice? (b) What are the prevention and intervention strategies that professional nurses employ to address these problems? (c) What is the impact on clients (individuals, families, select aggregates, or entire communities) that are attributable to these nursing activities? and (d) What are the actual and comparative costs of providing these nursing services? [2]

Answers to those questions and others will depend in large measure on the collection and analysis of comparable data from many different nursing practice settings. Faculty and staff of the University of Wisconsin-Milwaukee (UWM) Nursing Center have undertaken a community nursing center demonstration project with a focus on a program of research designed to explore these health policy related questions from a community health nursing perspective.

The development of computerized systems that will yield comparable data from multiple community nursing settings will be essential to the implementation of health services research programs able direct public policy. Although most acute care settings have been computerized for some time, community-based health care settings, particularly public health departments and community nursing centers, are being automated more slowly. One goal of the initial phase of the UWM Silver Spring Community Nursing Center (CNC) demonstration project was to develop a computerized data system which would facilitate the collection and analysis of data on various aspects of community nursing practice. The first phases of this project focused on two major objectives: (a) to establish a comprehensive, computerized, longitudinal database related to community nursing practice; and (b) to design a computerized information system which met the clinical and administrative data needs of a community health practice setting.

The initial phase of this project, begun in 1988, has resulted in the development of the Automated Community Health Information System (ACHIS), a relational database software application for community health practice. The resulting database consists of descriptive client data, nursing process data, and outcome ratings on over 15,000 visits of approximately 1,200 unduplicated Nursing Center clients served during a three year period at this writing. Data collection is on-going.

1.1 Conceptualization of the ACHIS System

In most community nursing settings, there is significant overlap in the questions posed by administrators, providers, and researchers. The form of data required by each may vary a great deal, however. Furthermore, some methods used to collect clinical or administrative data may not satisfy the researcher and vice versa. The ACHIS Project is testing data collection and computer programming strategies aimed at the development of a data management system that simultaneously will serve the clinical, administrative, research, and health care policy agendas of community nursing centers. Three criteria were considered critical in the conceptualization and development of the ACHIS: (a) conceptual fit, (b) efficiency, and (c) affordability.

1.2 The Conceptual Fit of ACHIS

It was important to the integrity of the project that the documentation system be developed from a nursing perspective. The data elements to be collected needed to include client demographics and the administrative and clinical data pertinent to tracking and billing clients; however, it was essential that documentation of nursing data (assessment, intervention, and outcome) be at the core of the database. Therefore, the selection of the data elements for inclusion was based on those identified in the Nursing Minimum Data Set [3]. The Nursing Minimum Data Set (NMDS) has been proposed as a system to facilitate the collection of comparable nursing data. The 16 elements of the NMDS considered the minimal items necessary for analysis of nursing practice across practice settings include the nursing elements of nursing diagnosis, nursing intervention, and outcome [4]. After a review of the literature on the existing taxonomy systems under development for use by professional nurses, the Omaha System was selected for the coding of the nursing diagnosis and nursing intervention data elements.

The Omaha System is a nursing classification system developed and tested by staff at the Omaha Visiting Nurses Association over a 15-year period [5,6,7]. It includes (a) a broad, community health focused client problem classification scheme, and (b) a two level system for coding nursing interventions. In addition, the Omaha System has developed a 5-point rating scale for client outcomes specific to each nursing diagnosis in three categories: knowledge, behavior, and health status.

The Omaha System includes 42 client problem classifications which serve as "a taxonomy of nursing diagnoses valuable to community health nurses, other community health providers, supervisors, and administrators [7]. These diagnoses are categorized into four broad domains: Environmental, Psychosocial, Physiological, and Health Related Behaviors. Each of these nursing diagnoses can be defined with more specificity through the use of a list of four to ten signs and symptoms. The Omaha System also allows the provider to code whether the identified nursing diagnosis is a potential or actual health problem or is a concern related to health behaviors of the client. Further definition of the problem is provider through the use of either an "individual" or "family" modifier.

Nursing intervention coding is classified in four major areas: health teaching, guidance and counseling; treatments and procedures; case management; and surveillance. Within each of these four major intervention categories, the provider is able to specify one or more of 62 target areas related to the intervention (e.g. medication administration, caretaking/parenting skills, or sickness/injury care).

Selection of the Omaha System for use in the development of the ACHIS centered on three major factors: (a) the comprehensive nature of the Omaha classification scheme; (b) the applicability to community-based nurse practice settings; and (c) the adaptability of the Omaha System to computerization.

The availability of an integrated, tested documentation system that systematically codes both nursing diagnoses and nursing intervention elements mandated serious consideration of the Omaha System at the onset of the ACHIS Project. In addition, the system includes an outcome rating scale that holds great potential for documentation of outcomes related to nursing intervention. It is, in the opinion of this author, the most comprehensive classification scheme currently available for documentation of nursing practice and its impact on clients.

A second reason for seriously considering the Omaha System as the classification system of choice for the ACHIS Project was the ability to computerize the system easily. The Omaha System has been developed as a mutually exclusive set of items with systematic and numerical coding of items. Therefore, as noted by Martin over a decade ago, the scheme can be adapted for computerization without difficulty [8].

A third advantage of the Omaha System is its ability to provide flexibility and adaptation to specific practice settings while still permitting the ability to compare data across multiple sites. This is accomplished through the use of "other" categories in both the Problem Classification Scheme and the Intervention Scheme of the system. Discussion of specific augmentations of the Omaha System categories incorporated into the ACHIS for CNC practice settings will be outlined in future publications.

The most important reason for adapting the Omaha System for this project, however, was the applicability of system categories to the community setting. This classification system has been developed and tested and refined through a series of studies conducted by and with community health nurses in practice. Recent refinement of the client outcome rating scales has further increased the applicability of the Omaha System for community health practice and research [7]. A comparison of the Omaha System to other existing nursing classification schemes was done by UWM nursing faculty developing the ACHIS Project and the master's prepared nurse clinicians who would act as nurse clinicians and data collectors at the CNC demonstration site. The review resulted in a unanimous decision by the UWM Nursing Center faculty and staff that the Omaha System best fulfilled the criterion of conceptual fit for the community practice settings.

1.3 The Affordability of ACHIS

Most community nursing practice settings are limited in the fiscal and personnel resources that can be allocated to data management. This may be especially true for parish nurses, mental health nurses, nurse practitioners and midwives, schools of nursing, and small groups of entrepreneurs who are developing community nursing center models, but it also the case for many VNAs, public health departments, schools, and other more traditional settings. Any community nursing data system that might have applicability to these settings must be developed with an eye to the costs of both system implementation and maintenance. The development and testing of the ACHIS has, therefore, been undertaken at the Nursing Center's inner city urban site where resources are severely limited.

The ACHIS was developed using an affordable personal computer technology. Due to security concerns at the practice site, currently all data is entered and stored on an IBM compatible personal computer with a 486 microchip. Clinical and administrative reports can all be generated from this unit. Extensive statistical analysis for research purposes may be done through the transfer of data files to the University mainframe.

1.4 The Efficiency of ACHIS

Collection and processing of the data must be kept simple if the system is to be well accepted and used in the clinical setting. Client demographic data is collected on a simple initial encounter form by the CNC receptionist and updated as necessary during subsequent visits. All clinical data is collected directly at the time of each visit by the nurse provider. The nurse clinician documents the nursing diagnoses, nursing interventions, and client outcome ratings specific to each problem according to a numerical scheme of 2-digit Omaha System codes. These codes are entered directed into the computer from the daily log and ultimately generate the computer printout which documents the client visit. Other pertinent data is recorded by the nurse in the client record as appropriate to augment these codes, although nurse clinicians are able to keep the narrative process recording to a minimum.

The data recording process has been relatively easy for the nurse clinicians to learn and use. Although the delivery model developed at the UWM Silver Spring CNC relies primarily on a team of master's prepared nurse clinicians, student nurses and School of Nursing faculty who see clients on site also collect and code data using ACHIS [9]. Pilot testing of the system with non-nurse providers, including community outreach workers, is currently underway. Data entry is also kept efficient due to the development of entry screens that closely mirror the data collection forms. Currently, entry is maintained entirely by an undergraduate nursing student. Point of contact entry is being considered for 1994.

Finally, efficiency for both clinical and administrative purposes is being increased through the development of a menu-driven report generation format for standard administrative and clinical reports. This facilitates the rapid generation of management reports, the printing of individuals client records as they are updated, and chart review for quality assurance purposes. Customized reports can be generated enabling specific grant reporting requirements, quality assurance concerns to be met with greater efficiency. In addition, the relational nature of the database links all client profile data with nursing diagnosis, intervention and outcome data, thus allowing faculty staff and students to retrieve data in a format that facilitates research activities.

1.5 Applications of ACHIS

Currently, a number of applications of the ACHIS are being tested. These include administrative, clinical, and research uses. Although further evaluation is necessary, preliminary discussion of applications that appear promising will be presented briefly.

1.6 Administrative Applications

There is a growing need for more relevant administrative management data in community health agencies. This need has increased as revenue sources have decreased in many communities. Comprehensive information is needed in order to develop and monitor programs that seek to balance the cost and quality of services in these settings effectively. The data requirements of payers, funders, and policy-makers for program evaluation purposes have increased in sophistication beyond previous "head count" levels. Frequently, programs that are funded by multiple sources are required to produce client encounter, intervention and outcome data in many different formats and to analyze this data for many different reporting periods throughout the calendar year. Direct billing for nursing services requires yet another system for processing claims in most agencies. There is a critical need for the development of data systems that will integrate and streamline these very costly reporting activities which constitutes a constant drain on personnel resources in community health agencies.

1.7 Clinical Applications

There are on-going needs for clinical data analysis in community health settings that will improve practice, aid clinical supervision, and provided the basis for quality assurance programs. Such data, which is frequently collected in the course of normal practice documentation activities, should be processed and returned to clinical staff in a timely manner. Many research questions are best addressed from a clinical perspective. Clinical settings must develop mechanisms that integrate data collection activities into the process of established and continuous clinical documentation. At the same time, the data collection process must not become unduly cumbersome for clinicians.

The nursing services that can be provided to community-based clients are vital health and safety of many of the nation's neediest population groups, but the availability of community nursing services falls far short of the need. The development of data collection systems that will generate not only meaningful statistical reports, but simultaneously collect elements of the clinical record for community nursing services will be necessary if the comprehensive reporting requirements of both private and public payers are to be satisfied while still upholding the highest standards of excellence in the delivery of client services.

1.8 Research Applications

There is a continuing need to capture and analyze both client and nursing intervention data in community practice settings so as to contribute to the body of nursing knowledge about the nature of nursing practice in these settings, and the impact of nursing practice on non-institutionalized clients and the communities in which they live. Such research requires that multiple data elements be collected on many clients in these settings over long periods of time.

Computerized relational data management systems that combine on-going clinical reporting with management and research applications will serve community nursing settings in important ways. The institutionalization of such systems will facilitate the development of longitudinal studies in community nursing settings. Analysis of the rich data provided by such systems can provide rapid and relevant feedback to the nurse clinicians who actually collect and record these data. This can serve to develop and reinforce an important dual role of clinician/clinical research associate.

Finally, integrated community nursing data systems will facilitate the timely integration of research findings into the existing clinical environment for continued testing and refinement of intervention strategies.

1.9 The UWM Silver Spring Community Nursing Center as a Testing Site

The development of a computerized data system for community health nursing practice that addresses the multiple clinical, administrative, and research agendas requires a setting that values each. The UWM Silver Spring Community Nursing Center is a collaborative, primary care demonstration project serving economically disadvantaged individuals and families on Milwaukee's northwest side. This setting proved an ideal site to develop and test the integration of these multiple agendas.

In an academic nursing center, the multiple missions of research, teaching, and practice necessitate the constant search for a balance between these competing agendas. The various funders, both private and public, who support the Silver Spring CNC require extensive reports. This has necessitated a streamlining of complicated administrative data collection and analysis procedures. In addition, the UWM Nursing Center also seeks to link new knowledge generated through the CNC and other Nursing Center projects as directly as possible to policy initiatives at the local, state and national levels. This computerized data system can assist in the organization of timely information necessary to policy makers as they consider issues of importance in the area of community nursing practice and primary care. This was an important objective in the conceptualization of the system.

It is important to note that the development and refinement of ACHIS is occurring within the CNC practice environment. Therefore, several critical clinical issues have been balanced with the desire to develop and test a useful research tool. First, if longitudinal data are to be available for analysis without constant disruption of the practice environment for data collection purposes, that data must be collected as a matter of course by the clinical team and support staff in the course of normal client encounters. The data system has been designed and implemented with these issues in mind. Continued testing and revision continues so as to limit the burden of data collection and management on both the client and the nurse provider even further.

2. Summary

On-going research on issues of access, quality and cost are critical to the establishment of professional nurses as key players in the determination of the health care policy agenda for the coming decades. The focus of much of nursing's impact on that agenda will be through community based settings such as home care agencies, neighborhood health centers, public health facilities, and community nursing centers. It is important that computerized data systems be developed that facilitate the effective management in these settings and document the nursing practice provided, while simultaneously providing comparable data for nursing research across various practice settings. The Automated Community Health Information System provides a mechanism to meet the clinical and administrative needs of a community nursing practice site while also contributing to the implementation of a longitudinal program of health services research that seeks to address important policy issues.

3. References

[1] American Nurse's Foundation. *Nursing's agenda for health care reform.* Kansas City, MO, 1991.

[2] Lundeen SP. *The Nursing Minimum Data Set for Nursing Centers.* Paper presented at the American Public Health Association Convention. New York, 1990.

[3] Werley HH and Lang NM. *Identification of the Nursing Minimum Data Set.* New York: Springer Publishing, 1988.

[4] Werley HH, Devine EC and Zorn CR. *Nursing Minimum Data Set Collection Manual.* Milwaukee: University of Wisconsin-Milwaukee, 1990.

[5] Simmons DA. *A Classification Scheme for Client Problems in Community Health Nursing.* Hyattsville, MD: DHHS, Bureau of Health Professions, Division of Nursing, 1980.

[6] Martin K, Scheet N, Crew C and Simmons DA. *Client Management Information System for Community Health Nursing Agencies: An Implementation Manual.* Rockville, MD: Division of Nursing, US DHHS, PHS, HRSA, 1986.

[7] Martin KS and Scheet NJ. *The Omaha System: Applications for Community Health Nursing.* Philadelphia: W.B. Saunders, 1992.

[8] Martin KS. A Client Classification Adaptable for Computerization. *Nursing Outlook* 1982, 30:515-517.

[9] Lundeen SP. Comprehensive, Collaborative, Coordinated, Community-based Care: A Community Nursing Center Model. *Family and Community Health* 1993, 16(2): 57-65.

Nursing Informatics: An International Overview for Nursing in a Technological Era
S.J. Grobe and E.S.P. Pluyter-Wenting, eds.

The Omaha System:
A Model for Nursing Care Information Systems

Martin KS

Formerly Visiting Nurse Association of Omaha, Omaha, Nebraska; presently Health Care Consultant, Omaha, Nebraska, U.S.A.

The Omaha System offers direct delivery providers, educators and students, and researchers a useful model for classifying client data. The System provides an efficient, research-based, reliable and valid method for capturing, sorting, and analyzing that data. The three components of the Omaha System are designed to address nursing diagnoses, interventions, and client outcomes. The language of the Problem Classification Scheme, Intervention Scheme, and Problem Rating Scale for Outcomes enables health care professional to accurately describe diverse clients, their needs, and their progress over time. Health care professionals who are beginning to use the Omaha System as part of their nursing minimum data set and data management systems are located throughout the United States, Canada, United Kingdom, Denmark, and The Netherlands.

1. Introduction

The practice of community health nursing is as varied as its clients and nurses. The conceptual umbrella has traditionally included home care or bedside nursing services, public health home visits and clinic services, and school nursing. More recently, community health nurses have begun to practice in prisons, ambulatory care facilities, migrant sites, and homeless shelters [1][2]. Regardless of the setting, one goal of community health nurses is to provide holistic, sensitive, and economical services to all. A second goal is to provide service to the client as an individual, family, group, or community [3].

The Omaha System language and codes represent the dynamic and complex practice of community health nursing, while facilitating documentation and data management. As nurses throughout the world begin to transform data into information and, then, into knowledge, their interest in the Omaha System is escalating.

2. Description of Research

Using research methods, the Omaha System was initiated and continues to be refined in the service setting [4][5]. Four research projects were conducted by the Visiting Nurse Association (VNA) of Omaha staff between 1975 and 1993. The purpose of the first three projects was to develop, pilot test, and field test a model. That model consists of the Problem Classification Scheme, Intervention Scheme, and Problem Rating Scale for Outcomes. The current prospective study extends the previous research by measuring the reliability, efficiency, and utility of the Omaha System in diverse settings. Data from shared home visits, time studies, and questionnaires submitted to experts, clients, family members, supervisors, and staff nurses are included in the study. Furthermore, extensive research data were abstracted from more than 2,000 client records. Data have been analyzed using frequencies and discriminate analysis. The current study is intended to increase the generalization potential of the Omaha System.

2.1 Conceptual Framework

The nursing process was used as the conceptual framework for the four studies. Similarly, others have selected the nursing process for practice-based projects and research involving automated data bases and client management information systems. Examples include the Technicon System (California) [6] and the Cross Association (The Netherlands) [7] projects.

2.2 Participants and Goals

Nurses employed at the VNA and other agencies in Iowa, Wisconsin, Nebraska, Texas, Indiana, and Delaware participated in the research projects. These staff were valuable as reliability and validity were established through extensive testing and retesting activities. In addition, the studies were designed to emphasize empirical data and inductive reasoning and to produce a system characterized by simplicity, practicality, unity, and taxomonic principles. Throughout the research, the importance of clinical significance was recognized [8].

2.3 Further Research

Research based on portions of or the entire Omaha System is being conducted by other service providers, faculty members, and students enrolled in masters and doctoral programs. Their research settings include home health and public health home visit programs, school health programs, ambulatory care clinics, nurse-managed clinics, and community-wide programs.

3. Description of Computer-Compatible Schemes

The products of the research are referred to as the Omaha System and are three standardized schemes of nursing diagnoses, interventions, and ratings of client problems. A brief description of those schemes follow.

3.1 Problem Classification Scheme

A non-exhaustive, mutually exclusive taxonomy of four domains, 40 client problems or nursing diagnoses, two sets of modifiers, and clusters of signs/symptoms. The Scheme provides consistent client-focused language for collecting, sorting, classifying, documenting, and analyzing data about the individual or family's health-related concerns.

3.2 Intervention Scheme

A taxonomy of four general nursing actions or intervention categories and 62 targets or objects of intervention. Categories and targets are usually accompanied by client-specific information. The Scheme is used as the basis for planning and interviewing. It offers a method of describing client services associated with specific nursing problems.

3.3 Problem Rating Scale for Outcomes

A five-point, Likert-type scale involving the concepts of knowledge, behavior, and status. The Scale is an evaluation framework designed to measure client progress in relation to specific problems or nursing diagnoses at regular or predictable intervals. Suggested times include: admission, specific interim points, and dismissal.

4. Nursing Information Systems

Why are classification schemes such as the Omaha System so essential to nurses? Because nurses are beginning to recognize that classification schemes are required before data can be transformed into information and, then, into knowledge. This transformation of data into database systems represents power for nurses. Power is inherent in the ability to describe and count the clients nurses serve, the information used with those clients, and the clients' progress over time. Power is related to communicating information to others and to interfacing nursing data with other data in the management information system for practice, educational, and/or research purposes. Power is linked to the potential for increasing the visibility of nursing and obtaining reimbursement for practice. For these reasons, Hettinger and Brazile [9] and others are developing relational data bases and using the Omaha System or other classification systems.

Nursing organizations are also recognizing the value of classification systems. The American Nurses Association established a database task force in 1991. The ANA and the task force enabled the Omaha System and three other classification systems to be incorporated into the U.S. National Library of Medicine's metathesaurus [10][11]. In a related effort, the Canadian Nurses Association sponsored a large national nursing minimum data set conference in 1992 [12]. The conference addressed many of the basic information system issues relevant to community health and other settings.

5. Summary

Community health nurses, their agencies and nurses in general are concerned about practice, documentation, and data management issues. Public pressure and governmental regulations are exerting increasing demands to provide evidence that services are appropriate, high in quality, and beneficial. Nurses and their agencies need reliable and valid research-based instruments to collect and analyze such evidence. The Omaha System is an example of an instrument designed to address such concerns in the community health setting. Nursing diagnoses, interventions, and client outcomes are synthesized into a user-friendly framework to produce the Omaha System. The Omaha System can help community health nurses name, describe, and measure the important services they provide to clients throughout the world.

Funded by National Center for Nursing Research, National Institutes of Health, Grant # R01 NR02192; previously funded by Division of Nursing, U.S. Department of Health and Human Services.

6. References

[1] Stanhope M and Lancaster J (eds). *Community Health Nursing: Process and Practices*. St. Louis: CV Mosby Co, 1992.

[2] Wagner J and Menke E. Case management of homeless families. *Clin Nurs Spec* 1992, 6:65-71.

[3] Stewart M, Innes J, Searl S et al (eds). *Community Health Nursing in Canada*. Toronto, Ontario: Gage, 1985.

[4] Martin KS and Scheet NJ. *The Omaha System: Applications for Community Health Nursing*. Philadelphia: WB Saunders Co, 1992.

[5] Martin KS and Scheet NJ. *The Omaha System: A Pocket Guide for Community Health Nursing*. Philadelphia: WB Saunders Co, 1992.

[6] Mayers MG. *A Systematic Approach to the Nursing Care Plan* (3rd ed). Norwalk, CT: Appleton-Century-Crofts, 1983.

[7] Jonkergouw PH. Computerisation of the nursing process. In: *Lecture Notes in Medical Informatics*. Rienhoff O, Lindberg DA (eds). Berlin: Springer-Verlag, 1991: 457-463.

[8] LeFort SM. The statistical versus clinical significance debate. *Image J Nurs Sch* 1993, 25:57-62.

[9] Hettinger BJ and Brazile RP. A database design for community health data. *Comput Nurs* 1992, 10:109-115.

[10] Zielstorff RD, Cimino C, Barnett GO et al. Representation of nursing terminology in the UMLS metathesaurus: A pilot study. In: *Proceedings of the Sixteenth Annual Symposium on Computer Applications in Medical Care*. Frisse ME (ed). New York: McGraw Hill Inc, 1992:392-396.

[11] Zielstorff RD, Hudgings CI, Grobe SJ and NICNIP. *Next-Generation Nursing Information Systems*. Washington, DC: American Nurses Association/National League for Nursing, 1993.

[12] Canadian Nurses Association. *Papers from the Nursing Minimum Data Set Conference: 1992*. Edmonton, Alberta: Canadian Nurses Association, 1993.

Nursing Informatics: An International Overview for Nursing in a Technological Era
S.J. Grobe and E.S.P. Pluyter-Wenting, eds.

Developing a computerized program for activities of community health practitioners

Lee CY

Department of Community Health Nursing, College of Nursing, Yonsei University, C.P.O. Box 8044, Seoul, Korea 120-752.

The purpose of this study was to develop a computerized program for the activities of the Community Health Practitioners (CHPs). CHPs have provided primary health care to people in the rural area since 1981. About 2,039 CHPs are working in Community Health Post at the Lee (village) level, which is the lowest national administrative unit, each serving around 400 families. At the present, there is no computerized program to collect population-based data in Korea. Therefore, this study will contribute to the collection of population-based data which can, in turn, contribute to health policy development. This study shows the whole process of developing a computerized health service program from the planning phase to programming and to the actual application phase. Also it shows the detailed contents of the computerized program for the CHPs: family record, clinic activities, home visits, education, and environmental services. The results of the study will serve as a model for future development of computerized programs in community health.

1. Background of the Project

Health care in Korea is delivered from the Ministry of Health and Social Affairs to the provincial health departments, the county health centers, sub-county health centers, and to the community health posts which are located at the distal level. Public health nurses are working in the health centers and CHPs who are registered nurses are working in the community health post. The CHPs have been the representative primary health workers in Korea since 1981. There are about 2,038 CHPs in Korea.

The Korean government started computerization in the Ministry of Home Affairs in 1986. Therefore, most of the work can be done by computerization even in the distal level. However, the Ministry of Health and Social Affairs has just started to pay attention to computerization of work in the health centers. Currently one health center in an urban area is demonstrating computerization using the LAN system. In the rural area, Kang-Hwa County, county and sub-county health centers have been carrying out demonstration projects to computerize the activities of the health center. However, these demonstration projects have focused on the people who visit to the health center. This means their health information is only for the numerator data on the people who seek out the health center. To assess the health problems in the community, it is not only necessary to have numerator data but also to have denominator data. Having only data on how many people having certain problems does not provide incidence or prevalence data. To do that, it is necessary to have data from population-based registry systems. Without the population-based registry system, it is impossible to get any valid health data. The target population of one CHP is about 1,500 to 2,000 people (around 400-500 families). Since there are 2,038 CHPs working in the nation, the population covered by CHPs is about 10% of the total Korean population. The CHPs have family health records for all families in their area. Therefore, if the computerization of the CHPs' activities could be done, it would serve as a population-based registry system which covers 10% of the total population.

2. Process of computerization of CHPs activities

The process of this project followed the System Development Life Cycle (Davis, 1974) which consists of five states as followings.

1) Planning: Selection of target area, equipment establishment, understanding the services of Community Health Post, analyzing the activities of the CHPs, and deciding the range and the priority of Computerization.
2) System analysis: Detailed analysis of each activity of the CHPs, analyzing all record forms, need assessment for the CHPs, selection of input and output information, and standardization of the information for activities.
3) System design: Design of logical flow of the system, design for input and output screen, design of logics for each program, program design, unit testing for each program, testing for the whole program, development of a user's manual.
4) System installation: Set up of system, education for users, and demonstration of the system.
5) System evaluation: Selection of the indexes and methods for system evaluation,   evaluating the system, and editing the system.
    The research team was consisted by one professor, one research assistant, two CHPs who are actual program users, one programmer, and two assistant programmers.

3. Results

The results are illustrated according to the stages of the System Development Life Cycle.
1) Planning: Target areas, two community health posts, were selected in Kang Hwa county which is located near Seoul, the capital of Korea. Two CHPs were involved in the   research team. Their input was very useful in all aspects of the development process. A IBM AT compatible computer of 640K byte, with a 40M byte hard disk, 1.6M byte floppy disk drive, 12 inch monochrome monitor, and a 132 column dot printer were purchased for one community health post. The other community health post already had a similar computer and printer. The data on activities of CHPs were gathered by forms from the CHPs, and from law related CHPs activities. Also, a simple survey was done to identify the activities done by the CHPs. Following this, the range and priority of the computerization was set up by the research team.
2) System analysis: In the system analysis stage, all the forms which the CHPs are using were collected and analyzed. To assess user needs, a workshop was held with 16 CHPs who work in one province. They gave ideas on what forms should be computerized and what kind of computer program they want for their work. Information on the activities of CHPs was standardized. The activities to be computerized were divided into three main areas: family health record keeping, direct health care, management of community health post. The activities of each area are illustrated in figure 3.1 and 3.2.

404

Figure 3.1 Content Analysis of Family Health Record

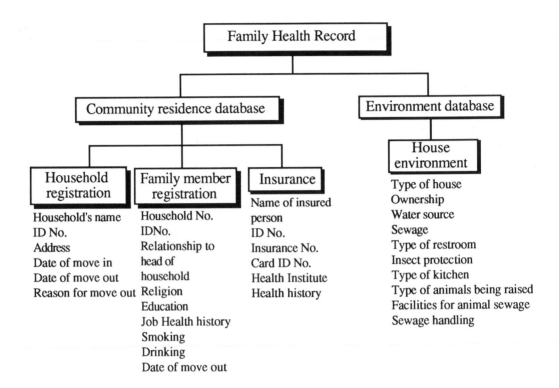

Figure 3.2 Content Analysis for Direct Health Care Activities

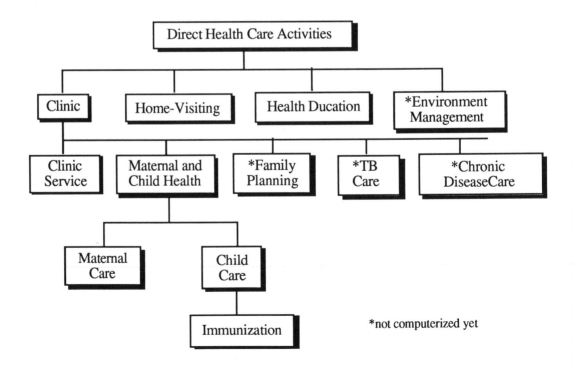

Management activity records for the community health post consisted of the following forms: CHP daily record, drug record medical insurance record, financial record, yearly plan sheet, quarter report, monthly report, equipment record, meeting record, cashbook, willage worker record.

The contents of family health record were completely computerized. Among the direct care activities, the activities of four area (environment management, family planning, tuberculosis control, chronic disease control) were not computerized within the research period. Regarding the management activities of the community health post, only two records were computerized: the drug record and the medical insurance record.

3) System Design: The research team designed input and output data and screens. In the system design stage, the research team met every week and discussed the design of the program and gave suggestions to the programmers. Two CHPs tested each unit program right after the program was designed. The programming language was clipper which can be utilized in the MS/DOS system. Input data and output forms according to the specific activities are as follows in Table 3.1.

Table 3.1 Input data and Output form

Area	Input data	Output form
Family registration	Household registration Family member registration Medical insurance Home environment	Family health record Family registration ledger Community diagnosis data Home environmental characteristics Demographic characteristics Health problems, etc.
Clinic activities	Clinic activities data Client refer data	List of chronic disease patients Client referral sheet Medical insurance request form Daily patient log
Maternal care	History of pregnancy First visit data Prenatal care Delivery data Postnatal care	New patient ledger Schedule for pre-postnatal care
Child care	Data on child born Follow-up care Immunization	New child ledger Schedule for child care Schedule for immunization List of immunization child
Education	Group health education data	Group health education ledger
Home visit	Home visit data	Home visit ledger
Drug management	Drug use data	Drug disbursement record

4) System installation : The whole program was too wide to fit on one diskette. Therefore, the program was reduced by compact program to fit on a diskette. When the user installs the program in A drive, the program is automatically extended to the original size. Two CHPs who were involved in the development team are using this program to make sure that the programs run without any problems.

5) System evaluation: This is the last stage in the System Development Life Cycle. This stage was not completed in this project. The followings can be considered for evaluation for this project: Information management function of the system, efficacy, feasibility, effect to the CHPs' activities, CHPs' satisfaction with the system, reliability of the system, time consumption, etc.

4. Conclusion

To computerize the activities of the CHPs, a research team consisting by one professor, one research assistant, three programmers, and two CHPs were set up. The process of the project followed the System Development Cycle which was consists of five stages. The last evaluation stage was not included in the project due to a time limit. The total research period was one year. When the project was started, it focused on which activities of the CHPs should be computerized. Therefore, as many activities as possible were included. However, after the project was completed, one lesson had been learned that there are another approaches for this project. For example, instead of trying to include as many activities as possible, consideration should be given to what the actual users want immediately. Although the frame of this system was very broad and public health oriented, it will take time to complete the whole program so that it runs without any problems. The immediate needs of user were not completely matched with the outcome of the project. Present plans call for spending another year to edit this program and to consider the user's immediate needs, so the users can utilize the program as soon as it is completed.

5. References

[1] Davis GB. Management Information Systems: Conceptual Foundations, Structure and Development. New York, McGraw-Hill, 1974.

[2] Kim ES. Analysis of Activities of Community Health Practitioner and Development of Curriculum of Community Health Practitioner. Final Report to International Development Research Centre, 1988.

[3] Kim JS. Evaluation of Activities of Community Health Practitioner. Korean Population and Health Research Institute, 1982.

[4] Kin JS. Analysis of management of Community Health Post. Korean Population and Health Research Institute, 1987.

[5] Korean Nurses Association. Medical Law: Special Law for Community Health Practitioner, 1980.

[6] Park HY. Development and Evaluation of Medical Information System in Urban area. Presentation at the Seminar on Medical Informatics, August 30-31, 1989.

[7] Lee IS. Strategy for Developing Medical Information System to Improve Community Health Practitioner's Activities. Master Thesis, School of Public Health, Yonsei University, 1991.

Nursing Informatics: An International Overview for Nursing in a Technological Era
S.J. Grobe and E.S.P. Pluyter-Wenting, eds.

ComputerLink: An Innovation in Home Care Nursing

Brennan P F

Associate Professor of Nursing and Systems Engineering, Case Western Reserve University, Cleveland, Ohio 44106

The ComputerLink is a specialized computer network designed to provide home-based nursing support to caregivers of persons with Alzheimer's Disease in a manner that is timely and convenient. ComputerLink has three functional components: a communications area, a decision support module, and an electronic encyclopedia. 102 AD caregivers participated in a randomized field experiment evaluating the effects of ComputerLink on caregivers' sense of social isolation, decision making skill, and confidence in decision making. ComputerLink provide a viable medium for nurses to deliver social support, education, and clinical interventions to home-bound AD caregivers.

1. Background and Research Objectives

Nurses of the late 20th century face many challenges as they diagnose and treat human responses. Some of these challenges arise from the complexities of life and disease processes which confront humans. Other challenges arise from the psychological, temporal, geographical, or physical barriers to reaching and intervening with persons in need. The purpose of this project was to determine the feasibility of using commonly available computer technology to circumvent barriers to the delivery of nursing care, and to deliver services in a timely and convenient manner.

Caregivers of persons with Alzheimer's Disease (AD Caregivers) were selected as an important target group in need of nursing care and for whom barriers arising from time constraints, shame, and distance presented formidable obstacles for obtaining necessary services [1]. Over five million family members and friends provide home care support for persons with AD. Most of these caregivers find meaning and fulfillment in the caregiver role; yet, due to the stress and demand of caregiving, many become vulnerable to physical health decline and psychological distress [2]. Thus, nursing care is needed to aid the AD caregiver in meeting the caregiving role expectations and to help this population avoid the negative consequences of caregiving.

The nursing care required by AD caregivers include social support, professional counselling, and assistance with the challenges of caregiving, such as gaining information about or confidence in the decisions they make for themselves and the person for whom they provide care [3]. Traditional methods of providing these types of service require face-to-face contact between the caregiver and nurse at meetings and counselling sessions. Notwithstanding the benefits of face-to-face encounters, many AD caregivers cannot avail themselves of these services because they lack the time or ability to travel to the meetings, or because the caregiver suffers from shame or embarrassment. Therefore, nursing care is needed, and nurses must examine and creatively employ technology to insure the delivery of the service. One technology with great potential for transcending physical, psychological, temporal or geographic barriers is computer networks.

Computer networks, electronic links between remote sites, provide a mechanism for nurses to reach AD caregivers in their homes in a manner that is timely and convenient. Computer networks support asychronous communication; that is, the sender and receiver need not be present simultaneously. This aspect permits a caregiver to leave a message for a nurse, and review the response, when it is convenient for the caregiver to do so. Conversely, the nurse need not wait for a mutually convenient time to respond to the caregiver's request for information; rather, he/she can respond as needed at a time convenient to the nurse. Additionally, computer networks allow caregivers to communicate with each other in the same timely and convenient fashion, thus mimicking many of the features of a support group without requiring the caregivers to leave home and come to a central site.

Computer networks also support a "broadcast" communication; messages relevant to many individuals can be posted once and delivered to all involved persons. Computer network also provide pathways into repositories of information, such as electronic data bases and encyclopedias. Nurses can prepare materials for caregiver education and teaching once, and then make these materials accessible to the caregivers as they need so. Computer networks provide portals into specialized programs that can guide the caregiver through complex decisions and analyses, thus facilitating nurse's use of adjuvants to individual counselling strategies.

A team of nurses and social scientists developed the ComputerLink, a specialized computer network having three functional components: a communications area, a decision support system, and an electronic encyclopedia. Built within an existing free, public-access computer network, the ComputerLink provided a pathway for nurses to reach individuals at home, in a timely and convenient manner. ComputerLink also provided a central repository for programs and information resources likely to be helpful to the person at home.

2. Presentation of Methods

2.1 The ComputerLink

The ComputerLink consists of hardware, phone lines, software and nursing interventions. The ComputerLink was designed to provide three major types of nursing services to AD caregivers: social support, clinical advise and information and decision support. Caregivers accessed these services through computer terminals placed in their homes. ComputerLink was available 24 hours a day for an 18 month period, and caregivers could access the system as often as they desired. One nurse served as nurse moderator; she logged onto the system daily, read and responded to caregiver comments as needed, and maintained the currency of the information available through the network.

Social support, defined as both peer and professional support, was available through the communications area. The communication area permitted several options for public and private communication among caregivers and between caregivers and the nurse moderator. In an unrestricted bulletin board (The Forum) any user could read, post and respond to issues of concern and interest. Private electronic mail afforded one-to-one interaction away from the scrutiny of others. In a special feature combining private mail with The Forum, called Q & A, caregivers could send questions anonymously to the nurse moderator, who posted the answer to the question for all to read.

In addition to responding to specific requests for information through the communications areas, the nurse moderator also provided structured information through the Electronic Encyclopedia. The Electronic Encyclopedia included over 150 short articles designed to enhance self care, understand issues about Alzheimer's Disease and about the experience of caregiving, and promote home-based management of the person with Alzheimer's Disease. Caregivers could browse through the Electronic Encyclopedia in a screen-by-screen manner, selecting topics from a key-word listing, or search using specific words and phrases for the information of their choice.

Supporting caregivers through complex decisions can occur through interpersonal interaction, either individually or in the open bulletin board discussions. In addition, in the decision support module, caregivers could work though a decision problem on their own. English-language questions guided users in an analysis of a self-defined decision problem. For some users, the decision problems focused on selecting living arrangements. For other users, intimate questions of relationships served as the focus of the analysis. The analysis strategy, decision modelling [4], helped the user focus on the values and trade-offs that occur during difficult choices. The decision support module permitted caregivers to explore their values, and to select choices that best meet their own stated values.

2.2 Research Design and Procedures

Subjects in the 18-month randomized field experiment included 98 individuals who considered themselves to be the primary caregiver of a person with AD, sixty-six females and 32 males. Caregivers were randomly assigned to a placebo or experimental (ComputerLink) conditions. Subjects also completed self-report inventories at the beginning and end of the study. Research nurses visited the homes of caregivers, installed the necessary equipment, and trained caregivers in the use of the ComputerLink. Caregivers accessed ComputerLink via Wyse 30 terminals placed in their homes. A 1200 baud modem provided the connection between the terminal and the standard telephone line. Caregivers entered the ComputerLink through the CWRU modem bank. Successful access occurred in over 95% of desired encounters.

Because the present report deals only with caregivers who used ComputerLink, Table 1 summarizes the profile for ComputerLink users. Care recipients were predominantly spouses (60%) and parents (31%), and required care for an average 34.5 months (s.d. 26.8). This sample is representative of other study samples of caregivers of elderly patients [5]. Thirty-two percent of the subjects stated that they care for someone in addition to person with AD. Twenty-six of the subjects (26%) in this sample placed their loved one in a nursing home made during the one-year period of involvement. This incidence represents substantial evidence that caregivers are making decisions about health service use, such as nursing home placement.

Table 1
Demographic Summary of ComputerLink Caregivers

		Caregiver Relationship	
Age	60.8 years (s.d. 14.92)	Spouse	26 (57%)
Gender	Male 14 (33%)	Daughters or daughters-in-law	11 (24%)
	Female 33 (66%)	Son	3 (6%)
		Other	7 (13%)
Race	Black 14 (33%)		
	White 33 (66%)		
Years of School	<12 years 14 (33%)		
	>12 years 33 (66%)		

3. Results and Discussion

The ComputerLink was active for 540 days. Caregivers accessed the system on 3875 occasions (median 2.5 uses per week). All caregivers used the system on at least three occasions; one caregiver accessed ComputerLink on over 575 occasions. A typical encounter lasted 12 minutes, and included use of two or more functions. Table 2 summarizes the use of ComputerLink by feature.

Table 2
ComputerLink Feature Uses (Note: Caregivers use one or more function of each access)

Feature	# of Uses	Duration in Minutes (SD)
Forum	3312	9.87(12.15)
Private Mail	2019	5.78 (9.34)
Q & A	878	3.14 (4.95)
Electronic Encyclopedia	541	9.34 (10.32)
Decision Support	106	7.65 (7.92)

The communications area was used most often; in this area caregivers could interact with each other in a public, "bulletin-board", a private mail service or through a nurse-advising service in which caregivers could post confidential questions. The Forum received the most attention from the caregivers. The nurse entered the Forum daily and posted messages whenever necessitated by direct request or professional judgment that such comments would enhance peer support .

Caregivers sought direct contact with the nurse in several ways. First, they sent 27 private mail messages to the nurse, with topics ranging from requests for assistance with the computer system to questions about managing specific problems with the person with AD. Second, of the 749 messages posted in the Forum, 50 made a direct reference to the nurse moderator. The nurse moderator posted 88 messages in this area. Finally, caregivers asked thirty questions in the Q & A area. Interestingly, the caregivers accessed this section to read questions and responses 20 times more often than they did to ask questions.

The Electronic Encyclopedia and the decision support module received less attention by the caregivers than did the more interactive functions of the system. Within the Electronic Encyclopedia caregivers sought information on the care of the person with AD more often than any other topical area. The 106 uses of the decision support module included analysis of such decisions as placement of a mother in a nursing home or return to work.

3.2 Discussion

The evidence presented here demonstrates that ComputerLink provided a vehicle for nurses to reach and support AD caregivers. The system proved easy for caregivers to access and use. Communication services, moderated by the nurse, receive the most attention by the caregivers. The surprizing pattern of caregiver use of the Q & A section

410

suggested that in addition to using ComputerLink to reach peers, caregivers also employed it as a pathway to professional contact.

The disproportionate access to the Forum relative to the private mail section of the ComputerLink suggests that the most extensively valued nursing intervention was the provision of social support. While peer contact was available under both "public" (Forum) and "private" (private mail) conditions, the caregivers participant in this study sought the more public environment. Because support groups are a common, but under-used mechanism for facilitating peer support among AD caregivers [6] it is likely that these caregivers were seeking out similar types of experiences in the electronic media.

Caregivers made most use of those parts of the system supporting interaction among peers or between caregivers and the nurse. It is possible to consider such nursing strategies as providing information on request and facilitating social support as "active" interventions. In contrast, then, the construction of an information utility (Electronic Encyclopedia) or the provision of adjuvant programs (decision support) may be considered indirect nursing strategies (indirect because the nurse is instrumental in providing access, but not directly involved in implementing the nursing strategies than of the indirect nursing strategies available through ComputerLink.

Preliminary evidence indicates that ComputerLink enhances caregiver decision making confidence, and serves as a viable medium for nurses to provide social support, education, and clinical interventions to home-bound AD caregivers in a manner free of time and space boundaries. Caregiver are more likely to use the interactive rather than the broadcast features. ComputerLink represents and efficient use of technology to support a new approach to nursing care.

3.3 Generalizability of ComputerLink Nationally and Internationally

Certain features of the ComputerLink suggest that this intervention is likely to be successful in a variety of communities in the US and world-wide. First, although the participants in this project were AD caregivers, their performance suggests that ComputerLink may be desirable whenever nurses need to reach individuals in remote areas who face ongoing complex health management challenges. The success of ComputerLink with individuals of all age groups indicates that advancing age is not a barrier to successful use. The nature of the services provided here (information, decision assistance, social support) were tailored to the needs of this particular group; it is possible that other groups may require different mix of services. While not all nursing interventions can be delivered in an electronic medium, many may be effectively delivered so. The challenge remains to nursing to evaluate the needs of the target population and determine how to best employ existing technologies to delivery nursing care.

Some aspects of the technology may preclude its use in certain developing countries. For example, a stable electrical supply and access to phone lines is required to implement a home-based electronic pathway for nursing care. Telephone service, whether satellite-mediated or not, is also necessary to make the link between the remote sites and a central site. Finally, the ability to insure privacy of telecommunication transmission is a necessary precursor to the effective use of technology in delivering nursing care to remote sites.

Supported by a grant from the National Institute on Aging, #AG8617, Patricia Flatley Brennan, PhD, RN, FAAN, Principal Investigator.

4. References

[1] U.S. Congress, Office of Technology Assessment. (1990). Confused minds, burdened families: finding help for people with Alzheimer's Disease & other dementias. (Report No. OTA-BA-403).

[2] Brody EM. Patient care as a normative family stress. *Gerontologist* 1978, 25:19-29.

[3] Haley WE, Brown SL and Levine EG. Experimental evaluation of the effectiveness of group intervention for dementia caregivers. *Gerontologist* 1987, 27: 376-382.

[4] von Winterfeldt D. and Edwards W. *Decision Analysis and Behavioral Research.* Cambridge: Cambridge University Press, 1986.

[5] Stone R, Cafferata GL and Sangl, J. Caregivers of the frail elderly: a national profile. *Gerontologist.* 1987, 37:616-626.

[6] Noelker LS and Bass DM. Home care for elderly persons: Linkages between formal and informal caregivers. *J Geron : SocSci* 1989, 44:S63-70.

1994 Elsevier Science B.V. All rights reserved.
ursing Informatics: An International Overview for Nursing in a Technological Era
J. Grobe and E.S.P. Pluyter-Wenting, eds.

Healthy people 2000: Nursing informatics project

Reinhard SC   Moulton PJ   Davis JC

gers, The State University of New Jersey, College of Nursing, University Heights, Newark, New Jersey 07102

The purpose of this project was to provide students in the Master's Program in Community Health Nursing with opportunities to develop skills in managing and processing information related to the health patterns of communities. Students used advance nursing knowledge, in conjunction with the *Healthy People 2000: National Health Promotion and Disease Prevention Objectives*, to develop indicators that measure a community's health patterns. Through collaboration with community health nursing faculty and computer specialists, students designed an automated community assessment tool and created a database capable of describing relationships among the Healthy People 2000 objectives. Students collected and analyzed data the described relationships among the Healthy People 2000 objectiveswithin communities. This is an ongoing project with each cohort of students working with the database to strengthen its capacity as a community health assessment tool.

Introduction

Advanced practice nurses in community health must be more than computer-literate. To effectively practice at the ggregate level, they must be able to design and use databases that capture a nursing perspective of the community. Working with community members, nurses seek information about a community's health patterns and resources. They ompare this information with regional, state, and national health statistics to document the need for programs that romote self-help at the individual, family and community levels. To efficiently and effectively monitor these programs nd evaluate outcomes, community health nurse specialists need to create appropriate databases. Based on national studies f the essential content of graduate programs in community health nursinng [1], the need to integrate learning pportunities in nursing informatics as it relates to community assessment and program management is compelling.

Funded in part by the Division of Nursing, Public Health Service Department of Health and Human Services, the 'ollege of Nursing at Rutgers, The State University of New Jersey developed the "Healthy People 2000 Nursing nformatics Project" to meet five purposes. First, the project was designed to help students apply advanced theory in ommunity health nursing. Since the primary goal of specialists in community health nursing is to promote the health f the community as a whole [2][3], they must be able to create tools to assess the community-as-client [4]. Second, to e consistent with the conceptual framework of the graduate nursing curriculum, the project focused on assessment of *atterns* closely related to health promotion, and relevant to all students regardless of their selected population focus (ie, :nior citizens, pregnant adolescents, or young adults on a college campus). Third, the learning experience was ntentionally linked to the current and future policy-relevant national health objectives detailed in *Healthy People 2000: 'ational Health Promotion and Disease Prevention Objectives* [5]. Fourth, consistent with adult learning principles that mphasize experiential learning, the project was developed *with students* who had no formal preparation in computers. inally, the project was designed to promote the use of nursing informatics in non-structured settings. Through the use f note book computers, modems, and file servers, students could bring computers into the community and learn how) use file servers or telecomputing to aggregate and analyze data.

Project Description

The project involved the development and implementation of a computerized community health assessment data base, ased on the health promotion objectives presented in the Healthy People 2000 document. These objectives address a road spectrum of health related needs for individuals, groups, and communities. Participants included four Master's students in Community Health Nursing, two faculty members, and one programming consultant. Two experts in the fie of nursing informatics also served as consultants to the project. At the inception of the project, students were direct to select one of the eight objectives as the foundation for initial tool and software development. The original gro selected the nutrition objective. Subsequent cohorts of students have expanded the data base by incorporating questic and indicators pertaining to the remaining health promotion objectives. To facilitate learning, students receiv didactic content pertaining to the classification, ordering, understanding, and importance of data. As the proje progressed, barriers encountered included students' lack of knowledge in developing automated assessment tools, the lack of experience in actual computer use, and the programming consultant's lack of familiarity with health related da For the students, the barriers were addressed through seminar discussion, demonstration of software, and hands-experience with computer hardware. Working with the programmer involved sharing information regarding the purpo and outcome expectations of the project. The programming consultant played an essential role in keeping the studer focused on collecting the right amount and type of data to support the project.

The completed Healthy People 2000 Health Assessment Software Program is a record handling editor with utiliti Subject records can be added, located, edited, deleted, or listed individually or in groups. Data are collected based the criteria listed in the Healthy People 2000 health promotion objectives. Examples of demographic data include ag weight, living arrangements, disability, educational level, and economic status. Other data collected refer specifica to the criteria listed in each health promotion objective. For example, data collected for the nutrition objective descri subjects' body mass index, the calcium, iron, and fat contents of their diets, and the calories derived from the major fo groups. The relational factors present in the software package allow comparisons and contrasts of data with cases a across cases. Consistent with the goals of the project, data can be aggregated to form a community. Comparisons a contrasts of data are carried out based on the criteria in the objective.

The hardware environment includes IBM PC clones with DOS 3.0 or higher, 3.5' disk drive, and a minimum of 3 MB of memory. The hardware decisions were based on availability of equipment to he school and to the programme Given the nature of the project, the majority of the programmer's work was done away from the school. Programmi for the database was done using the Paradox 3.5 Personal Programming Package.

Testing of the software package involved a two-part process. A paper and pencil questionnaire was develop simultaneously with the software. Since the questionnaire was completed several weeks prior to the software packag students were able to pilot test the tool on select populations. This testing provided the opportunity for editorial chang which enhanced the tool's usability. Members of the Community Health Advisory Committee, composed of local leade and experts in the field of community health nursing, participated in the pilot testing by arranging to have t questionnaire administered to select populations within their agencies.

The initial software package was completed and installed on the office hardware (PC-486) and on three notebo computers. approximately six months after the inception of the project. Confidentiality is maintained by physical cont of the disks and by controlling access to the microcomputers through passwords. The system is designed so that the P 486 functions as a file server. Students take the notebook computers with them on practicum experiences and a encouraged to enter data while interacting with clients. The software package is designed with an import-export featu so that data entered on the notebook computers can be exported to the PC-486 for aggregate analysis. The repo generated by the package enable students to analyze the health status of their communities based on the Healthy Peo 2000 nutrition criteria.

3. Summary

In summary, the HP 2000 has been developed as a prototype for community assessment and evaluation as set forth the *Healthy People 2000: National Health Promotion and Disease Prevention Objectives*. It is a forerunner in t community health information systems arena. HP 2000 has served as an innovative vehicle for advanced communi health nursing education. Through its development, cohorts of students have contributed to its development, expansio utilization, and refinement. The involvement of the Community Health Advisory Committee has strengthened the li between education and service and enhance collaboration among professionals. This experience has facilitated continu student learning in the areas of computer acceptance, awareness of hardware, software, and student capabilities; an potential for management and processing of community health nursing information utilizing a system designed f community health nursing.

4. References

[1] Selby, M., Riportella-Muller, R., Salmon, M., Legault, C., & Quade, D. Master's degree-level community health nursing ducational needs: A national survey of leaders in service and education. *J Prof Nurs* 1991, 7:88-98.

[2] American Nurses Association *Standards of community health nursing practice.* Kansas City, MO: The American Nurses Association.

[3] American Public Health Association *Definition and role of public health nursing in the delivery of health care.* Washington, DC: the American Public Health Association, 1980.

[4] Williams, C.A. Community health nursing-What is it? *Nurs Outlook* 1977, 25:250-254.

[5] *Healthy people* 2000: *National health promotion and disease prevention objectives.* Boston: Jones and Bartlett, 1992.

Nursing Informatics: An International Overview for Nursing in a Technological Era
S.J. Grobe and E.S.P. Pluyter-Wenting, eds

414

A Proposed Computerized Information System for Primary Health Care Rendered from Mobile Clinics

Mc Donald T

Dept of Computer Science, University of the Orange Free State, P.O. Box 339, Bloemfontein, 9300, Republic of South Africa.

Primary Health Care (PHC) services in the Republic of South Africa stand at the dawn of massive extensions. Demands by disadvantaged people for accessible and affordable health care will have to be met. As it stands now, a shortage of qualified nurses exists and the service is provided on a tight budget. Those providing health services are further burdened with an enormous administrative task. The only way in which effective PHC can be provided in the future, is to enable the nurses to spend more time with their patients. This must be done without detracting from an efficient information system. A redesigned computerized information system is the answer to the problem. A model for such a system is proposed.

1. Introduction

The health service of the Republic of South Africa is in the process of dramatic change. The emphasis is to shift from a high quality medical service for the few, to an accessible and affordable service for the masses. Hundreds of new clinics are envisaged in the near future. This will not only increase the responsibility to manage the service properly, but at the ground-level a service must be provided by under-staffed and over-worked nurses. In addition, all this must be done on a tight budget. To accomplish this with any measure of success, a well-designed information system is required.

The World Health Organization says that inadequate information support is a major constraint for the managerial process in practically all countries. The same organization feels that "the road towards health for all by the year 2000 passes through information". The role that computers can play in this regard is well-documented [1,2]. Many of the information systems reported in the literature, however, are only partly computerized [3] and do not include mobile clinics. In this paper a model for a fully computerized information system is proposed. The model covers the spectrum from data collection at the ground-level, to a decision support system for management.

2. Background

The object under investigation is community health as provided by the Provincial Administration of the Orange Free State, a province roughly in the center of the Republic of South Africa. The province is divided into four regions. Each region is divided into several areas, each area roughly corresponding to a managerial district. A registered nurse with a nursing assistant is responsible for PHC in an area. The health service is provided by means of a mobile clinic in the rural areas. In the cities and towns the same service is provided from stationary clinics. The focus will be mainly on mobile clinics as that is the most difficult to computerize.

A recent study [4] reports on the workload and attitude of nurses, rendering PHC from mobile clinics, towards their work. The activities that comprise a nurse's task and the time spent on each activity were additionally determined. The study showed that only 24% of a nurse's time is spent on direct patient care, while the administrative activity that consists mainly of completing forms and preparing reports account for 23% of the time. It was also found that computer and communication technology can be effective in activities that represent 35% of a nurse's time.

2.1 Attitude towards computers

No computer system can be implemented without an analysis of the attitudes and information needs of the people involved. For a description of the sample and methods used see [4]. The findings of the 95 nurses that completed the questionnaire are reported in Table 1. Eighty-seven percent of the nurses are frustrated with the time wasted by all the administrative work. Computer technology is seen as a solution to the information processing problems by 77% of the nurses. Most of the nurses (73%) agreed that computers will improve their productivity .

Just more than half the number of nurses have fears that computers may interfere with the nurse-patient relationship. On the question whether they have reservations about the use of computers, they were evenly distributed. They were slightly more positive regarding their concern that there are more urgent needs in PHC than the purchasing of computers. The above fears and reservations may be attributed to a lack of experience in the use of computers (79%), a poor knowledge of available computer technology (86%) or an uncertainty whether the computer system will actually help them in their care and their administrative responsibilities. Cognisance should, however, be taken of these factors in the needs assessment and design of any computer system in which education, training and a friendly and easy to use user interface should play a major role.

Table 1
Attitude towards computers

	Strongly Disagree	Disagree	Neutral	Agree	Strongly Agree
Frustrated by all the administrative work	2 (2%)	7 (7%)	4 (4%)	34 (36%)	48 (51%)
Computers solution to information problems	2 (2%)	3 (3%)	17 (18%)	29 (31%)	44 (46%)
Computers will improve productivity	3 (3%)	5 (5%)	18 (19%)	35 (37%)	34 (36%)
Computers may interfere with relationship	11 (12%)	41 (43%)	27 (29%)	12 (13%)	4 (4%)
Have reservations to computers	5 (5%)	27 (28%)	31 (33%)	30 (32%)	2 (2%)
More urgent needs in PHC	8 (8%)	28 (30%)	19 (20%)	26 (27%)	14 (15%)
Have previous experience in computer usage	53 (56%)	22 (23%)	5 (5%)	11 (12%)	4 (4%)
Wish had more knowledge of computers	1 (1%)	2 (2%)	10 (11%)	63 (66%)	19 (20%)

2.2 Problems identified by nurses

To identify what the nurses found to be problem areas in their work, several open-ended questions were asked. Their response as to which activities they saw as the biggest time wasters, ordered by the number that responded, was as follows:

* Administrative work (all paper work). More specifically: the duplication of information on cards and forms to be completed, calculating statistics and obtaining family history from illiterate people.
* Movement of people from an area. There is presently no way of transferring information from one area to the next.
* Travelling time in a mobile clinic and the transporting of patients between a hospital and a farm.
* Trying to understand people who are only able to speak an African language.
* Numerous meetings

The activities which they found to be most frustrating were:

* Administrative work.
* Not understanding the language of the patients.
* Waiting for patients to come to the clinic.
* Working from a car (some nurses do not have mobile clinics as yet).
* Searching for people and records.

The main response to the question of any other comments, was as follows:

* More nurses were needed so that the area they work in can be smaller.
* Support is needed in the form of a driver for the vehicle, a secretary for the administrative work and in the future an operator for the computer.
* A reduction in the amount of data to be collected.
* Better communication between all people involved in PHC.

From the above it is clear that the administrative activity is seen as the main problem by nurses providing PHC from mobile clinics. The study does not differentiate between administrative tasks (statistics, reports, etc.) and the recording of vital patient data, although from the above responses it seems that problems exist with both kinds. No research data is being collected at this stage, but it will have to be incorporated in a new system. Whatever data is to be collected, it should be reduced to the absolute minimum. Health information is important and ultimately it leads to better health for the population. The time of nurses for direct patient care is even more precious in this instance and should be maximized. A well designed computerized information system with a skeleton data requirement may be the solution.

3. Model of a computerized information system

Each region should have its own database (see Figure 1), containing information about all the PHC patients in the region. The movement of people is usually within a region because of a lack of transport and will therefore not affect the information in the database. This approach will also keep the database in manageable proportions. The design of the database should take cognisance of the following facts: it must contain only information that will be utilized, no duplication of information, relationships between family records, also relationships between individual patients and community/environmental factors should exist and it should be possible to group individuals according to region, area and farm.

Each mobile clinic serving an area should be issued with a computer, possibly a pen-based or notebook computer with communications facilities. Data of new patients seen during a visit will be captured directly on this computer by the nurse or his/her assistant. Data of existing patients can be updated with whatever intervention takes place. The application program handling the data capturing and updating must be simple and easy to use with minimum effort. Nurses should be deeply involved in the selection of an user interface they are comfortable with. Some means to enter community information (living conditions, economic status, etc.,) must also exist. Communication of information between the clinic and community hospitals, district surgeons (and other doctors) and laboratories are more difficult. If the same identification is used in all the cases and the region and area can be determined from the identification number, then information concerning the patients can be sent to the clinics.

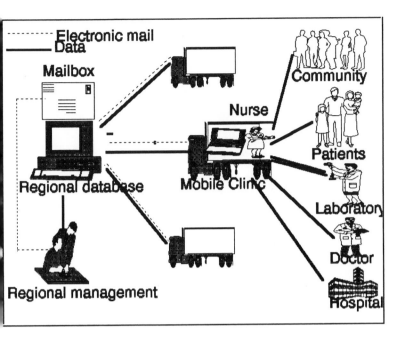

Figure 1 Regional Database Model

To keep the regional database up to date, several possibilities exist. In the first world countries the computers in the clinic can be integrated with wireless technology like radio and cellular. In this case the regional database is accessible directly from the clinic in realtime and therefore always up to date. In the poorer countries a different approach is needed. If the nurse has access to a telephone, then the regional database can be downloaded from the database server during the night to the portable computer used in the clinic. This database is then used during the day in the mobile clinic. At the end of the day this database can be uploaded to the regional database to have it updated. If this is done by all the clinics in the region then the regional database will never be more than one day out of date. If the movement of people from the areas are mostly at specific times, then this up and down loading needs to be done less frequently. It is possible for this process to work even in the absence of telephone lines. In this case the clinics will be provided with a copy of the database on magnetic media.

From the regional database all the necessary reports (statistics of patients, monitoring of health worker, usage of resources, etc.) required by management may be generated by application programs. This time consuming task for nurses is thus completely taken out of their hands. Another advantage is that information on individual patients exists in the database and is available for various queries from regional management. In this way problem areas can easily and speedily be identified. The application program is also able to send information back to the areas so that a nurse may see what is happening in her area.

Apart from the database the system should also include electronic messages. In this way, problems or patterns identified in an area by management may be communicated to a nurse's electronic mailbox as also new information may be sent to the nurse in each area. This will save nurses precious time in travelling to meetings, holding meetings, travelling to training sessions and receiving training. Time spent on telephone conversations will also be saved.

On the provincial level, all the regional databases must be linked to a central database server (see Figure 2). Here all the regional databases are merged into one provincial database. It is important to note that even at this level information on individuals will be available. A decision support system based on this database will assist management through reports, graphs and queries to make optimal decisions regarding the health services. An electronic mailing system must also be available on this level. By this means, top management can relay important information to the regions.

418

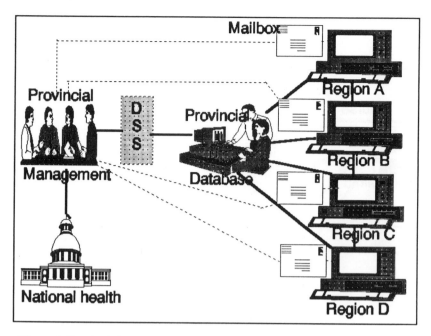

Figure 2 Provincial model

4. Conclusion

Nurses spend a lot of time on administrative work at the expense of direct patient care. A computerized information system covering all levels of the information hierarchy is proposed. Data is captured directly on computers in the mobile clinics. These computers are linked to a regional database server. All the regional databases are then linked to a provincial database server that contains information of all the patients in the province. This system will make more time available for nurses providing health services on ground-level. At the same time quality information is provided to management for control and planning.

5. References

[1]   Sinclair V G. The Impact of computer support on social and political dynamics in health care organizations. *Nurs Admin Q* 1990, 14(3), 66-73.

[2]   Barry C T and Gibbons L K. Information Systems Technology: Barriers and challenges to implementation. *J Nurs Adm* 1990, 2(2),40-42.

[3]   Robey J M and Lee S H. Information System Development in Support of National Health Programme Monitoring and Evaluation: The case of the Philippines. *Wld Hlth Statis Quart* 1990, 43,37-43.

[4]   Mc Donald T, Chapman R C and Mackenzie J E. Primary Health Care rendered from Mobile Clinics: Can Computers Help? *Submitted for publication.*

Nursing Informatics: An International Overview for Nursing in a Technological Era
S.J. Grobe and E.S.P. Pluyter-Wenting, eds.

Computer assisted learning for use in the education of renal patients on continuous ambulatory peritoneal dialysis - results of an evaluation study

Luker K A[a] Ackrill P[b] and Caress A-L[a]

[a] Dept of Nursing, University of Liverpool, PO Box 147, Liverpool, L69 3BX, England

[b] Artificial Kidney Unit, University Hospital of South Manchester, Withington, Manchester, M20 8LR, England

This paper presents results from a 3-year Department of Health funded study involving the development and evaluation of computer assisted learning (CAL) material for use with patients training to undertake continuous ambulatory peritoneal dialysis (CAPD). An in-depth descriptive study involving 30 patients from a single study centre was undertaken. CAL was well received and was especially useful for presenting complex material such as anatomical and physiological information. The results suggest that the medium is worthy of further investigation and has considerable potential for use with other patient groups.

1. Introduction

The rising prevalence of such chronic illnesses as end-stage renal disease (ESRD) has increasingly necessitated patient participation in and self-management of therapeutic regimens. Since inadequate management of ESRD can have distressing, costly and potentially life-threatening consequences, considerable emphasis is placed upon adequate pre-discharge preparation of patients. Patient education can, however, be complicated by a number of physical and psychological factors [1]. The education of renal patients is rendered especially difficult by the deleterious effects upon cognitive ability of uraemia and the lethargy and tiredness which arise from anaemia. Organisational features, such as lack of available staff time and pressure to increase the throughput of patients can also impair the process of patient education.

2. Computers in Patient Education

Computer assisted learning (CAL) is gaining increasing popularity in schools and in professional education. However, to date, its use with patients has been limited. The small number of studies conducted in this area appear to suggest that CAL can be successfully used in patient education and may offer a number of benefits, including increased patient control over the learning process [2]; improved knowledge outomes as compared with traditional educational formats [3]; more satisfying and enjoyable learning experience for patients [3,4,5]; and more efficient and cost-effective use of staff time [2].

3. CAL in CAPD Patient Education

Continuous ambulatory peritoneal dialysis (CAPD) is a self-care therapy which is increasingly used for the treatment of ESRD. Its greatest risk is the potential for development of peritonitis as a result of technique failure. In the United Kingdom, training of patients to undertake CAPD is typically undertaken in hospital by specialist CAPD nurses over a period of as little as a week, and requires that patients learn a large amount of information and numerous technical procedures. CAPD patient education is challenging. Learners are typically uraemic and anaemic, and many are visually impaired. CAPD patient populations are demographically diverse, and therefore have very varied educational needs; older patients form a large proportion of those on CAPD and are reported to have especial learning needs [6]. Not surprisingly, therefore, considerable problems experienced both in preparation for discharge [7] and in post-discharge outcomes [8]. The reported benefits of CAL appeared to make it well suited as an educational means of overcoming some of these deficits and, since it was untried in the field, a study of its usefulness and acceptability was deemed worthwhile.

4. The Study

A 3 year study, funded by the Department of Health, was undertaken at a single centre in the North West of England. The aims of the study were:-
 1. to develop CAL material for use in CAPD patient education
 2. to evaluate its usefulness and acceptability to patients and nursing staff
The CAL software was specifically developed for the study, and was a series of six tutorials with high graphics content, incorporating multiple-choice questions. A multiple-choice format game invloving subjects in simulations of real-life situations was also devloped.

The first eighteen months of the study were spent in program development and in selection, preparation and piloting of instruments. The small numbers of patients involved precluded the use of an experimental design, and an in-depth descriptive study was therefore undertaken. Data was collected to fulfil four purposes:-
 1. To provide demographic information and allow for acomparison of subjects' responses to CAL by such features as age, sex and occupation
 2. To explore the influence upon response to CAL of a number of considerations identified in the literature as influencing learning ie mood state, intellectual ability and health locus of control
 3. To obtain the opinions of patients and nurses as to the usefulness and acceptability of CAL as a patient education tool by means of an interview schedule designed for the study and exploring issues relating both specifically to the software and more generally about the medium of CAL.
 4. To examine the educational usefulness of CAL by exploring its effect on subjects' levels of knowledge about their condition and its treatment and their ability to apply this knowledge as indicated by their transfer of learning, compliance and the incidence of dialysis related complications
A large volume of data was produced; useful application of inferential statistics was limited owing to the small sample size and uneven distribution of subjects' responses. The most valuable material was qualitative data relating to the subjects' opinions of CAL; this paper will therefore concentrate on this data.

4.1 Piloting

Pilot work was undertaken with a group of 12 patients already trained in CAPD techniques. The pilot was designed to explore the acceptability of the software to patients and to deal with such issues as screen design and complexity of program content. Development of instruments specific to the study and testing of pre-existing tools was also undertaken at this time. Pilot work suggested the need for adaptation of the user interface from the standard QWERTY keyboard, and this was undertaken before commencement of the main study.

4.2 The Sample

The sample was drawn from the total patient population accepted for CAPD training over one calendar year (N=45); 33 subjects were recruited into the study and 30 complete data sets obtained. The sample was found to be generally representative of the overall CAPD population at the study centre. Mean age was 50.9 years (median =54.0 yrs), ages ranging from 19-71 years. There were 18 males and 12 females and all socio-economic groups were represented. The occupational and educational experience of subjects was very varied and, notably, more than half of the sample had last had any educational experience more than 20 years ago. 18 of the 30 subjects had no prior computer experience, whilst 6 had used one regularly. 22 of the 30 subjects had some degree of visual impairment, 4 being registered blind or partially sighted.

4.3 Subjects' Response to CAL

Subjects' response to both the software and the medium of CAL was overwhelmingly positive, all reporting having benefited from their experience of using the computer and considering it useful as a tool for CAPD patient education. 96.3% (N=32) of the sample reported that they would be willing to use the computer again to learn from, with only one individual considering that he would "not really" like to do so; 53.3% (N=16) stated that they would "very much" like to use CAL in the future.

Exposure to CAL had a positive impact upon subjects' appraisal of the medium, 20% (N=6) considering it to be more useful than they had anticipated.

The software was considered by all subjects to be of a high standard and to have presented useful information. The use of graphics was greatly welcomed, with only one individual disliking the graphics, finding this method of presentation too simplistic. Animations of, for example, anatomical and physiological details were very popular with subjects and were considered to add greatly to their enjoyment of the programs and their understanding of the information taught.

The potential benefits of CAL for visually impaired individuals are graphically illustrated by the finding that 29 of the 30 subjects experienced no difficulty seeing the material on screen, despite the fact that 22 of the 30 subjects had some degree of visual impairment; the ready visibility and clarity of the material was widely commented upon. Four of the 30 subjects were registered blind. None of these four was able to see printed material, even when emboldened and of double height. Only one of these four individuals reported any difficulty reading on-screen text and this was only intermittent and typically occurred after some time at the computer when his eyes became "tired".

The most popular material presented was - to the surprise of both the researchers and the nursing staff - anatomical and physiological information, which subjects reported as having been useful in helping to put the stringencies of their regimen into context.

Such information had previously been missing from the CAPD programme at the study centre, owing to the need to concentrate upon imparting practical skills. The benefit accruing to patients from being in possession of such information, however is readily apparent in the number of patients who commented positively upon the introduction of this material into their education. The popularity of anatomical and physiological information appeared to be derived from the vivid and uncomplicated manner in which it could be presented using CAL. The potential for extension of this benefit of the medium is clear, since many areas of patient education require that individuals learn to understand physiological processes. Work is currently in progress to extend the medium to haemodialysis training at the study centre.

A number of advantages of the medium were highlighted by subjects, most common of which were the facility it provided for learning in privacy and at one's own pace. A number of subjects noted that they felt less awkward learning from the computer than in the presence of a nurse, since the computer was an uncritical judge of their progress and of any mistakes. Other advantages were cited as being the greater choice given to subjects over what they would learn and the potential for repeating teaching material as often as required without making extra demands upon nurses' time - something which subjects appeared loathe to do partly because of a perception of nurses as being very busy individuals and partly because of anxieties that any such queries would result in prolonged hospitalisation, an outcome universally dreaded by subjects.

Few disadvantages of CAL were detailed by subjects and those which were mentioned related to the lack of humanity in the computer, which was considered to make it unsuitable for providing individualised information. Subjects also commented upon the importance of the "human touch" provided by interaction with nurses in the teaching of practical skills.

5. Conclusions

The introduction of a novel medium such as CAL requires careful attention to detail during program development. It is possible to successfully utilise CAL in patient education, the medium best serving to supply contextual information and re-inforce messages given elsewhere. The diverse needs of patients as learners make the process of their education a complex one. However, the present study appears to suggest that CAL can usefully be employed even to teach such a widely diverse and particularly challenging group as renal patients.

422

6. References

[1] Close A. Patient Education: A Literature review. *J Adv Nurs* 1988, 13:203-213

[2] Bell JA. The Role of Microcomputers in Nursing *Comput Nurs* 1986, 4:6:255-258

[3] Deardorff WW. Computerised Health Education: A Comparison With Traditional Formats *Health Educ Q* 1986, 13:1:61-72

[4] Fisher LA, Johnson TS, Porter D, Bleich HL and Slack WV. Collection of a Clean Voided Urine Specimen: A Comparison Among Spoken, Written and Computer-Based Instruction *Am J Public Health* 1977, 67:640-644

[5] Rippey RM, Bill D, Abeles M, Day J, Downing DS, Pfeiffer CA, Thal SE and Wetstone SL. Computer- Based Patient Education for Older Persons with Osteo-Arthritis *Arthritis Rheum* 1987, 38:8:932-5

[6] Johnston S and Phillipson C. *Older Learners: The Challenge to Adult Education* 1983, London; Bedford Square Press/NCVO

[7] Luker KA and Box D. The Response of Nurses Towards the Management and Teaching of Patients on Continuous Ambulatory Peritoneal Dialysis (CAPD) *Int J Nurs Stud* 1986, 23:1:51-9

[8] Steinberg SM, Cutler SJ, Nolph KD and Novak JW. A Comprehensive Report on the Experience of Patients on Continuous Ambulatory Peritoneal Dialysis for the Treatment of End-Stage Renal Disease *Am J Kidney Dis* 1984, 4:3:233-41

© 1994 Elsevier Science B.V. All rights reserved.
Nursing Informatics: An International Overview for Nursing in a Technological Era
S.J. Grobe and E.S.P. Pluyter-Wenting, eds.

YUMIS :
Computer Assisted Instruction for Diabetic Patients
Using Multimedia Environment on a Macintosh Computer

Nishimoto M[a] Kobayashi Y[a] Kuribayashi S[a]
Takabayashi K[b] Yoshida S[b] and Satomura Y[c]

[a]*Division Of Diabetic Care , Shinyahashiradai Hospital, 1-8-10, Higurashi, Matsudo, 270, Japan*
[b]*Department of Internal Medicine II , School of Medicine, Chiba University*
[c]*Division of Medical Informatics, Chiba University Hospital,*
1-8-1 Inohana, Chuou-ku, Chiba, 260, Japan

A computer-assisted instruction program for diabetic patients was developed on a Macintosh computer with a card-ware called "SuperCard" in which colour graphics and sounds are available. In this module the patients learn how to use a pen-type insulin injector by themselves. The only manipulation of the computer required by patients is the mouse, and no difficulties in manipulation were found. All the volunteers showed some interests with this method during the trial test. Use of the program reduces the instruction time for patients and may lessen the nurses' work load.

1. Introduction

In the treatment of diabetes, self-management education is one of the most important aspects for patients. To achieve self-management, a patient must learn not only a considerable amount of knowledge concerning diabetes but also the use of various equipment necessary to measure his blood glucose level, and of course his/her self-injection of insulin. The purpose of a diabetes teaching school is to motivate patients to learn accurate medical knowledge about diabetes and perform treatment independently. From this point of view, Computer Assisted Instruction (CAI) is a valuable tool which encourages diabetic patients through active participation in the learning process.

The application of CAI is gaining popularity in the medical field, such as simulation tests for medical students and nurses. Patients have more difficulties to manipulate a computer than medical students. Therefore we developed YUMIS (Yahashira-University Medical Instruction System) which can handle colour pictures and sounds by using SuperCard [1] to provide the extremely user-friendly environment for patients. In this system patients can easily benefit from it.

The goal of YUMIS is for patients to use it easily for self-management and at the same time reduce the redundancy of the nurses' explanation to each and every patient. As for the first part of this CAI program, we developed the module for teaching patients' self-injection with a pen-type insulin and started to use it in practice.

2. System Configuration

YUMIS was developed using the SuperCard version 1.6 (Silicon Beach Software) on Macintosh IIci (Apple) with 8M RAM and a 150M internal hard disk. Graphics were installed from the original pictures with a Scan JX image scanner (Sharp). Thirty-two bit colour pixcel PICT form was created and evolved into an eight bit colour format in an Adobe Photoshop ver. 2.0 and transferred to the SuperCard. A musical passage and verbal instructions were digitalized with the MacRecorder (Fallaon) and transferred to YUMIS by way of a Hypersound (Fallaon).

The CAI program explaining for the pen-type insulin injector is composed of 64 cards with pictures and sounds. Each card has a drawing to explain one action continuing systematically. The only manipulation of the computer required in this program is performed with a mouse, and the patients can continue their learning by clicking the objects. Many buttons are prepared in the pictures to give hints or explanations for easier understanding.

The size of this module is 9.4 M bytes. This module is composed of five sections; 1) how to use this computer, 2) explanation of the pen-type insulin injector and various kinds of insulin, 3) how to prepare to inject insulin, 4) how to exchange an insulin cartridge, 5) other requirements. The contents of each card originated from an experienced nurse's ideas. Rather than photos we adapted drawings in order to explain the contents because drawings seem much more intimate and easier for the patients to understand.

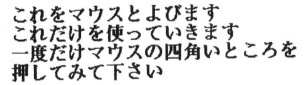

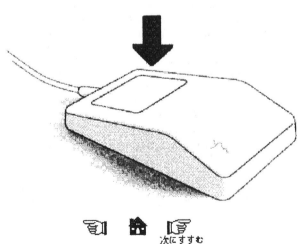

Fig. 1. One of the introduction cards in YUMIS. In the above, both written and verbal instructions are included on the operation of the mouse. In this sentence it is described the use of a mouse. By actually using the mouse the user can go on to the next card.

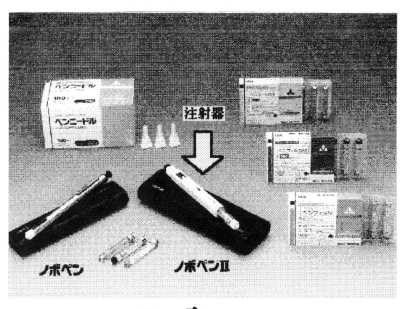

Fig. 2. This picture is showing all the necessary equipment. Some cards have colour photo pictures with verbally explaining for the use of a pen-type insulin injector. The equipment is introduced one by one with an arrow and at the same time, verbally.

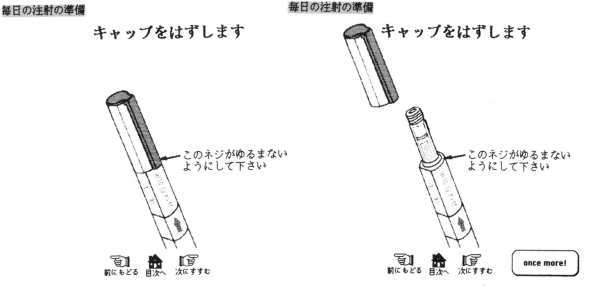

3. These pictures explain how to take off a cap. The right picture shows the cap on and then the picture automatically changes to the left picture which shows the cap off. Normally, one maneuver is presented on one card. A patient is supposed to follow the same procedure as shown on the monitor. The same action and verbal explanation can be repeated on the monitor as often as necessary until he understands.

3. Objects and Validation Test

We tested YUMIS on volunteers composed of patients and medical staff. Ten volunteers ranging from 18 to 57 years old (34±15; mean±SD) manipulated the insulin injector via computer by themselves for the first time and then showed how to use the pen-type insulin injector to a nurse.

We also re-evaluated the previous way of teaching in seven patients (63±14 years old) for calculating the nurse's instruction time and assessing their comprehension. They learned how to manipulate the insulin injector without the computer directly from nurses and then demonstrated how to use it afterwards.

4. Results and Discussion

As for users' manipulation, we did not find any major problems, and this system was welcomed especially by young adults because it was easy to understand. All the volunteers showed at least some interest in this method. A verbal explanation was very helpful in explaining necessary medical knowledge to patients. For patients especially the elderly who are not accustomed to computers, a mouse is not the ideal device, and a more direct input method such as a touch screen might be better. At the present time however, touch screen monitors are rare, so it is much more practical to use a mouse device in the YUMIS system in order to gain widespread popularity.

It seems apparent that YUMIS contributes to time saving. Our previous way of teaching can be divided into three parts. First, explanation of the insulin injector by a nurse, actual execution by the patient, and lastly the completion test. By using YUMIS, the first two parts could be performed almost without a nurse, thus reducing the actual nurses' instruction time (42.6±7.0 (mean±S.D.) minutes). By using YUMIS, it took only 26.4±4.4 (mean±S.D.) minutes. In addition to that, patients could use it at their own pace.

We can not simply compare the time difference between the two groups with or without YUMIS because there is a difference in regards to their ages, and also the time required for CAI naturally depends on the length of the program. These figures however, are encouraging to apply CAI in this field and the important point is that patients could handle it and understand the contents well. We first considered using YUMIS as an introduction to learn about insulin. Seven out of ten volunteers to our surprise indicated that they could understand the information without any further explanation from nurses and they actually demonstrated their good comprehension.

We learned that it was impossible for patients to use the computer completely by themselves and a nurse should advise patients during this CAI. It does not seem to make sense in terms of time saving for nurses. However, since a computer instructs patients standard knowledge in order, only things to do for a nurse is to teach them additional knowledge that they do not understand from the computer. Therefore YUMIS can give a more in-depth and accurate understanding in a shorter time than the previous way and actually reduce the nurses' work load. Furthermore we found that the program is also beneficial for educating nurses themselves before teaching.

The results from YUMIS were comparable to those of DIACIN[2] which was produced in Germany to instructs diabetic patients on the use of insulin by computer. These findings support the practicality of CAI programs such as YUMIS for patients throughout the world.

References

[1] Clancey, W.J. and Letsinger, R. NEOMYCIN: Reconfiguring a rule-based expert system for application to teaching, in WJ Clancey and EH Shortliffe (Eds.), Readings in Medical Artificial Intelligence : The first decade (Addison-Wesley, Reading, MA,) 1981:361-381

[2] Takabayashi,K. et al. Computer Assisted Instruction for Diabetic Patients with SuperCard (DIACIN) : A User Friendly Environment For Patients of All Ages. Health Systems. (Omnipress, Prague) 1992:1459-62

1994 Elsevier Science B.V. All rights reserved.
ursing Informatics: An International Overview for Nursing in a Technological Era
J. Grobe and E.S.P. Pluyter-Wenting, eds.

Multimedia Interventions in Maternal-Infant Community-Based Clinics

Sweeney M A Mercer Z Lester J Oppermann C

The University of Texas Medical Branch, Galveston, Texas 77555, U.S.A.

The Healthy Touch™ Series of multimedia programs has been developed, implemented, and evaluated in selected maternal-infant clinics. A high-tech, high-touch effort in carrying out the design and evaluation of the programs has resulted in a new intervention in clinical care with positive outcomes for both patients and staff. Utilization of the technology has opened up the opportunity to provide consistent, individualized, and enjoyable programs that attract patient participation. The technology is also useful in recording responses to various instruments,and producing a tracking record of the learner's progress.

The purpose of this paper is to describe three aspects of a multimedia series designed to provide health care for new mothers nd their infants: 1) Program development, 2) Implementation in community-based clinics, and 3) Impact Evaluation. The Healthy Touch™ eries, was developed by a team of educators, researchers, and clinicians at The University of Texas Medical Branch in Galveston as part f a health promotion program for community-based clinics with the support of the W.K. Kellogg Foundation.

The interactive courseware is designed for a PC-based platform with a touch-sensitive monitor. Program operation is at an deal level for novices since it requires no technical skills, reading skills, or prior experience with computer programs. The bilingual rograms provide up to six hours of interaction, simulation, and testing of concepts related to pregnancy, infant nutrition, and issues related o infant and childhood safety and immunization.

Interactive multimedia uses technology to bundle together multiple collections of information into a single program or pplication. The collections of information can be full motion video, computer data, animation, graphics, still-frame slides, and stereo audio 1]. Although there are numerous examples of the usefulness of multimedia applications in various teaching functions for professional ducation in the health care field such as nursing education [2], medical education [3], and dental education [4] there are few applications nentioned for patient utilization. The patient-based applications consist of varied applications in rehabilitation medicine [5], and clinic-ased health promotion programs [6],[7]. The development and implementation of The Healthy Touch™ Series is a current example of the ew directions that nursing can take to integrate multimedia applications with sound clinical practice. As Carol Lindeman predicted, Nursing practice in the 21st century...is a vision of the knowledgeable worker using the cutting edge of technology to provide patients, lients, and families with the best of high touch and the best of high tech (p.10.)"

1. Program Development

The multimedia programs were designed from the outset to provide a comfortable, non-threatening, learning environment that vould put the patients at ease; an overall approach of enjoyment or fun so they would be motivated to continue to learn; and a style that vould appear to be non-technical and would provide assistance for learners who may lack basic skills in general literacy, or in dealing with igh technology equipment. The program was also designed to accommodate bilingual patients with comparable versions in Spanish and n English.

The artwork, the screen colors and the navigation system were carefully crafted to meet the overall design. The opening sequence ncludes a colorful animated quilt that was used to enhance the "low-tech" appeal of the program. The quilt icons are used throughout all he programs to provide continuity such as with the teddy bear who appears in the safety program with his arm in a sling.

428

The computer screen in Figure 1 exemplifies many of the design features we sought to include. One section of the program, *Feeding Your Baby*, includes a visit to a computerized grocery store. Colorful foods are pictured for the shelves, and the learner can navigate in any direction around the 3-D grocery store. A discovery learning experience has been constructed in which the patient can touch the sign above the food (to hear the label rather than read it); touch the food (to hear animated audio sounds such as sizzling bacon and get information on nutrient values or age-appropriateness of the foods); or touch the animated grocery cart and move to a new aisle. Screens were created with PC Paintbrush, imported as PCX files directly into the authoring system, Quest 4.0, and combined with digital audio files to be delivered via Soundblaster Pro. The files were mastered on a CD-ROM disc because of the large file size of both the digitized graphics and audio files. (The version of the grocery store with the English version print and audiotrack was nearly 100 MB alone.)

A second example from the series shows how the flexibility in the design can accommodate varied learning needs and styles. In the safety program, entitled *Home "Safe" Home* , the learner is offered a choice of relational courseware formatting or linear formatting. The relational format is the best choice when learners are encouraged to explore all factors affecting the task or concept being taught [1] .

In the "safety house," learners choose between a "browsing" mode and a "tour" mode. In the browsing mode, learners wander into the locations of their choice in the 3D house, garage, or yard, and select any items they want to explore. For example, if they touch the medicine cabinet in the bathroom, the door opens to dislay medicines and many of the other usual items. Each item in the cabinet will respond with an animation or an audio file of information about the particular substance. The "tour" mode offers a selection of tours that have been developed in a linear format to assist in providing organization and structure for the new information. For instance, the Fire Safety tour visits only the locations in the house that

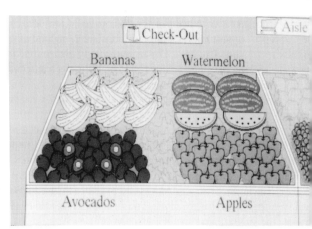

Figure 1 Computer screen from the browsing animation in the program, *Feeding Your Baby*

contain items related to fire or burns. The learner has the opportunity to touch the items to see the animation or hear the fire safety audio message that relates to it, but they cannot move to other non fire-related items in the room if they are on the tour.

One factor that creates added instructional capability in the linear or tour mode is the inclusion of digital video in scaled windows by means of a video digitizer card and video compression technology [9]. A fireman conducts the Fire Safety tour of the 3D graphic safety house. He coordinates the linear instructional approach and gives moving video demonstrations of safety techniques such as the operation of a home fire extinguisher. Thus learners have a wealth of options to meet their educational needs.

2. Program Implementation

The Healthy Touch™ Series was installed in two community-based clinics that are satellite clinics of the university OB-GYN Department operating in conjunction with the County Public Health Department. The clinics handle an annual combined patient load of 14,773 maternity patients, and one has a specialized clinic that was initiated exclusively for pregnant teenagers. Each clinic has a designated area for the interactive learning stations which are housed in kiosks or stationary units. In addition to providing security, the kiosks set forth a friendly, non-threatening environment while exposing only the touchscreen portion of the monitor to the learners. The top portion of the kiosk pictured in Figure 2 stores the computer, the videodisc player, the CD-ROM drive, and the major bulk of the monitor. The end result is a decidedly "low-tech" look for a learning station repleat with the latest of high-technology hardware and software. The learners are largely unaware of the level of sophistication of the hardware since they interact only with the touch-sensitive monitor.

The learning stations have been in operation in the clinics for more than two years and there has been continuous upgrading of both hardware and software as the technology world has changed and matured. The hardware has migrated from 286 processors (and slower) to the present-day world of 486 and greater. The monitors have undergone a transition from EGA to VGA, and the moving images have slowly moved to a CD-ROM platform as that device has been nearing the 30 frames per second rate of video technology. The two onstants of the delivery system to date have consisted of: 1) the ouchscreen method of data entry which mitigates technological know-ow, and 2) the bilingual English and Spanish soundtracks. The authoring software used in program development and implementation consists of a combination of Quest 4.0 and Multimedia Toolbook 1.5, oth of which were supplemented by in-house programming for specific application enhancements written in Pascal.

Gaining cooperation of patients and families in utilizing and evaluating the instructional programs has been extremely easy. The patients often volunteer on their own to take the programs, and most ask o return to the learning station to finish their lesson if it has been nterrupted by a session with the health care provider. They tend to keep their attention on the program despite the usual array of noises and distractions of a busy clinic. We have learned to keep toys and other materials available for the entertainment and educational enhancement of the young children of the patients to provide a diversion if needed.

The multimedia learning stations have been set up to run as efficiently as possible while requiring a minimum level of hands-on nvolvement from the staff. A built-in tracking program records the earners' choice at each decision point, thus providing a digital file of each session. This form of "electronic record keeping" provides a record of the earning choices throughout the use of the program, and stores re-ponses to machine-administered tests and program evaluation instruments.

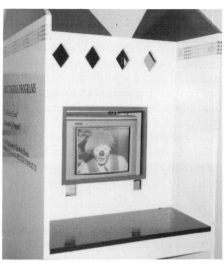

Figure 2 The multimedia learning station or kiosk is designed for security and ease-of-use the community-based clinics.

. Evaluation

The overall program evaluation is assessed in regard to three areas: impact on patients, impact on clinic staff, and utilization of the technology for delivering patient care. The most important data at the front-end evaluation phase is viewer feed-in[10], and it was collected by means of observation, self-report questionnaires, computer-based learner tracking systems, and computer-managed nterviews. Formative evaluation results in all three areas are summarized as follows:

1. Patients like to interact with the program and control the type of information they obtain. We have observed the undivided attention of the patient's program in spite of noisy environmental distractions. After all, the interactive program requires a response from the learner in frequent time intervals in order to move forward to the next phase.

2. The multimedia program appeals to the entire family unit as a learning tool. We have observed a high level of interest from prospective fathers as well as the mothers. Many fathers seem especially interested in the technology. The clinics we are utilizing are attempting to increase the involvement of males in pre and post-natal care. The multimedia technology-based learning is definitely the right step in this direction.

3. Patients are motivated to learn from the program as evidenced by:

a. Requests to return to the place where they left off if they get interrupted while taking the program for an examination by the health care provider.

b. Returning at a later appointment time with a request to see the program again.

c. Returning with another individual (such as a relative, friend or the baby's father) with a request to use the program again. Approximately one-third of the patients bring someone else to use the program.

d. Requests to view the program at times other than routine clinic visits.

e. Requests for printouts of some of the information.

f. Writing down information that appears on the monitor. (Due to this response, we are planning to add a printing option to specific parts of the program.)

4. A positive evaluation of the program as evidenced by responses to a computer-managed "inteview." The authors designed a unique computer-generated program to "interview" patients in a standardize format with minimal response bias. By combining features of a digitized audio card, the touchscreen response system, and a computerized tracking system, subjects are allowed to choose the language of the interview, and whether to *read* or *hear* the questions. For those who experience any difficulty with reading either the questions or response mediaum provides privacy for patients during the session and reduces errors by directly transcribing patient answers to a digital file.

3.1 Staff

1. The programs have been carefully incorporated into the routine educational activities of the clinic. Availability of the programs is advertised in conjunction with other clinic classes and programs.

2. The utilization of the program by the patients is charted. It becomes a part of the patient's permanent health record.

3. Some staff are learning how to operate the equipment in order to provide educational opportunities for patients when our project staff are not available on site.

4. Staff critique programs and make suggestions for adding or modifying content for the patient versions. Advanced level versions which will provide Continuing Education Units for staff will be available in the near future, and should provide increased attention to the interactive equipment.

3.2 Technology

1. The patients were unsure about what to call the interactive program. They began referring to it as the "little video" which prompted us to place a sign on the side of the learning station that labels it as " MULTIMEDIA PROGRAMS, The Healthy Touch™, From the University of Texas Medical Branch, Sponsored by the W.K. KELLOGG FOUNDATION PROJECT

2. Patients are not intimidated by the "high tech" equipment and program. The easy-to-use touchscreen interface makes it seem like a specialized "television monitor" is being used rather than a computer and other components of the technology.

3. Security was an issue before the use of the kiosks. There were minor problems with missing parts such as knobs from the monitor.

4. Technical problems with the hardware and software have been minimal during our pilot-testing as well as the actual implementation of the program. In the experience we've had with operating multimedia units in a total of six community health clinics over a four year period, we have experienced no technical failures to date.

4. Conclusions

The multimedia programs have attained "high marks" from a variety of respondents. The professional staff in the clinic view the high-technology equipment as an adjunct to their clinical care. Patients and families learn specific information by utilizing the multimedia programs and the programs they have completed are listed in their permanent medical record. Clinic staff apply the learning concepts from the multimedia programs to specific aspects of the patient's situation, thus increasing the comprehensiveness of high-touch clinical care.

. References

1] Anderson, C., and Veljkov, M. *Creating Interactive Multimedia.* Glenview, IL. Scott, Foresman and Company, 1990.

2] Becchio, D., Cavicchioli, A., Magnino, M.E., Berra, I., Zara, G.P., Narduzzo, G., and Eandi, M. Multimedia and hypertext programs for nursing education. K.P. Adlassnig, G. Grabner, S. Bengtsson, and R. Hansen,(Eds.). *Lecture Notes in Medical Informatics, Medical Informatics Europe, 1991.* Berlin: Springer-Verlag,1991.

3} Carson, N.E., Kidd, M.R., Cesnik, B., Connoley, G., and McPhee, W.J. Hypermedia medical education programmes. K.C. Lun (ed.). *In MEDINFO '92, Proceedings of the Seventh World Congress on Medical Informatics.* Amsterdam: North-Holland, (1992).

4] Richards, B. and Khoury, D. The use of a touch-screen computer for dental charting. K.P. Adlassnig, G. Grabner, S. Bengtsson, and R. Hansen, (Eds.). *Lecture Notes in Medical Informatics, Medical Informatics Europe, 1991.* Berlin: Springer-Verlag, 1991.

5] Delouis, S., Kouloumdjian, J., Taterode, H., Mohan-Said, H., and Bonnet, C. The use and implications of multimedia systems to help the mentally disabled: A tool to rehabilitate memory. K.C. Lun (ed.). *In MEDINFO '92, Proceedings of the Seventh World Congress on Medical Informatics.* Amsterdam: North-Holland, 1992.

6] Sweeney, M.A., Gulino, C., and Small, M.A. Videodisc technology: Teaching underserved populations about infant feeding. *Journal of Tropical Pediatrics,* 1990, 36, 40-42.

7] Sweeney, M.A., Mercer, Z., Oppermann, C., McHugh, D., and Murphy, C. Innovative designs in multimedia programs for clinical teaching. *In MEDINFO '92, Proceedings of the Seventh World Congress on Medical Informatics.* Amsterdam: North-Holland, 1992.

8] Lindeman, C. Nursing and technology: Moving into the 21st century. *Caring Magazine,* 1992, 9: 5-10.

9] Luther, A. *Digital Video in the PC Environment.* New York: McGraw-Hill Book Company, 1989.

10] Sneed, L. *Evaluating Video Programs: Is it Worth It?* White Plains, NY: Knowledge Industry Publications, Inc., 1991.

Section III

RESEARCH

Nursing Informatics: An International Overview for Nursing in a Technological Era
S.J. Grobe and E.S.P. Pluyter-Wenting, eds.

Research Plan for Implementation of a Nursing Information System

Button PS Hall PD Joy JA Slattery MJ

Dartmouth-Hitchcock Medical Center, Lebanon, NH 03756

This paper will explore the various aspects of a research plan for an automated Nursing Information System. The paper will initially discuss the role of individual and institutional motivation and commitment to research as a component of information systems planning and implementation. Critical to a research plan is the inclusion of specific research activities in the overall nursing information system plan. The dearth of well conducted and reported research in the current literature serves to both motivate and discourage potential researchers. While it is very clear that both quantitative and qualitative work regarding systems, their implementation and their impact is needed, there are relatively few good studies available to use as models. A positive factor for potential researchers is the growth of interest and early research efforts and the willingness of those involved to share ideas, tools, and preliminary findings. Networking is critical.

The initial step in developing a research plan is a thorough assessment of a variety of factors: (1) the scope of current research, including identification of those areas which have been neglected; (2) the needs of the institution, as defined by project tools and objectives; (3) available resources within and external to the institution, such as graduate students and grants; (4) potential researcher interest and expertise. There is no prescription for the appropriate content of a particular institution's research plan.

The remainder of the paper will focus on description of the research plan at one institution, including the development of motivation and commitment, the specific plan, and the current status of the plan, including results to date. Three research studies will be described in detail.

1. Overview

The purpose of this paper is to describe the development and content of a research plan that is an integral part of a clinical information system development project. In 1991, DHMC contracted with the Cerner Corporation to install several of Cerner's market ready software packages and to function as a co-development partner with Cerner for applications to address the functions of care planning, provider documentation, results reporting and display and physician order entry.

During the clinical information system selection process, nursing members of the project team conducted a thorough review of the published literature on clinical information systems. This review revealed many anecdotal articles but very few quality research studies. For this reason, the team decided that including research in the project plan would not only enhance the project but would make a contribution to the science of nursing informatics and the nursing profession as a whole.

In addition, there was significant expertise and motivation both within the project and the Nursing Department. The Director of Nursing Research provided consultation to the team throughout the project, as well as being the initial contact with the University of Iowa research team for the NIC work. Two project team members were doctorally prepared. Several others were part-time masters' students during the project and incorporated some of the research in their programs of study.

Another key motivating factor was the availability of networking opportunities. Through conferences, vendor reference calls and recruitment efforts, various team members established relationships with nurses involved in informatics. Many of these nurses had either completed studies that had not been published or had wonderful ideas. They served, and continue to serve, as a rich source of input related to research, as well as other aspects of the overall project.

Another factor which influenced the research plan was the team's analysis of the needs of the institution, as defined by the project goals and objectives. The three project goals which the team identified as particularly important to address include: direct on line entry of medical orders by physicians, measurable improvements in the quality of documentation, and measurable productivity improvements related to the processing of orders. The institutional significance of these goals is grounded in the strong commitment of the organization to improve the processes of patient care as the means of continuously improving quality, as well as appropriately reducing costs.

Based on the influence of the factors listed above, the project team agreed to include research as a formal component of the overall project plan. Next, the team brainstormed the potential content of the plan. The resulting number of studies was overwhelming given available resources and the other aspects of the project plan. It is of note that the institution strongly supported the concept of including research in the project plan, but did not fund additional positions to carry out the studies. The next step in the development of the actual plan was a careful assessment of priorities based primarily on the needs of the institution and researcher expertise, interest, and availability. The resultant list of studies included: Quality of Nursing Documentation, Amount of Nurse Overtime, Nursing Intervention Classification (NIC), Staff Nurse Response to the Process of Clinical Information Systems Implementation, Order Capture, Time Frames of Order Entry Process, Physician Attitudes related to Clinical Automation, Effect of Automation on Providers' Sense of Professionalism, Patient Attitudes Related to Clinical Automation, Cost Benefit Study.

The team has achieved the operationalization of this plan by means of insisting on including research activities as part of the formal project structure, role definitions, and daily operations. The research group of the project staff meets monthly for two hours as the primary means of facilitating the development and implementation of studies. The group members serve as consultants to each other on the content of studies.

2. The Impact of Automation on Nursing Documentation

Documentation is an integral part of patient care. Nurses have a legal and professional responsibility to document their ca' however the realities of current systems often result in documentation that is incomplete, illegible and redundant. Not only do documentation have medicolegal and reimbursement implications, it is one of the major modes of communication between health ca providers. Implementation of a computerized system designed to improve the quality of documentation and therefore facilita communication between providers should have a positive impact on patient care. The purpose of this study, therefore is to evalua the impact of automation on the completeness of nursing documentation.

The investigators developed a "completeness of documentation" instrument based on JCAHO standards for documentati and input from a paper of staff nurses. Items were selected for this measure based on the results of an in-house JCAHO "moc survey and include critical elements of the nursing process. Variables to be measured include documentation of admission assessmer nursing care plan, progress toward outcomes, discharge teaching/medications, and discharge planning. System variables which m reflect nursing workload, admission and discharge day of the week, patient acuity, census, and nursing models of practice on the un will also be measured.

For this study, data will be collected pre- and post-implementation of the nursing components of an automated Clinic Information System. A pilot study will be conducted in May 1993, prior to the JCAHO survey. Pre-implementation data will collected 3 months prior to the initial implementation of the system. Data will be collected by retrospective chart audit from clos records after patients have been discharged. Post implementation data will be collected from documentation completed 6 to 9 mon' after implementation of the system.

For the time period 3 to 6 months prior to CIS implementation, one data representing each of the seven days of the week w be randomly selected. Patients will then be randomly selected from the list of discharges on each of those seven days. Fifteen recor per day (for a total sample of 105 patients) will be selected from patients who, except for time spent in an intensive care unit (limit to one ICU), were only on one nursing unit during their hospital stay. Hospital records of employees and Short Stay Patients (< hours) will be excluded from the study.

Pilot study data will be analyzed using descriptive statistics. Results of the pilot study will be available for the Qualit Assurance Department to help identify areas of nursing documentation needing improvement prior to the JCAHO visit (fall of 199: Comparisons will be made between the pre and post CIS implementation data.

This paper will present the findings of the project to date including refinements of the instrument based on the pilot study a results of the first phase of data collection.

3. Staff Nurse Response to the Process of Clinical Information Systems Implementation

The manner in which an automated Clinical Information System (CIS) is implemented has the potential to affect the ultima success of the system. The purpose of this study is to examine how different factors influence implementation of such a system. T research questions for this qualitative study will be based on those used by Dr. Patricia S. Button in a study of clinical poli implementation.

The term Clinical Information System refers to automated order entry, nursing documentation, and nursing care planning nctions. Implementation refers to the actual process of "going live," making the transition from manual to the automated systems scribed.

The research questions will explore the perception of staff nurses of relevant implementation factors in the process of CIS plementation on their unit. Respondents will be asked, during semi-structured, open ended interviews, their perceptions of what ctors influenced the implementation of the CIS, and in what way. Results will be compared to Dr. Button's findings. Literature ated to change and to implementation of other changes in nursing will be utilized.

The methodology for sample selection, data collection, and analysis will be presented. The progress of the study up to the ne of the presentation will be shared.

Physician Order Entry Time Study

Research related to the benefits of computer based order entry by physicians has only recently begun to appear. Clinical and st benefits as a result of legible and complete orders, electronic communication of orders, and reduction in duplication and necessary examinations have been noted. Direct benefit to physicians in time savings or improved clinical information are not often ted or, on the contrary, note increases in order entry time as a result of automating the process.

The purpose of this study is to compare the time taken by a manual order entry and order communication process (to partmental computer systems) with the time taken to achieve the same objective following implementation of direct physician order try and electronic transmission of orders to the departmental systems.

The study will be hospital based and confined to orders written on active inpatient records. The sample will consist of at least house officers and 20 attending physicians who agree to participate and who will be available for both study periods. A trained server will accompany subjects individually on rounds at a time selected by the subject. The post-implementation observation will blicate the time selected for the pre-implementation period. Using operationally defined order entry time segments, and a data llection tool designed for the purpose, the observer will time all order entry behavior from initiation to completion in ten records m each subject.

In the pre-implementation data collection period (manual ordering system), the time segment to be monitored will be the time m the initiation of a chart search to entry of the order into the appropriate departmental systems. The order entry time segment to measured in the post-implementation study (automated system) will be the time period from initiation of a search for an available minal to the electronic signature of entered orders (roughly equivalent to the moment that orders would be queued to departmental stems). The order types studied will be limited to those with operational departmental systems: laboratory, pharmacy, and iology.

Nursing Informatics: An International Overview for Nursing in a Technological Era
S.J. Grobe and E.S.P. Pluyter-Wenting, eds.

438

The progress of computer supported health and nursing care information systems in Swedish hospitals

Rosander R, PhD and Bergbom Engberg I, RN, DMSc

University College of Health Sciences, P.O.Box 1038, S-551 11 Jönköping, Sweden.

During last decade, the rapid implementation of computer supported health care systems in Swedish hospitals has brought about quite radical changes in the daily work of many professional groups. In order to describe the progress and experience of computerization, we have carried out a survey study of most hospitals in Sweden. The aim was twofold, partly we wanted to present a quantitative picture of the different types of hardware, software and systems currently in operation, and we also wished to evaluate the extent of nursing involvement in the process of decision making and implementation.
A total of 361 computer users in 69 major hospitals / districts have contributed to the study by replying to a questionnaire, giving an extensive view of the level of, and the experience of the use of computers in Swedish health care. With the findings of this survey, we can, for the first time, describe the nursing use of computers, as well as the nurses' role and participation in the planning and implementation process of computerization in our country.

1. Background

Except for a small number of private hospitals, almost all hospitals in Sweden are publicly owned by the county councils, which are regional units of self-governement, mainly financed by local income tax. The 23 county councils are also responsible for outpatient medical care at hospital clinics and outpatient centers, as well as for public preventive health services. Up to now the county councils have also been in charge of nursing and related health care professional training programs within the higher education system.

The use of computer technology and information systems has increased considerably in Swedish health care work, bringing new demands to the nursing profession, as well as other para-medical staff. Although there have been a few attempts to establish nation-wide hospital information systems, most districts, hospitals or units choose their own computer strategy, based on locally developed systems or commercially available programme packages. Knowing that nurses are, to a great extent, end users of the new technology, we have carried out a study of the implementation of different information systems in the hospital environment, as well as an evaluation of the extent of nursing involvement in this process. Such survey studies have been reported from other countries or states [1, 2], but not yet in Sweden.

2. Methods and Data Collection

As a base for our survey we constructed a model or "structural map" of health and nursing care information systems available, see Figure 1, with five main areas: *A: Personnel management, B: Patient care management, C: Service and support, D: Patient care documentation and E: Expert systems.* This design was presented as a preliminary version at the Nursing Informatics`91 Conference [3].

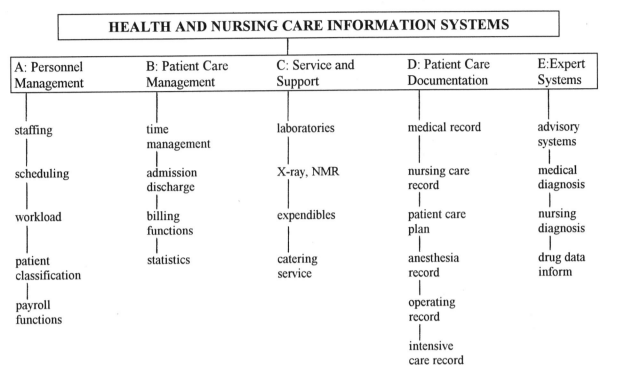

Figure 1. A "structural map" of health and nursing care information systems running in Swedish hospitals.

The data collection was performed by a semistructured, self-report questionnaire, developed to examine the following topics:

- *the level of computerization*
- *characteristics of users*
- *opinions and attitudes towards computerization.*
- *hardware and systems specifications*
- *benefits and drawbacks of installed systems*

The questionnaire was distributed to the 94 Swedish major hospitals/districts, covering all counties. Just a very few small units were excluded. A total of 361 computer users or user teams in 69 hospitals/districts contributed to the study, giving an extensive view of the level of and experience of the use of computers in Swedish health care, up to 1991. The hospital response rate was 73.4% and an average of 5.2 respondents or teams per hospital participated.

3. Some Results

The analysis of the research data gave partly a quantitative picture of the systems, software and hardware in operation, the time scale of computerization, characteristics of end users and so on. This will be described further in some detail. We also received a qualitative image of nurses´ participation in the decision making process and of their opinions, attitudes and educational needs. The result from this part is presented in another paper in this Proceedings [4].

The distribution of health and nursing care information systems in operation 1991 in Swedish hospitals can be seen in Figure 2. *Personnel management* and *Patient care management* are areas where the need of computer supported systems was established early and where the software solutions are similar to those of any effective business management. More than 90% of the hospitals have such systems in operation. Two rapidly developing areas are *Patient care documentation* and *Expert systems*, which in our study are used in more than half the number of hospitals.

440

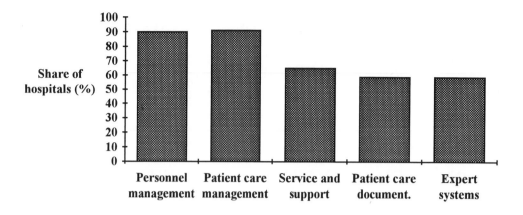

Figure 2. Distribution of health and nursing care information systems in operation 1991.

Furthermore, we have tried to describe a time scale for the computerization of Swedish health care, see Figure 3, which shows that the main areas in our model are implemented in different stages. In the graph we have combined system areas A and B, used in hospital management, and C, D and E, which are related to the operative health work. Systems concerning *A: Personnel management* and *B: Patient care management* were introduced a few years before systems in the areas of *C: Service and support, D: Patient care documentation* and *E: Expert systems.* Only 1% of computer systems running today were installed in the Seventies.

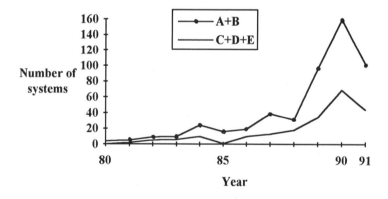

Figure 3. Number of new systems installed per year 1980 - 1990, plus part of 1991.

The most used computer applications is given in order in Table 1 as a percentage of all respondents (n=361).

Table 1
The five most used computer applications (% of respondents)

Patient time management	46.3
Personnel scheduling	34.6
Patient admission/discharge	31.0
Personnel staffing	25.8
Medical diagnosis	20.8

More than half of the systems (55%) are used by nurses, as can be seen in Figure 4, showing the distribution of end users among different health professional groups. The remaining group consists principally of ward secretaries and physicians.

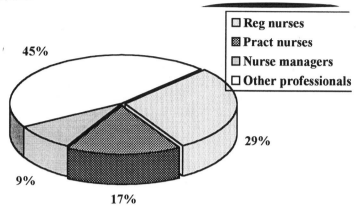

Figure 4. The distribution of end users among health professionals.

In the following applications *registered nurses* are the largest user group:

- workload
- time management
- communication with laboratories
- nursing care record

- patient care planning
- intensive care supervision
- patient advisory systems

4. Discussion

Summarizing our results we can distinguish a few *very simplified trends* in the process of computerization versus time in Sweden:

TIME PERIOD	End of Seventies	Eighties	Nineties
HARDWARE	some large computers with batch processing a few microcomputers	mainframes with "dumb" terminals	more PC's, Mac's and local networks
SOFTWARE	home-made by users	large expensive custom designed	more commercial packages
USERS	experts administrators a few physcians	administrators secretaries	most professional groups
TYPE OF PROBLEM	financial/administrative limited medical problem solving	all financial and most personnel administration	all financial, personnel and patient administration some care documentation some decision support

We have shown that after a slow start in the early Eighties, the computerization of Swedish hospitals is undergoing a rapid growth. The different nurse professionals are already the major end user group. In our opinion strategic planning for system development, supporting nursing work, has been weak. This depends partly on low computer literacy and inadequate training among nurses, and partly on too many different locally developed hospital systems. What we could need is a more general nursing system model, for example as described by Behrenbeck et al [5], designed for Swedish conditions, possibly on a national level.

In our survey study we have been able to catch a glimpse of current nursing use of computerized information systems in Sweden. Unfortunately, because of the very rapid development in this field, we may have been about two years early in our data gathering. Many respondents have remarked this as for example:

- "just started with computerization in our hospital"
- "you could have waited with your questions one year more"
- "we feel that we are still beginners"
- "in our hospital we have not yet realized our plans"
- "we have an intense preparation work going on".

However this makes a follow-up study desirable, as we can imagine that more experience of, and more influence on new technology will give increased benefits in the advance of nursing quality.

5. References

[1] Hausman JP and Grant JM. A New Zealand strategic plan to introduce nursing informatics on a national basis. In: *Nursing Informatics '91*. Hovenga EJS, Hannah KJ, McCormick KA, Ronald JS (eds). Berlin: Springer-Verlag, 1991: 35-39.

[2] Axford R and McGuiness B. Computerisation of nursing information systems in public and private acute care hospitals: The state of the art. In: *Nursing Informatics '91*. Hovenga EJS, Hannah KJ, McCormick KA, Ronald JS (eds). Berlin: Springer-Verlag, 1991: 231-233.

[3] Bergbom Engberg I and Rosander R. Health system development research: A survey of nursing use of information systems in Sweden. *Nursing Informatics '91*, Poster session 7. Melbourne, Australia 1991.

[4] Bergbom Engberg I and Rosander R. Nurses' participation in and opinions towards the implementation of computer based information systems in Swedish hospitals. In: *Nursing Informatics '94*, to be published.

[5] Behrenbeck JG, Davitt P, Ironside P, Mangan DB, O'Shaughnessy D and Steele S. Strategic planning for a nursing information system (NIS) in the hospital setting. Development of a nursing system model. *Comput Nurs* 1990, 8: 236-242.

Nursing Informatics: An International Overview for Nursing in a Technological Era
.J. Grobe and E.S.P. Pluyter-Wenting, eds.

Nursing Informatics: The Unfolding of a New Science

Ryan SA[b] and Nagle LM[a]

Gerald P. Turner Department of Nursing, Mount Sinai Hospital,
600 University Avenue, Toronto, Ontario CANADA M5G 1X5

School of Nursing, University of Rochester, Rochester, New York USA 14642

The essence of nursing in the 21st century will be most likely defined by our knowledge and science. The profession must capitalize on the potential of nursing informatics to advance nursing knowledge and expand the boundaries of nursing science. Accepting nursing informatics as an essential dimension of nursing science will be pivotal to demonstrating our unique and valuable contribution to the health care system. The authors discuss the science of information as it arises in the context of nursing informatics and interfaces with nursing science. Challenges and directions for expanding the science of information in nursing will be identified.

1. Introduction

In the 80's, the term "*information* society" was used to describe the disposition of the modern world [1]. The preponderance of activities directed to the management of unwieldy volumes of data and information warranted this characterization. More recently, Toffler [2] described the transformational effects of *knowledge*, the breakdown of conventional disciplines, and resulting power shifts:

> With the help of the computer, the same data or information can now easily be clustered or "cut" in quite different ways, helping the user to view the same problem from quite different angles, and to synthesize meta-knowledge [p.427].

An essential and core function of nursing, the ability to purvey, process, and manage information is largely determining the future of nursing as a practice discipline. The evolution of nursing informatics has provided nurses with opportunities to influence the design and selection of technologies to support practice. New tools for the manipulation of data and information beyond better management are rapidly becoming accessible to nurses in clinical settings throughout the world. The ability to electronically integrate and analyze data and information from diverse settings and populations provides an opportunity to enrich nursing science and generate nursing knowledge in ways heretofore unknown. Nursing informatics is rapidly emerging as the vehicle by which the science of "nursing" information will be elucidated for the discipline and vendor community.

2. What is a Science?

A discipline science is "a field of scholarly inquiry which expresses the entire domain of problems studied by that scholarly community" [3]. This is a metaterm mapping out the broad theoretical domain of problems and ideas which are unique to that particular discipline.

Nursing science has been described as a subset of the discipline of nursing [4] and distinguished from nursing research [5]. Nursing research is the systematic process of inquiry into the phenomena of interest and concern to nurses whereas nursing science has been defined as a representation of:

> "our currently limited understanding of human biology and behavior in health and illness, including

the processes by which changes in health status are brought about, the patterns of behavior associated with normal and critical life events, and the principles and laws governing life states and processes" [5, p. 180].

Distinguished from nursing practice and nursing knowledge, the science of nursing is purported to provide an empirical substantiation for nursing practice. Nursing knowledge is derived from the conduct of nursing science.

Refinetti [6] described the two predominant modes of knowledge development espoused by philosophers: analytical and dialectical. Proponents of the analytical approach support Cartesian notions and suggest that knowledge development is a cumulative process. Where as supporters of the dialectical view advance the position that knowledge development is a wholistic and integrative process. Historically, nursing science has been dominated by the tenets of logical positivism thus the analytical view. Within the context of this paradigm, knowledge development is a gradual process and based on the movement from simple to complex concepts. A majority of nurse researchers have attempted to develop nursing knowledge on the basis of findings from *multiple* studies, across *multiple* populations, using *multiple* measures of *multiple* concepts. Although the contributions of analytic nursing science have been substantial, the advancement of nursing knowledge from these cumulative studies has been limited.

An indepth discussion of philosophy of science and knowledge development in nursing is beyond the scope of this paper, but will be necessary in determining modes of information processing. New views of nursing science have emerged and multiple methods of knowledge discovery are being advocated by nurse scientists [7,8,9,10]. Acknowledging the philosophical and methodological diversity in nursing science will be fundamental to the design of knowledge yielding systems in the future.

It has been suggested that although divergent views of knowledge development might be complementary, convergence would not be practical in terms of information processing [6]. These authors suggest that in light of new technologies an intersection of analytic and dialectic modes of knowledge development should be quite possible. Furthermore, the responsibility for unfolding nursing knowledge need not be limited to the nurse scientist, but extended to nurses in all roles. New modes of knowledge generation will need to be based upon a reconceptualization of the requirements for data and information processing in nursing - an articulation of nursing's "science of information".

3. Information as Science

The concept of information is derived from the Latin *information* which means a process to communicate or the communication of something. According to Yuexiao [11], information may refer to messages, news, data, knowledge, documents, literature, intelligence, symbols, signs, hints, tips. The process and phenomenon of information exists in the realm of human societies, but can also be described in relation to philosophical concepts (e.g. time and space) and the mechanical and animal world [12]. In fact there is a multiplicity of definitions and classifications of information, each of which may have particular meaning and import to nursing.

Examining information schemes such as that described by Mikhailov [13] may provide direction for defining the nature and boundaries of nursing information. Subsequent to an analysis of the definitions and sciences of information, Yuexiao [11] concluded that consensual definitions within professions or sciences is important and necessary for precise communication and scientific progress. This appeal for concordance may be likened to the case for a minimum data set in nursing but expands the notion from data to information.

Information related fields such as cybernetics, semiotics, library science, computer science, cognitive science abound in academia. Many disciplines have identified the science of information as it relates to the particular practice or knowledge base of the practitioners: Information Sociology, Information Economics, Information Politics, Information Psychology. Further examination of these disciplines may provide insights to the process of explicating a "nursing" science of information.

4. Science of Nursing Information: Nursing Informatics

The science of information has been named *Information Science, Informatics, Informatistics, Informology, and Informatology* [14]. Informatics has been described as the convergence of information science, computer science, and discipline-specific science [15]. Applying this definition to the study of nursing informatics, Graves and Corcoran [16] discussed the interface of computer science, information science, and nursing science. A recent discussion of the interface added the notion that this merging of sciences allows for "informatization" to occur within the discipline [17].

Informatization is defined as the "synergistic use of computer, information, and discipline-specific science resulting in the generation of new knowledge that could be used as expert decision support" [17, p. 977].

Scarrott [18] described the need for a "science of information" and its ultimate value in leading to the development of a conceptual framework to guide system design at every level. He identified six criteria which could be used to ascertain the existence of a credible "science of information". The necessity and centrality of a "science of information" to all other dimensions of nursing science becomes apparent when examined in the context of these criteria. For the purpose of illustration, each criterion will be briefly discussed as directly relates to the practice and science of nursing.

• *Should be derived from observation of the functions, structures, dynamic behaviour, and statistical features of information and the symbols used to represent information.*

In nursing, data and information are derived from the practice of nurses, their observations, interactions, and their knowledge representations. Nursing information arises from the compilation of many data elements for one or several patients. The capability to accrue patient data and information over time, across multiple settings and populations from multiple sources (e.g. patient databases, monitors) should be the goal of systems to support knowledge development.

• *Should respect the distinction between limited symbol combinations and the rich human understanding they are used to represent.*

Increasingly, nurse scientists are enhancing or moving away from the traditions of the empiricist paradigm. This shifting of paradigms, in the Kuhnian sense [19], can be partially attributed to the need for methods of inquiry which capture the richness of human experience. Data and information as collected by nurses has limited capacity for quantification. Nurse scientists have begun to recognize the limited utility and generalizability of codified information. Nurse informaticists have begun to identify the need for information systems which allow for the capture of unique human experience.

• *Must fit with our established understanding of nature including the existence of complex living organisms, together with social groups of such organisms.*

To date, applications of information science and technology have been largely designed on the basis of the interdepartmental complexity of health care organizations. Accommodation of complex discipline-specific needs for information management is less apparent in the realm of current clinical information systems. However, nurse informaticists are providing vendors with insights to those complexities more than ever before.

• *Must offer a context into which established but hitherto isolated theoretical aspects of information engineering e.g. automation theory can be fitted.*

The science of nursing informatics supports the integration of information engineering principles into the context of nursing practice, administration, research, and education. As a matter of course, information engineering is being embraced and advanced by nurse informaticists as a mechanism to engineer new nursing knowledge.

• *Should offer useful guidance to those engaged in the design of information systems to serve organized groups of people in the most cost-effective way.*

Nurse informaticists have directed energy to the evaluation of existing system designs and components. Numerous studies report the impact of nurse involvement in the selection, implementation, and evaluation of information systems in practice and education. Evaluations of efficiency and effectiveness outcomes have largely focused on the potential cost-savings associated with hospital information systems and not direct consequences for nursing practice.

• *Should offer useful and verifiable evidence regarding the scope and limitations of AI and consequently should offer useful guidance to those engaged in selecting, supporting, and undertaking exploratory enterprises in the field of information engineering.*

Nurse researchers have investigated the potential benefits to be derived from the development of expert systems to support nurses in practice settings. Several nurse authors have acknowledged the limitations to developing and using expert systems in nursing [20,21,22]. Nevertheless, there are many opportunities for further research in understanding the nature of information processing among nurses.

5. Conclusion

New modes of knowledge generation will need to be based upon a reconceptualization of the requirements for data and information processing in nursing - an articulation of nursing's "science of information". Delineating a science of information is a challenge for all professions and disciplines, not just nursing. Nursing informatics is rapidly emerging as the vehicle by which the science of "nursing" information will be elucidated. The development of a schema for the identifying the dimensions of nursing information will provide a foundation for further explication of what and how knowledge engineering can evolve in nursing. Ideally, a science of information for nursing will evolve over the next decade such that technological opportunities can be used to illuminate the unique and essential role of the nursing profession.

6. References

[1] Naisbitt J. *Megatrends: Ten new directions for transforming our lives.* New York: Warner Books, 1984.

[2] Toffler A. *Powershift.* New York: Bantam Books, 1990.

[3] Schrader A M. In search of a name: Information science and its conceptual antecedents. *Library and Information Science Research* 1984, 6:227-271.

[4] Donaldson S K and Crowley D. The discipline of nursing. *Nurs Out* 1978, 26:113-120.

[5] Gortner S. Nursing science in transition. *Nurs Res* 1980, 29:180-183.

[6] Refinetti R. Information processing as a central issue in philosophy of science. *Information Processing & Management* 1989, 25:583-584.

[7] Tinkle M B and Beaton J L. Toward a new view of science: Implications for nursing research. *ANS Adv Nurs Sci* 1983, 5:27-36.

[8] Allen D, Benner P, and Diekelmann N L. Three paradigms for nursing research: Methodological implications. In *Nursing Research Methodology.* Chinn P (ed.). Rockville, MA: Aspen, 1986:23-38.

[9] Davidson A W and Ray M A. Studying the human-environment phenomenon using the science of complexity. *ANS Adv Nurs Sci* 1991, 14:73-87.

[10] Coward D. Critical multiplism: A research strategy for nursing science. *Image* 1990, 22:163-167.

[11] Yuexiao Z. Definitions and sciences of information. *Information Processing & Management* 1988, 24:479-491.

[12] Weiner N. *Cybernetics, or control and communication in the animal and the machine* 2nd ed. Cambridge, MA: MIT Press, 1984.

[13] Mikhailov A I et al. *Scientific communications and informatics* (English version translated by R H Burger). Arlington, VA: Information Resources Press, 1984.

[14] Wellisch H. From information science to informatics: A terminological investigation. *Journal of Librarianship* 1972, 4:157-187.

[15] Gorn, S. Informatics. In: *The Study of Information Interdisciplinary Messages.* Machlup F and Mansfield U (eds.). New York: Wiley, 1983:121-140.

[16] Graves J R and Corcoran S. The study of nursing informatics. *Image* 1989, 21:227-231.

[17] Shamian J, Nagle L M, and Hannah K J. Optimizing outcomes of nursing informatization. In *MEDINFO 92* Lun K C, Degoulet P, Piemme T E, and Rienhoff O (eds.). Amsterdam: North Holland, 1992:976-980.

[18] Scarrott G. The need for a "Science" of information. *J of Info Tech* 1986, 1:33-38.

[19] Kuhn T S. *The Structure of Scientific Revolutions*. Chicago: University of Chicago Press, 1962.

[20] Sinclair V G. Potential effects of decision support systems on the role of the nurse. *Comput Nurs* 1990, 8:60-65.

[21] Ozbolt J G. Developing decision support systems for nursing: Theoretical bases for advanced computer systems. *Comput Nurs* 1987, 5:105-111.

[22] Brennan P F and McHugh, M J. Clinical decision-making and computer support. *App Nurs Res* 1988, 1:89-93.

Nursing Informatics: An International Overview for Nursing in a Technological Era
S.J. Grobe and E.S.P. Pluyter-Wenting, eds.

448

High Performance Computing for Nursing Research

Meintz S L

Dept of Nursing, College of Health Science, University of Nevada, Las Vegas, 4505 South Maryland Parkway, Las Vegas, Nevada 89154, USA.

Nursing research has found a new source of power in the high performance computing and communication environment with the application of the CRAY Y-MP 2/216 supercomputer. The paradigm shift in statistical analysis to global analysis tera exploratory statistics redefines the statistical methodology for analysis of mega/tera databases using data visualization as a supercomputer completes computations in seconds or minutes. The avenue for including graphic user interfaces to link Global Analysis Tera Exploratory Statistics (GATES) with computer model simulations and data analysis networks provides for future directions. In the future, after establishing the foundational parameters of health, new applications may lead to a formula for predicting effects of nursing action and intervention on health trends; or application of virtual reality techniques for educating both lay persons and professionals about health parameters; or a means for analysis of acute care data as the data are being collected. The possibilities for discovery and advancement in Nurmetrics, Computational Nursing, and Nursing Informatics are significant when the high performance computing and communication environment is explored with a CRAY Y-MP supercomputer for analyses of mega/tera datasets in nursing and health.

1. Introduction

From the validation of supercomputing for nursing and health data research in 1991 to supercomputers powering nursing research discoveries in 1992, research efforts continue to maximize the utilization of supercomputers for data research in nursing, health science, and associated disciplines. A window of opportunity was opened for nurse researchers through the UNLV/CRAY Project for Nursing and Health Data Research (PNHDR) of the University of Nevada, Las Vegas, USA, to determine the viability of supercomputing for analyzing huge datasets of health data archived by government and nongovernment sources (Meintz, 1992). Analysis of such large samples of population could support or nullify the current theories supporting nursing practice and the foundations of health care. Although supercomputers seem necessary to analyze huge datasets of archived health data, the use of the supercomputer by nursing researchers demanded a break from traditional methodologies.

Nurse researchers typically use classical analysis to formulate theories--that is, they reduce data to a manageable size and form generalizations for larger populations and broader theories. Frequently the sample size is barely large enough to be statistically significant; however, the research results are added to the body of scientific nursing knowledge, and nursing practice is based on this theory without the benefit of validation from huge samples.

With a Cray Research grant to PNHDR, the supercomputer application was able to open new directions for analysis. For the first time, nursing science entered the high performance computing environment to confirm, nullify, and/or deduce new parameters in nursing and health science with the ultimate goal of providing better prescriptive and preventative health care within controlled economic boundaries. Parameters of health previously established with a sample size of 1,000 could now be evaluated with a sample size of 25,000 to 50,000 to 10 million.

2. Research and Development (R&D) Methodology

The PNHDR's R&D project involves seven phases of research and development. The phases include: (1) Conceptualization of complex problem resolution, (2) Design of product and/or process, (3) Development of product and/or process, (4) Dissemination of preliminary results and/or prototypes, (5) Alpha site application for testing and debugging, (6) Beta site application for refinement and further debugging, and (7) Dissemination of product and/or process through software, manuals, educational programs, publications and/or presentations. The phases are independent and interrelated resulting in a multilevel approach for supercomputing application to establishing the foundational parameters of health through mega/tera data base analysis.

To facilitate the R&D effort, a framework for application of supercomputing to nursing and health data research was developed as a means to clarify the input, throughput, output, and outcome of R&D phase one. Pioneer efforts by nursing scientists to enter the high performance computing environment with application of the CRAY Y-MP 2/216 Supercomputer were successful in validation of the supercomputer application. The validation Case Study utilized a manageable data base of 17,000 cases and analyses with the Statistical Package for Social Scientists (SPSS) using computer platforms including personal computer, Sun, and the Cray supercomputer. Needless to say, the personal computer was unable to process the analysis and the Sun was slower than the CRAY Y-MP which completed the analysis in approximately 127 seconds.

3. Research Progress

Although nursing professionals are relative latecomers to the high performance computing and communication environment, this path to discovery is well worth the effort. Through the use of the Cray Research system, databases with millions to trillions of bytes can be analyzed in seconds instead of hours or days. Critical elements related to humans and the nursing meta paradigm are available in many diverse databases---databases whose size demands the capabilities of supercomputing for analysis.

While the supercomputing solution seems like the only current option, barriers to this application also exist. Most nursing researchers need new skills to facilitate supercomputing applications, even with the assistance of engineers and computer scientists. Supercomputing standards, while generally familiar to traditional users, are not familiar to nursing professionals who are accustomed to a personal computer interface. Additionally, many of the available statistical software packages for high performance computing require programming, a skill not currently taught in nursing curricula, and very few nurse scientists understand the components or architecture of supercomputers. Although they may be skilled in the use of a personal computer and its role in secondary data analysis on small datasets, they need further knowledge to analyze large datasets with supercomputers.

Nurse researchers also are limited by existing tools. Because their personal computers are constrained by performance and lack of connection to important networks, nurse researchers using supercomputers often must "borrow" the workstation of a scientist or engineer, run the program, and print out the results which often consist of reams of paper for a relatively simple analysis in order to share these results with other researchers. Traditional users of supercomputers have ready access to a networked workstation and can often view results in graphical form and share them easily with others via an electronic connection.

The application of supercomputing in the nursing profession has generated a new branch of nursing science called *Nurmetrics* which incorporates the two specialties of Computational Nursing and Nursing Informatics (Meintz, 1992). Each is defined:

- *Nurmetrics*, the branch of nursing science applying mathematical form and statistical techniques to the testing, estimation, and quantifying of nursing theories and solutions of nursing problems.
- *Computational Nursing*, the branch of Nurmetrics using mathematical/computer models and simulation systems for the application of existing theory and numerical methods to new solutions for nursing problems or the development of new computational methods.

Nursing Informatics, the branch of Nurmetrics applying the principles of computer science and informatics to understanding the interplay of the architecture of information form (data, text, audio, visual) with information function (generating, processing, storing and transmitting) for the solving of problems in nursing administration, nursing education, nursing practice, and/or nursing research.

Nurmetrics with computational nursing and nursing informatics represents a new specialty area within Computational Health Sciences. Nursing has been identified as an appropriate alternative to expensive health care costs; therefore, nurse researchers utilizing the principles of nurmetrics can be expected to impact significantly the future of health care.

These new directions in nursing will form the foundation for new discoveries powered by supercomputing. The framework for application of supercomputing to nursing and health data research illustrates the components involved in the conceptualization of complex problem resolution for supercomputer application. A paradigm shift in statistical analysis to Global Analysis Tera Exploratory Statistics (GATES) has occurred. GATES provided the direction for development of a prototype software and the conceptualization of VuSTAT, a graphic user interface linking GATES with computer model simulations emphasizing trends.

Although there are many barriers to analyzing datasets with supercomputers, it is the only current resource that can support this nursing and health application. The PHNDR's goal is to address the outstanding issues, making the supercomputing solution easily accessible to nursing researchers. As identified by current PNHDR research, ease of access will not be possible until: (1) a new statistical program is created to analyze trends in massive datasets, (2) all interfaces required by nursing researchers are transparent and include a visual postprocessing package, (3) current social science statistical software packages are modified for mega datasets, and (4) nursing researchers are teamed with the traditional users of supercomputers--engineers, computer scientists, and computational scientists.

4. Importance of the Research

Nursing research utilizing mega/tera data bases typically applies one of two analysis pathways--either (1) to confirm or nullify what is existing or (2) to establish new relationships (or parameters) not previously discerned. To confirm or nullify what is existing can be accomplished by modifying current statistical analysis methodologies to run on the CRAY Supercomputer and by addressing technical problems related to handling the mega/tera data sets. However, to establish new relationships not previously discovered involved the development of a technical presentation of data in a visual format allowing the nursing scientist to see the new relationship. The primary importance of this phase of the PNHDR project was to conceptualize the path and design the tools necessary to result in a paradigm shift from models identifying specifics toward the general to models that present mega/tera data in a format allowing the nursing scientist to visualize new relationships. The paradigm shift in statistical analysis has resulted in the design of Global Analysis Tera Exploratory Statistics (GATES). The software prototype for GATES was designed using 249 megabytes of data from the Hispanic Health and Nutrition Examination Survey obtained from the National Center for Health Statistics. The prototype was a joint design effort with Vance Faber, Ph.D., Group Leader, Computer Research and Applications Group, Los Alamos National Laboratory. The application of GATES and other new methodologies will lead to the establishment of a scientific foundational baseline for the parameters of health across the life span through analysis of mega/tera data bases. Without establishing a foundational baseline, difficulty is experienced in monitoring trends, predicting intervention impacts, or controlling allocation of scarce resources--both human and fiscal. From the scientific foundation for parameters of health emerge the mechanisms for monitoring health trends, determining health cost control methods, identifying impacts on global health care, coordinating environmental data with health data, and providing the scientific information for the future biotech revolution.

Currently, approximately 250 gigabytes of nursing and health data exist in the United States alone. The supercomputer would allow for perusal of this data in about 10 hours. Because researchers benefit from the ability to access and analyze the mega/tera data sets, a Data Analysis Network Initiative (DANI) with a Health Interactive-Data Analysis Network (HI-DAN) is proposed. The DANI would provide a communication link from the researcher's location to the high performance computing capability with an interactive nursing and health data archive for access and analysis.

5. Summary

Nursing research has found a new source of power in the high performance computing and communication environment with the application of the CRAY Y-MP 2/216 supercomputer. The paradigm shift in statistical analysis to Global Analysis Tera Exploratory Statistics (GATES) redefines the statistical methodology for analysis of mega/tera databases using data visualization as a supercomputer completes computations in seconds or minutes. The avenue for including graphic user interfaces to link GATES with computer model simulations and data analysis networks provides for future directions. In the future, after establishing the foundational parameters of health, new applications may lead to a formula for predicting effects of nursing action and intervention on health trends, or application of virtual reality techniques for educating both lay persons and professionals about health parameters, or a means for analysis of acute care data as the data are being collected. The possibilities for discovery and advancement in Nurmetrics, Computational Nursing, and Nursing Informatics are significant when the high performance computing and communication environment is explored with a CRAY Y-MP supercomputer for analyses of mega/tera datasets in nursing and health.

6. Acknowledgements

This research is supported by Cray Research, Inc., National Supercomputing Center for Energy and Environment, National Center for Health Statistics, Advance Computing Laboratories, Los Alamos National Laboratory, and Silicon Graphics, Inc.

7. References

[1] Meintz S. Supercomputers Open Window of Opportunity for Nursing. *Computers in Nursing* in press for May 1993.

[2] Meintz S. Supercomputer Application to Nursing and Health Data Research. In *Communicating Nursing Research Vol. 25:489*. Boulder: Western Institute of Nursing.

[3] Meintz S. Supercomputer Application to Nursing Data Research. Podium Presentation: *First Japanese International Research Conference*. Japan: Tokyo, 1992.

[4] Meintz S. Supercomputers Power Discoveries in Nursing. *Cray Channels* 1992, 14:20-21.

Nursing Informatics: An International Overview for Nursing in a Technological Era
S.J. Grobe and E.S.P. Pluyter-Wenting, eds.

452

To what extent are student nurses attitudes influenced following a course on Nursing Informatics?

Hardy JL and Bostock EA

aSchool of Nursing and Human Movement, Australian Catholic University (NSW) 40 Edward Street, North Sydney, NSW 2060, Australia.

In 1994 the first graduates in N.S.W Australia with a BN degree will be eligible to enter the workforce. At the same time the Health Care System is undergoing major changes as a result of political and economic factors. As a consequence technology has been introduced to monitor and implement these changes. Hence the identification of information technology needs of nurses is of great significance in the development of an undergraduate nursing curriculum. The problems encountered by nurse educators in North America over a decade ago are now a reality to counterparts in the Southern Hemisphere. A positive attitude, user acceptance and willingness to use computer technology is related to the success of any computer system. One of the major objectives therefore in an undergraduate course is to develop "computer friendly" graduates. The paper describes a study undertaken to evaluate the effectiveness of a new course in Nursing Informatics, and its influence on student nurses attitudes towards Computing and Nursing Informatics, following a 12 month course in the first year of a Bachelor of Nursing degree (BN).

1. Background

1.1 Introduction: In 1989, the NSW government developed a strategic plan to develop information systems to meet the needs of the public health care sector [1]. Developments in Australian Health Information Systems, including training for healthcare workers, had lagged behind major countries such as the United Kingdom and the United States of America [2].

The new clinical systems in Australian hospitals will be mainly used by nurses and physicians, emphasis being placed on designing a framework to support educational requirements, including the need for varying degree of informatics input in all undergraduate and post graduate nursing curricula [2, 1]. The clinical systems should also meet the needs of nurses as well as those of healthcare consumers. It therefore becomes critical that nurses be more active and involved in all initiatives related to computer systems. Involvement includes participation in the development and design of computer applications in all aspects of nursing; clinical practice, administration, research and education [3].

The acknowledgment that nurse educators produce an informed and knowledgeable workforce is well recognized, as the following comment illustrates: "*An educated workforce learns how to exploit new technology, an ignorant one becomes its victim*" [4]. Likewise, those who control information are more powerful [5]. So if the nursing profession is to maintain ownership of its affairs and functions, participation in all facets of the implementation of computers to their practice is essential, nurses therefore need to be computer literate [6].

Dramatic changes during the 1980's occurred in baccalaureate nursing educational programs in North America. They included a growing awareness of the acceptance of computer technology programs as nurses became more involved in computer applications related to their profession. Thomas et al state that with the exposure to rapidly changing computer technology comes "*the realisation that attention must be paid to promoting positive attitudes toward computer technology.*" If research-based practice commands positive attitudes to encourage lifelong learning, the evolution of a "computer friendly" nurse requires positive attitudes toward computing [7].

Studies have been reported concerning nurses' attitudes toward computers; what factors cause anxiety; relationship between resistance or non acceptance and age, gender and computer exposure and the impact on users of educational and training designs [8, 9, 10, 11, 14, 15, 16, 7, 3]. Other studies have investigated attitude change as a consequence of some precise plan or intervention, for example, Ball, Snelbecker, and Schechter [16} used a questionnaire to assess change in attitudes toward computing in a group of student nurses before and after a computer literacy lecture. The instruments used in a number or studies have been questioned for not providing objective evidence of attitude change.

Thomas developed two parallel forms of an instrument to obtain such objective evidence [17]. In the clinical setting nurses have been hesitant to embrace computerisation because they were concerned that it would mean depersonalisation of nursing care [17].

Some resistance and lack of appreciation of computing in nursing educational settings results from; insufficient exposure; costs of hardware and software; lack of appropriate software and computer terminology. Nursing students see their objective as patient care and are unable to recognize the contribution of computers [17]. Therefore the course aimed to promote an awareness of, and receptivity to, the use of computers by health care workers [17]. The content included an introduction to basic computer technology, terminology, and an overview of nursing informatics. By adopting a procedure whereby acceptance and effectiveness of such a course can be measured ensures that content, teaching and learning strategies are appropriate.

2. General purpose of the study

The purpose of this study was to determine:
1. the effectiveness of a new unit in the first year of a Bachelor of Nursing course,
2. the extent to which specific objectives were fulfilled,
3. the extent to which students perceptions can be regarded as reflecting attitudes.

3. Procedures

The evaluation survey was conducted at the completion of the first year of the course. At the time, a total of 524 students were enrolled in a 3-year nurse education program. All first year students (175) were invited to participate, but 138 (79%) agreed to participate in the survey.

3.1 Development of the questionnaire. A 27 item questionnaire was developed using the response categories of "strongly agree," "agree," "undecided," and "strongly disagree" on a 5-point Likert scale.
Rationale: The instrument was not based on any specific theory.

To assure the inclusion of items that the students regarded as important and relevant, three focus group interviews were conducted. The students were volunteers from randomly selected tutorial sessions. The interview for the focus groups consisted of 5 semi-structured questions which attempted to obtain information concerning: (a) general feelings about the unit, (b) identification of the skills the students had learned, (c) the usefulness and relevance of the resources, (d) attitudinal change toward technology as a result of the unit, and (e) students expectations of the unit.

Each interview was taped and a transcription of the tape produced. The transcripts were explored for themes and questions constructed using the students' phrases with syntax corrections the only alteration. Other item content was based on the literature review and University evaluation policy procedures.

The questionnaire was constructed and given to two nurse educators experienced in research methodology for both content and construct validity. Alteration to format, number of items and presentation were made and the questionnaire trailed on a convenient group of second year nursing students. They were asked to complete the questionnaire and comment on clarity and ambiguity. The questionnaire given to the students asked for their perceptions related to skills and knowledge acquisition; availability and use of resources; expectations about the course and attitude change.

4. Results

4.1 Sample characteristics. Only 83% of the respondents completed the demographic section fully of these 67% were female, 16% male. The ages of the students ranged from 34% under 20 yrs of age, 22% between 20-25 yrs of age, 10% between 26-30 yrs of age and 10% between 31-48 yrs of age. The entry level varied: 43% direct from school, 18% registered enrolled nurses and 20% assistants in nursing, i.e. 38% had previous or current experience in nursing. Of those with nursing experience only 7% worked in a hospital with clinical computing systems.

4.2 Factor analysis. Factor analysis was used to ascertain whether or not a conceptual model was supported by statistical analysis. The items had been "grouped" under headings outlined in section 3.2 and the researchers tested the assumption that one set of student perceptions may affect another. Seven disparate factors were extracted using eigen values of greater than one (1) as the decision rule for significant factors. As a consequence of this analysis the responses to each question were treated as discrete constructs and a frequency analysis performed.

4.3 Analysis of variance (MANOVA). It has been identified that background factors may effect perceptions, hence an analysis of variance was performed which showed little significance. However a p<.05 was found with gender and exposure to clinical information systems. Both males and females agreed they had acquired the skill of entering data into a computer as a result of the unit, although the females were more positive than the males. However the males agreed more strongly when asked to respond to an interest in technology. Those students with some exposure to clinical hospital systems agreed more strongly to the items related to the use of the manual as a resource and the format of the assessment, as well as to the items asking the students about the importance of information systems in hospitals and an overview of applications of computers in health care.

4.4 Internal consistency of the scales was calculated using Cronbach's alpha. The total of 23 items measured had an acceptable value of alpha=0.722.

4.5 Frequency analysis. Table 1. illustrates the frequency analysis performed on each item relating to students perceptions of the computer content of the course.

Table 1.
Perception scores of 1st year nursing students related to skills, knowledge, resources, expectations and attitudes to computers.   **Response %**

Item	Skills and Knowledge	SA	A	U	SD	D
1.	Didn't learn enough to master word processing skills	20	34	21	19	5
2.	Learned to enter data into a computer	13	49	25	9	4
3.	Gained some word processing skills	16	61	16	4	2
4.	Learned how to use library facilities	24	53	16	4	2
5.	Acquired skills to use database software	8	36	33	16	7
	Resources					
1.	The printers were terrible	32	24	25	13	4
2.	It was difficult to print assignments	30	23	31	7	2
3.	It would be better to have a high speed printer	37	27	33	2	2
4.	Film on nursing applications of use of computers in hospitals was interesting	16	29	34	13	8
5.	Computer manual was useful because of step by step approach	32	47	17	2	2
6.	The best way to learn about computers is through assignments	19	25	27	22	7
	Expectations					
1.	I don't feel I learned as much about computers as I thought I would	29	35	15	17	2
2.	I don't feel as confident about using computers as I would like to	29	30	16	18	6
	Attitude Change					
1.	I found how to use CD-ROM useful	13	50	18	9	9
2.	The main reason I make mistakes when using the computer for word processing is because of nervousness	3	20	23	29	24
3.	Watching computers appearing in more and more places is frightening	8	13	23	32	24
4.	I now have the use of a computer at home	8	13	23	31	24
5.	I now use a computer at home	27	19	11	17	25
6.	I am now confident to use a computer in a hospital	20	37	25	9	6
7.	I have an overview of computer applications in hospitals	16	39	28	13	5
8.	I am aware of the importance of nursing involvement in computer implementation	32	40	15	9	5

strongly agree=SA, (1) agree=A, (2) undecided=U, (3) disagree=D, (4) strongly disagree=SD, (5)

5. Summary and discussion

First year undergraduate students, received instruction for two hours a week for two 12 week semesters on computer literacy skills and nursing informatics. The majority of students had no or very little computer literacy skills on entry to the course and 59% felt that there was not enough support in the computer laboratory for beginners.

The acquisition of skills and knowledge as perceived by the students revealed that many (75%) felt that although they had gained some word processing skills, 64% felt they had yet to master these skills, but 61% were able to at least enter data into a computer (competencies). The use of library facilities improved (68%) but the use of database software (34%) was not acquired. The resources offered by the University were not regarded by the students as being conducive to acquiring computer literacy skills. Nor were their expectations met (63%) concerning the amount of information presented about using computers and the gaining of confidence (58%) in their use. The majority (71%), expressed an awareness of the importance of nursing involvement in the development of information systems in hospitals.

In conclusion, the purpose of this study was to determine the effectiveness of a new unit in an undergraduate nursing program, to evaluate objectives and access the extent to which student perceptions reflect attitudes. Students acquired some knowledge and gained computer competencies, and were seen to have met the course objectives to a limited degree. Whilst the questionnaire strongly demonstrated the student perception that the course did not meet with their expectations, they did however acknowledge a significant change from their entering behavior. Therefore the course can be seen as being partly effective. Although a change in attitude was not measured, the students exhibited a strong positive attitude towards computers as seen by their increased use of computers and awareness of nursing applications. This information has been useful in course review and development. Further studies involving the use of pre- and post testing, semantic differential, performance indicators and longitudinal or retesting is needed to be confident of producing a "computer friendly" graduate.

6. References

[1] Cook R, Van der Weegen L, and Morris S. Nursing Information System: The NSW Experience. Australian Health Informatics Association and Nursing Informatics. Australia Inaugural State Conference Proceedings, 1992.

[2] Soar J. *Information Management Technology: Training and Education in Health Care. The Australian Experience,* 1992.

[3] Ronald JS and Skiba DJ. Computer Education for Nurses: Curriculum Issues and Guidelines. in *Preparing Nurses for Using Information Systems: Recommended Informatics Competencies.* Peterson HE and Gerdin-Jelger U (eds) National New York, League of Nursing, 1988.

[4] Stonier T. Changes in Western Society-Educational Implications. in *Recurrent Education and Lifelong Learning.* Schuller T et al (eds) London, Kogan Page, 1981.

[5] Hales GD. *Nursing Informatics.* in Ball MJ et al (eds). Berlin, Springer-Verlag, 1988.

[6] Royal Australian Nursing Federation, *Information Processing: A Practical Guide to the Use of Computers in Nursing.* Victoria, 1987.

[7] Thomas BS, Delany CW and Weiler K. The Affective Outcomes of Course Work on Computer Technology in Nursing. *J Nurs Educ.* 1992, 31: 165-170.

[8] Wilson BA. Computer Anxiety in Nursing Students. *J Nurs Educ 1991,* 30: 52-56.

[9] Burkes M. Identifying and Relating Nurses' Attitudes Towards Computer Use. *Compu Nurss* 1989, 14: 152-157.

[10] Coates VE and Chambers M. Teaching Microcomputing to Student Nurses: An Evaluation. *J Adv Nurs* 1989, 14: 152-157.

[11] Bailey JE. Development of an Instrument for the Management of Computer User Attitudes in Hospitals. *Methods of Information in Medicine.* 1990, 29: 51-56.

[12] Allen LR. Measuring Attitude Toward Computer Assisted Instruction. *Comput Nurs* 1986, 4: 144-151.

[13] Romano CA, Damrosch SP, Heller BR and Parks PL. Levels of Computer Education for Professional Nursing. *Comput Nurs* 1989, 7: 21-28.

456

[14] Fochtman MM and Kavanaugh SB. A Nursing Service—Education Model for Introducing Baccalaureate Nursing Students to Research and Computer Concepts. *Comput Nurs* 1991, 9: 152-157.

[15] Harsanyi BE and Kesley CE. Attitudes of Physicians Towards Computer Technology. in *MEDINFO* '92 Lum et al (eds) Amsterdam: North Holland, 1992: 1243-1248.

[16] Ball MJ, Snelbecker GE and Scnether SL. Nurses Perception Concerning Computer Uses Before and After a Computer Literacy Lecture. *Comput Nurs* 1985, 3: 23-32.

[17] Thomas B. Development of an Instrument to Assess Attitudes Toward Computing in Nursing. *Comput Nurs* 1988, 6: 122-127.

Nursing Informatics: An International Overview for Nursing in a Technological Era
S.J. Grobe and E.S.P. Pluyter-Wenting, eds.

Contemporary influentials in nursing informatics:
The lived experience of becoming computer proficient

Magnus M M

Hunter College of The City University of New York, Hunter-Bellevue School of Nursing, New York, New York 10010

Pioneers in Nursing Informatics were interviewed to determine knowledge patterns associated with becoming computer proficient. This paper presents the research design, data collection, and transcription methods used in this qualitative investigation.

1. Introduction

Nursing is an information-intensive practice discipline. Increasingly, information processing technologies, such as computer systems, are being used by professional nurses to generate information and nursing knowledge needed for decision support in health care environments [1]. Although individual nurses, such as those interviewed for this study, have been involved with electronic information processing technologies for decades, many nurses still lack proficiency in using computers in their work. Furthermore, nursing educators only recently have begun to examine ways to integrate the study of informatics into nursing curricula and programs of study. A clear mandate for nursing is the discovery of knowledge patterns which reflect proficiency in the ever expanding technological component of practice. Nurses working in all types of health care setting must have access to computers as practice tools and must use information and knowledge generated by computers to support decision-making in their areas of specialization.

The research question addressed by this qualitative research investigation was: What knowledge patterns are associated with becoming computer proficient for a select group of American nursing professionals? Study objectives flowing from the research question were to describe unfolding themes and patterns associated with: first, situational involvement with computers of a select group of nursing professionals; second, holistic similarities recognition, when using computers, of a select group of nursing professionals; and third, intuitive know-how, when using computers, of a select group of nursing professionals. These three themes served as the framework around which this study was organized and the interview guide was developed.

2. Significance of This Qualitative Inquiry

The purpose of this investigation was to describe the experience of becoming computer proficient, as lived over time, by a select group of American nursing professionals. An heuristic research design [2] was chosen as the best way to discover, from first hand accounts, the meanings of the experience of becoming computer proficient.

Since the underlying focus of this study was to uncover knowledge patterns, common meanings, and situational "know-how," the findings of this study might be helpful in the design and development of curricular experience in nursing informatics. The outcomes might also help nursing educators in decisions relating to the selection of instructional methods and strategies for teaching computer use in nursing.

Nurse educators, involved with continuing and staff development, might also use the findings of the study to teach nurses about information technology and computer use in a variety health care settings. Furthermore, the use of nursing knowledge gained through the analysis of practice in contextual situations will enhance nurses knowledge of what it means to become computer proficient and will expedite the preparation of nurses in nursing informatics [3].

Study partially supported by PSC/CUNY Faculty Research Award

This study is dedicated to the memory of nursing influential, Karen Reider, whose untimely death provided the investigator with an added impetus to proceed with this inquiry.

Finally, and very important for this investigator, the special privilege of knowing and interacting with the outstanding nursing leaders, nominated by their peers for this study, created an imperative to document the important life events of these pioneers, as they journeyed toward expanding the horizons of nursing informatics for all of us.

3. Conceptual Dimension of the Study

The phenomenon central to this study was that of becoming computer proficient. The works of Dreyfus [4] and Benner [5] were used as a framework to conceptualize the phenomenon. Dreyfus described a five-stage situational competencies model applicable in any practice discipline. The stages are: novice, advanced beginner, competent, proficient, and expert. The stage, which Dreyfus referred to as "proficient" reflected the nature of the phenomenon of the present study, i.e. nurses becoming computer proficient. Dreyfus described proficiency as performance exhibited by an individual because of deep situational involvement, ability to recognize similarities, and intuitive understanding or "know-how." Dreyfus stated that "intuition or know-how . . . . is neither wild guessing nor supernatural inspiration, but the sort of ability we all use all the time as we go about our every day tasks."(p. 29) The author further explained that the "intuitive ability to use patterns without decomposing them into component features may be called holistic similarity recognition." Wiler [6] characterized this holistic similarities recognition as making "empirical connections."

Benner tested the evolving situational model in nursing practice. She referred to "know-how" as the untapped knowledge which experts nurses accrue over time. She indicated that a wealth of untapped knowledge is embedded in the practice and the "know-how" of expert nurses, but that this knowledge will not be expanded or fully developed unless nurses systematically record what they learn from their own experience. (p. 37)

Using the theoretical perspectives of Dreyfus and Benner, the phenomenon of becoming computer proficient was operationally defined as individual American nursing professionals who, over time, had deep situational involvement with electronic information processing technologies, while automatically recognizing similarities and holistic patterns, and demonstrating a deep sense of intuitive know-how in an information-intensive technological environment.

4. Related Literature

To date, no research studies were reported in nursing which addressed the phenomenon of becoming computer proficient from the knowledge perspectives of situational involvement, holistic similarities recognition, and intuitive know-how. Other related literature, including an article by Skiba [7], supported the need for on-going research in nursing informatics. Graves and Corcoran [8] presented a framework for organizing the study of nursing informatics. They emphasized the importance of information, generated by information processing technologies, being transformed into knowledge supportive of nursing decision-making, as well as for the discovery of new knowledge. Armstrong [9], as part of a national study on computer literacy, identified a list of computer competencies needed by nurse educators teaching in basic and continuing education programs in nursing. Reynolds and Fennel [10] also focused on computer literacy from a continuing education perspective. Ronald and Skiba [11], in their formative work on basic computer education in nursing, presented a curriculum framework for developing computer competencies along a continuum.

In recent months, a plethora of scholarly articles appeared on nursing informatics, which supported the need to study nursing informatics and what Graves [12] referred to as "the knowledge worker in nursing."

5. Methodological Dimension of the Study

Parse et al [13] and Morse [14] recommended that the sample for this kind of investigation be drawn from a population living the experience of the phenomenon being studied. The sample for this study was derived by a reputational method of peer nomination from among individuals who were influential in advancing computer use in nursing over many years. For this study, nominations were elicited from 383 individuals who were active members of the National League for Nursing Council on Nursing Informatics at the time the study was planned. One-hundred and fifty postcard responses were received, which generated a 320 person list of names. A frequency distribution was conducted and a list of twenty-five names emerged as the potential study sample. The actual sample size, i.e. persons actually interviewed for the study, was ten American nurse influentials. Davis and

Cannava [15] reported on the development and utilization of protocols which they used successfully in their qualitative study on transcultural and tranlinguistic research. This investigator used a similar approach to structure data collection. Once the nomination list was achieved, a letter was sent to each individual nurse inviting him or her to participate in the study and explaining the anticipated interview methods. Nominees were asked to return a signed copy of an informed consent statement, which also indicated their willingness to participate in the study. Responses were enthusiastic and supportive, which provided the investigator with a high level of affirmation to forge ahead with the study. Once the subjects responded, appointments for taped-recorded interviews were set up. A brochure, which included an interview guide, an electronically scanned likeness of the investigator, and a confirmation of appointment date was sent to each nurse approximately one week prior to the agreed upon meeting time. Davis and Cannava indicated that guide questions provided time for the subjects to think about their responses, and a photo of the interviewer provided an advance recognition focus which enhanced the flow of communication. (p. 188) The individual taped interviews, each of which lasted approximately 50 minutes, were conducted by the investigator in either Washington, D.C., San Francisco, or New York City, over the course of one year. When all of the interviews were completed, the taped conversations were transcribed into electronic text files. Hardcopy transcripts were also generated in preparation for the anticipated two-pronged approach to data analysis.

6. Interpretative Dimension of the Study

At the time this paper was presented for inclusion in the conference proceedings, analysis of data was still in progress. Data analysis consisted to two steps: first, data reduction, which consisted of dividing the text into units of meaning; and second, search for latent meaning of the textual materials, which included delineation of natural meaning units, identification of recurring themes, and the synthesis of themes into knowledge patterns.

Two approaches were used to analyze the data: first, the Minnesota Contextual Content Analysis (MCCA) computer program, developed by McTavish, was used to analyze contextual orientation, and to discover manifest and latent meanings inherent in linguistic expressions. Kelly and Sime[16] found the MCCA program useful in their nursing study on the meaning of health. They recommended that other nursing investigators validate its usefulness in nursing research. Text files were transmitted electronically by Internet, according to prior instructions agreed upon by the investigator and program developer, McTavish. Investigator and program developer communicated frequently by electronic mail as this aspect of data analysis was conducted.

Second, an heuristic data analysis approach, which was a "timeless immersion" with data[17] was the second approach. Dwelling with data in this manner, until a creative synthesis was achieved, was an intense, time-consuming activity, which required returning again and again to printed transcripts in order to generate new insights and perspectives and in order to arrive at a creative synthesis.

Outcomes of the first data analysis approach, using the MCCA program, will be reported on at Nursing Informatics-'94. While the results of the "timeless immersion" with the recorded transcripts will be reported at a later date when that component of the study is completed.

7. Summary

The purpose of this qualitative investigation was to describe the experience of becoming computer proficient, as lived over time, by a select group of American nursing professionals. Ten American nursing influentials, as nominated by their peers, were interviewed for the study. As the investigator listened to the taped recordings, repetitive statements, reflecting the themes and patterns relating to situational involvement, holistic similarities recognition, and intuitive know-how, unfolded. This paper presented the first phase of the study, i.e. the research design, data collection, and transcription methods employed. The outcomes of the on-going twofold data analysis will be reported as the process is completed.

8. References

[1] Graves J and Corcoran S. The Study of Nursing Informatics. *Comput Nurs 1989, 21:227-231.*

[2] Moustakas C. *Heuristic Research: Design, Methodology and Applications.* Newbury Park: Sage, 1990.

[3] Graves J and Corcoran S. The Study of Nursing Informatics. p. 230.

[4] Dreyfus H and Dreyfus S. *Mind Over Machine: The Power of Human Intuition and Expertise in the Era of the Computer.* New York: Free Press, 1986.

[5] Benner P. *From Novice to Expert: Excellence and Power in Clinical Practice.* Menlo Park: Addison-Wesley, 1984.

[6] Wiler J. The *Social Determination of Knowledge.* Englewood Cliffs: Prentice-Hall, 1981.

[7] Skiba D. Priorities for Research in Nursing Informatics. *Connections* 1993, 2:1.

[8] Graves J and Corcoran S. The Study of Nursing Informatics, p. 230.

[9] Armstrong M. Computer Competencies Identified for Nursing Staff Development Educators. *J Nurs Staff Dev* 1989, 5:187-191.

[10] Reynolds A and Fennell M. Computer Literacy: A Mission for Continuing Education for Professional Nurses. *J Cont Educ Prof Nurs* 1989, 20:132-135.

[11] Ronald J and Skiba D. *Guidelines for Basic Computer Education in Nursing.* New York: National League for Nursing, 1987.

[12] Graves J. Data Versus Information Versus Knowledge. *Reflections* 1993, 19:4-5.

[13] Parse R, Coyne A and Smith M. *Nursing Research: Qualitative Research.* Bowie: Brady Communications, 1985.

[14] Morse J. *Qualitative Nursing Research.* Rockville: Aspen, 1989.

[15] Davis K and Cannava E. Elements of Transcultural and Translinguistic Research. *Nurs Sci Q* 1992, 5:185-189.

[16] Kelly A and Sime A. Language of Research Data: Application of Computer Content Analysis in Nursing Research. *ANS Adv Nurs Sci 1990, 12:32-40.*

[17] Moustakas C. *Heuristic Research.* pp. 50-51.

© 1994 Elsevier Science B.V. All rights reserved.
Nursing Informatics: An International Overview for Nursing in a Technological Era
S.J. Grobe and E.S.P. Pluyter-Wenting, eds.

461

Information features of clinical nursing information systems: A delphi survey

Carty B

Director, Center Career Advancement, National League for Nursing, 350 Hudson Street, New York N.Y. 10014

Ninety-seven nursing information specialists representing 37 states and Canada, the majority of whom practiced in hospitals, participated in a two Round Delphi Survey. The Nursing Information Feature Survey (NIFS) tool, developed by the researcher, identified elements for a nursing information system in the delivery of patient care. The elements were divided into 6 categories: 1) Patient Specific 2) Nursing Domain 3) Institution Specific 4) System Security 5) Miscellaneous 6) Future Features.

There was a total of 70 items which were rated on a 5-point Likert scale. Items within each category were analyzed and ranked according to highest mean scores. Of the 70 items, 38 had a consensus of 80% of the panelists. An analysis of the data support the strongest consensus among the specialists was in the Patient Specific category. The categories with the least amount of consensus were the Nursing Domain and Future Feature categories.

Two themes emerged from the findings of the study. One was that the majority of the information features be patient-focused and integrated with other data bases. The other was that the features preferred by the panelists were complex and reflected knowledge processing rather than simple data processing. Comments by the specialists indicated a wide variance of opinion on the use of nursing models, standards of care, nursing diagnosis and critical paths in automated systems. There was also lack of agreement on what constituted nursing domain data.

1. Purpose

The primary purpose of this study was to identify the scope of information features for Clinical Nursing Information Systems (CNIS) deemed important in the administration of nursing care. Additionally, the research proposed to identify important features of future nursing information systems that are necessary in the administration of nursing care.

2. Population and Sample

An expert pool of potential panelists was identified from two sources: (1) membership in a computer council affiliated with a national nursing organization, and (2) membership in a national organization of nurses devoted to computer applications in nursing practice. All participants were considered well qualified in Nursing Information Systems by nature of their educational credentials, professional nursing experience, nursing informatics experience, and reputation in the field. One hundred sixteen subjects were invited to participate in the study. Ninety-seven consented and participated in Round I, and 75 participated in Round II. This represented a national sample of nurses from 37 states and Canada.

3. Informatics Background of the Participants

A total of 77% (n=75) of the respondents had up to seven years employment with nursing information systems. Twenty-one percent (n=22) had eight or more years experience with information systems, and two panelists indicated they were not presently working with nursing information systems. However, these two panelists indicated they had previously taken courses in information systems, one of them on a doctoral level.

The participants were well experienced nurse professionals. Eighty-eight percent (n=85) had 12 years or more experience in nursing. The majority of the panelists (n=61) were employed in hospitals. Four participants were employed in community agencies, two were employed in home health agencies, and four were faculty members in schools of nursing. A large number (n=26) identified other as their agency. These included three in the military, nine employed by vendors, five consultants, and two full-time students. The remainder were employed by the Department of Defense, a professional organization, a federal agency, an evaluation center for hospital information systems, an ambulatory care unit, an HMO, and a software company.

4. Instrument

The Nursing Information Feature Survey, used to identify important information features of clinical nursing information systems, was developed by the investigator. An extensive review of the literature was performed to identify categories of information features cited as important for inclusion in clinical nursing information systems. This review generated six categories of information features. Four of the categories were adapted from the Graves and Corcoran study [1]. They were: (1) patient specific data, (2) nursing domain data, (3) institution specific data, and (4) procedure information. Two additional categories were added to the Corcoran and Graves model by the investigator. One addressed system security and a second listed miscellaneous elements identified by the investigator. Information features within each category were then identified based on a comprehensive review of the literature, an examination of three information systems by the investigator and discussions with experts in the field of Nursing Information Systems.

A panel of three experts, all specialists in nursing information systems and responsible for implementing information systems in large medical centers, reviewed and critiqued the instrument to assess content validity. The resulting Nursing Information Feature Survey (NIFS) Round I instrument contained two parts. Part I consisted of six information categories, with a total of 53 features within the categories. The patient specific category contained 26 features, including assessment data, nursing orders, and medication and laboratory data. Nursing domain data contained nine features including data on drugs and information on nursing and medical texts. Institution specific data contained eight features related to patient charges, policies, and conference schedules. Procedure information contained three features on research protocols and patient procedures. System security contained two features related to system access and communication. The last category, miscellaneous, contained five features related to patient acuity and nursing care costs. Each feature was rated on a 5-point Likert scale, ranging from strongly disagree (1) to strongly agree (5). Part II of the instrument contained six features addressing future applications of clinical information systems. In addition, each section had an "other" or open-ended category to allow respondents to include features they deemed important that were not included in the Round I survey.

As a result of the comments by the panelists in Round I, the Round II instrument expanded to 70 items. The largest category, Patient Specific Category expanded from 26 to 30 items. The Nursing Domain Data increased by 2 items, System Security by 3 items, and Future Features expanded by 2 items.

5. Findings

The Patient Specific category contained the largest number of items and was concerned with direct clinical applications. Most of the features in this category relied on access to other information sources, including diagnostic tests, laboratory information, prior admission data, and medication information. This category also specified access to information of other disciplines. All of the elements related to these functions had a high mean (4-5). In addition, 25 of the 30 elements in this category had a consensus of 80% in the 4-5 range. These findings strongly support two important characteristics of information systems. First, the system must be integrated and across a number of disciplines, and second, the system must support communication capabilities. To support the delivery of nursing care, a system must be dynamic, integrated, and contain patient and clinical indicators from a number of disciplines.

These findings are consistent with the categories of information Graves and Corcoran [1] found to be important in their study of nursing information needs. They identified prior history, assessment data, medication information, and lab reports as the most frequently occurring information needs of nurses.

The elements identified in the Patient Specific category also strongly indicated that nurses need access to medical information such as diagnostic tests, lab reports, and prior admission and medication data in order to effectively make decisions and deliver patient care. System design specifications should incorporate and integrate these features as well as nursing features such as standards of care and critical pathways. An item, added in Round II as a result of feedback from Round I specified that the "system provides outcomes against standards of care for critical pathways".This item had a mean of 4.54 and ranked 11th in the patient specific category. This high rating indicates that critical paths have a high priority among informatician specialists. Conversely nursing diagnosis capability was rated 28th and had a mean of 3.74. The item which provided for a standardized care plan had a mean of 3.82 and was ranked 27th out of 30. The comparatively lower rating of features which support nursing diagnosis and care plans indicates that these features may not be considered high priorities in system design for the delivery of nursing care. The lack of consensus by the panelists on standards, critical paths, nursing care plans, and nursing diagnosis may be representative of the current inability of the profession to identify and agree on methods of documentation. This area of system design warrants additional research and for the present time systems may have to support a variety of documentation methods.

The Nursing Domain category had the lowest mean scores (4.18 to 2.84) and the least amount of consensus of all the categories in Part I. This category focused on information nurses could access in the delivery of patient care which would enhance clinical decision making. The only consensus item in this category supported access to knowledge bases to enhance clinical decision making. However, there was lack of agreement on the specific data bases to support decision making. Panelists rated access to specific data bases to inform decision making such as journals, texts, and other bibliographic sources below 3.5.

The comments of the panelists varied on these items. Some stated that these sources should be in libraries; others stated they would be nice but not necessary; and a number stated they would be very expensive. In contrast, others panelists who had access to these features indicated they were used frequently and were very important in informing decision making. This conflict in opinion reflects two major issues related to Nursing Domain information. One is the lack of agreement within the profession on what constitutes Nursing Domain information and the other is the paucity of domain data in clinical information systems.

Current research is attempting to identify a classification of nursing interventions [2]. However, much research is needed to identify standards and models of care for information systems. The technology of today and tomorrow will enable informatics specialists to test the application of various models of practice and place that knowledge back into systems, establishing a wealth of clinical research.

The category of Institution Specific Data had moderately high means (4.78 to 3.10) and the highest ranked features supported communication capability with other departments and personnel. The System security category high mean scores ranging from 4.87 to 4.55 and supported a matrix security for users as well as an ability to correct error without loss of original data. The Miscellaneous category also had high means of 4.82 to 4.28. The features in this category supported management and operational functions such as patient acuity, nursing care charges and report capability.

Finally, the Future Features category had moderate to low scores (4.11 to 2.75). The three highest ranking features supported the communication of data across institutional lines, via smart cards and home care monitoring.

6. Consensus

The information needs identified in this study had a high degree of consensus, particularly in the Patient Domain and Miscellaneous categories. Of the 70 items in the survey, 38 had a consensus of 80% or greater. Twenty-nine items, although they did not have consensus, had high means. Ten had means between 4-5 and 19 had means between 3-4. These findings support a strong rate of agreement. The elements identified in the Nursing Information Feature Survey (NIFS) could be used as generic information elements in the planning, development, and evaluation of clinical information systems. Overall the consensus items supported communication and a patient-centered focus in all of the categories. The items which generated consensus should be considered essential features for inclusion in information systems used in the delivery of care.

7. Patient-Focused Systems

The findings of this study clearly supported the emphasis on a patient-focused data base which would cross disciplines as well as institution lines. The support for a patient-centered system was evidenced most clearly in the Patient Domain Category. Most of these items were features providing patient-focused information. In addition, one of the elements added from a panelist's comments stated that the system should be patient-centered and across all disciplines. This element had a mean of 4.62 and was rated seventh in the Patient Domain category in Round II. Another support for a patient-centered data base was in the frequent comments of the panelists that care plans should be interdisciplinary patient care plans rather than nursing care plans. Recent writings support the concept of a patient-focused information system with components from other disciplines, including a nursing subset [3, 4].

The emphasis on a patient-centered data system subsumes the system's ability to access and process data from a number of sources. Today's technology is capable of this and systems of the future promise to be even more dynamic in their handling of explosive data that will be used across multiple settings by multiple users. Nursing information systems should be viewed in this light. Although nursing may be able to identify a nursing information subset, it has to be integrated with other systems that provide information that is not nursing domain data. The nursing domain data may be impotent without the nucleus of a generic patient data base and, in fact, aspects of the nursing domain data may be part of the generic data base.

8. Recommendations for Future Research

There was a recurrent theme throughout all the categories that the nursing information system should be integrated. The identification of common elements of information across all disciplines is crucial for the design of successful systems.

The area of Nursing Domain data needs additional study and refinement. Findings from this study indicate there is lack of agreement on what constitutes Nursing Domain data. Does it consist of standards, nursing diagnosis, outcomes, critical paths, and nursing care plans? Can Nursing Domain data be separated out from Patient Specific data, or are they inextricably connected in some instances? Should systems accommodate a number of documentation models and a variety of Nursing Domain sets? The findings of this study have raised a number of research questions. Additional studies could seek to identify defining characteristics of this domain which could be incorporated into the NIFS.

9. Implications for Practice

The comments and findings in this study raised a number of issues for nursing practice. Based on the forceful comments of the panelists, a major issue was the nursing care plan. Serious questions have been raised about the efficacy and legitimacy of the nursing care plan in practice [5, 6]. A major criticism is the linear approach to thinking which the care plan promotes. Findings in this study indicated that the nursing care plan is not considered a priority in information systems. Rather, there is a shift to incorporate standards, outcomes, and critical paths into nursing systems and to focus on a multidisciplinary patient care plan. This shift may be due to the ability to have data presented in an integrated, interdisciplinary manner. For nursing, this may mean a rethinking of the appropriateness of the care plan in practice. More dynamic ways of accessing, processing, and presenting data are promoting other avenues of planning, delivering, and documenting nursing care.

Innovative models of practice being implemented today emphasize a patient-focused culture and integration of resources [7]. Integration of information with a patient focus was a consistent theme in the findings of this research. Systems now provide the capability to integrate many data sources and support interactive and integrated environments. System design features should support models that are being implemented in practice.

As information systems are developed, nurses in practice need to be consulted in design specifications. Their input is important in defining the types of information nurses use for the delivery of care and how this information varies in different practice settings. Another finding of this study raised the possibility that different practice settings may influence both the presentation and type of information nurses need. Design specifications may in some instances be setting specific. Research that uses the NIFS instrument in different clinical settings would provide more insight on how information features may differ in a variety of clinical settings.

Clearly, nursing information specialists should collaborate with nurse users, vendors, and system designers to set up system environments to develop and test different design features of information systems. As practice settings develop innovative models of care delivery, these models should feed into design specifications for clinical information systems. Clinical information systems should reflect the collaborative efforts of system developers, practicing nurses, and nurse informatics specialists.

10. References

[1] Graves J. and Corcoran S. Supplemental information-seeking behavior of cardiovascular nurses. *Res Nurs Health* 1990, 13:119-127.

[2] McClosky J. and Bulechek G. Classification of nursing interventions. *J Prof Nurs* 1990, 6:151-157.

[3] Zielstorff R. Hudgings C. and Grobe S. *Next-Generation Nursing Information Systems: Essential Characteristics for Professional Practice.* Washington D.C.: American Nurses Publishing, 1993.

[4] Turley J. A framework for the transition from nursing records to a nursing information system. *Nurs Outlook* 1993, 40:177-181.

[5] Sovie M. Clinical nursing practice and outcomes: Evaluation, evolution, and resolution. *Nurs Economics* 1989, 7:79-85.

[6] Tanner C. The nursing care plan as a teaching method: Reason or ritual. *Nurs Edu* 1986, 11:8-10.

[7] Tornabeni J. A model for redesigning the nursing environment. *NLN Annual Meeting*, 1992. Council for Nursing Practice. Pittsburgh: Pennsylvania.

Nursing Informatics: An International Overview for Nursing in a Technological Era
S.J. Grobe and E.S.P. Pluyter-Wenting, eds.

466

New Technology: An Australian Experience.

Gordon J L [a] & Griffiths W [b]

[a] Fairfield Hospital, P.O. Box 5 Sydney, 2165, Australia.

[b] Westmead Hospital, Hawkesbury Road, Westmead, 2145, Australia.

This research project was undertaken at a 224 bed Sydney metropolitan hospital which had selected to be a pilot site for the first Clinical Information System in a public hospital in New South Wales. The purpose of the study was to determine staff attitude towards change, computers, the benefits and problems associated with computers and the perceived impact computers would have on their work environment. These responses were compared to certain demographic details of staff members, to ascertain whether there was any statistically significant correlation between their experience with computers and their work environment using their responses to the thirty items in the questionnaire. Two separate studies were undertaken, the first before the implementation of the Clinical Information System and the second during training for the Clinical Information System.

1. Introduction

In 1991 Fairfield Hospital was selected by the New South Wales Department of Health to become a pilot site for a Clinical Information System (CIS). It has been well documented in the literature that implementation of computer systems can be greatly facilitated if staff can be encouraged to approach this change in a positive manner [1]. It was therefore essential that staff should feel like the system "belonged to them", that they were appropriately educated in its use and that they were involved in assessing the limitations and benefits of the system from the beginning [2]. This new C.I.S. was obviously going to have a major impact on both the clinical and administrative staff in the hospital. In order to identify the needs of staff in relation to this technology, the author, with the support of the other hospital executive, undertook a series of studies of the staff. The aims of these studies were :
* to determine staff attitude towards change, computers, the benefits and problems associated with computers as well as the perceived impact computers would have on their work environment.
* to compare demographic details of the staff, to ascertain whether there was any statistically significant correlations between experience with computers, and work environment, and their responses to the thirty item questionnaire.
The results of the initial study were to be used to formulate the basis of the education package for all staff. It was imperative that the attitudes of the affected employees be assessed adequately if the change is to be implemented successfully [3]. Medical personnel or clinicians often are "computerphobic" and become intimidated by the idea of using computers, often referring to them as a machine which dehumanizes their patients [4]. The second study was undertaken during the training phase of the implementation. The hospital executive recognized that there would not be any certainty or opportunity to correlate individual responses to both studies but the two results would indicate a general difference or change in attitude in the overall organization.

2. Literature Review

This review of the literature concentrated upon studies/questionnaires undertaken focussing on the attitudes of clinicians to computer systems. Houle [5] identified that variables such as age, previous computer experience and education have positively influenced the adoption of a new I.S. Chang [6] developed a "Computer Use Expectations Scale (C.U.E.S.)" which grouped subjects by age, sex, clinical area and compared these demographic details with their willingness to interact with computers. Significant correlations occurred with younger clinicians who had used computers more frequently. Theis [7]) utilized a Thurstone attitude scale to measure the attitudes of different staff to computers. Brodt and Stronge [3] tested eight hypotheses which related to nurses' attitudes to computerization as indicated by their age, sex, length of employment, education, clinical areas, shifts worked, interaction with indicated by their age, sex, length of employment, education, clinical areas, shifts worked, interaction with computers and length of service. Calhoun et al [8] surveyed one thousand and twenty two staff to also find that age, education and duration of employment resulted in statistically significant attitudes towards computers. It was based upon this research that the author developed a thirty (30) item questionnaire to evaluate the attitudes of staff in an Australian hospital about to undergo such a significant change in computer technology.

3. Method

3.1. Instrument

The purpose of this study was to develop a thirty item instrument which would evaluate attitudes towards, the impact of computers on the clinical area . These attitudes would be compared to two demographic questions; experience with computers, as well as their clinical environment. A Likert - type scale was designed to contain six questions relating to the same five attitudes (ie. attitude to computers). Each question was considered to be equal in value. The staff member was requested to read each item and circle the number closest to their own opinion. One = Strongly Agree through to Five = Strongly Disagree [3].

3.2. Subjects

Because the C.I.S. would have such a major impact on Fairfield Hospital, the hospital executive decided to perform a census. This meant that all five hundred employees were invited to participate in completing the questionnaire both before implementation and during training. Eleven work environments were covered which included ; Administration, C.S.S.D., Domestic Services, Catering, Nursing, Ward Orderlies, Medical, Allied Health and Area Health Service personnel. Sex was not included in the demographic details because gender is highly correlated with work environment at Fairfield Hospital. Confidentiality was ensured. The questionnaires did not have a section for the subject's name, even if the individual wished to complete such a section. The covering letters also reassured the subject re the confidentiality of his/her responses. These letters also encouraged each staff member to participate as it would allow them to be involved in the implementation of this system.

3.3. Setting

The research was undertaken at Fairfield Hospital. This hospital is located as a unit of the South Western Sydney Area Health Service. The hospital is only four years old and consists of 224 beds. The clinical areas within the hospital include all specialities found in district hospitals.

3.4. Procedure

A copy of the questionnaire and covering letter was distributed to each staff member via the internal mail. The first study resulted in a return rate of approximately sixty four percent. The second study resulted in a slightly higher return rate of sixty five percent.

The results of both surveys were then tabulated and transferred onto grid sheets. The data from these grid sheets was input to a word processing package - Word Perfect then transferred onto an ASCII file. Once the information was in this format the first study was analysed on an I.B.M. computer using the S.A.S. statistical package. The second study was analysed on a Macintosh computer using the Statview statistical package.

4. Statistical Analysis

The information collated from the surveys were analysed using the following methods.

4.1. Frequency Tables

Frequency tables were produced which examined the responses according to work/ computer experience. The researcher decided to concentrate her analysis of the questions according to existing levels of computer expertise as well as work environment.

Questions 1 - 6 examined staff attitudes towards the benefits of a C.I.S.
Questions 7 - 12 examined attitudes towards problems with computer systems.
Questions 13 - 18 examined attitudes to change.
Questions 19 - 24 examined attitudes to computers.
Questions 25 - 30 examined attitudes towards the impact this technology would have on staff.

4.2. Hypotheses

A number of hypotheses were tested using Chi square analysis. These included in the first study :

1. There is no association between attitude towards benefits of computer systems and work environment of staff. H_1 df 40 ∞ .05.
2. There is no association between attitude towards problems with computer systems and work environment of staff. H_2 df 40 ∞ .05.
3. There is no association between attitudes towards change and work environment of staff. H_3 df 40 ∞ .05.
4. There is no association between attitudes to computers and work environment of staff. H_4 df 40 ∞ .05.
5. There is no association between attitudes of the impact of technology and work environment. H_5 df 40 ∞ .05.

And in both studies :

6. There is no association attitudes towards benefits of computer systems and computer experience of staff. H_6 df 12 ∞ .05.
7. There is no association between attitudes towards problems with computer systems and computer experience of staff. H_7 df 12 ∞ .05.
8. There is no association between attitude towards change and computer experience of staff. H_8 df 12 ∞ .05.
9. There is no association between attitudes towards computers and computer experience of staff. H_9 df 12 ∞ .05.
10. There is no association between attitudes of the impact of technology and computer experience of staff. H_{10} df 12 ∞ .05.

5. Results

The response rate of the first study was 317 questionnaires, while the response rate of the second study was 320. The nursing returns were 162 and 150 respectively. The second study concentrated on the nursing response.

The results demonstrated that 42.43% of all staff have no computer experience at all, a further 22.22% have experience with home computers and the remaining 35.35% have received some form of computer training. Of the major work categories, nursing had more than 50% of respondents without computer experience as compared to the administrative area which had more than 77% of respondents with some or formal computer training. Both the medical and allied health areas have approximately 50% of respondents with either none or home computer experience and 50% with some or formal computer training. The remaining work areas have a fairly even distribution of computer training.

To ascertain if there was any significant differences in the responses given in the questionnaire from staff, the author performed a number of Chi - square analyses. When the initial Chi - square analysis was undertaken, it was identified that in a number of cells there were less than five subjects per cell. Therefore a decision was made to collapse the cells. In the section examining work environment, the cells were combined into divisional categories. This meant that Nursing and Ward Orderlies were combined, Medical, Allied Health and Area Health Services were combined and Administration, C.S.S.D., Domestic Services, Stores, Maintenance and Catering Services were combined. The hypothese did not change, But for the area of work, the degrees of freedom became 8. In the section of experience with computers, the cells of no experience and home computers were combined and the cells containing some training and formal training were combined. Again the hypothese did not change, however the degrees of freedom became 4. The results demonstrating a statistical significant difference in the tests for Study One were :

1. H_1 df 8 ∞ .05 X^2= 19.147 p<.025.

Therefore the author rejects the null hypothesis and accepts that there is an association between attitude towards the benefits of computer systems and the work environment of staff.

2. H_2 df 8 ∞ .05 X^2= 16.7615 p<.03.

Therefore the author rejects the null hypothesis and accepts that there is an association between attitude towards change and work environment of staff.

3. H_3 df 8 ∞ .05 X^2= 18.266 p<.02.

Therefore the author rejects the null hypothesis and accepts that there is an association between attitudes towards the impact of technology and work environment of staff.

4. H_4 df 4 ∞ .05 X^2= 23.863 p<.0001.

Therefore the author rejects the null hypothesis and accepts that there is an association between attitude towards the benefits of computer systems and the computer experience of staff.

5   H_5 df 4 ∞ .05 X^2= 12.857 p<.012.

Therefore the author rejects the null hypothesis and accepts that there is an association between attitudes of the impact of technology and computer experience of staff.

The statistically significant results for Study 2 were :

1. H_1 df 4 ∞ .05 X^2= 37.983 p<.0001.

Therefore the author rejects the null hypothesis and accepts that there is an association between attitude towards problems with computer systems and the computer experience of staff.

2. H_2 df 4 ∞ .05 X^2= 10.6 p<.002.

Therefore the author rejects the null hypothesis and accepts that there is an association between attitude towards change and the computer experience of staff.

3. H_3 df 4 ∞ .05 X^2= 41.35 p<.0001.

Therefore the author rejects the null hypothesis and accepts that there is an association between attitude towards computers and the computer experience of staff.

4. H_4 df 4 ∞ .05 X^2= 19.969 p<.0001.

Therefore the author rejects the null hypothesis and accepts that there is an association between attitude towards impact of technology and the computer experience .

6. Discussion

The main purpose of this study was to determine staff attitude towards , computer technology. In study One there was a statistically significant correlation between the area of work of staff and their attitudes towards change and the benefits of computer systems and the impact this technology will have on their work environment. There was also a statistically significant correlation between the computer experience of staff and their attitudes towards the benefits of computer systems and the impact this technology will have on their work environment. While in study Two there was a statistically significant correlation between computer experience of staff and their attitudes towards problems with computers, change, computers and the impact of technology on staff.

The results of these studies certainly supported the findings of the author in the available literature. Even though limited studies of this kind have been undertaken in Australia - the results are very similar to the findings overseas.

7. Conclusion

In this paper the author undertook a research program involving two studies at various stages of a C.I.S. implementation in a Sydney metropolitan hospital. These studies examined the attitudes of staff in various demographic categories, to computers. The entire 500 staff members were issued with a 30 item questionnaire at the beginning of implementation and then again during training, with a response rate of 317 or 64% in Stage 1 and 320 or 65% in Stage 2. The nursing area had the largest number of staff without any computer experience, while the administrative area had the largest number of staff with computer experience.

The results of the questionnaire demonstrated a statistically significant correlation between, where people worked and the amount of experience they had with computers, and how they perceived change, as well as the   benefits and problems of computer systems and how the introduction of this technology would impact on their work environment.

Further studies will be undertaken to examine staff attitudes to the same categories after the hospital has "gone live" with the pilot C.I.S.

8. References

[1] Brondt, A and Stronge, J. Nurses Attitudes Towards Computerization in a Midwestern Community Hospital. *Comput Nurs.* 1986, Vol. 4/No. 2. 82-86.

[2] Stronham, G. Computing in Practice-Information Management and Technology. *Nurs Times.* 1991, July 17, Vol. 18, No. 29, 47-49.

[3] Stronge, J and Brondt, A. Assessment of Nurses Attitudes Towards Computerization. *Comput Nurs.* 1985, July/August Vol. 3/No. 4, 154-158.

[4] Happ, B. Should Computers be Used in the Nursing Care of Patients? *Nurs Manage.* 1983, July, 31-35.

[5] Houle, C. *Continued Larning in the Professions.* 1980, Jossey Bass.

[6] Chang, B. Adoption of Innovations. Nursing and Computer Use. *Comput Nurs.* 1984, November/December, 229-235.

[7] Theis, J. Hospital Personnel and Computer Based Systems: A study of Attitudes and Perceptions. *Hosp Admin.* 1975, 20, 17-26.

[8] Calhoun M, Stanley D, Hughes L and McLean M. The relationship of age, level of formal education and duration of employment toward attitudes concerning the use of computers. *J. Med Syst.* 1989, Feb 13(1), 1-9.

Nursing Informatics: An International Overview for Nursing in a Technological Era
S.J. Grobe and E.S.P. Pluyter-Wenting, eds.

A Bibliometric Analysis of Published Maternal and Child Health Nursing Research from 1976 to 1990

D'Auria J P

Assistant Professor of Nursing, Dept of Women and Children's Health, The University of North Carolina at Chapel Hill, Chapel Hill, North Carolina 27599-7460, USA.

The purpose of this bibliometric study was to explore and describe evolving patterns of scholarly activity in the maternal and child health nursing subfield as represented in the citation patterns of published nursing research from 1976 to 1990. Citation data demonstrated that the clearest glimpses nurse scholars currently have of the evolving structure of nursing science in the maternal and child health subfield are patterns of foundational fields and the identities of nurse scientists and other scientists from across disciplines whose interests are shaping the generation of scientific information. Findings support the value of using research methodologies from information science to contribute working models of the development of nursing science that may assist in the evaluation of nursing's scientific progress and the dissemination of knowledge among nurse scholars.

1. Overview of Bibliometrics

Alternative research methodologies for describing and visually representing the communication structure of a scientific field of interest have been successfully used in other fields to evaluate such things as emergence, change, and communication networks [1]. Specifically, bibliometrics has been a useful research methodology for studying the structure of science as represented in the literature of a disciplinary field. Two bibliometric techniques that have been helpful in tracing the evolution of a new field of inquiry include: (1) the identification of scientists or scholars influencing the intellectual development of a field and (2) the identification of a new field's foundational fields (i.e., other scientific fields which have driven the genesis of the new science).

Bibliometrics is the application of mathematics and statistical methods to published scientific communication in a disciplinary field [2]. Research questions addressed by bibliometric studies generally fall into one of four categories: (a) characterization of the scholarly community, (b) evolution of a scholarly community, (c) evaluation of scholarly contributions, and (d) diffusion of ideas from within and across disciplines [3]. In bibliometrics, authors, citations, and texts found in the scholarly literature of a field are used as empirical indicators.

Citation analysis is the best-known form of citation-based bibliometric research. It includes descriptive as well as multivariate statistical strategies for graphically representing linkages between and among citation data. The counting of citations is the basic mathematical unit for determining whether citation data will be included in subsequent statistical procedures. Citation counts are the summation of certain identified bibliographic characteristics. Descriptive strategies of citation patterns of interest in this paper include citation rate and citation source. A *citation rate* refers to how often an author is cited. Citation rates are most useful in identifying the productivity of scientists and emerging networks in scientific communities [4]. *Citation source* refers to the form of a publication and the discipline it represents. Journals are generally the primary communication media and the largest reference source in scientific fields [5]. The broad subject categories of citations may provide evidence of the degree of reliance of nursing on its own body of information and the degree of articulation of the field of nursing with other disciplines.

2. Purpose of the Study

The purpose of this *ex post facto* bibliometric analysis was to explore and describe the evolving patterns of scholarly activity in the maternal and child health nursing (MCN) subfield as represented in the citation patterns of published nursing research from 1976 to 1990. This paper will focus on the following two subquestions: (a) What are the patterns of citing and cited authorship in the 325 source articles published from 1976 to 1990? (b) What are the changes in citation characteristics of cited journal references from 1979-1981 and from 1988-1990? The unit of analysis for this study was the individual research article.

3. Limitations of Citation Data

Bibliometrics as a research methodology is generally considered to be highly reliable for two reasons: (1) it relies on unobtrusive measures of readily available data, and (2) results of bibliometric studies can be replicated. When conducting bibliometric studies, errors in measurement can occur in data sources. However, these sources of potential error can be identified and corrected by the researcher. A major assumption of bibliometric research is that bibliographic data are a reflection of the influence of prior works and/or authors. In citation analysis, frequently cited authors or documents are assumed to be of some importance in the scholarly literature of a disciplinary field. In order to interpret data meaningfully, the researcher must consider the state of scholarly communication in the disciplinary field at a designated point in time. In addition, it is critical when using citation-based measures that data be collected over a significant span of time to allow for the identification of trends or changes over time.

4. Instrumentation

The Bibliometrics Toolbox [6] was used for the editing and counting of bibliographic data, e.g., author citation counts and journal citation counts. This program is specifically designed to facilitate calculations in bibliometric studies. *Pro-Cite* ® [7] and *Microsoft ®Excel* [8] were used to manage bibliographic data and calculate descriptive statistics.

5. Procedure

This bibliometric analysis was confined to published MCN research articles whose first author was a nurse. This was determined by the qualifications of the primary or single author listed in the published articles. A published research article had to be relevant to the subfield of MCN as defined by the study, collect and analyze data to answer a research question, and have a reference list.

A total of 325 research articles in *Journal of Advanced Nursing (JAN), Nursing Research (NR), Research in Nursing & Health (RINAH)*, and *Western Journal of Nursing Research (WJNR)* were the source of citation data. Citation data for three of the four nursing research journals were electronically reproduced from Social SCISEARCH® (the on-line version of the *SSCI*).   The *WJNR* is not presently on Social SCISEARCH®; bibliographic references from research articles published in *WJNR* were manually entered into database workforms. The above procedure created the citation index for the study.

Three subsets of text files were created from the 15-year computer data set. The first subset contained counts of recurring and nonrecurring citing nurse authors at 5-year intervals (1976-1980, 1981-1985, 1986-1990). A second subset of text files included all primary authors cited in the 325 source articles at 5-year intervals (1976-1980, 1981-1985, 1986-1990). Due to the emergent nature of nursing science and the large number of total citations ($\underline{N}$ = 8345) in the MCN published nursing literature, the third subset included text files of journals cited in the source articles from 1979-1981 and 1988-1990. The journal citations were classified with Ulrich's periodical classification system [9]. This classification system gives the general subject category of the journal an article is published in, not of the article itself. In addition, the field of nursing is included under the broad subject heading of *Medical Sciences (MS)*: *Nurses And Nursing*. Journals that changed serial titles were merged under their most current serial title.

6. Data Analysis and Interpretation

The findings of the study demonstrate the increasing trend of recurring authorship patterns among MCN researchers. The number of recurring citing authors increased from 0 (0%) in 1976-1980, to 12 (13.6%) in 1981-1985, and to 29 (20.3%) in 1986-1990. There was also an increasing trend in the numbers of source articles published by a single recurring nurse author in a 5-year time period. The range of source articles published by a specific recurring author ranged from 2 to 3 in 1981-1985 and from 2 to 6 in 1986-1990. The number of recurring nurse authors contributing at least 2 source articles in a 5-year period increased from 10 authors in 1981-1985 to 21 authors in 1986-1990. The number of recurring nurse authors contributing 3 or more source articles increased from 2 authors in 1981-1985 to 8 authors in 1986-1990.

These trends in recurring authorship patterns represent an important scientific resource for MCN scholars. These data indicate that nurse researchers are establishing publication histories in their own publication channels. The works of these published nurse researchers assist in the dissemination, building, and challenging of scientific knowledge in the MCN subfield. In addition, these authorship patterns support an increased frequency in the number of reports by individual nurse researchers over each of the 5-year periods. These trends indicate that the work of certain individual MCN researchers is becoming more visible and accessible to scholars who share an interest in their phenomena of interest. This is important because scholars in a disciplinary field must build communities around substantive areas to receive support and build a recognized body of knowledge. Scholarly communities must build a body of knowledge that promotes cohesion and consensus around disciplinary problems [10]. Further investigation as to whether or not these data support the development of such communities is warranted.

Author citation counts were used to provide an initial glimpse of the prominent individuals and their range of influence as evidenced through their body of works (*oeuvre*) in the emergence of MCN science. These data support the absence of a core of authors responsible for a high proportion (10% or more) of the total citations in each of the 5-year time periods. The two most frequently cited authors from 1976-1980 (Klaus MH and Rubin R) were responsible for only 1.4% of the total number of citations. The two most frequently cited authors from 1981-1985 (Brazelton TB and Klaus MH) were responsible for only 1.8% of the total number of citations. Again, the two most frequently cited authors (Mercer R and Lazarus RS) from 1986-1990 were responsible for only 1.8% of the total number of citations. Presently, scholars in the MCN subfield demonstrate a minimal level of consensus on the contribution of nurse scholars and scholars from other disciplinary fields in the development of knowledge.

It is critical to note that general trends in cited author patterns supported the emergence of increasing numbers of nurse authors into the citation networks of MCN research literature. Four of the 15 authors cited 10 or more times from 1981-1985 were nurse researchers. Eleven of the 39 authors cited at a frequency of 10 or more from 1986-1990 were nurse researchers. These data support that nurse researchers are increasingly being cited by other nurse scholars. This is an important trend in the field of nursing because it suggests that these nurse researchers are contributing a relevant and credible body of information to the endeavor of science [11]. Contextual analyses of these citations would assist in determining how nurses are building and challenging the work of other nurse scholars.

The proportion of journal citations in the literature of a field is a measure of the scholarliness of the field of interest [12]. Of the total number of 840 citations (43 source articles) from 1979-1981, 544 (64.8%) were journal citations. Of the total number of 3510 citations (128 source articles) from 1988-1990, 2398 (68.3%) were journal citations. The high percentage of journal citations in the MCN research literature suggests evidence of scientific activity among its scholars [13]. In addition, the sharp increase in total citations from 1979-1981 to 1988-1990 parallels the surge in the publication of the nursing research literature in the mid-1980s.

The total number of journal citations from 1979-1981 was distributed among a total of 173 journals. Twenty-one of these journals accounted for 50% of the journal citations. The subject dispersion of these 21 journals was high, with 77.2% classified outside of *MS: Nurses And Nursing*. The total number of journal citations from 1988-1990 was distributed among a total of 451 journals. Of these 451 journals, 24 accounted for 49% of the journal citations. The subject dispersion was again high, with 75% of the 24 journal serials classified outside of *MS: Nurses And Nursing*. This finding is indicative of an emergent and unstable body of scientific literature [14]. This finding, however, is to be expected in a new field of inquiry. MCN scholars must look to other disciplines for direction in developing a relevant body of scientific information. Ultimately, nurse scholars must synthesize and integrate information from across disciplinary fields into a body of relevant scientific information for nursing.

Over 60% of the journal literature cited by MCN scholars was classified as Medical Sciences (MS) in both 3-year periods. These trends resembled the trends identified by Garfield [15] in a journal citation analysis of core nursing journals from 1981-1983. The MCN research literature in this study demonstrated an increasing trend in the use of the journal literature from the *Medical Sciences*, *Psychiatry And Neurology* and the subject area of *Psychology*. These data demonstrate the shared interests MCN researchers have generally had with scholars in the fields of *Children and Youth* and *Medical Sciences* (pediatrics, obstetrics and gynecology). These fields have been useful as foundational bases for early research among MCN scholars.

The 21 journals cited from 1979-1981 were cited at relatively low frequencies (range: 7-35). The subject analysis showed that the core journal from 1979-81 was *Child Development*. *NR* (fourth most frequently cited journal) and three MCN specialty journals were also in the top 21 journals. The core journal from 1988-1990 was *NR*. The dramatic rise of *NR* (citation frequency = 215) in the citation networks of published MCN research must be viewed cautiously. *NR* was the first journal dedicated to the dissemination of nursing research findings and has been an important medium (and for many years the only medium on the general field and specialty levels) for the generation, dissemination, and advancement of research activity in the field of nursing, especially the MCN subfield. These data also parallel the tremendous explosion in research publications among MCN scholars in the 1980s. Finally, the majority of source articles in this 3-year data set were published in *NR* and it is common practice for published authors to cite the journal they are publishing in on their reference list.

Two additional nursing journals appeared in the top 5 most frequently cited journals from 1988-1990: *RINAH* and *Journal of Obstetric, Gynecologic, and Neonatal Nursing*. Many of the most active and influential nurse scholars in the MCN subfield have had shared interests in the prenatal, pregnancy, and early postnatal periods. Specialty MCN research journals have played an important role in the dissemination of knowledge useful to MCN scholars across both 3-year data sets. As increasing numbers of nurse researchers seek to publish their scientific findings, the specialty nursing journal network will gain in importance for the dissemination of knowledge in the MCN subfield.

7. Conclusions and Implications

Nursing science in the MCN subfield can be characterized as pre-embryonic. The clearest glimpses nurse scholars currently have of the evolving structure of nursing science in the MCN subfield appear to be (a) patterns of influence of foundational sciences on the development of nursing knowledge and (b) the identities of nurse scientists and other scientists from across disciplines whose interests are shaping the generation of scientific information in nursing. By examining common bases of information exchange across sciences, nurse scholars can better develop classification systems to facilitate the networking of scientists and research information. By discovering trends in interdisciplinary linkages, nurse scholars can identify underdeveloped or neglected areas of research in nursing science. By identifying emerging networks of nurse researchers, nurse scholars may more efficiently access scientific information and thereby prevent the loss of information generated in the MCN subfield.

Understanding how information and knowledge in the field of nursing evolve is critical to the advancement of theory, research, and practice. Nurse scholars must be able to efficiently locate information generated by other nurse scientists to facilitate the accumulation as well as the advancement of nursing knowledge. As the nursing research literature continues to grow, rigorous and systematic bibliometric research of citation data will contribute working models of the development of nursing science. These models will assist in the evaluation of nursing's scientific progress as well as the dissemination of knowledge among nurse scholars.

8. References

[1]   Culnan MJ, O'Reilly III CA and Chatman JA. Intellectual Structure of Research in Organizational Behavior, 1972-1984: A Cocitation Analysis. *J Am Soc Inf Sci* 1990, 42:453-458.

[2]   Pritchard A. Statistical Bibliography or Bibliometrics? *J Doc* 1969, 25: 348-349.

[3]   Borgman CL. Editor's introduction. In *Scholarly Communication and Bibliometrics*. Borgman CL (Ed). Newbury Park: Sage Publications Inc, 1990: 10-27.

[4]   Lindsey D. Further Evidence for Adjusting for Multiple Authorship. *Scientometrics* 1982, 4: 389-395.

[5]   Saracevic T and Perk LS. Ascertaining Activities in a Subject Area through Bibliometric Analysis. *J Am Soc Info Sci* 1973, 24: 120-134.

[6] Brooks TA. *The Bibliometrics Toolbox*. Version 2.8. Seattle, Washington: North City Bibliometrics, 1987.

[7] *Pro-Cite® for the Macintosh*. Version 1.3. Ann Arbor, MI: Personal Bibliographic Software Inc, 1988.

[8] *Microsoft® Excel*. Version 3.0. Redmond, Washington: Microsoft Corporation, 1991.

[9] Pierce SJ. Disciplinary work and interdisciplinary areas: Sociology and bibliometrics. In *Scholarly Communication and Bibliometrics*. Borgman CL (Ed). Newbury Park: Sage Publications Inc, 1990: 46-58.

[10] Bowker RR (Ed). *Ulrich's International Periodicals Directory 1989-90 Volume 3: Indexes*. New York: Reed Publishing (USA) Inc, 1989.

[11] Gortner S. The History and Philosophy of Nursing Science and Research. *ANS Adv Nurs Sci* 1983, 5: 1-8.

[12] Frohman B. A Bibliometric Analysis of the Literature of Cataloging and Classification. *Libr Res* 1982, 4:355-373.

[13] Kanasy J. Citation Characteristics and Bibliographic Control of the Literature of Microbiology [Dissertation]. Pittsburg, Pennsylvania: University of Pittsburg, 1971.

[14] Ibid.

[15] Garfield E. Citation Patterns in Nursing Journals, and their Most-Cited Articles. In *Essays of an Information Scientist* Vol 7. Philadelphia: ISI Press, 1985: 336-345.

Nursing Informatics: An International Overview for Nursing in a Technological Era
S.J. Grobe and E.S.P. Pluyter-Wenting, eds.

Computer assessment by nurse therapists of motivation to quit in problem drinkers: the virtual page is treated differently to the real page.

Mc Mahon J and Jones B T[a]

[a]*Department of Psychology (Nurse Information Processing Group), University of Glasgow G128QQ, Scotland UK*

Although the NAEQ (Negative Alcohol Expectancy Questionnaire) which has been developed as a tool to measure motivation for recovery in problem drinkers has been found to be highly reliable, it contains many questions of a sensitive nature which may promote reactance in clients leading to under-reporting of problems. It has been well-demonstrated that when giving sensitive information, subjects are more 'truthful' in a computer interview than a face to face interview. Since computer hardware and software is expensive, can reactance be avoided in the same way by simply using a paper and pencil questionnaire? To test this empirical question, the NAEQ and a similar questionnaire with no sensitive questions (the AEQ, Alcohol Expectancy Questionnaire) were presented to 30 subjects using both a computer and paper and pencil method. The results show that subjects reliably under-report when using the paper and pencil as compared with the computer method with the NAEQ but not the AEQ.

The implications that this might have for assessment by nurse therapists are discussed.

1. Background

"The virtual demise of the medical model in alcoholism has opened the floodgates for nurses to adopt a more responsible role in treatment, heralding the emergence of nurse-therapists: a role which puts nurses at the sharp end of treatment delivery as counsellors and health educators" Mc Mahon and Jones [1].

Whilst there have always been those who recover from problem drinking without help, there are also many who do not. It has become part of the rhetoric of the treatment of problem drinkers that client-motivation is at the heart of recovery [2] and the inference is that those who recover on their own must have generated sufficient motivation to stop and that those who continue problem drinking have not. The majority of contemporary treatment in the UK is directed towards raising the motivational levels of clients and the seriousness with which the motivational approach to treatment is taken world-wide was marked by the three-yearly International Conference on the Treatment of Addictive Behaviors (ICTAB-6, Santa Fe 1993) being entirely dedicated to 'Motivation for Change'.

The difficulty that confronts therapists is (i) knowing what motivation to quit *is,* (ii) knowing how to *measure* it and, once the measure of motivation is known, (iii) knowing how to *use* the measurement to effect appropriate care. Jones [3]) sees this difficulty as a general one and has argued that the (i) heeding (ii) measuring (iii) utilising dimensions referred to above is one of the most useful way of systematically approaching any activity in healthcare. (He has called this the 'informatics template', preferring to harness the term 'informatics' to informing rather than computing)

As Mc Mahon and Jones [4] have argued elsewhere, this is a difficulty with which the nurse is very familiar for it embeds quite comfortably within the conceptual schemes used in contemporary nursing. Knowing what motivation to to quit *is,* requires the nurse therapist to know what sources of information should be *heeded* when addressing problem drinking in general and is tantamount to a nursing model for problem drinking. Knowing how to represent or *measure* each of these sources of information requires the development of an assessment tool so that, through the use of the nursing model of problem drinking, the nature of the client's specific problems can be identified. Knowing how to *utilise* the information thus collected (the assessment) is tantamount to planning client-specific care or therapy.

If therapy is designed to raise the motivational levels for stopping or restraining drinking, then within the normal processes of systematic nursing there are the opportunities to periodically evaluate the effects of the therapy until some goal has been reached and the therapy can be discontinued or until the evaluation suggests that the plan of care needs to be modified. Central to assessment and assessment/evaluation procedures such as this is a valid and reliable assessment tool designed to measure motivational level. Mc Mahon and Jones have designed such a tool: the Negative Alcohol Expectancy Questionnaire (NAEQ).

2. The Negative Alcohol Expectancy Questionnaire

This 60-item assessment tool is designed to identify an individual's expected negative consequences of drinking alcohol. It comprises a series of statements about the expected negative consequences and subjects are asked to respond by indicating on a 5-point Likert scale the likelihood of each one happening to them. It is designed to measure within three temporal contexts and the following questions illustrate this: (i) What negative consequences would you expect to occur to you if you went out for a drink NOW (21 items)? (ii) What negative consequences would you expect to experience TOMORROW if you went for a drink now (18 items)? (iii) What longer-term negative consequences would you expect to occur to you if you were to CONTINUE drinking at your current rate (21 items?). The NAEQ is available for photocopying along with extensive psychometric/reliability data [5,6]. The NAEQ was designed to be used as the framework for a structured assessment interview with the therapist writing down the client's responses.

For assessment purposes, the NAEQ represents two related but functionally different aspects of the problem drinker. First a measure of the motivational level to stop is provided by aggregating the scores within each of the three temporal contexts described earlier. This can then be assessed against norms that we have established over the past three years. Second, and much more important for problem-identification and appropriate careplanning, the client's answers to each of the 60 items of the NAEQ give *precise* information about what specifically needs to be done to RAISE the client's overall motivational level. This is important because it is well-established that recovery is a function of motivational level and it is Mc Mahon and Jones' contention that measuring expected negative consequences of alcohol use (negative expectancy) is tantamount to measuring motivation to recover [4,7].

The problems that the client *already* recognises and is prepared to discuss are easily identified from the NAEQ (because the client, him/herself, has declared them) and these can be used to begin to gently address the other problems that (s)he must surely be experiencing (or they would not be in treatment) but is recognising *less well*. This 'easy-to-hard' approach is designed to ensure that the reactance that is so much a feature of any form of interviewing (particularly when personal details are in focus), is avoided.

3. The Problem

Although the predictive validity of this tool is high both with problem drinkers [8,9] and with the drinking behaviour of social drinkers [10], we have begun to suspect that a number of the particularly sensitive statements to which clients are asked to respond may be treated differently to the remainder. Although this does not matter very much in terms of assessing their scores against norms (for the norms would also be biased) it *does* matter in terms of relative problem assessment and the development of a plan for the motivational interview. Although appropriate training might be thought to begin to help therapists avoid this difficulty, we have little evidence that it does.

Of course, one possible solution is that the clients could be asked, themselves, to fill in the NAEQ: either presented on paper to be filled in with a pencil or on a computer screen to be filled in using a mouse-driven cursor to press screen buttons. Both could, potentially, avoid the reactance difficulty.

Indeed, there is no shortage of evidence that for sensitive information, computer-based questions are answered more 'truthfully' than are *interview-based* questions [11]. There are a wide range of domains in which this appears to be the case: psychological [12], sexual [13], marital [14] and suicide [15] problems as well as personnel selection [16]. There is also good evidence to show that alcohol-related problems and self-report of consumption fall into this category, too [17]. Moreover, with respect to alcohol consumption, clients report 33% more to the computer than to the interviewer [18].

This brief review of what is a very large body of evidence begs the question: Since computer-gear is more expensive, cumbersome and difficult to use than is paper-and-pencil and since paper-and-pencil might be regarded as just as distant from the interviewer as is a computer, might it not be as effective to present the NAEQ as a paper-and-pencil test than a computer-test? For if there is good evidence that a computer-based questionnaire is 'better' than an interview, should this not also extend to paper-and -pencil. There might be grounds, though, for suggesting that a client might be more ready to commit responses to sensitive questions to a *virtual page* on a screen within which responses are to mouse-driven radio buttons than to *hard copy* on paper written with a pencil by their own hand. One method is clearly more remote, less concrete, apparantly more accesible to others than is the other.

These speculations are easily tested with respect to the NAEQ and this is what the experiment below is designed to do. With the following information, (i) high NAEQ scores represent a highly-motivated client and low NAEQ scores represent a poorly motivated client and (ii) our suspicions that on a number of sensitive items, scores within the context of a structured interview are lower than they 'should' otherwise be; the hypotheis to be tested is:

$$\text{NAEQ (computer) scores} > \text{NAEQ (paper/pencil) scores}$$

4. Method

4.1. Subjects
Fifteen male and 15 female volunteers aged between 21 and 60 served as subjects. None were abstainers and had no self-reported history of problem drinking.

4.2. Assessment tools
The NAEQ as described earlier was used. In addition the AEQ was administered (the Alcohol Expectancy Questionnaire is a 90-item tool, 60 items of which assess an individual's expectation of the positive, rather than negative, consequences of alcohol use [19]). Unlike the NAEQ, it contains *no* sensitive items and because of this represents a useful control for it should not be subject to the same 'under-reporting' as would an assessment tool which contained sensitive items. It all senses it can be regarded as complementary to the NAEQ.

4.3. Design
Two conditions were used: Paper/pencil (P) in which the NAEQ and AEQ were administered as printed questionnaires to be completed at a table, alone in a room; Computer (C) in which they were administered as a computer program (written using the Apple application HyperCard taking advantage of the mouse-driven, screen-button utility to replace keyboard use). An Apple Macintosh LC with 14" BW screen was used. The HyperCard program has also been run on a PC compatible 386SX using the conversion utility of PLUS2 and subsequently run under Windows3.

Half the subjects received condition P first followed by Condition C seven days later (a within-subjects design) and half C followed by P. Seven days is, in fact, the length of time we allow to elapse before ressessment with the NAEQ in the clinical setting and we already know that over this length of time there are no reliable carry-over effects. The data from the two orders of presentation were combined.

Within these two groups, approximately half of the subjects received the NAEQ first (at each of the times of presentation) followed almost immediately by the AEQ and half the AEQ followed by the NAEQ. The data from these two orders of presentation were combined.

5. Results

The mean AEQ scores for conditions P and C were 170 and 173, respectively, and the mean difference was not reliable (related t-test p>0.50). The mean NAEQ scores for conditions P and C were 95 and 105, respectively and the mean difference was reliable (related t-test p=0.035 2-tail test p=0.0175 1-tail test). The NAEQ scores were approximately 10% higher in condition C than P. For some individuals this was 20%.

6. Conclusions

NAEQ scores were reliably higher when it was administered via the computer than paper/pencil. The AEQ scores showed no difference between these two methods of presentation. If there was some irregularity in the procedures for administering the tests that was responsible for the NAEQ difference, then one would expect there to be an AEQ difference, too. There is not. Since there are few *(if any)* sensitive items in the AEQ and *many* sensitive items in the NAEQ, this suggests that it is the sensitive nature of these items embedded within the two different methods of presentation that is responsible for the difference.

We continue to speculate that the attitudes that surround the *virtual* as opposed to the *real* page underpin this result. But we now speculate with more confidence! We are currently extending this experiment to use heavy drinkers and problem drinkers (both in-treatment and otherwise) as subjects and where NAEQ scores routinely reach 200-250 (maximum 300). If subjects such as these show a 10% difference between the two methods of administering the NAEQ (as do social drinkers), it would be an important finding because 'losing' 20-25 points at assessment could represent 'losing' as many as half a dozen of the twenty or thirty *potential* problems that a problem drinker in treatment might have and that the NAEQ is capable of detecting. This is serious. It is even more serious if one considers that not all of these twenty or thirty problems will apply to any one individual, under which circumstances a mis-assessment that loses a half dozen is, in fact, losing much more than it appears.

The *practical* impact of computer assessment and computer feedback to the post-discharge outcome of clients admitted to an alcohol problems treatment unit is currently being explored in a two-year follow-up project.

7. Acknowledgements

The first author is supported by Scottish Office Home and Health Department Nurse Research Training Fellowship K/OPR/2/3/82 supervised by the second author. The support of Alcohol Education and Research Council grant R6/92 is also gratefully acknowledged. The follow-up project is supported by Scottish Office Home and Health Department Clinical Biomedical Research Committee grant K/MRS/50/C2071.

8. References

[1]   Mc Mahon J and Jones B T.   Negative expectancy: An assessment measure of motivation for use by nurse therapists in the treatment of problem drinking. *J Assoc Nurs in Subst Abuse* 1992, 11:20-23.

[2]   Prochaska J O and DiClemente C C.   Common processes of self-change in smoking, weight control and psychological distress. In: *Coping and Substance Abuse: A Conceptual Framework.* Shiffman S and Wills T. (eds) New York: Academic Press, 1985: 345 - 363.

[3]   Jones B T. Heeding, measuring, utilising: the informatics template. *Int J Health Inf* 1993, 2: in press.

[4]   Mc Mahon J and Jones B T.   The change process in alcoholics: client motivation and denial in the treatment of alcoholism within the context of contemporary nursing. *J Adv Nurs* 1992, 17:173-186.

[5]   Mc Mahon J and Jones B T. The Negative Alcohol Expectancy Questionnaire. *J Assoc Nurs in Subst Abuse* 1993, 12:17.

[6]   Jones B T and Mc Mahon J. The reliability of the Negative Alcohol Expectancy Questionnaire and its use. *J Assoc Nurs in Subst Abuse* 1993, 12:14-16.

[7]   Mc Mahon J and Jones B T. Negative expectancy and motivation. *Addiction Res* 1993, 1:144-155.

[8] Jones B T and Mc Mahon J. (1992) Negative and positive expectancies in group and lone problem drinkers. *Br J Addiction* 1992, 87:929-930.

[9] Mc Mahon J and Jones B T. The negative alcohol expectancy questionnaire (NAEQ), an instrument to measure motivation for recovery from problem drinking: reliabilty and validity. Presentation at the *Sixth International Conference on the Treatment of Addictive Behaviors*, Santa Fe US.

[10] Mc Mahon J and Jones B T. Comparing positive and negative alcohol expectancies in social drinkers. *Addiction Res* 1993, 1:in press.

[[11] Evan W M and Miller J R. Differential effects on response bias of computer vs, coventional administration of a social science questionnaire: an exploratory methodological experiment. *Behav Sci* 1969, 14:216-227.

[12] Farrell A D, Camplair P S and McCullough L. Identification of target complaints by computer interview: evaluation of the computerized assessment system for psychotherapy evaluation and research. *J Consult Clin Psychol* 1987, 55:691-700.

[13] Greist J H and Klein M H. Computer programs for patients, clinicians, and researchers in psychiatry. In: *Technology in mental health care delivery systems.* Sidowski JB, Johnson JH and Williams TA (eds). Norwood: Ablex Publishing, 1980: 109-202.

[14] Olson D H. Microcomputers for couple and family assessment: ENRICH and other inventories. *J Psychother Fam* 1985, 1:105-115.

[15] Greist J H, Gustafson D H, Strauss F F, Laughren T P and Chiles J A. A computer interview for suicide risk prediction. *Am J Psych* 1973, 130:1327-1332.

[16] Grant D. Automating the selection procedure. *Pers Man* 1987, 15:29-31.

[17] Lucas R W, Mullin P J, Luna C B X and McInroy D C. Psychiatrists and a computer as interrogators of patients with alcohol-related illnesses: a comparison. *Br J Psych* 1977, 131:160-167.

[18} Duffy J C and Waterton J J. Under-reporting of alcohol consumption in sample surveys: the effect of computer interviewing in fieldwork. *Br J Addiction* 1984, 79:303-308.

[19] Brown, S. A, Christiansen B A. and Goldman, M S. The alcohol expectancy questionnaire: an instrument for the assessment of adolescent and adult alcohol expectancies. *J Stud Alcoh* 1987, 45:483-491.

Nursing Informatics: An International Overview for Nursing in a Technological Era
S.J. Grobe and E.S.P. Pluyter-Wenting, eds.

Critical Care Nurses' Reasoning in Practice and Associated Indicators of Patient Outcome

Fonteyn M E [a] and Fisher A A [b]

a, bUniversity of San Francisco, School of Nursing, 2130 Fulton St., San Francisco, California, 94117-1080, USA.

Proficiency in clinical reasoning and the capacity to make reliable judgments are essential to nursing practice. Higher patient acuity levels and the complexity of their clinical status demand that nurses possess the domain knowledge and reasoning skills necessary to solve patient problems quickly and accurately. In critical care, expert nurses are extremely valuable because of their ability to solve patient problems by making sound and efficient decisions for problem resolution before their patients' condition deteriorates. Less experienced nurses frequently rely on these experts for advice and assistance with patient care dilemmas. But expert critical care nurses are a rare commodity, and thus are in great demand. In other fields where the demand for expertise exceeds the supply, decision support systems have provided a means to make expertise routinely available. Prior to the development of decision support systems for use in critical care nursing practice, the reasoning processes and strategies used by expert critical care nurses' must be better described and understood. Additionally, the relationships between nurses' reasoning, decision making, and patient outcomes must be better explained. Using a triangulated method (incorporating think aloud technique, participant observation, and in-depth interviews) we designed a study to describe expert nurses' clinical reasoning in practice, the nature of their expertise, and the indicators of patient outcome that were associated with and effected by their reasoning.

1. Problem Statement

Critical care nursing practice is undergoing profound change. Increasingly complex health care problems, high patient acuity, and greater dependence upon technology characterize the current critical care environment. To avoid patient deterioration and promote positive outcomes, nurses must possess the knowledge and reasoning skills necessary to solve patient problems quickly and accurately.[1, 2]

An initial understanding of the clinical reasoning and decision-making associated with expert nursing practice in critical care has been provided in studies by numerous investigators.[3-15] None of these previous studies, however, have identified or described the specific indicators of patient outcome that are associated with nurses' reasoning, even though research has shown that nurses' reasoning and decision making have a significant effect on patient outcome.[16-20] Bond and Thomas[16] remind us that research examining nurses' impact on outcome should aim to identify the nursing interventions [and the associated reasoning] which result in optimal patient outcomes. Jennings[17] noted the importance of viewing patient outcomes on a continuum that can be broken into increments, each representing advancement toward more long-term outcomes, some of which may not even be achieved by the time of discharge. Marek[19] recommended that nurses use outcome indicators as measures of progress towards long term goals regarding patient outcome.

Acknowledgments

This study was partially funded by the Beta Gamma Chapter of Sigma Theta Tau International and the Faculty Development Fund of University of San Francisco, School of Nursing.

In this paper, we identify the specific indicators of patient outcome that were associated with and effected by our expert nurse subjects' reasoning and decision making during their care provision to patients representing a particular type of clinical case about which the subjects possessed extensive knowledge and experience.

2. Sample and Setting

Our sample consisted of three registered nurses who volunteered to be in our study after being identified by both the nurse manager and their peers as expert (in terms of their knowledge and experience) on their nursing unit. One subject had been identified as being able to function as expert on both the cardiovascular surgery and the neurosurgery unit (S1); a second subject was identified as expert on the neurosurgery unit (S2); and a third subject was identified as expert on the cardiovascular unit (S3). This small sample was appropriate for our study because our primary goal was not to generalize across subjects, but rather to examine in detail the reasoning strategies of individuals.

We conducted our study at a 600-bed tertiary care medical center, where we identified two intensive care units with distinctively different postoperative patient populations: neurosurgical and cardiovascular. After obtaining informed consent, we collected data from subjects during their nursing shifts when they were providing immediate post operative care for patients within their area of expertise (using think aloud technique and participant observation) and during scheduled times with each subject when they were not on duty (using in-depth interview techniques).

3. Data Collection and Analysis

We used a triangulated method that included: think aloud technique, participant observation, and in-depth interviews. Combining collection of verbal protocol data at the bedside while care is being given, with a field research approach designed to reveal the complexity of the clinical environment and the routine and problematic aspects of clinical practice, provided a richer and more detailed description of expert nursing practice and its associated patient outcomes than could be obtained using simulation outside the clinical setting.

In a pilot study, we obtained verbal protocol data at the bedside while subjects were caring for patients either immediately after open heart surgery or after a craniotomy, depending on each subject's area of expertise. We found that using think aloud method in the clinical setting caused no disruption to unit function, nor was patient safety compromised. Subsequent to our pilot study, we conducted our full study incorporating the three components described below.

Think aloud technique. During data collection in the clinical setting, subjects carried a small portable tape recorder in their pocket, and wore a voice-activated microphone on their lapel. We prompted them to "think aloud" while they were reasoning and making decisions about their patient's care. These taped verbalizations were transcribed and subsequently analyzed, using a type of protocol analysis previously described by Fonteyn, Kuipers, and Grobe[9].

Participant observation. During data collection sessions, we took field notes regarding subjects' patient care activities. At intervals, when subjects were not thinking aloud, we asked them questions that helped us to clarify their reasoning strategies and to understand their actions. We asked subjects to identify their goals [expected outcomes] for patient care, and the data [outcome indicators] they were using to assess progress towards meeting these goals. These verbal interactions were tape-recorded, transcribed, and later analyzed using dimensional analysis that has been described by Schatzman[10] and Fisher[11].

In-depth interviews. We conducted in-depth interviews with each subject at a scheduled time in a small office near their units. We asked questions designed to identify the dimensions and range of each subjects' expert nursing practice, to determine how they had acquired, enhanced, and maintained their knowledge and reasoning skills, and to substantiate and verify findings that we had obtained during the think aloud and participant observation data collection sessions. The in-depth interviews were tape-recorded and subsequently transcribed and analyzed using dimensional analysis. This paper provides a report of our findings related to subjects' heuristic use, that was identified through protocol analysis of the think aloud data.

This paper provides a report of our findings related to patient outcome indicators, that were identified through protocol analysis of the think aloud data, and were verified and further explained through questioning subjects during participant observation and guided interviews.

4. Results and Discussion

During data collection episodes, we asked S3 (the expert on the cardiovascular unit) to identify the primary outcomes that nurses expected during the immediate post-operative period of care for patients who had open heart surgery. The primary outcomes anticipated during the immediate postoperative period remained constant, regardless of the specific type of operation that each patient had, such as coronary artery bypass and graft or valve replacement: 1. The patient will stabilize hemodynamically; and 2. The patient will remain hemodynamically stable. An excerpt from one of S3's transcript substantiates this:

I: *Are we right in thinking that your primary goals with these* [open heart, immediately
        post-op] *patients is to achieve and maintain stability?*

S3:   *Right...[we're] trying to avoid catastrophes by keeping them stable moment to moment.*

Using protocol analysis, we identified the indicators of these outcomes that subjects S3 and S1 (the expert on both the cardiovascular and the neurosurgery unit) articulated during multiple data collection episodes. The indicators that we identified, in order of frequency were: mean arterial pressure (MAP) and blood pressure (BP); heart rate and rhythm; serum magnesium and potassium levels; partial pressure of oxygen (PO_2) and oxygen saturation (O_2 Sat); breath sounds; temperature; cardiac output; chest tube drainage; serum calcium level; expired carbon dioxide level (ECO_2); urine output; and hematocrit and hemoglobin levels.

We were able to verify the importance of these indicators by questioning our subjects during participant observation and the in-depth interviews:

I: *What is the primary indicator that you use to know whether you are maintaining stability in these patients?*

S3:   *"The mean arterial pressure, the MAP. It tells me how the heart is pumping and how well it's perfusing the
        brain and the rest of the body.*

Likewise, we asked S2 (the expert on the neurosurgery unit) to identify the primary outcomes nurses expected during the immediate post-operative period of care for patients who had a craniotomy. The primary outcomes anticipated during the immediate postoperative period remained constant regardless of the specific type of operation that each patient had, such as repair of cerebral aneurysm or resection of tumor, were: 1. The patient will become responsive; and 2. The patient will remain hemodynamically stable. An excerpt from one of S2's transcript substantiates this:

I: *What are your overriding goals for these* [craniotomy, immediately post-op] *patients?*

S2:   *My overriding goal for this initial post-op period is that, by the end of my shift, the patients will wake up
        enough to be responsive, although I don't expect them to be alert.*
        My second goal is that they will be hemodynamically stable.

Using protocol analysis, we identified the indicators of these outcomes that subjects S2 and S1 articulated during multiple data collection episodes. The indicators that we identified, in order of frequency were: Level of consciousness (LOC) and neurological status; MAP and BP; breath sounds; temperature; ability to control own secretions; central venous pressure (CVP); heart rate and rhythm; pulse pressure; and arterial blood gases.

Again, we were able to verify the importance of these indicators through questioning during participant observation and in-depth interviews:

I: *Because when we analyzed data from you, it seemed like the thing you mentioned over and over was the MAP
        and the blood pressure; and then the level of consciousness and the neuro status.*

S2:   *Well, you know what? If you're standing here* [at the foot of the patient's bed] *it's hard to tell neuro status.*
        So, you might mention the changes on the monitor first [MAP and BP]
        that make you want to go over and talk to him [assess LOC].

During participant observation we noted that our expert nurses subjects consistently exhibited a high level autonomy when reasoning and making decisions about the care of their critically ill patients. They used protocols for therapy (such as titrating the intravenous drips of various hemodynamic medications, adjusting the level of oxygen flow, and obtaining a variety of laboratory tests as indicated by the patient's condition) as a means to meet their expected patient outcomes. Throughout the immediate post operative period, these subjects vigilantly monitored their patients, using the outcome indicators mentioned above to guide their reasoning and decision making about patient care.

Data from subjects' transcripts exemplifies both their autonomy in making decisions regarding therapy, and their use of outcome indicators to guide those decisions:

I: *Do you feel autonomous in changing and adjusting anything that's ongoing therapy?*

S3:   *Yeah, pretty much. Sometimes on the drips, they'll* [MDs] *write a minimum* [i.e., maintain a minimum
        nitroprusside drip rate of 5 mcg/kg/min].
        But if they wrote a minimum, and the patient's blood pressure was too low .on the minimum
        dose of nitroprusside],
        I would just change it [decrease it further] *and then call and report what had happened.*

S2:   *If something happens to this patient, like say his intracranial pressure goes up,*
        what can I do at the bedside before I call the doctor?
        I can look at the vital signs; I can go up or down on my drips.
        And the next thing I can do is bag the patient [hyperventilate the patient with
        the ambu bag to decrease their CO_2 level, which will decrease intracranial pressure].
        And the other thing I can do is I can put the head of the bed up a little bit so you'd have proper drainage.

5. Summary and Conclusion

Previous studies of nurses' clinical reasoning have failed to provide an understanding of the relationship between nurses' reasoning, decision making and patient outcomes. Research investigating this relationship has been hampered by an inadequate description of the outcome indicators that nurses' use to guide their care so as to achieve specific patient outcomes. Viewing patient outcomes as longitudinal, and breaking them down into increments that represent advancement toward more long-term goals, makes it easier to identify the outcome indicators that can be directly associated with nurses' reasoning and decision making during select periods of time on a continuum.

In this study of expert critical care nurses' clinical reasoning, we used a triangulated method to identify and describe the goals for patient outcome during the immediate post operative period with two types of patient cases. We then identified the specific indicators of these patient outcomes that could be associated with our expert nurse subjects' clinical reasoning and decision making.

Results from our study would be useful in developing decision support systems for use in critical care nursing practice. Such systems would be particularly helpful as educational tools to assist less-experienced nurses to learn to identify patient problems and to reason about the care of specific populations of critically ill patients, modeling their reasoning strategies of expert nurses. Improvement in nurses' reasoning and a better understanding of how reasoning affects patient outcome would assist in achieving optimal long-term outcome.

References

[1] Clochesy J. Implementing the commission recommendations. *Dimensions in Crit Care Nurs* 1989, 8:131-132.

[2] Dente-Cassidy A M. Predictions for critical care nursing. *Nurs* 1992, 92:43-45

[3] Benner, P, Tanner C and Chesla C. From beginner to expert: Gaining a differentiated clinical world in critical care nursing. *Adv Nurs Sci* 1992, 14:13-28.

[4] Bourbonnais F and Baumann A. Stress and decision making in nursing: an administrative challenge. *Nurs Admin Q* 1985a, 9:85-91.

[5] Bourbonnais F and Baumann A. Crisis decision making in coronary care: A replication study. *Nurs Papers Perspectives in Nurs* 1985b, 17:4-19.

[6] Bruya M and Demand J. Nursing decision making in critical care: traditional versus invasive blood pressure monitoring. *Nurs Admin Q* 1985, 9:19-31.

[7] Corcoran-Perry S and Graves J. Supplemental information-seeking behavior of cardiovascular nurses. *Res Nurs Health Care* 1990, 13:119-127.

[8] Fonteyn M. Clinical reasoning in critical care nursing *Focus on Crit Care* 1991a, 18:322-327

[9] Fonteyn M. A descriptive analysis of expert critical care nurses' clinical reasoning. *Doctoral dissertation* 1991b.

[10] Fonteyn, M. & Grobe, S Expert nurses' clinical reasoning under uncertainty: Representation, structure, amd process. Proceedings of the Sixteenth Annual Symposium on Computer Applications in Medical Care. Los Alimitos, CA: IEEEE, Computer Society Press, 1992.

[11] Guyton-Simmons J and Mattoon M. Analysis of strategies in the management of coronary patients' pain. *Dimensions Crit Care Nurs* 1991, 10:21-27.

[12] Pyles S and Stern P. Discovery of nursing gestalt in critical care nursing: The importance of the gray gorilla syndrome. *Image: J Nurs Scholar* 1983, 15:51-57.

[13] Rew L. Intuition in critical care nursing practice. *Dimensions Crit Care Nurs* 1990, 9:30-37.

[14] Sims K and Fought S. Clinical decision making in critical care. *Crit Care Nurs Q* 1989, 12:79-84.

[15] Thompson D and Sutton T. Nursing decision making in a coronary care unit. *Internat J Nurs Studies* 1985, 22:259-266.

[16] Bond S and Thomas L. Issues in measuring outcomes of nursing. *J Adv Nurs* 1991, 16:1492-1502.

[17] Jennings B. Patient outcome research: Seizing the opportunity. *Adv Nurs Sci* 1991, 14: 59-72.

[18] Knaus W, Draper E, Wagner D and Zimmerman J. An evaluation of outcome from intensive care in major medical centers. *Ann Int Med* 1986, 104:410-418.

[19] Marek K. Outcome measurement in nursing. *J Qual Assur* 1989, 4:1-9.

[20] Naylor M, Munro B and Brooten D. Measuring the effectiveness of nursing practice. *Clin Nurs Spec* 1991, 5:210-215.

[21] Kuipers B and Kassirer J. Causal reasoning in medicine: Analysis of a protocol. *Cog Sci* 1984, 8:363-385.

[22] Fonteyn M, Kuipers B and Grobe S. A description of the use of think aloud method and protocol analysis. *Qual Health Res* 3(4), 430-441.

[23] Schatzman L. Dimensional analysis: Notes on an alternative approach to the grounding of theory. In D. maines (ed.) *Social Organization for a Natural Sociology*, pp.303-314. Aldine de Gruyter, New York, 1991.

[24] Fisher S. Dimensional analysis as a vehicle for the study of dangerousness. Unpublished paper presented at the Western Society for Research in Nursing Annual Conference in Seattle, WA, April 30,1993.

Nursing Informatics: An International Overview for Nursing in a Technological Era
S.J. Grobe and E.S.P. Pluyter-Wenting, eds.

Using the Actigraph to Measure Activity-Rest in the Acute Care Setting

Wykpisz EM[a] Redeker NS[b] Mason DJ[c] Glica B[c]

[a]Robert Wood Johnson University Hospital, 1 Robert Wood Johnson Place, New Brunswick, NJ, 08903 USA.

[b]College of Nursing, Rutgers, the State University of New Jersey, Newark, NJ, 07102 USA.

[c]Beatrice Renfield Division of Nursing Education and Research, Beth Israel Medical Center, 1st Ave at 16th Street, New York, NY, 10003 USA.

Patterns of activity and rest are disrupted by illness and treatment, while improvements in activity and rest may lead to enhanced recovery and well-being. Despite the importance of activity and rest in nursing, there have been few appropriate objective clinical measures. The wrist actigraph provides continuous, non-invasive objective measurement of activity-rest. The purpose of this paper is to describe the use, reliability, validity, advantages and disadvantages of the wrist actigraph in the medical-surgical acute care setting.

1. Introduction

Patterns of activity-rest, are of central importance in acute care nursing. Alterations in activity-rest may be symptomatic of disease. Activity-rest patterns "can play significant roles in the prevention, cause and alleviation of fatigue," [1,p.192] a common symptom of illness and treatment. Improvement in activity is an important component of recovery and quality of life.[2,3] Studies have shown that an improvement in activity after surgery is related to greater perceived health status and enhancement in quality of life.[4,5] Redeker, Mason, Wykpisz, Glica, and Miner[6] found that rhythm and positive linear trend in activity predicted self-reports of dysfunction and length of stay in women who had undergone coronary artery bypass surgery. In another study[7], adherence to the critical path for activity was an important determinant of length of hospital stay in coronary bypass patients.

There has been relatively little systematic research into the outcomes of activity or its use as an intervention, and few instruments available to objectively measure activity. Researchers have relied on subjective methods, such as observation and questionnaires, or polysomnography, which is cumbersome and expensive, to measure sleep. None of these methods allows continuous measurement of the complete activity spectrum.[8,9] Recent advances in electronic technology and computers have made objective measurement of activity-rest practical in the acute care setting.

2. Wrist Actigraph

The wrist actigraph or motionlogger (tm), distributed by Ambulatory Monitoring, Inc., Ardsley, New York, is an electronic accelerometer. It senses motion via a ceramic bimorph beam arranged to generate a signal or charge when subjected to the force of acceleration; it processes and quantifies the sensed motion over a pre-programmed period of time; and stores that information. It operates on a lithium battery that is easily replaced and can last from days to weeks. Two forms of the motionlogger are available: the 16K actigraph (2.5 X 3.5 X .75 inch; weight 3 ounces) and the 32K Mini-Motionlogger (about the size of a divers' watch - 1.5 X 1.3 X .375 inch; weight 2 ounces). Both actigraphs produce equivalent measurements and have event markers that allow marking of the activity record to note timing of events, such as preparation for sleep, onset of specific activities, or symptoms.

The actigraph is sensitive to movement ranging from 0.05 to 0.10 g (g=9.81 meters/second^2) at sea level and senses movement in three dimensions. Two units of measurement are produced: The zero crossing mode counts the number of times that the displacement of the sensor beam generates sufficient voltage to cross a pre-set zero point during a pre-programmed epoch of time. The threshold mode indicates the amount of time per epoch that activity above a certain threshold is sensed. Units of measure in the threshold mode are seconds of activity per epoch length of time, while units of measure in the zero-crossing mode are number of movements/epoch of time. Use of the threshold mode is helpful for eliminating fine movement, such as tremors, or vibrations from an automobile.[8,10] The zero crossing mode is used for general activity monitoring and is required for use with available sleep algorithms. The motionlogger contains a microcomputer that permits programming of start-stop times, data collection intervals, or epochs, and storage of data.

3.   Reliability and Validity

The motionlogger is highly reliable and valid. Reliability is demonstrated by the virtually identical measurements produced by recording the repeated swings of a laboratory pendulum. Validity is determined by comparing the decay in the amplitude of the pendulum swing with the data recorded by the actigraph.[10] Validity in healthy human subjects was demonstrated in a recent series of studies.[11] In the first study, fifteen healthy, young adult males and females wore actigraphs on the non-dominant wrist while performing a set of non-sedentary and a set of sedentary activities. Differences between actigraph counts among treadmill levels and speeds and among two levels of stair stepping were statistical significant ($p < .0001$). Differences among various sedentary activities were also significant ($p < .0001$). Although overall differences between actigraph counts for the sets of sedentary and non-sedentary counts were statistically significant, the author noted that sedentary activity requiring a great deal of wrist activity (eg. playing video games) produced higher activity counts than knee bends or stair stepping. This finding highlights the importance of considering the site of attachment when planning activity studies or interpreting the results. The authors also found that average and high levels of activity computed from an activity diary were correlated with activity counts ($r = .81$ and $r = .80$, respectively, $p < .0001$). The 16K actigraph has also been reported to have higher subject acceptability than an activation-deactivation checklist.[12]

The actigraph has been shown to be a valid measure of sleep in the sleep laboratory and in health persons. Computerized programs for calculating sleep parameters from actigraphic data have been developed. Most recently, Cole, et al.[13] reported that their sleep algorithm distinguished nocturnal sleep parameters from wakefulness (as defined by polysomnography) approximately 88% of the time. Actigraphic sleep percentage and sleep latency estimates were correlated $r = .82$ and $r = .90$, respectively, with parameters obtained from polysomnograms ($p < .0001$). Several researchers have reported that actigraphy overestimated sleep time.[13,14] However, this may be due to methods of scoring of polysomnography and the presence of a sleep onset spectrum.[10]

4.   Site of Attachment

Site of attachment will influence the type of data obtained.[10] The actigraph can be used on the wrist, waist, ankle, or trunk. Webster et al.[15] compared the sites of attachment of a piezo-ceramic accelerometer over 22 nights of activity recording. They found that the non-dominant wrist reflected the greatest amount of bodily activity. This site has become the standard site for distinguishing sleep/wake and activity using actigraphy.

5.   Downloading of Data

Data are retrieved, and the motionlogger is programmed through an interface unit that connects to an IBM compatible personal computer. Action (tm) software is available from Ambulatory Monitoring Inc., Ardsley, N.Y. This DOS-based program is used to manipulate and partition data; calculate descriptive statistics; perform sleep analysis; and graphically display and print the data. In addition, the software is used to initialize the actigraph. A more advanced program, Action3 (tm) performs full and daily cosinor analysis, autocorrelation, cross-correlation, and maximum entropy spectral analysis and multiple channels for graphically displaying and printing the data, allowing multiple parameters to be assessed simultaneously. Although marketed for use with the Actillume (tm), Action3 can be used with data obtained from motion loggers.

6.   Uses of Actigraphy

Actigraphs have been used in a variety of populations, including patients with sleep disorders, children with attention deficit disorders, adult psychiatric patients, and patients involved in drug studies. Tryon[10] provides a detailed review of these studies. To our knowledge, our study of activity patterns and levels in women who had undergone CABS is the first use of the actigraph in adult surgical patients. The implications of using actigraphy in critical care have been described previously.[16]

Figure 1 presents data obtained with the Motion-logger actigraph and the Action3 Software program on one female CABS patient for one week from the immediate post-operative period to hospital discharge. The channel labeled "PCDACT" displays the raw activity data, measured in one minute epochs, the standard epoch length used for sleep scoring. The lower channel for each day of recording displays sleep scoring for the activity data. The scale to the left of the activity bar (Y axis) indicates activity counts. Each horizontal mark indicates 100 counts of data. The X Axis, ranging from 0 to 24 indicates hours of the day. The data presented have been reduced to fit on one page. However, larger data plots are available to allow more detailed inspection of data. Evident in this display is this subjects' increase in daytime activity over the course of the week and consolidation of sleep during the night time hours as the week progresses.

7.   Advantages of the Wrist Actigraph

The actigraph provides continuous, objective data on activity-rest. Measurement of the relative decrease in motion associated with sleep can be incorporated into the assessment of 24 hour rhythms and patterns as patients progress through stages of recovery and move from critical care to medical-surgical settings, and then are discharged to the home environment.

The actigraph requires minimal subject attention to data collection, an attribute of particular importance in patients who are beginning to return to normal patterns of ambulation and self-care, but may be experiencing pain, fatigue, and emotional distress. Many of the women in our study[6] preferred the 32K to the 16K motionlogger because of its smaller size and lighter weight. The unobtrusive and non-restrictive nature of the actigraph is a factor that prevents interference with post-operative activity progression such as might occur when using a larger device, direct observation, or a device involving wiring or leads (ie, polysomnography).

The actigraph requires little manipulation by the research team, aside from initialization and downloading. The nursing staff and research team were vigilant about noting that subjects were wearing the actigraphs throughout the study period, to guard against loss. Nurses were also instructed to avoid using the non-dominant wrist for intravenous catheter insertion. If that was impossible, actigraphs were moved further up the forearm or placed on the dominant wrist. Patients were instructed not to immerse the device in water while bathing, to guard against water damage.

8.   Disadvantages of the Wrist Actigraph

The primary disadvantage of the actigraph is its cost. Currently the interface unit is listed at a cost of $4000.00. Each actigraph is $2100.00.

We experienced some data loss because of moisture accumulation inside the actigraph due to environmental humidity and perspiration. Since the completion of our study, Ambulatory Monitoring, Inc. has upgraded the device to provide a better seal against moisture. Several subjects also complained of perspiration underneath the arm band. This problem can be solved by placement of a gauze pad or terry cloth athletic wristband between the actigraph and the skin.

9.   Summary

The actigraph is an effective, reliable, and valid means of measuring activity in the acute medical-surgical setting. It has the potential to greatly enhance knowledge of activity-rest patterns. The use of this new technology, along with computer hardware and the software described, will lead to the development of new

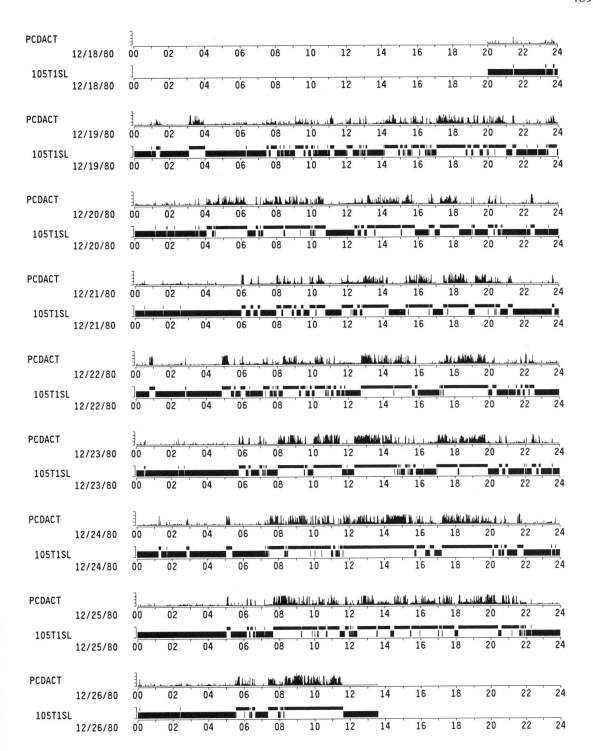

Figure 1. Seven Day Data Obtained from one Subject Using Wrist Actigraphy and Action3 Software

knowledge that will result in more effective means of promoting recovery and quality of life in patients recovering from illness and surgery.

10. References

[1] Piper BF. Fatigue: Current bases for practice. In SG Funk, EM Tournquist, MT Champagne, LA Copp, & RA Wiese (Eds.). *Key Aspects of Recovery: Management of Pain, Fatigue, and Nausea* (pp. 187-198). New York: Springer, 1989.

[2] Andreoli KG. Key Aspects of Recovery. In SG Funk, EM Tornquist, MT Champagne, LA Copp, & R Wiese (Eds.) *Key Aspects of Recovery: Improving Nutrition, Rest and Mobility* (pp. 22-31). New York: Springer, 1990.

[3] Schron EB and Shumaker SA. The integration of health quality of life in clinical research: Experience from cardiovascular clinical trials. *Prog Cardiovasc Nurs* 1992, 7:21-28.

[4] Allen, JK, Becker, DM and Swank, RT. Factors related to functional status after coronary artery bypass surgery. *Heart Lung* 1990, 19:49-55.

[5] Permanyer-Miralda G, Alonso J, Anto JM, Alijardo-Guimera M and Solen-Solen J. Comparison of perceived health status-conventional functional evaluation in stable patients with coronary artery disease. *Qual Life Coronary Dis* 1990, 12:779-786.

[6] Redeker N, Mason DJ, Wykpisz EM, Glica, B, and Miner C. Activity patterns, mood, and recovery in women after coronary artery bypass surgery: The first post-operative week. Manuscript in review.

[7] Strong A and Sneed, NV. Clinical evaluation of a critical path for coronary artery bypass surgery patients. *Progr Cardiovasc Nurs* 1991, 6:29-37.

[8] Mason DJ and Redeker, N. Measurement of Activity. *Nurs Res* 1993, 42:87-92.

[9] Redeker NS and Mason DJ. Perspectives on Activity. Manuscript in review.

[10] Tryon WW. *Activity measurement in psychology and medicine.* New York: Plenum, 1991.

[11] Patterson SM, Krantz DS, Montgomery LC, Deuster, PA, Hedges, SM and Nebel, LE. Automated physical activity monitoring: Validation and comparison with physiological and self-report measures. *Psychophys* 1993,30:296-305.

[12] Mason DJ and Tapp W. Measuring circadian rhythms: Actigraph versus activation checklist. *West J Nurs Res* 1992, 14: 358-379.

[13] Cole RJ, Kripke DK, Gruen W, Mullaney DJ and Gillin JC. Automatic Sleep/Wake Identification from Wrist Activity. *Sleep* 1992, 5: 461-469.

[14] Mullaney DJ, Kripke DF, and Messin S. Wrist-actigraphic estimation of sleep time. *Sleep* 1980, 3: 83-92.

[15] Webster JB, Messin S, Mullaney, DJ, and Kripke DF. Transducer design and placement for activity recording. *Med Biol Engineering Comput* 1982, 20: 741-744.

[16] Redeker NS, Mason DJ, Wykpisz EM, and Glica B. Using the Wrist Actigraph to Measure Activity in Critical Care. Abstract presented for the National Critical Care Nursing Research Conference, May 1993.

© 1994 Elsevier Science B.V. All rights reserved.
Nursing Informatics: An International Overview for Nursing in a Technological Era
S.J. Grobe and E.S.P. Pluyter-Wenting, eds.

Computer Support for Power Analysis in Nursing Research

Paul, S M[a]

[a]*Office of Research, School of Nursing, University of California, San Francisco, CA 94143-0604, USA*

A primary concern in the design and implementation of nursing research is the determination of the sample size needed to ensure adequate power to detect hypothesized treatment effects and relationships. The sometimes tedious calculations necessary to perform statistical power analyses have been dramatically simplified with the advent of computer applications that assist the researcher in manipulating the components of the process in an interactive fashion. This paper describes the use of computer assisted power analysis. Power analysis has become a mandatory component of the research proposal process. Fortunately, statistical packages have been developed that incorporate all of the necessary power and sample size tables and computational formulas that enable the researcher to calculate the power requirements of many different design scenarios that will help in the choice of an efficient and feasible research plan. Two such programs are: *Statistical Power Analysis: A Computer Program* by Michael Borenstein and Jacob Cohen and *SOLO Statistical System Power Analysis* by Jerry Hintze. The four parameters involved in a power analysis; sample size, alpha level, power, and effect size, and their interrelationships are discussed. One of the biggest advantages of computer assisted power analysis is the ability to make minor adjustments to any one of the four parameters and instantly see the consequences. Power calculations should be examined for every statistical test that will be performed in a study. Multiple power calculations become easy with computer assistance. With knowledge of the sample size necessary for each specific analysis, the sample requirements for the entire study can be efficiently determined.

1. Introduction

One of the most frequently asked questions during the planning stages of any research study is how large a sample is needed. The basis for such a decision must take into account a power analysis. That is, the systematic determination of the probability that the statistical tests proposed for the study will lead to the rejection of stated null hypotheses. The sometimes tedious calculations necessary to perform statistical power analyses have been dramatically simplified with the advent of computer applications that assist the researcher in manipulating the components of the process in an interactive fashion. This paper describes the use of computer assisted power analysis.

The power of a statistical test can be thought of as its likelihood of detecting a significant effect, if one indeed exists. A well designed and thoughtfully planned research study should have a good chance of detecting clinically relevant and meaningful relationships or perhaps of detecting differences between contrasting treatments. The ability to generalize sample results to the population that a study sample is intended to represent is often based on statistical hypothesis testing procedures. Achieving statistical significance is a common criteria by which the merit of many research projects are judged. Although many other factors must be considered, it is vital that research in nursing be carried out with a full understanding of the power of statistical tests to detect significant findings.

Power analyses have become mandatory requirements for any research proposals that compete for funding at a federal, state, or local institutional level. A grant proposal that does not include considerations of statistical power when attempting to justify the proposed project's sample size will most likely be dismissed as incomplete. Funding agencies need to know that their money will be well spent. They want to be assured that there is a reasonable chance that the project will be able to detect what it is intended to find.

2. Hypothesis Testing and the Parameters of Power

To understand how computers have become invaluable aids to the researcher concerned with power estimations, a brief description of hypothesis testing procedures and the parameters involved in power calculations is required.

A null hypothesis is "the hypothesis that the phenomenon to be demonstrated is in fact absent [1]." One does not hope to support this hypothesis. In fact, typically the researcher hopes to reject this hypothesis in favor of the alternative that the phenomenon in question is in fact present [2]. Results from a random sample drawn from a population will only approximate the characteristics of the population. Consequently, even if the null hypothesis is, in fact, true, a given sample result is not expected to mirror this fact exactly. The researcher must consequently set appropriate probability standards, i.e., significance criteria, for research results which provide a basis for rejection of the null hypothesis. The significance level is selected before the sample data are gathered. The researcher selects an appropriately small criterion value, such as the typical .05, so that the following statement may be made. If the null hypothesis is true, the probability of the obtained sample result is no more than 5%, a statistically significant result. The idea being that the probability of the sample result is so low as to bring the truth of the null hypothesis into question. The null hypothesis is rejected at the stated probability significance level, also referred to as the alpha (α) level or Type I error rate. If the probability of the sample result is greater than the stated alpha level, the researcher has failed to reject the null hypothesis at that particular significance level. The alpha level is the risk of mistakenly rejecting the null hypothesis when it is true, that is, drawing a spuriously positive conclusion (Type I error). The beta (β) value is the probability of failing to reject the null hypothesis when it is false (Type II error).

Any given statistical test of a null hypothesis can be viewed as a complex relationship among the following four parameters [3]:

1. The power of the test, defined as $1-\beta$ (the probability of rejecting the null hypothesis).
2. The region of rejection of the null hypothesis as determined by the α level and whether the test is one-tailed or two-tailed. As α increases, power increases.
3. The sample size, n. As n increases, power increases.
4. The magnitude of the effect in the population, or the degree of departure from the null hypothesis. The larger the effect size the greater the power.

These four parameters are so related that when any three of them are fixed, the fourth is completely determined. Consequently, when a researcher decides for a particular research scenario, the α level, estimated effect size, and desired level of power, the sample size is determined. The most common level of desired power found in nursing research is .80. The investigator would like to have an 80% chance of detecting a statistically significant effect. Unfortunately, the power analysis process is most typically hindered by the fact that the researcher does not know the magnitude of the effect size in the population. Without this restriction, power analyses would not be too much more than a series of strait forward mathematical calculations.

Jacob Cohen, the authority on power analyses for the behavioral sciences, suggests three general strategies for determining the size of the population effect that a researcher is trying to detect:

1. Previous research. Pilot work by the current researcher or studies that others have conducted involving the variables and relationships closely related to the study being planned can reflect the magnitude of effect that can be expected. Review of relevant literature or perhaps a meta-analysis of the issue can help suggest a reasonable range of expected values.
2. Practical significance. Conceptually different from statistical significance, in some research areas the investigator may be aware of some minimum population effect that would have either practical or theoretical significance. As an example, a nurse researcher may decide that the effect of a new procedure for reducing blood pressure in adolescents facing surgery would have to show an effect of at least 10 points before she would be willing to suggest changing current policy.
3. Conventional definitions. One can use certain suggested conventional definitions of small, medium, and large effects provided by Cohen in his classic text on power analysis [2]. These conventional effect size values may be used by choosing one or by determining power for all three population effect sizes. The researcher could then make revisions in the research plan based on his estimates of the various effect sizes to the particular problem at hand.

Although previous research and practical significance are preferred methods for estimating population effect sizes. The availability of computerized power programs enables an investigator almost unlimited options in calculating the power and sample size requirement for dozens of potential effect size estimates and research scenarios.

3. Procedures Available in Power Programs

Two power analysis computer programs that are currently available are *Statistical Power Analysis: A Computer Program* by Michael Borenstein and Jacob Cohen [4] and *SOLO Statistical System Power Analysis* by Jerry Hintze [5]. The Cohen and Borenstein program provides power calculations for t-tests for the difference between two means, correlations, the difference between proportions, one-way and factorial analysis of variance (ANOVA), and multiple regression and correlation. It does not, however, deal specifically with repeated measures analyses. Hintze's SOLO program includes all of the statistical procedures mentioned above and in addition includes the nonparametric analogues to the independent samples t-test (Mann-Whitney) and matched paired t-test (Wilcoxin), repeated measures ANOVA, the difference between two correlations, log-rank survival tests, logistic regression, matched case-control, and bioequivalence for means or for proportions. The Borenstein and Cohen program can generate Monte Carlo simulations. These simulations enable the researcher to run a study on the computer and determine whether or not the findings are likely to be significant, before gathering data on the actual subjects. In the simulations procedure the researcher uses the program to create populations that mirror the intended hypothesis. Both programs have the capability of producing graphic plots that show values of power for various alpha levels and sample sizes at specific effect size estimations.

4. An example

The most commonly used statistical test is the two-sample t-test. There are several variations of the t-test. The standard deviations of the two groups may be known or unknown, equal or unequal. The sample sizes of the two groups may be equal or unequal. The underlying distribution of the data may or may not be normal. The following example, based on a scenario presented by Cohen and Borenstein [4], will illustrate the use and flexibility of computer assisted power analysis.

A researcher plans to run a study in which patients suffering from muscle spasms will be treated with either Drug-A or placebo. After a month of treatment the level of spasms, defined as the rating on a 40-point scale, will be compared in the two groups. The analysis is initiated by providing the following estimates and values: Drug-A mean = 20, Placebo mean = 24; standard deviation for both groups = 10, sample size for both groups = 20. The test will be done at a two-tailed alpha of .05. Because the drug carries the risk of serious side effects, its use would be appropriate only if it could effect a clear and substantive improvement, that is a large effect. Cohen [2] defines the effect size, d, for the two-sample t-test as the difference between the two population means divided by the population standard deviation. He gives guidelines that suggest that a small d is .20, a medium d is .50, and a large d is .80. The power program would indicate that for the initial estimates the effect size is only ,.40, which is somewhere between small and medium. The researcher can elect to modify the population estimates. She decides to lower the estimate of the Drug-A mean from 20 to 18. She also decides that her initial estimate of the population standard deviations were too high and lowers them from 10 to 8. The program would indicate that the new estimated effect size is .75, which is just below large. The researcher may now decide that the effect is now large enough to be substantively important.

The program would indicate that the power for the current status of the parameters would be .64. The researcher desires the power to be at least .80. She changes the sample size estimates upward and watches as the program indicates the change in power that corresponds with the changes in sample size. When the sample size for both groups reaches 30, the power equals .81. When the sample size reaches 38 per group, the power equals .90. The sample size would have to equal 47 per group for the power to be .95. The researcher can then decide what sample size best fits with her needs, expectations, time constraints, and other factors that impact on the research process.

5. Practical Applications

The advantage of an interactive power analysis program is that one can see instantly what the effect of changing one parameter has on any of the other parameters. This is often most easy to see when one uses either the table presentation or graphic plot options of the programs. Often many different scenarios are investigated before a reasonable compromise between desired power and needed sample size may be reached. The ease and speed with which the computer can make the necessary calculations makes this intensive but necessary process feasible. Power calculations should be examined for every statistical test that will be performed in a study. With knowledge of the sample size requirements for each specific analysis, the sample requirements for the entire study can be efficiently determined.

Although the experience of many investigators is one in which their power analysis indicates that the sample size necessary to provide them with a reasonable chance of detecting what they are after is larger than they might have hoped for, it is also quite possible that the sample size requirements derived from a thorough power analysis may be much less than what was originally thought to be necessary.

If the sample size for a particular research study can not be increased, due perhaps to the limited availability of subjects that meet the study's entry requirements, a power analysis is still a worthwhile endeavor. Why would one go to the time and expense of conducting a study that has only a 50% chance of finding significance when significance actually exists and it is of practical importance? It would be better to know what the limitations of the study are at the outset of the process and cancel the project if need be, than to find out too late. Perhaps by considering alternative recruitment strategies or increasing the value of alpha, e.g., from .01 to .05, one could increase the likelihood of finding significance to an acceptable level.

While the most common use of power analysis is to determine sample size during the design phase of a study, it is also legitimate to conduct a post hoc power analysis after a study is concluded. Questions that can be answered include: What sample size would have been needed to detect a difference (or relationship) of the magnitude observed in the study with alpha = .05 and power = .80? What is the smallest difference (effect size) that could be detected with this sample size, at certain values of alpha and power?

Consider a researcher whose intent is not to reject the null hypothesis. In situations where an investigator would like to show that there are no differences between two treatments, for example, simply not rejecting the null hypothesis of no difference is not enough. Any critic of the study could claim that a significant difference does actually exist in the population in question, but that the study did not have the adequate power to detect it. If the researcher could determine the magnitude of the difference between the treatments that would be of practical importance, it would be possible to determine if the study could have detected this treatment effect. If the conclusion of the study is not to reject the null hypothesis, the researcher can be confident that no real important difference exists between the treatments.

Statistical power is only one of the many considerations that are part of developing the scientific merit of a research project. Researchers must also pull from their extensive clinical and practical experiences and the research of others when developing a study. The necessary power calculations, that can give a research proposal the justification that it deserves, have become easy and accessible through the use of computerized power programs.

6. References

[1]   Fisher, R.A. *The Design of Experiments*. New York: Hafner, 1949.

[2]   Cohen, J. *Statistical Power Analysis for the Behavioral Sciences*, Second Edition. Hillsdale, New Jersey: Lawrence Erlbaum, 1988.

[3]   Cohen, J. and Cohen, P. *Applied Multiple Regression/Correlation Analysis for the Behavioral Sciences*, Second Edition. Hillsdale, New Jersey: Lawrence Erlbaum, 1983.

[4]   Borenstein, M. and Cohen, J. *Statistical Power Analysis: A Computer Program*. Hillsdale, New Jersey: Lawrence Erlbaum, 1988.

[5]   Hintze, J. *SOLO Statistical System Power Analysis*. Los Angeles: BMDP Statistical Software, Inc., 1991.

Nursing Informatics: An International Overview for Nursing in a Technological Era
S.J. Grobe and E.S.P. Pluyter-Wenting, eds.

Computers and nursing research in acute care settings

DePalma, J A

Nursing Research, Allegheny General Hospital, 320 East North Avenue, Pittsburgh, Pennsylvania, USA

Computers are an integral part of nursing research in today's high-tech acute care setting. Computer applications play a vital support role when the goal is to facilitate research with nurses functioning in a metropolitan, regional referral hospital. Data analysis has long been recognized as a computer-based task, but *every* step of the research process can be correlated with a computer software application. The correlation can be discussed beginning with the initial review of literature by CD-ROM indices, through development of data collection tools with word processing and database programs, to the communication of research results with assistance from graphics programs and a desktop presentation toolkit. From a perspective of a rich, varied clinically-based nursing research background, a wide variety of examples can be offered to demonstrate the effective usage of computers in planning research and carrying out the daily tasks of research projects. Quality assurance of the research department itself can also be managed through on-site developed databases. A manger in the process of proposing a nursing research position or department, an information services specialist wondering what computer support nurse researchers need, an educator wanting to incorporate computer application into research content, or a nurse-investigator wondering how to better utilize computers in research studies--these varied audience participants can benefit from the discussion of the interrelationship of computers and the research process as it can function in an acute care setting.

1. Introduction

The association of computers and research has long been recognized, but primarily this relationship has been synonymous with data entry and analysis. Working with nursing research daily in a high-tech acute care setting provides a new perspective--computer involvement in *every* step of the research process. As any project progresses through the development, implementation, and analysis phases application of computer software is a vital determinant of whether the project is feasible and how smoothly it will progress. Lack of time is a commonly stated barrier to initiating research projects, especially in an acute care setting. Even when administration and nursing recognize the contribution that research and research utilization can contribute to quality practice and quality patient outcomes, time is always a deterring factor. Computer application can enhance efficiency and effectiveness in every step of the research process, from the initial literature review to the dispersion of results. Computer application packages that are essential for research facilitation are CD-ROM indices, word processing, databases, statistical analyses, slide design, and desktop publishing.

2. Literature Search

Generally the initial step in the research process is to review the available literature which assists in developing the research focus and research questions. CD-ROM databases have raised literature searches to a new level of ease and applicability. Search strategies can be established quickly with the assistance of thesaurus and index functions. The available sources in abstract or citation form can be viewed on screen, printed to hard copy, or downloaded to a disk to be viewed at a later time. Search strategies can be stored to facilitate frequent duplication which is especially valuable for those who have specific research interests and are constantly updating their resource files. Access to such biographical search services can be obtained through companies (i.e., Dialog, BRS) that provide nation-wide service to many on-line databases for network users or through subscriptions to individual CD-ROM databases. Such CD-ROM databases contain medical, health, nursing, psych, business, and education literature.

Presently to obtain the actual journal articles they must be photocopied or faxed from other libraries. The second generation of the computerized biographical search technology will provide the article in its entirety on publicly available online systems. This is available in a limited form at present for approximately 3000 journals and newsletters through Information Access Corporation [1]. The user will be able to view or print an article directly from the database search rather than merely having access to the citation or abstract.

Development of a professional library management system is possible with software such as Paradox. This is especially useful for a researcher who is developing resource files regarding particular research topics and does frequent searches to keep the resource literature current. The user can create a very individualized file with fields considered vital in describing the literature, to the extent of creating a memo file for a critique of the article. The user is then in control of a massive file of literature from innumerable searches and has the freedom to sort the reference material in the database by different key terms for specific reports.

3. Proposal/Questionnaire Development

A word processing package such as WordPerfect is invaluable when preparing the proposal and designing data collection tools. The endless revisions of a manuscript are facilitated with word processing capabilities. Creating text directly on the computer eliminates the need for transcription and recommended revisions from research review committees can be made easily. Frequently used forms for consent and declaration of confidentiality can be created as macros in word processing which allows for minimal revision across many projects.

The most frequently developed data collection form is the demographic sheet. Even when using a published research instrument the researcher my attach their own demographic sheet. A prototype with the most commonly collected information (i.e., age, gender, level of education) can be created and easily modified for each specific project by simply deleting unwanted fields.

4. Proposals for Funding/Budget Preparation

Proposals that are being prepared for submission to funding sources can be prepared on software packages that are particularly created for such preparation. They include the most frequently used forms (i.e., bibliographic, budget) and a function to prepare reference lists according to the widely accepted American Psychological Association (APA) format. Budget preparation and maintenance can be facilitated by such packages as Quicken, Lotus, or Excel. The proposed budget transfers to the spreadsheet function that then allows tracking of expenditures.

5. Data Collection/Data Entry

Data collection instruments will either be developed by the researcher or selected from published sources. The databases that will be utilized for data entry should be created simultaneously with the selection of the data collection tool. Looking at a research instrument such as a questionnaire from the perspectives of data collection and data entry simultaneously tests the coding of the instrument. This approach allows for many important revisions to the instrument that may not otherwise have been anticipated but would have complicated data entry and ultimately data analysis. Individual questions are sometimes identified that can be coded rather than presented as open-ended. A mock completed instrument provides a trial data entry exercise to estimate the time the total data entry will entail and to allow for more realistic budgeting of time and money for data entry on the project. The instrument being developed can be imported from a word processing package directly to a database package and then modified as needed. Transferring data from the paper instrument to the computer database is sometimes less time consuming when the database is the exact format as the original instrument. Databases designed for efficient data entry are especially important when large amounts of data are being collected or when the project in ongoing (i.e., patient satisfaction, exit interviews).

Database software has been available for a long period of time and has seen many upgradings, most recently the adaption to windows. Most database software (dBase, Paradox, EpiInfo) offers the same basic functions, differing in ease of querying, sorting, creating reports, and integrating multiple files.

Traditionally data has been collected on paper forms, but laptop computers and computerized hospital and patient information systems provide an alternative. Portable or laptop computers can provide a method to enter data immediately into the database on the clinical units when interviewing patients or doing chart reviews. This eliminates data entry errors that often occur and need to be controlled for when transcribing data from the paper forms into the computer. Data from existing information systems can be downloaded directly into databanks that can then be sorted and prepared for analysis. Objectivity and accuracy [2] are the advantages to this direct transfer of data and are especially pertinent to physiologic data collected on subjects over time [3] or data from longitudinal studies [4].

6. Quantitative Analysis

Once data has been entered into developed databases it can be accessed and analyzed via statistical software packages (i.e., BMDP, SPSS, SAS). Statistic packages allow for import of data and numerous parametric and nonparametric analyses. Quantitative statistical analyses programs have been available for many years but there has been continued upgrading to improve the "user friendly" aspect of such software. This especially relates to elimination of the programming language aspect of the software. Window versions of such software (i.e., SAS) has greatly improved usability. The user is prompted to describe the data and analysis desired and then is provided with a list of possible appropriate analyses from which to choose.

7. Qualitative Analysis

In comparison to quantitative data management computer application for qualitative data is in a rudimentary stage. Great advancement in qualitative data management and analyses programs has been seen in the past decade. This has been in response to the demand for rigorous qualitative analysis. Prior to the mid-1980's word processors and indexers were primarily used to code and retrieve themes from narrative text. Software packages now have been developed specifically to organize qualitative data (i.e., Ethnograph, Martin, GATOR). The major differences in qualitative text analysis programs are those designed for descriptive/interpretive analysis and those designed for theory building [5]. The descriptive/interpretive programs are most frequently used and they assist in the process of identifying and separating segments of the narrative data from the total text and then reassembling these segments into a thematic or conceptual summary [6]. As with any array of software, various features separate the programs especially the capacity to code, search, display, and recombine the text [7].

8. Communicating Results

Clinical nursing research conducted in an acute care setting can have impact on standards of practice and patient outcomes, but only if the results are disseminated to the profession at large. Personal communication between researchers is a luxury no longer limited to telephone conversations. With fax machines, EMAIL, and electronic bulletin boards research information can be disseminated over a wide geographic area instantaneously.

Publication of results would obviously involve word processing. Quality graphics enhance manuscripts and quality slides enhance research presentations and these can be easily created with computer software. Many spreadsheet and database packages allow for graphic representation of data, and word processing programs include pictorials that can be combined with text.

Slide design software (Persuasion, Harvard Graphics, Excel) has become continually more user-friendly and more powerful in creating quality images. Many of the packages now allow for the import of data and graphics and their editing capabilities have become less complicated. Window and mouse applications allow for more creative layouts. The higher-priced systems may include utilization of files created by other pc programs, 3D type bar graphs, placement of two graphs side by side, and transfer of completed graphs to other programs [8]. Persuasion's AutoTemplate automatically creates notes and handout masters with a miniature version of the corresponding slide represented on each. The presenter can organize notes to correspond with each slide on the note pages and the audience can take limited notes because they have a copy of the actual slide on the handout pages.

Another way to communicate research results and other general research-related information is through the design and distribution of a newsletter. Desktop publishing packages such as Pagemaker facilitate design and layout of such a printed periodical. Such a newsletter can be a one page flyer type format or a multi-paged issue. Text, photographs, and pictorials can be imported from word processing packages and scanners once the layout has been designed. Many variations of headers, type style, columns, and shading can be used to create a format and electronic templates that are consistent with the purpose of the periodical. The challenge is to create a periodical that reflects the desired image and establishes a strong identity for nursing research.

9. Research Quality Assurance

Quality assurance at the individual study level can be monitored via computer databases to tract missing data and variances in protocol, such as an alteration in the protocol due to an individual subject's situation or subject attrition. The nursing research department itself monitors its activities with the aid of spreadsheets and databases to facilitate tracking of resource utilization, budget allocations and expenditures, activity reports, and project progression. Quarterly and final reports are created from the information in these databases.

10. Summary

Computer application is imperative for cost effective and efficient quality research activities. Once a use for a particular computer software program is identified and the researchers become familiar with the capabilities of the software the use of the program mushrooms as everyone sees more and more potential for its use. Computer usage breeds greater reliance on electronic support. The initial orientation to the software may be time consuming but once everyone is familiar with the application there is a time savings and general feeling of quality productivity. The research process is time consuming and some areas are laborious, but computers can facilitate the process every step along the way and this is vital in the acute care setting.

11. References

[1] Finnigan G. Document delivery gets personal. *Online* 1992, 16:106-108.

[2] Harrison LL. Interfacing bioinstruments with computers for data collection in nursing research. *Res Nurs Health* 1989, 12:129-133.

[3] Gilkison C and Ploessl J. The impact of computers on patient care and research: The pentobarbital coma experience. *J Neurosci Nurs* 1986, 18:196-199.

[4] Parka PL. Development and use of a database management system for longitudinal research. *Comput Nurs* 1989, 7:110-111.

[5] Tesch R. *Qualitative Research: Analysis Types and Software Tools.* New York: Falmer, 1990.

[6] Walker BL. Computer analysis of qualitative data: A comparison of three packages. *Qual Health Res* 1993, 3:91-111.

[7] Richards L and Richards T. computing in qualitative analysis: a healthy development? *Qual Health Res* 1991, 1:234-262.

[8] Daly JM. Computer graphics for slide presentations. *Comput Nurs* 1991, 9:224-226.

12. Notes on Software

Paradox & dBase. Borland Int Inc, 1800 Green Hills Rd, PO Box 660001, Scotts Valley, CA 95067-001.

WordPerfect. WorkPerfect Corp, 1555 N. Technology Way, Orem, UT 84057.

Quicken. Intuit, 66 Willow Pl, Menlo Park, CA 94025.

Lotus. Lotus Develop Corp, 55 Cambridge Pkwy, Cambridge, MA 02142.

Excel. MicroSoft Sales & Service, 1 Microsoft Way, Redmond, WA 98052-6399.

EpiInfo. USD Inc, 2075 A West Park Pl, Stone Mountain, GA 30087.

BMDP. BMDP Stat Software Inc, 1440 Sepulveda Blvd, Suite 316, Los Angeles, CA 90025.

SPSS. SPSS Inc, 444 North Michigan Ave, Chicago, IL 60611.

SAS. SAS Institute Inc, Box 800, Cary, NC 27511.

Ethnograph. Qualis Research Assoc, PO Box 2070, Amherst, MA 01004.

Martin. Univ of Wisconsin-Madison Sch of Nurs, 600 Highland Ave, K6-113, Madison, WI 53792.

GATOR. Center for Social Sciences, Columbia Univ, 420 W 118th St, New York, NY 10027.

Persuasion & Pagemaker. Aldus Corp, 411 First Ave South, Seattle, WA 98104-2871.

Harvard Graphics. SPC, 1901 Landings Dr, PO Bos 7210, Mountain View, CA 94039-7210.

Disclaimer: The software cited in this article is the software with which the author is best acquainted. In no way is there intent to exclude other quality products or to advertize these specific products.

© 1994 Elsevier Science B.V. All rights reserved.
Nursing Informatics: An International Overview for Nursing in a Technological Era
S.J. Grobe and E.S.P. Pluyter-Wenting, eds.

A Database System for Storage and Retrieval of Nursing Care Plans Organized Around the Roy Model of Nursing

L. A. Curl

Information and Computing Science, University of Wisconsin - Green Bay, 2420 Nicolet Dr., Green Bay, WI 54311.

This project created the software for a database system that was used as an instructional tool for nursing education in a microcomputer laboratory setting for the storage, retrieval, and modification of nursing care plans based on the Roy model of nursing. The software tool dBASEIII+ and systems analysis and design techniques were employed to develop the system in an IBM-compatible Zenith microcomputer environment. Students in a nursing baccalaureate completion program at the University of Wisconsin-Green Bay tested the nursing care plan storage and retrieval system in a classroom setting. The care plans that were produced on the system were consolidated in a central storage location as a resource for future nursing research.

1. Introduction

The acquisition and interpretation of data followed by the generation and evaluation of more data is a primary nursing activity [1]. The earliest pioneers in the field of nursing called attention to the fact that these data were largely disorganized and unrecorded, to the great detriment of the art and science of nursing [2]. The inconsistent format and terminology and the irretrievable loss of nursing data have greatly impeded nursing research in the past.

The proliferation and accessibility of computer systems have made a new approach to nursing data possible. Nursing care planning and documentation by computer have become avenues of investigation and application during the past decade [3, 4]. Nursing students must be prepared to become pro-active in the design of these computer systems in order to avoid becoming the passive recipients of systems developed without considering the needs of either nurses or patients [5]. A recent NLN publication presents information on creating and using an automated care planning system in a nursing curriculum [6].

Some researchers have suggested using a relational database structure for the management of patient records [7]. Conceptually straightforward software for relational database management and affordable microcomputers for running this software are widely available today. One paradigm of nursing used in both academic and clinical settings that lends itself to relational database storage is the Roy model of nursing [8]. Database software using this model could provide nursing students with an educational experience with automated care planning in a laboratory setting.

2. System Design

The data generated during each phase of the nursing process constituted the information requirements for this system: demographic data about the patient, nursing assessment of the patient's condition, nursing diagnosis of patient problems, goals or objectives of nursing care, nursing interventions designed to help the patient pursue the goals, and evaluation of effectiveness of the current plan of care.

The main menu screen (Fig. 1) is the user's central point of reference in this program. The main menu options lead to pathways that are recognizable as parts of the nursing care plan.

To determine demographic information requirements, data sheets for patient admission forms from several Wisconsin health care agencies as well as numerous nursing care plans in journal articles and textbooks [9] and student care plans in use at the University of Wisconsin-Green Bay were examined. Harriet Werley's Nursing Minimum Data Set [10] provided some guidelines for selecting a group of 16 demographic data items for this project.

```
┌──────────────────────────────────────────────────────────────┐
│ ┌──────────────────────────────────────────────────────────┐ │
│ │      UWGB Professional Nursing Program  -  Care Plan System│ │
│ ├──────────────────────────────────────────────────────────┤ │
│ │                        MAIN MENU                           │ │
│ ├──────────────────────────────────────────────────────────┤ │
│ │              ▓ Demographic Information ▓                    │ │
│ │                                                            │ │
│ │                Nursing Problem                             │ │
│ │                                                            │ │
│ │                Objective                                   │ │
│ │                                                            │ │
│ │                Intervention                                │ │
│ │                                                            │ │
│ │                Print                                       │ │
│ │                                                            │ │
│ │                Enter Another Patient                       │ │
│ │                                                            │ │
│ │                Leave Care Plan Program                     │ │
│ ├──────────────────────────────────────────────────────────┤ │
│ │   Use Arrows to highlight       Use <Return> to select     │ │
│ └──────────────────────────────────────────────────────────┘ │
└──────────────────────────────────────────────────────────────┘
```

Figure 1. System Main Menu

The student has already made the decisions involved in the creation of a care plan before entering this program to store that plan. The patient's problems have been determined and their relationship to the assessment data is known and understood by the student. Since nursing models are developed around the groups of problems that they consider, every data item in this database is related to a patient problem number. The assessment entry screens are reached via the patient problem menu. Assessments are entered to conform to the Roy model.

The Problems menu permits the user to enter nursing problems, to inactivate problems, to update problem assessments, and to display a list of problems either active or inactive. Nursing problems are selected by number from a display of possible diagnoses (Fig. 2). The nursing diagnoses used in the program are the Roy nursing diagnoses in the four Roy modes: Physiological, Self-concept, Interdependence, Role-function as used at the University of Wisconsin-Green Bay with North American Nursing Diagnosis Association modifications.

The objectives submenu permits the student to add, modify, delete, or evaluate objectives, or to see a list of problems and their related objectives. Objectives for each problem are entered free-form from the keyboard. The current status of each objective is entered as Pending, Cancel, or Met. Interventions are entered in a pattern similar to that for objectives.

This project used the commercially available relational database management system dBASEIII+, a product of Ashton-Tate Corporation, because it is extensively documented, straightforward to use, and the product of an established company [11]. Hardware consisted of 18 Zenith Z-100 microcomputers with IBM style keyboards and monochrome monitors. The machines shared Epson FX-85 printers. The machines were located in an enclosed classroom and connected by a storage network which provided the dBASE III+ program.

System output specifications included screen formats, printed reports, and output to file storage. The program was created to be menu-driven with screens designed to accept entry of a nursing care plan in a pattern which is familiar to the nursing student and minimizes typing effort. An orientation message at the top of each screen identifies the user's current location in the program. A message at the bottom of each screen contains instructions to the user.

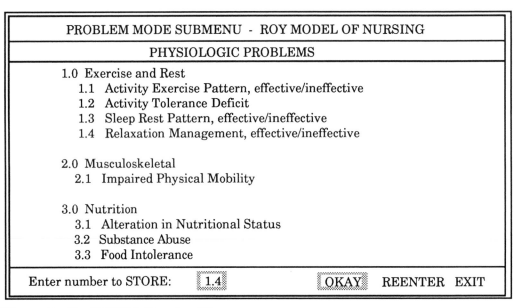

Figure 2. Roy/NANDA Nursing Diagnoses

All printed output contains the patient identifying number, the date on which the report was printed, and a descriptive heading. The printed nursing care plan is divided into 5 columns, one for each of the phases of the nursing process. The patient's current problems are printed in one column in ascending numerical order with associated assessments, objectives, interventions, and evaluations printed parallel to the problems in vertical columns across an 8 1/2" by 11" page in compressed (16.5 cpi) print. Lists of problems, assessments, objectives, interventions, or evaluations may be printed separately. Problems and their associated assessments may be printed together as one list.

Care plan data is automatically stored on the student's floppy disk as it is entered. No special steps need be taken by the user to save the data on the disk. Care plans are transferred to hard disk storage at the end of the semester. In order to estimate the storage space necessary for this project, a number of care plans were examined. Although care plans vary widely, a typical plan might contain 5-7 problems with 4-8 assessments per problem, 1-3 objectives per problem, and 3-5 interventions per problem. The amount of computer storage needed for these plans was estimated at about 4000-10000 bytes per care plan or about 50 care plans on one 5 1/4" floppy disk.

The database was designed as a series of separate files that could be accessed individually or in groups. One of the purposes of the file design was to avoid data duplication and wasted space in the database. Therefore, records were designed with a limited number of data fields. Another purpose of the database design was to provide unique access to data for investigation of the relationships among nursing diagnoses and the other parts of the nursing process: nursing assessments, objectives, and interventions.

To locate related data items, data fields may be used individually as key fields or they may be combined into a multi-item key field. Data files can be joined together via their key fields to search the database or to present a particular view of the data. The unique key for this project is composed of two fields: the patient identifying number and the code number signifying a specific nursing diagnosis. For example, in order to access the nursing assessments that supported the selection of a given problem for a patient, the key field would be a combination of the fields for the patient identifying number and the problem number.

Access to the data is controlled by identification numbers. The students's social security number serves as a password to enter the system. Individual patients are identified in the system only by the last six digits of their social security number.

3. System Implementation

The software system was written in dBASEIII+ as a series of 21 small, related modules. Top-down design enhanced the reliability and flexibility of the finished product. Easily understood and easily modifiable code were emphasized over rapid execution of program code. The completed program was alpha-tested using care plans from a community health agency. These plans were general in nature, easily available, and unrelated to previous computer system designs. Students in the nursing baccalaureate completion program at the University of Wisconsin-Green Bay beta-tested the program. The program system is relatively simple to use for students who are familiar with Roy model nursing care plans. However, a brief user's manual was created. Over a period of eight semesters beginning in fall 1987, students tested the program by using it to store, retrieve, modify, and print nursing care plans. The program served as an experiential learning device for a two-week period during a one-semester computer applications in nursing course.

4. System Evaluation

Students were asked to evaluate the program in the areas of ease of use, screen layout, work flow, and suggestions for improvement.

They reported that they understood the program system easily and rarely resorted to the documentation to find their way around the program or enter data in the appropriate spot. All users found the screens easy to read and to follow. However many students wanted more free-form space in which to type their entries. Students also frequently stated a preference for an input device other than a keyboard such as a touch-screen or a voice-activated system. User evaluations indicate a good level of competency with the program after two work sessions.

Most users found the work flow to be natural. Students who were uncomfortable with the work flow pattern fell into two categories: those who were unfamiliar with the Roy model of nursing and those who preferred to 'work on' one nursing problem exclusively at a time. The logic of the program considers the patient as a whole through each of the phases of nursing. That is, all of the patient's

Table 1
Student Care Plan Elements In Storage

	Estimated	Actual		
	Average	Low	High	Average
Care Plan Size	4000 bytes	3341 bytes	7508 bytes	3746 bytes
Problems	5 records	1 record	6 records	3 records
Asssesments/Problem	6	1	22	15
Objectives/Problem	2	1	6	5
Interventions/Problem	4	1	13	13

problems are considered at one time, all of the objectives are set, and then all of the interventions are ordered. The care plans stored by students averaged 3746 bytes in size (Table 1). The students recorded an average of 3 problems, 5 objectives, 15 assessments, and 13 interventions per care plan. Evaluations were entered to a lesser degree. This organization of the flow of work is consistent with the nursing process. To encourage the students to conceptualize their patients in a holistic fashion rather than as a series of discrete problems, the current program flow should be maintained.

Among suggestions from the students for future modifications were the ability to erase previously stored data, the ability to see the entire care plan on the screen at once and the ability to select objectives and interventions in the same manner that problems are selected.

5. Summary

The software package created with dBASE III+ functioned in an IBM-compatible microcomputer environment to give baccalaureate level nursing students an experience with storage, retrieval, and modification of nursing care plans based on the Roy model of nursing. The program has been tested and evaluated by students and used for eight semesters at the University of Wisconsin-Green Bay. Over 50 student care plans have been stored on hard disk for future nursing research.

6. References

[1] McHugh M and Schultz S. Computer Technology in Hospital Nursing Departments Future Applications and Implications. In:*Proceedings - Symposium on Computer Applications in Medical Care*. Blum, B (ed). IEEE, 1982: 557-561.

[2] Nightingale F. *Notes on nursing: what it is and what it is not*. London, Harrison and Sons, 1859.

[3] Brooks K. Computerized Nursing Care Planning Utilizing Nursing Diagnosis. In: *Proceedings- 3rd International Symposium on Nursing Use of Computers and Information Science*, Dublin. St. Louis: C.V.Mosby 1988 216-218.

[4] Strength D and Keen-Payne R. Computerized Patient Care Documentation. *Comput Nurs* 1991, 9(1): 22-28.

[5] Ronald J and Skiba D. *Guidelines for Basic Computer Education in Nursing*, NY:NLN Pub.No. 41-2177, 1987.

[6] *Computer applications in nursing education and practice*. NY:NLN Pub.No. 14-2406, 1992.

[7] Ozbolt J. Designing Information Systems for Nursing Practice: Data Base and Knowledge Base Requirements of Different Organizational Technologies. In: *Proceedings-Symposium on Computer Applications in Medical Care*. Ackerman, M (ed). IEEE, 1985:790-793.

[8] Roy Sr C. *Introduction to Nursing: An Adaptation Model* (2nd Ed.), Englewood Cliffs, NJ: Prentice Hall Publishing Co., 1984.

[9] Giger J, Bower C and Miller S. Roy Adaptation Model: ICU Application, *Dimens Crit Care Nurs* 1987, 6(4): 215-224.

[10] Werley HH and Lang NM. *Identification of the Nursing Minimum Data Set*. New York: Springer Publishing, 1988.

[11] Ashton-Tate Corporation, *Learning and Using dBASEIII+*.

Nursing Informatics: An International Overview for Nursing in a Technological Era
S.J. Grobe and E.S.P. Pluyter-Wenting, eds.

505

An Integrated Relational Database for Neonatal Care

Cho P J[a] and Donnelly M M[b]

Division of Neonatology, Department of Pediatrics, University of Cincinnati, Children's Hospital Medical Center and the Perinatal Research Institute, Cincinnati, Ohio 45267

We implemented a cohesive patient database for a large newborn nursery (3,500 births annually) and two large neonatal intensive care units (56 and 55 bed respectively, each with 800 admissions per year), organizing the data into a relational database (RDB). We integrated four disparate and non-compatible databases into a single system which allows clinicians to retrieve data, create reports, and analyze data sets using statistical tools for quality assurance (QA), clinical administration/management and clinical research. We studied and tracked the use of the database for two years.

1. Background

The Department of Pediatrics of the University of Cincinnati provides neonatal clinical services to the Full Term Nursery (FTN) and the Neonatal Intensive Care Unit (NICU) of the University of Cincinnati Hospital and the Regional Center for Neonatal Intensive Care (RCNIC) of the Cincinnati Children's Hospital. All surgeries are performed at the RCNIC which also functions as a regional neonatal referral center. Infants are routinely transferred between the NICU and the RCNIC thus creating the need for a single patient record system with access in either hospital. Annually, the University FTN has 3500 births and the NICU and the RCNIC each has 800 admissions. Neonatal data sets and computer files for each of the nurseries had existed in various forms since 1974. Definitions for diagnoses and other data fields were established and had undergone ongoing reassessment over a number of years by a committee of clinicians. Prior to 1991, data for the FTN, NICU and the RCNIC resided on four different systems, all incompatible, non-networked and accessible only by developing custom application software for each data set and data query. Output from the various systems was through standard computer printout. The data was abstracted from the medical record, manually entered by clerks, had little or no verification and reports were not available in a timely manner. The goal, therefore, was to implement a database that was timely, accurate and easily accessible to researchers and clinicians. The single, cohesive database should integrate the data from each of the three clinical units. The data fields selected for the database should be clinically relevant to the patient population and should be well defined. Automated acquisition, verification tools, and report generation would be used where possible.

2. Selection of Software and Hardware

We examined the suitability of Oracle, Focus and SmartStar to meet our data volume needs and the degree of their flexibility in manipulating relational data sets. We based our decision on programming environments and end-user applications, and selected SmartStar (SmartStar Corporation), primarily for their end-user products SmartReport (SR), SmartQuery (SQ) and 4GL programming tools. SmartStar (SS) served as the development tool and functioned as the interface between users and the underlying RDB database. We chose VAX RDB to run on a multi-user VAX 6210 (Digital Equipment Corporation). The

506

VAX 6210 has 2G bytes of on-line storage and 16M bytes of random access memory. An 8mm tape system (AVIV AB-8202) was selected for archiving. Project cycle time was approximately 14 months for database structure development and FORTRAN (3GL) programs. The new database was piloted in September of 1990 in parallel with the existing data sets and files. Debugging was completed in December 1990 and on January 1, 1991 the new RDB database replaced all prior data sets and files.

The VAX environment provides many local area network features. Data can be analyzed on the VAX or exported to networked personal computers via Ethernet or Token Ring where individual preferences for statistics and data presentation software are more readily accommodated. The system provides data entry checks and allows for efficient retrieval of information through indexing of common retrieval fields. System upkeep requires less than 5% of one system analyst's time. Hospital admissions computers and bedside 'point-of-care' systems which have been installed in the nurseries provide automated data entry for 72% of our data fields. The remaining data is taken from the patient chart and entered by clerks. The database is always current because data abstraction and entry are completed daily.

3.   Database Design

The underlying database structures were developed using the VAX RDB package. The relational database structure was selected as it allowed structural changes within the database, like adding or removing fields or tables, without degrading data retrieval performance. Using a relational database allowed placement of appropriate and logical data fields in separate tables. We normalized our database by eliminating the repetitive fields and placing functionally-related fields together within their corresponding relational tables [1].

Indices were used for faster data retrievals, and can be added, deleted, or modified as required. We used both hashed and sequential indexing algorithms for optimized retrieval performance [2]. Formerly, our database was a flat file system with each patient having one record and the same number of fields. Since patients had varying numbers of diagnoses and procedures, many empty fields existed, creating inefficient storage and degraded data record retrieval performance.

Relational Database Table Design

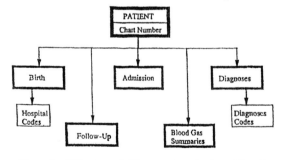

Figure 1   This schematic illustrates the major data tables. The patient chart number is the common join field.

Figure 1 is a schematic of the new database architecture. The primary key for each major table is the patient chart number. The *BIRTH, ADMISSION, DIAGNOSES, FOLLOW UP,* and *BLOOD GAS SUMMARIES* tables contain data corresponding to the patient profile, totaling 130 fields with a virtually unlimited number of records. The *BLOOD GAS SUMMARIES* table could contain several thousand records per patient. Two lookup tables, *HOSPITAL CODES* (transport, birth and admitting hospital codes) and *DIAGNOSES CODES* are read-only tables that display textual translations for the codes entered in the major tables. Neonates have one birth record yet may have multiple admissions with all admissions linked to a unique chart number. The number of diagnoses, follow-up data, and blood gas patient records are limited only by physical storage available.

When data from more than one table are displayed or reported, the separate relations are programmatically joined by a common unique data field using the Structured Query Language (SQL). This unique field matches the same patient among the major tables. The patient chart number is the primary key, while some lookup tables, such as diagnoses ICD9/HICDA translations or hospital transfer names, use code numbers as unique keys that will match the correct name with the corresponding code.

The SQL code used to search ADMISSION the BIRTH table for all infants dates whose birth weight is less than chart or equal to 1000 grams is shown 1000 below:

```
SELECT infant_name
FROM birth
WHERE birth_weight < = 1000;
```

The SQL code used to search both the BIRTH and tables for all infants and their respective admission on which the admission chart number matches the birth number, and the birth weight is less than or equal to grams is listed below.

```
SELECT infant_name
FROM birth, admission
WHERE admission.chart_no = birth.chart_no
AND birth_weight < = 1000;
```

We have developed screen designs using SQ and SR which allow multiple tables to be linked using join fields. The user can then easily select the fields to view, type qualifiers on specific fields, and retrieve the data. The SQL code is masked when using SQ and SR.

4. User Interface

Both RDB and SS have their own dialects of SQL, which is the standard programming language for database queries and reporting. SR and SQ provide front-end queries and report generation, masking the background SQL processing. SS allows for personalized screens and code to limit access only to the required database fields. SR has another advantage in that it generates modifiable SQL files. A clinician may type in the extra fields that are desired for the report. This file may also be modified later for a date change, type of diagnoses, or other qualifying fields.

SS allowed the database to become more user friendly and easily accessible, allowing a computer novice to retrieve data and create customized reports with very little instruction. We have networked the system with the hospital admissions computer, which initiates a birth and admission record for every patient using the Health Level Seven (HL7) protocols. This record contains all the available hospital admissions data, including demographic data. With the patient already in the system, the data clerk reviews the medical charts daily, entering specific birth data and diagnoses until patient discharge. This networking has resulted in the availability of complete and up-to-date patient information within hours instead of weeks.

A final review is performed on all patient files, to identify missing or incorrect data. Another quality check is performed by selecting a number of charts on a regular basis, and reviewing the data entered in the database from these charts. This technique has been helpful in identifying consistent data errors. Printouts which show missing data are also a valuable error checking tool. Files which identify missing data items are also generated and displayed as needed.

To prevent errors we customized SS to include procedures for range checking, calculated fields, default values, error handling, display-only fields, required-entry fields, help fields and screens, list fields for correct spelling, and automated field entry. RDB constraints are implemented as a data checking tool to prevent duplicate chart numbers from being stored. SS data entry features include testing of entries for reasonable values, city and state fields automatically derived from zip code entries, and pop-up list boxes which allow selection from a fixed set of entries.

We use both RDB and SS for two levels of data security. SS security guards against manual data entry errors while RDB protects table integrity and patient records from the other systems, such as the individual nursery on-line patient data management systems, which load data onto the network. Both SS and RDB feature data locking, which prevents simultaneous modifications of the same record. Also, each user has an individual account with appropriate security levels, allowing the system manager to monitor individual account usage levels.

508

5. Results and Evaluation

Our database is currently used by six different clinical and research groups. Each receives hard copy reports and on-screen displays of patient data. Batch files run each morning for the Cincinnati center of the National Institute of Health (NIH) Neonatal Network in the Department of Pediatrics and the Maternal/Fetal Network in the Department of Obstetrics, producing seven protocol-based research data files. The reports show new admissions, current network census and discharge information. The patients are selected by birth weight from both hospitals. Child and Family Health Services Pediatric Tracking (CFHS) data tables are provided as a subset of the neonatal database. The basic infant profile in the database is supplemented with specific CFHS data. Monthly QA Reports for the NICU, FTN, and RCNIC are generated for both hospitals. Major diagnoses, sorted by birth weight categories, are provided monthly and yearly. The clinicians in this administration group used the SR and SQ programs frequently, creating customized reports. The Regional Perinatal Statistics (RPS) group used the database for reporting, as well as verification of their own smaller database. The High Risk Clinic (HRC) clinicians had two batch files run each week, providing a list of patients that fit a specific birth weight criteria. This provided an efficient method for managing the follow-up clinic. We provided Faculty and Fellows (FF) interested in research with training on the use of SS and SR and assigned computer accounts as needed, but this research group used the database infrequently. The queries from the FF research group were limited to data which provided general indications of trends in our clinical population; there were no queries which focused directly on hypothesis testing.

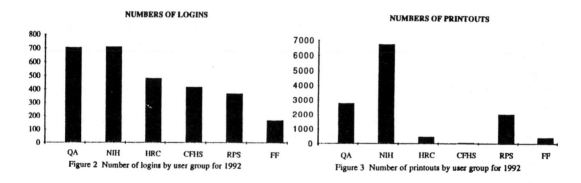

Figure 2 is the total number of logins annually for each of our user groups. The pattern of logins does not exhibit the same trend as that of the printout/reports usage summary. We have used logins as an indicator of system usage rather than CPU usage. We have tracked CPU usage but observed it to be a number indicative of the complexity and breadth of database query rather than the frequency of usage. Figure 3 shows the total number of printout/reports generated annually for each of our user groups. The NIH group had the greatest number of requests with QA functions being the next frequent user of the database. The combined total for all other users was less than that of the QA group alone. The FF group had an extremely low usage over the entire study period.

The timeliness and accuracy of the database increased since we first went on line. Clinicians generally enjoyed the independence of using the SS programs, and while some were fearful of attempting queries on their own initially, quickly learned, and use the system frequently. However, we continued to have requests to expand the database to encompass a greater number of laboratory tests and diagnostic information which would have the potential to expand the system's use for research.

By using range checking and gross error trapping, we maintained a consistent and accurate database. We generated reports for QA which track patient admissions, census, diagnoses and discharges. We have identified trends in data errors. For example, in the monthly reports we discovered that birth head circumference (OFC) and length was frequently not available in the medical records.

6.   Discussion

One of the primary goals in the development of the database was to increase the level of clinical research by expanding the scope of the database and by having patient data available within 24 hours of admission. This, as others have suggested, could expand the use of nonexperimental data sets to research [3]. However, like others, we were unsuccessful in increasing the research utility of the database [4]. Most of the querying for research has been to gather counts on patients with particular diagnoses, birth conditions, and mortality rates. As a research tool, clinicians used the database to establish a sense for the size of a particular subset of patients. The database generally acted as the initiator for research studies, and the study was conducted in a prospective basis with some very specific study-related variables which were not tracked as part of the normal clinical regimen.

The current neonatal database system has been in use for three years, and contains information on over ten thousand patients with three hundred thousand records and over four million data entries. Because we maintain   on-line the database of diagnostic summaries with patient demographics we have observed a significant increase in the use of the database for quality control and clinical administration. Patient charts are reviewed daily for up-to-date data capture, including laboratory results, initial birth data, admission and discharge information, diagnoses, as well as follow-up information.

We also observed the common difficulty in the development of databases that no database can meet the needs of all future users. While this may seem obvious, it is a fact that is often ignored, as some clinicians feel that collecting all diagnoses will answer any or most questions. Yet, invariably, as the volume of data is expanded, answers to new questions that are asked are not always found in the available data. Having very specific questions can help to insure that the data fields will be compatible with the types of questions that need answering. Prioritization is also an important consideration in determining the information available in a specific record. For example, birth weights in a neonatal database are very important in Neonatology whereas infant blood type is not as critical. Fields that are not being queried should be eliminated, instead of stored for some unpredictable future use.

Data accuracy should be reviewed on a regular basis. This can be achieved by randomly sampling charts on some schedule to identify errors. Clinicians also help in the identification of errors in their normal use of the data. As a result of this study, we have found that in our application a comprehensive database functions well as a quality control tool, offering a convenient means to analyze clinical trends. However, as a research tool, there are shortcomings, because research questions usually require data outside the normal clinical regimen to test hypotheses. This makes the use of a clinical practice based database unsuitable to answer questions retrospectively. However, as hospitals advance to the computerized medical record the availability of even larger databases than those currently in use may expand the opportunity for applying these databases in retrospective hypothesis testing [5].

7.   References

[1] Elmasri and Navathe. *Fundamentals of Database Systems*. Redwood City, California: Benjamin/ Cummings Publishing Company, Inc., 1989.

[2] Korth and Silberschatz. *Database System Concepts*. New York: McGraw Hill, Inc., 1991.

[3] Pryor D, Califf R. Clinical Data Bases Accomplishments and Unrealized Potential. *Med. Care* May 1985, Vol. 23, No. 5.

[4] Sechrest L, Perrin E. and Bunker J. AHCPR Conference Proceedings: Research Methodology: Strengthening Causal Interpretations of Nonexperimental Data. U.S. Department of Health and Human Services, May 1990.

[5] Byar D. Why Data Bases Should Not Replace Randomized Clinical Trials. *Med. Care Biometrics*, June 1980.

Nursing Informatics: An International Overview for Nursing in a Technological Era
S.J. Grobe and E.S.P. Pluyter-Wenting, eds.

510

From Barcodes to Bedpans: Use of Patient Data on Incontinence for Patient Management

Halloran EJ[a] Welton JM[a] England M[b] Whitman S[c] Williams T[c] and Kiley M[c]

[a]University of North Carolina, Chapel Hill, NC

[b]Wayne State University, Detroit, MI

[c]Case-Western Reserve University, Cleveland, OH

1. Introduction

In general, urinary incontinence is not documented as a significant functional problem in hospital medical records [1]. Nor is there a regular mechanism to store information about urinary incontinence in hospital computer files, as these files are most often abstracts of medical records. Inattention to the problem places incontinent patients at risk for incontinence related complications. Yet urinary incontinence has been long known to affect the quantity of nursing care delivered patients and is generally captured in computerized patient classification systems [2]. These systems, however, are used to deploy nurses, pulling them from wards with low demand for nurses to wards where the patients have high demand for care. This information can also be used productively in patient management.

More knowledge of urinary incontinence and its correlates among hospitalized patients is needed. With this data nurses can identify patients and implement clinical practice guidelines to manage the problem both in the hospital and the community [3].

Previous research has shown that urinary incontinence is associated with cognitive impairment and overall functional disability [1,5,6,7]. It is not associated with most medical conditions or with prescription medication use [1,6,8]. There is well established evidence that urinary incontinence is related to demoralization and to restrictions in social activities [4,6,9].

2. Purpose of Study

The purpose of this study was to use routinely collected patient classification data to describe the functional health condition of hospitalized medical/surgical adults who exhibit loss of bladder control. Our objective was to better understand a clinical condition using data commonly available in hospital nursing departments. Specifically, the study examined: the prevalence of urinary incontinence among hospitalized patients; the associations between urinary incontinence and age, gender, marital status, financial class, and discharge disposition; self-care and cognitive function disability; and the odds for extended care placement. The odds that incontinent patients would go to a nursing home were computed to determine the implications of incontinence on the decision to institutionalize for long term care.

3. Method

The sample consisted of consecutive patients admitted to an adult medical/surgical division of a large, midwestern health science center hospital during one calendar year. Nurses assigned to the care of each patient classified their patients using an instrument developed from nursing diagnoses [10]. They entered data on the presence or absence of 61 nursing diagnoses into hand-held portable computer terminals using bar code technology. These data, in turn, were transmitted via telephone to the hospital mainframe computer where they were stored in a relational database which could access other databases abstracted from the medical record [11, 12].

4. Findings

There were 14,717 adult medical/surgical patients admitted to the hospital during the study period. Their mean age was 55.06 ($\sigma = 19.59$) years, and their mean hospital length of stay was 7.75 days ($\sigma = 9.55$) Their average DRG relative cost weights were 0.908 ($\sigma = 1.036$).

4.1. Prevalence of Urinary Incontinence

The overall prevalence of urinary incontinence in the sample was 14.8% (Table 1); 6.1% of the patients (n = 896) were incontinent for one day and 8.8% (n = 1,298) were persistently incontinent, that is, they were incontinent for more than one day of hospitalization. The persistently incontinent patients were incontinent an average of 5.75 ($\sigma = 6.04$) hospital days.

Table 1. Age Distribution

	Continence		Incontinence		Total	
	N	%	N	%	N	%
>25	1,119	7.6	53	0.4	1,172	8.0
25-34	1,634	11.1	108	0.7	1,742	11.8
35-44	1,527	10.4	104	0.7	1,631	11.1
45-54	1,710	11.6	138	0.9	1,848	12.6
55-64	2,497	17.0	358	2.4	2,855	19.4
65-74	2,434	16.5	547	3.7	2,981	20.3
75-84	1,281	8.7	564	3.8	1,845	12.5
>85	321	2.2	322	2.2	643	4.4
	12,523	85.1	2,194	14.8	14,717	100.0

4.2. Correlates of Urinary Incontinence

Age and gender were strong correlates of urinary incontinence (Table 2,3). There was a greater proportion of incontinent patients in the greater than 64 year age range (N = 1,433, 65.31%. Table 4) than in other age groups ($\chi^2 = 875.2$, $\rho < .00001$). There were significantly more incontinent females (n = 1,355, 61.76%) than incontinent males ($\chi^2 = 28.8$, $\rho < .00001$, Table 4).

Table 2. Correlates of Urinary Incontinence

	Continence N=12,523		Persistent Incontinence N=1,298		Statistics	
	$\bar{x}$	σ	$\bar{x}$	σ	t	α
Age	43	19.0.	70	16.3.	48.8.	<.00001
Length of hospital stay	7	6.7.	18	18.6.	47.7.	<.00001
DRG relative cost weight	.859	.017	1.362	1.0.	54.8.	<.00001
Nursing dependency	18	9.9.	38	9.1.	69.8.	<.00001
Self-Care disability	1	1.0.	2	1.2.	44.9.	<.00001
Cognitive function disability	0.4	0.8.	2	1.2.	76.0.	<.00001

Incontinent patients in general were older ($t = 48.8$) and in the hospital longer ($t = 47.7$) than were continent patients (Table 2). Their DRG relative cost weight was higher ($t = 54.8$). In addition, the incontinent patients had higher self-care (t = 44.9) and cognitive function ($t = 76.0$) disability scores than did the continent patients – a reflection of their greater overall functional disability.

As noted in Table 3, the prevalence of persistent incontinence was 10.6% of the total sample (N = 825) for women and 7.8% (N = 473) for men ($\chi^2 = 30.28$, ρ <.00001). The prevalence of persistent urinary incontinence in those aged 65 or more years was 41.9% percent for women and 23.1% for men   ($\chi^2 = 20.679$, ρ <.00001).

Table 3. Demographic Data

	Continence		Persistent Incontinence*		Total		Statistics	
	N	%	N**	%	N	%	χ^{2***}	df
Total	12,523	90.6	1,298	9.4	13,821	100.0		
Sex							30.28	1
Male	5,560	44.4	473	36.4	6,033	43.7		
Female	6,963	55.6	825	63.6	7,788	56.4		
Marital Status							289.30	3
Married	6,186	49.4	488	37.6	6,674	48.3		
Widowed	1,803	14.4	423	32.6	2,226	16.1		
Single	3,306	26.4	278	21.4	3,584	25.9		
Divorced	1,228	9.8	109	8.4	1,337	9.7		
Financial Class							548.84	4
Standard Health Insurance	3,469	27.7	119	9.2	3,588	26.0		
Medicare	4,640	37.1	920	70.9	5,560	40.2		
Public Aid	3,168	25.3	211	16.3	3,379	24.4		
Self-Pay	580	4.6	36	2.8	616	4.5		
Missing Data	666	5.3	12	0.9	678	4.9		
Discharge Disposition							2842.00	5
Home	11,590	92.5	598	46.1	12,188	88.2		
Home Care	348	2.8	142	10.9	490	3.5		
Nursing Home	131	1.0	257	19.8	388	2.8		
Other Acute Care Facility	68	0.5	59	4.5	127	0.9		
Death	211	1.7	163	12.6	374	2.7		
Missing Data	175	1.4	79	6.1	254	1.8		

*   Urinary incontinence for more than one day of hospitalization.
**   The N reflects the deletion of 896 subjects with one hospital day of incontinence.
***   Chi Square tests of association between continence and persistent incontinence by variable; all tests significant at ρ < .00001.

Table 4. Distribution of Incontinence by Gender and Age

Age		Male		Female		Total	
		N	%	N	%	N	%
< 25		28	1.3	25	1.1	53	2.4
25-34		53	2.4	55	2.5	108	4.9
35-44		47	2.1	57	2.6	104	4.7
45-54		48	2.2	90	4.1	138	6.3
55-64		150	6.8	208	9.5	358	16.3
65-74		238	10.8	309	14.1	547	24.9
75-84		192	8.8	372	17.0	564	25.7
> 85		83	3.8	239	10.9	322	14.7
	Total	839	38.2	1,355	61.8	2,194	100.0
> 64		*513*	*23.4*	*920*	*41.9*	*1,433*	*65.3*

4.3. Urinary Incontinence and Discharge Disposition

As shown in Table 3, only 46.1% of incontinent patients were discharged to home unassisted compared with 92.5% of continent patients. Home care patients represented 3.5% of all patients but disproportionately 10.9% of incontinent patients (χ^2=496.68, ρ <.00001). These patients constituted 71% of those receiving home health care. Less than 3% of all patients were discharged to nursing homes. Proportionately more incontinent than continent patients were discharged to nursing homes (χ^2 = 1,840.96, ρ <.00001), but only 19.8% of all incontinent patients were discharged there. Finally, a greater proportion of incontinent patients expired while they were in the hospital (χ^2 = 562.96, ρ <.00001).

5. Discussion

In general, because urinary incontinence is not documented as a significant functional problem in hospital medical records, hospitalized patients are not routinely referred for diagnostic evaluation of this problem. Inattention to the problem places incontinent patients at risk for incontinence-related health complications. It also places them at risk for believing that the problem is an intractable one; frequently leading to institutionalization for long term care.

Because the hospital so often serves as the focal point for inpatient, outpatient, and home health care, it made sense to track the problem of urinary incontinence there. This study was a systematic attempt to document the problem of urinary incontinence and some of its correlates in a total medical/surgical population of inpatients.

Hospitalized incontinent patients clearly were more likely to be discharged to nursing home care than were continent patients. However, only one fifth of all persistently incontinent patients were actually discharged to nursing homes. These patients made up 66% of all patients who went to extended care. The odds of their going to extended care were 21 to one.

Urinary incontinence and functional disabilities appear to play an important role in the decision to institutionalize patients for long term care following hospital discharge. Although the incontinent patients in this study were more functionally impaired than were the continent patients, these factors did not necessarily determine their going to a nursing home. Even the presence of urinary incontinence did not necessarily determine this decision. The suggestion is that urinary incontinence in itself is not an intractable problem. It may become an intractable problem only when it is combined with other factors like nursing dependency and cognitive function disability. It may be a solvable problem when it is combined with other factors like mobility, compliant interpersonal behavior, information on how to manage the problem, and the availability, strain and willingness of professional, family and friend caregivers. Further research on clinical practice is needed to unravel the nexus of factors that combine with the incontinence to determine discharge disposition and rehabilitation potential[14].

514

Clinical data from nurses' patient classifications can be better used to promote optimal patient functioning than for nurse deployment. Clinical practice guidelines, when applied to incontinent patients, will reduce the need for long term care [3]. Behavioral techniques are low risk interventions that decrease the frequency of urinary incontinence in most individuals when provided by knowledgeable nurses. As illustrated with the problem of urinary incontinence, case finding for treatment is a far more appropriate use of the clinical data from patient classification exercises. As Nightingale said "... to the experienced eye of a careful observing nurse, the daily, I had almost said hourly, changes which take place in patients, and which changes rarely come under the cognizance of the periodical medical visitor, afford a still more important class of data, ...for... treatment of sick"[13].

6. References

[1]   Sier H, Ouslander J, Orzeck S: Urinary incontinence among geriatric patients in an acute-care hospital. *JAMA* 1987; 257:1767-1771.

[2]   Young, JP, Giovanetti, P, Lewison, D, Thoms, ML *Factors affecting nurse staffing in acute care hospitals.* DHEW Publication No. HRA 81-10, 1981. Hyattsville, MD: U.S. Department of Health & Human Services. p.77.

[3]   Urinary Incontinence Guideline Panel. *Urinary Incontinence in Adults: Clinical Practice Guideline.* AHCPR Pub. No. 92-0038. Rockville, MD: Agency for Health Care Policy and Research, Public Health Service, U.S. Department of Health and Human Services. March, 1992.

[4]   Noelker, L: Incontinence in elderly cared for by family. *Gerontologist* 1987; 27:194-200.

[5]   Ouslander JG, Uman GC, Uman HN, Rubenstein LZ: Incontinence among nursing home patients: Clinical functional correlates. *J Am Geriatr Soc* 1987; 35:324-330.

[6]   Ouslander JG, Morishita L. Blaustein J, Orzeck S, Dunn S, Sayre J: Clinical, functional, and psychosocial characteristics of an incontinent nursing home population. *J Gerontol* 1987; 42:611-617.

[7]   Williams ME, Hadler NM, Earp JAL: Manual ability as a marker of dependency in geriatric women. *J Chronic Dis* 1985; 35:115-122.

[8]   Sullivan DH, Lindsay RW: Urinary incontinence in the geriatric population of an acute care hospital. *J Am Geriatr Soc* 1984; 32:646-650.

[9]   Ory MG, Wyman JF, Yu L: Psychosocial factors in urinary incontinence. *Clin Ger Med* 1986; 2:657-671.

[10]   Halloran, EJ: Computerized nurse assessment of patient functional and social status. *Proceedings: Third International Symposium on Nursing Use of Computers and Information Science,* 20-23 June, 1988, 538-548.

[11]   Nosek, LJ: Use of a computerized nursing information system to support continuity of care between nurse caregivers. *Proceedings: Third International Symposium on Nursing Use of Computers and Information Science,* 20-23 June, 1988, 778-80.

[12]   Vandewal, D.: Nursing portable unit and barcodes: A useful technology on a nursing ward? *Proceedings: Third International Symposium on Nursing Use of Computers and Information Science,* 20-23 June, 1988, 498-505.

[13]   Nightingale, F. *Notes on hospitals.* London: Parker and Son 1859, p.3.

[14]   McGrother CW, Castleden CM, Duffin H, Clarke M: Provision of services for incontinent elderly people at home. *J Epidemiol Community Health* 1986; 40:134-138.

1994 Elsevier Science B.V. All rights reserved.
ursing Informatics: An International Overview for Nursing in a Technological Era
J. Grobe and E.S.P. Pluyter-Wenting, eds.

The Use of a Relational Database Management System for the Categorization of Textual Data

Reilly CA Holzemer WL and Henry SB

Department of Mental Health, Community and Administrative Nursing, University of California, San Francisco, CA 4143-0608

As part of an ongoing research project examining the quality of nursing care of persons with AIDS, various data sources were utilized to describe patient problems and nursing activities at five points in time. In order to prepare the textual data for analysis, a method for organizing and categorizing the data was necessary. Although the decision to utilize a qualitative software package had been made and two software packages had been tried, the research team began to question the usefulness and expediency of utilizing a qualitative software package for coding short answer textual data. A database management program seemed to offer a feasible alternative to utilizing a qualitative software package. For the purposes of this study, Paradox® provided a reliable data reduction method and allowed for the preservation of the original integrity of the data and was found to be the most efficient and effective software program for organizing and analyzing this data.

1. Background

As part of an ongoing research project examining the quality of nursing care of persons with AIDS, various data sources were utilized to describe patient problems and nursing activities at five points in time [1-4]. In order to prepare the textual data for analysis, a method for organizing and categorizing the data was necessary. This paper will first review the nature of the data generated and the tasks at hand. Secondly, the qualitative software programs the research team attempted to utilize to organize and categorize this data will be described. The usefulness and limitations of these programs for this particular data set will be presented. Ultimately the research team opted to utilized a relational database management system to prepare the data for analysis. The rationale for choosing a relational database management system will be discussed and the advantages and limitations of the software program selected will also be addressed. In conclusion, the value of utilizing qualitative software programs and relational database management system in the research process will be examined.

Acknowledgments: This study was supported by "Quality of Nursing Care of Persons with AIDS", NIH-NCNR-R01NR02215, W.L. Holzemer, Principal Investigator. We thank the members of the Quality of AIDS care team and our clinical collaborators for their continued support.

516

2. The Nature of the Data

Patients and nurses were interviewed by a nurse research assistant and asked to identify three or four major patient problems and the manner in which the nurse was helping the patient with their problems. The nurse research assistant also listened to the intershift nursing report and recorded patient problems and nursing activities identified by the nursing staff. Patient problems and nursing activities were also extracted from three additional sources in order to create a comprehensive view of patient problems and nursing activities. These sources included the nursing care plan, the patient activity record, and the nursing kardex. The textual data derived from the patient interview, the nurse interview, and the intershift nursing report were in the form of short narrative responses. The data extracted from the nursing care plan, the patient activity record, and the nursing kardex were in the form of brief written statements. The data collected on 201 subjects resulted in a file with over 7,000 patient problems and over 21,000 nursing activities.

Once the data had been collected a method for organizing and categorizing the data was required. The research team identified several fundamental criteria desired of a software program which were deemed necessary for preparing the data for analysis. First and foremost, a software program which provided a reliable data reduction method and allowed for the preservation of the original integrity of the data was necessary for the classification, the potential reclassification, and the subclassification of the data into contextual categories. It was important to maintain the integrity of the data in its original form, as the language people use communicate their construction of reality [5]. The need to tabulate the number of patients identified as having a particular type of problem, and the number of problems and nursing activities reported within in a particular contextual category was also important. The research team also wanted to have the ability to sort the data by the hospital site, the point in time that the data had been collected, and the source of the data. In addition, the ability to search the data in a variety of ways was necessary to answer several of the research questions proposed in this study. The option of importing numerical data into a statistical analysis software package was also a desired feature. Lastly, a software program which was easy to learn and to use, and would provide the most efficient and effective method for organizing and analyzing this data were important requirement.

3. Qualitative Software Programs

In 1984, software programs specifically designed for the management of qualitative data became available. Qualitative analysis programs provide the researcher with an automated data reduction technique. The software permits the researcher to assign codes to unstructured text and to retrieve text segments according to similarly assigned codes, allowing for the eventual classification of text in to a coding scheme [6]. All qualitative programs basically perform two major functions and differ in the available enhancement functions which include: automatic coding according to data structure, searching for co-occurring codes, selective searching, searching for a particular sequence of codes, and counting the frequency of the occurrence of codes in the data [7]. The majority of qualitative analysis programs are designed for descriptive analysis for research in which the main purpose is to achieve deeper insight, to search for commonalities across the study participants or sites, to explore uniqueness, and to interpret the meaning of patterns [6]. The major achievement of most current qualitative data analysis software has been the efficient coding of online data and the retrieval of coded segments [8].

Initially the research team decided to utilize The Ethnograph® software program [9]. The Ethnograph is a qualitative software package which enables one to code, recode, and sort data files into contextual categories. The program allows the user to review text, mark text segments, and to display, sort, and print text segments in any order or sequence desired. Five steps are required in order to prepare a file for searching on code words. First the data must be transcribed on a word processor according to specific formatting instructions. Next the file must be converted to a standard ASCII file in order to import the file into the Ethnograph® program. Once the data has been imported, the user instructs the program to number the lines of the entire file. A printout of the file is utilized to manually record notes which will aid the researcher in developing a code mapping scheme. Once a code mapping scheme has been identified, the user must assign code words to various lines of text. Up to twelve code words can be used to define a segment of text and overlapping text lines can be contained in up to seven code words. A search then conducted by entering specified code words. The lines of text associated with the code words are retrieved and the output can be sent to the screen, printer, or a disk. A template for face sheets can also be created which would allow the user to sort on both alphanumeric and numeric variables, such as sex and age, according to specified selection criteria.

The Ethnograph® program is useful for coding extensive text segments. Many lines of text can be attached to a single or multiple code words. In this study however, thousands of text segments were generated and individual text segments contained under 132 characters. The task of assigning thousands of line numbers to various code words seemed very labor intensive, considering the fact that the program does not tabulate the number of text segments retrieved. By utilizing the face sheet function, the ability to sort the data by the additional variables of interest was possible, yet once again manual tabulation was necessary once the data had been sorted. The option of importing numerical data into a statistical analysis software package is not a feature of this program. The Ethnograph® program is relatively easy to learn and use and the manual provides clear instructions. In the final analysis, the Ethnograph® program did not seem to provide the research team with an efficient and effective method for organizing and analyzing this data set.

After considering the limitations of the Ethnograph® program for the purposes of this study, the research team explored the possibility of utilizing a recently developed qualitative software program, MARTIN® [10]. MARTIN® was designed to allow for maximum flexibility in facilitating qualitative analyses. The program uses the Microsoft Windows' graphical environment and is essentially a Windows application which operates in accordance with the conventions of the Windows environment. MARTIN® is designed to make the process of reading text, extracting and organizing significant passages, and developing observations related to the text as efficient and flexible as possible. A MARTIN® project generates numerous icons in the course of the analysis and each icon is represented by its own window. Icons include texts, cards, folders and groups. Texts are the original documents imported into the program. Marginal notes can be added to texts. Cards are electronic similes of index cards on which you copy passages. Key codes can be attached to cards for searching purposes. Folders are electronic similes of files in which you can arrange and store cards with related themes or content. Cards may only be placed in one file. Groups are larger files which store related folders. Groups themselves can be categorized into related, larger groups. Detailed summaries can be attached to various cards, folders, and groups. The number of icons you can create and display is primarily limited by the availability of computer resources within the Windows environment. The printing of cards, folders, groups, and summaries can occur at any time.

MARTIN® did allow for the preservation of the original integrity of the data and provided a method for categorizing the data into contextual categories, yet the program did not provide a mechanism for subcategorizing major categories, while still retaining the broader categories. Since a card can only appear in one folder it was impossible to include text segments in two categories. Additionally, the maximum amount of text to be imported into MARTIN® is approximately 12.5 pages per project which severely limits the ability to work with a vast amount of text without partitioning the data. The program did not offer a means for tabulating the text segments or importing the numerical data into a statistical software package. The ability to sort the data by the other variables did not seem possible with this program. MARTIN® contains an online help menu and the manual provided dependable support for using the program. The generated output of this program did not seem to warrant the tremendous resources required to utilize this program.

Although the decision to utilize a qualitative software package had been previously made, the research team began to question the usefulness and expediency of utilizing a qualitative software package for coding short answer textual data. The ultimate purpose of any data management scheme is to facilitate a systematic process of data analysis that can be communicated to others [11]. These qualitative software programs may have facilitated the process of determining contextual categories, yet due to the enormous data set, the programs were of limited use for the purposes of this study.

4. A Relational Database Management System

Prior to the mid 1980s, researchers utilized word processing and database programs to aid in the organization and analysis of textual data. Database management programs allow the researcher the ability to create, store, search, sort and group phenomenologically valid units of data [12]. Several disadvantages of utilizing a database management program for organizing and categorizing qualitative data have been identified. Historically, powerful database programs have been difficult to learn and use. Pfaffenberger [12] noted that most database management programs do not permit changes in the structure of the database once the data has been entered. Those that do allow changes place limits on the scope of reorganization that is possible. Tesch [6] reported that when using database managers, the data must be structured before entry or the boundaries of the text passages are not indicated in the retrieved material, resulting in segments which consist of entire paragraphs or a specified number of lines or words instead of representing the meaning unit.

Due to the nature of the data which emerged in this study, a database management program seemed to offer a feasible alternative to utilizing a qualitative software package. As text segments to be coded and organized were in the form of short answer responses or fairly brief statements, an entire text segment could be contained in one field. Paradox®, [13] a full-featured relational database management system, was chosen for this project. All information in Paradox® is arranged in tables. Each table is comprised of fields designated by the user. Fields are defined by entering a field name, defining the field type, and indicating whether or not it is a key field. Field types include: alphanumeric, numeric, currency, short number, and date fields. A table can always be redesigned as fields can be modified, inserted, or deleted at any time. The user can work with data in a table or on a form, and changes in one are immediately reflected in the other.

Paradox®'s query ability is the heart and soul of the program. The user can create queries to find or select information from a table, combine information from more than one table, perform calculations on the data, insert new or delete old data, change selected values, and define groups and sets of information on which to perform calculations and comparisons. The user can query up to 24 concurrently open tables provided the tables contain identical key fields. In constructing query statements, one enters an example in a field, essentially telling the program to display only those records that have certain values in one or more fields. Paradox® provides 41 query operators which aid in the process of sorting the data by set conditions. Queries can be constructed according to any single parameter or by any desired combination or sequence of characters. Other fields are then selected to appear in the answer table by inserting a check mark via a function key.

For the purposes of this study, Paradox® provided a reliable data reduction method and allowed for the preservation of the original integrity of the data. The program accommodated the need for the classification of broader contextual categories, the subclassification of these categories, and the inclusion of additional variables of interest (Table 1). Paradox® provided a mechanism for tabulating data and importing numerical data into a statistical software package. The powerful query function allows for the retrieval of data in a variety of ways. Paradox® is simple to utilize and is designed for computer users with all levels of experience. Paradox® is highly visual and is a menu driven system. Context sensitive online help is available and the manual is well written and easy to use. In short, Paradox® provides novice and expert users with significant versatility and the power to perform complex functions. Paradox® appeared to be the most efficient and effective software program for organizing and analyzing this data.

Table 1.
An example of a Paradox® table with coded data.

PROBLEMS	PTID	TIME	SOURCE	TYPE	SUBTYPE
I can't breathe	1	1	1	1	1
Respiratory status	1	1	2	1	1
Diarrhea	1	1	2	2	
Activity intolerance	1	1	3	1	2
O2 Saturations down	1	1	3	1	1
Potential for hypothermia	1	1	4	1	3
Activity intolerance: ADLs	1	1	4	1	2
Potential for injury; safety	1	1	5	1	12
Disturbances of emotional well being	1	1	5	3	
Impaired gas exchange	1	1	6	1	1
Potential for hypothermia	1	1	6	1	3

. Conclusion

As Knafl and Webster [11] suggested, the purposes of a study and the research questions proposed dictate the manner in which data is organized and categorized for eventual analysis. In a descriptive study, coding is more efined and is a means to the researcher's ultimate intent of identifying and delineating major descriptive themes. Likewise, the intent of coding and the specifics of coding techniques vary according to the purposes of a study. If the purpose it to collect qualitative data for illustrating quantitative results of various categories, the coding scheme s derived from variables or constructs measured in the larger study. For the purposes of instrument development, the aim of the coding scheme is to classify the range of subjects' responses so they can be translated into structured questions or scales.

Therefore the appropriate class of software programs to be utilized for the purposes of organizing and categorizing data is dependent upon the purposes of the study and the research questions to be examined. In studies where lengthy segments of textual data need to be preserved in their original form, a qualitative software package appears to be most appropriate. For studies where the nature of the data is in short narrative responses or fairly brief written statements, a relational database management system offers the researcher additional functions and versatility.

A relational database management system appears to be an ideal software program for the purposes of instrument development. The responses to open ended questions can be entered into the program and then responses can be coded and tabulated. A relational database manager also holds great promise for examining the reliability of a coding scheme. The reliability of the coding scheme can be assessed in two ways. Interrater reliability and intrarater reliability can be determined by computing correlations on individual ratings. Querying on the particular derived categories and listing the associated textual data allows for a team of experts to review the data that has been assigned to a particular category. This method would also enhance the validity of a particular coding scheme. Paradox® provides the researcher with a powerful tool for coding analyzing short answer open ended responses while maintaining the original integrity of the data. Differences among individuals and or groups of individuals can be easily identified by performing a simple query. Once the coding has been completed, the data can easily be exported to a statistical package for additional analyses.

5. References

[1] Holzemer WL and Henry SB. Computer-supported versus manually generated nursing care plans: A comparison of problems, nursing interventions, and patient outcomes. *Comput Nurs* 1992, 10:19-24.

[2] Holzemer WL and Henry SB. Nursing care plans for people with HIV/AIDS: Confusion or consensus? *J Adv Nurs* 1991, 16:257-261.

[3] Henry SB, Holzemer WL, and Reilly C. Nurses' perceptions of the problems of hospitalized PCP patients: Implications for the development of a nursing taxonomy. In:*Proceedings of the Fifteenth Annual Symposium on Computer Applications in Medical Care*, 1991. Los Alamitos, CA: IEEE Computer Society Press.

[4] Janson-Bjerklie S, Holzemer WL, and Henry SB. Patients' perceptions of problems and nursing interventions during hospitalization for *Pneumocystis carinii* pneumonia. *American Journal of Critical Care* 1992, 1:114-121.

[5] Leonard VW. Heideggerian phenomenologic perspective on the concept of the person. *ANS Adv Nurs Sci* 1989, 11:40-55.

[6] Tesch R. Computer programs that assist in the analysis of qualitative data: An overview. *Qual Health Res* 1991, 1:309-325.

[7] Tesch R. Software for qulitative researchers: Analysis needs and program capablities. In:*Using Computers in Qualitative Research*. NG Fielding and RM Lee (eds). Newbury Park, CA: Sage 1991:16-37.

[8]   Richards L and Richards T. Computing in qualitative analysis: A healthy development? *Qual Health Res* 1991, 1:234-262.

[9]   Seidel JV, Kjolseth R, and Seymour E. *The Ethnograph®: A User's Guide (Version 3.0)*. Littleton, Colorado: Qualis Research Associates 1988.

[10] Diekelmann NL, Lam S, and Schuster RM. *MARTIN® (Version 2.0)*. Madison, Wisconsin: School of Nursing, University of Wisconsin-Madison 1991.

[11] Knafl KA and Webster DC. Managing and analyzing qualitative data: A description of tasks, techniques, and materials. *West J Nurs Res* 1988, 10:195-218.

[12] Pfaffenberger B. *Microcomputer applications in qualitative research*. Newbury Park, CA: Sage Publications 1988.

[13] Borland International. *Paradox® (Version 3.5)*. Scotts Valley, CA: Author 1990.

EDUCATION

A. Informatics education

Nursing Informatics: An International Overview for Nursing in a Technological Era
S.J. Grobe and E.S.P. Pluyter-Wenting, eds.

The Informatics Educational Needs of Graduate Nursing Students

dela Cruz FA[a] and Jacobs AM[b]

[a]*Professor/Program Director, High Risk Home Health Nursing Clinical Specialty Program,*
School of Nursing, Azusa Pacific University, Azusa, California 91702

[b]*Professor Emeritus/Program Evaluator, High Risk Home Health Nursing Clinical Specialty Program,*
School of Nursing, Azusa Pacific University, Azusa, California 91702

The purpose of the study was to assess the informatics educational needs of graduate nursing students at Azusa Pacific University (APU). A questionnaire was constructed for the study and mailed to all 90 enrolled graduate nursing students. Sixty-seven responded, for a response rate of 74%. The content validity index (CVI) of the questionnaire was .92, based on ratings of eight experts using Popham's method of average congruency. Test/retest reliability was .86, on a random sample of 30 of the respondents. Descriptive statistics were used in the analysis. The majority of the students have skills in word processing, but most of them lack skill in the use of spreadsheets, learning modules, decision analysis, and statistical analysis. In addition, many of them also lack skill in using computer applications in nursing practice. Findings supported the need for incorporating informatics content and experience in the curriculum.

1. Introduction

The purpose of this survey was to assess the informatics educational needs of graduate nursing students as a basis for integrating nursing informatics into the curriculum for the Master of Science in Nursing at Azusa Pacific University. Nursing informatics refers to the cognitive, information processing, and communication tasks of nursing practice, education, and research including the information science and the technology to support these tasks.[1] Impetus for the incorporation of informatics into the curriculum came as a result of the ongoing curriculum evaluation of a federally-funded master's-level clinical specialization in high-risk home health nursing at the School of Nursing. The need for informatics skills in home health care nursing, where traditional library services are generally unavailable, became increasingly evident because home health clinical nurse specialists must access and analyze important new information and knowledge as it becomes available in order to fully realize their roles as expert clinicians, educators, consultants, researchers, and clinical program managers.[2] Thus, a survey was designed to address computer and information technology skills needed for advanced nursing practice, education, and research, with special emphasis on seeking, retrieval and management of information from large data bases.

2. Method

2.1 Sample

A questionnaire was mailed to all 90 students enrolled in the graduate nursing program. It was completed by 67 students, for a response rate of 74%. The demographic characteristics of the respondents represented those of the graduate nursing student population as a whole: over half (51%) of the respondents were enrolled in

This project was supported by a grant from the Advanced Nurse Education Program, Division of Nursing, US Department of Health and Human Services (Grant D23 NU 00820).

clinical specialization options, while approximately 24% were enrolled in the nursing education option and 25% in the administration option. Sixty percent of the respondents had completed less than 23 semester units of the required 43 semester units of the Master of Science in Nursing program and the remaining 40% had completed 23 or more units. Seventy-six percent possessed BSN degrees and were enrolled in the regular BSN/MS track, in contrast to 24% who possessed non-nursing baccalaureate degrees and were enrolled in the articulated RN/MS track. The respondents' positions included clinical (46%), educational (24%), administrative (20%) and other positions (10%). Twenty percent were ages 22 to 29 years; 47%, ages 30 to 39 years; and 33%, ages 40 or more years. The years of nursing experience varied: 6% had 1 to 2 years, 16% had 3 to 5 years, 15% had 6 to 10 years, and 63% had 11 or more years.

2.2 Instrument

A questionnaire was developed for the survey, applying standard instrument development procedures: review of literature, drafting of the questionnaire by a team of content and curriculum experts, content validation, and reliability assessment. The questionnaire content included: (a) demographic and experiential characteristics of the students, (b) extent of use of computers, (c) types of computers and systems used by the student, (d) self-reported skill in 16 computer applications in practice and education settings, (e) types of word processing and spread sheet software used, (f) specific questions about competency in conducting literature searches and using computerized data bases, (g) an overall self-rating of extent of computer skills possessed, and (h) an open-ended general comment section.

A panel of eight informatics experts rated the content validity of the questionnaire, establishing a .92 content validity index (CVI)[3] based on Popham's method of average congruency.[4] A test/retest reliability was conducted on a randomly selected subsample (N=34) of the study population, a month after the final returns were received from the survey. A $10 honorarium was offered to the students for completing the second questionnaire. Based on a total of 30 returned questionnaires, a test/retest reliability of .86 was established.

2.3 Data Analysis

Descriptive statistics were used--frequencies, percentages, and measures of central tendency. Cross-tabulations and Chi square were used to determine whether there was any difference in the responses based on the following respondent characteristics: experience in the program as defined by the number of units completed; program track (whether the respondent was in the regular master's track or in the RN/MS articulated program); position (clinical positions versus all others); and program option (clinical specialization versus education and administration). Narrative responses were content analyzed and summarized.

3. Findings and Discussion

Congruent with a National League for Nursing[5] report and other related literature,[6-9] our survey revealed that an educational need exists among our graduate students in most areas of computer application (see Table 1). This need was related to the number of units completed in the program (those students completing more than 23 units toward the degree reported a greater degree of skill). The need was also related to the students' program options and employment positions. Those students enrolled in clinical specialization options and holding clinical positions generally had more skill in clinical applications and less in administrative applications. The need was not related to the students' program track (whether they were enrolled in the regular BSN/MS track or in the articulated RN/MS track).

While a majority of the students have skills in word processing, most of them lack skill in the use of spreadsheets, learning modules, decision analysis, and statistical analysis. Of greatest concern is the absence of skill in using computer applications in nursing practice, including patient monitoring (79%), accessing medical information (79%), making medicine calculations (83%), care planning (82%), and documenting (77%). While it is understandable that 90% of the graduate nursing students would lack computer skills related to patient accounts (an administrative function), the students' inability to perform computer tasks that are basic to patient care is of significance in a health care delivery system that is becoming computer-dependent. Although only 42% of the students were unable to access patient information, this is significant in that patient information is the lifeblood of clinical decision making. Given the projected master's-prepared nursing shortage, with its consequent increased client caseload for nurses, it is no longer reasonable to expect nurses in advanced practice to manage

Table 1
Graduate Nursing Students: Self-reported Skill in Computer Use

| Skills/Application | Number of Respondents | Frequency and Percentage of Respondents | | Total | |
		Beginning Skill	Advanced Skill	Some Skill	No Skill
• Word processing	67	27 (40%)	28 (42%)	55 (82%)	12 (18%)**
• Spread sheets	66	12 (18%)	4 (6%)	16 (24%)	50 (76%)*
• Learning modules	66	8 (12%)	6 (9%)	14 (21%)	52 (79%)
• Decision analysis	65	1 (1.5%)	1 (1.5%)	2 (3%)	63 (97%)
• Statistical analysis	66	15 (23%)	7 (10%)	22 (33%)	44 (67%)***
• Practice applications					
Patient accounts	63	3 (5%)	3 (5%)	6 (10%)	57 (90%)
Patient monitoring	66	7 (10.5%)	7 (10.5%)	14 (21%)	52 (79%)
Patient information	66	19 (29%)	19 (29%)	38 (58%)	28 (42%)
Med. information	66	8 (12%)	6 (9%)	14 (21%)	52 (79%)
Med. calculation	66	5 (8%)	6 (9%)	11 (17%)	55 (83%)
Care planning	66	4 (6%)	8 (12%)	12 (18%)	54 (82%)*
Documenting	66	7 (11%)	8 (12%)	15 (23%)	51 (77%)
• Literature search					
Do own search	67	12 (18%)	8 (12%)	20 (30%)	47 (70%)
Ask others to do	59	22 (37%)	21 (36%)	43 (73%)	16 (27%)**
Choose search words	57	18 (32%)	23 (40%)	41 (72%)	16 (28%)
• Use of DOS	65	--	--	29 (45%)	36 (55%)**
• Use of IBM PC	66	--	--	43 (65%)	23 (35%)**
• Use of Macintosh	64	--	--	18 (28%)	46 (72%)

Chi Square between the students who had completed more than 23 semester units and those who had completed less than 23 semester units: *p < .05; **p < .01; *** p < .001

Adapted from: A.M. Jacobs and F.A. dela Cruz, The informatics education needs of graduate nursing students, In: Arnold, JM and Pearson, GA (eds). *Computer Applications in Nursing Education and Practice.* New York: National League for Nursing, 1992, p. 341.

complex patient care data by hand. Master's-degree students therefore must be able to use computers and information technology in order to have the time to give quality care to patients. The respondents' general comments also indicated their support of the integration of nursing informatics into the graduate nursing curriculum.

The lack of skill in using the computer to access patient information by nearly half of our graduate nursing students has significant implications for the use of various types of information collected and stored in information systems. The types of patient information collected in information systems serve as a primary basis for governmental health policies at the local, regional, and national levels. Because the majority of home health care agencies depend on government funding, if graduate home health care students do not have the skills to access available information, then these practitioners remain unaware of policy developments that directly affect nursing practice and ultimately the quality of patient care. Hence, there is a need for our graduate nursing students to become "proficient users"[10] of computers, not only in patient care applications, but also in accessing large data bases in existing information systems. These skills are critical to the exercise of professional leadership functions inherent in the clinical nurse specialist role. For the nursing profession to be autonomous, it must be able to influence policies bearing on all domains of professional nursing practice.

With the current knowledge explosion, the ability to search the professional literature independently is a reasonable expectation for graduate level education. However, 70% of our students are currently unable to do their own computerized literature search and must rely upon others. Given that home health care nurses practice independently in the home setting, and most frequently do not have a librarian available, graduate students in home care nursing must demonstrate competency in searching computerized bibliographic data bases. The lack of skill in this area, from the majority of the respondents, is a clear indication of the need for integrating information seeking, retrieval and management into our current curriculum.

In summary, the survey underscored the need to incorporate nursing informatics into our graduate program. Although the findings are limited to the study sample, they bring up issues relevant to graduate nursing education: What is the best placement of informatics in the graduate nursing curriculum? How should it be incorporated? How much time should be allocated? Is there a sufficient number of graduate nursing faculty competent in nursing informatics who will be instrumental in making graduate nursing curricula responsive to the demands of an information-dependent society? Is there adequate support for acquiring up-to-date computer and information technology? At no other time are these issues more compelling for nursing education to resolve in order for graduate nursing students to fully realize their professional growth potential.

4. Acknowledgements

Portions of this report were excerpted from: Jacobs AM and dela Cruz FA. The informatics educational needs of graduate nursing students. In: *Computer Applications in Nursing Education and Practice*. Arnold JM and Pearson GA (eds). New York: National League for Nursing, 1992: 334-345. Permission to use the excerpted portions has been obtained from the National League for Nursing.

5. References

[1]   Greenes RZ and Shortliffe EH. Medical Informatics an Emerging Academic Discipline and Institutional Priority. *JAMA* 1990, 263:1114-1120.

[2]   dela Cruz FA, Jacobs AM, Nelson KA, Villegas LM and Collins CM. *High Risk Home Health Nursing Clinical Specialty Program: Phase I Final Report.* Submitted to the Advanced Nurse Education Program, Division of Nursing, U.S. Department of Health and Human Services. Azusa: CA, 1992.

[3]   Waltz CF, Strickland OL and Lenz ER. *Measurement in Nursing Research*. Philadelphia: F.A. Davis Company, 1991.

[4]   Popham WJ. *Criterion-referenced Measurement.* Englewood Cliffs: Prentice-Hall, 1978.

[5]   National League for Nursing. *Nursing Data Review 1987.* New York: National League for Nursing, 1988.

[6]   Newbern VB. Computer literacy in nursing education: An overview. *Nurs Clin North Am* 1985, 20: 549-556.

[7]   Parks PL, Damrosh SP, Heller BR and Romano CA. Faculty and student perceptions of computer applications in nursing. *J Prof Nurs* 1986, 2:104-113.

[8]   Saba V. The computer in public health: Today and tomorrow. *Nurs Outlook* 1982, 30:510-513.

[9]   Schwirian P, Malone JA, Stone VJ, Nunley B and Francisco T. Computers in nursing practice. *Comput Nurs* 1989, 7:168-177.

[10] Ronald JS and Skiba D. Computer education for nurses: Curriculum issues and guidelines. In: *Preparing Nurses for Using Information Systems: Recommended Informatics Competencies*. Peterson HE, Gerdin-Jelger U (eds). New York: National League for Nursing, 1988: 15-23.

© 1994 Elsevier Science B.V. All rights reserved.
Nursing Informatics: An International Overview for Nursing in a Technological Era
S.J. Grobe and E.S.P. Pluyter-Wenting, eds.

Curriculum Integration of Nursing Informatics Within the Context of a Regional Health Information System

Ronald JS[a] Finnick M[a] Glenister AM[a] and Werner MA[a]

[a]State University of New York at Buffalo School of Nursing, Kimball Tower, Buffalo, New York 14214

This paper describes the initial development of a model to integrate nursing informatics into a Nursing Administration graduate program that exists within the context of a regional health information system. The information system will provide information support for a regional system of health science education and health care delivery for Western New York. The goal of the graduate nursing administration program is to prepare nurses who have sound knowledge of the concepts and methods of informatics, and can apply and integrate them into their daily administrative practice. Development was funded by the Division of Nursing, Advanced Nurse Education Training Grant # 1D23NU01044-01.

1. Regional Health Information System

The Western New York Regional Health Information System is a collaborative information network of the Western New York Health Sciences Consortium. The Consortium formed in 1987 and initially included the School of Medicine, its eight teaching hospitals and a rural health care cooperative. It has expanded to include the Schools of Nursing, Dentistry and Health Related Professions as well as other rural, urban and suburban health care agencies. Its goal is to provide information support for a regional system of health science education and health care delivery for Western New York (WNY). The information network will perform functions such as: giving members access to patient medical records, latest scientific articles, and learning tools; tracking treatment decision-making; and providing on-line instruments for continuous quality assurance and improvement. [1] All of the clinical facilities (e.g., hospitals, long term care facilities, home health care agencies) in the Western New York area are in various stages of automating their information systems. Some are just beginning to explore systems that are available, while others are well along in the implementation of a system. Many hospitals have a nurse designated as a part-time coordinator of the nursing information system.

The first phase of the Health Information System development was networking the Buffalo Health Sciences Center to its eight major teaching hospitals via fiberoptic, microwave or modem connections. Several information systems projects are currently operational with others under development. A Resident Credentialling System that records the procedures a resident is qualified to do under general supervision has been implemented for 663 residents in 27 programs scattered over the eight teaching hospitals. This development and successful implementation represent a major effort to standardize terminology and agree on standards across eight hospitals that have traditionally been in competition with one another. In addition, highly successful interactive video tele-consultation is being done between two Buffalo hospitals and a small rural hospital.

Another consortium project is the development and implementation of the Hospital and University at Buffalo Library Resource Network (HUBNET) which features information resources that support patient care, biomedical research and educational programs at seven teaching hospitals and the University at Buffalo Health Sciences Center. It provides computer access to bibliographic databases, full text journals, clinical manuals, textbooks, drug information resources, expert systems, and communication tools for faculty, staff and students. The resources can be accessed either onsite in the library or through remote access from home, office or laboratory. This project has expanded to provide clinician access to information resources, including an instructional computer laboratory in the School of Medicine, at the site of patient-provider interaction. [2] The workstation is in limited use in one teaching hospital.

The architects of the Western New York Regional Health Information System are committed to interdisciplinary collaboration in the design, implementation and evaluation of the System. Although the Consortium was initiated by the medical school, the School of Nursing is actively involved on the major planning committees. These Committees focus on support applications for clinical practice, administration, education and research. In addition, a WNY Nursing Informatics Group was formed to serve as a vehicle for networking and information sharing among nurses who are involved with automated nursing information systems within the Consortium. This group also serves as an advisory body for the informatics component of the School of Nursing Administration Program.

2. Need for Informatics Knowledge

The development of the WNY Health Information System brought to the forefront the need for nursing administrators who have a solid background in Nursing Informatics. Development of nursing information systems has lagged behind those of medicine. Nursing applications have been the last planned for and implemented in most hospitals. Many hospitals still do not have a nursing information system, and systems that are in place often do not meet the needs of nursing.

Informatics knowledge will become increasingly important as hospitals follow the lead of other organizations and change their structure to one that is flat and team oriented rather than hierarchical. In such an organizational structure, information technology becomes the key factor in the success of the organization as a whole and its component parts. Tapscott and Caston describe this new structure as open and networked with a new paradigm of Information technology to support the structure. Open, networked information technology "technologically empowers, distributing intelligence and decision making to users." [3] The application of this technology to nursing must be controlled by nursing. This will occur only if knowledgeable nurses are involved at the highest levels of decision making.

The need for administrators to have informatics knowledge is not new. It was identified by a 1988 International Task Force on Education in Nursing Informatics convened in Stockholm, Sweden. According to this international group, nurse administrators should be able to use automated information systems for innovative decision making and strategic planning. The administrative role with respect to information included: directing the organization of information, accessing information, using a system's data and information, and communicating and networking inside and outside the organization. [4] Simpson supported this view when he stated that knowledge of the concepts of Nursing Informatics is rapidly becoming essential to function in any administrative role. [5]

Currently, many nurse administrators do not have adequate knowledge and skills in automated nursing information systems to participate fully in decision-making at top administrative levels or to provide leadership and guidance to their staff in these areas. Although most graduate nursing programs now require some degree of competency in using a computer, the needs of nurse administrators extend beyond computer skills to information management and processing.

Based on this premise, the State University of New York at Buffalo School of Nursing wrote and was awarded a three-year grant to significantly revise and expand its present nursing administration graduate program by integrating nursing informatics into all aspects of the curriculum. The goal of the revised program is to prepare nurse administrators who have sound knowledge of the concepts and methods of informatics, and can apply and integrate them into their daily administrative practice.

The project is a natural extension of the School of Nursing's commitment to integrating information technology throughout the Graduate and Undergraduate curricula. The School requires all Undergraduates to take Computer Science as a prerequisite course. This course teaches basic concepts and skills of word processing, databases, spreadsheets and telecommunications. In the School of Nursing, students have opportunities to apply these skills. In addition, they are introduced to the concept of Nursing Informatics and various applications of the computer to clinical practice in the classroom and clinical agencies.

3. Curriculum Development

It is the belief of the University at Buffalo nursing administration faculty that the unique knowledge requirements for nurse administrators in the area of nursing informatics mandates a new approach to the conceptualization of nursing administration. They also believe that it is important to do this without compromising the essential components of the current strong nursing administration program. The first step in the process was to develop a definition of informatics and a framework within which to revise the curriculum. Following this, the objectives, content and methods of each of the administration courses were reviewed in light of the pervasive use of technology to manage and process information in health care settings. The review served as the basis for revising and expanding current courses so that informatics could be integrated in a logical and appropriate way.

3.1. Curriculum Model

Graves and Corcoran's definition of nursing informatics as "a combination of computer science, information science and nursing science designed to assist in the management and processing of data, information and knowledge to support the practice of nursing and the delivery of nursing care" was selected to support the development of the informatics component of the curriculum. [6] Following this, a framework within which to revise the administration program was developed. After considerable discussion and research, the faculty adopted a curriculum model based on the flow of information in nursing administration. The model is an adaptation of Graves and Corcoran's model for the flow of symbolic content in the discipline of nursing. [7]

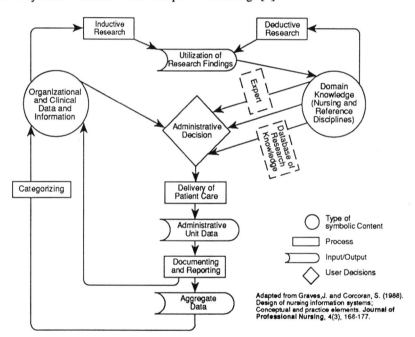

Figure 1. Model for Flow of Information in Nursing Administration

The heart of Graves' and Corcoran's model is the "Clinical Decision" which leads to the process of Patient Care" and then to the output of "Individual Data". For nursing administration, the core of the Model has been modified so that the central decision is an *"Administrative Decision"*. The administrative decision leads to the *"Delivery of* Patient Care" (rather than Patient Care) since the role of the administrator is to provide appropriate and effective structures to support patient care. The output from the process of delivery of care is *"Administrative Unit* Data" (rather than Individual Data) reflecting the administrative role in analyzing group data to support the delivery of care.

Graves' and Corcoran's model is further modified with respect to specific areas included under the two types of symbolic content flowing through the system. In nursing administration, "Domain Knowledge" expands to include: concepts and principles of nursing administration, budgeting and forecasting, program planning and evaluation, health care systems, administrative issues, and nursing informatics. The Curriculum is organized to provide students with an opportunity to gain domain specific knowledge and skills, integrate this new knowledge into their current nursing knowledge, and apply both to administrative decision making. The second type of symbolic content identified on the original model is "Clinical Data and Information". In our modification, this content expands to include organizational data and information. The culminating course of the administration program is an internship experience that provides the student with the opportunity to apply domain knowledge in an organizational setting.

3.2. Curriculum

Informatics related program objectives fall into three major areas. Graduates of the program are expected to apply information technology to manage and process information needed for administrative decision-making and strategic planning. This includes the ability to analyze nursing management information needs at the technical, operational and strategic levels, as well as to evaluate different types of software to meet these information needs. Graduates are also expected to be active, informed participants in the selection of an information system and to provide the structure for the system's selection, implementation, maintenance, evaluation and continuing development. This includes the evaluation of health care information systems for their ability to support nursing practice, assessment of nursing's role at each stage in the life of a health care information system, and application of principles related to the diffusion of technological innovation in an organization. In addition, nursing administrators need to analyze legal, ethical, and professional issues related to the application of information technology to nursing and health care.

Because information management is fundamental to all aspects of nursing administration, basic concepts and methods of informatics are incorporated into each administration course. All students are expected to have basic computer skills in word processing, database management and spreadsheets before enrolling in the program, so that the focus of learning experiences can be on information rather than the computer. Individual administration courses give the students an opportunity to apply basic concepts of information technology to specific nursing information management problems at the technical, operational and strategic levels. Assignments relate directly to the theory focus of the course. For example, in the course on budgeting and forecasting students develop a budget using a spreadsheet and then export data to a forecasting program to provide information needed for strategic planning. In other courses, students use a decision analysis program to assist them in choosing among alternatives. The applications range from selecting among several applicants for a position to selecting a hospital information system that best meets the needs of nursing. Students use electronic mail, internet, and access remote databases regularly. A seminar in nursing and health care informatics focuses on the nursing administrator's role at each stage in the life cycle of a health care information system and analysis of significant issues related to health care informatics.

4. Evaluation

The accomplishment of the objectives of the grant is conceptualized as a chain-of-events in which several levels of objectives are identified and the connections between these objectives are specified. These are identified as follows: 1) Through an increase in faculty complement and strengthening of their expertise, existing courses will be expanded and new courses developed; 2) Through expansion and development of courses, the number of students admitted to the Nursing Administration Program can be increased; 3) Through an increase in the number of students, there will be an increase in the number of graduates who are prepared to function as nursing administrators who are knowledgeable about nursing informatics; 4) Through an increase in the number of graduates the critical need for nurse administrators prepared to function effectively in an increasingly automated environment will be addressed and nursing will influence the development of the Regional Health Information system to better meet the needs of patients and nurses.

The methodological approach for evaluating the project objectives is primarily descriptive in nature. Characteristics of the students, faculty and curriculum at the beginning of the project comprise the baseline data. For each year of the project, the status of student enrollment, faculty expertise and curriculum revision/expansion are to be compared to baseline data and the data from the preceding year of the project to insure that growth is occurring.

The nature of the project and the time frame restrict evaluation of the input-process-outcome relationship to a pre-experimental design. Input and operational (process) factors are to be carefully delineated and examined in relation to outcome factors. In many instances, during data analysis, students will be divided into groups based upon their incoming characteristics in order to look for differences in performance or satisfaction.

5. Conclusion

Unfortunately, the program evaluation will never be completed because grant funding was withdrawn from the Program after the first year. According to the letter received from the funding agency, the Nurse Education and Practice Improvement Amendments of 1992 deleted the authority to make Advanced Nurse Education grants to meet the costs of maintaining graduate programs and to meet the costs of programs that prepare nurses to serve as administrators or researchers.

This withdrawal of funds after only one year has affected our ability to carry out the program on the timetable projected. It has also impeded our progress in further developing and testing the curriculum model presented above. However, the faculty is committed to proceeding with its original plans as resources permit. The delay in our progress will adversely affect the preparation of nurses who are able to function effectively in a health care system in which nursing practice will be strongly influenced by decisions made about Information Technology.

6. References

[1]   Information Management: New York hospital consortium takes high-tech turn. *Hospitals*. August 5, 1992. 43-44.

[2]   Loonsk, J., Lively, R., TinHan, E., Litt, H., (1992). Implementing the medical desktop: tools for integration of independent information resources. *Proceedings of the Fifteenth Annual Symposium on Computer Applications in Medical Care*. Washington D.C. New York: IEEE Computer Society Press. November, 1992; 574-577.

[3]   Tapscott, D. and Caston, A.. (1993). *Paradigm Shift*. New York: McGraw Hill, p.xiii.

[4]   Petersen H. and Gerdin-Jelger, U. (1988). *Preparing Nurses for Using Information Systems: Recommended Informatics Competencies*. New York: National League for Nursing.

[5]   Simpson, R. (1990). Nursing's voice in selecting an HIS. *Nurs Mgmt*, 21(7), 46.

[6]   Graves, J. and Corcoran, S. (1989). The study of nursing informatics. *IMAGE: Journal of Nursing Scholarship*. 21(4), 227-231.

[7]   Graves J. and Corcoran, S. (1988). Design of nursing information systems: conceptual and practice elements. *J Prof Nurs*. 4(3), 168-177.

Nursing Informatics: An International Overview for Nursing in a Technological Era
S.J. Grobe and E.S.P. Pluyter-Wenting, eds.

Necessity and Utilization of Computer Education for Nurses

Miura K[a], Handa I [a], Murakami T[a] , Moriya Y[a], Shimoda H[a], Takemoto Y [a] and Narita Y[b]

[a]Akita Red Cross Hospital, 1-4-36 Nakadori, Akita City, Akita 010 Japan

[b]Department of Information Engineering, Mining College, Akita University, 1-1 Tegata Gakuen-cho, Akita City, Akita 010 Japan

A clinical information system utilizing small-sized computers and distributed processing is now under development at the Akita Red Cross Hospital. Hospital workers are designing and developing the system. One nurse each year is attending Akita University to acquire the skills necessary for contributing to the design and development of information technology. As a consequence, nurses who have received this computer education have been able to offer development suggestions, perform computer system maintenance, and make system changes. Because of the efforts of those nurses who are now well-versed in computer operating skills, this computer knowledge is being successfully diffused to other nurses. As a result, the computer system has been developed to run smoothly for practical nursing jobs. Thus a computer system has been developed and put to practical use; a system that can improve nursing jobs by effectively using various kinds of clinical information.

1. Introduction

In both Europe and the USA, it is popular that computer education is provided for nurses [1] and that computers are used for nursing tasks [2]. In Japan, some computerization of nursing practice is in progress in large-sized hospitals, such as university-affiliated hospitals, where hospital information systems (hereafter abbreviated to HIS) using expensive mainframe computers have been introduced under the guidance of a computer vendor [3]. However, in medium-sized hospitals, often managed on a self-paying basis, nursing practice tasks have rarely been computerized [4]. Most computer systems in medium-sized hospitals are designed to deal primarily with the accounting and business management aspects of hospital operations. Furthermore, because systems are already developed using the vendor's own techniques and specifications which cannot be altered, it is difficult for hospital workers to modify these systems for their own purposes . However, since 1988, the Akita Red Cross Hospital has had computer system engineers (hereafter called SEs) and has begun development of an information system utilizing small-sized computers such as personal computers (PC) and work stations (WS). It has successfully completed a clinical survey system employing a personal computer, a food service system, and a medical affairs system using UNIX [5]-[10]. With respect to nursing, several nurses who acquired computer education began to contribute their expertise to the design and development of the system. In this report, we describe the computer education made available to nurses, the levels of computer competencies and the results of these nurses' efforts.

2. Present situation of computerization

Akita Red Cross Hospital's clinical staff are comprised of 78 medical doctors, 319 nurses, and 34 nursing clerks together with 194-member general personnel as non-clinical clerks. The hospital has 440 beds, and serves 1300 outpatients daily for diagnosis and treatment. However, the HIS has not been fully established. Currently, the largest system is an accounting system for medical affairs that uses X-terminals connected with a minicomputer and UNIX via Ethernet. For other purposes, a system using PCs is being developed and utilized in the individual working sections where computerization of the work is desired. Approximately 40 sets of PCs are in use. In the nursing division, 10 PCs are connected via Ethernet. These computer systems are now in use for creating and utilizing working schedules, nursing manuals, a database about nurses and for nursing worksheets.

3. Practical situation of computer education

3.1 Necessity of computer education

In Japan, although very few hospitals have full-time SEs, 3 SEs work for Akita Red Cross Hospital. These SEs are in charge of planning and operating the computer system for the entire hospital. However, they cannot direct the computerization of medical jobs in each clinical site. Therefore, users in each site raise problems and then try to implement a computer application to solve them. The computer systems currently in use are not clever enough to comply easily with the demands of those who are not familiar with computers. Rationalization of nursing jobs, effectiveness and rapid utilization of clinical information from computers cannot be expected however until nurses develop computer expertise.

3.2 Fundamental policies of computer education

Since 1990 Akita Red Cross Hospital has had one nurse per year acquire information technology knowledge and skills. And, because the hospital uses a distributed processing system and multi-vendors' PCs , each site can design its own applications and define the necessary data for an application. The data are given to the SEs who willingly convert the data into a database for the system and create files using ASCII format. Thus, nurses who understand the basic technology of PCs can effectively put this knowledge to practical use. Several abilities have been identified as important for nurses. These include the ability to:

(1)   Systematically conduct analyses from the viewpoint of computer science so that discussions can be held with SEs for developing computerized applications for nursing. Thus, the ability to determine what kind of jobs are suitable for computer processing rests with nurses.
(2)   Comprehend the fundamentals of the computer-operating technologies such as MS-DOS manipulating and data structure of files.
(3)   Code a program using BASIC language or C-language.
(4)   Comprehend how to use or adapt existing software applications that are commercially available.
(5)   Use software applications that are commercially available .
(6)   Perform fundamental operations using computers including keyboarding skills and database manipulation skills.

Three ability levels can be derived using these previously listed abilities. The highest ability level (Level A) includes (1), (2), (3), (4), and (6). The moderate ability level (Level B) is composed of (1), (5), and (6) while the ability level of general users (Level C) is made up of only item 6. In Japan, very few opportunities exist to train nurses to achieve ability level A. In hospitals where an HIS has been adopted, only a few nurses are at the ability level B.

Akita Red Cross Hospital is striving to have several of the nurses attain ability level A. Furthermore, the hospital intends to increase the number of the nurses at level B to support of the nurses at ability level A. Finally, it wishes to raise all nurses' abilities to level C when the computerization for the entire hospital is accomplished. For students of nurse-training schools affiliated with the Akita Hospital, the practice-priority computer education component is aimed at students achieving level B status every year.

Several steps are necessary for nurses who wish to achieve ability level A. These include:

(1)   Successful applicants are admitted to Akita University as auditors.
(2)   The term is one year. Thus, the hopefuls are allowed to attend classes in the university one day every week.
(3)   Subjects are taught the fundamentals of hardware and software along with an analysis method for examining nursing applications using the computer science viewpoint. Practical exercises are aimed at coding a program and utilizing the ASCII format files and C-language.
(4)   Program attendees state their own purposes. The hopefuls propose problems that can be improved using a computer, and they solve the problems by coding their own programs as solutions.

4. Educational effect

At present, five hospital nurses have been provided with computer education. Nurses 1 and 2 are at ability level

534

A, whereas Nurses 3, 4 and 5 are at the ability level B. Each is described next.

4.1 Ability Level A (Nurses 1 and 2)

Nurse 1 has 14 years experience in nursing and belongs to the human dry dock section. She found it a problem that more than ten sheets of test tube labels were needed and printed [11]. She is now engaged in maintaining the software and in guiding users about how to use this system. Furthermore she has proposed problems that allow computer processing to support nursing tasks. For example, with the aid of a dock diagnosis system, she developed a corpulence-prevention classroom system [12]. This is the computer system that offers a group of corpulent people the advice on how to make an appropriate habit of living and the prescription for how to do physical exercise according to the physical and/or medical examination data. She also has started developing programs for creating chief nurses' work schedules, with the result that great labor-elimination effects have been obtained [13]. This system was put into operation in April, 1992. The nurse now assists eleven chief nurses in the use of the system, edits their data individually, and assists them to interpret the data for practical purposes, without assistance of in-hospital SEs.

Nurse 2 has 8 years experience in nursing and works in the first-aid medical section. She has proposed creating first-aid nursing manuals and keeping them up to date. Current manuals have not been used effectively for training of nurses fresh from schools or for the re-education of partially skilled nurses. The new manual is usable only with PCs using MS-DOS. Since the manual has a simple data structure and has versatility, it is used for a first-aid manual and also for various kinds of medical business manuals or electronic textbooks that are in progress [14]. The manual can also be used on any PC on the networks.

4.2 Ability Level B (Nurses 3, 4 and 5)

Nurse 3 has 24 years of experience in nursing and is a chief nurse. She has created a database system about all the nurses in the hospital since 1992, using the idea of NMDS [15], where NMDS stands for Nursing Minimum Data Set. The NMDS concept has been proposed as minimum required clinical data for each patient with a field that contains a unique caregiver (nurse) identification number. The database contains nursing experience for each individual nurse and the kind of training experience they possess. The system as designed is certain to be put to practical use for the future in nursing sites.

Nurses 3 and 4 are currently in training to acquire information technology. They both work in the internal department of the hospital.

4.3 Roles of personnel with ability level A

Figure 1 shows a flow of operating jobs, from design to application, in developing the system utilizing computers.

And, while many of today's

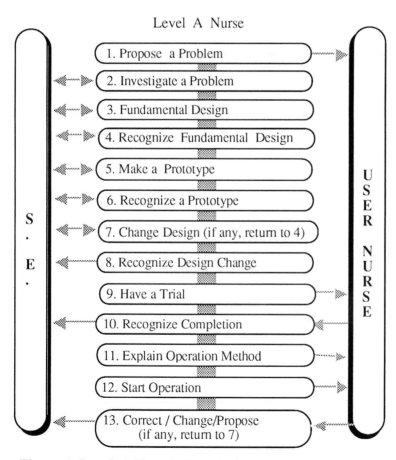

Figure 1 Level A Nurse's Roles in System

HISs have been developed using a top-down method, development has been achieved in our hospital by means of a user-dominant bottom-up method with the aid of the users at the ability level A. In our present computer system, differences between SEs and personnel with ability level C are narrowed through the use of users at ability level A. As a result, systems become good enough to satisfy the people working in clinical sites. Existence of personnel at the ability level A in clinical sites makes communication between the sites and SEs smoother and allows for better systems to be developed rapidly and inexpensively, and with excellent sensitivity to the needs of users.

5. Conclusions

Availability of nurses who have acquired computer knowledge has facilitated the introduction of computers to nursing sites, and has contributed to improvements in the quality of nursing care. On the one hand, computerization of nursing tasks by means of a bottom-up method cannot easily be accomplished to provide health care professionals with computer education. On the other hand, it must be acknowledged that none of the achievements in computer education would have occurred, had there been no opportunity to develop applications with open system small-sized computers. Also, the existence of education agencies such as universities, colleges, etc., as well as in-hospital SEs that are willing to cooperate in promoting health care professionals' computer education is a very important factor in the success of developing nursing applications at Akita Red Cross Hospital.

6. Acknowledgments

The authors wish to express their sincere gratitude to Mr. Kazuhide Ando and Ms. Yukari Itoh, of our hospital who have been willing to extend the project of computerization to nursing jobs. We are also thankful to Professor Hideo Tamamoto of Akita University who has been very helpful by offering valuable suggestions.

7. References

[1] Thomas BS, Delaney CW and Weiler K. *The Affective Outcomes of Course Work on Computer Technology in Nursing.*J Nursing Educ 1992,31(4):65-170.

[2] Eaton N.*Computers as an aid in nurse education.* Nursing Standard 1991,5(42):36-39.

[3] Uto Y. *Present Situation and Subject in Introduction of Computer System for Improving Nursing Service.* The Japanese Journal of Nursing Science 1993,18(2):7-51.

[4] Okajima Y, Wakita E, Inuzuka K, Tomomatsu J, Kumazaki S, Taketani H and Yagami J. *Beneficial Effect of Computerization on Nursing Management.* 12th Joint Conference on Medical Informatics 1992:765-768.

[5] Andou K, Takemoto Y, Narita Y, Tamamoto H, Tateoka M and Ohba H. *A Trial to Structure a Medical Information System by Means of LAN, Various Type Small Computers.* 9th JCMI 1990: 421-424.

[6] Narita Y, Tamamoto H, Takemoto Y, Miyasita M, Murakami T , Andou K and Ohba H. *Human Dry Dock Diagnosis System Operating under the Personal Computer.* 10th JCMI 1990: 815-818.

[7] Narita Y, Tamamoto H, Takemoto Y, Miyasita M and Ohba H. *Unification of Program Execution under a Multi-Vendor Environment for Personal Computers.* Japan Journal of Medical Informatics 1991,11(1):43-52

[8] Ito Y, Andou K, Sato K, Kume M, Hirakawa H, Takemoto Y and Narita Y. *A Subject for Food Service Section of Computer System by Self Development.* 11th JCMI 1991: 423-426.

[9] Narita Y, Tamamoto H, Miura K, Andou K and Takemoto Y. *Improvement of Human Dry Dock System by Introducing Open MS-DOS Concept and Object-Oriented Data Structure.* 11th JCMI 1991: 221-224.

[10] Narita Y, Tamamoto H, Ando K, Shimoda H, Takemoto Y and Ohba H. *Aiming at Building up Hospital Information System by Midget Computers --The 1st Report.* 12th JCMI 1992: 223-226.

[11] Miura K, Murakami T, Miyasita M, Ito Y, Andou K, Takemoto Y and Narita Y. *Improvement of Handwriting Works using Tagform Design System.* 10th JCMI 1990: 415-418.

[12] Miura K, Yamaguchi T, Murakami T, Miyasita M, Takemoto Y and Narita Y. *The System for the "Corpulences" with Personal Computer.* 11th JCMI 1991: 779-782.

[13] Miura K, Konno R, Karasu T, Moriya Y, Andou K, Takemoto Y and Narita Y. *Development and Evaluation of a Nursing Service Schedule System giving Importance to Operability and Versatility.* 12th JCMI 1992: 745-748.

[14] Handa I, Karasu T, Ito Y, Andou K, Takemoto Y and Narita Y. *A Trial for an Electronic Manual Drawing System for an MS-DOS Personal Computer.* 12th JCMI 1992: 439-442.

[15] Werley HH, Devine EC, Zorn CR, Ryan P, and Westra BL. *The Nursing Minimum Data Set:Abstraction Tool for Standardized, Comparable, Essential Data.* Am J Public Health 1991,81:421-426.

Nursing Informatics: An International Overview for Nursing in a Technological Era
S.J. Grobe and E.S.P. Pluyter-Wenting, eds.

536

Summer Institute: Providing Continued
Learning in Nursing Informatics

Gassert C A

Department of Education, Administration, Health Policy, and Informatics, University of Maryland at Baltimore, School of Nursing, 655 West Lombard Street, Baltimore, Maryland 21201.

A summer institute in nursing informatics was implemented to prepare administrators and nurses working in informatics for information system selection, implementation and evaluation. The curriculum and teaching strategies utilized are described. During the first two years of the institute participants were surveyed to identify their demographics, their educational and experience backgrounds in informatics, and the primary responsibility of their current positions. More nurses employed in informatics positions than nurse administrators attended the institute, even though basic content was taught. Institute evaluations were very positive. Results indicate that the summer institute is meeting a need for providing continued learning in nursing informatics.

The increasing use of information technology in nursing practice has prompted nurses to seek education in the area of nursing informatics. Until recently educational opportunities in nursing informatics in the United States have been primarily from regional workshops and national conferences. Meetings have been sponsored by professional nursing organizations with informatics interest groups, such as the American Nurses Association and National League for Nursing, or by informatics organizations, such as the American Medical Informatics Association and the Healthcare Information Management Systems Society. Additional conferences in nursing informatics have been held annually by New York University Medical Center and by Rutgers College of Nursing.

The University of Maryland at Baltimore (UMAB) School of Nursing added a new dimension of educational opportunity within the field of nursing informatics by opening the first master's program in the fall of 1988 [1]. This program prepares nurses to analyze nursing information requirements, design system alternatives, manage information technology, develop and implement user training strategies, and evaluate the effectiveness of clinical and/or management information systems for patient care. By facilitating master's specialization in the field of nursing informatics, this program has prepared more than 40 graduates to serve as nursing informatics specialists within healthcare agencies, vendor corporations, and consulting firms [2].

In July 1991 UMAB again increased educational opportunities by establishing a doctoral emphasis area in nursing informatics [3]. While the master's program prepares nurses to be information system modifiers, doctoral study prepares nursing informatics scientists to be innovators of information systems for nursing and to conceptualize nursing information requirements, design effective nursing information systems, create innovative information technology, conduct research regarding integration of technology with nursing practice, and develop theoretical, practice and evaluation models for nursing informatics.

Although the master's and doctoral programs provide formal learning opportunities in nursing informatics, a number of nurses expressed interest in a more informal and time limited educational program. In response to this need, an annual summer institute was established at the School of Nursing in 1991. Since that time the institute has been offered each July, with the help of the Information Resources Division, the University of Maryland Medical System, and the Veterans Affairs Medical Center on UMAB's campus.

1. Overview

The institute is designed for nurse managers, nurse executives, nurses interfacing with information system departments, managers of information systems for nursing, and other healthcare providers interested in nursing informatics. To allow participants opportunity to network and exchange information with the experts and among themselves, enrollment in the institute is limited.

The purpose of the six-day summer institute is to prepare nurses through a continuing education program for information system selection, implementation and evaluation. Therefore, the institute focuses on information technology and its effects on administrative and clinical nursing practice, information system selection and evaluation, strategies for system implementation, and nursing informatics perspectives. Experts in nursing and healthcare informatics expose participants to didactic sessions, group discussion, software/hardware demonstrations, field observation of selected systems, workshops teaching informatics techniques and computerized information management tools, and networking opportunities through various social events. More than 40 faculty from academic centers, healthcare agencies, vendor corporations, and consulting firms throughout the United States provide the learning opportunities.

2. Educational Strategies

Several teaching strategies are used during the institute. Four didactic sessions, each with a theme, are interspersed throughout the six days. Four or five topics relating to the theme of nursing informatics issues, system evaluation, system selection, or system implementation are offered during the didactic session. Faculty welcome questions from participants and are generally available for individual discussion at the conclusion of their session.

Workshop sessions are used to provide small group learning activities. If a workshop's objectives include interacting with software, the session is taught in one of several computer laboratories available on UMAB's campus. Workshops focus on techniques and tools used in nursing informatics activities. Examples are strategic planning, identifying information system requirements, cost/benefit analysis, decision support systems, and project management.

Field observation is also used to provide learning opportunities. Small groups of participants are transported to at least two different healthcare facilities in Maryland, Virginia, or New Jersey to see administrative, clinical and educational information systems that are operational. A variety of settings are visited, including small and large facilities, and civilian and military installation sites. In addition to interacting with the systems in place, participants discuss selection and implementation strategies used by agency personnel.

Networking opportunities are provided throughout the institute. Several social events are planned to facilitate interaction among participants, faculty and institute administrators. Student volunteers from the nursing informatics graduate programs at UMAB also facilitate participants' networking. As a follow-up, institute participants receive a group photograph and names and addresses of other attendees. To promote continued information exchange an updated list is mailed each year to institute participants .

3. Participants

To describe participants, demographic information and information about their work experience and educational background in nursing informatics were collected by surveying all summer institute attendees. As of this writing, two summer institutes have been held. A total of 150 surveys were distributed to participants from throughout the United States and Canada in July 1991 and July 1992. Eighty percent of participants (n=121) returned surveys. Most participants (88%) were female and averaged 41.5 years of age. More than half of the participants received a baccalaureate degree as initial educational preparation in nursing and almost half of them have obtained either a masters degree or a doctorate as their highest level of educational preparation. Most of these nurses (90%) had received no computer or information systems content in their basic educational program, but nearly half of them had completed some informatics courses since their basic education.

Most participants (89%) were employed in hospitals that had an average of 449.4 beds. A majority of participants (78%) worked for the nursing department and had been in their current position from 1 to 324 months (mean=3.7 years). Participants were asked to indicate the primary responsibility of their current position. As indicated in Table 1, nearly one fourth of the participants were in assistant director, associate director, or director of nursing roles. Half of the participants were involved with informatics activities as a primary responsibility. The largest group (29.2%) identified themselves as nursing information specialists. Nearly one fourth of participants selected the "other" category to explain their primary responsibilities. Many of them then listed nursing informatics responsibilities under this category. The question will be modified for future surveys.

The survey also found that in their present position more than 64% of respondents used computers on a daily basis. An additional 20% of participants used the computer sometime during every week. More than 80% of the participants rated their level of information systems expertise as either above average or well above average.

538

Table 1
Primary Responsibility in Present Position*

	N	%
Staff nurse	0	
Staff nurse assigned to a computer project	0	
Staff nurse in charge of a computer project	2	1.7
Nurse educator for a computer project	7	5.8
Head nurse/supervisor	0	
Head nurse/supervisor assigned to computer project	5	4.2
Head nurse/supervisor in charge of a computer project	3	2.5
Nursing information specialist	35	29.2
Clinical nurse specialist	1	0.8
Assistant or associate director of nursing	22	18.3
Director of nursing/top level nurse executive	6	5.0
Director of information technology	5	4.2
Other	31	25.8

* N=120

Questions were included to determine whether participants' employing agencies were actually using information systems (IS). Results indicated that 55% of employing agencies were currently using some IS functionality to process nursing information. Reflecting the changing nature of systems 46% of the agencies were involved in improving the existing IS. Participants also indicated that 60% of their agencies were in the process of selecting an IS.

4. Evaluation

Summer institute participants were asked to evaluate the general program, learning objectives and speakers. A tool, used for continuing education evaluation at UMAB, was used to measure the total program on eleven items using a nine point semantic differential scale, with 1 being poor and 9 being excellent. The vast majority of participants (83%) returned completed evaluation tools. General program results are summarized in Table 2 for both 1991 and 1992. Overall participants evaluated the summer institute very favorably and most felt they learned "much new information." Discussion time was increased in the 1992 institute, a change that was favorably reflected in the evaluation. The setting for the institute was also changed after the first year, but even though more space was available, temperature and seating factors caused participants to rate the physical environment lower in 1992.

Participants were asked to evaluate the organization, delivery and content of all speakers. The faculty were highly rated in all three categories. Comments regarding the institute were sought from participants throughout the week. Immediately after the institute concluded, the student volunteers and the planning committee met to discuss problems they had encountered during the week and to make suggestions for the next year's institute. Comments written on the evaluations were reviewed. Topics suggested for further study were used in planning subsequent institutes.

5. Discussion

The summer institute in nursing informatics has been very successful in meeting an educational need. During initial planning the audience was expected to be primarily administrators and those nurses new to informatics positions. Findings indicate that although some participants from the target audience attended the institute, a larger number of participants were employed in positions that are primarily responsible for information systems for nursing and that they had been in those positions for more than 3 years. When initial enrollments were received, there was concern that the content planned would be too basic for most participants. The evaluation results indicated, however, that the content was relevant and contributed to participants' professional knowledge in nursing informatics.

During the institute participants developed professional networks that they described as being very helpful. They expressed a desire to stay in touch with each other and to continue increasing their informatics knowledge. In response UMAB began offering a 4 day advanced summer institute in 1992. The advanced institute is open to UMAB nursing informatics graduates and to those participants who have attended previous summer institutes in Baltimore.

Based on survey and evaluation findings plans for both a summer institute and an advanced institute for 1993 have been completed. UMAB is committed to providing continued learning in nursing informatics as long as the need continues to exist.

Table 2
General Program Evaluation Data

Item	Statement	1991* Mean	1992** Mean
1.	The workshop content was relevant to the announced topics.	8.1	8.1
2.	The presentations were appropriately sequenced.	7.9	7.8
3.	The time allotted to each of the presentations was adequate.	7.1	7.3
4.	There was adequate time for discussion.	5.8	7.3
5.	The sophistication of the content was appropriate for me.	7.5	7.3
6.	Audiovisual materials effectively supplemented the content.	7.6	7.6
7.	The quality of audiovisual materials was good.	7.7	7.7
8.	Audiovisual materials were easily visible.	7.3	7.8
9.	The handouts appropriately complemented the content.	7.3	7.8
10.	The content presented in this workshop will be professionally useful.	8.7	8.1
11.	The physical environment was conducive to my learning.	7.6	6.6

* N=55
**N=70

6. References

[1] Heller BR, Romano CA, Moray LR and Gassert CA. The Implementation of the First Graduate Program in Nursing Informatics. *Comput-Nurs* 1989, 7: 209-213.

[2] Gassert CA. Preparing for a Career in Nursing Informatics. In:*Nursing Informatics '91 Post Conference*. Marr PB, Axford RL, and Newbold SK (eds). New York: Springer-Verlag, 1991: 163-166.

[3] Gassert CA, Mills ME, and Heller BR. Doctoral Specialization in Nursing Informatics. In:*Symposium on Computer Applications in Medical Care*. Clayton PD (ed). New York: McGraw-Hill, 1991: 263-267.

Nursing Informatics: An International Overview for Nursing in a Technological Era
S.J. Grobe and E.S.P. Pluyter-Wenting, eds.

540

After the School of Nursing Strategic Plan for Computing, Then What?

Joos I R[a]

[a]School of Nursing, University of Pittsburgh, 465 Victoria Building, Pittsburgh, PA. 15261

The School of Nursing at the University of Pittsburgh undertook the task of developing a five year strategic plan for computing. While that task was accomplished within a year, the most trying of the tasks was the implementation of the plan. This paper presents a brief overview of the plan, but focuses on the process, problems and solutions in the implementation of the first two years of the plan. Key areas that require attention during implementation are presented.

1. Introduction

Most schools of nursing are faced with tough decisions about how to allocate scarce resources. In 1991, a Computer Resource Planning Committee (CRPC) was formed to develop a five year strategic plan for the School of Nursing. This plan was to address the computer needs of the faculty, students and staff as well as to set the direction for computing in the School. This paper focuses on the process, problems and solutions in the implementation of the first two years of the plan. An overview of the computing plan is presented followed by a discussion of implementation. Seven key areas are presented as they relate to implementation.

2. Strategic plan

The strategic plan developed by the CRPC was the end product of months of meetings, data collection and data analysis. A review of the literature revealed a lack of models adequate for this type of planning. The chair of the committee developed and the committee accepted a three dimensional model to assist in the development of the computer plan. This three dimensional model was used to identify data sources and content for the plan. This model had as one dimension the users (students, staff, faculty and administration), as the second dimension the activities (teaching/learning, research/publication and administration/service) and the plan (philosophy, administrative structure, hardware, software, maintenance/supplies, training/support and budget/resources) as the third dimension.

Two broad goals where identified: create an environment where computers, technology and information systems are effectively used as tools that support the ongoing educational, research and service functions of the school and secondly, establish a fertile environment where evolution of nursing informatics as a specialty can flourish. Part 1 of the plan included an introduction to computing in the school, recommendations, budget and position descriptions. Part 2 of the plan contained the data sources, findings and implications. Recommendations and budget covered the areas of administrative structure/personnel, hardware, software, connectivity and finances.

This plan was presented to the faculty and the Dean for approval and support in December, 1991. Once the CRPC presented and had the plan approved, this committee was dissolved since its charge was met.

3. Implementation

While a plan provides direction to the school, someone or some group needs to assume responsibility for its implementation. Left with no leadership, a plan will self-destruct. Therefore, one of the earliest decisions to be made is who is responsible for seeing the plan implemented. Early on it became clear that critical to the effective implementation of a plan is the composition of personnel to manage the plan. Composition of personnel vary with institutions and financial resources, but should include a key person or persons vested with the power and resources to make it happen. In our case, an implementation committee (Computer Resources Committee) was appointed by the Dean. This committee consisted of the Director of the LRC (chair), the Director of Budget and Facilities and the Assistant Dean for Student Affairs. The charge to this committee was to implement the plan, make the alterations suggested by the Dean and stay within the allocated budget.

Implementation of Year 01 occurred from January 1, 1992 to June 31, 1992 and Year 02 went from July 1, 1992 to June 31, 1993. What is presented here are seven areas that need tending throughout the implementation phase: revisions, personnel, finances, procedures and policies, hardware/software, training and communications.

3.1 Revisions

As everyone who works with computers knows, this is a rapidly changing area. Since YR01 ended with fiscal year 91-92, the committee had six months to implement the first year of the plan. While a budget was included in the original plan, some revisions were necessary based on feedback from the faculty and Dean. Each responsibility center was charged with refining their budget requests to identify priorities and confirm prices. It is amazing how requests change once people know what the dollar amount is!!! To ensure fairness in the process, each area had to justify its requests and costs to the committee. Negotiations then occurred to finalize each areas budget. While implementing YR01, we began relooking at YR02. Priorities shifted and everything from YR01 was not purchased in YR01. As we began evaluating our progress, it became clear that the recommendations identified in the plan needed to be pulled out and operationalized to include clear strategies for achieving them.

Six goals were developed with strategies identified for each one. For example, one goal was to organize for effective computer utilization and support in the School. Four strategies were identified to achieve this goal: designate one administrator to oversee computers; establish an advisory School Computing Committee responsible for revising the plan, setting priorities and assisting with development of policies and procedures; continue the Computer Resource Committee (CRC) as an operating committee; and offer quick "need to know" courses on software and services supported by the School. These six goals and related strategies now serve as a guide to the work of the CRC.

3.2 Personnel

In addition to the committees listed above, other personnel needed to provide computer support varies with the number and configuration of the computers, the work being done on the computers, the level of computer literacy of the users and the budget. One of the major decisions here is whether the school will have in house personnel, utilize computer service contracts or depend on University computer personnel (CIS) for meeting their computing needs. If the school decides to have in-house personnel, how many and what composition are the next questions to be answered. If the school goes with service contracts or University computer personnel, the questions needing answers relate to services, response times and costs. Since there is a cost to each of these options, the decisions are not easy ones. What you do not want to do is duplicate services offered by the University at no or nominal cost.

In our case it was decided that we needed three levels of personnel. Position descriptions were written for a computer administrator, programmer/analyst and technical expert. Since the Director of the LRC in addition to nursing/education degrees also has a graduate degree in information science and experience in setting up and managing a microcomputer lab, the administrative role was assigned to the LRC Director. A programmer/analyst was hired to assist faculty with database design and management for their research projects. Since we were undergoing major computer purchases, networking and designing a database in the Student Affairs Office, installing ethernet ports as each department was renovated, it was also decided that we needed a three day a week CIS contract for a network person for at least the next two years. We already had on board a technical expert who took on the responsibility of setting up, trouble shooting and maintaining the computers in the student computer lab. With the reassignment of some of the technician's other responsibilities to LRC staff, this job was expanded to include servicing computers in the school.

3.3 Finances

A major issue to resolve early is how will the costs of implementation be covered? How will funds be found to ensure successful implementation? In our case, YR01 and YR02 funds were appropriated from a variety of sources: unfilled faculty positions, Fuld grant, research grants, indirect costs from grants, University infrastructure grants and health center funds. Someone needed to encourage and assist faculty to submit University related computing grants available to all faculty and departments. We received ten computers, four laser printers, 1 VCR/monitor for an interactive computer station and two ethernet ports from such University computing grants. In addition, two faculty received CAI development grants from Health Science Consortium. These grants included three computers, one laser player and one printer. All research grants submitted should have computer and related software in the budget when appropriate.

The next question that arises is how will decisions be made on the priorities when adequate funds are not available? Sometimes straight percentage cuts across the areas can't be made because the systems require all the components to function. Sometimes you need to focus on one area or group first with the idea that next year another area takes priority. For example, our Student Affairs Office undertook a major overhaul to streamline their operations through networking, downloading student data from the mainframe and tracking the admission through graduation process. In making these decisions you will be more successful if you pay attention to two principles: fairness and need.

The last area to consider under finances is to make sure the budget is realistic and reflects what is needed to complete the job. This means that the budget needs to include not only the purchase of new equipment, but also money for software, hardware and software upgrades, repairs and supplies. Don't overlook such items as port activation charges, monthly port charges, cables and ethernet cards. Most Deans don't appreciate continued requests for money when a budget that was thought to be adequate did not include essential items.

3.4 Procedures and Policies

Effective implementation requires the development of some key policies. Basic principles guiding the development of these policies should be fairness, efficiency and clarity. Remember the intent of policies and procedures is to communicate how things work. These policies should cover some of the issues that need to be resolved: ordering equipment/software, reassigning equipment, illegal software, maintenance, location and storage of master disks, maintenance of an inventory, etc. For example, how will ordering of equipment/software be handled? Will each department be responsible for ordering equipment and tracking orders or will it be done through a centralized source? In our case the decision was made and a policy written to centralize this process with the Director, LRC. Streamlining this process has saved us time and money. It also helps to keep the hardware and software inventory current. What software will be supported by the school and what software will be purchased for each new and reassigned computer? Each faculty member with a computer is entitled to three software packages. Faculty are encouraged to request software that is supported by the school and university. In addition, they are to request only software they intend to use. Twice a year faculty can submit requests for additional software with justification. The exception to this is our faculty with grants. They may purchase more software.

3.5 Hardware/Software

This area covers not only the acquisition of new hardware and software but the management of these resources. Early on it became critical to get a handle on equipment (computers, printers etc). It is not possible to manage reassignment of equipment without an inventory of what is available for reassignment. A database of hardware and software is needed. When you have only 30 computers, you can manage them fairly well; when you now have 150, a database is essential. Other hardware decisions needed relate to what platform(s) will be supported by the school, what system configuration is minimally acceptable to do the work now, what configuration is anticipated in 2 years, at what point do you not put money into upgrading older computers and how do you handle printers and other peripheral devices? Regarding software, the issues become what software will the school support, how do you handle upgrades and what software will be placed on all machines?

Since the University maintains an asset database, early thoughts led to downloading this data. It turned out not to be helpful. A hardware and software database using Paradox was designed for tracking our hardware and software inventory. Expandable folders are used to store requisitions, warranty and related hardware pamphlets. Each folder also contains a printout of the system configuration, maintenance done and system problems with solutions. Special filing cabinets were purchased to store all master disks. These are filed by computer ID and department. All software license agreements and purchase requisitions are also stored in appropriate folders for easy referral along with a list of all software owned by the school. A system was developed for tracking all hardware and software orders.

3.6 Training

The key issues here are what training is needed for users to effectively and efficiently use the equipment/software to do their work, who should provide the training and what form should the training take? Training needs vary with the users and their level of computer expertise. We, therefore, offered courses at beginning, intermediate and advanced levels. We encourage more experienced users to assist less experienced users on an impromptu basis. The LRC also provides some individual training at time of need. Undergraduate students are required to take a Nursing Informatics course that has literacy woven in it. Graduate students have the option to take a computer course that teaches literacy skills. Additional skills are included in courses as needed.

Scheduled training session should be provided by experienced trainers and should not duplicate services offered free at the University. The University Office System Services (OSS) provides free classes on select software. They also customize programs for departments and schools. Each term they provide four custom classes for our faculty and staff. The LRC provides additional training on software not supported by OSS and custom task oriented training. For example, how to create slides and transparencies using Harvard Graphics, how to create an electronic grade sheet using Lotus and how to access internet and bulletin boards. Users are also encouraged to use the tutorials and training videos, but these seem to take too much time and may or may not cover the topics needed by the user. They have not been as successful as the sponsored training sessions.

Successful programs relate to hands-on, location, length, readiness and timing of the programs. All programs require hands-on exercises completed by the learner. Each program provides the user with a handout or "cheat sheet" to take back to their office. The programs are 2-3 hours in length, held in the school's computer lab and timed around term schedules.

3.7 Communications

The key issue here is keeping users informed about computer policies/procedures, support services available and progress being made. Communications can take a variety of forms: announcement/reports at faculty meetings, memos, newsletters, flyers, etc. Since all policies must go to the policy committee for development and the faculty for approval, that is the mechanism used to communicate policies. Procedures not included in policies are sent to each department and service center administrator for communication to their faculty/staff.

We found announcements at faculty meetings and memos regarding support services not to be effective. What worked best for knowing where to turn for help was a computer service information card that contained a list of services, how to use them and phone numbers. In addition a Computer Service Request Form was developed to request services and track assistance provided. As more staff/faculty have access to E-mail, reminders and information are shared via E-mail.

4. Summary

Major factors to successful implementation of a computer plan include commitment from administration that automating work through computers is a priority, a realistic budget backed by funds, effective policies and procedures, automated inventory, appropriate personnel, excited users and a dedicated, hardworking implementation committee.

5. References

[1]   Computer Resources Planning Committee. Plan for Computing Part I and Part II. Pittsburgh: University of Pittsburgh School of Nursing, 1991.

[2]   Computer Resources Committee. Computer Plan for 1992-1994. Pittsburgh: University of Pittsburgh School of Nursing, 1992.

© 1994 Elsevier Science B.V. All rights reserved.
Nursing Informatics: An International Overview for Nursing in a Technological Era
S.J. Grobe and E.S.P. Pluyter-Wenting, eds.

544

Using a Faculty Practice Model in Nursing Informatics: An Australian Perspective

McGuiness B[a] and Carter B E[b]

a Centre for Nursing Practices and Therapies, Dept of Nursing, LaTrobe University, Locked bag 12, Carlton South, Victoria 3053, Australia

b Information Technology Services, Alfred Hospital, Commercial Rd, Prahran,Victoria 3181, Australia

In 1990 a faculty practice arrangement was formed between an Australian university and a major teaching hospital to provide mutually beneficial exchange of experiences and information. This arrangement provided a framework for establishment of a forum between educators involved in nursing informatics and nurse informaticians employed in the development and maintenance of clinical information systems. In 1991/92 university faculty taught in-patient systems to new hospital staff, had input into systems development and hospital informatics policy. Nurse informaticians participated in curriculum development and delivery of informatics education to nursing students. By working together faculty were exposed to the problems and successes associated with systems implementation, while clinicians were exposed to current academic endeavours. The result has been a richer curriculum, including the development of educational software, that reflects both academic inquiry and clinical practicalities. This paper describes the outcomes of an informatics faculty practice model.

1. Introduction

As Australian nurses are required to use information technolgy in all facets of their practice the demands upon educational institutions to provide appropriate preparation for such practice is increasing. Whilst faculties are cognisant of the need, there exists a deficit in the knowledge and experience needed to provide this type of instruction. Efforts to over come this deficit are hampered by the service-education gap [1,2,3]. To compensate two approaches are commonly used. The first is to contract a computer scientist to design and provide the necessary curricula content. This tends to result in content that focuses on general-business applications (word processing, spread sheets and data bases) or the intricacies of the hardware. The second approach is to use a "computer buff", usually a nurse, who may either have an interest in computers and a desire to teach, or have completed a formal course e.g. a computer science degree. With the latter, content tends to be much the same as the first approach but some attempt is made to link the technology to nursing related applications. However, without practitioner level experience, the content does not replicate the complexities of information needs in the practice environment. The result is that in Australian Nursing Informatics a substantial service-education gap exists.

As faculty practice has often been cited as a method of reducing the service-education gap [4,5,6,7], it was decided to develop a faculty practice model for nursing informatics A collaborative link between LaTrobe University and the Alfred Hospital was established in order to:

1. provide faculty members with the opportunity to work with information technology in the practice environment,
2. enable practitioners, experienced in using information technology, to contribute to curricula design and delivery, and
3. to facilitate research in the area of nursing informatics.

2. Informatics faculty practice defined

The process began by establishing a working definition. A search of faculty practice literature revealed that consensus for a single definition has yet to be achieved. Two central themes were evident, direct patient care and the pursuit of scholarly activity [8&9]. Nursing informatics, similarly accepts the pursuit of scholarly activity, but presents a broader view in relation to patient care activities. It was felt that as nursing information systems include aspects of both direct and indirect patient care, a faculty practice definition should include both. As a result, informatics faculty practice was defined as:

Faculty having access to direct and indirect patient care nursing information systems for the purpose of:
1. obtaining knowledge and experience that can be articulated to students of nursing and
2. stimulating informatics research inquiry.

3. Expected Outcomes

Having established an operational definition expected outcomes were then identified. Several benefits of a faculty practice model have been cited in the literature. Herr [4] provides a succinct overview:

"Enhancing clinical instruction (Chicadonz, Bush Korrthuis, &Utz, 1981; Christman, 1979;Mauksch, 1980; Parson & Felton, 1987), improving quality of patient care (Christman, 1979; Dickens, 1983; McClure, 1987), strengthening relationships between nursing service and nursing education (Chicadonz et al,1981; Cook & Finelli, 1988), and giving credibility to the professional role in a practice discipline (Algase, 1986; Royal & Crooks, 1986)".

Just, Adams and DeYoung [3] point out however, that the majority of benefits documented are purely speculation, with little empirical evidence to support them. They also purport that two schools of thought exist . One believing that faculty practice is designed for the good of teachers and students by enabling educators to maintain their clinical skills, which inturn enhances the legitimacy and accuracy of their teaching. The other believes that it is the profession and client who benefit most from faculty practice. By enabling faculty to practise, they can identify and research more appropriate questions, thus enhancing professional practice and improving patient care.

It appeared that our informatics faculty practice model was congruent with both schools of thought as it was intended to increase awareness among educators, facilitate research, and provide opportunity for clinical practice. Using this eclectic approach the following outcomes were expected:

1. Increased awareness, amongst the faculty, of the issues confronting clinicians using information technology.
2. Increased awareness, amongst clinicians, of current academic thinking in regards to nursing informatics.
3. Provision of education experiences that are closely aligned to the clinical setting.
4. Furthering the development of nursing informatics through research stimulated by collaborative educator-clinician inquiry.

4. Operationalising the model

From the outset it was agreed that the following practice opportunities would be provided.

For faculty:
- conducting clinical practice in ward areas currently using information systems;
- participation in informatics education provided for new hospital staff;
- buddying with the informatics nurse to experience day to day issues of liaison between clinicians and the department of Information Technology Services, and
- participating in policy formulation meetings in regards to nursing information systems.

For clinicians:
- participation in curriculum design meetings to gain insight into current academic thinking and influence curricula

content;
- provide input into the development of educational materials to ensure congruency with practice, and
- conduct education events for both undergraduate and postgraduate students.
The model was implemented in January 1992 and invitations issued to both faculty and clinicians to participate.

5. Actual outcomes.

At the time of writing this paper the opportunities offered by this model have been taken up by one faculty member. and one clinician. The faculty member was the co-coordinator of the Nursing informatics subjects offered at Latrobe University, and the clinician was the informatics nurse at the Alfred Hospital. All opportunities have been utilised by both participants with several identifiable benefits being achieved.

The nursing informatics curriculum has undergone a number of fundamental changes. The original focus of familiarisation with common business applications (word processing, spread sheets and data bases) has moved to a nursing application focus. Nursing information issues provide the foundation for class discussion with participants being encourage to explore ways in which computers may enhance more efficient use of this information. Often students identify common applications as possible options, but they are no longer the focus of the learner's endeavours. The same curriculum has been offered as a short course in the University's continuing education program and is proving to be extremely popular.

Discussions and explorations of nursing informatics issues have been further enhanced by the inclusion of actual clinical representatives. For example, when students are examining the implementing of nursing information systems, the discussions are chaired by the Director of Information Technology Services and the relevant clinician from the Alfred hospital. Any questions or concerns can be addressed directly to the people confronting the issues on a daily basis. The inclusion of representatives from clinical agencies have also provided closer liaison with relevant vendors enabling demonstrations of current hardware and software.

Laboratory sessions have been improved by the development of computer aided instruction packages. At the time of writing, access to vendor systems had been frustrated by the absence of appropriate hardware and funding for software purchases. Computer aided instructional packages have been designed to mimic the features of existing systems and to provide a platform for development of new features. The latter being derived from the experience of the clinicians and the postulation of the faculty member. The involvement of clinicians has meant that packages more closely represent those of clinical settings.

Individual benefits articulated by the faculty participant include an increase in job satisfaction related to direct involvement with the clinical setting, a closer relationship between curricula content and clinical realities, and an increased motivation to devote time to research in the area of nursing informatics. Benefits articulated by the clinician similarly include an increase in job satisfaction related to role expansion, professional development through exposure to current academic thinking and a stimulated desire to promote informatics across the nursing discipline.

Both formal and informal feedback from students indicate that they have little difficulty linking the theory to practice. Of the many students who indicated a fear of using computers in practice, all agree that they have sufficient confidence to explore the use of information technology at the completion of the subject. A high percentage have gone on to implement nursing information systems in their own work places.

A major benefit to the university has been that students have been able to gain insight into the clinical setting without the expenses that accompany placing students in the field. By having the clinicians come to the students, and being able to providing laboratory experiences that mimic existing systems the need for actual field experiences has been greatly diminished. The major benefit realised by the hospital has been in the area of in-service education. Contributing to informatics education prior to graduation has meant that new staff require less extensive in-service education in this area. Finally, by having university faculty conduct some of the in-service teaching sessions the amount of resources needed in the area have also been reduced.

At the time of press, no formal collaborative research has resulted from the informatics faculty practice model but a number of studies have been planned and funding is being sought.

6. Conclusion

If a service-education gap exists in nursing, within Australia, it is more that likely to be in the area of Nursing Informatics than else where. Contributing factors to this gap include educators who lack the rudimentary experiences of using information technology in the clinical arena, the cost of hard and software support needed to teach this material and the developing nature of this sector of the nursing discipline. If the gap is to be breached, education and service will need to establish formal collaborative links. It has been proposed that an informatics faculty practice model is one option available. Enabling collaboration between education and service by providing faculty with opportunities to experience nursing information issues first hand, and allowing clinicians the opportunity to have input into educational activities, the service-education gap can be dramatically reduced.

7. References

[1]   Christy T. Clinical practice as a function of nursing education: An historical analysis. *Nurs Outlook* 1980, 28:493-497.

[2]   Mauksch I. Faculty Practice: A professional imperative. *Nurse Educ* 1980, 5:21-24.

[3]   Just J, Adams E, and DeYoung S, Faculty Practice: Nurse Educators' views and proposed models. *J Nurs Educ* 1989, 28 (4):161-168.

[4]   Bennett S. Blending the entrepreneurial and faculty roles. *Nurse Educ* 1990, 15(4):34-37.

[5]   Herr K.A. Faculty Practice as a requirement for promotion and tenure. *J Nurs Educ* 1989, 28   (8):347-353.

[6]   Stainton M, Rankin J, and Calkin J. The development of a practising nursing faculty, *J Adv Nurs* 1989, 14:20-26.

[7]   Starck P, Walker G, and Bohannan P. Nursing faculty practice in the Houston linkage model: Administrative and faculty Perspectives. *Nurse Educ* 1991,16(5):23-28.

[8]   Kent N. Evaluating the practice component for faculty rank tenure. In *Cognitive dissonance: Interpreting and implementing faculty practice roles in nursing education.* New York: National League for Nursing (pub. No 15-1831), 1980.

[9]   Anderson E, and Pierson P. An exploratory study of faculty practice: Views of those faculty engaged in practise who teach in an NLN accredited baccalaureate program. *West J Nurs Res* 1983, 5:128-143.

Nursing Informatics: An International Overview for Nursing in a Technological Era
S.J. Grobe and E.S.P. Pluyter-Wenting, eds.

Teaching nurses computer skills: It can be fun

Russell B

Nursing Department, Fremantle Hospital, Fremantle, Western Australia.

Training of approximately 600 nursing staff in the use of the first application of the computerised Patient Care System (PCS), is both challenging and rewarding. This paper describes the implementation and training process for the Nurse Management System (NMS), involving Allocation and Leave modules. A brief description of the hardware and mainframe networking process will be given, along with some background to the System. Methods used to facilitate data uptake and ensure data integrity along with the problems encountered will be presented. The reasons why NMS is important as a Human Resource planning tool will also be discussed.

1.   Introduction

This paper is to inform conference delegates and readers of exciting and challenging experiences that can be obtained from training approximately 600 nurses in the use of a computerised allocation and leave system. Exciting from the point of view of observing these nurses, many of whom have never used any sort of computer at all, start their training sessions with fear and trepidation. By the end of 3 hours of instruction, they leave the training room with smiles, looks of relief and the capability of being able to control their individual personnel data and leave. Challenging from the point of view that most of these nurses are on rotational varying shifts and it is therefore a logistical nightmare to schedule for training sessions. Challenging also from the point of view of breaking down the barriers that are thrown up against the introduction of any change to existing ways of life.

2.   Background

Fremantle Hospital is a 403 bed general hospital and is situated in the sea port of Fremantle, 12 miles from Perth, the capital of Western Australia. As well as general Medical and Surgical beds, other specialities include Paediatrics, Psychiatry, Gerontology, an Obstetrics unit, an Emergency Department, four Operating Theatres plus a Diagnostic Suite and ancillary services. The Hospital was the pilot site for the computerised Nurse Management System (NMS) and it was involved in modifying the system prior to implementation. NMS is part of the Patient Care System (PCS) that was purchased by the Health Department of Western Australia. After some delays due to modification to the system, NMS was implemented in November 1989. Since implementation at Fremantle, four other teaching hospitals and eight non-teaching/country hospitals have also successfully implemented and are at various stages of educating staff in the use of the system. NMS is based on a centralised mainframe computer and is accessed by DUMB TERMINALS equipped with light pens. It is envisaged that in the future, dumb terminals will possibly be replaced by disk-less workstations incorporating a windows type environment and equipped with a mouse. There is a belief that this would provide a more reliable and possibly cheaper alternative to the present dumb terminal network. NMS has been designed to operate as either a Centralised or Decentralised management system. To this end, NMS was implemented at Fremantle Hospital with Decentralisation in mind. In December 1990 the first training sessions for ward based nursing staff at Fremantle Hospital were commenced. Nurse Managerial and clerical staff were involved with the use of NMS during the modification and implementation phases and therefore they were already competent in the use of this system.

3. Data uptake

Major information needed to set up NMS came from the Nursing Staff Personnel files. The information needed was keyboarded by data processors from a private data bureau, onto tape and then uploaded onto the mainframe. This method proved most unsatisfactory and the problems associated with this type of data uptake were many. Problems included inaccurate interpretation of written information from personnel files, typographical errors from keyboarding, interpretation problems from the data on the data forms and the removal of edit checks, (field checks) for the upload of data. The removal of edit checks caused the biggest problem as this allowed numerical data to be entered into alphabetical fields and vice versa. Edit checks must be in place when an uptake is in progress to preserve the integrity of data. It is only recently that a conversion program has been written to check data for corruptions. This has enabled some incorrect data to be automatically corrected, and other corrupt data to be identified on a print error report. The User Co-ordinator can make appropriate corrections based on the error report.

4. Data integrity

Employees work history was the greatest concern for data integrity. Checking individual records proved to be a tedious and time consuming task, when the work history error report, previously spoken about, was written and run through Fremantle Hospitals data, the enormity of the problem was realised. Many calculation errors in the Work History Length of Service were evident, along with other incomplete information resulting in inaccurate information. These problems have, in the main, been resolved with the aid of the conversion program. Other problems encountered were incomplete or missing information in other fields resulting in corrupt data. To assist in identifying errors, all nurses check their own data during training sessions. As mistakes or missing information are pointed out to the instructor, the data set is corrected. Although slow, this method will, in the long term, ensure data is reliable and valid.

5. Training

Training commenced with one ward at a time. It was predicted that each nurse would need approximately 4 hours to be deemed competent. The training sessions were broken into 2 sessions of 2 hours duration each. This was, however, reviewed after 18 months because only 44% of the nursing staff had been trained. One session of 3 hours duration with a minimum of 2 people and a maximum of 6 people was found to be more effective. This not only sped up the training, but also eliminated the difficulty of scheduling nurses back for the second session with a short time after the first session. To prevent being accidentally missed, all nursing staff commencing employment at Fremantle Hospital receive training during their orientation (induction) period. Constant liaison with the ward Staff Development Nurse and the Nurse Manager was necessary to ensure all other staff were rostered for training sessions. An obvious incentive for the Nurse Managers to assist in rostering staff for training sessions is that once staff are trained in the use of NMS, the Nurse Managers work load decreases, because employees under their control enter leave requests directly into the computer. Instead of collecting and processing written leave requests, the nurse Managers generate one leave report each week and approve or deny leave from this. This leave report is generated from within NMS and captures any OPEN leave that is inputted into NMS, i.e. leave that requires to be APPROVED. When individual employees request leave it can only be entered into the system as OPEN and the managers will APPROVE leave only if their establishment numbers allow.

During training sessions, nurses are instructed in elementary keyboard skills, how to view their personnel data and how to request leave of any form, be it Annual Leave, Accrued Days Off, Study Leave, etc. There are 19 different types of leave that NMS can cater for including "OTHER". To help break down the barriers of fear of computers and resistance to change, an application program called "BIGBIRD" is used during the training sessions. The benefit of this is the ability to provide a hands on application and allow nurses who had never used a computer before to become familiar with the position of the most frequently used keys. This time is when the fun begins. It is very rewarding to see nurses smiling, laughing and obviously looking quite at ease using the keyboards by the end of their lessons. This is opposite to how the nurses looked as they entered the training room before the lesson begins. Most nurses, when they first come in for training look very nervous and tense. With gentle guidance and close instruction this soon passes. Approximately 3/4 of an hour is allowed for BIGBIRD and the rest of the session is used to familiarise the nurses with accessing their personnel data held in NMS. This is followed by comprehensive instruction on how to use the leave request function. To supplement training, a User Manual, developed by the User Co-ordinator, is handed out to everyone who attends training. The manual gives a brief introduction and rationale of why it is necessary to learn the use of NMS, a description of all the functions available in NMS (at the user level), a step by step guide on how to request leave and the conditions that apply to these requests, e.g. that all leave requested by individuals is in "OPEN" status until "APPROVED" by a Nurse Manager. All leave is "APPROVED" by a Nurse Manager, using the ENTER/UPDATE LEAVE REQUEST FUNCTION so that this leave will appear on the "APPROVED LEAVE REPORT". This report is generated by the Salaries Department each week to prepare leave entitlements.

Another important condition is that, for managerial planning purposes, "OPEN" leave can only be requested with a leave start date greater than 28 days in advance. This means that nursing staff can only put a leave request into the computer if their leave starts in the next month or later. Leave with a start date of less than 28 days in advance can only be entered on NMS with a managerial access type menu by the Nurse Managers.

Part of the training process requires nurses to complete an exercise which allows them to enter a leave request into NMS and cancel this leave with no instruction. Only rarely has the instructor had to intervene and assist in the entry or cancellation of leave by the end of training sessions. An evaluation questionnaire was developed and is given to all nurses who attend training sessions. This anonymous survey asks for basic demographic details such as age, gender, ranking (type of nurses, e.g. Registered Nurse, Enrolled Nurse) and the ward/unit they are allocated to. Other questions are designed to obtain information on:

1. Whether the teacher imparted enough knowledge to enable nurses to use NMS effectively.
2. The appropriateness of the training method.
3. Nurse confidence level in using NMS effectively.
4. Ways that training could be conducted in a better or more appropriate manner.

As of December 1992 approximately 600 forms have been returned and most provided positive answers to all questions. Six months after training a second questionnaire is distributed to staff. As of December 1992 a return rate of 54% has been achieved for this questionnaire with indications that most staff who have been trained are still using NMS to request leave. The main reasons given by nursing staff who have not used NMS since being trained were:

1. Not enough terminals or difficulty of access to a terminal.
2. Not enough time to use NMS.
3. No incentive to use NMS as Nurse Managers were still prepared to accept leave forms.

To counter-act some of these problems leave forms have been withdrawn from the areas where training has been completed. This ensures nurses use NMS because it is the only method they can now use to request annual leave. With Rostering (staff scheduling) to be introduced at a later stage, nurses will need to be able to use NMS to request shifts they want for following rosters. Because the User Co-ordinator is unable to commit more time to training due to the developmental side of the project, e.g. testing new screens/functions, creating/modifying new screens, another person was seconded to the project in June 1992 to take over the training role for six months. The number of nursing staff who have completed training has increased from 44% to 89% (100% as of June 1993) since training resources were increased.

6. Human resource planning

In these days of shrinking health budgets, there is intense pressure on the Nurse Managers to provide safe nursing coverage with a minimum of nursing staff. This demand requires that Nurse Managers have access to accurate, timely information on the total contracted hours of nursing coverage available for their areas. This information is provided by NMS. Before an employee commences at Fremantle Hospital information, including their contracted hours, is entered into NMS. NMS has the ability to automatically accommodate all planned changes that are entered for an employee, e.g. changes in contracted hours for the entire hospital, or one ward, up to 15 weeks in advance. Batch reports may also be generated for whatever date the Nurse Manager wishes, either current, prospectively or retrospectively. This information is crucial in assisting Nurse Managers to make decisions on recruitment, transferring nurses from one clinical area to another and reducing or increasing an individual employees contracted hours. Resignations are also accommodated in similar fashion in that, once a resignation date is inserted into NMS for an employee, the contracted hours are deducted from the nursing establishment as from that date. This data from NMS has proved to be accurate, reliable and readily accessible for the Nurse Managers.

7. Summary

NMS has been in use at Fremantle Hospital since November 1989 and has provided accurate and timely information to Nurse Managers. Nursing Staff are currently using NMS to request leave. Other functions used by the Nurse Managers include updating Personnel data, entering planned changes, alterations to contracted hours and generating reports from NMS. Dumb terminals connected in a mainframe environment provide the platform for data entry at present, however in the future a more flexible platform may be introduced to replace these dumb terminals. The method of data uptake when converting from a manual system to an electronic information system can have serious impacts on the integrity of data and a source of corruption to data residing within a management system. To assist with the success of a data upload, edit checks must not be removed. Yet, beyond the accuracy of data held, and the usefulness of the system for the Nurse Managers, has lain another dimension. That which can assist in employee empowerment, by enabling them to have better control over their own data and which gets them to leave a training session smiling.

EDUCATION

B. Technology for education

Nursing Informatics: An International Overview for Nursing in a Technological Era
S.J. Grobe and E.S.P. Pluyter-Wenting, eds.

Multimedia Patient Case Study Simulations: Considerations for Their Evaluation and Use

Mary Anne Rizzolo, EdD, RN

Director, Interactive Technologies, American Journal of Nursing Co., 555 West 57th St., New York, NY 10019

Patient case study simulations using videodiscs have been commercially available for a few years and have received an enthusiastic reception by nurse educators. At this time many nurse educators are grappling with the problem of how to evaluate programs that are currently available and integrate them into the curriculum. This paper focuses primarily on the evaluation of fidelity in multimedia patient case study simulations and discusses a variety of ways that these programs can be used. Relevant research related to evaluation and use is cited and some ideas on the future of simulations are discussed.

1. Introduction

Patient case study simulations are unique applications of multimedia technology. These programs combine video, audio, graphics and the branching power of the computer to permit the creation of learning experiences that have never before been possible. They can allow learners to practice patient care management and decision-making in a risk-free environment. They can provide all students with an experience caring for patients with common problems, as well as conditions that are rarely seen. A patient case study simulation can place the learner in a variety of environments. And, they can provide the ideal learning sequence by presenting a patient with a condition that matches the content that is being studied. Ever since the early days of multimedia technology, experts overwhelming urged developers to focus their efforts on simulations to meet educational needs in nursing [1].

When used for evaluation and testing, multimedia patient case study simulations can facilitate mobility and progression through learning experiences. The potential of these programs to test decision-making led the National Council of State Boards of Nursing to initiate the Clinical Simulation Testing (CST) Project. A videodisc has been produced, some field testing has been completed, and additional research will be done to determine if programs of this type are a feasible, valid and reliable method to assess the clinical decision-making of RN licensure or re-licensure candidates [2].

Multimedia patient case study simulations using videodiscs, usually referred to as interactive video (IAV), have been commercially available for a few years and have received an enthusiastic reception by nurse educators. However, due to the complexity of these programs, many nurse educators are grappling with the problem of how to evaluate programs that are currently available and integrate them into the curriculum. Certainly educators are experienced in evaluating many types of educational materials and do not need assistance to determine if the content of a product is accurate, if it meets their objectives and is presented at an appropriate level for their learners. However, computer-based programs require additional consideration. Jonassen [3] wrote that there are at least 144 ways to vary each instructional event. Since a patient case study simulation will have numerous events within a program, evaluation can become a formidable task.

When evaluating multimedia patient case study simulations, the nurse educator must consider such factors as instructional design, branching capability, screen design, learner control, user interface and navigational issues. Many evaluation tools are available to assist educators in this process, and some instruments are specifically geared to IAV [4]. A good tool should facilitate consideration of all relevant features and help educators come to a conclusion about whether or not a program uses each multimedia capability appropriately and to its fullest extent. However, few instruments alert educators to consider fidelity in the evaluation process. This chapter will focus on the evaluation of fidelity in multimedia patient case study simulations, discuss a variety of ways that the programs can be used, and speculate about the future of simulations.

2. Evaluation of Fidelity

One aspect unique to patient case study simulations that must be carefully examined is fidelity. Fidelity refers to how closely a simulated experience imitates reality. In general, low fidelity simulations produce the highest level of learning for novice students, while high fidelity is required for more experienced learners who wish to perfect their skills [5]. It is useful to consider five aspects of a program to determine its value as a patient case study simulation and if the degree of fidelity fits the intended student: realism, level of decision-making, user input, feedback and balance of video and text.

2.1 Realism

Patient case study simulations must involve the user. The designers of these programs usually accomplish this by creating characters that the learner can relate to. While the characters and the event may be somewhat exaggerated in order to establish a feeling of involvement in a short period of time, they must stay within a sphere of realism. Certain techniques, such as having the characters look directly into the camera, create the impression that the character on the screen is talking directly to the user. This approach can increase the learner's sense of involvement in the simulation and make it a more realistic and meaningful experience.

If the intended audience for the program is practitioners who have a solid grasp on content, then the patient case study should mimic reality as much as possible. It should include such features as subtle changes in the patient that require good observation skills, time clocks, a patient whose condition changes over time in response to presence or absence of nursing intervention, and the random inclusion of chance events that affect decision-making.

On the other hand, low fidelity simulations designed for novice learners should keep the patient's condition static to give the learner time to determine appropriate nursing diagnoses and interventions. The environment, the variables and amount of irrelevant data included in the scenario should be limited. In fact, some low fidelity simulations may not require video to accomplish involvement. *SOS - Strategies for Problem Solving* [6], is a wonderful example of a low fidelity simulation that uses only graphics to prepare students for their first experience on a hospital unit. The limited choices that are available to users can help them develop the confidence they need to make decisions that are expected of student nurses on their very first morning of patient care.

Most of the nursing programs that are commercially available fall between the two extremes and provide an experience similar to a real situation, but with limited imitation of real events. Therefore, they are classified as moderate fidelity simulations.

2.2 Level of decision-making

Thiele and Holloway [7] developed a decision-making taxonomy that can be used to help focus on the level of cognitive processing required by learners as they use a computerized simulation. It describes four levels of decision-making and the type of decision-making skill required at each level. Level One, for example, requires only recall of facts to resolve a problem, while Level Four involves multiple complex events and priority setting. This tool was designed and tested with computer-based programs (not multimedia programs), but the descriptions of cognitive processing required at each level should be helpful for determining the decision-making aspect of a multimedia patient case study simulation as well.

Since nurses use the nursing process to make decisions, Klaassens [8] developed an instrument to determine if an interactive video program contains adequate percentages of the essential components of the nursing process. In her research, 75% inclusion of the steps of nursing process indicated that a program could adequately teach problem-solving. Both the Thiele and Holloway and Klaassens tools can be useful to nurse educators, especially during initial attempts to evaluate patient case study simulations.

2.3 User Input

The way learners make choices after seeing a patient scenario is another design feature that should be dictated by the level of fidelity. Low fidelity simulations lend themselves to multiple choice questions where the numbers of options are limited. Moderate fidelity simulations may employ menus and submenus that list more extensive choices and require some priority setting. High fidelity simulations may require free text entry without any prompts.

2.4 Feedback and Record Keeping

Low fidelity simulations should offer immediate feedback to correct inappropriate actions and prevent unfavorable outcomes. Generally, gentle reminders are most appropriate for novices. As programs increase in fidelity, feedback should be progressively delayed and learners should experience the consequences of their choices [5].

Reports of how well a student performed do not need to be very detailed for low fidelity simulations, since novice learners are expected to make many mistakes and since extensive remediation is delivered throughout the program at each decision point. As programs increase in fidelity, record keeping should be more extensive and broken down into subsections that reflect the program's areas of concentration.

2.5 Balance of video, text, and graphics

Generally, video is used to present patient scenarios and, sometimes, to show outcomes of decisions made by the user. Text and graphics are used for supplemental information about a patient (a patient chart, for example), in a library or resource section where supplemental information is available, to display information requested by the user, and for feedback. The literature does not reveal any studies on the appropriate balance of text and video, but based on personal experience watching learners use patient case study simulations, it has become evident that learners do not like to be distracted from the events that are taking place with the patient for too long a period of time. Spending too long reading text dilutes the sense of involvement and, therefore, the fidelity. Feedback and remediation should be brief, with more extensive explanations in text and graphics saved for the conclusion of the case study.

2.6 A Final Word on Evaluation

Because many multimedia patient case study simulations are exciting and involving, it is useful to keep asking the following questions frequently throughout the evaluation process: Does this program meet a curricular need? Will it assist in content areas that are difficult to teach and evaluate? Could these objectives be met just as efficiently and effectively with a less costly media such as a videotape or a CAI? No matter how good a program is, unless the answers to these questions are "Yes," money might be better spent elsewhere.

3. Using Multimedia Patient Case Study Simulations

There are many factors to consider regarding integration and use of multimedia patient case study simulations. The evaluator must view an entire program with all its branches to decide how it can be used. Most library or resource sections of programs are tutorial in nature, and may be appropriate for novice learners, while the case study simulation may be used for higher level students. *Nursing Educator's MicroWorld* reports regularly on innovative approaches to integration of all types of computer-based programs, and educators are increasingly presenting papers detailing their success at conferences. Although each educational program has its own unique curriculum and instructional needs, reading and hearing about the success of others can generate discussion and ideas.

3.1 Individual vs. groups

While multimedia patient case study simulations can be used by individuals for independent learning, several studies indicate that viewing a program in a group may be more beneficial for some students. Camber and Castner [9] reported that students preferred working in small groups. Battista-Calderone [10] had students work through *Intravenous Therapy* [11], an IAV tutorial program. Some worked individually, some in groups of 2 or 3, the rest in larger groups of 7 to 10 students. Study results revealed no significant differences in learning and attitude.

This author compared the pre and post-test scores of students who worked though *Nursing Care of Elderly Patients with Acute Cardiac Disorders* [12], a moderate fidelity simulation, in a large classroom situation to those who worked through the program individually. Both groups achieved significant increases (p<.0005) in scores from pre to post-test. When pre and post-test scores were compared between groups, there was no significant difference in the pre-test scores of the two groups (p.592), but there was a significant difference in post-test scores (p .031). The group of students who viewed the program in the classroom setting scored significantly higher on the post-test then those who viewed the program alone [13]. It appears that additional learning occurs as a result of the discussion that takes place among the viewers. Two dissertations in progress [14,15] may provide additional data on this issue.

3.2 Small clinical groups

Nurse educators can use patient case study simulations to evaluate students or newly hired nurses. While having the user work through the program individually can provide some evaluation, consider the possibilities with an instructor present. The educator can interject additional patient data and question individuals in the group. This approach quickly reveals to the instructor such things as individual strengths and weaknesses in observation skills, knowledge of background pathophysiology, and decision-making ability. The instructor can then make more informed decisions about the type of experiences to provide for each student or staff member in the clinical area.

This author can report considerable personal success using this type of approach with senior level nursing students. It was much easier to make patient assignments for a new group of students and make decisions on how to best use my time while supervising those students in the clinical area.

3.3 Classroom use

An approach similar to that described above for small clinical groups can be used in a large classroom setting. Sections of a program projected onto a large screen can bring a patient into the classroom to illustrate the application of theoretical material. The teacher may interject additional data for students to consider in addition to the information already presented in the program. The instructor can ask students to imagine different scenarios and how they would respond differently. Patient data that would alter nursing diagnoses and interventions can be discussed and explored.

3.4 As a Research Tool

The quality and acceptance of multimedia case study simulations are indicated by the fact that they are beginning to be used as a research tool. Predko [16] used *Nursing Care of Elderly Patients with Acute Cardiac Disorders* [12] to measure both process and outcome components of decision-making in her study which examined the effect of knowledge level, clinical experience and education on clinical decision-making skills of cardiac care nurses. McAlindon [17] used vignettes from two IAV programs, *Therapeutic Communication* [18] and *Nursing Care of the Elderly Patient with COPD* [19] to determine the effect of abstract and concrete examples on two aspects of learning the process of Quality Assurance -- knowledge and valuation.

4. The Future of Multimedia Patient Case Study Simulations

If developers and educators work through a reasoned development and evaluation process, today's programs will have a profound influence on the patient case study simulations of the future. As it becomes more feasible to link together multiple data and visual storage devices, more complex simulations can be designed for individuals and groups of students. Consider the ability to move a learner through a simulation, with the degree of realism and complexity increasing as the learner's knowledge and skills increase. He/she would begin by managing a fairly simple patient, with a limited number of variables present. As the learner progresses, the patient's condition can change unexpectedly and the learner will have to deal with additional data, some relevant, some irrelevant. Once he/she has achieved proficiency with one dynamic patient simulation, the learner can be challenged to manage the care of two patients, then an entire group - prioritizing, delegating responsibility to others in the health care team. Interpersonal problems with other professionals, as well as unexpected emergencies, can complicate patient care situations. Groups of learners could all participate in the same scenario, with each playing a different role. The next set of circumstances and problems in the simulation could be determined by the input from each individual learner, as well as the composite input of the group.

Programs of the future will not remain tied to computer screens and keyboards. Advances in virtual reality will enable us to create entire hospital units, complete with patients, staff and equipment. Advances in miniaturization and voice recognition technology will make it possible to build programmable humanoids. Pop in a cartridge and our humanoid/simulator will exhibit signs and symptoms that require intervention; another cartridge, another nursing problem.

While all these marvelous learning activities are going on, the computer is collecting data and analyzing the learner, so that it can design the next simulated experience that can advance the user to a more challenging problem, or, remediate, reevaluate problem areas, and better meet the learning style of the user.

Although the applications described above are in the future, what we learn about the design and use of today's technology will greatly influence the applications of the future. We must take advantage of current technology and influence its development, use, and evolution. We must evaluate the current state of the art, then take action to move beyond existing models and roles to create new arenas for exploration and development.

5. References

[1] Rizzolo MA. Factors Influencing the Development and Use of Interactive Video in Nursing Education: A Delphi Study. *Comput Nurs* 1990, 8(4), 151-159.

[2] Brady D. A New Generation in Competence Assessment in Nursing: Computerized Clinical Simulation Testing (CST). *Issues*, (National Council of State Boards of Nursing, Inc.), 1993 14(1), 1+.

[3] Jonassen DH. Interactive Lesson Designs: A Taxonomy. *Educational Technology* 1985, 25(6), 7-17.

[4] Sparks SM and Kuenz MA. *Interactive Instruction in Nursing and Other Health Sciences: Review of Evaluation Instruments.* National Library of Medicine, Lister Hill Monograph LHNCBC 93-1, February 1993.

[5] Alessi SM. Fidelity in the Design of Instructional Simulations. *J of Comput-Based Instr* 1988,15(2), 40-47.

[6] C & D Enterprises, Inc. *SOS - Strategies for Problem Solving*, Glen Ellyn, IL 1991.

[7] Thiele JE and Holloway JR. Development of a Taxonomy of Decision-Making Properties of Computerized Clinical Simulations. In Arnold JM and Pearson GA (eds). *Computer Applications in Nursing Education and Practice*, New York: National League for Nursing, 1992: 351-362.

[8] Klaassens EL. Evaluation of Interactive Videodisc Simulations Designed for Nursing to Determine Their Ability to Provide Problem-Solving Practice Based on the Use of the Nursing Process. Unpublished doctoral dissertation, Northern Illinois U., De Kalb, 1993.

[9] Cambre MA and Castner LJ. *The Status of Interactive Video Technology in Nursing Education Environments.* Athens, OH: Fuld Institute for Technology in Nursing Education, 1991.

[10] Battista-Calderone A. Investigation of the Effect of IVI with Three Modes of Instruction on Learning and Attitude towards the Instructional Media. Unpublished doctoral dissertation, Widener University 1992.

[11] Hocking Technical College. (Producer). *Intravenous Therapy* [videodisc program]. Athens OH: Fuld Institute for Technology in Nursing Education, 1989.

[12] American Journal of Nursing Company (Producer). *Nursing Care of Elderly Patients with Acute Cardiac Disorders* [videodisc program]. New York NY: American Journal of Nursing Company, 1989.

[13] Rizzolo MA. (ed.) *Interactive Video: Expanding Horizons in Nursing.* New York: American Journal of Nursing Co. (in press).

[14] Garcia BR. Effect of Group Size on Learning via Interactive Video Instruction in Nursing Education. Doctoral dissertation in progress, Texas A & M University.

[15] Moyer BA. The Effect of Interactive Video in Group Settings on the Problem Solving Abilities of Senior Nursing Students. Doctoral dissertation in progress, Lehigh University.

[16] Predko JE. Effect of Knowledge Level, Clinical Experience and Education on Clinical Decision Making Skills. Unpublished doctoral dissertation, Michigan State U. 1992.

[17] McAlindon MN. A Study to Determine the Effectiveness of an Interactive Video Instruction Program in Teaching Registered Nurses in the Clinical Setting the Process of Quality Assurance in Nursing. Unpublished doctoral dissertation, Wayne State U. 1992.

[18] Fuld Institute for Technology in Nursing Education. (Producer). *Therapeutic Communication* [videodisc program]. Athens OH: Fuld Institute for Technology in Nursing Education, 1990.

[19] American Journal of Nursing Company (Producer). *Nursing Care of the Elderly Patient with COPD* [videodisc program]. New York NY: American Journal of Nursing Company, 1988.

© 1994 Elsevier Science B.V. All rights reser

Nursing Informatics: An International Overview for Nursing in a Technological

S.J. Grobe and E.S.P. Pluyter-Wenting,

558

Meeting Communication Needs with an Electronic Bulletin Board

Davis KE[a] and Hassett MM[b]

[a]*Compucare, 12110 Sunset Hill Road, Reston, Virginia 22090*

[b]*Department of Nursing, WHT116, Massachusetts General Hospital, Fruit Street, Boston, Massachusetts 02114*

The Nursing Informatics (NI) program at the University of Maryland at Baltimore (UMAB) provided a unique opportunity to utilize information technology to improve communication between students, alumni, and faculty. Increased program enrollment, student utilization of multiple campuses, and relocation of graduates created a complex communication environment and poor access to information. The campus utilized a technological infrastructure enabling the use of computers in solving the problem of poor access to information. A local area network (LAN) over which much computing is accomplished, and a state-of-the-art microcomputer lab were made available for students in the NI program.[1] An electronic bulletin board system (BBS) was established and is maintained by students. The BBS provides a means for conferencing on a variety of topics while teaching students about the application of network technology.

1. Problem

Communication at UMAB is accomplished in a number of ways. Individual student mailboxes are provided in the Schoo Nursing on the Baltimore campus. A video monitor in the lobby of the school displays general information about the school campus and specific departmental information is posted on a bulletin board in the NI department. While effective, these tools accessible only when the buildings are open. Other methods of communication including in-class announcements, telephone, mail are limited by proximity to informatics classes, and cost, particularly for those students and alumni living outside the lo region.

Student contact with the main campus or the primary source of information is limited by several factors. The student popula resides in locations across Maryland and the surrounding states of Virginia, Pennsylvania, and Washington, DC. The progra cirriculumn provides for both full and part time study. The nature of the University of Maryland system enables and at times requi students to take classes on different campuses. The program's growth increases demand on faculty time and reduces facu availability. Finally a majority of students completing the program relocate out of the area and away from the main campus.

The objective of this project was to evaluate communication needs and develop a tool to increase access to information for students, faculty and alumni of the NI program. An assessment was performed to document perceived deficiencies using current communication methods. As a result of this initial assessment, an evaluation of resources and participant interest, the determination was made that an electronic bulletin board system (BBS) would meet this population's communication needs. The following is a discussion of the planning and implementation process for the BBS.

2. Literature Review

Information technology (IT) and its ability to enhance information access and exchange have brought new focus on the subj of communication. The more recent influence of IT has created the concept of electronic communication which enhances pers to-person networking in many ways. Information is meaningful and useful only if it is easily accessible, relevant, timely, reliab secure, and cost effective[2].

Peters and Waterman[3] discuss the benefit of increased contact among individuals in an organization. For example in academic setting, increased contact among students, faculty, and alumni promotes improved collaborative efforts, resulting in r information exchange, new learning opportunities, and improved problem solving.

Electronic communication provides timely information whose availability is not limited by work schedules. The communicat is not dependent upon location or proximity. There is no restriction to the amount or types of information a user may seek

puter networks support the information exchange process by accessing specialized resources, colleagues, and information
ough a personal resource sharing network or a large computer data base[5].

Electronic bulletin board systems (BBS) running on computer networks have been used effectively to increase access to
ormation for a wide variety of users[6],[7]. These systems allow participants to interact with others on an unlimited variety of
ics. Information may be sent locally, nationally, and internationally[8]. Skiba and Warren[9] see the BBS as a way to create an
ended nursing community. This community is not bounded by geographical regions and couples computing power with
communication and networking capabilities.

BBSs change the nature of communication. They enable many people with many different perspectives to interact and permit
rs to read, write, send, and receive messages in complete privacy at a convenient time[10].

Planning

Successful implementation of a computer-based system to solve a problem requires that a systematic approach be taken. This
roach is called the systems life cycle (SLC). McLeod[11] defines four phases of this evolutionary process: (1) planning, (2)
tem analysis and design, (3) implementation, and (4) operations.

An additional approach taken by many system developers is prototyping. Prototyping is an iterative approach to the SLC which
ws the developer to take small steps, test the product with the user, and go back and make changes and enhancements. The
pleted prototype then becomes the production system if it contains all the elements necessary; otherwise it serves as a blue print.
project to implement a BBS for the NI program at UMAB used this prototype model.

Once the problem had been identified and a solution proposed a preliminary project plan was developed. Flexibility in any project
n is important. Prototyping demands that revisions be made throughout the development process as additional needs and
uirements are identified.

The initial project plan included an outline of necessary tasks and an estimated time table. Specific tasks included development
a communication needs assessment to survey the intended BBS participants, determination of system requirements including
sonnel and maintenance, hardware and software selection, implementation, and plans for training and marketing of the BBS.
A project log was maintained by the authors to track task completion and identification of additional tasks or obstacles as the
ject progressed. The log was maintained by noting the tasks, completion dates, and changes in project plan dates. These notations
re then compiled in a table format which enabled the listing of dates, activities, and prototype development stages.

System Analysis

The information needs of the students, faculty, and alumni in the NI program at UMAB and their ability to access information
re determined by conducting a survey. Data obtained from the survey was used to determine the effectiveness of current systems,
ds for access to specific information, and the ability of current systems to meet these needs. The need for implementation of a
S to improve access to information was assessed.

Methodology

Sixty-four surveys were distributed to 55 students currently enrolled in the program, 4 faculty members working directly with
program and its students, and 5 alumni of the program. Thirty surveys were returned for a 47% response rate. Of the 30 surveys,
(80%) were from students, 3 (10%) from faculty, and 3 (10%) from alumni.

The survey, developed by the authors, was divided into two sections. Section one was comprised of a questionnaire using a 5-
nt Likert-type scale to score responses. Higher scores reflect a more positive response. Questions asked respondents to assess
current communication environment. Respondents were then asked to identify the importance of knowing about various
tinent academic topics and evaluate the effectiveness of available systems to meet their need for this information. Interest in using
nputers to meet communication needs through use of a BBS was also evaluated.

Section two asked for demographic information, whether or not subjects had access to a computer and modem, and information
ut their knowledge and use of current computer communication tools.

Surveys were distributed through campus mailboxes, and the U. S. mail. Respondents returned the questionnaires by way of
npus mailbox, U.S. mail, or hand delivery. Indication of the respondent's name and address was optional.

Results

All respondents stated that they had convenient access to a computer, 87% having access to an MS DOS computer and 13% to
Macintosh computer. Fifty-seven percent had access to a modem. When asked about use of the computer as a communication
l, only 48% had used a BBS, however, 97% were interested in using a BBS. Ninety percent of the respondents believed that an

educational program on *communication via computer* would be useful and 93% were willing to participate in such a program.

Generally, respondents perceived the current communication systems as being effective (N=30, M=3.19) (see Figure However, the current communication methods were inadequate in meeting needs for specific information such as departmental ne and upcoming workshops and conferences (see Figure 2). Participants stated that they would be interested in communica electronically with nursing informatics students in other programs (M=4.5), and in using electronic communication after gradua (M=4.47).

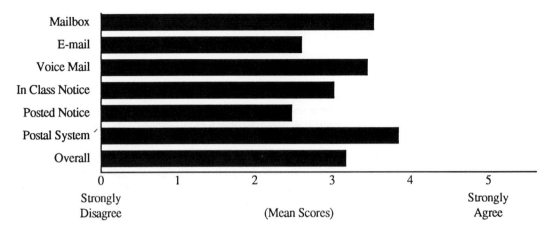

Figure 1. Effectiveness of Current Communication Systems

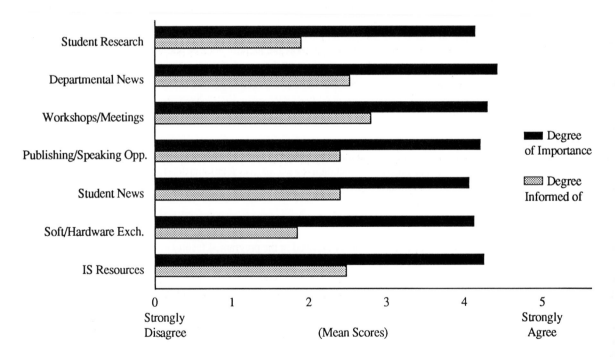

Figure 2. Topics of Interest

4.3 Discussion

There is a need in the NI program to augment the current methods of communication to increase access to information. Stude of nursing informatics must evaluate and use technological solutions to problems as part of the learning process. Finally, ther a strong interest in using a BBS for communication by students in the program.

In addition to interest in using the bulletin board while in school, respondents are eager to correspond not only with students faculty from their own program, but also with nurses in other informatics programs. This is an area that will allow the bulletin bo to grow as the program grows and other students become involved in its operation.

System Requirements

. number of experts both within the UMAB Information Services department and outside the UMAB system were contacted
heir expertise in networks and telecommunications. This information, and an extensive literature search, were the basis for
tification of the following minimum system requirements: a microcomputer with at least an 80286 processor, 2 megabytes of
A, a 20 megabyte hard drive, and the MS DOS operating system; a 2400 baud modem; communication software; bulletin board
ware; a dedicated telephone line; and screen design software.

Development & Implementation

lardware needed for the this project was evaluated. An IBM AT with an 80286 processor and the necessary memory and hard
e already owned by the department was available and did not need to be purchased. A Hayes-compatible 2400 baud modem,
ever, was purchased for the project.

wo new telephone lines were installed in the NI lab, one line dedicated for the BBS project. The establishment of an 800 number
o-cost access by students and alumni living outside of the local region was not feasible at the time of implementation but will
considered as the BBS becomes established and more students and alumni use it.

our key factors in the BBS software selection process were: (1) low cost, (2) ready availability, (3) ease of use both by the system
ator (sysop) and end users, and (4) capacity for several security features. The security features were: password protection,
rent levels of access, and the ability to maintain a closed system. It was also important that the developers be able to test the
ware before making a final, potentially costly, decision.

hree BBS software products, QuickBBS, RBBS, and WILDCAT! were considered. Because cost was one of the primary issues,
earch was begun by looking at the shareware version of each product. After examination of each of the products, WILDCAT!
chosen for the project. This product was readily available, relatively inexpensive, easy to use, and had the necessary security
ares.

dditional equipment was required to test the communication link up to the BBS. That equipment included a microcomputer,
xdem, communications software, and a telephone line. PROCOMM communications software which was available in the NI
was used.

he screen design process was initiated using TheDraw and Harvard Graphics software. Screens were designed for the
ductory screen with the BBS name, NIBBS (Nursing Informatics Bulletin Board System), and for conference screens
LDCAT! divides user interest areas into conferences). Initial conference topics, determined from the survey, were alumni news,
rtment news, and employment opportunities.

olicies and procedures are important steps in the development and implementation process. The system developers met with
faculty advisor to make recommendations as to the policies and procedures needed to set-up, operate, and maintain the BBS.
ortant issues included security, sysop responsibilities, faculty advisor responsibilities, and set-up parameters. Policies and
edures were written with the realization that they would need to be revised as future sysops become more familiar with operating
BBS and user needs change.

Conclusions

Access to information is an important aspect of communication. Innovative ideas to improve information access must be tried,
icularly in an academic setting where creativity and experimentation are encouraged. Information technology and a great interest
tudents and faculty of the NI program at UMAB prompted the authors of this paper to develop and implement a BBS. It is
cipated by the developers that this tool will be widely accepted and used by participants of the program to ensure they receive
rmation critical to their success as students and NI professionals.

Development of a BBS using the prototype model of the systems life cycle accomplished a number of goals. The very basis of
sing informatics demands that students learn to use technology to solve problems whenever possible and feasible. By embarking
his type of project, students learn first hand the "agony and the ecstasy" of system development as they apply theory learned in
classroom to the real world. Development of the BBS taught the authors a great deal about the process of development, and
forced the principles of project management: project identification, resource determination and allocation, project planning,
lementation, and evaluation.

An area of great frustration to the developers was the lack of formal technical support for the project. Electronic communication
computer networking were areas in which the developers had little if any working knowledge. This meant that they were
endent upon others to provide this expertise. Busy schedules and too few available technical experts caused delays in the project
a realization that securing this expertise up front is important for development of this type of technical project.

562

7. Implications for Nursing

Students entering the field of nursing informatics must understand the concepts of electronic data communication, and be able to manage and develop nursing and health care information systems that utilize this technology. Use of a BBS in an academic setting teaches and reinforces these concepts. Students can be exposed to a practical application of a complex subject. This type of "learning by doing" can be a very effective tool used by faculty in an NI program.

Nurses entering the field of informatics are expected not only to manage information systems, but to develop systems. Knowing the principles of the systems life cycle is fundamental to the process. By developing and implementing a working system, students put into practice the theory they have learned in class. The lab is a very good place to learn what works and what does not work when developing a system.

A successful BBS in the NI program at UMAB will eliminate many of the barriers to accessing information that are present in the current environment. This includes students living substantial distances from the Baltimore campus, differing schedules with classes on a variety of campuses, and personal priorities that make it difficult for students to be on campus on a regular basis. This electronic form of communication will enhance the exchange of information, ideas, and research. Students and faculty will communicate differently than they do today. Those with a personal computer, modem, telephone line, and communication software will be able to access the BBS at any time. As participants become more dependent upon this type of communication, it will be vital that the system be managed properly to ensure that it is operative and contains information that is usable, timely, and of interest to the users.

8. References

[1] Heller BR, Romano CA, Moray LR and Gassert CA. The implementation of the first graduate program in nursing informatics. *Comput Nurs* 1989, 7(5):209-13.

[2] Cook M. The identification of communication flow patterns and information needs of an organization. In: *Nursing Informatics '91*, Hovega EJS, Hannah KJ, McCormick KA and Ronald JS (eds). New York: Springer-Velag, 1991:59-6

[3] Peters TJ and Waterman RH. *In search of excellence*. New York:Macmillian, 1982.

[4] Hekelman RP. The electronic city: A vehicle for providing patient information. *Comput Nurs* 1988, 6(4):183-4.

[5] Armstrong ML. Techniques for networking in the computer world. *Nurs Clin North Am* 1985, 20(3):517-25.

[6] Kittle PW. Putting the medical library online: Electronic bulletin boards...and beyond. *Online* 1985, May:25-30.

[7] Skaggs BJ. Moving from corkboard to an electronic bulletin board for nursing. *Am J Nurs* 1989:858.

[8] Keller P. Nurses, computers and "What is a BBS?". BBS Message download, *Nurselink*, April 18,1991.

[9] Skiba DJ and Warren CN. The impact of an electronic bulletin board to disseminate educational and research information to nursing colleagues. *Nursing Informatics '91*, Hovega EJS, Hannah KJ, McCormick KA and Ronald JS (eds). New York: Springer-Velag, 1991:704-9

[10] Brennan PF. Home care nursing via computer networks: Justification and design specifications. In: *Proceeding for the Twelfth Annual Symposium on Computer Applications in Medical Care*. Greenes RA (ed). Los Angeles, CA: IEEE Computer Society, 1988:805-9

[11] McLeod R. *Management information systems*. New York: Macmillian. 1990.

Nursing Informatics: An International Overview for Nursing in a Technological Era
S.J. Grobe and E.S.P. Pluyter-Wenting, eds.

An Effective Approach for Providing Nursing Students with HIS Access

Mascara CM[a] Bartos CE[a] Nelson R[b] and Rafferty D[c]

Nursing Informatics Specialist, University of Pittsburgh Medical Center, DeSoto at O'Hara Streets, Pittsburgh, Pennsylvania 15213.

Manager, Nursing Informatics Department, University of Pittsburgh Medical Center, DeSoto at O'Hara Streets, Pittsburgh, Pennsylvania 15213.

Assistant Clinical Administrator, University of Pittsburgh Medical Center, DeSoto at O'Hara Streets, Pittsburgh, Pennsylvania 15213.

Many hospitals have been hesitant in providing access to the hospital information system for non-employees who have a short-term relationship with the organization. Nursing students are one group of caregivers who may be denied access to the hospital's computer system. The practice of limiting a student's access to clinical information can be incongruent with the educational mission of the hospital. As the use of information technologies in nursing expands, nursing students must be given the opportunity to learn the use of electronic data and information as they learn to care for patients. This paper describes a pilot project that addresses this problem in a large university medical center.

1. Introduction

The mission statements of health care institutions state their service, education and research responsibilities. In achieving their educational mission, many institutions provide clinical experiences for nursing students. Often these hospitals hesitate to provide these non-employees with computer access.

Nursing students learn how to care for clients by providing patient care. To provide this care, students require access to general health care information, hospital policies and procedures, supplies and patient data contained in the medical record. All of these requirements can involve access to a computer. The increasing use of computers in health care settings makes it imperative that these institutions now address a whole new range of educational issues.

The Institute of Medicine's recent report, The Computer-Based Patient Record: An Essential Technology for Health Care [1], demonstrates that decisions related to student access are imperative. The report recommends that health care professionals and organizations adopt the computer-based patient record as the standard for medical records related to the patient. Students need access to the patient's automated medical records in the same way that they have access to traditional paper records.

The increasing use of automation to support nursing tasks or procedures further demonstrates the need for student access to hospital computers. This includes the use of bar codes for the identification of patients as well as supplies, automated medication administration records, automated order entry and results reporting. Without access to these automated systems, students are unable to learn many of the responsibilities inherent in nursing care. In addition, the student may not learn to integrate computer use with caring for patients.

While the need for this access is clear, the process whereby students are given computer access is poorly described in the literature. Soja and Lentz [2] describe the process used in one hospital in 1987. Through a cooperative effort between this hospital and two baccalaureate schools of nursing, a nine hour course was developed. The course covered the use of the computer for order entry and charting. Completion of the course and a competency test were necessary before a student was given access to the computer system.

Faculty at the University of Pittsburgh School of Nursing identified that student nurses completing their clinical experiences at the University of Pittsburgh Medical Center (UPMC) did not have access to any of the hospital computer systems. The UPMC includes two adult medical/surgical hospitals having a total of 1236 beds and a psychiatric hospital with 279 beds. A cooperative endeavor between the School of Nursing and the Medical Center was undertaken to develop and implement a four step process providing computer system access to student nurses at the medical/surgical hospitals. This paper describes that pilot project.

In the pilot, access was given to fifty-five senior nursing students prior to a six week clinical rotation. These students were precepted by a clinical nurse at the Medical Center. The students often had clinical experiences with a preceptor at times when a School of Nursing faculty member was not available. As a result, these students were in the position of asking the clinical nurse to perform all computer activities, or even to allow the student use of the nurse's computer access. These inappropriate solutions to this problem inhibited the student's ability to learn all aspects of the nursing role or violated the institution's policies regarding data security.

2. Collaborative Planning

The first step in developing this process involved collaborative planning between the School of Nursing faculty, the Medical Center's Information Services Division and the Nursing Informatics Department. These groups identified five key issues. Table 1 outlines the issues, potential approaches and key discussion points identified by this group.

Table 1
Issues and Approaches in Providing Students with HIS Access

Issues	Approaches	Discussion
1. Level of Access	a. Students receive the same access as professionals.	a. May allow functionality that is not appropriate for students. Minimal programming effort is required.
	b. Students receive a more restricted access previously developed for other personnel.	b. May or may not appropriately limit student access. Minimal programming effort is required.
	c. Students receive a more restricted level of access using a unique access developed for them.	c. An appropriate level of access for students can be developed, but analysis and programming time is required.
2. Data Security	a. Assign each student a unique user ID.	a. Provides close control over access. Ongoing use of this system may be time consuming, with frequent changes in the student population due to clinical experience rotations. Must be maintained by hospital programming personnel.
	b. Use generic student user IDs that can be temporarily assigned to one student.	b. Involves less time for ongoing maintenance as students rotate. Requires maintenance of a separate data base of student information.
	c. Documentation of student agreement of HIS confidentiality policies.	c. Employee confidentiality statements may need to be rewritten in order to be appropriate for students and faculty.

Table 1
Issues and Approaches in Providing Students with HIS Access

Issues	Approaches	Discussion
3. Responsibility for Student Instruction	a. Provided by hospital employees using hospital facilities.	a. Information regarding the HIS would always be current. May not be feasible for employees to always perform these additional duties.
	b. Provided by school of nursing faculty.	b. The faculty must be kept informed of changes to the HIS. Computer instruction could be integrated with curriculum.
4. Instruction Format	a. Lecture.	a. Does not allow students to see the HIS, making learning difficult. Does allow flexibility and easy update of information.
	b. Demonstration.	b. May provide adequate information, depending on the complexity of the HIS.
	c. Self-Learning.	c. May provide the best use of the instructor's time and the hardware. Students may learn at their own pace.
	d. Hands-on Experience.	d. Students learn computer skills most easily with hands-on experience. Requires that each student have access to the hardware.
5. Evaluation	a. Evaluation of student learning.	a. Students should demonstrate competency before they are given access to the on-line hospital computer.
	b. Evaluation of the benefits of student access.	b. Obtained following a student's clinical rotation.

3. Pilot Implementation

The first issue is defining the appropriate level of access for students. This access should allow them to obtain pertinent patient information while restricting their functionality with inappropriate activities. At UPMC, the Licensed Practical Nurse functionality provided access to all patient data but did not allow order entry. This fit the needs of the students, since students in this setting are not responsible for transcribing orders.

The second issue involves data security. The approach should maximize the ability to track student access of patient information while minimizing programming time. It was decided that each student would be assigned an individual computer system account or user ID. Since each student would only be using their user ID for a short time, generic student user IDs were established. These are temporarily assigned to a student for use during the clinical rotation, then reassigned to another student during the next clinical rotation. Students select their own passwords. A data base of students assigned to UPMC is maintained. This record includes the student's name, school of nursing, instructor, dates of the clinical rotation and the generic student user ID assigned.

In addition, it was determined that the UPMC Receipt of Computer Password/ID document needed to be revised. This document is signed by employees upon receipt of access to the HIS and indicates agreement to the organization's guidelines for maintaining the confidentiality of patient information. Consequences of misuse of patient information may result in disciplinary action including termination of employment. Since these consequences are not appropriate for students or faculty, two additional documents were developed.

The third issue is the approach to providing the necessary concurrent computer education. Training was initially provided by the Medical Center's Nursing Informatics Department. The Medical Center's training facilities were utilized. Plans call for shifting these responsibilities to School of Nursing faculty at a later point. In this way, the computer instruction can be incorporated into the curriculum.

The format for instructing the students is similar to the format used when instructing hospital employees. This includes a combination of lecture and self-learning. Hands-on experience is also provided, with each student having access to a computer terminal throughout the class. A two hour class was developed that reviews all of the HIS functions available to the students.

The final issue is the evaluation of the pilot project. Evaluation was performed from several perspectives. The extent of student learning was measured with a post test. The test required that students use perform specific functions using the HIS to locate patient information. Students were also given a course evaluation form to complete following their computer instruction. A final evaluation of the students' perception of the benefit of computer access was performed following the clinical rotation.

4. Pilot Evaluation

The average student score on the post test was 99.9%, indicating that the students were able to use the HIS effectively. The results of the course evaluation indicated that 88% of the students felt that the instructional methods used were excellent, while 12% felt that they were satisfactory. None of the students believed that the instructional methods were poor. Students were also asked to rate the usefulness of the computer course on a scale from 1 to 10, with 1 indicating no usefulness and 10 indicating maximum usefulness. Fifty-six percent of the students indicated a usefulness score of 9 or 10, with a mean usefulness score of 7.7.

Following their clinical rotation, 39% of the students indicated that they used the computer access on a daily basis. Another 39% indicated that they never used this access during the entire six week rotation. The remaining students indicated that they used this computer access seldom or occasionally. When asked if having HIS access was beneficial, 68% of the students responded affirmatively, while 32% responded negatively. It is interesting that some of those students who never used their computer access still indicated that having this access was beneficial.

5. Ongoing Student Access

The final step of the four part process is providing nursing students with HIS access on an ongoing basis. This pilot project demonstrates that it is feasible to provide students with hospital computer access. The approaches used regarding level of access and data security can easily be transferred into a method for providing computer user IDs for a larger group of students. School of Nursing faculty can use the same training facilities and instruction methods to teach other students how to use the hospital computer system. In this way, all nursing students may be given the computer access that is vital to their role in the clinical setting.

6. References

[1] Dick R and Steen E (eds). *The Computer-Based Patient Record: An Essential Technology for Health Care*. Washington, D.C.: National Academy Press. 1991.

[2] Soja M and Lentz K. Development of a Hospital-based Computer Users' Course for Student Nurses. *Comput Nurs*. 1987, 1:15-19.

Nursing Informatics: An International Overview for Nursing in a Technological Era
S.J. Grobe and E.S.P. Pluyter-Wenting, eds.

567

Development of Technological Access
for RN Degree-completion Students at Distant Learning Sites

Hodson K[a] Hanson A[b] and Brigham C[c]

[a]Coordinator of Instructional and Computer Resources, School of Nursing, Ball State University, Muncie, IN

[b]Assistant Professor, School of Nursing, Ball State University, Muncie, IN

[c]Assistant Professor, School of Nursing, Ball State University, Muncie, IN

The presentation describes a plan to provide technological access for approximately 400 RNs enrolled in six televised nursing courses in an outreach program that spans a number of strategic areas of a Midwestern state. Portable computers will allow students to search and retrieve library resources, communicate with instructors, advisors, and classmates as well as other health care personnel, and use multiple on-campus resources via datalink access. It is anticipated that successful implementation of the project will provide a usable blueprint as well as a communication channel for other distance learning programs throughout the nation.

1. Introduction

The growth of national electronic networks for education and research will significantly impact the nursing profession [1]. Increased electronic connectivity will improve the ability of the end-user researcher and educator to access data processing capabilities and other researchers/faculty electronically to advance scholarship and educational activities [2,3,4]. The significance of the trend can be a reconceptualization of the research and educational process. It is, therefore, critical that nursing students and nurse clinicians become knowledgeable users of electronic networks which focus on quality health care delivery.

2. Problem Statement

It is critically important that the practicing professional, such as the registered nurse, be prepared to plan and deliver client services which utilize all the capabilities of our increasingly technological age. Improving technological access for students at the distance learning sites who, for the most part, received their basic education in a pre-computer era is critical to enabling these students to retain their current positions of leadership in their profession and to become active participants in a world increasingly networked through communication channels.

3. Background

Ball State University is a major provider of distance education programs to the State of Indiana, offering full degree programs and numerous general studies and in-service courses by one-way television and two-way audio. The Indiana Higher Education Telecommunications System (IHETS) has been the primary carrier of distance education services in the state and has been successful in delivering higher education directly to the employment site or to an educational site near the student's home.

The distance learning program of the School of Nursing illustrates the effect of this television/audio transmission of coursework on the lives of professional nurses across the state. With a total enrollment of approximately 500 students, the BS in Nursing completion program serves about eighty registered nurses each semester. The majority of people enrolled in these televised degree programs are in their late twenties to early forties, have family and home responsibilities, and still need to complete their degrees for professional growth and job security. The opportunity for televised courses has been a most effective and efficient method for the transmission of didactic content.

The University has adopted as a general goal that distance learning students should have, through electronic media, a learning environment that is comparable to the on-campus technological environment. They should have electronic access to services, resources, faculty, and other students, including at least the following: library card catalog and indexes, state and national databases, electronic mail and bulletin boards to communicate with other students, instructors, advisors, administrators; on-line access to instructional software; assistance with software and hardware questions; and on-line access to administrative procedures, including advising, registration, and career counseling.

4. Project Description

A proposed solution to the delivery of computing and networking services to this distance learning student will be pilot tested in the Spring semester, 1993-94 with Nursing 309, the first of five courses in the RN-Completion program. Each of the approximately 30 students in the course will be provided with a suitable laptop computer fully configured with all necessary storage, applications software, instructional software, and communications capabilities. They would be able to do much of their course-related computing communication in a stand-alone environment. However, for data communication two approaches will be considered. First, the student laptops will be equipped with data-compression, error-checking modems that permit baud rates of up to about 40,000, compared to the 2,400 to 9,600 commonly available now. Ball State will provide 800 numbers and networked modems so that students can dial into university computer systems as needed. Second, where greater network speed is needed, other institutions could, at very low cost, provide a small number of ethernet ports, in a library, for example, where distance learning students could simply attach their laptop computers and log into Ball State networks over Internet and the IHETS Data Network. Most of Indiana's higher education institutions are equipped to make such network access available at moderate cost to the institution.

5. Projected Outcomes

The project has a direct effect on improving the classroom learning environment for students. Implementation of this project will create a futuristic reconceptualization of the classroom learning environment for the distance learning student. They will have unprecedented electronic access to services, resources, faculty, and other students, including at least the following: library card catalog and indexes, state and national databases; electronic mail and bulletin boards to communicate with other students, instructors, advisors, administrators; on-line access to instructional software; assistance with software and hardware questions; and on-line access to administrative procedures including advising, registration, and career counseling. The improved technological access for students at the distance learning sites who, for the most part, received their basic education in a pre-computer era will enable them to become active participants in a world increasingly networked through communication channels.

The project is an innovative approach to deal with an existing problem or issue. Nurse educators must address the issue of technological access for the distance learning student [5,6]. Currently, Ball State University broadcasts classes to ninety-seven different locations throughout Indiana and Kentucky. Ball State currently reaches 38% of the 253 sites in Indiana that are set up to receive classes via the state's educational television system. The potential for growth in the area is evident from these figures. In fact, the office of Continuing Education reported enrollments for the 1990-91 year to be 678 full time equivalents (FTEs). Continuing Education plans to increase enrollments by ten percent each year to reach 1499 FTE by the academic year 2001-02.

The proposed model for computer and information resource access at the distance learning sites eliminates most of the site support problems experienced in the past and reduces considerably the costs for computing support at the remote sites. Successful completion of the pilot project would establish protocols for technological access sharing across the state of Indiana. It is an innovative approach in line with university, state and federal incentives. Information processing skills will become an integral component of the student's approach to learning.

The project involves collaboration among faculty. This project is the culmination of work completed by a university-wide, multi-disciplinary committee. Faculty members from the two disciplines with a large number of distance education students, College of Business and the School of Nursing, will work collaboratively with personnel from University Computing Services to successfully implement the pilot phase of the project during 1993-94. The pilot project will then establish the framework for further implementation of the university-wide plan to other disciplines involved with distance education learning.

The project has potential for initiating long-term change. For example, implementation of the pilot project will facilitate student access to the State University Library Automation Network. It will foster complete development of computer aided instruction software to instruct students how to access on-campus computers. The pilot project will establish the framework for the university to provide distance learners with adequate computing resources without requiring a trip to campus.

6. References

[1] Gore A. The Information Infrastructure and Technology Act. *EDUCOM Rev* 1992, September-October, 27-29.

[2] Krumenaker L. Electronic Universities: Learning on your time. *PCToday* 1991, October, 57-60.

[3] Carr CWN. On the Leading Edge. *OUTPUT* 1992, 12:9-13.

[4] Sholes W and Edwards V. Distance Learning: Innovative Applications of Telecommunication Technology. *J Med Technol* 1992, 3:28-30.

[5] Twigg CA and Brennan, PF. Distance Learning and Support through Computers. *Nurs Educ Microworld* 1991, 5:9,11.

Nursing Informatics: An International Overview for Nursing in a Technological Era
S.J. Grobe and E.S.P. Pluyter-Wenting, eds.

570

Descriptive Study of Computer Mediated Communication of Graduate Nursing Students: Implications for Nursing Practice and Life Long Learning

Lyness AL[a] Raimond JA[b] and Albrecht SA[c]

[a,b,c]School of Nursing, University of Pittsburgh, Pittsburgh, PA 15261, USA

This descriptive study sought to reveal satisfaction and behavioral outcomes of graduate nursing students as a result of computer mediated experiences in course assignments. The subjects were a convenience sample consisting of 45 graduate nursing students at a large northeastern university. Based on instructions about computer mediated communication and an orientation to the computer system, students initiated exchanges to attain learning objectives through specified electronic communication. During the term, students entered a series of email messages to their classmates related to the assignment via a computer based group alias. When the assignment was completed, students responded to an Evaluation Survey instrument to gauge their agreement about the effectiveness of computer mediated communication for attaining the learning objectives and their satisfaction with the method. Quantitative data were analyzed using descriptive statistics. Qualitative data from the communicated messages and the responses to the open ended questions in the Survey were analyzed by content analysis. Students have responded to the assignment positively. They appreciated the time and location independence for sending and receiving class messages. In addition to being able to attain the learning objectives by computer mediated communication, students showed an awareness of self pacing and self direction. Collaboration among classmates was supportive while also showing critical thinking and leadership skills. Implications for nursing practice and life long learning can be identified from the findings of this study.

1.0 Background

A master's course on applying nursing theory to practice has been offered at a northeastern U.S. university school of nursing for more than a decade. This was a core course taken early in the student's program; often during the first or second term of enrollment. This was the first time that students in this course had an assignment using computer mediated communication.

2.0 Computer Mediated Communication

Computer mediated communication has been gaining attention among educators because of the potential benefits suggested by early research efforts. In a Speech Communication Project at the Pennsylvania State University, a traditional group discussion course was re-designed to operate via computer mediated communication. Findings indicated more frequent student contact with instructors, high level of course approval by students, and group output that equalled or excelled that of the traditionally taught course [1]. The investigators of the present study had used computer mediated communication for discussion previously and had found it an effective format and strategy for student learning [2], [3], [4], [5].

3.0 Descriptive Research

3.1 Specific Aims. The purpose of the study was to determine the subjective experiences of graduate nursing students as they participated in class communications with classmates toward learning objectives on a group email system. The communication assignment was carried out after the subjects had an opportunity to study a self learning module about using the email system. The study aimed to: 1. Identify cognitive, affective, and situational components of the experience perceived by students who were involved with computer mediated instruction and 2. Reveal students' perceptions of satisfaction and effectiveness in developing communication skills via the computer.

3.2 Methodology. This study used a descriptive design to provide an accurate portrayal of events and to discover meanings and frequencies of occurrences surrounding the experience of computer mediated communication. A descriptive design is particularly useful when little is known concerning the research area. The study was approved by the institutional review board. In the present study, two sections of the course offered in the fall of 1992 were included for a total of 45 subjects. The subjects represented a convenience sample. After students voluntarily agreed to participate, the investigators explained the procedure involved in the study.

3.3 Instruments. The instruments included two researcher designed surveys: a Computerized Information Management Assessment and an Evaluation Survey. The Computerized Information Management Assessment provided an objective measure of the participants' familiarity with computer hardware and computer software, as well as providing demographic information. The Evaluation Survey consisted of 26 questions using a Likert type scale. In this study, 4 choices were given: strongly disagree (1), disagree (2), agree (3), and strongly agree (4). The last part of this survey included several open ended questions. Participants also received a set of instructions that outlined the assignment and a self-learning module on using electronic mail.

3.4 Treatment of Data. All subjects' replies on the Evaluation Survey were coded to assure anonymity. The data were entered and verified on a computer. SPSS-PC was employed for the objective questions. The open ended questions and the content of the email messages were entered into the computer using word processing software and underwent content analysis to generate themes.

3.5 Procedure. At the beginning of the course, subjects were given printed instructions of an assignment which involved sending four rounds of email messages to classmates for purposes of discussion. Each message sent by a student was sent to a class alias. This meant that when a student sent a message to the alias, every student in the class and the instructors received the message. If a student was uncertain about the procedure, an individual message could be sent to the instructor for clarification.

The printed instructions explained that a video, *Discovering the future: The Business of Paradigms* [6], concerning change and innovation would be shown to the class. After seeing the video in class, the students were to consider this question adapted from the video: "What today is impossible to do but if it could be done would change fundamentally the use of theory in nursing practice in the future?" After reflecting on this question, there were four rounds of communications to classmates for discussion using: a) brainstorming; b) prioritizing; c) summarizing; and d) extracting key ideas or themes. Each round of communication began on a specified date that was given in the printed instructions. At the end of the term a debriefing was held to summarize the experience and to answer any questions of the subjects.

3.6 Email Assignment. During the four rounds of messages, a number of themes emerged. In the first round, brainstorming, students gave many ideas; often innovative ones, about how theory could be used more effectively in nursing practice. Examples included: a) videotaping nursing interventions to playback and to study where theory had been applied; b) use of computerized communication forms to provide frequent continuing education offerings to nurses in relating theory to practice; these communications could be interdisciplinary; c) making a concerted effort to have respect for others' new ideas and encouraging innovation in nursing; and d) encouraging nursing staff to read research articles focusing on testing nursing theories in the work place. In the second round, prioritizing, the list of priorities centered on: a) having more independence in practice; b) educating nursing students from the beginning with many examples of the use of theory in practice; c) viewing change as positive; and d) applying a pluralistic approach to the use of theory in practice.

In the third round, summary, these ideas emerged: a) the importance of studying relationships among autonomy in practice, education and research; b) need to overcome the inertia about entry into practice; and c) open and increased communication between nursing and society. The fourth round, theme identification, yielded these ideas: a) the importance of supporting the use of theory in nursing practice; b) the importance of increasing communication among nurses and others regarding conceptualizations and their use.

4.0 Results

The Evaluation Survey was administered to the 45 subjects at the end of the course. The Likert type items could be categorized into three parts: instructional emphasis, email emphasis, and learning transfer potential, that is, ability to use this learning in other situations. Students responded favorably to these items. For the 9 items addressing the assignment as an instructional method with clear objectives and so forth, the mean was 3.1. For the 10 items addressing the assignment with an email emphasis the mean was 2.99. For the 7 items addressing ability to transfer this learning to other situations, the mean was 2.79. Since the range of the response set was 1 (strongly disagree) to 4 (strongly agree), a moderately favorable overall response to the assignment can be concluded.

The results of the open ended questions were analyzed with an independent content analysis by each researcher followed by a group meeting to verify the themes. The resulting themes from these questions included the following: Question One - What did you particularly like about this assignment? *Themes*: a) Communication for purposes of discussion via the computer was new learning; b) Time and location independence to do the assignment was appreciated and convenient; c) The use of email is very relevant to nursing today. Question Two: What improvements need to be made? *Themes*: a) The large number of messages from all of the students in the class had some repetition; perhaps break the topic into parts for subgroups to work on to reduce repetition; b) Give more expansive instruction on email. Following the second open-ended question some students made additional comments such as these: a) It was fun; b) Stimulated thought; c) It [the assignment] made me sit in front of a computer and use it.

In this class the majority of the students had little experience with computers. Additional questions dealing with computer use prior to the computer mediated communication assignment revealed the low experience. Responses showed that only 20 % (n=11) of the students used a computer one time a week or more. Only 13 % (n=7) of the students had access to a home computer with a modem. Only 9 % (n=5) of the students used communication software one time a week or more.

4.1 Interpretation. The researchers determined that even though most of the subjects had little experience with computers, with some preparation they could achieve a discussion via email. The use of a group alias for the class made possible the messages going to all the subjects and researchers at once. Brainstorming, prioritizing, summarizing and theme extracting was also possible. Besides the moderately favorable view by the subjects about the assignment, there was an appreciation of the need to learn more skills of this type by the subjects. In response to the suggestions made for improving the assignment, the researchers have strengthened the email orientation and are working on ways to divide the topics for subgroups to discuss.

5.0 Implications for Nursing Practice

5.1 Collaboration. Much of the work of nursing involves collaboration. With the help of an email system, nurses on a unit, within a hospital, or other locality could communicate easily about areas of practice where problems or questions exist. They could have a goal oriented discussion with inputs given at a time and place that is convenient. Nurses could collaborate on research projects directed toward clinical practice with other nurses and with members from other disciplines.

5.2 Information Intensive Environment. The work setting in which nurses practice is becoming increasingly information intensive. Nurses must have knowledge of electronic technology to manage information concerning care of patients effectively. Every opportunity nurses have to engage in electronic communication will strengthen skills in dealing with masses of information.

6.0 Implications for Life Long Learning

6.1 Electronic Capability of the Future. In the future, electronic communication will travel over the Integrated Services Digital Network (ISDN). The ISDN is essentially digital telephone links, capable of 64,000 bps communication [7]. The ISDN will eliminate the need to convert data for transfer over phone lines and will provide end to end digital connectivity [8]. This increased capability will provide great access to information over a life's career to persons prepared in the knowledge and skills of electronic communication.

7.0 Summary

This descriptive study of computer mediated communication by graduate nursing students showed that learning objectives can be achieved through this format. Given adequate preparation, students can have a productive discussion via the computer. The spin offs are in the increased computer skills that are acquired by the students and their increased confidence that is developed. The recognition by students of the benefits of time and location independence to communicate with others, is important for adult learners. This form of communication will increase in the future as nurses gain skills in this area and find more applications for practice.

8.0 References

[1]   Phillips, G.M. and Santoro, G.M. Teaching group discussion via computer-mediated communication. *Communication Education* 1989, 38: 151-161.

[2]   Lyness, A.L., Albrecht, S.A. and Raimond, J.A. *Social learning and electronic communication: Development of a conceptual framework.* Annual Convention of the Association for Educational Communications and Technology, Showcase of Achievement, AECT '92, Capture the Vision, Washington, D.C., 1992, 1-8. ERIC Pub. No. ED344580.

[3]   Lyness, A. and Raimond, J. Computer mediated communication of graduate nursing students: Implications for enhancing the diffusion of new knowledge in nursing. In: *Proceedings of the West Virginia Nurses' Association 1992 Research Symposium: Creating Excellence, Nursing's Agenda for Change.* Wang, J.F., Simoni, P.S., Borgman, M.F. & Nath, C.L. (eds.). Charleston, WV: WVNA, 1992: 17.

[4]   Lyness, A. and Raimond, J. Electronic communication to promote concensus building skills: An innovative teaching strategy. *Journal of Nursing Education* 1992, 31: 331-334.

[5]   Lyness, A., Raimond, J. and Albrecht, S. Electronic consensus building: Implications for nursing education and research. *MEDINFO '92.* Lun, K.C., Degoulet, P., Piemme, T.E. & Rienhoff, O. (eds.) Amsterdam:North Holland, Elsevier Science Publishers, 1992: 1016-1020.

[6]   *Discovering the future: The business of paradigms* (2nd ed.), Charthouse Learning Corporation, 1989: video.

[7]   Dvorak, J.C. and Anis, N. *Dvorak's guide to PC telecommunications.* Berkley, CA: Osborn McGraw-Hill, 1990.

[8]   Wigand, R.T. Integrated services digital networks: Concepts, policies, and emerging issues. *Journal of Communication* 1988, 38: 29-49.

Nursing Informatics: An International Overview for Nursing in a Technological Era
S.J. Grobe and E.S.P. Pluyter-Wenting, eds.

574

Intercollegiate Electronic Networking Among Nursing Graduate Students

Mikan KJ[a] Hodson KE[b] and Thede L[c]

[a]*School of Nursing, University of Alabama at Birmingham, Birmingham, AL 35394-1210, USA*

[b]*School of Nursing, Ball State University, Muncie, IN 47306, USA*

[c]*School of Nursing, Kent State University, Kent, OH 44242-0001, USA*

Opportunities for electronic networking are rapidly becoming available at many academic institutions. This paper reports the results of an exploratory research project which was designed to evaluate the use of electronic communication networking among nursing graduate students located at three different universities in the United States. Subjects were enrolled in a computer course and were expected to use electronic communication networks to access on-line databases and discussion groups through the use of Internet. Data were collected using researcher-developed instruments. The multiple uses, problems, and issues of intercollegiate electronic networking among graduate students identified in this exploratory study have relevance for other nursing programs which are considering the initiation and integration of electronic communication for scholarly interactions within and between graduate nursing education programs.

1. Background

Many opportunities for networking among professional colleagues are now possible with the recent advances in computer technology. Electronic communication networking is a rapidly growing field that provides opportunities for scholarly interactions [1]. A major advantage of electronic communication is its ability to facilitate interaction between individuals who have similar interests but who are geographically separated. Advances in technology and participation in networks by academic institution in the United States have made it possible for academicians to have free-access to wide-area (even global-area) networks [2] [3]. While these electronic resources are now available in most academic institutions, electronic networking among professional nurses is in its infancy [4] [5]. Uses of electronic communication by nurses on a regular basis for scholarly purposes have just started. The reasons for this are many, but the net results are that very few nurses in the United States use electronic communication for scholarly interactions.

2. Purpose

The purpose of this exploratory research project was to initiate and evaluate the use of electronic communication networking among nursing graduate students located at three geographically distant universities in the United States. The three universities that participated in this study were Ball State University at Muncie, Indiana; Kent State University at Kent, Ohio; and University of Alabama at Birmingham in Birmingham, Alabama. Collectively, the researchers wanted to (a) explore the use of electronic communication networking; (2) provide intercollegiate sharing of information between graduate students; (3) identify uses, problems, and issues associated with intercollegiate student exchange of electronic information; and (4) identify ways to promote intercollegiate graduate student electronic communication in the future.

3. Participants

Three nursing professors, each located at a different school of nursing in a different state, were responsible for teaching a graduate course on the use of computers in nursing at their respective institution. Part of the "course" expectations was for students to learn to communicate electronically. It was hoped that once graduate students learned how to use electronic communication as students, they would continue to use it as graduates.

Each of the academic institutions participating in this study had access to Internet, a worldwide electronic communication system that is available 24 hours a day, 365 days a year. Thus, Internet became the electronic linkage between and among the three groups of graduate students. Because of the vast public distribution (in the United States) of microcomputers, modems and Internet, students at all three schools were encouraged to access `Internet from their home, work, or school--wherever and whenever they wished. Designated terminals were available within each institution for students who did not have an Internet access outside of the academic institution.

4. Methodology

Subjects for this study were graduate nursing students enrolled in an introductory computer course offered at each of the three participating institutions by three different nursing professors. All three institutions, beginning in 1993, included content and hands-on learning exercises on the use of electronic communication in their respective computer course. At two of the sites, the course was an elective while it was a required course at the third institution. Data reported in this paper were collected from subjects enrolled in the nursing computer course offered at one of three participating institutions between January and September 1993.

All students who enrolled in the computer course were expected to communicate via electronic mail (E-mail). Students' and instructors' E-mail addresses were shared among the participating institutions and students. Students were taught to send, receive, save and delete electronic messages as well as how to upload, download, and perform "housekeeping" tasks with their files. The graduate students were encouraged to communicate with their student colleagues electronically.

In addition to personal E-mail communication, all students were expected to use electronic communication networking to access two different on-line databases: Sigma Theta Tau International Nursing Library whose purpose is to make nursing research available to the nursing community, and ETNet, a national conference network which is a part of the National Library of Medicine in Washington, DC. Additionally, one of the professors created, using the ListServ software, a private on-line discussion group for practicing nurses. Although other ListServ electronic nursing interest groups did exist, none of them focused on situations encountered by practicing nurses.

5. Data Collection

Data were collected using researcher-developed instruments which focused on the uses, problems, and issues of electronic communication by graduate students. A questionnaire was administered to all subjects at the beginning of the course. This instrument (Electronic Networking Technologies) collected data about the subjects' use and knowledge of electronic networking technologies and their ideas about electronic communication purposes and applications. Another questionnaire was administered at the end of the course.

The second data collection instrument was the Electronic Communication Access Record which the students were asked to complete whenever they accessed the electronic network. This log identified the type of networking activity they engaged in during each network access. Depending on which network the student accessed, additional data were collected about the nature of the type of information exchange. For example, if they accessed an on-line database, graduate students were asked to indicate if, during that interaction, they sought information (read only), gave information (answered a question), prosed a problem (opinion), or shared solution to a problem (solution). Students could check multiple activities per network interaction.

At the conclusion of each network interaction, students were asked to indicate if they were able to complete their interaction without having electronic difficulties, if they were able to "sign off" without difficulties, and the amount of time spend on the computer during each interaction. Students were also asked to identify any problems they had encountered during the electronic interaction and what they gained from their interaction. These data were collected immediately following the students' electronic communication network interactions.

6. Data Analysis

Data collected at all three sites were combined for purposes of data analysis. Between January and September, 1993, a computer "course" for graduate students which contained a section on electronic communication was offered a total of five times at the three participating institutions. The total graduate student enrollment during the five times the "course" was offered was 43. Due to differences in length of the computer "course" at each of the participating institutions, no between institutional comparisons were made with the data.

Analysis of the pre-course questionnaire data revealed that a high percentage of the nursing graduate students had no prior experience in using electronic communication, but they had had experience in using computers for clinical practice, self-instruction, word processing, library searches, and statistical analysis. A few students reported prior use of a computer to communicate with friends or family (E-mail) using a commercial service while even a fewer number of students reported any prior experience with E-mail with professional colleagues, electronic document/file transfer, electronic conferences or discussion groups. A few students reported using electronic resources such as the local on-line library. None of the students reported prior experience in searching off-campus libraries or accessing electronic publications or journals. Only a few indicated they had every used Internet/BITNET before. None of them had ever accessed ETNET, Sigma Theta Tau, or ListServ prior to taking the course. The pre-course questionnaire indicated that students were able to identify uses for electronic communication within their individual health care institutions. The post-course questionnaire revealed that the learning experiences provided in the graduate computer course expanded the students' understanding of electronic communication to include information available outside their health care institution and provided them with beginning skills in how to access this information. Additionally, the course strengthened the students' beliefs in the value of electronic communication within an institution and created a desire to have the ability to access informational resources beyond those available at their local institution.

The forty-three graduate students accessed electronic communication a total number of 232 times during the course. Data analysis of the Electronic Communication Access Record revealed that the most frequent use of electronic communication was for E-mail. Reading personal messages was the most frequent activity followed by sending messages to known colleagues. Reading messages sent by the ListServ groups to which they subscribed was the next most frequent activity.

Most students were able to complete their interaction without any electronic difficulties and were able to sign off. The average amount of time spend on the computer during a session was 53.86 minutes ($\underline{SD}$ = 52.064). The number of times students accessed the network ranged from 5 minutes to 360 minutes. The averaged number of reported uses of electronic communication by students was 4.3 and ranged from 1 to 15 ($\underline{SD}$ = 2.2882).

7. Findings

The findings indicated that a high percentage of the nursing graduate students had no prior experience in using electronic communication, encountered technical problems (after they were once on Internet) infrequently, accessed a variety of information items on the network, and generated numerous potential uses for electronic communication within nursing.

The types of problems students encountered during the networking sessions related to learning the mechanical operation of the communication software and computer/modem at the local level, the slowness of the computer response time (baud rate of transmission plus slow mainframe response time), and information anxiety [6], i.e., understanding the structure of information in different databases, comprehending the vast amounts of information systems already available, and being orientated to where the student was in the electronic information universe. Students also had difficulty relating the available electronic information networks and resources to the practice area of nursing, i.e., most electronic information sources did not directly relate to nursing practice. Overall, the types of problems students encountered were user, not technical problems.

As novice users of on-line electronic communication databases, students found electronic sources of information to be "unfriendly", i.e., on-line "help" was either not available or the user directions were unclear. The students reported gaining insight into the variety of electronic information sources available, being pleased to learn that they could communicate electronically, and being able to engage in collaborative scholarship with other nurses.

Incidental findings during the study were that students who lived and worked at some distance from the participating institutions were enthusiastic about the possibilities of electronic communication being a help in meeting some of their personal and professional communication needs. Those who could access the network using a home computer used electronic communication more than those who did not have network access from their homes. Nevertheless, all students saw electronic communication as a means to contact other nurses, decrease their feelings of isolation, and solve nursing problems. Students were positively motivated toward the use of electronic communication and became aware of the wealth of information available with the touch of a key. Students seem to appreciate the fact that their professors were nurses who were able to translate the world of electronic networking into something that was relevant to the professional practice of nursing.

During the initiation and evaluation of the electronic communication learning experiences, the professors identified some problems and issues that needed to be addressed when teaching graduate students the use of electronic communication systems in the future. The professors found that students needed (1) assistance in arranging for access to Internet off-campus without having to pay for long distance phone calls (i.e., many of the graduate students lived at a distance from campus), (2) a comprehensive orientation to electronic communication, (3) to be supported during their initial interactions on the networks, and (4) to be encouraged to share questions, concerns, items of interest, or problems with others whom they did not know personally. Detailed handouts (often in the form of manuals) were needed for each of the networks the student were expected to access. Frequently the guides supplied by the "Network" agencies were confusing and had to be re-written for local use. The professors found that students who had some familiarity with word processing, although beneficial, had to switch to line, rather than text editing when using many network systems. Participation in on-line conference was not done as frequently as the instructors wished; there seemed to be a reluctance on the part of the graduate students to either offer advice or ask questions of others on the network. Also, because it is difficult for students to absorb so many new things that are so different, students needed learning and processing time. To become comfortable with the concepts, methods, processes, and usages of electronic communication takes time. The professors learned that electronic communication can not be accomplished in one or two class sessions.

From an intercollegiate standpoint, minimum difficulties were encountered outside of differences in course scheduling (two institutions offered the computer course on a semester basis and one institution offered the computer course on a quarter basis). This meant that some graduate students only had ten weeks in which to interact with the network while the majority of the students were able to interact with it over a 16 weeks time span. However, in the future as more nurses become comfortable with networking, electronic interactions by nurses will not be confined to the length of a "academic computer" course, but rather they will be on-going discussions of nursing situations that all nurses can use as they wish 24-hours a day. Now that nurses can communicate electronically worldwide, it is hoped that graduate nurses (and students) will consider requesting and offering help to colleagues all over the world.

Another incidental outcome of this exploratory research study was that once the electronic communication activities of the students became known to other graduate nursing programs in the United States, the authors received requests from other schools of nursing to allow their graduate students to also participate on GRADNRSE. As a result of this project and the interest of nurses both in education and practice, the GRADNRSE discussion group has been made public.

Other issues that the professors found that needed to be addressed when developing an intercollegiate electronic communication course were: (1) socializing students into the use of electronic communication for scholarly interactions, (2) teaching electronic communication netiquette [7], and (3) helping students get access to Internet after the course was completed so that they could continue to use the knowledge and skills learned and apply them in nursing practice.

8. Summary

Electronic communication offers many opportunities for nurses to share scholarly information worldwide. The technology is in place. The information sources are available. What is missing are nurses who are knowledgeable users of electronic communication. Based on the researchers' successful preparation of a cadre of knowledgeable electronic communication users at each of their respective institutions, it is hoped that the findings of this study will inspire other nursing programs worldwide to consider the initiation and integration of electronic communication within and between nursing education programs. Then and only then will nursing have a true worldwide electronic network of scholars.

9. References

[1] Harrison TM and Stephen T. On-line Disciplines: Computer-Mediate Scholarship in the Humanities and Social Sciences. *Computer Hu* 1992, 26:13-25.

[2] Krol E. *The Whole Internet User's Guide & Catalog*. Sebastopol, CA: O'Reilly & Associates, Inc. 1992.

[3] Lynch DC and Rose MT. *Internet System Handbook*. Reading, MA: Addison-Wesley Publishing Company, 1993.

[4] Schneider D. Internet: Linking Nurses, Scholars, Libraries. *Reflections* (Sigma Theta Tau International Newsletter, Spring, 1993) 19:9.

[5] Skiba, D. Collaborative Tools. *Reflections* (Sigma Theta Tau International Newsletter, Spring, 1993) 19:10-12.

[6] Wurman RS. *Information anxiety*. New York: Doubleday, 1989.

[7] Kehoe BP. *Zen and the Art of the Internet A Beginner's Guide*. Englewood Cliffs, NJ: Prentice Hall, 1993.

Nursing Informatics: An International Overview for Nursing in a Technological Era
S.J. Grobe and E.S.P. Pluyter-Wenting, eds.

Development of a thesis via electronic mail at a remote educational site

Thiele JE

Intercollegiate Center for Nursing Education, Washington State University, West 2917 Ft. Wright Drive, Spokane, WA 99204, USA

1. Introduction

In 1990, the University of Guam (UOG) contracted with Washington State University (WSU) to offer the WSU Master of Nursing (MN) program to a single cohort of students at the University of Guam School of Nursing, Mangilao, Guam, USA. The program was offered over four consecutive summers to accommodate the academic year workload of the prospective students. As on the home campus at the Intercollegiate Center for Nursing Education (ICNE) in Spokane, Washington, a total of 39 semester hours of credit was required to complete a Master of Nursing degree. A core element of this program is a strong research component, culminating with a required thesis.

The original plan was that faculty from WSU would travel to Guam each summer to provide the classroom instruction. During the fall and spring semesters, the students were to continue to develop their thesis with guidance from the home campus faculty. Development of a thesis requires multiple interactions between students and faculty from proposal stage to completed thesis. The 6,000 miles distance between the students and faculty increased the complexities of this difficult process. Other difficulties encountered with a site so distant from the main campus included differences in cultures which effected perceptions of time and priorities [1]. Lack of face-to-face communication during the time faculty were on their home campus hampered efforts to reinforce classroom instruction and introduce new information. Geographic isolation of students enabled other more immediate concerns to take priority over available study and research time. Full-time employment of all of the students also further limited their time to continue their studies in a self-directed manner after completing a summer session. Ten graduate students completed the first component of 10 semester credits of course work during the 1990 summer session. The first day of class revealed that the students were not sufficiently computer skilled to write their papers using a word processor. The vision of electronic transmission of messages and files seemed like an impossible dream. The instructor who taught the research course spent time with individual and groups of students helping them with word processing.

The faculty who traveled to Guam that first summer quickly realized that continuing communication with the students during the academic year was going to require monumental efforts. Mailed information required up to 12 days to reach Guam. Telephone and Fax use quickly consumed the allocated budget for communications. In addition, the 32 hours time difference (eight clock hours, plus a day gained or lost by crossing the international date line) made telephone calls very difficult to plan at a time that was convenient for both parties. To facilitate more effective communications, funds for an international program development project were obtained from WSU. The purpose of this project was to establish technological links for critique, collaboration, and dissemination of research between students on Guam and faculty in Spokane. A major portion of these funds were to be used for training of students and faculty at both sites in use of electronic communications.

Faculty were available to the students for a maximum of eight weeks of the summer, a factor which further compounded the communications difficulties. In addition, when a student is in the final phases of a thesis and preparing for presentation of the finished research study, multiple revisions are often required within a time span of five working days. Electronic transmission via computer between Spokane, Washington, USA and Guam was envisioned as a means for expediting thesis development and revisions and meeting graduate school deadlines. Computer naivete on the part of both faculty and students emphasized the need for training to facilitate use of computers in education [2].

2. Barriers to the Project

At the time of the project, BITNET was identified as "THE international academic network linking higher education and research organizations together"[3]. Communications to Guam required Spokane based faculty to access BITNET and address their E-mail to Cupertino, California where the connection was made to a commercial system named PORTAL. From there, messages were transmitted to Hawaii and then on to Guam. While a seemingly easy electronic task, the system experienced frequent malfunctions [4].

During the first year of using this system, the electronic address of UOG changed three separate times. On the other hand, once students on Guam completed the initial training session, they were literally left on their own to cope with changes in the electronic addresses and transmission routes.

3. Training of Faculty

Staff members in the libraries at University of Guam and the ICNE were identified as being skilled in use of electronic transmissions. At both sites, these individuals provided a portion of the instruction in sending electronic mail. Eight faculty in Spokane were taught to use BITNET to communicate with colleagues. Although these individuals grumbled, participation in the training sessions was followed by sending messages such as meeting notices to one another. As each person became more comfortable with this process, they expanded their sphere of communications to include colleagues at other universities [5].

4. Training of Students

As part of the ICNE's effort to provide instruction and direction for research by the students, the ICNE library provided many needed research articles. Lists of needed materials were sent electronically between the two libraries. At the start of the second summer session, one of the librarians provided instruction to the Guam students in use of an international network. Following several sessions, the students were able to send a message electronically if someone assisted them. One student became quite skilled in this process and aided other students with their learning. The vision at this time was that students would expand their computer use to include accessing other data bases and electronic resources [6].

To continue these communications, students enrolled in a special topics course which required electronic communications during the academic year when faculty were back on their home campus. While not an "on-line course", computer exercises and reporting of activities were incorporated into the course design [7]. However, between the second and third summers, UOG moved equipment into a new computer facility. During this time, electronic communications capabilities were totally unavailable to the students.

5. Results

As a result of the training and practice provided, faculty in Spokane began using electronic communications. From this small core of eight faculty, the use of E-mail has expanded to approximately 30 faculty. A second series of training was required when the ICNE connected faculty computers by means of a local area network. However, the training required consisted of approximately 30 minutes. Today, these individuals are accustomed to arrange meetings, sending notes, and communicating with one another on a daily basis by E-mail. An increase from 2 to 30 users in 2 and one-half years is significant progress in learning to communicate electronically.

Of the students, one became very proficient and four others became comfortable users of electronic mail. The remaining five improved their skills in using a microcomputer, but did not venture forth into electronic mail. As a major goal of this endeavor was to establish computerized communication linkages, success is indicated by the number of messages transmitted. The individuals who learned to use e-mail acquired a skill which they now use to communicate around the world. To date, however, not a single thesis has been transmitted electronically. For the fourth and final summer session, the nine students who remained in the program traveled to Spokane, Washington. There they completed clinical specialization training at various regional hospitals and finished writing their theses under the direction of the faculty. While in Spokane, the students who learned e-mail were be able to communicate directly and inexpensively via computer with friends in Guam. Graduation occurred for six of the remaining nine students.

6. Implications

As the ICNE plans to establish its MN program at distance education sites within the state of Washington, the lessons learned in Guam are being studied. Current projections are that the first course to be offered at a new distance education site is to be computer usage, including mainframe communications between sites. In addition, computer conferencing by students and faculty is planned as part of the initial course. The faculty have become strong supporters of computer messaging and are developing a wide range of innovative uses for electronic communications. In addition,. faculty are no longer willing to leave the learning of computer usage to chance. Deliberately teaching students the skills needed to program success is viewed as a critical first step in planning and implementing distance education, even for distances less than 6,000 miles.

7. References

[1] Thiele J, Higgs Z and Busch K. Have program, will travel! *NursEducator* 1993, 18:1, 21-25.

[2] Davie, LE. Facilitating adult learning through Computer-mediated distance education. *J Distance Ed* 1988, 3:2, 55-69.

[3] Bowers, M. *BITNET user guide*, 1990. Eastern Washington University: Client services.

[4] Solomon MB. E-mail: A primer for academics. *THE Journal* 1990, 18:10, 64-65

[5] McKenzie R and Santoro G. A guide to establishing mainframe computer-mediated communication between a host and a remote site. *THE Journal* 1990, 18:10, 63-66.

[6] Kilby S, Fishel C, and Gupta, A. Access to nursing information resources. *Image: J of Nursing Scholarship* 1989, 21:1, 26-30.

[7] Harasim L, Teaching and learning on-line: Issues in computer-mediated graduate courses. *Can J Educ Commun* 1987, 16:2, 117-135.

Nursing Informatics: An International Overview for Nursing in a Technological Era
S.J. Grobe and E.S.P. Pluyter-Wenting, eds.

582

The Development of a Large Local Area Computer Network in a School of Nursing

Slaughter R E

School of Nursing, University of California at San Francisco, 500 Parnassus Ave., San Francisco, California, 94143-0604, USA.

This paper discusses the rationale for, and design and implementation of a large local area computer network (LAN) within a school of nursing. Approximately one year before the project began, school administration undertook a study of communication within the school. With four academic departments and a Dean's Office housed on different floors in the same building, it was determined that interdepartmental communication was hindered by the physical characteristics of the building itself. In its central supportive role, the Dean's Office proposed a study of intra- and interdepartmental electronic linkages to coincide with the remarkable growth of personal computing activity within the school. After a full year of hardware and software evaluation by the school's Office of Research, a recommendation was made to school administration to implement a Token Ring LAN. Because of the university's yearly funding limitations, the project was designed with a phased installation plan. In the first year of implementation, a prototype or "pilot" network was installed to further evaluate the LAN hardware/software choices that had been made. The pilot network consisted of 25 workstation nodes and spanned five floors within the school. In short, LAN performance exceeded expectations, and those involved in the pilot program were highly enthusiastic. The current network connects approximately 185 workstations. The primary network application is electronic mail, which has greatly enhanced and continues to facilitate communication within the school. Shared database applications and ease of software maintenance are further benefits of the current LAN. While present applications are primarily administrative, plans are currently being made for educational applications as well as wide area network linkages.

1. Introduction

During the Summer of 1987, the dean of the University of California, San Francisco (UCSF), School of Nursing, asked for a study of communication within and outside the School. It was the perception of School faculty, staff and administration that the physical architecture of the six-story building, on UCSF's main Parnassus campus, was limiting the flow of information and general communication both within the School and between the School and other campus schools, departments, and facilities. Concurrent with this study, the School was in the midst of expanding its use of microcomputer technology, which began some five years earlier, in 1982. At that time, the advent of the IBM Personal Computer and its proliferation into higher education markets, brought the opportunity to provide faculty and staff with powerful new tools which promised to increase productivity and generally enhance the educational and administrative environments. Because the UCSF School of Nursing was one of the first schools of nursing in the world to integrate microcomputer technology into curriculum, administration and faculty productivity on a large scale, the IBM Corporation took great interest in the activities that were taking place within the School. Toward the end of the Summer of 1987, IBM sponsored a full-day retreat for School of Nursing faculty and administration at its San Francisco headquarters. The purpose of the retreat was to assist the school in planning for the continuing growth and utilization of computing technology in its academic and administrative endeavors. It was during this retreat that IBM representatives discussed the development of mini- and microcomputer-based local area computer networks as powerful tools for increasing productivity and as potential solutions to the School's communication problems. As a result of the retreat, there was widespread agreement within the school to determine the feasibility and cost of developing a local area network within the school. The School's Office of Research, Evaluation and Computer Resources was given the task of developing a feasibility study.

2. Comparison and Evaluation of Network Architectures

Because of the School's early entrance into the microcomputer technology arena, the predominant computing platform within the school was IBM/Compatible. It should be noted that the School of Nursing was the first of the four schools on the UCSF campus (the others being Medicine, Pharmacy and Dentistry) to embrace the widespread use of microcomputer technology. To some extent, this situation was problematic, in the sense that there was no expertise on campus for network development, and certainly no resources. The campus' own Computer Center, in fact, had not yet begun investigating local area networks.

The two predominant local area network architectures were (and still are, to a large extent) Ethernet and Token-Ring[1]. The latter had only recently been introduced by IBM, who announced that the Token-Ring network architecture would be the strategic choice for networking its computer systems. While Ethernet networks were somewhat plentiful in academic environments[2,3], and tended to be associated with Unix-based systems, Token-Ring networks were rapidly being developed in business environments with multiple computing platforms[1,4,5].

The choice between the *tried and true* Ethernet architecture and the relatively new Token-Ring architecture was an extremely difficult one. The two architectures were fundamentally different in many respects[1,2,3,4,5]. First, the cabling strategies used for each system were quite different. Ethernet networks used coaxial cable, and were typically arrayed in a linear, bus-type topology. In order to build a cost-efficient cable plant, the network developer had to make very specific long-range decisions about the future growth of the network. Token-Ring networks, on the other hand, used twisted-pair cable, which was similar to regular telephone cable. Further, most Token-Ring networks were cabled in a *ring* or *star* topology, which made it very easy to design the cable plant in a modular, somewhat dynamic fashion.

Second, the protocols used to transport information throughout the network were extremely different in the two network architectures. Ethernet networks used a *collision detection and avoidance* protocol[2,3]. Under this protocol, network requests were handled on an ad-hoc basis. If two workstations, for example, requested the same network service at exactly the same time — reading a file from a file-server, for example — the network would detect a collision and instruct each workstation to resubmit its request with a tiny random hardware delay imposed, which would have the effect of avoiding the collision upon resubmission of the request. When network traffic was light, very few collisions occurred, and things proceeded smoothly. When network traffic was heavy, however, numerous collisions were possible, and the entire network segment would potentially slow down while trying to manage all the collisions. Token-Ring networks, on the other hand, handled network traffic in a considerably more orderly way[4,5]. A *token* (or special data packet) was circulated around the network, from workstation to workstation. When a workstation needed a network service (e.g., requesting a file to be read from a file server), it would wait for the token to pass by. When the token arrived, the request was attached to the token, which would then circulate around the ring until it reached its destination, at which point the request was delivered, and the token was freed and sent on its way around the ring again. In this way, there were absolutely no collisions, because no request would ever be made without the token. Further, because of this token-passing protocol, network performance was extremely predictable since it was not a function of random network traffic[5].

Third, network speeds differed greatly between the two network architectures. Ethernet networks ran at 10 Megabits per second (MBPS), which was 2.5 times faster than the 4MBPS rate of Token-Ring networks. It was widely speculated, however, that although Token-Ring networks ran at a slower speed, the orderly token-passing protocol would provide greater throughput in large (>200 workstations) networks because the Ethernet protocols would be necessarily dealing with the chaos that would ensue from massive numbers of collisions[1].

Fourth, the costs associated with the two architectures were different. Because of the relative simplicity of the Ethernet hardware and protocols, and the relative complexity and novelty of the Token-Ring hardware and protocols, Ethernet hardware was approximately half the cost of Token-Ring hardware. This was further exacerbated by the fact that only two vendors offered Token-Ring hardware at the time, IBM and Ungermann-Bass, who co-developed the technology.

Despite all of the inherent differences in the two architectures, the end result was virtually identical from the end-user's perspective. Both Ethernet and Token-Ring appeared to deliver network services comparably well. The decision was made to adopt the Token-Ring architecture for several reasons. First, all cabling contractors that examined the School of Nursing building felt that it would be far more cost-effective and flexible to install twisted-pair cabling in a ring/star topology. Each room in the School would be directly connected to a central *patch panel*, or wiring console, located in the existing telephone wiring closets located on every floor of the building. Then, each patch panel would be connected to a central patch panel on the third floor of the building, in the rear of the Dean's Office. In this wiring configuration, each floor could run independently of the others, or as a part of the entire school ring. This arrangement would offer excellent trouble-shooting capabilities, in that each floor could be taken out of the ring in an effort to isolate a problem to a specific floor. Additionally, the cable plant design was highly modular, allowing for different areas to be cabled at different times, and as budget allowed, without affecting network performance.

Second, because of the inherent orderliness of Token-Ring networks, they are generally thought to be considerably easier to maintain and trouble-shoot than Ethernet networks which must be carefully balanced to distribute network traffic evenly. Further, in the event of a cabling problem, Token-Ring networks are known to be extremely robust because the protocols will actually reverse transmission of the data in an effort to reach a destination on the other side of the cable break — something that Ethernet networks cannot do.

Third, the size of the School's local area network was projected to be slightly over 200 nodes. Without the widespread use of Ethernet repeaters, bridges and careful balancing, it was felt that network traffic might saturate the bandwidth of an Ethernet network, and degrade the overall performance of the network as it grew. Token-Ring, on the other hand, seemed to provide adequate bandwidth for the School's needs well into the future.

Fourth, despite the short-term difference in hardware cost favoring Ethernet, it was felt that the inherent ease of maintenance in a Token-Ring network would result in a smaller level of long-term personnel support — a fact, incidentally, which has indeed proven true relative to other UCSF campus networks. In short, the School's needs and physical characteristics seemed to be well matched to the Token-Ring architecture.

3. Development of Prototype Network

Before committing to the expense of cabling and networking the entire school, a small 20 node network was constructed in the school. This prototype network was designed to involve all of the School's academic and administrative departments. This was done for two reasons: first, it provided an opportunity to generate interest and commitment to the project throughout the school; and, second, it provided a way for building the cabling infrastructure for the entire building at one time, which was considerably more cost-efficient.

The hardware chosen for the prototype network was manufactured by Ungermann-Bass, primarily, and IBM secondarily. The network operating system chosen was Novell Advanced NetWare 286. Although several other operating systems were evaluated, including IBM's PC Lan Program, Ungermann-Bass' NetOne, and 3Com's 3+, NetWare proved to be the most reliable and delivered better performance than any of the others tested.

One of the early successes of the prototype network was the implementation of an electronic mail system. cc:Mail software was chosen, as it was clearly the best product of its kind on the market at the time. Within the first week after installation, the 20 workstations on the prototype network had passed over 800 e-mail messages! Almost instantly, faculty and staff began to see the improvement in intra- and interdepartmental communication. After only three months of operation, the prototype network proved so beneficial and reliable that a decision was made to expand the network throughout the School. The original cabling contractor was brought back in to finish cabling every office and conference room in the School of Nursing building. All of the cabling was financed by Dean's Office central administrative monies in an effort to provide the academic departments with a network infrastructure, or backbone, onto which they could attach their microcomputers at whatever pace was needed. Once the cabling project was completed, the Dean's Office, and two of the four academic departments made a decision to fully network all of their faculty and staff. The third academic department chose to attach approximately 20% of their faculty and staff to the network. The fourth academic department chose not to participate beyond what had been installed for the prototype network.

4. Current Network Configuration

During the first two years of full operation, the School's strategic network hardware vendor, Ungermann-Bass, proposed replacing the first-generation Token-Ring hardware with state-of-the-art hardware because of some reliability problems with the original products. The School was offered, and accepted, an extremely favorable arrangement to upgrade all of the original network hardware. All of the 4MBPS Token-Ring network adapters were replaced with 16MBPS adapters. All wiring concentrators were replaced with the Ungermann-Bass Access One intelligent network hub system. After the upgrade took place, the already successful School of Nursing network saw a phenomenal increase in speed and reliability. In addition, the network hardware management system installed with the upgrade, entitled "Net Director," was nothing short of amazing. The entire network is now maintained by the equivalent of one full time person, largely because it is so reliable and easy to maintain.

The number of Novell NetWare file servers has risen to six. All of the file servers are Dell 386 and 486 class systems with a combined disk storage capacity of approximately 2 gigabytes. One file server is located in each of the academic departments, one is in the Dean's Office and the other is in the School's computer laboratory. Each of the departmental file servers holds the licensed network software used by that department as well as thousands of user files and databases. The Dean's Office file server is the home of a school-wide information system called "Columbus," which contains faculty, student, and course information as well as grant tracking data, inventory, vendor information, and numerous other databases.

Electronic mail continues to be the most heavily used network application. Faculty and staff regularly use e-mail to communicate information and exchange files. The widespread use of e-mail has greatly diminished the physical barriers to communication that existed before the network was installed. The School's e-mail system has grown to 5 cc:Mail post offices — one in each academic department, and one master post office located in the Dean's Office, which routes mail between itself and the other departmental post offices using a cc:Mail Gateway router. The cc:Mail Gateway router also provides asynchronous access to and from other external cc:Mail Post Offices. This is used primarily to exchange technical support e-mail between the School and various vendors such as cc:Mail, Dell and Novell.

A major benefit of the network has been the ability to share resources, especially laser printers. In most departments, a few strategically placed laser printers have been attached to the network in an effort to make them available to a group of faculty and staff. One laser printer typically serves anywhere from 5 to 15 people. Additionally, a number of tape backup systems have been placed on the network. These backup systems are primarily used to backup network file servers, although they are also used to backup individual PC hard disks through the network. These tape backup systems have proven themselves absolutely invaluable, and have averted many potential data-loss crises, including a very large earthquake! Many faculty researchers frequently keep their current, critical data on the network file servers because of the safety and security provided by the nightly tape backups.

Network management is accomplished through the use of several critical applications. First, as previously mentioned, Ungermann-Bass' NetDirector software is used to monitor and manage the network hardware. This software keeps a database of the location and performance of every piece of network hardware. Using a graphical interface, NetDirector displays performance problems and network hardware faults with color changes in the icons representing the problematic hardware elements. This makes it extremely simple to isolate and correct problems within minutes of their occurrence. Second, a network-based menu system, developed by Saber Software, is used throughout the school. This ingenious system utilizes a matrix of application menus arrayed by users. In order to give a network user access to a new network application, for example, the network administrator simply places a check-mark on an application menu for a particular user, and re-generates that user's menu. At that moment, the user will see the newly added application added to their network menu choices. This process is normally accomplished remotely, from the network administrator's workstation, without ever having to make changes to the user's workstation. Finally, a suite of other software products are used to accomplish such tasks as counting and monitoring software licenses, taking inventory of network users' microcomputer hardware and software configurations, as well as many others.

Recently, the School's Computer Resources Laboratory was brought onto the school-wide network. The laboratory is widely used by UCSF students and faculty for instruction as well as independent study and computing. With the Computer Resources Laboratory on the network, the laboratory and network administrators can easily work with faculty and students in an effort to provide instantaneous access to a wide variety of software, including computer-assisted instruction, available on the entire network. The laboratory has proven extremely beneficial as a staff development facility, as well, and has enabled the school to provide training to virtually everyone in the school without incurring the expense of having to send faculty and staff to external courses and facilities.

586

5. Future Plans

In the last two years, the UCSF campus has begun development of a campus-wide fiber-optic network backbone. This backbone will, upon its completion, connect all of the campus' schools, laboratories, libraries, clinical facilities and administrative entities. Plans are currently underway to attach the School of Nursing network, which is, to date, the largest and most fully developed network on campus, to the campus backbone. The attachment will allow School of Nursing faculty, staff and students access to the multitude of new information sources that have been built into the new campus library, which opened in 1992, as well as unfettered access to the Internet, an international network of computer networks. Faculty will be able to communicate and exchange information and ideas with colleagues around the world as easily as they would with a colleague down the hallway.

Within the School of Nursing network, itself, new databases are being added and will continue to be added almost weekly. Faculty and staff can use the School's Columbus Information System to access information on a wide array of subjects. Because all of the databases are linked, a faculty or staff member can look up a faculty member's name and see such things as addressing information, grants on which the faculty member is involved, either as a Principal Investigator or as a co-investigator, committee assignments, student advisees, course information and teaching assignments, etc. Access to all information is controlled through an intricate security system which controls access to certain databases, and even fields within a database, depending on the identity of the faculty or staff member. Because the data is kept centrally, on the network, it is current and up-to-date.

6. Summary

The UCSF School of Nursing network is a vital and integral part of the School's academic and administrative environment. It is difficult, if not impossible, to envision not having it. Originally designed to improve the internal communication problems imposed by an "unfriendly" physical building structure, the network has far exceeded its original goals. The careful hardware and software evaluation undertaken by the School's Office of Research proved beneficial in the development of the network, as it averted a number of potentially costly mistakes. All of the hardware and software choices made early in the development of the network proved to be the right ones for the UCSF School of Nursing.

7. References

[1] Pujolle G. (Ed.). *High-capacity local and metropolitan area networks: architecture and performance issues*. Berlin; New York: Springer-Verlag, 1991.

[2] Hancock B. *Designing and implementing Ethernet networks*. Wellesley, MA: QED Information Sciences, 1988.

[3] Shotwell R. (Ed.). *The Ethernet sourcebook*. New York: North-Holland, 1985.

[4] Abrahams J. R. *Token ring networks: design, implementation and management*. Manchester: Blackwell, 1991.

[5] Townsend C. *Networking with the IBM Token-Ring*. Summit, PA: TAB Books, 1987.

Nursing Informatics: An International Overview for Nursing in a Technological Era
S.J. Grobe and E.S.P. Pluyter-Wenting, eds.

Creating a Twenty-First Century Learning Lab Environment for Nursing

Jones A [a] Skiba D J [b] and Phillips S [c]

[a]CliniCom, Inc., 4720 Walnut Street, Suite 106, Boulder, CO.

[b]School of Nursing, University of Colorado Health Sciences Center, Campus Box C-288, 4200 E. Ninth Ave., Denver, CO 80262 USA.

[c]School of Nursing, University of Colorado Health Sciences Center, Campus Box C-288, 4200 E. Ninth Ave., Denver, CO 80262 USA.

The creation of a Twenty-First Learning Lab environment for nursing students represents a colloboration between a School of Nursing and CliniCom, Inc., a clinical information system company. This collaboration has made it possible for our students to practice nursing within an automated clinical environment. Students enrolled in the Nursing Doctorate Program have the opportunity to document nursing assessments and care planning via a point of care terminal located within our Learning Laboratory. This Twenty-First Learning Lab environment clearly represents a first step toward the reconceptualization of the nursing curriculum and an exploration of new instructional techniques to facilitate the teaching-learning process.

1.   Background

In practice, nurses provide holistic and humanistic nursing care for patients. Over the last decade, nursing practice has become more diverse, information-intensive, and highly dependent upon a technologically advanced environment. A major component of this technological environment is the use of an automated information systems. Hospitals view clinical and management information systems as necessary components of providing quality, cost-effective patient care. The Secretary's Commission on Nursing strongly recommends the use of information systems in the clinical arena to better support nurses and to ameliorate many problems identified with the nursing shortage. Thus, nurses' knowledge of electronic information access, retrieval, management, and manipulation are critical components of contemporary professional nursing practice.

Other publications in recent years have strongly emphasized the need to effectively access and manage the ever increasing quantity of professional literature and patient-related information. According to the Pew Health Profession Commission [1], the quantity and quality of patient-related information available to, and required by health care organizations and professionals are exponentially increasing. More patient data is being collected as patients are now living longer and require longitundinal computerized records. According to the Commission, "the challenge for the future is in mastering information:finding effective ways to gather, store, retrieve, evaluate, distill and select information in ways that enhance cognition and support action rather than increase confusion and indecision" [1].

Nursing education has been responsive to this call for information mastery. In many instances, literature review skills, information management skills and computer skills have been incorporated into either pre-requisites or as part of the baccalaureate program. In most instances these skills are taught in research courses. Although there are several attempts to address this issue, many schools do not teach information mastery within the context of the clinical practice. There are exceptions. Several schools have been addressing the issue of preparing nurses to practice in an automated clinical environment. Some have incorporated the use of clinical information systems as part of the student's clinical rotation. This solution is very effective for those schools whose clinical sites have clinical information systems with nursing documentation and care planning. Some supplement this experience with "hands on" experiences with customized pc-based clinical databases.

For some schools, there is either a lack of clinical information systems available at clinical sites or the sites do not allow students to enter patient data into the automated system. For these schools, many have developed pc-based exercises that simulate clinical databases or have purchased the CAI program that simulates a hospital information system. For these students, the experience is less than desirable but it may be the only opportunity for practice in an automated environment. In all likelihood, these experiences are probably incorporated into the computer applications course or informatics electives being offered at the baccalaureate levels.

There are a few schools of nursing who have established learning centers with access to clinical information systems. The Columbia School of Nursing established a Technology Learning Center in 1991 that uses Hewlett-Packard equipment for basic clinical education in critical care, neonatal and anesthesia programs [2]. A similar center has been opened at the University of Iowa College of Nursing. The Informatics programs at the Universities of Maryland, Utah and Case Western Reserve all offer similar experiences for their students. These universities have established liaisons with various information systems vendors.

2. 21st Century Learning Lab Concept

In response to this growing demand, the School of Nursing recently formulated a long-range plan to prepare nurses to practice in the 21st Century. One curriculum long-range objective focuses on the increased use of instructional technologies as teaching-learning tools. An outcome of this objective is the preparation of nursing students at both the baccalaureate and nursing doctorate (N.D.) level to practice in an automated health care environment and to function in an information-intensive society.

This objective is an extension of the School's current computer focus. The School of Nursing course offerings incorporate computer exercises related to literature retrieval and data processing. Students also use computer assisted instruction (CAI) as an instructional methodology and use the computer as a productivity tool (word processing and spreadsheets). The focus has been on computer literacy and computer comfort. Although this approach previously met the student needs, it is time to move beyond the comfort level. A needs assessment conducted in the Spring, 1990 documented the demand for clinical information systems in the curriculum and increased access to computers. An elective, Nursing Information Systems course has been added to the curriculum. Although this is a well-received elective, there is still a need to incorporate this area into the curriculum. Information processing concepts and skills, critical thinking, and clinical decision-making in an automated health care delivery system need to be the focus for educating future nurses.

The establishment of a 21st Century Learning Lab clearly represents a reconceptualization of the nursing curriculum and the initiation of new instructional techniques to facilitate the teaching-learning process. Nursing students have an opportunity to learn clinical practice in an environment similar to their future work environment. Practicing in an automated nursing unit is simulated through the use of a bedside clinical information system and by remote access to a HIS. Students learn to complete nursing assessments, nursing notes, and care planning using clinical information systems. Students simultaneously learn to sustain the principles of caring by fostering a positive and supportive interaction with patients while using an automated-information system. In addition, students learn the economics of health care and the organizational context of the health care delivery system through access to a HIS.

To accomplish these tasks, the School of Nursing has been working cooperatively with CliniCom Incorporated, a Boulder-based clinical information systems company. The Clinicare system is a patient centered, client-defined clinical information system that offers a fast, accurate method for data input and retrieval at the point-of-care with the objective of improved clinical provider productivity and quality of patient care. CliniCom provides a comprehensive set of application software designed for use in the acute (medical/surgical, obstetrical, pediatric and respiratory) and critical care areas.

The company was a bit apprehensive about this collaborative effort but after numerous meetings with the nursing staff at the company, an agreement was reached. The University of Colorado Health Sciences Center, School of Nursing would purchase the touch screen hardware and remotely connect to the company's minicomputer to gain access to the CliniCom software and demonstration unit. In order to make this connection, a phone line with a modem was installed at both sites. The training and use of the software expenses as well as technical support would be the responsibility of the CliniCom company. One system was puchased initially to begin the project. After a few months, a second system was purchased. At the time of the second purchase, a new communication connection was needed to handle the newly designed wireless terminals. The new communication connection required the following items: a WINport (Wireless Interactive Network port device that receivers and transmits radio frequency communications) and a multiplexor (allow multiple devices to run concurrently over a single phone line and communicate between the WINport and the modem).

3. CliniCom System

The CliniCare point-of-care computer system allows a nurse to input and retrieve valuable and necessary patient data at the point-of-care rather than at the nursing station. CliniCom provides a comprehensive set of application software. Functionality of the software includes: vital sign documentation, medication and IV administration, admission history and assessment, on-going assessment, plan of care documentation, as well as review of all laboratory and radiology results and physician orders, with the proper interfaces.

The CliniCare software uses the following hardware: CliniView RF (radio frequency) portable terminal and an accompanying integrated bar code wand. The CliniView RF is a wireless, interactive terminal that combines radio frequency communications and full size, touch screen technology. According to CliniCom, the wireless technology allows providers working in different areas of the hospital instantaneous access to patient data not confined to a stationary terminal. The CliniView RF has been designed for care providers to input and retrieve information at the point of care. The bar code wand is used to screen medication administration and consumption of patient supplies, both of which are directly related to billing.

4. Nursing Doctorate Program

The bedside computer technology is currently integrated into the newly developed nursing doctorate (ND) program. The ND program prepares advanced practice nurses who are second degree students with baccalaureate degrees in disciplines outside of nursing. This innovative program provides a fruitful ground for curriculum development. The ND program is a four year program of study and clinical practice. The first three years combine rigorous academic study with exploration of traditional and non-traditional practice roles in health and human caring. The fourth year is a full-time professional clinical residency in sponsoring clinical agencies [3] .

The program is partially supported by the Helene Fuld Health Trust as a national demonstration program along with corporate sponsors throughout Colorado. The graduates of the program are being prepared to provide advanced clinical practice in a caring/healing professional practice model. The curriculum is designed to prepare graduates to demonstrate the competency to provide complex leadership, care management, advanced caring and healing modes, critical clinical and ethical judgments, and advanced technological decisions both in and out of institution.

The curriculum is designed to emphasize clinical practice. Students progress through a curriculum balanced with exploration of art and humanities and their role in care as well as the basic sciences and "state of the art" bio-technology. Emphasis is placed on processing complex information, the critical analysis and implementation in a new caring/healing delivery model. The faculty has piloted a variety of teaching-learning models in an effort to stimulate and reinforce critical thinking and self initiated learning. Diverse clinical models have been utilized (i.e. preceptors, clinical teaching associates, masters prepared clinical scholars, doctorally prepared clinical role models) as well as diverse classroom models (i.e. case studies, experiential laboratories in healing models, clinical exemplars, competency based skills learning, and computer databases for care management).

Within this curriculum, the point-of-care system is used in a variety of courses. For example, individual faculty have developed clinical cases that students use on the CliniView system and students also document their health assessments on the system. The students use the body system review component of the Care Planning System to document their health assessments conducted in the learning lab environment. The purpose of this exercise is twofold: to learn documentation skills and to practice the use of an automated clinical information system. The faculty are trying to eliminate the need for students to write 25 pages of care planning notes (a nursing education tradition) and to teach the students how to document in an automated environment. Faculty are also using the CliniView system as an automated version of their paper copies of case studies. Case studies of selected patients have been incorporated into several different courses. The students are even investigating methods to use the system for their residency requirements. These are just a few general examples of curriculum integration. Specific curricular materials will be shared at the presentation.

5. Future Plans

Although this is our current focus, an increasing number of faculty and baccalaureate students desire the same educational opportunities. At present, access by other classes is limited because the current hardware configuration and remote access connection is sufficient for a class of 12, not for classes of 30 students. In addition, several schools of nursing would like to have a similar system for its students. In order to accommodate these requests, the University of Colorado Health Sciences Center School of Nursing is writing a grant to establish a hospital unit with a full CliniCom system that would be available to other schools of nursing via the Internet.

6. Summary

In summary, the 21st Century Learning Lab supports our current nursing curriculum and complements the School of Nursing's philosophy of providing patient care within a humanitarian paradigm. To usher in the 21st Century, the University of Colorado Health Sciences Center School of Nursing, a leader in nursing education, has created a vision that balances human caring and technology. That vision would not have been possible without the collaboration of CliniCom, Inc. This collaboration represents a new venture for both organizations. This venture is a successful and fulfilling experience. Both organizations learned a lot about each other goals, cultures, values and environments. Cooperation, knowledge sharing, risk-taking and mutual respect for each other have been key ingredients for this fortuitous venture.

7. References

[1]   Shugars D, O'Neil E and Bader J. *Healthy America: Practitioners for 2005, an Agenda for Action for U.S. Health Professional Schools.* Durham, NC: The Pew Health Professions Commission, 1991.

[2]   Students Gain a Head Start with Technology Labs. *Nurs and Tech*, 1992, 3:3-6.

[3]   Watson J and Phillips S. A Call for Educational Reform: Colorado Nursing Doctorate Model as Exemplar. *Nurs Outlook* 1992, 40:20-26.

Section IV

EDUCATION

C. Attitudes toward computerization

Nursing Informatics: An International Overview for Nursing in a Technological Era
S.J. Grobe and E.S.P. Pluyter-Wenting, eds.

The Effect of Implementation of a Computer System on Nurses' Perceived Work Stress Levels and Attitudes Toward Computers

Diekmann J[a] Metoff D[b] Wanzer M[c] Zwicky D[d]

[a]Department of Health Restoration, School of Nursing, University of Wisconsin-Milwaukee, P.O. Box 413, Milwaukee, Wisconsin, 53201

[b,c,d]St. Joseph's Hospital, 2000 Chambers Avenue, Milwaukee, Wisconsin, 53210

Change is not always easily accomplished. In spite of the advantages of computers in saving time, nurses may not readily accept this technology. Finding out about nurses' attitudes before and after computerization is implemented could help to identify areas where education could be provided to nurses on other units to ease the transition to this new technology. The purpose of this study was to determine nurses perceived work stress levels and attitudes toward computers before and after implementation of a bedside computer documentation system. A pretest-posttest quasi experimental design was used in this study. The study took place on a 35 bed oncology unit at a Midwestern Hospital where computerization was implemented. A convenience sample of approximately 60 Registered Nurses who worked on a unit where computerization was implemented composed the experimental group. The control group consisted of approximately 60 nurses who work on randomly selected units at the same hospital where computerization was not implemented at this time. After human subjects approval, nurses in both groups completed: The Staff Burnout Scale for Health Professionals (SBS-HP), the Nurses' Attitude Toward Computerization Questionnaire (NATCQ), and a self-report questionnaire designed by the investigators to assess selected sociodemographic information. They repeated this procedure six months later. Descriptive statistics were used to describe the sample. The student's T-test and the Pearson product-moment correlation and the analysis of variance were used to determine answers to the research questions.

1. Background of Study

The expanding computer technology in hospitals has implications not only for patient care but also for the documentation of that care. In the next decade, computers in the clinical area will become common place. Computer technology will expedite data entry and data retrieval. Although the implications to nursing are not yet fully described, it is expected that nurses will have more time to focus on providing nursing care thus it is possible that the level of perceived job stress might be altered.

2. Statement of the Problem

Change is not always easily accomplished. In spite of the advantages of computers in saving time, nurses may not readily accept this technology. Resistance to computers may be based on simple resistance to change [1], apprehension of the unknown [2], impractical expectations of the computer [3], fear that the computer will replace human touch with rigid depersonalization [4], or a sense of powerlessness [5]. Finding out about nurses' attitudes and their work stress levels before and after computerization is implemented could help to identify areas where education could be provided to nurses on other units to ease the transition to this new technology.

3. Theoretical Framework

The conceptual framework for this study is an adaptation of Lewin's change model by Urban [6]. Kurt Lewin [7] described a model of conscious change having three stages; unfreezing, moving, and refreezing.

4. Research Questions

The following research questions were addressed in this study: 1. Will there be a difference in pre and post attitudes toward computer scores for nurses who work on units in which a computer documentation system is implemented? 2. Will staff nurses who work on a unit in which computer technology is implemented have a more positive attitude toward computers than staff nurses in a control group? 3. Will there be a difference in pre and post work stress scores for nurses who work on a unit in which a computer documentation system is implemented? 4. Will staff nurses who work on a unit in which computer technology is implemented report less work stress than staff nurses in a control group? 5. Is there an association between selected sociodemographic characteristics of staff nurses and the frequency of self-reported work stress levels? 6. Is there an association between selected sociodemographic characteristics of nurses and their attitudes toward computer technology?

5. Method

A pretest-posttest quasi experimental design was used in this study.

6. Sample

A convenience sample of 49 Registered Nurses who worked on two units where computerization was implemented composed the experimental group. The control group consisted of approximately 61 nurses who worked on randomly selected units at the same hospital where computerization was not implemented at this time. The names of the nurses were obtained from the head nurses of the various units. After human subjects approval, nurses in both groups completed: The Staff Burnout Scale for Health Professionals (SBS-HP), the Nurses' Attitude Toward Computerization Questionnaire (NATCQ), and a self-report questionnaire designed by the investigators to assess selected sociodemographic information. They repeated this procedure 6 months later.

7. Instrumentation

The research instruments included: The Staff Burnout Scale for Health Professionals (SBS-HP), the Nurses' Attitude Toward Computerization Questionnaire (NATCQ), and a self-report questionnaire designed by the investigators to assess selected sociodemographic information.

7.1 Staff Burnout Scale for Health Professionals [8].

The SBS-HP was used because it measures the current psychological, behavioral and physiological dimensions of the work stress syndrome. The score on this 30-item forced choice scale can range from 20 (absence of work stress) to 140 (a severe degree of work stress). Twenty items comprise the work stress scale and 10 items form a lie scale. The reliability for the work stress scale has been reported to be å 0.93 [9] and å .87 [10]. All items on the scale correlate with the total work stress score at the 0.001 level of confidence or less; the average item correlation with the total work stress score is 0.71. Several validation studies reveal relationships which statistically indicate that the SBS-HP identifies the presence or absence of work stress syndrome [8],[9],[11],[12].

7.2 The Nurses Attitude Toward Computerization Questionnaire [13] .

The NATCQ[11] consists of a 20 item Likert-type scale of statements related to computers and nursing. Content validity of the questionnaire was determined with the Index of Discrimination test. Of the 20 items selected for the questionnaire, 19 had index of discrimination scores greater than .48. These scores were considered acceptable by Stronge and Brodt for inclusion in the final questionnaire. The items are evenly distributed between six areas, identified from a literature review conducted by the authors of the instrument. These topic areas include: a) job security; 2) legal ramifications; 3) quality of patient care; 4) capabilities of computers; 5) employee willingness to use computers; and 6) benefit to the institution.

7.3 Sociodemographic Information Questionnaire.

This 17 item questionnaire, designed by the investigator will elicit data on selected demographic characteristics of the respondent including: (a) age, (b) gender, (c) educational preparation, (d) number of years in nursing, (e) present unit worked on, (f) length of time worked on present unit, (g) present staff position, (h) number of assigned hours to work per week, (i) number of overtime hours per week in the last month, (j) number of shifts worked in the past month, (k) number of missed days of work in the past month, (l) work related stress level, (m) overall feeling toward using a computer, (n) rate if exposure to a computer, (o) whether there is a computer at home, (p) level of comfort in taking a computer course, and (q) level of comfort in having a computer in the workplace.

8. Results

Members of the experimental and control group were, on the average, of a similar age, 32 years. They did not differ significantly in number of years in nursing, length of time on present unit, present staff position, number of assigned work hours per week or number of days of work missed. The two groups were similar in the highest degree obtained, in the shifts worked, and in gender. Similar numbers in each group reported owning home computers and taking computer courses.

Study questions 1 and 3 concerned possible differences between pre and post NATCQ and SBS scores for nurses who worked on a unit in which a computer documentation system was implemented. These questions were addressed using a paired t-test technique and with data only from the units which underwent computer implementation. There was no significant mean SBS change over time ($t=-.45$, $p=.66$) Levels of burnout did not change significantly during the computer implementation. There was, however, a significant decrease in mean NATCQ scores over the study period ($t=-4.85$, $p=.001$).

Study questions 2 and 4 concerned possible differences between NATCQ and SBS scores for nurses who worked on units in which a computer documentation system was implemented, contrasted with scores from a control group of nurses. These two questions were addressed with using a two-way repeated measures ANOVA technique. SBS scores for the computer units increased slightly over time, while those for the non-computer units decreased by approximately the same amounts. That is, stress levels increased on the experimental units and decreased on the control units. This difference between units was significant ($F=4.63$, $p=.04$). There was no significant effects due to time, or to the interaction of time and unit. Differences between the units' mean NATCQ scores were confounded by a significant interaction with the time factor. Mean differences existed between the units, but only prior to implementation (experimental = 74.51, control = 68.98). At the posttest period, the mean unit scores were much closer: 62.28 for the experimental units, and 66.23 for the control units.

Questions 5 and 6 concerned the possibility of relationships between selected sociodemographic variables and the dependent measures: work stress (SBS) and attitudes towards computer use (NATCQ). Relationships between the scores and all but a few of the sociodemographic variables were assessed using Pearson product moment correlation as the variables were fairly well distributed. Relationships between the scores and gender, educational preparation, present staff position, and experiential variables were examined using a one-way ANOVA technique.

There was an inverse correlation between age and stress. The more years subjects practiced nursing, the less stress they experienced. In addition, at the second measurement point, subjects were more willing to take a computer course. This correlated positively with the subject's attitude toward the computer. At measure one, subjects who had more stress had a more positive attitude toward computers. However, at measure two, the more stress subjects had, the less they liked computers. Also, the more positive attitude subjects had toward computers the more positive they were about using it. Those subjects who were more comfortable with computers in the workplace had a more positive attitude toward computers.

9. Discussion

A significant finding of this study is that nurses' attitudes towards computers became more negative over time on both the experimental and control units. One may speculate that this may have happened for those in the experimental group because learning this new method of documentation takes time. For those subjects who were in the control group, they may have heard about the difficulties in learning this new documentation system from nurses who were in the experimental group and this may have influenced their attitudes. Another interesting finding is that nurses in the experimental group felt significantly more stress six months after implementation of the computer documentation system. The reason for this is not clear. A third measure was attempted to determine SBS one year after computer implementation. However, due to attrition, the number of subjects with three complete sets of data was so small that data from the third data collection period could not be analyzed.

Implementing a computer documentation system represents a major change for staff nurses. Even though nurses in the experimental group had intensive training in how to use the new system, it appears that after six months of use, they continued to experience significantly more stress than those subjects in the control group. However, it is important to recognize that many other factors that were not assessed in this study may have contributed to their stress.

10. References

[1] Ball M and Hannah K. *Using Computers in Nursing.* Reston, Virginia: Reston Publishing Company, 1984.

[2] Hannah K. The Computer and Nursing Practice. *Nurs Out* 1976, 24:555-558.

[3] Beckmann E, Cummack B and Harris B. Observations on Computers in an Intensive Care Unit. *Heart and Lung* 1981, 10:1055-1057.

[4] Tamarisk N. The Computer as a Clinical Tool. *Nurs Mange* 1982, 13:46-49.

[5] Zielstorff R. Nurses Can Affect Computer Systems. *J Nurs Adm* 1978, 8:49-51.

[6] Urban N. *Critical care nurses' attitudes towards computers and change in these attitudes over time.* Unpublished Master's Thesis, Medical College of Wisconsin-Milwaukee, 1986.

[7] Lewin K. Group Decision and Social Change. In: Readings in Social Psychology. Macoby E, Newcomb T, Hartley E (eds). New York: Holt, Rinehart and Winston, 1958.

[8] Jones J. *Preliminary Manual: The Staff Burnout Scale for Health Professionals (SBS-HP).* Park Ridge, Illinois, London House Management Consultants, 1980.

[9] Jones J. Dishonesty, Staff Burnout and Unauthorized Work Break Extensions. *Pers Soc Psych Bull* 1981, 7:406-409.

[10] Paustian A. *Self-reported coping behaviors and responses to psychological stress in hospital staff nurses.* Unpublished Master's Thesis, University of Wisconsin-Milwaukee, 1988.

[11] Jones J. A measure of staff burnout among health professionals. Paper presented at a meeting of the Annual Convention of the American Psychological Association. Montreal, Quebec, Canada, September, 1980.

[12] Jones J. Attitude Correlates of Employee Theft of Drugs and Hospital Supplies among Nursing Personnel. *Nurs Res* 1981, 30:349-351.

[13] Strong H and Brodt A. Assessment of Nurses' Attitudes Toward Computerization. *Comp in Nsg* 1985, 3: 154-158.

Nursing Informatics: An International Overview for Nursing in a Technological Era
S.J. Grobe and E.S.P. Pluyter-Wenting, eds.

598

Nurses' participation in and opinions towards the implementation of computer based information systems in Swedish hospitals

Bergbom Engberg I, RN DMSc[a] and Rosander R, PhD[b]

[a]Borås College of Health and Caring Sciences, P.O.Box 55140, S-500 05 Borås, Sweden.

[b]University College of Health Sciences, P.O.Box 1038, S-551 11 Jönköping, Sweden.

The development of computer supported health and nursing care information systems can be both promising and threatening to new user groups. From a survey study of computer users in 69 major hospitals/districts in Sweden, we have analyzed user characteristics, computer education and influence on the implementation process. The majority of the users were nurses. They had been given little education and training, but had a positive attitude to the new technology. They had to a certain extent participated in the decision making process of computerization. The nurses have obtained valuable experience of systems in operation, which must be recognized in future development of health information systems.

1. Introduction

Nursing is a very information intensive profession. It is therefore quite logical that computer technology has provided effective and useful tools in daily nursing work all over the world. The development of computer supported health care systems in Swedish hospitals has, particulary during the last four - five years, involved and influenced nursing care. The system selection process, personnel training and the implementation of computerized systems are of great importance regarding the impact on nursing [1]. According to Glancey et al [2], the promotion of nursing's integral role in computerization, being the largest user population, will ensure the success of the system. The entire process is, however, not finished after implementation as stated by Allen [3]. She claims that after implementation the system belongs to the staff who are using it, and every effort to satisfy the staff's needs must be identified and used consistently in future plans.

A training and education program is compulsory before implementation in order to achieve user competence [4, 5]. The nurses must also be participants in the decision making process if the system is designed to facilitate their work and/or change the content of the work and their role in this. Many investigators have tried to assess the attitudes of nurses towards computerization, giving very important information for the development of future systems [6, 7].

During the last few years, clinics in hospitals in Sweden have become units with responsibility for their own budget. The medical and administrative head manager for a clinic is a physician. The nurse managers are usually participants in the management of the clinics - but not always. The nurse manager's role has also changed, from personnel administration for one clinic, to management development, usually for more than one clinic, with sometimes overlapping or undefined responsibilities. During the same period we have experienced rapid transition from manual to computer supported information handling in nursing care.

We have therefore carried out a survey study of the progress of computerization in Swedish hospitals as reported in another paper in this Proceedings [8]. The part of the study presented here focuses on the users and especially the nurses' opinions and their perception of participation in the decision making process and their possibility to influence the implementation and development of computer based systems.

The study also aims to describe the users suggestions for change and increased computerization which in their opinion should facilitate their work.

2. Method and subjects

A semi-structured self-report questionnaire was designed, consisting of questions about the level of computerization, system specifications, users′ participation in the decision making and implementation process, and their opinions about the advantages and disadvantages of computer based systems. The users' suggestions for future computer support were also requested.

The questionnaire was sent to 94 hospitals i.e. university, regional and county hospitals and a few minor hospitals. Some primary health care centrals are associated with hospitals and these therefore are also included.

The response rate was 69 hospitals (73.4%) from which 361 questionnaires were obtained. The questionnaries received were answered by a total of 377 individuals (25% males and 75% females). Of these 55 worked at primary health care centrals and 322 at hospitals.

Of the respondents, 127 were nurses or head nurses, 75 were nurse managers, 96 assistants or clerks to nurse managers, 32 physicians, and 47 had different kind of professions.

3. Results

3.1 User characteristics

Most of the respondents (n=283) had worked in their professions more than 11 years. Of these, 130 had more than 21 years of experience in their professions and about 16% of the respondents had less than 10 years.

More than half of the nurses had participated in short training programmes which focused on the application of the software, used in the system, see Table 1.

Table 1
Educational level among four user groups.

professional group	n	software training program, n(%)	basic computer training, n(%)	formal computer education, n(%)	auto-didact, n(%)
Nurses	127	74 (58)	39 (31)	12 (9)	2 (2)
Nurse managers	75	32 (43)	33 (44)	9 (12)	1 (1)
Assistants, clerks	96	43 (45)	43 (45)	9 (9)	1 (1)
Physicians	32	12 (38)	8 (25)	1 (3)	11 (34)

When a system or programme had already been implemented the respondents had usually been trained by staff who had been using the system in their work. The *software training program* before the application of a system or programme was usually from a few hours up to 7 days. The *basic computer training* included general knowledge of hardware and software, DOS functions and some programming. This training was usually paid for by the employer.

Formal computer education refers to education at college or university level and are not offered by the employer. The users expressed dissatisfaction with the short training programmes. No-one expressed satisfaction with the training programmes in the comments.

About half of the users reported that they had taught themselves to use the system or programme. Only those who were employed as computer coordinators and already had an education did not express discontent. The same was found among respondents who created their own programmes, for example some physicians.

3.2 Decision making

Physicians and computer coordinators also had, to a much greater extent, the possibility to decide whether or not a computer/PC and the necessary software should be bought and implemented. Of 361 computer users or user teams 30% (n=109) reported that the decision was made at the clinic level in the organization. Of all these decisions 57% were made by the physicians alone and 43% (n=47) by the physicians together with representatives from the nursing staff and/or from the administrative or financial area.

Forty-two (12%) respondents reported that users of the computers and software participated in the decision making process. Twenty of these included the head physician of the clinic, and 22 said that the users decided. The management group of a clinic was also found to be involved in the decision making process together with the management group for the entire hospital (30%). This group were usually the sole decision makers (70%).

Most of the respondents, 161 of 361, stated however that decisions about implementation of computers and software were made at a central level i.e. the county council. Of these 161, 15 said that physicians participated in this process, and 9 of the intended users. Eighty-seven of the respondents stated that decisions were made in different boards and committees within the county council.

As can be seen in Table 2, 63% of the respondents reported that they had no influence about the selection of computers/PC. About 33% (n=120) stated that they had influenced the selection of software. Development and change of the software in operation were by 57% (n=205) of the respondents seen to be possible. Of these, 28 said by continous contact with the producer or supplier they could develop and change the software to adapt them to the work. Seventy of the respondents stated that by giving their opinions and suggestions to a co-ordinating group for computers and software they could influence the development of the products used.

Thirty-one stated that by giving ideas to the head physician of the clinic or to a person with a co-ordinating responsibility they could influence development. Those who stated that they could not influence the software said that it was impossible due to lack of financial resources, or that they had tried, but nothing happened.

Thirteen of the respondents stated that they participated in the development of software and a further eight participated in the planning of purchases of software. A total of eight respondents produced their own software.

Table 2

The respondents opinions about their influence on decisions about selection of computers, software and the development or changes of systems and software (n=361).

	yes n (%)	no n (%)	partly n (%)	do not know n (%)	unanswered n (%)
influenced selection of computers	93 (26)	229 (63)	10 (3)	1 (0)	28 (8)
influenced selection of software	120 (33)	203 (56)	13 (4)	1 (0)	24 (7)
influenced changes/deve-lopment of software in operation	205 (57)	107 (30)	13 (4)	5 (1)	31 (8)

Of all the respondents 139 (39%) were engaged in different kind of groups or teams who co-ordinated, developed, planned for training and implementation, or participated in groups who evaluated the usage and adaptation of computers and software.

3.3 Opinions and suggestions

The respondents were also asked about their opinions about the way computers could be used to facilitate their work. About 30% (n=109) suggested that hospital information systems including patient classification, workload measurement, scheduling and staff planning could do so. Financial support systems were wanted by 43 of the respondents. Patient information systems were wanted by 53, and patient record systems including medical and nursing care records, care and operation planning, anesthesia report and bedside systems were wanted by 67 (19%) of the respondents. Service systems were seen to support the activities for 99 persons. Most of them, 53, suggested systems for facilitating communication between laboratories, kitchen, x-ray units, different stores, pharmacies and the units/wards.

Two respondents wanted expert systems such as advice service to patients given by nurses in an outpatient setting. Mainframe systems were usually criticized because of the inability to change and develop the system and that they were slow and time-consuming with poor overall comprehension. Others claimed that these systems were closed several hours per day and this did not help in working activities. Some of the advantages were the useful statistics and reports and that it was possible for more than one person to work with the system at the same time. Several respondents stated that these systems were out of fashion.

PC based programmes were criticized if the user had to shift distances between different parts of the programme and if the supplier did not give efficient and quick service. The respondents also wanted programmes which were adapted to their specific work, if they were supposed to facilitate and support the user activities. Some programmes were seen as time saving while others were not. However, the respondents sometimes found it more enyoyable to use computers compared to manual routines.

Lack of information, preparation before implementation, and support during and after implementation were the most common comments by the respondents. More basic education and training programmes were also suggested and needed. Several users expressed the need for small, flexible programmes which are capable of development. The manuals or handbooks were by the respondents found to be difficult to use and not written for ordinary users.

4. Discussion

The response rate, 361 questionnaires from 69 different hospitals/districts in Sweden, can be expected to give a fairly good picture of the computerization level at the present time.

Most of the respondents had more than 11 years of professional experience, which reflects the selection of respondents made by nurse managers. The respondents are mostly in positions as head nurse, nurse manager or assistant. Among the physicians, there is probably a preponderance of clinic head managers.

Physicians are to a greater extent participators in the decision process at several levels in the organization, than nurses and nursing staff. Decisions about hardware and software purchasing are mostly done at central level, where the nurses do not have any possibility to participate. It seems to be easier for the users to influence the decisions made at the clinic level.

The respondents perceptions about their possibilities to influence changes in, and development of, operational software are however higher. This was usually accomplished by supplying ideas and opinions to members of different co-ordinating groups or by contacts with the suppliers. This type of group aims to co-ordinate training, development and adaption of the system, taking users demands and requirements into consideration, which is vital as Bongartz [9] has stressed.

The training and computer education for the users is inadequate and unsatisfactory, which increases the risk for negative opinions and attitudes to system applications in nursing, and leads to limited use of the programmes [4, 5]. However, the respondents have given many valuable suggestions for further development and computerization of daily health and nursing care work.

602

The most important suggestions or requirements from our computer users concerns the level of competence and *the need for continued learning.*

As a challenge for the future, our nursing colleges and hospitals must provide an effective computer education at for example four levels, as suggested by Romano et al [10], in order to increase the nursing staff's level of knowledge about computers, computer applications and information technology.

5. References

[1] Hasset M. Computers and nursing education in the 1980's. *Nurs Outlook* 1984, 32:34-36.

[2] Glancey TS, Brooks GM and Vaughan VS. Hospital information systems. Nursing's integral role. *Comput Nurs* 1990, 8:55-59.

[3] Allen S. Selection and implementation of an automated care planning system for a health care institution. *Comput Nurs* 1991, 9:61-68.

[4] Plummer CA and Warnock-Matheron A. Training nursing staff in the use of a computerized hospital information system. *Comput Nurs* 1987, 5:6-9.

[5] Pulliam L and Boettcher E. A process for introducing computerized information systems into long-term care facilities. *Comput Nurs* 1989, 7:251-257.

[6] Burkes M. Identifying and relating nurses´ attitudes toward computer use. *Comput Nurs* 1991, 9:190-201.

[7] Scarpa R, Smeltzer SC and Jasion B. Attitudes of nurses toward computerization: A replication. *Comput Nurs* 1992, 10:72-80.

[8] Rosander R and Bergbom Engberg I. The progress of computer supported health and nursing care information systems in Swedish hospitals. In: *Nursing Informatics' 94*, to be published.

[9] Bongartz C. Computer-oriented patient care. A comparison of nurses´ attitudes and perceptions. *Comput Nurs* 1988, 6:204-210.

[10] Romano CA, Damrosch SP, Heller BR and Parks PL. Levels of computer education for professional nursing. Development of a prototype graduate course. *Comput Nurs* 1989, 7:21-28.

Nursing Informatics: An International Overview for Nursing in a Technological Era
S.J. Grobe and E.S.P. Pluyter-Wenting, eds.

Attitudes to and experiences of intensive care technology:
A study on nurses in Sweden

Wojnicki-Johansson G [a] and Bergbom Engberg I [b]

[a] *Intensive Care Unit, Dept of Anaesthesiology, Länssjukhuset Ryhov, S-551 85 Jönköping, Sweden.*

[b] *University College of Health Sciences, P.O Box 1038, S-551 11 Jönköping, Sweden.*

Intensive care nursing involves a daily use of a substantial set of high technology equipment. This study was designed to explore nurses experiences of and attitudes to this "high-tech" environment. A questionnarie, including 34 structured and three open questions, was administred in three intensive care units. It was found that the technical equipment was percieved to facilitate nursing. The majority also felt safe and secure working with the equipment and thought that they had enough knowledge for this work. The technology was not seen as stress evoking. The computerized patient monitoring system was generally seen as satisfactory from the nurse viewpoint.. However, it was found to worry next of kin. Most nurses held favourable attitudes toward the intensive care technology, although many were hesistant to more technique. Noteworthy, the majority reported that their professional role as a nurse was not enriched or further developed by the technology. It is suggested that the success in incorporating new technology is affected by the nurses experiences from the daily use of present technology and their attitudes created in that setting.

1. Introduction

Intensive care represent a hospital setting with a high technological standard and where recent advancements in medical technology are likely to be introduced. The implementation of new and more advanced technology, for both treatment and patient monitoring, has generally improved the ability to care for patients who require intensive care because of serious threats to their fundamental life process.

This "high-tech" intensive care setting affect the entire staff working with the patients. Because of their legal responsibility for nursing and patient monitoring, registered nurses (RN) are particulary exposed to the demands raised in this care setting. The 24-hours-a-day patient monitoring, includes the monitoring of the patients' vital functions using a substantial amount of technical equipment and apparatus such as a ventilator, pulse-oximetry, hemofiltration and infusionpump. In addition, information from the computerized patient monitoring system (PMS) have to be interpreted and used for interventions.

Although significant issues concerning the effects of the complex "man-machine" interaction are likely to be adressed in the intensive care setting, few studies have been conducted to explore these issues from a nursing perspective. The nurses' overall attitudes to and experiences of intensive care technology, including computerized PMS-systems, are likely to influence the implementation of new technology. Besides, negative experiences and attitudes may also influence an effective use of current technology (1,2). When computerized systems do not meet the requirements and fullfill the needs of the RNs, the actual use may also be influenced (2). Stronge and Brodt (3) found that nurses working in different hospital settings showed different attitudes towards computerization and that nurses with a higher educational level and more years employed in health care expressed more positive attitudes. Bongartz (2) stressed the need for further research concerning nurses attitudes toward computerization in hospital settings. The lack of studies concerning the effects of computerization and the use of other technical equipment therefore makes it important to evaluate nurses experiences of and attitudes to intensive care technology, including the impact this may have on both the nurse and the patient-nurse relationship. A study aimed to explore these issues is briefly presented here.

604

2. Aim of project

The aim of the study was to evaluate the RNs attitudes to and experiences of the medical technology, including patient monitoring systems (PMS), used in contemporary intensive care units.

3. Subjects and Methods

3.1. Sample

The sample comprised three sub-samples of RNs, all directly involved in nursing of intensive care patients. The sub-samples were drawn from three intensive care units (ICU), one representing a county hospital, the second a regional hospital, and the third a university hospital. These three levels of hospital care correspond to the general organization of the Swedish health care system.

The datacollection was conducted during January and February 1993. All eighty-nine RNs at work at the three sites during this time period were invited to answer a questionnarie. The response rate was 100 percent which means that everyone participated in the study. The demographics of the sample is shown in Table 1.

Table 1
Demographics of the RN sample at the three sites (N=89).

	County	Region	University
Mean age	38.1	35.4	37.4
Age range	27-51	22-52	25-48
Gender(% women)	100	81	96
Mean years as RN in intensive care	9.5	6.9	7.7

There were no significant differences between RNs at the three sites on the background variables described in the table, nor for educational background or in reponses to the question whether a personal interest in medical technology once had motivated them to apply to intensive care. A total of 44 percent answered that such a personal interest in medical technology was a reason for their application.

3.2. Methods

A 37-item questionnarie, containing 34 structured and three open questions, was administred, following verbal explanation about the purpose of the study. The general response format for the items on experiences and attitudes was: 1 = Yes, to a high degree, 2 = Yes, to a rather high degree, 3 = No , to a rather low degree, and 4 = No, to a low degree.

Although the overall reponse rate was 100%, a few items in the questionnaires were sometimes left unanswered. Data were analyzed using the Chi-square test, analysis of variance (ANOVA) and Spearman´s correlations coefficient. The significance level for differences between or across groups and correlations between items were set at p<.05.

4. Results

The results presented next focus on experience from the use of general medical technology, the patient monitoring system (PMS), and the RNs attitudes to medical technology in the intensive care setting. A general finding here was that of no differences in attitudes and experiences between RNs at the three ICUs, exept for different experiences of PMS.

4.1. General technology

The responses to some of the questions concerning the nurses experience with intensive care technology are shown in the following table.

Table 2
Responses (in percent) to questions about how technology affects the RN (N=89)

Topic	Yes, high degree	Yes, rather high degree	No, rather low degree	No, low degree
Percieved stress	1	9	55	35
Self-reported knowledge of medical technology	12	79	9	--
Security and safety in technology use	18	76	6	--
Facilitates nursing	17	68	13	2
More time for patient	3	29	48	20
Enriched work role	2	37	60	1

The analysis revealed significant correlations between the responses to these items. Nurses who percieved low stress also reported high security and safety in their use of the medical technology, a better self-reported knowledge of this technology, and attitudes and experiences that technology facilitated nursing. The RNs who reported an enriched work role due to technology also thought that more time could be devoted to the patients because of this technology.

4.2. Patient monitoring

The main questions concerning the RNs experiences from the patient monitoring were: "Is the computerized patient monitoring system well-functioning from a RN perspective?", and "Have you percieved that patients and next of kins are worried about the information from the monitor?".

Table 3
Responses (in percent) to questions about patient monitoring systems, PMS. (N=89).

Topic	Yes, high degree	Yes, rather high degree	No, rather low degree	No, low degree
PMS satisfactory	20	67	11	2
Worries patients	2	24	58	16
Worries kins	14	60	23	3

The three ICUs had a different PMS. Significant differences between the three sites were also found in response to the first and second question about PMS, but not to the third topic. Independent of system, nurses percieved that the PMS worried next of kins equally, whereas different PMS were viewed as more or less favourable from the nurses´ viewpoint.

4.3. Attitudes

There were two general attitude items: "Do you question the value and usefulness of certain equipment at your site?" and "Do you question the value and usefulness of more medical technology?" The reponses are shown in table 4.

Table 4
Respones (in percent) to questions about the value and usefulness of technological equipment (N=89).

Topic	Yes, high degree	Yes, rather high degree	No, rather low degree	No, low degree
Present technology	7	45	38	10
More technology	9	39	40	12

Significant correlations were found between a more hesistant attitude to technology and older age, lower self-reported knowledge and worries that the "clinical eye and skill" could fade with more technology.

5. Discussion

The background for this study was that RNs experiences of and attitudes to medical technology is an overlooked factor in the context of hospital implementation of technical equipment. The high response rate seems to confirm the great importance of this issue among the nurses themselves. The finding of no differences in attitudes and few differences in general experiences between RNs at different ICUs support the notion that they are largely exposed to similar experiences.

The results showed that few nurses felt stressed by the medical technology used in contemporary intensive care units. Most nurses experienced that it facilitated their work. Younger and better well-trained RNs had more favourable attitudes to and experiences of the intensive care technology, which is in disagreement with Sultana's (1) study about nurses attitudes towards computers in clinical practice. The technology at focus in the present study, however, involved not only computers but all "high-tech" equipment used in intensive care. New technology and equipment are often assumed to be stress evoking and anxiety not to control the equipment is assumed to contribute to stress reactions (4). This study showed that a vast majority of the nurses reported rather low or even low percieved stress. This could be explained by a selection of nurses applying for intensive care work, as well as a satisfactory system for educating and training RNs how to use the technology. In addition, RNs who remain in intensive care are likely to become adapted to the high stress imposed by critically ill patients and the equipment used for the treament(4). This should be taken into account as the vast majority of nurses participating in this study had rather long experience from ICU´s (mean = 8 years). A majority (68%), however, expressed that the technical equipment implied less time for direct care of patients, which is in agreement with Sultana's finding (1) but not with Hendrickson and Kovner (6). Nurses who claimed that less time could be devoted to the patients also felt that the "clinical eye and skill" could fade due to this technology involvment.

Older nurses and those who reported less knowledge of the medical technology expressed more negative attitudes to the technical equipment in ICU. This finding may reflect that older and more experienced nurses thought that other caring interventions may be more useful in relation to the patients needs and condition, and perhaps that a technological environment also can contribute to problems in the care (5). It is noteworthy that 61 % of the nurses expressed that the technology had not enriched or developed their professional RN role. It is likely that less time for direct patient care is seen as an unfavourable trend among the nurses themselves and that technology in this context is recognized as time demanding and that computerized systems do not fullfill the needs of the nurse (2).

The computerized patient monitoring system was for a majority of the nurses percieved as a well-functioning technological equipment. Only twelve nurses out of 89 (13.5%) thought that the PMS was not a satisfactory device. Seventy-four percent of the nurses had experiences of negative reactions in next of kins due to the PMS. An equal proportion, however, claimed that there were no perceived worries in the patients concerning the information displayed by the PMS. While the patients, when in such a state, continously can be informed about different signals and sounds from the PMS, the need for information among next of kins are perhaps overlooked, especially in acute phases where it becomes an issue of lack of time.

6. Conclusions

Many of the intensive care nurses (44%) reported that they once had applied to intensive care because of a personal interest in medical technology. However, a majority experienced that the medical technology in their contemporary intensive care settings had not enriched their work role. A majority also showed a hesistant attitude to more technical equipment in the ICU. This attitude was especially pronounced in older nurses and in those who reported less knowledge about the medical technology. A majority had not experienced that the medical technology increased the amount of time that could be devoted to direct patient care even when it facilitated other domains of the RNs work. Many RNs also expressed a worry that the "clinical eye and skill", in the care of critically ill patients, could fade when the "technical part" of caring dominates. A majority of the nurses perceived worries among next of kins when faced with PMS. Such specific experiences, as well as other experiences from the RNs themselves must be further explored to provide a better feedback for the development and adjustment of intensive care technology.

The success of incorporating new technology in intensive care is dependent on human factors such as experiences from daily use of previous technology, which are likely to have created certain perceptions and attitudes. More knowledge is needed to resolve these issues, especially how to prepare RNs for intensive care nursing and how feedback from present users of medical technology should be utilized in the construction as well as in the implementation of new technology.

7. References

(1). Sultana N. Nurses attitudes towards computerization in clinical practice. *J Adv Nurs* 1990, 15:696-702.

(2). Bongartz C. Computer-Oriented Patient Care. A Comparison of Nurses' Attitudes and Perceptions. *Comput Nurs* 1988, 6:204-210.

(3). Stronge J. and Brodt A. Assessment of Nurses' Attitudes toward Computerization. *Comput Nurs* 1985, 3:154-158.

(4). Sundström-Frisk C. and Hellström M. Vad blev det av svaren? Exempel på resultatåterföring från en enkät om medicinteknisk säkerhet: "Att lära av misstagen". National Institute of Occupational Health, Stockholm. Undersökningsrapport 1993:18.

(5). van Bemmel J.H.: Computer assissted care in nursing. Computers at the bedside. *Comput Nurs,* 1987,5:132-139.

(6). Hendrickson G. & Kovner C.T.: Effects of computers on nursing resource use. Do computers save nurses time? *Comput Nurs,* 1990, 8: 16-22.

Nursing Informatics: An International Overview for Nursing in a Technological Era
S.J. Grobe and E.S.P. Pluyter-Wenting, eds.

608

Computer Self-Efficacy in Professional Nurses: An Analysis Selected Factors Using Latent Variable Modeling

Coover D

Fairfield University School of Nursing, Fairfield, Connecticut 06430-7524

1. Introduction

The primary objective of this research was the formulation of a structural equation model (SEM) that estimates the degree to which certain factors influenced judgments of self-efficacy related to computer use. The sample comprised 1200 randomly-selected critical-care nurses. A combination of social cognitive, educational, and attitudinal theories (Bandura, 1986; Fishbein & Ajzen, 1975; Kolb, 1984; Schunk, 1985) were employed in the creation of the SEM that depicted relationships among the latent variables: cognitivestyle aptitudes, math ability aptitudes, life experiences, computer attitudes, and computer self-efficacy. The influence on individual's perceptions of self-efficacy relative to using computers in the work setting was examined using multiple indicators derived from scores on three standardized measures and demographic data.

2. Focus and Research Questions

The focus of the study was to assess the influence of multiple, selected factors that contribute to positive computer attitudes and perceptions of computer self-efficacy among a sample of professional nurses. Research questions that guided the conduct of this investigation were 1) to specify and test the measurement model that best explains the relationships among the exogenous latent variables Active-Reflective Cognitive Style Aptitudes, Abstract-Concrete Cognitive Style Aptitudes, Math Ability Aptitudes, Life Experiences and the endogenous variables Computer Attitude/Use and Computer Self-Efficacy; the measurement model, showing the hypothesized relationships among the latent variables and their respective indicators, along with correlated measurement error is illustrated in Figure 2; and 2) to identify and test a structural model that is consistent with the data collected in this study and that best explains the causal relationships among the latent exogenous latent variables (as above), and the endogenous latent variables (as above). The proposed structural equation model is shown in Figure 1.

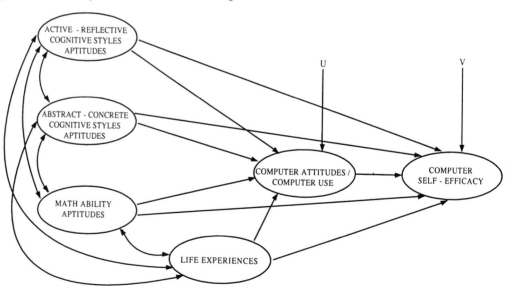

Note. U, V depict variable disturbance
Figure 1. Hypothesized Structural Equation Model of Computer Self-Efficacy.

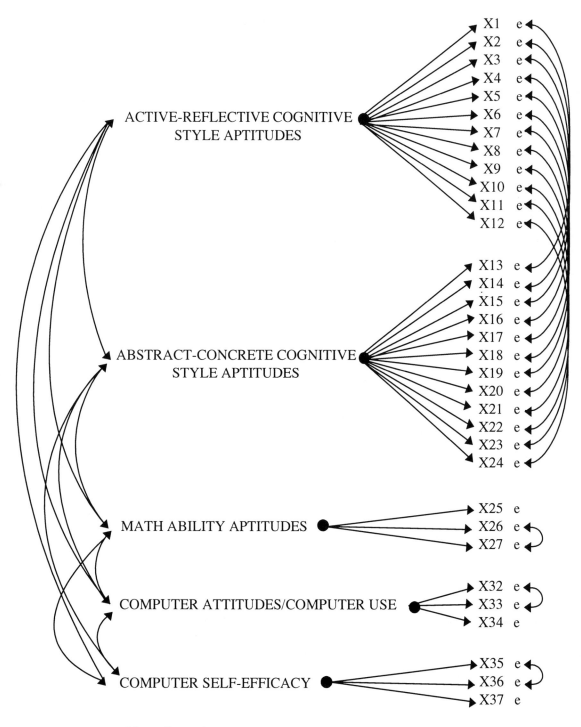

Note. Curved arrows denote correlated measurement error.

e = error

Figure 2. Hypothesized Measurement Model of Computer
Self-Efficacy

3. Sample and Methodology

Questionnaires were mailed to 1200 nurses working in the Northeastern region of the United States who were then current members of the American Association of Critical-Care Nurses. A total of 512 (43%) questionnaires were returned; 498 (42%) responses met the inclusion criteria, and therefore were included in the analysis. Three standardized instruments were employed for data collection: 1) the Computer Self-Efficacy Scale (Murphy, Coover & Owen, 1989),
2) the Attitudes Toward Computers Adult Form Survey (Delcourt & Lewis, 1987), and the Learning Style Inventory (Kolb, 1985) along with survey items related to assessment of math ability, computer history and frequency of use, and demographics. The proposed structural equation model with 37 observed variables was specified, estimated and tested through the use of LISREL VI (Joreskog & Sorbom, 1986).

4. Characteristics of the Study Sample

The *study sample* comprised 470 nurses; 413 females and 57 males; the average age of the nurses was 35 years old (SD = + 7.6 years).

The mean number of *years experience* as a professional nurse was 12 years. Professional experience ranged from less than one year to more than 41 years for the subjects. Average *educational level* was the Baccalaureate Degree with the range extending from RN Diploma to Doctoral Degree.

This sample of nurses regarded their work wetting as *fairly technical* (equivalent to 4 on a scale of 1 to 5 with 5 = highly technical). These professionals employed computers in the work setting (*frequency of use*) an average of 8.5 hours per week with a range of one to 36 hours per week. In the work setting, study subjects had gained more than two years computer experience (*duration of use*), with a range of two months to more than eight years of experience.

Considering *math ability aptitudes*, subjects on the average had completed Basic College Math with a grade of "B" and regard themselves moderately high (4 on a scale of 1 to 5 with 5 = very high) on the average with respect to math competency.

Study subjects were *very interested* in the use of computers (4 on a scale of 1 to 5, with 5 = most interested). Yet, these same nurses were less than moderately *comfortable* when actually involved in the use of computers (average on 2.8 on a scale of 1 to 5 with 5 = very comfortable).

Subjects indicated a moderately high sense (4 on a scale of 1 to 5 with 5 = high) of *computer self-efficacy* for performing *basic computer skills*. Their feelings of computer self-efficacy for *advanced* and *mainframe skills* were low (M = 2.4) and moderate (M = 3.0), respectively.

This sample of critical care nurses characterized themselves as *Doers* and *Thinkers* in relation to the four basic *learning styles* described by Kolb (1984), i.e., feeling, observing, thinking, and doing.

The *attrition sample* (N=28) included subjects whose scores on one or more study measures were greater than two SD. These individuals did not vary significantly from the study sample. The 21 women and 7 men spent more hours per week in their *use of computers* at work (M = > 9.5 hours/week), and had a longer *history of computer use* (M = > 3 years) compared to an average of just two years for the study subjects.

5. Significant Findings

The Respecified Structural Equation Model of Computer Self-Efficacy (Figure 2) produced a Chi Square (20, N=470)=33.00, p=.034 and demonstrated a Tucker-Lewis (1973) non-normed fit index of .971 which is indictive of a satisfactorily-fitting model.

There were *four significant parameter estimates* in the respecified structural equation model of computer self-efficacy:
- Computer Attitudes and Frequency of Computer Use were strong predictors of Computer Self-Efficacy
  (b=.821, p<.001).
- Duration of Computer Use is a signficant predictor of:
  - Positive Computer Attitudes and Frequency of Computer Use (b=.167, p<.05).
  - A strong sense of Computer Self-Efficacy (b=.114, p<.05).
- Math Ability Aptitudes was a significant predictor of positive Computer Attitudes and the Frequency of
- Computer Use (b=.569, p<.001).

The findings of this study clearly show there are some factors that strongly influence an individual's sense of competence to perform various levels of computer skills.

- An interest in computer use.
- Frequent (daily) use of the computer in the work setting.
- A sense of comfort in the use of computer technology more than likely gained from
- A significant history of computer use.

A *sense of capability to do math problems* and *prior achievement in math* were strong indicators of positive Computer Attitudes, but only *indirectly* influenced perceptions of Computer Self-Efficacy. The Computer Self-Efficacy Scale and Attitudes Toward Computers Survey were shown to be valid from a statistical perspective, and also, to have high reliability estimates, thus providing evidence of their value for use in computer training program evaluation.

Further, these outcomes support the tenets of self-efficacy theory that suggests computer training is most effective if the program is:

Designed so that skill acquistion is sequenced in a hierarchial fashion, and
Skill acquistion is reinforced and maintained with frequent computer use.

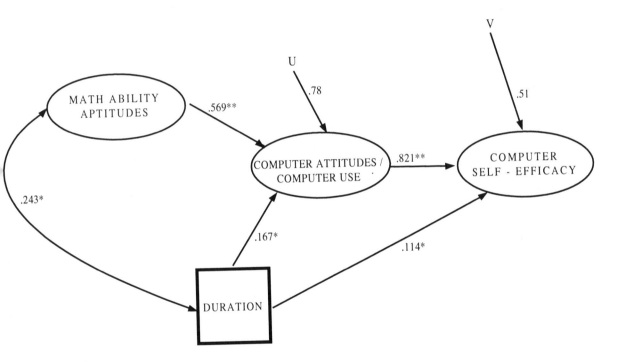

Note. *p < .050 **p < .001. U, V√= 1 - R Square. Chi Square (20, N=470)=33.00 p=.034

Figure 3. Respectified Structrual Equation Model of Computer Self-Efficacy

6. References

Bandura A: *Social Foundations of Thought and Action* Englewood Cliffs, NJ: Prentice-Hall 1986 390-448

Delcourt MAB and Lewis LH: Measuring Adults' Attitudes Toward Computers: An Initial Investigation A paper presented at the Lifelong Learnign Research Conference, University of Maryland 1987

Fishbein M and Ajzen I: *Belief, Attitude, Intention and Behavior: An Introduction to Theory and Research* Reading, MA: Addison-Wesley Publishing 1975

Joreskog KG and Sorbom D: *LISREL VI: Analysis of Linear Structural Relationships by Maximum Likelihood Instrumental Variables and Least Squares Methods* 4th ed. Mooreville, IN: Scientific Software, Inc. 1986

Kolb DA: *Experiential Learning: Experience as the Source of Learning and Developmentt* Englewood Cliffs, NJ: Prentice-Hall 1984

Kolb DA: *Learning Style Inventory: Self Scoring Inventory and Interpretation Booklett* Boston, MA: McBer and Company 1985

Murphy CA Coover D and Owen SV: Development and Validation of the Computer Self-Efficacy Scale *Educ & Psych Meas* 1989 49:893-899.

Schunk D: Self-Efficacy and Classroom Learning *Ann Rev of Soc* 1985 2:161-207.

Tucker LR and Lewis C: A Reliability Coefficient for Maximum Likelihood Factor Analysis *Psychometrika,* 1973 38:1-10

Nursing Informatics: An International Overview for Nursing in a Technological Era
S.J. Grobe and E.S.P. Pluyter-Wenting, eds.

Cyberphobia and the Learning Process

Honey M L L

Nurse Lecturer, Faculty of Health Studies, Manukau Polytechnic, PO Box 61-066, Otara, City of Manukau, New Zealand.

This paper will examine cyberphobia, the fear of computers, and the effect this can have on the learning process with particular regard to nurse lecturers learning computer skills. The group of people this will be applied to is nurse lecturers. Nursing Informatics is still fairly new to many of us involved in nursing education. There is a need for students to learn computer skills, but there is a real need to acknowledge the fear that many nurse lecturers may have with regard to the rapid implementation of computer technology in the areas of administration and clinical practice.

This paper attempts to recognize those who are experts in their own areas of work who feel threatened by computers, and the effect this has on their ability to learn how to use the new technology.

Finally strategies and practical suggestions will be offered for dealing with cyberphobia.

1. Cyberphobia

The concept of computer anxiety first began to appear in the literature in the early 1980's [1, p. 52]. Cyberphobia is a term used for `fear of computers' or `computer anxiety'. This has been defined [2] as "subjective feelings of fear or apprehension experienced by persons when using computers".

Reasons for this fear or anxiety with computers may be due to a lack of familiarity with computers, fear of their dehumanizing potential and, for female nurses, the sex-role stereotype relating to maths-associated tasks [3,4]. More commonly mentioned reasons are a fear of losing work, ruining a system or doing permanent damage to the hardware.

It is thought [4, p. 271] "that nurse educators may feel anxiety about computers more acutely because of cognitive dissonance over their failure to model the progressive behaviour of computer use for students".

2. Nurse Lecturers

There is a clear need for students of nursing to learn computer skills, but their educators should not be forgotten. Nurse lecturers may be among those for whom computer literacy was not part of their nursing education. There is a perceived responsibility for all nurse lecturers to be computer literate, not only to manage their own work, but to show competence in their role and as an example to other nurses.

As well as the clinical use of computers, nurse lecturers can use the computer for administrative details, including student records. Then there is the actual teaching. As Procter [5, p. 5] states, a well designed computer-assisted learning package, can assist in determining the learning style of the student. Such opportunities are not available to the nurse lecturer unversed in computer based teaching strategies.

The use of computers in education has grown dramatically since the early 1980's, in primary and secondary schools and in schools of nursing. Many of the students entering nursing have computer skills, and a number have access to a home computer. This may mean a class of students with a high entering level of knowledge about computers and practical experience with them as well. Knowing this does not help the nurse lecturer contemplating learning computer skills and may well magnify their anxiety.

3. Effect on the Learning Process

Change of any description can cause anxiety and nurse lecturers in New Zealand are seeing change on two significant fronts. The first is in the health sector and the structural changes to our health system. Secondly there are concurrent changes within education. Amidst these changes are rapid technological advances. Nurses, in general, seem to cope well with new technology. Wolfe [6, p. 352] feels that it would seem logical to predict that nurses would embrace computer technology. This is because nurses often use other technology in the course of their work, from clinics, community health care settings to intensive care units. Nurses are renowned for their empathy with people -getting on well with machines requires a different approach and mental attitude [7]. This mental attitude may lead to some strong emotions.

It is interesting that computers seem to evoke diverse feelings. These feelings have been described as varying from anxiety to actual intimidation [8].

3.1 Time

Colleagues commonly report difficulties related to time. This included a lack of time, the need to work at one's own pace when learning a new skill, the time it took for some trial and error learning and the time it took to look up directions as needed. The additional time to complete work that involved computer use was such that it could seem easier to not bother, thus affecting the opportunities for learning.

3.2 Awkwardness

Nurse lecturers have experience and expertise in their own areas of practice but may find themselves in the position of being a novice with computers. Adult learners who have already gained expertise in a field usually want to be proficient and do not like experiencing the awkwardness associated with learning a new skill [9, p. 133]. This leads to nurse lecturers feeling uncomfortable and stressed.

3.3 Stress

Stress causes certain responses in the body and these can be both physical and psychological. Draper [10, p. 415] writes about the effects of stress and states, "When a person is under pressure or experiences stress, the limbic system becomes highly activated and learning is subsequently inhibited". It is important to appreciate and make allowances for the individual manner nurse lecturers may express and deal with their stress. For example a person can be unusually talkative, or quiet, or mood changes may be apparent.

3.4 Tunnel Vision

Another effect of stress can be a form of tunnel vision [6, p. 352] where an awareness of possible options is distorted or diminished. This means an inability to apply the strategies that would normally be used. A nurse lecturer who normally applies the problem solving process, and teaches this to students may find they are unable to utilize this strategy for themselves. Another example is not reading the instructions clearly, either on the screen or from a manual, when one normally would.

Clearly, teaching strategies that address cyberphobia and display a special sensitivity to the feelings of the nurse lecturer are required.

4. Strategies

The strategies offered here are practical suggestions for nurse lecturers learning computer skills. They are particularly suitable for nurse lecturers who exhibit anything from cyberphobia to mild reticence towards computers.

4.1 Acceptance

It is important to remember one's own introduction to computers and those initial feelings when first facing the screen. Sharing those emotions can be beneficial and reinforces that feelings of fear or anxiety are normal when facing something new [9]. When working with colleagues it is helpful to acknowledge their expertise in a particular area, and to recall other new learning experiences. For example, learning to drive can be extremely stressful, but it is only practice that makes it all come together in the end. The car analogy [11,9] can be usefully applied as not all drivers need to be mechanics, or racing drivers. Similarly in computing it is not necessary to understand all the electronic componentry, nor be the fastest on the keyboard or with the mouse!

4.2 Positive Thinking

Focusing on the positive aspects of what computers can do for you, makes it much easier to continue to try when those first attempts don't go as well as hoped. It seems that colleagues find it easier to learn a computer skill if it is something that they want or need to know, or can use right away. This may be because of time constraints and a busy work load.

For example, creating computer-generated overhead transparencies is a relatively simple skill to learn which provides wonderful results that can be highly effective in use. Ensuring examples that are manageable and where success is attainable leads to a more positive feeling towards the computer.

4.3 Privacy

If a nurse lecturer is in any way fearful of learning computer skills then privacy is essential. Either working alone, or with another colleague of their choice, is ideal. It is useful to ensure privacy for two main reasons. The first is consideration for the feelings of ones' colleagues. Secondly, it allows for practice in a safe environment without interruptions or observers.

4.4 Encouragement

Encouragement and positive reinforcement, not only for achievements but also for the effort and energy expended is something naturally offered to our students. It is easy to forget that our colleagues need it just as much.

Ongoing assistance to nurse lecturers can be given when working alongside each other. Queries can be answered and immediate feedback given. This informal education is sometimes more relevant and better appreciated than setting separate time aside.

4.5 Hands-off

A hands-off approach when teaching is essential. While some theory may be needed it is practice with the computer that leads to understanding, and from that, confidence. There is the danger of a too rapidly executed demonstration, where nothing is really seen. A verbal explanation and time to work it through is a better alternative.

An example, from nursing education, is teaching students how to do a dressing. It is necessary to provide some background information, but the important part is the practice. A demonstration is helpful initially, but the student has to practice the skill to gain understanding and confidence in perfecting a safe dressing technique. Similarly practical computer skills need a hands-off approach by the educator. The person learning must do it themselves, at their pace, so that their understanding is maximized.

4.6 Thinking Aloud

Another strategy that can be very effective is the use of what is sometimes called a scaffolding technique [12, p. 28]. A simple term for is `thinking aloud'.

When asked a question, it is possible to show the way one thinks about the problem and possible solutions verbally. It allows others to "see" the way you think.

For example, if someone is editing a word processed document and is having trouble with deleting or adding extra space where they want to, it can be helpful to verbalise what they are attempting.

Not only does this strategy solve the question of how to perform a task, it shares the mental processes or thinking behind the actions. This can assist with trouble-shooting other problems later.

4.7 Humour

A sense of humour seems essential for maintaining perspective in this area. To the nurse lecturer learning computer skills an ability to see the funny side of actions like talking to the computer or ascribing it a personality allows a release of emotions. Sharing that humour makes learning co-operative and reduces the isolation of learning `alone with the computer'.

5. Future

There is no one solution to cyberphobia as people experience and exhibit it differently. The above strategies are practical suggestions that are particularly suitable for assisting nurse lecturers learn computer skills. That there is a need for nurse lecturers to be computer literate is undoubted.

Computers are here to stay in nursing education and should be seen as an opportunity for nurse educators to enhance their practice. As Procter [5, p. 66] states, the computer in education should not be viewed as a replacement for teachers, more as a tool to aid teachers in educating their students. If the focus is kept on improving nurse education, in all the facets that nursing education entails, then the motivation is there for nurse lecturers to overcome their reluctance to learn about computers.

6. References

[1] Wilson BA. Computer Anxiety in Nursing Students. *J Nurs Educ.* 1991, 30:2.

[2] Maurer M & Simonson M. Development and Validation of a Measure of Computer Anxiety. In: *Association for Educational Communications and Technology.* Dallas: Texas, 1984.

[3] Grobe SJ. Conquering Computer Cowardice. *J Nurs Educ.* 1984, 23:6.

[4] Jacobson SF, Holder ME & Dearner JF. Computer Anxiety Among Nursing Students, Educators, Staff, and Administrators. *Comput Nurs.* 1989, 7:6.

[5] Procter PM. *Nurses, Computers and Information Technology.* London: Chapman & Hall, 1992.

[6] Wolfe K. Getting a Grip on Computerphobia. *AAOHN J.* 1991, 39:7.

[7] Honey MLL. The Challenge in Teaching Computer Skills. In: *Nursing Informatics In New Zealand: An Impetus for Learning.* Auckland: New Zealand, 1991.

[8] Ball MJ, Snelbecker GE & Schecter SL. Nurses' Perceptions Concerning Computer Uses Before and After a Computer Literacy Lecture. *Comput Nurs.* 1985, 3:1.

[9] Reynolds A & Ferrell MJ. Computer Literacy: A Mission for Continuing Education for Professional Nurses. *J Contin Educ Nurs.* 1989, 20:3.

[10] Draper W. Emotional Development. In Thomas RM, (ed) *The Encyclopedia of Human Development and Education: Theory, Research and Studies.* Oxford: Pergamon, 1990. pp. 415-421.

[11] Rushby NJ. *An Introduction to Educational Computing.* London: Croom Helm, 1979.

[12] Rosenshine B & Meister C. The Use of Scaffolds for Teaching Higher-Level Cognitive Strategies. *Educational Leadership.* 1992, 49:7.

Nursing Informatics: An International Overview for Nursing in a Technological Era
S.J. Grobe and E.S.P. Pluyter-Wenting, eds.

618

The effects of individual and group characteristics on innovation adoption within the context of nursing informatics

Kim IS and Kim MI

School of Nursing, Yonsei University, C.P.O. Box 8044, 134 Shin-chon-dong Seodaemun-ku, Seoul, 120-752, Korea

This study investigated the effects of efficacy and cooperativeness on innovation adoption at the multiple levels--I.e., person and nursing unit. the data showed that an individual's willingness to adopt innovation was determined by his or her self-efficacy and the nursing unit's efficacy that was associated with the unit's innovation adoption. However, the data showed that a cooperative individual was willing to adopt innovation regardless of whether the nursing unit was cooperative or noncooperative or regardless of whether the unit was willing to adopt or reject innovation. From the overall results, we concluded that nursing administrators should consider both individual and nursing unit characteristics--e.g., efficacy--in order to diffuse innovation.

1. Theoretical Background

Within the context of nursing informatics, diffusion of innovation has been widely investigated at single level (e.g., person, nursing unit or organization, see Somano, 1990, for a review). For example, at the person level, it has been found that personality characteristics and demographic variables are significantly associated with computer-use willingness (Brodt & Strong, 1986; Burkes, 1991; Chang, 1984; Melhorn, Legler, & Clark, 1979). At the unit level, interpsersonal networks, group norms, and leadership have been found to be major factors for determining diffusion of innovations (Anderson, Joy & Hackman, 1982; Becker, 1970; Coleman, Katz, & Manzel, 1965; Davis, Bagozzi, & Warshaw, 1989). At the organizaational level, structural variability, authority system, decision strategy, and contextual variables have been found to influence hospital adoption of technological innovations (Kimberly, 1978; Kimberly & Evanisko, 1981 and see Demanpour, 1991; Rice & Aydin, 1991 for innovation adoption of business organizations).

Nevertheless, very few studies have attempted to examine diffusion of innovation at the multiple levels of analysis (i.e., person and nursing unit). The advantage of multiple level of analysis is clear: We are able to build several competitive hypotheses and decide which one is more plausible (Dansereau, Allutto & Yammarino, 1984). Accordingly, the purpose of this paper is to investigate innovation adoption at the person and nursing unit levels. To accomplish this purpose, two variables that are viewed as potentially important for diffusion of innovation in literature and that can be constructed at the person and nursing unit levels are considered. Before discussing these two variables, we will start with innovation adoption.

1.1 Innovation Adoption

Innovation adoption consists of five steps in innovation decision process: Knowledge, persuasion, decision implementation and confirmation (Rogers, 1983). In this process, an individual's decision for innovation adoption or rejection is determined by his or her behavioral intention to emit the behavior, which is in return determined by favorable or unfavorable attitudes toward the innovation (Ajzen & Fishbein, 1980); Fishbein & Ajzen, 1975). Thus, if we know an individual's attitudes toward innovation and/or his or her behavioral intention to adopt or reject the innovation, we can see whether he or she adopts or rejects the innovation. In a similar vein, a nursing unit's willingness to adopt innovation will be determined by the unit's intention and attitudes toward the innovation. Now the question is who or which type of nursing unit will adopt or reject innovation. An attempt to solve this question is made by introducing individual and group characteristics.

1.2 Efficacy

Self-efficacy as a person level variable is defined as one's belief in one's capability to perform a secific task (Bandura, 1986). A number of studies have found that self-efficacy is strongly associated with difficult career-related tasks (Stumpf, Brief & Hartman, 1987) and adaptability of new technology (Hill, Smith & Mann, 1987). That is, individuals with high self-efficacy have an optimism for performing a specific task and even new tasks. Accordingly, they are more willing to adopt new technology. In contrast, individuals with low self-efficacy have a low efficacy expectation and a fear of failure (Bandura, 1982; Gist, 1987). Thus, they are not willing to adopt new technology.

The concept of self-efficacy can be extended to groups or nursing units (Gist, 1987). If a group or nursing unit is characterized by high efficacy, it is more likely to adopt new technology. In contrast, a nursing unit with low efficacy is less likely to adopt innovation because of a fear of failure.

In sum, we can hypothesize that efficacy will be positively related to innovation adoption at the person and nursing unit levels.

1.3 Cooperativeness

Rogers (1983) proposed that the rate of innovation adoption is associated with the degree of interconnectedness of units in a social system. In a similar vein, when unit members show a lot of internal agreement and cooperativeness and are attracted to each other, the degree of interconnectedness willl increase and thus unit memters are more likely to adopt innovation (cf., Weenig & Midden, 1991). Further, if unit members share information about innovation because of high degree of cooperativeness, they could reduce uncertainty about new technology. Accordingly, a cooperative nursing unit is willing to adopt innovation.

A cooperative individual also tends to share information of new technology with coworkers and is less likely to be threatened by innovation. Thus we can hypothesize that cooperativeness will be positively related to innovation adoption at the person and nursing unit levels.

2. Method

2.1 Sample

The study was conducted in 64 nursing units of a university hospital in Korea. Four or five nurses from each unit were randomly selected as respondents. 275 nurses actually participated in the study. The average age of respondents was 29 years (s.d. = 5.7) and the average tenure was 5.9 years (s.d. = 5.1).

2.2 Measures

Innovation Adoption. In order to measure innovation adoption, attitudes toward computer and willingness to use computer were assessed by the respondents. The 7 items were factor-analyzed and produced one factor. The items were then added to form a total score that was divided by the number of items in a scale to form the average scale score for the measure. This measure was then aggregated to the nursing unit level. The intraclass correlation, ICC(1), was computed in order to estimate whether nurses within the unit agreed in the responses. Icc(1), which compares the between-unit sum of squares to the total sum of squares (James, 1982), was 0.3. This value indicates acceptable level of "agreement" (Ostroff, 1992).

Self-Efficacy. Self-efficacy was assessed with general/achievement subscale of the self-efficacy scale developed by Sherer et al. (1982). As Earley and Lituchy (1991) reported, the 17 item scale showed four factors with eigen values of 7.56, 1.32, 1.28, and 1.13. We selected the first factor as the self-efficacy scale because it accounted for 60% of the variance and the other three factors accounted for only an additional 7% of the variance. The 5 item scale was then aggregated to the nursing unit level. The ICC(1) was 0.25. This value indicates acceptable level of "agreement."

Cooperativeness. To measure cooperativeness, respondents assessed 5 items (e.g., "I tend to trust my coworkers;" "I am very friendly and approachable to coworkers;" "I tend to help coworkers in their solving difficult problems") in terms of 4 point Likert type scale. The 5 item scale was then aggregated to the nursing unit level. The intraclass correlation was 0.35. This value indicates acceptable level of "agreement."

3. Results

3.1 Person level of analysis

Table 1 presents the means, standard deviations, reliabilities, and intercorrelations of innovation adoption, self-efficacy, cooperativeness, and demographic variables. The data show that innovation adoption is positively related to self-efficacy and cooperativeness.

Table 1
Means, standard deviations, reliabilities, and intercorrelations of measures (N = 275)

	Mean	SD	1	2	3	4	5	6
1. Innovation adoption	3.33	.44	(.80)					
2. Self-efficacy	2.95	.32	.26**	(.76)				
3. Cooperativeness	3.12	.38	.23**	.11	(.80)			
4. Age	29.01	5.72	-.02	-.03	.05	-		
5. Tenure	5.9	5.10	-.05	-.02	.04	.94**	-	
6. Position	1.86	.61	.01	.04	.06	.48**	.45**	-

*p<.05   **p<.01   Numbers in parenthesis are reliability estimates

Table 2 presents the results of the regression analysis predicting innovation adoption. Self-efficacy has a significant effect (β = .30, p<.01). Cooperativeness also has a significant effect (β = .16, p<.05) on innovation adoption. These results indicate that innovation adoption is determined by individual personality characteristics (i.e., self-efficacy and cooperativeness). To test that innovation adoption is influenced by nursing unit characteristics, a correlation analysis was performed at the nursing unit level.

Table 2
Regression analysis predicting innovation adoption

Independent variables	β
Self-efficacy	.30**
Cooperativeness	.17**
Age	.008
Tenure	-.001
Position	.04
(Constant)	1.06
R squares	.16
d.f.	52
F-ratio	6.67**

*p<.05   **p<.01

3.2 Nursing unit level of analysis

Table 3 shows that intercorrelations among innovation adoption, efficacy, and cooperativeness aggregated to the nursing unit level. Nursing unit efficacy is significantly related to innovation adoption. However, nursing unit cooperativeness is not significantly related to innovation adoption.

Table 3
Intercorrelations among measures at the nursing unit letel (N = 64)

	Innovation adoption	Efficacy	Cooperativeness
Innovation adoption	x		
Efficacy	.41**	x	
Cooperativeness	.14	.08	x

**p<.01

The results of the regression analysis show that efficacy has a significant effect ($\beta = .64$, $p<.05$), but cooperativeness has a nonsignificant effect in innovation adoption ($\beta = .13$, $p<.05$).

The data also showed that a nurse's willingness to adopt innovation was not significantly correlated with age ($r = .02$, $p<.05$), tenure ($r = -.05$, $p<.05$), and position ($r = .01$, $p<.05$). These results are not different from those of previous studies (Aydin, 1987; Bongartz, 1988; Brodt & Stringe, 1986; Ischar & Aydin, 1988; Krampf & Robinson, 1984).

4.   Discussion

This study investigated the relationship between innovation adoption, efficacy, and cooperativeness at the person and nursing unit levels. First, the data supported the hypothesis that efficacy would be positively related to innovation adoption at the person and nursing unit levels. These results indicate that both individual and nursing unit characteristics (i.e., efficacy) are important factors in determining innovation adoption. That is, whether an individual or a nursing unit adopts or rejects innovation is determined not only by the unit's efficacy but also by the unit member's self-efficacy.

Second, the data showed that cooperativeness was positively related to innovation adoption only at the person level. This result indicates that a cooperative individual is willing to adopt innovation. However, this willingness to adopt innovation was not influenced by the nursing unit's cooperativeness.

The overall results suggest that an individual's self-efficacy and willingness to adopt innovation reflect the nursing unit's efficacy and willingness to adopt innovation. In other words, an individual's willingness to adopt innovation is the function of both his or her self-efficacy and the nursing unit's efficacy that is associated with the unit's willingness to adopt innovation. Accordingly, even an individual with high self-efficacy would not adopt innovation, if the nursing unit is not willing to adopt innovation because of low efficacy.

Nevertheless, an individual's cooperativeness and willingness to adopt innovation do not reflect those of the nursing unit. That is, an individual's willingness to adopt innovation is determined only by his or her cooperativeness. Accordingly, a cooperative individual is willing to adopt innovation regardless or whether the nursing unit is willing to adopt innovation or regardless of whether the unit is cooperative or noncooperative.

Accordingly, from a practical perspective, nursing administrators should consider both a nurse's self-efficacy and the nursing unit's efficacy in order to diffuse inovation. However, they should consider a nurse's cooperativeness rather than the nursing unit's cooperativeness in order to diffuse innovation.

5.   References

[1]   Romano CA. Diffusion of Technology Innovation. *Adv Nurs Sci* 1990, 13:11-21.
[2]   Brodt A and Stronge JH. Nurses' Attitudes Toward Computerization in a Midwestern Community Hospital. *Comput Nurs* 1986, 4:82-86.
[3]   Burkes M. Identifying and Relating Nurses' Attitudes Toward Computer Use. *Comput Nurs* 1991, 9:190-201.
[4]   Chang BL. Adoption of Innovations: Nursing and Computer Use. *Comput Nurs* 1984, 2:229-235.
[5]   Melhorn JM, Legler WK and Clark GM. Current Attitudes of Medical Personnel Toward Computers. *Comput Biomed Res* 1979, 12:327-334.
[6]   Anderson J, Joy S and Hackman E. The Role of Physician Networks in the Diffusion of Clinical Applications of Computers. *Int J Biomed Comput* 1982, 14:195-202.
[7]   Becker MH. Factors Affecting Diffusion of Innovations Among Health Professionals. *Am J Public Health* 1970, 60:294-305.
[8]   Coleman JS, Katz E and Menzel H. *Medical Innovation: A Diffusion Study.* New York: Bobbs-Merrill, 1965.
[9]   Davis F, Bagozzi R and Warshaw P. Users Acceptance of Computer Technology: A Comparison of Two Theoretical Models. *Manag Sci* 1989, 35:982-1003.
[10] Kimberly JR. Hospital Adoption of Innovations: The Role of Integration into External Information Environments. *J Health Soc Behave* 1978, 19:361-373.

622

[11] Kimberly JR and Evaniski MJ. Organizational Innovation: The Influence of Individual, Organizational, and Contextual Factors on Hospital Adoption of Technological and Administrative Innovations. *Acad Manag J* 1981, 24:689-713.

[12] Demanpour F. Organizational Innovation: A Meta-Analysis of Effects of Determinants and Moderators. *Acad Manag J* 1991, 34:555-590.

[13] Rice RE and Aydin C. Attitudes Toward New Organizational Technology: Network Proximity as a Mechanism for Social Information Processing. *Adm Sci Quart* 1991, 36:219-244.

[14] Dansereau F, Alutto JA and Yammarino F. *Theory Testing in Organizational Behavior: The Varient Approach.* New Jersey: Prentice-Hall, 1984.

[15] Rogers EM. *Diffusion of Innovations.* New York: Free Press, 1983.

[16] Ajzen I and Fishbein M. *Understanding Attitudes and Predicting Social Behavior.* New Jersey: Prentice-Hall, 1980.

[17] Fishbein M and Ajzen I. *Beliefs, Attitudes, Intenton and Behavior.* Massachusetts: Addison-Wesley, 1975.

[18] Bandura A. *Social Foundations of Thought and Action.* New Jersey: Prentice-Hall, 1986.

[19] Stumpf SA Brief AP and Hartman K. Self-efficacy Expectation and Coping with Career-Related Events. *J Voca Beh* 1987, 31:91-108.

[20] Hill T Smith ND and Mann MF. Role of Efficacy Expectations in Predicting the Decision to Use Advanced Technologies: The Case of Computers. *J Appli Psy* 1987, 72:307-313.

[21] Bandura A. Self-efficacy Mechanism in Human Agency. *Am Psy* 1982, 37:122-147.

[22] Gist ME. Self-efficacy: Implications for Organizational Behavior and Human Resource Management. *Acad Manag Rev* 1987, 12:37:122-147.

[23] Weenig WH and Midden JH. Communication Network Influences on Information Diffusion and Persuasion. *J Person and Soc Psy* 1991, 61:734-742.

[24] James LR. Aggregation Bias in Estimates of Perceptual Agreement. *J AppliPsy* 1982, 67:219-229.

[25] Ostroff C. The Relationship Between Satisfaction, Attitudes and Performance: An Organizational Level Analysis. *J Appli Psy* 1992, 77:963-974.

[26] Earley PC and Lituchy TR. Delineating Goal and Efficacy Effects: A Test of Three Models. *J Appli Psy* 1991, 76:81-98.

[27] Sherer M Maddux JE Mercandante B Prentice-Dunn S Jacobs B and Rogers RW. The Self-efficacy Scale: Construction and Validation. *Psy Reports* 1982, 51:663-671.

[28] Aydin CE. The Effects of Social Information and Cognitive Style on Medical Information System Attitudes and Use. In: The Eleventh Annual Symposium in Computer Applications in Medical Care. Stead WW (ed). Washington, DC: IEEE Computer Society, 1987: 601-606.

[29] Bongartz C. Computer-oriented Patient Care: A Comparison of Nurses' Attitudes and Perceptions. *Comput Nurs* 1988, 6:204-210.

[30] Ischar R and Aysin CE. Predicting Effective Use of Hospital Computer System. In: The Twelfth Annual Symposium on Computer Applications in Medical Care. Greenes RA (ed). Washington, DC: IEEE Computer Society Press, 1988:862-868.

[31] Krampf S and Robinson S. Managing Nurses' Attitudes Toward Computers. *Nurs Manag* 1984, 15:32-34.

STANDARDS

A. Standards; terminology

Nursing Informatics: An International Overview for Nursing in a Technological Era
S.J. Grobe and E.S.P. Pluyter-Wenting, eds.

Using nursing standards as a basis for reporting care using a computer

Taylor M E[a] Scholten R[b] Cassidy D A[c] and Corona D F[d]

[a]*Administration, R. E. Thomason Hospital, El Paso, Texas, U.S.A.*

[b]*Administration, R. E. Thomason Hospital, El Paso, Texas, U.S.A.*

[c]*Administration, R. E. Thomason Hospital, El Paso, Texas, U.S.A.*

[d]*Nursing Administration, R. E. Thomason Hospital, El Paso, Texas, U.S.A.*

The purpose of this paper is to describe the process, content and evaluation of Nursing Standards as the foundation for giving and documenting patient care. Computerizing nursing documentation utilizing defined standards requires a nurse who can both conceptualize and use Nursing Process to provide care. Selecting nursing diagnoses, defining and developing standards, and fitting standards into a computer software template is complex. This report chronicles activities of a group of nurses who developed Nursing Standards, fit them into a computer format, used the computer to document their actions and evaluated the relationship between actions and patient achievement of the desired outcomes. Nursing practice standards were then compared with McCloskey and Bulechek Nursing Interventions Classification (NIC) [1], with the hope that the standards could contribute to development of "Nursing Minimum Data Set" (NMDS) as recommended by Werley and Lang [2].

1. Introduction

The Nursing Department of a 335-bed county hospital, located on the United States/Mexico border, was committed to the aggressive use of technology to improve the efficacy of patient care and minimize the time professional nurses spent documenting patient care activities. Shared Medical System (SMS) computer products were in use in the hospital for financial, admission/discharge/transfer (ADT), order entry, and results reporting functions. The SMS nursing product line, Unity 21, was acquired to computerize patient care documentation. The professional nursing staff, working in a Standards Committee format, developed and approved standards of patient care which provided the structure for data entry into the system. Support for this project was provided by a part-time nursing consultant and a non-nurse computer application specialist.

2. Content

Using NANDA Nursing Diagnosis, the Standards Committee developed patient care standards (patient outcomes) and nursing practice standards (nursing interventions)* as a step toward total integration of nursing

---

*N.B. Taking cognizance that the American Nurses Association (ANA) may have chosen to define standards/guidelines differently, we have defined standards in keeping with the usage of the Joint Commission on Accreditation of Healthcare Organizations (JCAHO).

documentation in the form of a computerized (electronic) medical record. Nursing diagnoses were selected based on needs of the population the hospital served. (Many clients are Hispanic, fall below the poverty level, and speak only Spanish or speak English as a second language.) Each clinical department selected the NANDA diagnoses appropriate to their patient population. Patient outcomes included socioeconomic factors as well as other patient considerations. Nursing actions were described as interventions which focused succinctly on outcome attainment. Illustration number 1 demonstrates how a care plan for "Urge Incontinence" looked in the coded format. In this format, nursing diagnosis was substituted for patient problem, patient outcome for goal and nursing intervention for activity. In the care plan, provision was made to identify the intervention by mnemonic. Also coded was whether the intervention was to be printed on the Patient Care Activity Record (PCAR) and if it was to be printed on the nurses' work list. Frequency was the ordered number of times an intervention was to occur. The PRN frequency indicated that no amount of time was described for the intervention. The term "ongoing" permitted a specified amount of time to be allocated. The time factors were defined in a program of patient classification. The target date by which time a patient might be expected to meet the outcome was stated and the time frame for the nurse to evaluate the outcome was required. The target date and evaluation date defaults mandated documented evaluation of outcome attainment.

```
DEPT: NSG              Nursing Department
PROBLEM: 24           NO DESCRIPTION
                      URGE INCONTINENCE
                      MNEM: MS20

GOAL:          1      INCONTINENCE WILL BE MINIMIZED
                      MNEM:  TRGT DFLT: 3  EVAL DFLT: @ 8H

ACTIVITY:
MON 28         1      ASSESS VOIDING PATTERN TIME AMOUNT SENSATION PRIOR TO VOIDING
                      FREQ DFLT:PRN  AOC:MUS        PCAR:Y  CLASF:N          WRK:Y
NSG 38         2      REMOVE ROOM BARRIERS THAT PREVENT REACHING BATHROOM QUICKLY
                      FREQ DFLT:PRN  AOC:NC PCAR:Y  CLASF:N          WRK:Y
NSG 39         3      DO NOT USE INTRICATE FASTENERS WHEN DRESSING
                      FREQ DFLT:PRN  AOC:NC PCAR:Y  CLASF:N          WRK:Y
ELM 20         4      PROVIDE BEDSIDE COMMODE
                      FREQ DFLT:ONGOING      AOC:ELM        PCAR:Y  CLASF:N          WRK:Y
ELM 21         5      RESPOND TO CALL LIGHT FOR ASSISTANCE IN BATHROOM
                      FREQ DFLT:ONGOING      AOC:ELM        PCAR:Y  CLASF:Y          WRK:Y
NSG 40         6      OBTAIN ORDER FOR URINE C AND S TO RULE OUT UTI AS CAUSE
                      FREQ DFLT:PRN  AOC:NC PCAR:Y  CLASF:N          WRK:Y
DCH 24         7      CONSULT MD FOR BLADDER TRAINING PROGRAM
                      FREQ DFLT:PRN  AOC:DCH        PCAR:Y  CLASF:N          WRK:Y
ELM 22         8      ESTABLISH TOILETING HABIT TRAINING PROGRAM
                      FREQ DFLT:ONGOING      AOC:ELM        PCAR:Y  CLASF:Y          WRK:Y
MED 10         9      ADMINISTER DIURETICS EARLY IN THE DAY IF ORDERED
                      FREQ DFLT:PRN  AOC:MED        PCAR:Y  CLASF:N          WRK:Y
ELM 23         10     LIMIT DIURETIC FLUIDS IE CAFFEINATED BEVERAGES ALCOHOL ETC.
                      FREQ DFLT:PRN  AOC:ELM        PCAR:Y  CLASF:N          WRK:Y
```

Illustration 1. Coded Format

Registered nurses were required to develop an individualized plan of care within eight hours of admission for every patient. Then, nurses were to document in the computer on the patients' progress notes. Doctors, nutritionists, social workers, and physical therapists had access to the use of progress notes as well.

3. Process

Orienting nurses to use of the system was a two-fold process; first, the nurses were introduced to how computers work, and what they can and cannot do, and second, the nurses were required to document using nursing process-based care plans. The first problem on the surface seemed the most troublesome. Based on reports in the literature and our actual experience, nursing personnel had varying degrees of computer literacy and skill. This problem was comparatively simple to handle. Classes on computer and software capability were held by the computer specialist and practice in the lab was required of all who were expected to use the computer. The second problem was much more complex to rectify, because it involved a change in how nurses think about patient outcomes and the relationship of outcomes to interventions, which is the work of nursing. Nurses were not always able to relate the interventions to the patient outcome. Because the conceptual orientation of nursing process eluded some nurses, the relationships among the factors associated with nursing process were not evident in the documentation. (Supposedly, nurses were using nursing process to chart manually, but this proved not to be the case.) Forcing computerized documentation of the patient plan of care graphically demonstrated problems in providing or reporting independent and interdependent nursing care which should focus on the accomplishment of a patient outcome versus doing isolated procedures or a nursing intervention. The lack of use of nursing process far exceeded the difficulty of using a computer. It required one-on-one exposure not only to the computer, but also one-on-one assistance in using nursing process. It was problematic for nurses to see how nursing diagnoses drove patient outcomes which necessitated certain nursing actions whether intellectual or skill-based. Emphasis on clinical decision-making judgements using standards was fundamental.

A model was developed to demonstrate the relationship between the nursing process and its use in computerized documentation. Illustration number 2 shows the initial model of nursing process used to develop computerized patient care plans. It shows a generally accepted systems model of nursing process. Our experience led us to further refine this model for greater clarity.

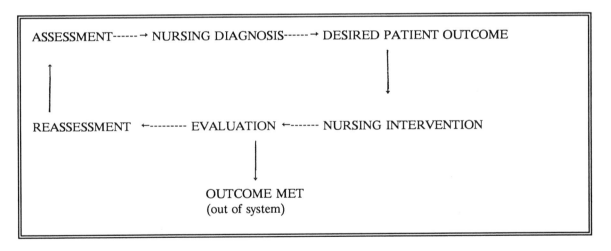

Illustration 2. Nursing Process

The next illustration depicts the relationship of interventions and outcomes (nursing standards) to each other and to the type of documentation needed for computerization. Assessment screens were built containing admission demographic requirements and assessment parameters. It was expected that all nurses would apply their own skill, knowledge, and judgement rather than accepting the standardized care plans. Some nurses were unable to do this. The software provided the opportunity to suggest nursing diagnoses which might be appropriate. The nurses were expected to judge if the suggested diagnoses were appropriate for their individual patients. Each nursing diagnosis had stated patient outcomes which described the desired state of an individual patient. The nurse was expected to decide which intervention would be appropriate for achieving the patient outcomes and select only those which were pertinent. A target date was suggested and it required the nurse to affirm that date as reasonable to accomplish the outcome(s) or to re-assign a suitable date. If the outcome was not achieved, the nurse was expected to re-evaluate the care plan based on re-assessment.

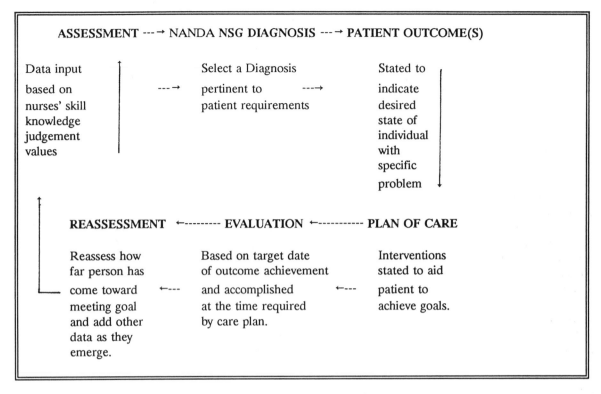

Illustration 3. Nursing Process and Required Nursing Documentation

4. Evaluation

To provide improved patient care was one stated goal for implementing a computerized patient care planning. A second advantage of the computerized system of patient care planning, was decreased time spent documenting and increased legibility of the record.

Those nurses who were able to conceptualize and apply the nursing process in planning and giving care, found that documenting using a computerized patient care plan was easier and a significant time saver. A follow-up study to an earlier one in which nurses reported that they spent up to an average of three hours per shift recording, now reported that they spent no more than 45 minutes total in the recording function. This left two hours and fifteen minutes to re-allocate to direct patient care. At first, no time savings were noted but as nurses became familiarized with the process, time savings became a significant factor.

Upon analysis, it was found that there was remarkable consistency between the interventions stated by hospital nurses and those articulated by McCloskey and Bulechek. The same verbs were frequently used and the content was similar, giving credence to the hospital list and the McCloskey and Bulechek list.

NMDS related to nursing care elements were consistent with those recommended by Werley and Lang. However, we expanded the client demographic elements to include not only race and ethnicity, but the culture of poverty and issues of nationality and entitlements as these elements are not addressed by NMDS.

Finally, the system provided other assets to support nursing administration and management. It provided a Work List from the intervention and nursing order files which was directed to the appropriate level of assistive personnel. This work list was ordered by skill level, patient, and time (frequency). Each nursing order or intervention had an associated time factor that was down loaded into a staffing and scheduling module to aid in determining number and skill level of staff needed.

5. Summary

When evaluating care based on patient outcomes, it was increasingly clear that a classification or taxonomy of patient care standards or patient outcomes must be developed so that the entire construct of nursing process can be articulated as has been done with nursing diagnosis and nursing intervention classification. This would enable outcome based care to be communicated and generally understood by nurses. It would finish what is necessary to complete a minimum nursing data set. It would also provide the last piece required to initiate changes for nursing care based on identifiable, justifiable results.

6. References

[l] McCloskey, J. and G.M. Bulechek. *Nursing Intervention Classification.* St. Louis: Mosby, Inc., 1992.

[2] Werley, H.H. and N. M. Long. *Identification of the Nursing Minimum Data Set.* New York: Publishing Company, 1988.

We acknowledge and thank Maria Luisa Bogan, Computer Application Specialist, for her assistance with the project.

© 1994 Elsevier Science B.V. All rights reserved.
Nursing Informatics: An International Overview for Nursing in a Technological Era
S.J. Grobe and E.S.P. Pluyter-Wenting, eds.

630

Maintaining Standards of Nursing Care Documentation Through Use of a Critical Care Bedside Clinical Information System

Colson A

Hewlett-Packard Company, 2101 Gaither Road, Rockville, Maryland 28050 USA. Formerly from Nursing Service, Department of Veterans Affairs Medical Center, 50 Irving Street NW, Washington D.C. 20422

Utilization of a Critical Care Bedside Clinical Information System (CIS) provides a mechanism for maintaining standardized documentation of nursing care in the intensive care units (ICUs). CIS automates the critical care patient flowsheet and enables nursing staff to follow a standard charting format. A Graphic User Interface (GUI) and point-and-click technology provide nursing staff with a means to efficiently and effectively meet documentation requirements in less time than manual charting. On-site configuration tools allow change and development of CIS software as standards of nursing practice change.

1. Introduction

Many hospitals have implemented bedside clinical information systems (CIS) in response to an increased focus on quality improvement (QI), the demand for accurate and concise documentation, as well as the need to reduce health care costs. Bedside CISs are ideal in critical care areas where the increase in patient age and severity of illness has lead to a notable escalation in the amount of data required on a critical care flowsheet [1].

This paper will discuss the use of a critical care bedside CIS at the Department of Veterans Affairs Medical Center in Washington D.C. (DVAMC-DC). A description of CIS, an explanation of Joint Commission on Accreditation of Health Care Organizations (JCAHO) and DVAMC-DC Nursing Service standards, and information on how documentation standards of nursing care have been maintained through use of the CIS will be discussed.

2. Description of CIS

The DVAMC-DC implemented a bedside CIS in the Medical and Surgical Intensive Care Units (MICU and SICU). CIS automates the critical care flowsheet which includes documentation of vital signs, intake and output, laboratory results, nursing and respiratory therapists' assessments, interventions, and evaluation of care. There is a beside cardiac monitor and laboratory interface in place. Interfaces for ventilators, intravenous infusion pumps, and electronic urimeters are planned. CIS operates on a Local Area Network (LAN) connecting 27 workstations to two sets of redundant Reduced Instruction Set Computing (RISC)-based minicomputers (one set located in MICU, the other located in SICU). The workstations are movable carts placed in patient rooms or immediately outside patient rooms, depending on the room size.

CIS's operating system is UNIX based, written in C++ and X-windows. A trackball, which allows users to point-and-click on structured-text entries, is used for the method of data entry. On-site configuration tools enable the Intensive Care Unit (ICU) Systems Coordinator, or the CIS project manager, to customize the software without the need for knowing a programming language. The system is maintained by personnel within the DVAMC-DC's Nursing Service.

3. JCAHO and DVAMC-DC Nursing Service Standards

In the 1993 Accreditation Manual for Hospitals (AMH), JCAHO refines quality assurance requirements to focus on systematic quality assessment and improvement, emphasizing patient outcomes [2]. AMH's standards indicate that the medical record must include documentation of assessments, interventions, and patient outcomes. Additionally, the AMH regroups patient and family education standards into a separate chapter to ensure this area is routinely addressed.

In response to JCAHO, the Department of Veterans Affairs, and VAMC-DC's Nursing Service incorporated documentation standards that center on the following outcomes: documented assessment of patient needs; reassessment of needs based on the patient's condition; documentation of the Nursing Plan of Care; documentation and evaluation of nursing interventions and patient outcomes.

Assessments and nursing care interventions must be documented a minimum of once a shift in the Intensive Care Units (ICUs). Evaluation of patient response to interventions and achievement, or lack of achievement, of expected outcomes must also be documented once a shift.

4. Standardizing Documentation Through CIS

Nursing documentation of assessments, interventions, and evaluation of patient care are standardized to meet JCAHO and DVAMC-DC Nursing Service requirements in the ICUs through use of structured-text entries and customization of CIS software. CIS's Graphic User Interface (GUI) and point-and-click technology provide a means for the nursing staff to meet documentation criteria in less time than manual charting. Please refer to Figure 1 to view the data entry screen within the CIS.

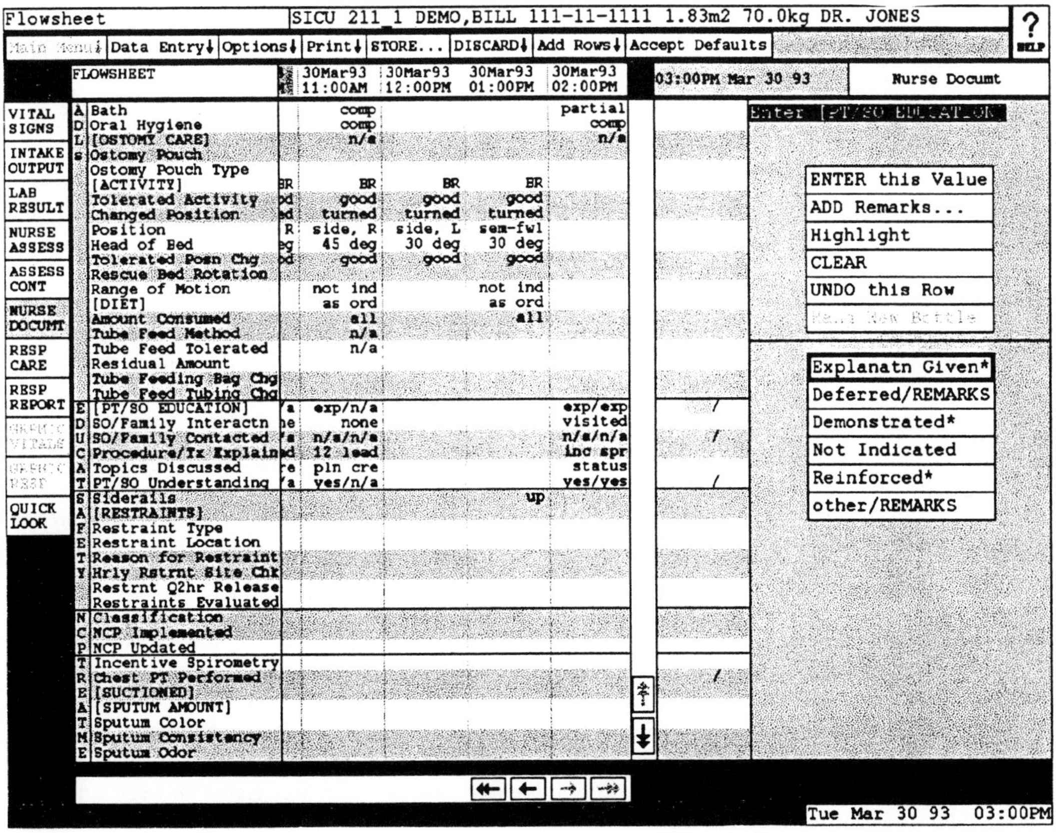

Figure 1. Data Entry Screen within the CIS Illustrating Row Labels in Nurse Documt Section.

Figure 1 illustrates how documentation criteria is structured in the CIS flowsheet. The top middle portion of the screen displays the patient's name, social security number, admission body surface area, admission weight, and doctor's name. On-line help is located in the top right corner. The left side of the screen displays the various sections of the flowsheet. To the right of the sections is a single column which lists the subsections in the chosen section. Immediately to the right of the subsections, row labels are displayed. The middle portion of the screen displays time columns where previous entries have been made. The right side of the screen shows the time column the user has selected to enter data. The user can change the time by using the trackball to point-and-click on the displayed time and can scroll the trackball to the desired time.

The user can use the keyboard or trackball to select the preferred row label. Once a row label is chosen, the user can select one of the structured-text entries that are displayed in the right lower corner of the screen. Users can further explain an entry by selecting "Add Remarks", which displays a window where the user can type supplementary comments. When a structured-text entry displays a " /REMARKS ", this indicates the user must add a remark to further explain the entry. Additionally, the user can highlight an option red by selecting the "Highlight" option. An entry may be highlighted if abnormal or if there is a change in patient status. For example, an abnormal lab result or deteriorating lung sounds.

DC-VAMC ICU policy indicates that the nurse must address each row label when documenting an initial assessment and must document any changes throughout the shift. Nurses can tailor individual patient flowsheets by adding or deleting row labels. For example, a cardiac surgery patient's flowsheet is more complex than a patient who is admitted for gastric pain. By using the trackball to point-and-click on the "Add Rows" option on the menu bar, a pop-down window displays additional row labels that can be added. Certain row labels are mandatory and cannot be deleted. Examples of mandatory row labels include temperature, heart rate, heart rhythm, respiratory rate, blood pressure, lung sounds, and code status.

5. Refining CIS Software to Meet Standards of Care

CIS flowsheets provide easily accessible information for QI monitoring. QI monitors reveal areas of compliance with charting policies regarding nursing assessment and documentation. Aspects of care that have been monitored in the ICUs include patient education, ventilator management, pain management, use of restraints, and IV site maintenance.

Configuration tools allow change and development of the CIS flowsheet as standards of practice change or if QI monitoring shows lack of documentation in certain areas. For example, one QI monitor revealed that patient and significant other education was not routinely documented in our ICUs. As a result, row labels related to this topic were created and customized into the CIS flowsheet. Subsequent patient and significant other education QI monitors show marked improvement.

Designing row labels necessitates creativity, especially when software character limits must be considered. Table 1 displays the patient and significant other education row labels and examples of structured-text entries. The capital letters and square parenthesis in first row label [PT/SO EDUCATION] indicates to the user that this is a new grouping of row labels within the subsection. Therefore, the subsequent row labels below [PT/SO EDUCATION] pertain to this topic. Notice that the [PT/SO EDUCATION] row labels include nursing interventions as well as evaluation of the intervention(s).

CIS row labels have a twenty character maximum. Row label choices have a sixteen character limit. The area in the flowsheet where row label choices are entered is called a "cell". Row labels can have a one cell property or two cell property. One cell properties have a seven character limit while two cell properties have a three character maximum. An example of a row label that comprises a two cell property is [PT/SO EDUCATION]. The first cell gives choices pertaining to the patient. The second cell displays choices pertaining to the significant other.

Row labels are designed by the ICU Systems Coordinator with input from the ICU nurse manager, nursing staff, and other appropriate personnel such as a nurse clinical specialist or QI coordinator. Row labels are entered into CIS's test environment where the ICU nurse manager and staff review them and give feedback. Additional personnel, such as QI representatives or the clinical nurse specialist may also review the row labels. New row labels are kept in the test environment until they are "activated" into CIS's live environment. The time frame between activation periods depends on how urgent the need for the new row labels. Routinely, activations are done once a month. Activations require ten minutes of CIS down time.

Table 1
CIS Patient and Significant Other Education Row Labels and Structured-Text Entry Choices

CIS Row Labels:	Cell Property	1st Cell Choices:	2nd Cell Choices:
[PT/SO EDUCATION]	2 Cell	Explanatn Given* Deferred/REMARKS** Not Indicated Reinforced* Other/REMARKS	Explantn Given* Deferred/REMARKS Not Indicated Reinforced* Other/REMARKS
SO/Family Interactn	1 Cell	No Interaction SO/Family Phoned SO/Family Visitd Other/REMARKS	
SO/Family Contacted	2 Cell	Not Applicable Yes/REMARKS Other/REMARKS	Not Applicable Physician Nurse Other/REMARKS
Procedure/Tx Explain	1 Cell	Not Indicated Arterial Line Bronchoscopy Cardioversion Cat Scan Central Line Chest Tube Dialysis Extubation	
Topics Discussed	1 Cell	Not Indicated Activity Level Chest Pain Scale ICU Environment Meds/REMARKS Plan of Care Status/Condition Visiting Hours	
PT/SO Understanding	2 Cell	Not Applicable No/REMARKS Yes/Understood Other/REMARKS	Not Applicable No/REMARKS Yes/Understood Other/REMARKS

* if the user selects an item with an asterisk he/she must chart on additional appropriate row labels.

** /REMARKS indicates a user must enter remarks via "Add Remarks" explaining this entry.

6. Conclusion

Use of a CIS in the ICUs at the DVAMC-DC has allowed standardization of nursing documentation. Point-and-click technology through use of a trackball has enabled ICU staff to document more efficiently and effectively in less time than manual charting. On-site configuration tools allow the project manager to update the CIS software based on changes in clinical practice or on QI monitor results.

7. References

[1] Leyerle B, LoBue M and Shabot M. Integrated Computerized Databases for Medical Management Beyond the Bedside. *Int J Clin Monit Comput* 1990, 7:83-89.

[2] Joint Commission on Accreditation of Health Care Organization. *Accreditation Manual for Hospitals.* Vol. 1 Standards, 1993.

Nursing Informatics: An International Overview for Nursing in a Technological Era
S.J. Grobe and E.S.P. Pluyter-Wenting, eds.

Educating Nurses to Maintain Patient Confidentiality on Automated Information Systems

Hebda T[a] Sakerka L[b] and Czar P[c]

[a]Dept of Nursing, Waynesburg College, Waynesburg, Pennsylvania 15370, USA

[b]Clinical Manager, Information Systems, Sewickley Valley Hospital, Sewickley, Pennsylvania 15143, USA (formerly Nurse Leader, Information Services, Washington Hospital, Washington, Pennsylvania 15301, USA).

[c]Project Sup, Clinical Systems, St Francis Medical Center, 45th Street, Pittsburgh, Pennsylvania 15201, USA.

Privacy and confidentiality have long been concerns in healthcare. Once, the patient's written record was kept and accessed at a centralized location. Now, computerized information systems (IS) permit access at decentralized points. Decentralized access reduces wait time for record access, but increases opportunities for unauthorized access. The best means to safeguard the privacy and confidentiality of automated patient records and guard against professional liability is through education of IS users. Education encompasses the following areas: responsibilities and rights of system users; legitimate uses of patient information (by health care providers and other users); legal consequences of violations of patient privacy and confidentiality, ways to safeguard the IS from intrusion, and providing computer pathways that promote confidentiality. Subsequent to a discussion of these areas, the measures established to protect patient confidentiality at two institutions are chronicled.

1. Privacy and Confidentiality

Privacy and confidentiality are concerns in health care. Once access to the patient's record was limited by its location and physical form. Now 75 or more persons have access to a patient record.[1] And, computerized information systems (IS) permit decentralized access. This reduces wait time for record access, but it increases opportunities for unauthorized access.[2,3] This paper defines confidentiality, discusses legal safeguards, reviews related literature, and outlines measures at two institutions to protect confidentiality.

While the terms privacy and confidentiality are used interchangeably, they are different. Privacy is defined as a state of mind, a specific place, freedom from intrusion, or control over the exposure of self or personal information.[4,5] Information privacy refers to the individual's ability to choose the extent to which, and the time and circumstances under which his attitudes, behavior, and beliefs will be shared with others. Information privacy includes the right to insure accuracy of records, and the right to confidentiality of information that has been collected by an organization.[6]

Confidentiality connotes a relationship in which information is disclosed.[7] It is dependent upon the loss of privacy. Unlike privacy, which is controlled by individual choice to reveal information, confidentiality is controlled by the person(s) to whom information is disclosed. Confidential information can be sensitive if disclosed to inappropriate persons. Inappropriate disclosure of confidential information may result in harm to employment, reputation, or personal relationships, and possible exploitation.[5] In the case of medical records, health care professionals are morally obligated by their professional code of ethics to maintain confidentiality of information as there can be no privacy of medical records without confidentiality.[8] Some states have regulations, statutes, and case law recognizing the confidentiality of medical records and limiting their access. Breach of confidence may lead to disciplinary action inclusive of revocation of license.[9] Such disciplinary measures generally apply only to physicians.[10] Confidentiality is essential to the relationship between health care provider and recipient. Anything that threatens confidentiality may keep people from seeking care or making disclosures required for treatment.[11]

2. Legal Protection in the U.S.

Laws to protect automated records cannot keep pace with technology.[12] Legal literature reveals an increased awareness of threats to medical record privacy but limited protection. In 1980 proposed federal legislation called for a time limit on consent to release information, standardized procedures for record access, a log of all parties accessing any medical record, and stiff penalties for obtaining records under false pretenses. Unfortunately the Privacy of Medical Information Act bill was defeated.[13]

Protection of medical records varies from state to state. Only some states have privacy laws which include private record keepers such as insurance companies and hospitals.[10] Some states provide criminal sanctions for the violation of confidentiality statutes and have monitoring agencies in place. But even with criminal sanctions and monitoring agencies, enforcement is generally up to the patient whose privacy was violated. Quantifying damage is difficult. Specific security measures for the possessors of confidential health care information are not required in all states.[5] Ohio case law has found unauthorized disclosure of medical information by anyone in a confidential relationship with the patient an actionable tort.[9]

3. Review of the Literature

Given the limited legal protection for patient records, the health care institution and professional must maintain patient confidentiality.[1] Unfortunately, weak data protection policies encourage information abuse. Any, and all elements of the IS can threaten its security including all levels of nursing personnel. Nonprofessionals are not bound by a professional code of ethics. But, even many RN's revealed that they had accessed information on patients not under their care.[14-17]. This has implications for the structure of IS and treatment of personnel.

Data protection must be built into the system. Institutions need clearly stated security policies that are enforced.[7,18-20] Everyone with IS access should sign a statement that pledges to uphold patient confidentiality and acknowledges the consequences for failure to do so. Data protection can also be achieved through limited access to hardware and software. Access to software can be achieved through user specific sign on codes that are changed frequently, eliminated upon employee departure from a unit or the institution, and limit access to a need to know basis. Codes should not be borrowed or exchanged. Unattended terminals should have an automatic sign off feature. And, tracking user access and changes must be possible. But perhaps the best way to safeguard patient information is through the creation of a structure that supports privacy and confidentiality. Users tend to ignore access rules and ignore possible ethical and legal implications. Personnel need periodic reminders of what constitutes professional, legal, and ethical practice and behavior, and their responsibility to safeguard patient confidentiality. [2,7,14,15,17,21,22]

4. A Tale of Two Institutions

St. Francis Medical Center is a Technicon Data System (TDS) hospital in Pittsburgh, Pennsylvania. St. Francis emphasizes the importance of patient confidentiality in several ways. First, all staff sign a form upon issue of their access code. This document states that violation of patient confidentiality constitutes grounds for dismissal. Staff are told that their access code is their legal signature and that it should be treated accordingly. Codes are distributed in sealed envelopes. Many staff keep their codes with them until transcription area.

Automated information systems also provide the technology to easily violate patient confidentiality. In recognition of this fact, the basic concepts of patient privacy and confidentiality must be even more heavily emphasized in the basic education of nurses and training of ancillary personnel. Continuous reinforcement of these concepts must be an integral part of IS training. Periodic reminders about patient confidentiality must also be a part of ongoing education for all employees. IS professionals must still recognize that humans will be curious. The successful IS strategy must address ways to maximize utilization of computer technology wile planning ways to promote patient confidentiality. Steps to reduce temptation to inappropriately access records must be addressed through institutional policy and IS structures.

6. References

[1] Calfee, B. Confidentiality and Disclosure of Medical Information. *Nurs Manage* 1989, 20 (12):20-23.

[2] Eleazor, PY. Risks Associated with Clinical Databases. *Top Health Rec Manage* 1991, 12 (2):49-58.

[3] Haddad, A. The Dilemma of Keeping Confidences. *AORN* 1989, 50 (1):161-164.

[4] Kmentt, KA. Private Medical Records: Are They Public Property? *Medical Trial Technique Quarterly* Winter 1987, 33:274-307.

[5] Winslade, WJ. Confidentiality of Medical Records: An Overview of Concepts and Legal Policies. *Journal of Legal Medicine* 1982 3 (4):497-533.

[6] Murdock, LE. The Use and Abuse of Computerized Information: Striking a Balance Between Personal Privacy Interests and Organizational Information Needs. *Albany Law Review* 1980, 44, (3):589-619.

[7] Romano, C. Privacy, Confidentiality, and Security of Computerized Systems: The Nursing Responsibility. *Comput Nurs* 1987, 5 (3):99-104.

[8] Maciorowski, L. The Enduring Concerns of Privacy and Confidentiality. *Holist Nurs Pract* 1991, 5 (3):51-56.

[9] Johnston, CE. Breach of Medical Confidence in Ohio. *Akron Law Review* Winter 1986, 19:373-393.

[10] Miller, M. Computers, Medical Records, and the Right to Privacy. *J Health Polit Policy Law* 1981, 6:463-488.

[11] Fry, S. Confidentiality in Health Care: A Decrepit Concept? *Nurs Econ* 1984, 2 (6):413-418.

[12] Nasri, W. Legal Issues of Computers in Healthcare: Liabilities of the Healthcare Provider. Paper presented to the Tri-State Nursing Computer Network Pittsburgh, Pennsylvania. March 19, 1992.

[13] Morihara, J. Computers, the Disclosure of Medical Information, and the Fair Credit Reporting Act. *Computer/Law Journal* Summer 1982, 3:619-639.

[14] Curran, M and Curran, K. The Ethics of Information. *JONA* 1991, 21 (1):47-49.

[15] Regan, BG. Computerized Information Exchange in Health Care. *Med J Aust* 1991, 154 (2):140-144.

[16] Solomon, T. Personal Privacy and the '1984' Syndrome. *Western New England Law Review* Winter

1985, 7:753-780.

[17] Wogan, MJ. New Technologies Raise Concerns about Protecting Patient Confidentiality. *Hosp Patient Relat Rep* 1991, 6 (2):1-2

[18] Barber, B. Guardians or Gizmos. *Health Serv J* 1991, 101 (5262):33-34.

[19] Lochner, MA. Legal Issues Pertaining to Clinical Record Systems. Paper Presented at the Medical Information Systems Association, Incorporated Spring 1991 Meeting: Achieving the Competitive Edge. April 24, 1991.

[20] Williams, FG. Implementing Computer Information Systems for Hospital Based Case Management. *Hosp Health Serv Adm* 36 (4): 559-570.

[21] Grady, C, Jacob, J and Romano, C. Confidentiality: A Survey in a Research Hospital. *J Clin Ethics* 1991, 2 (1):25-30.

[22] Powell, D. Plugging the Leaks in Data Networks. *Networking Management* 1992 10 (6):29-32.

Nursing Informatics: An International Overview for Nursing in a Technological Era
S.J. Grobe and E.S.P. Pluyter-Wenting, eds.

Nursing, Midwifery and Health Visiting Terms Project

Casey A

NHS Centre for Coding and Classification, Woodgate, Loughborough, LE11 2TG, England

A two year Project is underway in England to develop a comprehensive thesaurus of the terms nurses, midwives and health visitors use to record and communicate care. This project is closely related to Medical and Professions Allied to Medicine (PAMS) Terms Projects creating an agreed thesaurus of healthcare terms coded for use in clinical computer systems. This paper summarises the background to the Project, its aims, scope and working methods, and the structures put in place to ensure consultation and professional ownership of the work. A review is given of progress to date with discussion of the implications of the Project for nursing.

1. Background

The English National Health Service (NHS) Management Executive and its Information Management Group recognise the need for the Service to be supported by improved information at all levels. A major aspect of the Strategy for Information Management and Technology (IM&T)[1] for England is the development of a common infrastructure to facilitate computerisation and sharing of clinical information across the service. This infrastructure includes a thesaurus of coded clinical terms which is being developed by the Clinical Terms projects based at the NHS Centre for Coding and Classification.

Nursing was able to influence the IM&T Strategy and its programme of work through a body called the Strategic Advisory Group for Nursing Information Systems (SAGNIS). This group includes representatives from the service and the professional bodies: the Royal College of Nursing, the Royal College of Midwives and the Health Visitors Association. The project is a fully funded collaboration between the Centre for Coding and Classification and the nursing professions in the United Kingdom.

The starting point for the Terms Project was the Read Codes, a comprehensive, hierarchically arranged thesaurus of medical terms mapped to ICD9 and other main classifications, adopted by the NHS in 1990 as the standard coding system in General Practice. Over 40 Working Groups representing every medical specialty have contributed to the project, refining and extending the existing Read Codes. This work was completed in April 1994, with the incorporation of terms used by Professions Allied to Medicine (PAMS) in October 1994.

The recommendations of a scoping study completed in February 1993 form the basis of the plan for Nursing, Midwifery and Health Visiting Terms Project which will be completed in April 1995.

2. Aim of the project

Accurate, timely and comprehensive clinical information is essential for the provision of seamless, high quality patient care. As patient-based, integrated information systems are developed, a clinical thesaurus assumes central importance. A coded clinical thesaurus with agreed synonyms makes available medical, nursing and PAM's terms for use in clinical computer systems. It facilitates the sharing of information between health carers, purchasers, providers, managers and others. Terms agreed between professionals provide the basis for exchange and analysis of information on every aspect of patient care[2]. They satisfy the clinical data requirements for care plans, protocols, decision support, research, audit, central planning, management and epidemiology.

The aim of the Nursing, Midwifery and Health Visiting Terms Project is to produce an agreed thesaurus of Nursing, Midwifery and Health Visiting Terms incorporated into the Read Codes, and a plan for the maintenance and further development of that thesaurus.

This will allow the keeping of health care records on computer and, together with the Terms produced by the Medical and Professions Allied to Medicine Terms Projects will offer the potential for a shared, multidisciplinary computerised record.

The thesaurus being produced is a collection of terms used by nurses, midwives and health visitors to record and communicate the care of their patients/clients.

Patient terms are included in the project to the extent that are used in client-held or shared records and used in patient information documents such as admission letters or discharge advice.

Nurses, midwives and health visitors use medical and other terms such as medical diagnosis, operative procedure, and drug names. Close liaison with the medical and PAMS project working groups is essential to identify overlapping or shared terms and reduce duplication of effort. **Shared terms** will include those used by social workers, especially in community settings.

The project is NOT about monitoring or constraining practice, defining nursing or developing computer systems. Other projects within the strategy initiatives are working on issues such as clinician/computer interface, electronic patient records and the confidentiality and security of patient data. The project is also NOT about how the terms are used, such as for developing datasets, classifications, outcome measures or nursing diagnoses. There is already work in this area,[3] and more will be possible with the results of this project. As the terms become available the professions must decide how they can use them in groupings or classifications. Because the thesaurus is grounded in the practical language used by nurses in their daily work it has tremendous potential to add to our understanding and description of nursing practice.

3. Organisation and project management

The project is managed using PRINCE project management methodology, the NHS Management Executive's recommended standard for the management of large projects to ensure they produce what is required, to time and within budget. The organisational structure ensures appropriate management and quality control at all levels of the project.

The **Project Board** provide overall direction and guidance to the project at a high level and includes senior members of the professions including representatives from the Royal Colleges of Nursing and Midwifery and the Health Visitor Association. An independent **Project Assurance Team** are responsible for providing quality review of the terms listed.

Co-ordination of the work of the project across the working groups, and with the work of the other terms projects, is the responsibility of the **Project Working Team**. Day to day administration of the project is the responsibility of the **Project Management Team**. With the Project Support Office at the Centre for Coding and Classification they provide all the necessary administrative back-up to the project including technical and financial support.

Six **Working Groups** have been established to revise and expand the lists of terms and synonyms required by nurses in the main fields of Nursing:

Mental Health Nursing   Midwifery
Paediatric Nursing   Community Health Care
Learning Disability Nursing   Adult Nursing

These groups are made up of clinical practitioners and include representatives of relevant patient groups. **Specialty Working Groups** representing the many nursing sub-specialties will further refine and expand terms before they are piloted in a range of settings, including acute and community units, regions and special settings such as controlled environments and the forces.

4. Work Plan

The scoping project demonstrated that nursing records did not always reflect the full range of terms used to communicate nursing, especially in relation to the psychosocial needs and care of patients. Whereas the medical project had lists of terms (e.g. earlier versions of Read and ICD-9), there were no equivalent lists available to UK nurses. It was decided that the project would need to create initial lists from fieldwork term collection in hospital and community settings.

During the initial collection exercise a first list of terms was produced from patient records and spoken communications. This was organised into logical groups for easy access and refined by the working groups. The next stages include further expansion and review of the lists and relevant medical lists. The comprehensiveness and accessibility of the final list of terms will be tested at a range of sites not previously associated with the project. Figure 1 is an overview of the methods being used.

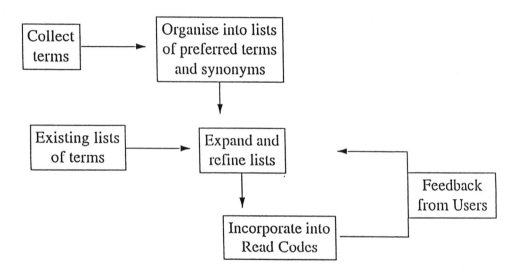

Figure 1.   Working Methods

On completion of the pilot and following further revision, the final lists of terms will be incorporated into the Read Codes for distribution. The Nursing, Midwifery and Health Visiting terms will be maintained and updated as an integral part of the complete Health Care Thesaurus. Communication to the professions and beyond about the Terms and related projects is continuing throughout the project. Educational material is being produced as part of the project to raise awareness in the nursing professions about Read Codes, terms and information issues.

4.1 Creating lists of terms

Fieldworkers collected statements made in patient records and in tape recorded conversations between nurses and patients: statements about the patient or client and their circumstances; about what needs to be done or has been done and so on. These statements were developed into lists of terms by first identifying the clinical concepts contained in them. A preferred term was selected to represent that term and any synonymous terms identified during the review processes. Additional information in statements was added in the form of qualifiers.

As an example, one statement found in a record was "patient is able to walk short distances with assistance". The clinical concept, in the nurse's words, was "is able to walk", and that was the preferred term. Synonymous terms included "can walk". Examples of qualifier attributes which gave additional information in this case were: "extent of walking ability" and "aids to walking".

5. Conclusion

The Nursing Midwifery and Health Visiting terms project is an example of a national infrastructure initiative which is essential for the realisation of the potential that Information Technology could offer. Seamless care across provider services and geographical boundaries is a long term goal in Europe. Without standards, the systems, security safeguards, and networks, to support such care will not be developed. This project is providing the United Kingdom standard for terms that are used by professionals and patients and is the cornerstone of NHS IT development.

6. References

(1)   Information Management Group. IM&T Strategy Overview. Leeds: NHS Management 1992.

(2)   Moores Y. Keynote address to British Computer Society Nursing Specialist Group Conference, Eastbourne. November 1992.

(3)   Grobe S. "Nursing Intervention and Taxonomy Study: Language and Classification Methods", Advances in Nursing Science. December 1990, pp 647-649.

Nursing Informatics: An International Overview for Nursing in a Technological Era
S.J. Grobe and E.S.P. Pluyter-Wenting, eds.

Nursing Information in Patient Records
Towards Uniform Key Words for Documentation of Nursing Practice

Ehnfors M

Dept of Social Medicine, Uppsala University, Akademiska Hospital, S-701 85 Uppsala, Sweden.

A model for documentation of nursing care, the so called VIPS-model was introduced in seven wards at two hospitals. Patient records (N 140) were reviewed for content and comprehensiveness before and after this intervention. The result showed that all categories of the nursing interventions were used and the documentation increased except for educational interventions. After the intervention nine out of ten records had notes representing five or more components of the nursing process model compared to slightly more than half before. The recording of problems which had some information on the progress or the outcome of the patient's situation for that particular problem was found for one third of the problems before the documentation intervention and in four-fifths after. The study is a national continuation of the International Council of Nurses (ICN) project, Standards of Nursing Regulation.

1. Nursing documentation in patient records

Nursing documentation is an integral and important part of nursing practice, although many studies have shown deficiencies in documentation practice or a strong medical orientation of the nursing records [1, 2, 3, 4, 5, 6, 7]. Inadequate recording may be partly due to a lack of understanding of the reasons for documentation [8, 9], lack of a unified system of documentation [9, 7] or insufficient time allocation and the nurse's experience of stress and decreased job satisfaction, in which case the recording is regarded as too demanding [10, 11] and probably also due to the strong tradition of reporting orally at least in Sweden.

In a complex and changing health care system the need for the development of documentation practices in nursing that facilitate both recording and communication becomes more and more obvious. There are many reason for practicing careful documentation, the most important being that the record is necessary for the delivery of good and secure care. This is crucial both for the patients and for the health care professionals. Professional nursing requires the recording of assessment, planning and evaluation of the patient's situation and the care delivered, to facilitate communication within the health care system, and to increase the possibility of advancing nursing knowledge and research. In addition, the documentation is a legal and regulatory responsibility.

Swedish authorities have emphasized that the record is intended to support the health care professionals in the delivery of care, to serve as a basis for quality care, and to be the reference point for judgements and choice of interventions to be implemented by personnel who had not met the patient prior to the actual situation, to be a tool in quality assurance activities, to be the basis for audit and control and to give the patient insight into the treatment and care he or she has received. Nursing documentation is also emphasized as a prerequisite for quality assurance in nursing [12]

2. Nursing interventions

According to Grobe ... "Nursing interventions are the actual practice terms nurses use in describing care and thus have the potential for representing all relevant aspects of nursing care" [13, p. 22]. A common definition of nursing interventions is that they are nurse initiated treaments in response to nursing diagnoses [14, 15], a statement that demonstrates the close connection between nursing diagnoses and nursing interventions as part of the nursing process model. Some authors relate nursing interventions to a health-illness continuum on which interventions are designed to promote, maintain or restore high-level wellness and health, as well as protect against illness. Other authors have an even wider perspective which includes society, in describing nursing interventions as actions intended to achieve environmental change, socio-cultural change, social systems change and individual personal change in patients. Likewise, different terms are used to describe nursing interventions, such as: action, activity, intervention, nursing care implementation, order, strategy, therapeutic or treatment.

Health teaching and information provision are often included in interventions as are counselling and supporting, including psychosocial and emotional support. Basic nursing intervention in relation to daily living, and the management of the environment are included as interventions, together with monitoring and surveillance, coordinating interventions and case management. Some "systems" have wordings like "acting/doing for" or "dependent/ independent" nursing interventions as broad categories, while others have long lists with a great amount of discrete actions

In an earlier study, criteria and guidelines as a model for nursing documentation were developed [16] using a systematic approach. The development consisted of different steps, such as an extensive literature review focusing on empirical findings, review of nursing records, use and asessment in clinical practice by nurses and students, expert panel judgment, and refinement of the key words including an examination of semantic accuracy of the Swedish key words by an expert in Nordic languages. The entire process can be described as a dialogue between researchers, practitioners and experts as an initial step towards an uniform nursing language suitable for documentation in patient records.

The documentation model was adapted after the nursing process concept with key words at two levels. The first level corresponds to the nursing process model with the following key words *nursing history*, *nursing status*, *nursing diagnoses*, *goals*, *nursing interventions*, *nursing outcomes* and finally a *nursing discharge note*. A second level of key words was also established with subdivisions for nursing histtory, nursing status and nursing interventions.

The key words for nursing interventions in the documentation model used in this study are: "Participation" (that is to promote the patient's participation and communication), "Information," "Education," "Support," "Environment" (that is the adaptation of the environment), "General Care," "Training," "Observation," "Special care," "Continuity" and "Coordination."

The concepts for nursing interventions in the documentation model covered the recording of planned and/or implemented nursing interventions and both independent and dependent nursing interventions. The what, when, where, how and sometimes also by whom was noted. Several different interventions were often needed to treat or resolve a patient's single problem or diagnosis.

Different opinions exists about which nursing activities should be included as nursing interventions. Activities carried out in connection to prescriptions by physicians —often called dependent nursing activities—have not always been included. Bulechek and McCloskey state: "The core of nursing interventions should be nurse initiated treatments, but any listing of nursing interventions [as for a computerized system] must also include physician-initiated treatments and the daily essential function activities [17, p 24]. The key words for interventions used in this study include physician prescribed interventions, primarily under the key words "Observation" and 'Special care."

3. Aims

The aims of this research were to study the effects on patient records of implementing a model for nursing documentation based on key words, with respect to the content and the comprehensiveness of nursing recording, especialy nursing interventions.

4. Methods

The study was conducted on four medical wards and three wards for infectious diseases at two hospitals in Sweden, where manual recording systems were used. The model for documentation was introduced in seminars when the nurses were released from their regular work for participating in a half-day seminar. Further seminars were held twice during the subsequent six months. The teaching methods used were lectures and group discussions using actual cases and records from the wards. The documentation model with the suggested key words was explained and examplified. The relationship of the key words with the nursing process model components were also emphasized. Discussions were held with the aim of improving critical reviewing skills and increasing nurses' awareness about content and comprehensiveness of nursing documentation. In addition to the seminars, on-site discussions at the wards were held with the nurses at work. A publication in Swedish presenting the documentation model and guidelines for critical examination of records [18] was available at the different wards. The nurses were encouraged to read this and reflect upon their nursing documentation. Also a small folder for use in practice with the key words and explanations was made available for individual nurses' use..

Nursing documentation in patient records was reviewed before and after the documentation intervention. Records of consecutively discharged patients were sampled retrospectively, in all 140 records, ten before and ten after the intervention from each participating ward. Copies of all permanent nursing documentation were obtained, including all notes that were recorded by nurses (except the routine medication prescriptions). The unit of analysis for the records was the smallest part of every written sentence that contained a separate piece of information. The notes were examined using two instruments developed and tested with good results based on interobserver agreement.

The recording for a single nursing problem was scored on a five point scale using the following criteria:

1. The problem is described (in nursing history, nursing status or nursing diagnosis) *or* intervention(s) planned *or* implemented.
2. The problem is described, *and* intervention(s) planned *or* implemented.
3. The problem is described, intervention(s) planned *and/or* implemented. Outcome is recorded (in outcome or nursing discharge note).
4. The problem is described, intervention(s) planned *and* implemented. Outcome is recorded.
5. All first level key words of the documentation model are recorded. Good description of the problem. Recording of relevance to nursing.

To be meaningful the notes in the records had to be interpreted in relation to their context, both when coding the units of analysis in the content analysis and when assessing the comprehensiveness of the recording for single nursing problems.

In addition to a detailed analysis of content and comprehensiveness, the mere occurence of an admission assessment and of a nursing care plan was identified. An admission assessment was defined as information on nursing history together with information on nursing status, recorded as a unit at the beginning of the care episode. A nursing care plan was defined as the recording of individually planned nursing interventions prescribed by a nurse, based on a recorded assessment. In all, the records reviewed represented 70 records before the intervention with 546 days of care, slightly more men and a mean age of 64.2 years, and 70 records after the documentation intervention representing 721 days of care with slightly more women and a mean age of 69.2 years.

5. Results

After the intervention both the number of records with notes and the mean number of notes per record increased with respect to all components of the nursing process except goals (Table I.). The greatest increases were found for nursing discharge notes with almost five times as many records with notes after as before the documentation intervention. The occurrence of nursing diagnoses increased three times and nursing outcomes increased to more than eight out of ten, compared with their occurrence in slightly more than half of the records. Nursing history and nursing status increased from a very high level of occurrence in nine out of ten records before, to almost every record after the intervention. The mean number of notes were about twice as many after the documentation intervention as before. This increase could not be explained only by the increased proportion of records containing notes in different areas. It also reflected a more extensive recording in the individual cases.

All key words of nursing interventions were found in the records. The recording of *nursing interventions* as shown in Table II increased to a mean of 38.5 number of notes per record after the documentation intervention compared to about half of this before the intervention. All categories showed an increase except for educational interventions which were seldom recorded even before the intervention. The highest level of notes was found on "special care" (that is nursing in connection with prescribed interventions such as drug administration and treatments) both before and after the documentation intervention. With respect to number of records with notes, the largest change was found for "participation" and "coordination" which increased 35 percent. The recorded interventions on "coordination" was to a high degree notes made in connection with transfers to another level of care. Other interventions with a large number of records with notes after the intervention compared to the situation before were "information" and "training." Recording of "observation" and "special care" were found in about 90 percent of the records both before and after the intervention. Special care notes constituted more than half of all intervention notes before and decreased slightly to about half after the intervention. Notes on temporary prescribed drug administration as a share of all special care notes was about the same before and after the intervention.

The nursing notes were analyzed to see if there was any correlation between the patient's length of stay and the recording. The occurrence of the studied components of the nursing process model increased with increasing length of stay in almost all records. By the use of indirect standardization it was found that the differences could not be explained by differences with respect to the distribution by the patient's gender, age or length of stay before and after the documentation intervention.

Table I.
Recorded nursing notes on certain components of the nursing process.

Part of the nursing process	Percentage of records with notes	
	Before	After
Nursing history	89	97
Nursing status	90	99
Nursing diagnoses	16	50
Goals	14	9
Nursing interventions	100	100
Nursing outcome	56	84
Nursing discharge note	9	41
TOTAL	100	100

Table II.
Recording on nursing interventions by certain key words, percentage of records with notes and mean number of notes per record.

Keyword	Percentage of records with notes		Mean number of notes per record (n=70)	
	Before	After	Before	After
Participation	16	51	0.2	1.3
Information	24	50	0.6	1.6
Education	7	4	0.1	0.1
Support	13	30	0.2	0.5
Environment	24	36	0.4	1.0
General care	56	69	1.9	3.9
Training	14	34	0.3	1.6
Observation	90	91	3.6	4.1
Special care [a]	90	94	12.2	20.2
Continuity	61	67	1.6	3.2
Coordination	1	36	0.0	0.9
TOTAL	100	100	21.1	38.5

[a] Notes on temporary prescribed drug administration comprised 36.4 percent of all special care notes before and 33 percent of all special care notes after.

Some components may be considered as more important than others in achieving of good nursing care. For example, the recording of an admission assessment and the identification and recording of the patient's current problem or nursing diagnosis, and individual planning of the patient's care are very important. Study results showed improvements in all these areas of recording. The records were also reviewed to find out how many of the studied components of the nursing process model were found in the same record. After the intervention nine out of ten records had notes representing five nursing process components or more, compared to slightly more than half before. The recording of problems which had some information on the progress or the outcome of the patient's situation for that particular problemwas found for one third of the problems before the documenetation intervention. This increased to four-fifths after.

In conclusion, the introduction of the new documentation model and the documentation intervention was followed by improvements in the nurses' recording in patient records both quantitatively and qualitatively.

References

[1] Weeks L and Darrah P. The Documentation Dilemma: A Practical Solution. *J Nurs Adm* 1985, 15:22-7.

[2] Lindencrona C. *Kontinuitet i omvårdnaden av äldre patienter. Studier av utskrivningen från sjukhus till hemmet samt attityderna till äldre bland sjuksköterskor.* Uppsala Dissertations from the Faculty of Medicine, 4. Uppsala: Uppsala University, 1987. (In Swedish).

[3] Hamrin E and Lindmark B. The Effect of Systematic Care Planning After Acute Stroke in General Hospital Medical Wards. *J Adv Nurs* 1990, 5:1146-53.

[4] Tunset AB and Øvrebo R. *Sykepleierapporter —idealer og realiteter.* Aurskog: Gyldendal Norsk Forlag, 1988. (In Norwegian).

[5] Rinell Hermansson A. *Det sista året. Omsorg och vård vid livets slut.* Medicinska fakulteten vid Uppsala universitet. Uppsala: Uppsala University, 1990. (Dissertation). (In Swedish).

[6] Ulander K, Grahn G, Sundahl G and Jeppsson B. Needs and Care of Patients Undergoing Subtotal Pancreatectomy for Cancer. *Cancer Nurs* 1991, 14: 27-34.

[7] Ron R and Bar-Tal Y. Quality Nursing Care Survey, 1988-1990.*Quality Assurance in Health Care* 1993, 5:(1), 57-65.

[8] Edelstein J. A Study of Nursing Documentation. *Nurs Manag* 1990, 21:(40).

[9] Ehnfors M. *Quality of Care from a Nursing Perspective. Methodological Considerations and Development of a Model for Nursing Documentation.* Acta Universitatis Upsaliensis. Comprehensive Summaries of Uppsala Dissertations from the Faculty of Medicine 415. Uppsala: Uppsala University, 1993.

[10] Mallinson M. The Shortage that Destroys. *Am J Nurs* 1987, 8: 899.

[11] Tapp RA. Inhibitors and Facilitators to Documentation of Nursing Practice.*West J Nurs Res* 1990, 12: 229-40.

[12] Socialstyrelsen. *Socialstyrelsens allmänna råd (SOSFS 1990:15) i omvårdnad inom sluten somatisk vård och primärvård.* Stockholm: Socialstyrelsen, 1990. (In Swedish).

[13] Grobe SJ. Nursing Intervention Lexicon and Taxonomy Study: Language and Classification Methods. *Adv Nurs Sci* 1990, 13:(2), 22-34.

[14] Bulecheck GM and McCloskey JC (eds). *Nursing Interventions. Treatments for Nursing Diagnoses.* Philadelphia: W. B. Saunders Company, 1985.

[15] Snyder M. Humor. In: Snyder M, (ed). *Independent Nursing Interventions.* New York: John Wiley & Sons, 1985.

[16] Ehnfors M, Thorell-Ekstrand I and Ehrenberg A. Towards basic nursing information in patient records.*Vård i Norden,* 1991, 21:(3/4), 12-31.

[17] Bulecheck GM and Mc Closkey JC. Nursing interventions. Treatments for Potential Nursing Diagnoses. In: Carrol-Johnson, RM (ed). *Classification of Nursing Diagnoses. Proceedings of the Eight Conference. North American Nursing Diagnosis Association.* Cambridge: JB. Lippincott Company, 1989: Chapter 6: 23-36.

[18] Ehnfors M and Thorell-Ekstrand I. *Omvårdnad i patientjournalen. En modell för dokumentation av omvårdnad med hjälp av sökord.* FoU-rapport nr 38. Stockholm: SHSTF, 1992. (In Swedish).

Nursing Informatics: An International Overview for Nursing in a Technological Era
S.J. Grobe and E.S.P. Pluyter-Wenting, eds.

Computer support for Nursing process and documentation

Sahlstedt S

Department of Development, Stockholm County Council, South Health Care and Nursing area
Box 17914, S-11895 Stockholm, Sweden.

A paperbased individualized nursing careplan was developed in Sweden 1984. It was mostly used by nursing students. The idea was to educate students and let the knowledge be brought in to the wards as they graduated. The intention was good but it was very hard to get nurses to accept new ideas. One reason we found was that nurses are lacking a common language. Six years later we got the opportunity to develop computer support for the same careplan. Our aim was to see if computer support could help introducing nursing process as a routine method in the ward. The response from the nurses was positive. Discussions then concentrated on nursing language and what definition and terminology should be used. The prototype was tested and evaluated in four different areas: acute care in hospitals, primary care in the community and in a psychiatric- and geriatric ward. A decision to develop a complete system was taken 1992. The problem with a lack of common language among the nurses can now be solved. Swedish nurse researchers have produced a set of key words for nursing documentation in patient records. The request from the nurses for the nursing careplan with computer support has been very encouraging and about 200 installations have been made all over Sweden.

1. Background

This development project, initiated by Spri, had as its purpose the support of nurses in planning the care needed by individual patients and its subsequent evaluation.

In the last decades a number of social changes have occurred in Sweden such as shrinking resources, internationalisation, a labour market characterized by unemployment and structural change, a demand for the leveling out of differences between sexes, social classes and geographic regions. All these changes mean that the organizations of work and the various types of education offered had become outdated and irrelevant.

In the health care and nursing sector, a new outlook gradually emerged, which of course, was influenced by changes in the community. One of the results of the emerging new policy was a new legislation on health care and nursing which took effect in 1983. The changes led to acceptance of the fact that to the extent possible, care and treatment should be planned and carried out in consultation with the patient. A patient has the right to be informed about medical status and methods of treatment available. The new law defines good health care and nursing. It must:
- be of good quality and cater to the patient's need for safety and security in care and treatment
- be easily available
- be based on respect for the patient's integrity and right of self determination and
- further good contacts between the patient and the nursing staff.

The nursing process was introduced as a model to guide care and collect data about the health status of the client/patient. Basically, the nursing process is an organized, systematic method of giving individualized nursing care that focuses upon identifying and treating unique responses of individuals or groups to actual or potential alterations in health. It consists of five steps - assessment, diagnosis, planning, implementation and evaluation - during which the nurse performs deliberate activities to achieve the ultimate goals of care.

The introduction of the nursing process did not infiltrate the health care the way the commissions had intended. It was very hard to get nurses to accept new concepts. In the records the assessment phase of the nursing process model was fairly well documented, usually under the heading "admission interview."

This part of the process reflected experience and routine among the nurses. The documentation of the following phases of the nursing process - planning, diagnosing, implementation and evaluation - were less developed. No nursing diagnoses were formulated in the records. Notes on evaluation were scanty and seldom related to goals or interventions. The meaning of keywords appeared but without any consistency. All the notes were handwritten, sometimes illegible and with informal abbreviations.

The reasons for the nurses' lack of interest in Sweden are probably no different from what has been found in other countries. [1][2] Brendan has analysed the problems nurses experience when using the Nursing Process and found:
- to use manual, paperbased careplans takes time and nurses do not have that time
- there is a fear of expressing yourself in writing that can be read by many and where you can be subject to criticism
- the manual careplan is difficult to read because of its limited space for writing. As time goes by and changes are done it can be hard to see the context
- careplans have not been regarded as a document of value to be filed as part of the patient record, the implementations have been erased as they are completed and thereby made evaluation impossible
- the issue of responsibility has not been clarified and many notes have therefore not been signed
- there has been little or no response to individual careprovider through lack of signatures.

The above mentioned statements have contributed in giving the documentation of nursing process a low priority and valuable knowledge have been lost. Cengiz says that if the manual careplan exists at all, it is often incomplete, out of date, and not used for guidance in nursing care. [3]

2. Nursing Resarch

Sweden also lacks a standardized nursing terminology for use in describing nursing practice. In 1986 a new Patient Record Act was adopted which made documentation compulsory for nurses. Nurses' documentation has usually been incomplete, unspecific and mostly concerned with medical prescriptions such as drug administration and other dependent nursing actions. [4] Ehnfors' nursing research has in a project produced a list of key words with definitions to serve as a tool that is easy to use and which gives content, language and structure to nursing documentation in patient records. [5]

3. The development project

A question aroused: *How can we help nurses to use nursing process in the safest, most efficient, and most effective way?*

In 1989 we got the opportunity to develop computer support for the nursing careplan. The aim was to see:
(a) if computer support could help introducing the nursing process as a routine method in the ward; (b) if computer support would help nurses to document nursing care more specific by using key words, and (c) if computer support could help quality assurance of care given by nurses.

The prototype was developed step by step in close contact with nurses involved in the project. The nursing process was used as a foundation and the aim was to allow nurses to write free text using key words. Two wards were initially involved at two hospitals in Stockholm. The nurses feared that the technique would put a restrain on their possibility to individualize the care-plan if they could not use free text. At one hospital the nurses had no experience in using the nursing process in their daily work. A teacher of nursing was assigned to the project to support the nurses in formulating care-plans and teach the principles of the nursing process.

At the other hospital the nurses had been using the nursing process on and off for some time. The pressure on the nurses to treat patients was higher than merely to write care-plans; the paperbased documentation made it difficult to get a good view of the patient's progress. At this hospital the head nurse was in charge of the project.

When the prototype was tested and evaluated a decision was taken to develop a complete system. To evaluate if the system could be used in more areas of nursing, the program was introduced in 4 different wards: acute care, psychiatric and geriatric care in hospitals and primary care in the community.

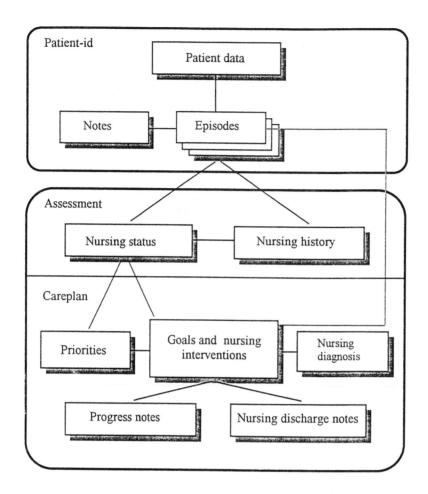

Figure 1. Layout for computerised Nursing Care Plan

The key words presented from the nursing research were used in the computer program. The structure was modelled based on nursing process. Key words in the first phase of the model, the assessment phase, include *nursing history* and *nursing status*. From this information *nursing diagnoses* are formulated. The planning phase consists of *goals* and *nursing interventions*, planned as well as implemented, and is followed by nursing outcomes. Finally there is a *nursing discharge note*.

Four key concepts in nursing are being used. They are: *well-being, respect for integrity prevention* and *safety*. The key concepts serve as a foundation for setting goals for nursing practice - optimal well-being, respect for integrity, prevention of health problems and optimal safety - and, as essential in the evaluation nursing process.

Nursing history contains the key words: *admission, health situation, hypersensitivity, previous health care, social history.* and l*ife style.* The key words used for nursing status are: *communication, breathing/circulation, nutrition, elimination, skin, activity, sleep, pain, sexuality, psychosocial, spiritual* and finally w*ell-being.*

Nursing interventions aim to promote and maintain health and well-being and prevent illness and discomfort. There is evidence that nursing interventions based on research can result in better outcomes than routine procedural nursing care. Several different interventions might be needed to treat a single patient's problem or diagnosis. The keywords suggested to be used for interventions are: *participation, information, education, support, environment, general care, observation, special care, continuity* and c*oordination.* [4]

4. Result of the development project

The computer support for nursing process can be used in the different areas of nursing where it has been tested. In the primary care unit the nursing process is used mostly when caring for the sick in homecare settings.

The interest from the nurses to participate in the development project has been positive. However, structural changes in health care and nursing, have made it hard for nurses to find time to develop their skills. A questionnaire was presented to nurses in the participating wards evaluated the nurses' views of the project and their work. Nineteen nurses responded (sixteen females and three males). Only seven of the nineteen participants could word processing before the project, and only five out of eighteen (1 missing) had any previous experience with computers. Thirteen respondents (6 missing) were positive about the new experience. Only twelve out of nineteen had previous experiences with nursing careplans prior to the project. Eighteen out of nineteen are convinced that individualized careplans will improve nursing care and that their knowledge of the patient needs has increased. Respondents also feel that the patients' self-determination has increased and that the nursing care is now carried out in consultation with the patient.

Fifteen of the nineteen feel that their workload has increased but no one can see how the nursing process and careplanning can improve the planning of their daily work. Six of the fifteen (4 missing) felt that their jobs were more satisfying, 5 reported that it is no different and 4 did not know.

The researchers also wanted to find out if the nurses found the program easy or difficult to learn, and how long they needed to learn the program.

Table 1
Nurses attitude to program

Evaluation		Time to learn the program	
Very easy	3	4 h	4
Easy	6	1-2 days	5
Rather difficult	9	3-7 days	4
Very difficult	0	> 1 week	4
Missing	1	Missing	2

The use of key words was found very positive or positive by sixteen of seventeen respondents. Twelve nurses say their documentation has improved since the start of the project. Writing nursing notes with help of computer support has been very positive or positive for fifteen of seventeen (2 missing). Nine nurses feel that their professional roles have improved to a certain extent.

5. Future developments

The program "Computer support for nursing process" is less than one year, and yet has been sold to about 100 different wards all over Sweden. The nursing schools can use the program free of charge for their students. The program will continuously improve as its developers and evaluators gain more experience.

In the future we are going to focus on evaluation and on possibilities of using the program for quality assurance. So far we have had a limited number of nurses involved in the project and we want to extend the number and clinical areas for a more extensive study. The next phase will start after summer 1993 and continue over 2 years. The nurse researchers will participate with their knowledge and together we hope to develop a computer-based support system that can help nurses use the nursing process in a safe, more efficient and more effective way.

6. References

[1] Ball M.J & Hannah K.J., *Using computers In Nursing*, Reston, 1984. pp 19-21

[2] Brennan L.E., *"The nursing care plan: Computerized, Professionalized, utilized"*, Symposium on computer application in medical care (1984). pp 556

[3] Cengiz M. and others, *"Design and implementation of computerized nursing care plans"* Symposium on computer application in medical care, 1984. pp 561

[4] Ehnfors M & Thorell-Ekstrand I. & Ehrenberg A., *Towards Basic Nursing Information in Patient Records;* Vård i Norden 3/4 1991 Vol 21. Årg 11, pp 12-21

[5] Ehnfors M., Quality of Care from a Nursing Perspective. Methodological Considerations and Development of a Model for Nursing Documentation. ACTA UNIVERSITATIS UPSALAIENSIS, Uppsala, 1993

STANDARDS

B. Quality improvement

Nursing Informatics: An International Overview for Nursing in a Technological Era
S.J. Grobe and E.S.P. Pluyter-Wenting, eds.

Nursing Informatics: The Key to Managing and Evaluating Quality

Harsanyi BE[a] Lehmkuhl D[a] Hott R[a] Myers S[a] and McGeehan L[a]

[a] *SMS, 51 Valley Stream Parkway, Malvern, PA 19355*

The nursing profession's commitment to meeting the health care needs of an ever-changing society requires the continual reshaping of nursing clinical practice to address those needs. Nursing's leadership role in the designing, implementing, and evaluating of evolving technology for health care delivery is the key to the accomplishment of nursing's mission. This paper addresses the use of current and evolving information technology for the managing and processing of information for quality patient-centered care delivery. A technological quality care delivery framework with the educated consumer at the center is used to illustrate the use of information technology for managing and evaluating quality.

1. Nursing's Mission

Nursing's mission is "...the diagnosis and treatment of human responses to actual or potential health problems" [1]. Nursing's Agenda for Health Care Reform, emphasizing quality, access, and cost, is an excellent example of the nursing profession's efforts to address the health care needs of an ever-changing society and a national health care system in crisis [2]. Continuous quality improvement (CQI) efforts in nursing are also a direct reflection of the profession's response to society's challenge of traditional views of quality health care delivery [3]. To fulfill nursing's mission as defined, nursing is continually reshaping clinical practice to address society's health care needs.

2. Technology's Value for Mission Accomplishment

One key to enhancing the accomplishment of nursing's mission is the assumption of nursing's leadership role in the design, implementation, and evaluation of rapidly evolving technology for the management and processing of nursing information leading to the evolution of nursing knowledge-based management tools [4]. Nursing's recognition of the value of technology in health care delivery is evident by the American Nurses Association's Congress of Nursing Practice's recognition of nursing informatics as a distinct area of specialty nursing practice. Graves and Corcoran (1989) defined nursing informatics as "...a combination of computer science, information science and nursing science designed to assist in the management and processing of nursing data, information and knowledge to support the practice of nursing and the delivery of nursing care" [5]. The focus of this paper is the use of current and evolving information technology for the managing and processing of information for quality patient-centered nursing care delivery.

3. A Technological Quality Care Delivery Framework

At the center of the framework is the educated consumer expecting quality patient-centered health care delivery. The consumer represents diverse populations with lifelong health needs spanning the health care continuum. The consumer requires access to services across windows of time, episodes of care, and organizational and geographical boundaries. The three components of the framework, philosophy, model, and evaluation, represent the circular pathway in the quality patient-centered care delivery process. Just as in the nursing process, the circular nature of the framework reflects a dynamic and cyclical process. The ongoing exchange of information required for managed change of patient care processes, treatment patterns and patient outcomes is reflected by the arrows (See Figure 1) [6]. The integration of health care informatics into patient-centered quality care delivery impacts each component of the model.

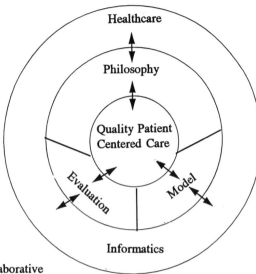

Figure 1. Technological Collaborative
Care Delivery Framework

The philosophy component is the foundation cornerstone for the defining, measuring, and evaluating of quality patient-centered health care delivery. It reflects the health care network's beliefs, values, assumptions, and culture regarding health care delivery. Furthermore, it guides the determination of consumers' access to multi-disciplinary services and care providers. It also guides the care providers' and payors' access to the patient's total health care picture. This health care composite portrays the patient's life-span and ranges from wellness and prevention to long term and hospice care. The philosophy also influences information technology selection, and the integration of technology with health care delivery. Data standardization, data movement, operational solutions, and service are also influenced.

The coordination and integration of care, cost, and resources comprise the model component of the framework. The care delivery model sets the stage for the delivery of the health care philosophy. A goal of the care delivery model is to enhance the expected qualitative and cost-effective patient care outcomes while including the patient, family, and multi-disciplinary care providers as an integral part of the associated delivery process. Case management provides the best example of this type of model. Case management also provides for care delivery standards with associated time frames and the evaluation of variances between the expected and actual care, cost, and resource utilization.

Successful accomplishment of patient-centered quality health care delivery in the first two components of the pathway can only be validated if evaluation is the third component of the circular pathway. The evaluation component addresses the determination of the ongoing process of movement towards excellence. It also addresses compliance with internal and external standards and requirements. Health care informatics of which nursing informatics is a part of provides an avenue for enhancing each component of the framework as well as the overall pathway of quality patient-centered health care delivery [7].

4. Technology As An Avenue for Quality Philosophy Implementation

Technology provides the avenue for the translation of the organization's and/or health care network's philosophy from paper into actual practice. For example, the implementation of philosophical statements regarding belief in universal consumer access results in increased demand for health care. This can be enhanced through the use of information technology. A current problem is the quick determination of a consumer's eligibility and availability for health care financial coverage. The consumer also enters the health care system from multiple locations such as surgi-centers, physicians' offices, and emergency rooms. In addition, the process of claim transmission and reimbursement is a slow and labor-intensive activity which impacts the organization's financial picture. An electronic data interchange provides a technological avenue for accessing patient-centered data from a national health network of employers, payors, government agencies, financial institutions, and other providers. A patient would present an electronically read standard health insurance card. A patient's eligibility from public and/or private plans and the coverage parameters can be quickly determined using an electronic data interchange thus expediting consumer access to health care delivery. The ability to obtain a comprehensive overview of the consumer's coverage also reduces risks for the organization as well as for the consumer. With the eventual development of a consumer comparative health care data base, the consumer can also determine where to go for the desired quality for the best price. An open systems concept, supporting system-to-system interconnection and interoperability, also provides for technological integration of an electronic data interchange and the organization's existing information system capabilities.

Support for the offering of a standardized core of essential health care services across the patient's life-span, windows of time, and in multiple, non-traditional, convenient, and familiar locations may also appear in philosophical statements. To accomplish this, the care providers must have access to integrated patient-centered information. The movement towards an electronic patient record, as outlined by the Institute of Medicine, provides a technological avenue for this to occur. The concept of integration does not just include the integration of information system functionality and applications. It also includes the use of open systems capability for the integration of multiple current and evolving information technologies across the horizontally and vertically integrated health care network. Most importantly is the strategic, tactical, and operational integration of the technology to provide integrated multidisciplinary patient-centered quality care delivery across a continuum. The electronic patient record, including images and video, can support multiple care providers' access from diverse locations to timely, complete, and standardized patient care data. Equally as important, the electronic patient record should provide user defined display and report formats for ease of data interpretation by the clinician. The ability to integrate imaging systems into information systems is a key component in the evolvement of the electronic patient record as opposed to the automation of a paper medical record. Technological capabilities exist for the inclusion of diverse image capabilities for such departments as patient accounting, medical records, and diagnostic imaging. Implementation of philosophical statements regarding wellness, prevention, and consumer satisfaction can be enhanced through the use of automated multi-resource scheduling integrated with outpatient and order processing. This provides for the quick, effective and efficient use of the health care network's resources across the health care continuum. Through report mechanisms, an integrated and comprehensive view, including productivity statistics, is provided for the analysis of consumer demand, consumer profiles, resource utilization and allocation, and multi-disciplinary practice patterns.

5. Model Implementation

Relational data base technology can provide for a single point of entry into a comprehensive data repository providing tracking of the patient's usage of services, the involvement of care givers and payors of care, and a summary of the episodes of care no matter where the patient entered the health care network. This same technology can also provide for a comprehensive online 24-hour available repository, including diagnostic imaging, of clinically significant patient-centered information reflecting an integrated longitudinal care provider view of the patient. This type of online repository also facilitates education and research efforts of care providers by providing a source spanning the entire patient population of an organization. The use of this technology in conjunction with expert care rules, knowledge-based systems, and structured clinical observations and results provide the clinician with a user-defined comprehensive view. This view includes the patients' previous and current problem lists, diagnostic tests, treatment regimes, clinical outcomes, patient/family education needs and discharge dispositions across the acute care and ambulatory perspective. This availability of data expedites patient centered treatment, decreases length of stay, increases accuracy and quality of the care needed, decreases cost, and improves clinical outcomes positively.

Data communication such as fiber optic networks joining separate institutions, local area networks within each institution, single software standards, a single data base, and workstation technology with CD-ROM capability can provide for successful model implementation. For example, the implementation of a case management model integrated with order processing, acuity, and patient accounting provides for the concurrent documentation of clinical care as well as incurred cost. The online critical path measurement, and documentation of plan of care variance provides feedback for standards and clinical protocol revision, patient and personnel education needs, and acuity and resource allocation relationships. Variance data can be analyzed at the patient level or at an aggregate level to improve quality and efficiency of care. In keeping with JCAHO standards, the automation of standards of care and protocols can be used as a basis for all forms of charting with the ability to also individualize critical paths to meet the patients' unique needs. The ability to assign target dates for goals and evaluation frequencies provides for the concurrent monitoring of patient care outcomes.

A proactive, quantitative, and objective quality assurance approach can be achieved through current information technology. Concurrently, quality assurance indicators can be identified as part of the clinical documentation process. Accepted clinical protocols and practices can be incorporated to prevent clinical problems before their occurrence. This significantly reduces patient risk and historical retrospective analysis. The use of automated exception charting, structured progress notes, integrated physiological monitoring with documentation assures standardized, accurate, consistent, and complete clinical documentation for later quality assurance and risk management evaluation. As the educated consumer becomes more responsible for wellness and prevention maintenance across a life time, online patient education and discharge planning activities become essential. Through awareness of tailoring tools, patient education can be individualized and compliances with standards for discharge planning, documentation, disposition, and continuity of care referrals to home health agencies can be captured throughout the care delivery process. To comply with internal policies and standards, the required capturing of "reason for procedure" for specified radiology examinations, or the required capturing of the location site and reason for the administration of a PRN medication provides a proactive approach to quality assurance documentation. The integration and presentation of required results such as blood sugar levels into the order entry pathway enhances the accuracy of the insulin order. To assure completion of patient care delivery upon discharge, unresolved problems or uncharted orders can be immediately displayed and action taken at the time of discharge summary completion.

6. Evaluation Implementation

As the nation moves toward a Health Care Agenda for Reform, the health care network's evaluation of compliance with internal and external standards, guidelines, and regulations will become more important. Decision support technology provides a technological avenue for evaluating the delivery of the most cost-effective and therapeutic options in the most familiar and convenient locations for consumer access. For example, analysis of cost variance provides for the identification of cost problems quickly through comparisons to historical performance, or health care network standards. If higher than expected costs are identified, technology can determine whether it is a result of treating more patients, treating a more complex case mix, the use of additional or more expensive services, cost center inefficiency, or higher prices and wages. The key to cost control and managed change is the analysis of variance and comparative evaluation against internal and external standards. Decision support capabilities such as product line management also provide nursing with insight into the possible reasons for revenue and cost problems, potential solutions, and evaluation of change implemented. Quality of care indicators can also be combined with financial and demographic information for the monitoring of such aspects as mortality rates and infection rates.

By integrating clinical and financial operational data into a comprehensive relational data base, decision support technology can facilitate quality initiatives. These quality initiatives can address process and utilization improvement, clinical protocol evaluation, and outcomes measurement. The use of these comprehensive data bases generated by information technology from diverse institutions in size, types of patient populations, and geographical locations opens up new doors for nursing research. For example, these comprehensive data bases have been used to answer such questions as "Does patient treatment of AIDS in a hospital experienced with AIDS patients impact the likelihood of the patient being discharged alive?" A methodology including the screening of computerized records from 15 participating hospitals for a designated time period provided evidence that experience with treating AIDS patients with pneumocystis carinii pneumonia impacted mortality [8]. These comprehensive data bases used in conjunction with standardized data elements such as the nursing minimum data set and automated taxonomies provide new opportunities for nursing research regarding patient outcomes management across diverse settings, geographical areas, and patient populations.

7. Summary

The understanding of current and evolving information technology for the management and processing of nursing information enables the nursing profession to assume a leadership role in the nation's pursuit of health care reform. Nursing must move beyond an understanding only of information system technology, functionality, and applications. "The core of the science of informatics is the commodities that computers process (data, information, and knowledge) and not the computer itself" [9,10]. Nursing must also understand the integration of information technology into nursing practice for managed change of patient care processes, treatment patterns, and patient outcomes for continuous quality improvement.

8. References

[1]   American Nurses Association. *Nursing A Social Policy Statement*. Washington, DC: American Nurses Publishing, 1980: 9.

[2]   American Nurses Association. *Nursing's Agenda for Health Care Reform*. Washington, DC: American Nurses Publishing, 1992.

[3]   Dienemann, J. (Ed.). *CQI Continuous Quality Improvement in Nursing*. Washington, D.C.: American Nurses Publishing, 1992.

[4]   Graves, J. R. and Corcoran, S. The Study of Nursing Informatics. *IMAGE: Journal of Nursing Scholarship*, Winter 1989, 21: 227-230.

[5]   Graves, J. R. and Corcoran, S. The Study of Nursing Informatics. *IMAGE: Journal of Nursing Scholarship*, Winter 1989, 21: 227.

[6]   Harsanyi, B.E. Use of Information Systems to Facilitate Collaborative Healthcare Delivery. In: *Proceedings of the 1993 Annual HIMSS Conference Healthcare Information and Management Systems Society*. Chicago, IL 1993: Vol 2, 229-240.

[7]   Harsanyi, B.E. Use of Information Systems to Facilitate Collaborative Healthcare Delivery. In: *Proceedings of the 1993 Annual HIMSS Conference Healthcare Information and Management Systems Society*. Chicago, IL 1993: Vol 2, 229-240.

[8]   Bennett, C. L., Garfinkle, J. B., Greenfield, S., Draper, D., Rogers, W., Mathews, W. C., and Kanouse, D.E. The Relationship Between Hospital Experience and In-Hospital Mortality for Patients With AIDS - Related PCP. *JAMA* 1989, 261: 2975-2979.

[9]   Graves, J. R. and Corcoran, S. The Study of Nursing Informatics. *IMAGE: Journal of Nursing Scholarship*, Winter 1989, 21: 227-230.

[10] Blois, M. S. What is it that Computers Compute? *Clinical Computing*, 1987, 4: 31-33.

Nursing Informatics: An International Overview for Nursing in a Technological Era
S.J. Grobe and E.S.P. Pluyter-Wenting, eds.

Clinical Databases And Total Quality Improvement

Lee J L [a,b]

[a] Medical-Surgical/Physiological Section, UCLA School of Nursing, 10833 Le Conte Avenue, Los Angeles, CA 90024-6918.

[b] The research described in this paper was supported by a UCLA School of Nursing Minigrant and by the PACE program, Sepulveda VA Medical Center.

The emphasis of healthcare quality has now shifted from the traditional quality assurance model to a more encompassing framework of total quality improvement. This paper describes a clinical nursing research study, focused on health services utilization and patterns of care in a chronically ill veteran population, and its usefulness in examining the influence of structure and process variables upon system, provider, and patient outcomes. A Nursing Effectiveness and Patient Outcomes Matrix illustrates the interface between nursing research and a total quality improvement program with improved patient outcomes as a primary objective. Health policy implications are presented.

1. Introduction

With the establishment of the Agency for Health Care Policy and Research, the United States formalized attention on research to assess and improve medical effectiveness and outcomes of care [1]. Subsequently, the National Center for Nursing Research convened an invitational conference to critically examine the state of the science and research base needed to guide the deliberative process of achieving particular patient outcomes, i.e., nursing effectiveness [2].

Nursing has a long tradition of developing, implementing, and evaluating high standards of clinical performance. However, in a review of health services and outcomes research in nursing, Ingersoll and colleagues identified several research gaps, including the evalaution of innovative care delivery approaches. These authors stressed the need for nurses to access existing databases for health services research [3]. McCormick has identified national databases, both federal (including those from the Veterans Administration (VA), which are available to health services researchers, including nurses [4].

This paper describes a clinical nursing research study, focused on health services utilization and patterns of care in a chronically ill veteran population, and its usefulness in examining the influence of structure and process variables upon system, provider, and patient outcomes. A Nursing Effectiveness and Patient Outcomes Matrix will illustrate the interface between nursing research and a total quality improvement program, with improved patient outcomes as a primary objective. Health policy implications will then be presented.

2. The Context of Total Quality Improvement

For the purposes of this paper, total quality improvement is focused on entire patient care episodes and recognizes the importance of synergy between the system and the provider in affecting quality outcomes [5]. Thus, total quality improvement is conceptually very congruent with the current outcomes research movement. This is in keeping with Hegyvary's concept of "a new mentality", that outcomes research in nursing be viewed as the complex study of defining the contribution of nursing in the context of an increasingly integrative health care services environment [6]. This perspective goes beyond the traditional structure-process-outcome approach to encompass the reality of multiple applicable levels of analysis, from the micro-level individual client or individual provider level to the most complex macro-systems constellation, such as alternate national healthcare delivery models.

This movement toward a more integrative, complex total quality improvement perspective is certainly not unique to the U.S. The international journal, Quality Assurance in Health Care, illustrates the similarities and differences in health quality concerns across national boundaries. In the first issue, authors represented several countries in Europe and the United States. Article foci included aspects of health quality at the macro societal level [7], the macro societal and provider level [8], and the micro patient/client level [9].

Section 3 of this paper will now describe a clinical research study undertaken to identify baseline data regarding health services utilization and patterns of care for a chronically ill veteran population prior to a major organizational change in the delivery of healthcare services. The study is presented as proposed and implemented. Then in Section 4, the study is re-conceptualized through an alternative framework, the Nursing Effectiveness and Patient Outcomes Matrix.

3. The Study: Health Services Utilization and Patterns of Care in a Chronically Ill Veteran Population

3.1 Specific Aims

This study had four specific aims: (1). To determine the number and describe the characteristics of veterans, with a medical diagnosis of diabetes mellitus, discharged from the Sepulveda VA Medical Center (VAMC) during federal fiscal year 1990: October 1, 1989 through September 30, 1990. (2). To examine the influence of sociodemographic (e.g., age, race, marital status) and case-mix (e.g., comorbid conditions) variables on number of hospital episodes and total number of hospital days. (3). To determine the patterns of care (e.g., clinic visits, walk-in care) for a subsample of these veterans to assess coordination of care and potentially unnecessary or avoidable admissions. (4). To identify the treatment and organizational variables associated with readmission of veterans with diabetes mellitus.

3.2 Background and Significance

Health care delivery is shifting from an inpatient focus to an outpatient focus [10,11]. This shift is spurred by economic pressures, technology advancements, and the rise in the consumerism/self-care movement. The Veterans Administration (now the Veterans Health Administration) has also responded to these changes [12]. The Pilot Ambulatory Care and Education project (PACE), implemented at Sepulveda VAMC in October 1990, shifts the focus of care and health professional educaton from acute hospital to ambulatory care services, with specific improvements in quality and continuity of care projected [13].

The results of this study were intended to provide baseline data regarding utilization of health services and patterns of care for a specific patient population, those with diabetes mellitus, which is the third most frequent medical diagnosis associated with hospitalization at this VA facility and which results in great morbidity and disability. Subsequent studies could then investigate whether, and to what degree, the implementation of PACE, a major structural change, has had an impact on the health services utilization and patterns of care in the diabetic population.

3.3 Conceptual Framework

The conceptual framework for this study was drawn from Andersen's determinants of health services utilization model [14,15] and from Donabedian's classical quality of care assessment approach [16]. Andersen's model suggests that a person's decision to seek medical care and the volume of services received depends on: 1) the predisposition of the individual to use services (predisposing), 2) the ability to secure services (enabling), and 3) the need for medical care (need). Donabedian's approach to quality of care assessment defines three aspects: structure, process, and outcome. Variables selected for inclusion in this study were limited by those available within two VA dabatases: the Patient Treatment File (PTF) and the Decentralized Hospital Computer Program (DHCP), in addition to data abstracted from the health care record.

3.4 Methodology and Results

The study population were all veterans who received health care at the Sepulveda VAMC and who had a medical diagnosis of diabetes mellitus. The sampling frame were those veterans who, upon discharge from an inpatient episode, had an ICD-9 code in the 250.00 range (diabetes mellitus), in any position (i.e., from diagnosis responsible for length of stay to diagnosis #9), during fiscal year 1990. To meet the patterns of care study aim, a subsample of 51 charts were randomly selected for review.

This study used a descriptive exploratory design. Data were obtained from several sources: PTF, DHCP, and medical records. Validity and reliability of the existing data sources (PTF, DHCP) could only be assumed. For the two Data Abstraction Forms developed specifically for this study, a Content Validity Index of 100% was achieved; interrater reliability was achieved at 100% agreement.

Data were analyzed at both the discharge episode-level (n=846) and the client level (n=538), as appropriate to meet study aims 1,2, and 4. Data from the retrosopective health record review (Study Aim 3) were quantified where possible and linked with the client-level dataset. Qualitative (narrative descriptions) from the record review were also recorded. All quantitative data was eventually stored in SAS datasets for statistical manipulation. Descriptive statistics, ANOVA, multiple regression, and logistic regression were used, as appropriate to level of measurement, to meet study aims. Specific study results have been reported elsewhere [17].

4. The Nursing Effectiveness and Patient Outcomes Matrix

Holzemer's Nursing Effectiveness and Patient Outcomes Matrix [18] offers a more comprehensive approach for conceptualizing this study within a total quality improvement perspective. This three-by-three matrix allows the researcher to identify relevant variables according to quality parameters: structure, process, outcome, and according to level of analysis parameters: client, provider, system. (See Figure 1.) Thus, the Matrix illustrates the interface between relevant clinical variables, a total quality improvement approach, and an outcomes research (i.e., nursing effectiveness) perspective.

To be more specific, the Matrix allows the investigator to identify many relevant variables, and further to classify them according to quality parameter, as well as the level of analysis. This can help clarify for the investigator the domain of relevant variables for consideration. The schematic representation of the Matrix can assist the investigator in the process of decision-making regarding which research questions to ask in which study, which resources to expend answering how complex a research question. For example, in the study presented here, Study Aim 1 asks only about patient-level characteristics, while Study Aim 2 asks about the influence of two types of patient-level variables (sociodemographic and case-mix) upon two types of patient-level outcomes (number of hospital episodes and total number of hospital days). Thus, the Matrix is helpful in conceptualizing the study, planning a program of research, and returning the investigator to the complexity of the task of implementing and evaluating outcomes research and eventually improving the quality of service provided and the quality of care received.

Nursing Effectiveness and Patient Outcomes Matrix	Structure	Processes	Outcomes
Patient/Client			
Provider			
System			

Figure 1. The Nursing Effectiveness and Patient Outcomes Matrix, modified from Holzemer [18].

5. Implications and Conclusions

Clinical databases, such as those used in this study, possess certain advantages and disadvantages when used for research purposes. Advantages include accurate and timely data, rich in clinical detail, some with continuous parameters, while disadvantages include missing data and possible bias and recording errors [19-21]. Nurses are in a position to influence development and refinement of these clinical databases. Werley and Lang has long advocated adoption of the Minimum Nursing Data Set [22]. Advocacy for development and adoption of clinical databases must occur in a deliberate fashion, tempered by overriding concerns of validity, reliability, sensitivity, and utility [23]. As nurses, we must remain vigilant to our societal mission: that nursing makes a difference in patient outcomes and that difference must be measurable and discernable from the contribution made by other healthcare disciplines.

In conclusion, this paper has described a clinical nursing research study and its usefulness in examining the influence of structure and process variables upon system, provider, and patient outcomes. A Nursing Effectiveness and Patient Outcomes Matrix has been presented which illustrates the interface between nursing research and a total quality improvement program with improved patient outcomes as a primary objective. Health policy implications for nurses, particularly in the area of clinical databases, have been presented.

6. References

[1] DeFriese GH. Outcomes research: Implications for the effectiveness of nursing practice. In: Patient Outcomes Research: Examining the Effectiveness of Nursing Practice. US Department of Health and Human Services, Public Health Service, National Institutes of Health: NIH Publication No. 93-3411, October 1992:11-15.

[2] Patient Outcomes Research: Examining the Effectiveness of Nursing Practice. US Department of Health and Human Services, Public Health Service, National Institutes of Health: NIH PUblication No. 93-3411, October 1992.

[3] Ingersoll GL, Hoffart N, and Schultz A. Health services research in nursing: Current status and future directions. *Nurs Econ* 1988, 8:317-326.

[4] McCormick KA. Nursing effectiveness research using existing data bases. In: Patient Outcomes Research: Examining the Effectiveness of Nursing Practice. US Department of Health and Human Services, Public Health Service, National Institutes of Health: NIH Publication No. 93-3411, October 1992: 203-209.

[5] Dienemann J (Ed.). *Continuous Quality Improvement in Nursing*. Washington, DC: American Nurses Publishing, 1992.

[6] Hegyvary ST. Outcomes research: Integrating nursing practice into the world view. In: Patient Outcomes Research: Examining the Effectiveness of Nursing Practice. US Department of Health and Human Services, Public Health Service, National Institutes of Health: NIH Publication No. 93-3411, October 1992:17-24.

[7] Calltorp J. The "Swedish model" under pressure -- How to maintain equity and develop quality? *Qual Assur Health Care* 1989, 1:13-22.

[8] Donabedian A. Institutional and professional responsibilities in quality assurance. *Qual Assur Health Care* 1989, 1:3-12.

[9] Reizenstein P. The quality of care of the elderly. *Qual Assur Health Care* 1989, 1:31-38.

[10] Coile RC. Health care 1990: Top 10 trends for the year ahead. *Hosp Strat Rep* 1989, 2(3):1-8.

[11] Smith D. (Ed.) *Nursing 2020*. New York: National League for Nursing, 1988.

[12] Abbott AV, and Lee PV. Medical student education in ambulatory care. *Acad Med* 1989, 64:S9-S15.

[13] Mission Statement, Pilot Ambulatory Care and Education Center. Sepulveda, CA: Sepulveda VA Medical Center, 1990.

[14] Andersen R, Kravits J, and Anderson OW (Eds.). *Equity in health services: Empirical analyses in social policy.* Cambridge, MA: Ballinger, 1975.

[15] Andersen R, and Newman JF. Societal and individual determinants of medical care utilization in the United States. *Milbank Q* 1973, 51:95-124.

[16] Donabedian A. Criteria and standards for quality assessment and monitoring. *QRB* 1986, 12:99-108.

[17] Lee JL, Jones KR, Johnson FN, and Hoenshell-Nelson N. Health services utilization in a chronically ill veteran population. Sigma Theta Tau International Nursing Research Conference, Columbus OH, May 19-22, 1992.

[18] Holzemer W. Nursing effectiveness research and patient oucomes. Western Society for Research in Nursing Postdoctoral Clinical Research Seminar, San Diego, CA. April 29, 1992.

[19] Pryor DB and Lee KL. Methods for the analysis and assessment of clinical databases: The clinician's perspective. *Stat Med* 1991, 10:617-628.

[20] Safran C. Using routinely collected data for clinical research. *Stat Med* 1991, 10:559-564.

[21] Tierney WM and McDonald CJ. Practice databases and their uses in clinical research. *Stat Med* 1991, 10:541-557.

[22] Werley HH and Lang NM. *Identification of the Nursing Minimum Data Set.* New York: Springer Publishing, 1988.

[23] Ozbolt JG. Strategies for building nursing data bases for effectiveness research. In: Patient Outcomes Research: Examining the Effectiveness of Nursing Practice. US Department of Health and Human Services, Public Health Service, National Institutes of Health: NIH Publication No. 93-3411, October 1992: 210-218.

The Clinical Application of Computer Information Systems
to
Continuous Quality Improvement

Romano Carol A.

Clinical Center, National Institutes of Health, Bethesda, Maryland, USA

The wave of change crashing into modern health care institutions is the movement from traditional quality assurance programs to initiatives focused on continuous improvement to the quality of care. This paper describes the application of a hospital-wide computerized information system, with an extensive nursing component, to the development and implementation of the new paradigm of Continuous Quality Improvement (CQI). The evolving concepts of quality assessment, quality assurance, and quality improvement as they relate to use of information systems is presented first. Specific clinical computer applications are then discussed in relation to the defined need for improvement, the description of the application, and the health professional's response to the implemented innovation. Different methods of incorporating improvement initiatives and standards with an automated information system are also proposed.

1. The Quality Paradigm

Berwick [1] discusses two theories of quality that describe the climate in which health care is delivered. The first suggests that quality is achieved through inspection in which thresholds for acceptability are established. The theory implies that the cause of trouble is people who do not care enough to do what they can or what they know is right. This "Bad Apple Theory" can be contrasted with the Theory of Continuous Quality Improvement. From this alternative perspective, improvements in quality care are said to depend on understanding and revising the systems and processes within an organization by a constant effort to reduce waste, rework, and complexity [2]. Historically, quality programs have focused on the Bad Apple Theory but are beginning to embrace the new paradigm.

The new quality paradigm embraces several key principles [3] usually referred to as Continuous Quality Improvement (CQI). These principles suggest that quality improvement requires the involvement of top management, a definition of quality in terms of customer satisfaction, examination and continuous improvement *of the key processes* by which services are delivered, and the pursuit of quality through teamwork. For a system to be improved, it must be assessed and understood.

2. Role of Clinical Information Systems

From the perspective of CQI, a hospital information system (HIS) to support the practice of medicine and nursing can be viewed both as a vehicle for improving communication within an organization and as a mechanism through which other processes can be improved. This is accomplished by decreasing the variance in how information is handled and extracting data for systematic quality assessment. On-line access to information regarding the quality standards for specific clinical functions facilitates continuous improvement and triggers collaboration in problem solving related to the use and management of patient information.

For the past 15 years, the Clinical Center of the National Institutes of Health has used an integrated hospital-wide computerized information system to support patient care and provide an electronic record [4,5]. Several clinical applications for an HIS were developed to improve quality for this 500 bed teaching-research hospital and are presented below.

2.1 Advance Directives

An advance directive is defined as a written document that specifies a person's preferences concerning medical treatment. In 1991, health care legislation required that the existence of such a directive be assessed on each patient admission and that requests for further information be accommodated [6]. The HIS was designed to cue an admission clerk to solicit and record this information during the admission process. Advance directive information is also incorporated into the computerized nursing admission note and reflects standards of practice regarding nursing responsibilities. This note automatically triggers a written request for Bioethics consultation in the Hospital Office of Ethics if appropriate.

The status and type of advance directive for each patient is programmed to print on specified patient documents. On-line retrieval of the information after discharge is also available to provide access on subsequent patient admissions. Physician and nurse response to this application has been favorable. Implementation of the legislation was facilitated and provider responsibility was clarified through the HIS.

2.2 Blood Administration

The need to communicate criteria for using irradiated blood components, to streamline medical ordering, to clarify nursing certification requirements for blood administration, and to simplify the reporting and recording of adverse reactions were identified as improvement opportunities. In response, several revisions were made to the HIS. First, criteria for use of irradiated blood components were established in policy and incorporated into the medical ordering of blood through the HIS. Second, medical ordering pathways were revised to differentiate between requesting type and cross match of blood from the blood bank, and the medical orders for time and rate of administration. This information was reorganized to print as a separate category of medical orders on the patient's plan of care (Kardex). Third, nurse certification requirements for blood administration were automatically programmed to print on care plan documents with the standards of practice and medical orders for managing a potential transfusion reaction. If an adverse reaction occurs, the HIS facilitates documentation in the patient record as well as the required regulatory reporting through one data entry process. The professional standards for symptom management were also programmed into the documentation pathways.

The HIS eliminate the duplication of effort and communication and automatically provides required specimen collection requisitions in the nursing area. The medical and nursing response has been favorable. Extra clerical work was streamlined, consistency in the information management was achieved, and compliance with standards of care was facilitated.

2.3 Patient Allergy Identification

The need to provide consistent and updated medical and nursing assessments regarding a patient's sensitivities or allergies across inpatient and outpatient encounters was identified as a quality improvement opportunity. In response, the HIS was designed to enforce a standardized assessment of patient allergies/sensitivities on each admission. This information includes identification of the allergy/sensitivity, the source of information, the history, and the supporting data and prints on key patient documents. This information is stored on-line so that a review on each subsequent patient encounter is possible.

Medication or diet ordering via the HIS is designed to prompt the prescriber with a review of current patient allergies. Customer response to this application was evaluated and found to be positive. The inconsistency between nursing and medical assessments was eliminated, the availability of information across patient encounters provides continuity of information and hence continuity of care, and the accessibility of the information to other departments (i.e., nutrition and pharmacy) is available.

2.4 Infection Control

A mechanism to provide annual education regarding Universal Precautions to all physicians was needed. In addition, the need to communicate a patient's infectious status to hospital escort personnel when requesting patient transportation services was identified.

The HIS was used as the vehicle to provide improvements in both these areas. Educational content related to Universal Precautions was identified and programmed into the HIS so that the physician can access the information at his/her convenience. An interactive on-line evaluation of learning was also designed so that a self assessment is conducted by the physician and feedback on incorrect responses is provided. Upon completion, a written verification prints to confirm compliance with the annual review requirement and is sent to the credentialing office. Physician response has been positive as the logistics and paper work of annual educational review are simplified.

To provide communication of a patient's infectious status to hospital escort personnel, standards for gown/gloves/mask use for patient transport were clarified and an HIS application was designed to provide an electronic request to patient escort service from nursing. The request includes the patient's isolation status as well as precaution information. This information is used by the patient escort service to assign employees with specific disease immunities to certain patient care situations. The HIS also differentiates and communicates patient transportation time and patient appointment time. Interdisciplinary evaluation was very favorable as employees felt their safety needs as well as the patient's were being addressed.

2.5 Medication Administration

The need to decrease medication errors and provide safe emergency drug administration were identified as targeted areas for improvement. The HIS was used to reformat patient medication documents such that medications were categorized according to the type of administration schedule. The printout subgroups information into medications with a scheduled time for administration, medications to be given on request (prn), and medications to be given according to a conditional schedule (i.e. on call). Because of the volume and complexity of medication orders, this reorganization allows the nurse to easily verify information and synthesize patient requirements. Response has been very favorable.

The HIS was also used to provide more accurate and timely information on emergency drug dosages. Recording of a pediatric patient's weight on admission automatically triggers a computerized printout of emergency medication dosages specific for that patient's weight. This application eliminates the need for complex calculations during an emergency situation. It also allows for the availability of this information at all times at the patient's bedside.

2.6 Continuity of Care

The need to avoid duplication of effort and inconsistency in recording discharge instructions and patient telephone encounters after the patient is discharged were identified as improvement opportunities. To address these needs, the HIS was programmed to facilitate the recording of the standards of practice for patient discharge instruction in the patient record. Recording this information in the patient record automatically generates a printout for the patient to take home. This patient document is formatted for readability. The information is designed to stay on-line 60 days after a patient's discharge so that retrieval of the information is available for easy reference and follow up if needed.

Content on the HIS was developed also to accommodate documentation of telephone encounters between patient visits. This application allows the nurse to enter on-line an assessment, planned interventions and patient outcomes resulting from any telephone interaction. Information is kept on line for 60 days and then automatically printed on a permanent patient record document in the Medical Record Department.

A patient's name is never removed from the HIS; thus, the ability to access the record and to record information on-line is always available. All information for inpatient and outpatient encounters is integrated into one electronic patient record. Access to information across care settings has been very well received. The fragmentation found with separate inpatient and outpatient charts is eliminated and accessibility to information from prior patient encounters is available.

While the development of any clinical computer application is important, the implementation process determines the success and effectiveness of the application. The introduction of computer systems and applications requires a change in how information is acquired, processed, and managed. Because information and its communication are critical to organizational and individual work, changes affecting these must be managed. Empirical evidence shows that technology can either replace or complement roles [7]. Organizational roles that focus on moving and processing information may need to be redirected as technology better accomplishes these types of activities [8,9]. Understanding implementation strategies related to the adoption of computer information systems is needed for clinical application to be successful.

3. Innovation Adoption

3.1 Resistance

Dowling [11] notes that recognizing resistance to computer-based information systems is critical to effective implementation. His study demonstrated five types of resistance: passive resistance; defaming the computer by complaining and spreading rumors; declaring inability to learn; actively interfering by sabotage; and overt refusal to use computers.

Several theories of resistance to automated information system implementation in organizations have been proposed [10]. They focus on resistance as it relates to either people factors, to software characteristics, or to the interaction between people and technology. This interaction can be from the sociotechnical perspective of division of labor as well as from the political perspective of organizational power.

No one theory in isolation can adequately describe the complexity and dynamics of modern organizations as they relate to resistance encountered in organizational change. The introduction of computer-based information systems, though, is more than an organizational change. It can be viewed as the introduction of an innovation. An innovation is defined as an idea, practice, object or knowledge perceived as new by individuals or groups [12]. While not all change is considered an innovation, all innovations are considered changes.

The diffusion of an innovation is the process by which an innovation is communicated via channels over time among members of a social system. Adoption involves a decision process through which one becomes aware of, is persuaded to try, and adopts or rejects continued use based on perceived characteristics of the innovation. These attributes include advantage, complexity, compatibility, trialability, and observability of effectiveness. From this perspective, resistance can be viewed as rejection of an innovation based on unawareness, negative evaluation of attributes, or incompatibility with the dynamics of the social system.

The critical question, however, is how can an organization plan for the systematic introduction of a clinical information system as an innovation, so as to enhance organizational effectiveness, efficiency, and employee satisfaction. To this end, several strategies for implementing such systems can be considered.

3.2 Strategies

Several authors have proposed strategies for implementing change which can be applied to the implementation of technology innovations. Sathe [13] references the work of Kotter and Schlesinger and suggests the following strategies: education and communication; participation and involvement; facilitation and support; negotiation and agreement; manipulation and cooperation; and implicit and explicit coercion. While each approach has its strengths and weaknesses, one is cautioned to carefully match the strategies to the particular situation.

Davis and Salasin [14] propose seven interacting factors that play a part in influencing human responses to change, and are considered both necessary and sufficient to account for people responses. These multiple factors incorporate the theories of resistance as well as the change strategies.

Computer systems are frequently introduced into an organization as a solution looking for a problem to solve. Organizations that are trying to "be modern", should first focus on triggering a felt *need* for the technology and its application as well as *awareness* through training. A computer system must "fit" the organization's culture or *value*. Davis & Salassin suggest developing a cadre of zealous participants who can network within and outside the organization to facilitate acceptance and adoption of the innovation. Mobilizing resources, timing the implementation appropriately, *anticipating resistance* by addressing legitimate concerns, and emphasizing the *benefits derived* all facilitate implementation. In summary, the introduction of information systems should be acknowledged as an organizational change that may affect all members of an organizational unit. The type and extent of the technology will determine the degree of organizational impact.

4. Summary

Integrating implementation strategies within the new Quality Paradigm can provide the mechanism not only to facilitate the adoption of valued and needed information system innovations, but also to enhance the continuous evaluation and improvement of the quality of care delivered and received. It is noted that the principles of CQI provide an organizational framework that focuses on executive level administrative support and customer involvement on the front end and customer satisfaction and evaluation at the other end. An HIS provides the vehicle to improve clinical information management and consequently the improvement of organizational processes and systems.

5. References

[1] Berwick, D. (1989) Continuous Improvement as an Ideal In Health Care, *N Engl J Med*, 53-56, 230.

[2] Deming, W.E. (1982) *Quality, productivity, and competitive position*, Cambridge, Mass: Massachusetts Institute of Technology, Center for Advanced Engineering Study.

[3] Appel, F. (1991) From Quality Assurance to Quality Improvement: the Joint Commission and the New Quality Paradigm, *JQA*, 13, 5, 26-29.

[4] Romano, C. (1984) A Computerized Approach to Discharge Care Planning, *Nurs Outlook*, 32 (1), pp 23-25.

[5] Romano, C., Ryan, L., Harris, J., Boykin, P., & Power, M. (1985) A Decade of decisions: Four perspectives of Computerization in Nursing Practice, *Comp in Nurs*, 3 (2), pp 64-76.

[6] Dimond, E.P. (1992) Oncology Nurses Role in Patient Advance Directives, *Oncol Nurs Forum*, 19 (6), pp 891 -896.

[7] Boddy, D. and Buchanan, D. (1982) Information Technology and the Experience of Work, In L. Bennon, U. Barry, and O. Holst (Eds.), *Information Technology Impact on the Way of Life*, Dublin, Tycooly International Publishing, pp. 144-157.

[8] Ahituv, N. and Neumann, S. (1990) *Principles of Information Systems for Management*, Dubuque, IA: Wm. C. Brown Publishers.

[9] Gorry, G.A. and Morton, M.S. (1989) A Framework for Management Information Systems, *Sloan Management Review*, Spring 1989, pp 49-61.

[10] Markus, M. (1983) Power, Politics, and MIS Implementation, *Communication of the ACM*, 26 (6), 430-444.

[11] Dowling, A. (1980) Do Hospital Staff Interfere with Computer System Implementation? *Health Care Manage Rev*, 5 (4), 23-32.

[12] Rogers, E. (1983) *Diffusion of Innovations* (3rd ed.), New York: The Free Press.

[13] Sathe, V. (1985) *Culture and related corporate realities*, Homewood, IL: Richard D. Irwin, Inc.

[14] Davis, H. and Salasin, S. (1982) Computers and Organizational Changes/Factors that Influence Useful Adoption of Computer Applications, in B. Blum (Ed.), *Proc Annu Symp Comput Appl in Med Care*, (371-379), New York: IEEE.

Nursing Informatics: An International Overview for Nursing in a Technological Era
S.J. Grobe and E.S.P. Pluyter-Wenting, eds.

670

Total quality management and maximized use of automation: the keys to success

Fredericksen LA

Independent Healthcare Information Systems and Management Consultant, 10425 50th Avenue, Kenosha, Wisconsin 53142.

Providing quality healthcare in a cost effective manner is a preeminent goal in all hospitals today. Achievement of this target has become an urgent necessity internationally as resources become more scarce. Managing and evaluating nursing care is an integral part of this goal achievement. This involves assuring ordered treatments are done in the most streamlined manner by the most appropriately educated staff member, treatments are initiated most expediently at the correctly prescribed times in the most courteous manner, and variances from expected outcomes are noted at the first sign of change. This paper will address two keys to achieving this initiative: the combining of the principles of total quality management and automation benefit achievement.

1. Introduction

Opening the doors to achieving this great initiative of providing high quality, cost effective healthcare requires two keys. Key One is application of total quality management principles. Key Two is maximization of automation benefit achievement principles. Both keys must be used together in a planned change process to open the door to business success and achievement of:
- Improved quality of nursing care delivery
- Stretching of scarce professional nurse resources
- Increased staff satisfaction with the work environment
- Cost containment

2. Key One: application of total quality management principles

The principles of total quality management are fundamentally those of effective management[1,2]. These principles include:
- Having a documented guiding vision
- Holding all staff accountable for work performance outcomes
- Using open and direct communication
- Empowering staff to be able to make decisions at point of service
- Basing decision making on facts
- Focusing on continually striving to provide service of higher quality more quickly
- Removing "walls" between departments and supporting "seamless" patient care delivery systems
- Supporting risk taking within the organization
- Placing a strong emphasis on education

Success begins with the hospital administration identifying their vision related to customer service expectations and business direction. This vision is then operationalized through the hospital strategic plan, service delivery strategies, qualitative and quantitative goal setting, and supportive information system decisions. Decisions are based on facts, not intuition. Time is devoted to data collection before decisions are finalized.

Once this vision is documented and the operationalizing process begun, assigning responsibility for achieving a specific outcome and holding staff answerable is imperative for achievement of successful outcomes. Without assigned responsibility and follow up, due dates slip as other assignments are received, outside factors receive blame for the failure, or the assignment target becomes unclear or lost.

Underlying the process of operationalizing the vision are key principles of human resource management. These include open, honest communication and empowerment of staff. Both of these principles are cornerstones of successfully operated, customer focused hospitals. The vision and end targets for the hospital are clearly communicated to all staff. Issues not in the best interest of the vision are addressed as they arise. These issues are not allowed to multiply, increase in intensity, or interfere with delivery of high quality service.

To provide rapid customer service, staff must be able to make customer related decisions at point of service. Service delivery is delayed anytime a staff member must seek a higher authority before rendering that service. Setting up situations where decisions are made away from the point of service introduces opportunities for errors as information must be passed on between staff. Each time the originating information is exchanged the information may be misinterpreted or altered. Any decisions based on this information may be incorrect.

A constant vigilance to seek more efficient methods to provide higher quality service delivery is fundamental to a total quality improvement environment. Staff inherently want to do their jobs well. What keeps them from achieving this end result are task interferences. Removing these roadblocks is key to improving service delivery efficiency. Roadblock removing involves assessing the entire process related to the issue. All relevant facts are gathered prior to resolution and decisions are based on fact not on intuition. These facts may include time, place, occurrence rate of the issue, and precipitating factors to the occurrence. Without proper data collection, changes may be initiated unnecessarily for one time occurrences, the root cause of the problem may never be addressed, or staff not involved with the issue may be penalized.

In total quality management environments, what is best for the patient is the preeminent factor in all decision making situations. No longer is decision making that supports one department over another condoned. Work processes and information systems are developed to support delivery of high quality care in the most expedient manner. Staff work responsibilities are designed for maximum utilization of a staff member's education within licensure parameters. Cross-training of staff moves them out of traditional department roles.

Mistakes are viewed as opportunities to improve process in total quality management environments. Each mistake is assessed from a viewpoint of what step in the process or outside factor caused the error to happen. Management establishes parameters within which staff are allowed to alter processes to decrease the chance of the error reoccurring. For new endeavors, targets and achievement timeframes are established. At each checkpoint, endeavors are evaluated. Endeavors are either continued, altered, or stopped without punitive action.

For any process change to be success, there must be a strong emphasis on education. Staff need to know what their job expectations are and how to do the tasks within those expectations. Along with knowing the tasks of the job, the staff must also be taught how to approach their work in an efficient manner. Time management and principles of streamlining work processes must also be included in staffs' education.

3. Key Two: maximization of automation benefit achievement principles

Achieving quality and productivity improvement targets is the cornerstone to providing high quality, cost effective nursing care[2]. Automation supports achievement of improvement targets in the following three ways:
- Streamlining of work practice
- Tracking of clinical and quality indicators
- Project management

Qualitative and quantitative benefits from automation do not "fall out" by "turning on" a system. The system must be designed and implemented in a manner supporting streamlined workflow and minimum data handling steps. For automation to play an integral part in achieving quality and productivity improvement targets, as identified in the above three ways, proper design and use of automation must be in place. As an information system consultant for over ten years I have observed there are certain system design and use principles utilized at hospitals achieving maximum benefits from automation[3,4,5]. These principles include:
- Maintain reliable overall system performance and system response times of less than 1-2 seconds per action
- Maintain consistent, reliable system security measures

- Provide all staff with direct system access to all relevant data needed to perform their job duties
- Establish system user access and procedures to support entry of data by the first person to acquire the data
- Setup system access and procedures so the person who has the greatest knowledge about the subject gathers and enters the data
- Set up screens and system displays in terminology familiar to users
- Maintain consistent system logic and format between various screens and pathways
- Set up the system to support one time entry of data elements
- Build pathways to support entry of data in smaller segments
- Use 80:20 rule on screens with data element selection lists
- Present data outputs in formats that meet the needs of the end user
- Print system documents at point of use

Achieving qualitative and quantitative benefits from automation, begins by having a system that technically functions correctly. The system must be available to staff at all times and respond rapidly to users' actions. A "down" or "slow" system is of no benefit to a user. The system must be functioning well for service delivery to be done since the computer system is the location of the most current patient information . If a system functions poorly or is "down" frequently, users retain old or create new manual methods to support handling of pertinent information needed to perform their work. Along with functioning correctly, the system must also be secure to maintain patient confidentiality and retain trust of the staff.

The automated system will replace other means of obtaining information. Thus, all staff must be provided access within the system to the information they need to perform jobs or document patient response to treatment. If access is not provided, staff will rely on others to obtain or record data. Limiting access forces users to set up procedures requiring staff members to seek or record data for one another. Each time this occurs an opportunity for error or misinterpretation is introduced.

For the most accurate collection of data, the person collecting the data should have the greatest knowledge related to use of the information and when incorrect or incomplete information has been received. The best scenario is to have the person who will be using the information collect and enter in the system. This may not always be feasible. If someone other than the person who will be using the information must collect the data, the collector of the information must be taught how information they are collecting will be used, how to gather correct and complete information, and what to do if questionable or incomplete information is received.

To promote more accurate data collection, set up screens and system displays in terminology familiar to the user. Maintain consistent system logic and format between various screens and pathways. This will not only promote accuracy but increase speed of data entry.

Systems should be set up to promote minimum handling of the data. Data elements should be entered in the system one time only. The system should be configured to transfer data to users in the format best suited for their needs. Hard copies of data should be printed at point of use not printed in one department and manually distributed.

Including the above principles in an information system installation promotes data collection and processing accuracy, increases timeliness of data availability, enhances user decision making, and streamlines workflow for staff. All of these results are integral to being able to provide higher quality service more cost effectively.

3.1 Role of automation in streamlining of work practice

Automation is designed to store, sort, collate, and transfer information. It is for these reasons maximizing the use of automation is key to streamlining work practice and reducing manual effort required of staff to provide nursing care[2,4,5]. Automation can process data far more efficiently than any manual process.

Several steps need to be completed to maximize the role of automation and streamline work processes. First, a review of all work practices in every area of nursing needs to occur. Nursing staff, with the assistance of "outside eyes", need to step back and assess all nursing care delivery procedures. These "outside eyes" help the nursing staff identify duplicative, manual processes the staff may be too involved with to notice. These "outside eyes" can be anyone who does not routinely work in the area being assessed.

Second, after the assessment is completed, a quality improvement process must be completed. Each process should be reviewed in light of seeking a more efficient, effective way to complete the process. The team reviewing each process needs to ask and seek answers to questions such as:

- Is automation used to process all information involved with the issue?
- Where are terminals located in relation to the location of the procedure?
- Are there any process steps that are completed both manually and in the automated system?
- Are the steps to enter information in the automated system streamlined?
- Is the process set up to support the collection and recording of information by the first person to receive the information?

Streamlining of work practices reduces duplicative, error-prone manual information processing steps. It the elimination of these unnecessary steps that leads to improved quality of service delivery and reduction in required staff hours per procedure.

3.2 Tracking of clinical and quality indicators

As stated earlier, automation is designed to store and process data. The key features of automation support the tracking of clinical and quality indicators. Maximizing the use of automation includes setting up all automated systems to track variances, provide warnings, and produce trending information.

Automated tracking produces more accurate management information in a more timely manner. Quicker turn-around on pertinent variances from the expected plan of care or outcome supports more timely initiation of corrective action. It is the initiation of corrective action in a more timely manner that reduces costs and improves quality.

3.3 Project management

Automation provides a mechanism in which to accurately and quickly track progress on quality and productivity improvement activities. Project management is key to on time completion of projects and achievement of the project outcome within budget. Automation is ideal for tracking improvement team activities.

Automated tracking can be done as simply as having an automated project outline in a word processing file to as elaborate as an exclusive project management software package. Either can be effective. The key is to document the specific tasks of a project, the due dates, and who is accountable to assure the completion of the task.

Responsibility for administrative follow-up and project work increases daily for nurse managers. This increase in follow-up necessitates having processes in place to track due dates and accountability across multiple scopes. Automation is the best solution and support for managers in this all important but time consuming task.

4. Conclusion

Managing and evaluation nursing care is a major component of improving the quality of the total healthcare delivery system. Implementing the principles of total quality management and maximizing the use of automation designed with a benefit achievement focus are the two major initiatives that will lead to decreased total healthcare costs. As consumers become better informed about healthcare outcomes and cost containment becomes a greater issue, these key initiatives will no longer be something nice to do, but a requirement of all hospital administrators.

5. References

[1] Choppin J. *Quality through people: a blueprint for proactive total quality management*, San Diego: Pfeiffer, 1991.

[2] Weaver CA. Realising the benefits from information technology: applying new wisdom to quality improvement practices. In:*Conference proceedings Health Informatics Conference*. Brisbane, Australia, August 1993.

[3] Fredericksen L. Benefits from automation: a myth or reality. In:*Proceedings of the 1993 Annual HIMSS Conference*. San Diego, California, 1993:105-113.

674

[4] Blask D, Cleary J and Dux L. A computerized medical information system sustaining benefits previously achieved. *Healthcare and Computers* Dec. 1985,60-64.

[5] Kahl K, Ivancin L and Fuhrman M. Realizing the savings potential offered by use of bedside terminals. In: *Proceedings of the 1992 Annual Healthcare Information and Management Systems Society Conference*, Orlando, Florida February 1992, 175-194.

Nursing Informatics: An International Overview for Nursing in a Technological Era
S.J. Grobe and E.S.P. Pluyter-Wenting, eds.

A Study to Determine the Effectiveness of Repurposing Interactive Video Discs in Teaching Registered Nurses in the Clinical Setting the Process of Quality Improvement

McAlindon M N

Assistant to the Vice President for Nursing Informatics, McLaren Regional Medical Center, 401 S. Ballenger, Flint, Michigan, 48532, USA.

The purpose of this study was to develop an interactive video instruction program (IVI) to teach registered nurses in the clinical setting concepts of quality improvement, and to test the effectiveness of the program. The Smith Author System was used to combine text and video sequences repurposed from videodiscs developed for nursing education in order to describe and illustrate concepts of quality improvement. A sample of 55 registered nurses from a midwest regional medical center who used the program had a significant increase in knowledge ($p > .05$) from pre to post-program Opinionnaire and expressed willingness to apply concepts of quality improvement to patient care activities.

1. Objectives

Quality improvement (QI) is the process of monitoring and evaluating patient care to ensure that the standards established by the professional organizations and the hospital accrediting and licensing agencies are met. Because of the constraints of time and availability of staff, it has become difficult to teach the concepts of quality improvement to the nursing staff in a timely, efficient, and cost-effective manner. In addition, the accrediting and licensing agencies frequently change requirements and terminology for this process, necessitating a means of keeping the nursing staff current. The first purpose of the study was to develop an interactive video instruction (IVI) program to teach registered nurses in the clinical setting concepts of quality improvement. The second purpose was to (a) determine whether these registered nurses would demonstrate a gain in knowledge and valuation of the QI process as a result of using the IVI program, and (b) express willingness to apply concepts of QI to patient care activities.

2. Study Sample

There were two versions of the IVI Program; both contained the same text and questions, however, one version contained video sequences illustrating abstract examples of the concepts to be learned, the other contained video sequences illustrating concrete examples. A sample of 55 registered nurses was randomly divided into two groups; one group used the IVI program containing concrete examples, the other group used the program containing abstract examples. Following a brief orientation to the computer and the program, participants completed the program and instruments and returned to work.

3. Methods

Methodology for the study included the development of the IVI program, the use of instruments to gather data, and analysis of the data.

3.1. Development of the IVI Program

The process of developing the IVI program involved the selection and use of (a) videodiscs suitable for repurposing, (b) an authoring system, and (c) an instructional model to serve as the framework for the program.

Six videodiscs developed for undergraduate nursing education were previewed and two were chosen from the variety of programs available. This choice was based on content analysis for sequences that would illustrate the concepts to be learned. The Fuld Institute of Technology in Nursing Education (FITNE) offered the use of their videodisc *Therapeutic Communication* to illustrate abstract examples of the concepts for quality improvement. The American Journal of Nursing Company permitted the use of their videodisc *Nursing Care of the Elderly Patient with Chronic Obstructive Pulmonary Disease* to illustrate concrete examples of the concepts.

Demonstration discs of authoring systems were reviewed and the Smith Author System was chosen to integrate video sequences with text to illustrate the concepts to be learned. The Smith Author System is an authoring language developed in 1985 to support the development of interactive video instruction. This system was chosen because it (a) was easy to use, (b) provided the frames necessary for formatting questions contained in the text, (c) was compatible with the available hardware and videodiscs, and (d) could retain participant responses for future analysis (Smith, 1989).

The Yordy and Nelson (1991) model for instructional design was used as the framework for the program. This included (a) a needs analysis, (b) an analysis of the learning environment with the establishment of instructional goals, (c) the design of learning requirements including the learning objectives, (d) the implementation of instruction, and (f) evaluation of the instruction. Principles of adult education and interactive screen design were also used in the development of the program. The sequencing of instructional content was from simple to complex with frequent summarizing. A handout summarizing the concepts included in the program was distributed to enhance retention and transfer of learning to patient care activities.

Once the instructional design process was completed, the videodiscs were previewed for sequences to illustrate the concepts being taught. Videodisc sequences were to be removed from the context for which they were intended and used to illustrate the abstract and concrete concepts of quality improvement. Content for the program was gathered from JCAHO materials and text was written following the instructional design (Monitoring, 1991). Learning objectives were to be measured by multiple-choice and open-ended questions contained in the IVI program. Multiple choice questions were designed to measure the learning of information presented in the program or to estimate valuation of the process. The open-ended questions were written to encourage the learner to analyze, synthesize and evaluate what they had learned, as well as to value, conceptualize and organize the concepts so that they could incorporate them into their daily practices.

Screen design was important since the learner did not have the benefit of teacher support. Consistency was used in the placement of information on the screen to simplify the process of reading and comprehension, allowing the learner to locate and interpret information without confusion. Frame numbers for the video sequences were written into the text using the Smith Author System so that they would be brought into the program by the computer in the proper sequence.

The instruction was tutorial, the learner was given information that was reinforced by a video presentation, followed by questions used to measure the acquisition of knowledge and valuation. Feedback to learner responses was either positive or neutral; for incorrect answers the correct response was provided with additional information for reinforcement. Periodic summaries of information in the text provided opportunities for retention and transfer of knowledge.

3.2. Instrumentation

Three instruments were used to collect data: (a) the Leuze Pre-Program and Post-Program Opinionnaires, (b) the Interactive Video Instruction Program and (c) the Exit Opinionnaire.

The Leuze Opinionnaires were originally developed by Edwardson and Anderson (1983) and used by Leuze (1990) to measure knowledge and valuation of the QA process. Validity and reliability were established by the authors of this instrument. The Leuze Opinionnaire was adapted for use in this study by eliminating four statements that did not reflect QI activities at the study site. The Opinionniares contained 12 knowledge and 14 valuation statements that required a yes or no response.

Two versions of the Interactive Video Instruction Program were developed from the same outline and considered one type of instrument. Multiple-choice and open-ended questions contained in the IVI program were used to measure knowledge and valuation of the concepts being taught. There were 17 knowledge-type questions and 12 valuation-type questions contained in the program. Seven open-ended questions were designed to measure higher levels of the cognitive and affective taxonomies. The Cochran Test of Reliability was used to measure the extent to which items measured the same construct. Item were shown to measure different constructs by an unequal length Spearman-Bowman of .9954.

The Exit Opinionnaire contained five questions to measure the expressed opinions of the participants toward the IVI Program. This instrument was designed by the researcher and evaluated by the directors of nursing and administrative personnel during the pilot process. Their suggestions for improvement were used in the formative evaluation of this instrument.

3.3. Analysis of the Data

This was primarily a descriptive study with data at the nominal and ordinal levels of measurement. Non-parametric statistics were used to test hypotheses concerning (a) a change in knowledge and valuation of the quality improvement process as a result of using the IVI program, and (b) willingness to apply the concepts of quality improvement activities to patient care activities.

The change in knowledge and valuation was measured through participant responses to the Leuze Pre-Program and Post-Program Opinionnaires and through answers to questions in the IVI Program.

The Sign Test was significant ($p <$ .05) for an increase in acceptable responses to knowledge questions from Pre-Program to Post-Program Opinionnaire as measured by the Leuze instrument for those participants using the concrete version of the IVI Program. For the items measuring valuation, there was no change from Pre-Program to Post-Program Opinionnaire for 51% of the participants using the abstract version of the program, and no change for 53% of those using the concrete version. This is consistent with the intuitive expectation that valuation systems are difficult to modify through brief episodes of instruction.

There were two versions of the Interactive Video Instruction Program, one contained abstract illustrations to demonstrate the concepts, the other used concrete illustrations. Both versions of the program contained the same multiple-choice and open-ended questions to measure knowledge and valuation. A greater number of participants using the abstract program scored above the median. The Wilcoxon Matched Pairs Signed Rank Test was significant ($p <$ .05) for the disparity between knowledge and valuation scores with more participants having knowledge scores greater than valuation scores.

Another area of interest was the willingness of the study participants to internalize and apply the concepts of QI illustrated in the program. Willingness was measured by an acceptable response to a question in the Exit Opinionnaire asking the participants how they planned to use what they had learned from the program. Based on their responses to the question, 81% of the nurses were considered to be willing to incorporate the concepts learned into their daily patient care activities. The Sign Test was significant ($p <$ .05) for the difference in expressed willingness to incorporate quality improvement concepts into patient care activities.

4. Discussion

The results of the study suggest that interactive video instruction can be an effective means of education for nurses in the clinical setting. An interactive video instruction program was developed for this study by repurposing videodiscs developed for undergraduate nursing education. Video sequences were removed from the context for which they were intended and combined with text in the program to teach registered nurses concepts of quality improvement. A desired benefit of the study was that these nurses would understand and value the process of QI. Although this study was limited to nurses in one setting, nurse participants gained a significant increase in knowledge as a result of using the IVI program and a slight but insignificant gain in valuation. In addition, a significant number of them expressed willingness to apply what they had learned to their patient care activities.

The development of IVI programs by repurposing videodiscs developed for nursing education should be useful for nursing education, practice and research. Any instructor with access to the necessary equipment can combine text and video sequences to supplement education, and for enrichment and remediation. In the practice setting, this medium for education reduces the need for an instructor, is portable, can be used anywhere that equipment is available, and is accessible 24 hours per day. Some means of identifying learner style and a preference for concrete and /or abstract examples might also be useful if this study is replicated. The advantages and uses of multimedia concepts and interactive video in the healthcare setting as well as the use of different strategies in instructional design should be topics for future research.

5. References

[1] Smith GR. *Smith's Author System to Create Interactive Videodisc Instruction.* Detroit: Wayne State   University, 1989.

[2] Yordy L, and Nelson C. A Model for Instructional Multimedia Design. *CBT Directions* 1991, 20-26.

[3] *Monitoring and Evaluation Process for Quality Improvement.* Chicago: Joint Commission on Accreditation of Healthcare Organizations, 1991.

[4] Edwardson S, and Anderson D. Nurses' Valuation of Quality Assurance. *J Nurs Admin* 1983, 7/8:33-39.

[5] Leuze MS. Correlation of Nurses' Knowledge and Valuation of the Quality Assurance Process. *J Nurs QA,* 1990, 2:37-50.

Nursing Informatics: An International Overview for Nursing in a Technological Era
S.J. Grobe and E.S.P. Pluyter-Wenting, eds.

Continuous Quality Improvement through effective planning.
PAtient Related Ressource management & Information System - PARRIS.

Buch TF, Jørgensen P, Bardrum B, Wejlgaard G, Mikkelsen F.

Dept. of Cardiology and Neurosurgery, Rigshospitalet the National University Hospital, 9 Blegdamsvej, DK-2100 Copenhagen Ø, Denmark

STRUCTURA Management & IT Consultants A/S, Rugmarken 27A, DK-3520 Farum, Denmark

Based on the WHO definition of Quality and Leavitt's organizational model the PAtient Related Ressource management & Information System - PARRIS is developed as a tool for patient-, staf- and departmentally planning. General in structure, flexible and applicable for different departments. Based on the Patient Care Recording method estimating the amount of ressources needed for a patient, *model plans* for each *patient type* are developed. Developing PARRIS is a multiprofessional (nurses, physicians, surgeons and EDP-engineers), multicenter (Heart- and Neurosurgery center) project at Rigshospitalet, the National University Hospital, Copenhagen. Developement and outcome of PARRIS is descriped during this presentation.
Succeeding the development and implimentation of PARRIS the staff members expectations, knowledge and qualifications for using computer systems are taken into account.

1. Introduction

Quality, Costs and Effectiv management are major problems in hospitals of to-day. Politically, there is increasing demand for effective management of the departments, aimed at decreasing waiting times and increasing "quality" in treatment as well as in nursing. The patients and their relatives, the hospital users, likewise make increasing demands to the health care system generally.

Our problem is: we have never described the costs of a defined level of quality or the different components in the concept "quality".

Another question is, do we have usable methods as computer systems taking our discription of "quality" into account ?

WHO defined the content "quality" as:

patient satisfaction, maximum security, technologically as well as in treatment and nursing, entirety during the hospital stay as well as between the primary and secundary health service, a high level of quality standards and finally effectively utilization of the resources.

Using Leavitt's organizational model it seems to be difficult to fulfill this definition, figure 1:

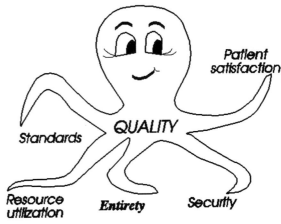

In 1986, the Danish system for classification and resource management in Intensive Care Units (ICU), the Nursing Care Recording system (NCR), was developed and tested on 393 patients in an ICU for adult patients [2,3]. The study involved developing methods as well as testing reliability, validity, sensitivity, cost-effectiveness, flexibility and acceptability of the NCR system [4].

The classification system is a retrospective classification of ICU patients and nursing activities (signs and interventions) into one of four patient categories (Table 1). This is achieved by using a point system in which each of ten indicators assigns the patient one to three points per indicator. The estimated nursing care time is an average per patient category taking into account the department's aims and standards of nursing care as well as the physical and psychological care and the care for the relativies.

Table 1

Classification of the patient according to TISS and NCR scores, and the estimated nursing time for each NCR patient category per 8-hour shift.

Category of patient	TISS points/24h	NCR points/8h	Estimated nursing time (h)
I	< 10	3 - 9	2
II	10 - 19	10 - 15	6
III	20 - 39	16 - 23	12
IV	> 40	24 - 30	16

The classification system has been correlated with an internationally well known system, the Therapeutic Intervention Scoring System (TISS). The correlation coefficient is 0.66 $p = < 0.05$. Interrater tests show fine agreement (range 90,5 - 100 percent), Kappa 0.9. The estimated nursing times have been validated by observational studies showing good agreement (range in mean -0.3 - 2.6).

Since 1988 the system has been used in Malmö, Sweden and in 1990 it was revised to our Critical Care Unit (CCU) at Rigshospitalet. The system is easy to use and flexible. Accordingly, it can be applied to different ICUs/CCUs. And it can be used to calculate: 1. the number of nursing staff per shift, per month and totally. 2. the adjustment of nurse staffing following new activities such as heart- and lungtransplantations. 3. the costs in the department or more specific of a defined level of quality standard.

Since January 1993 the departments of Cardiology and Neurosurgery at Rigshospitalet, Copenhagen Denmark have taken part in a collaboration project developing a PAtient Related Resource management & Information System (PARRIS) for patient, staff and departmental planning. The project is multidisciplinary including physicians, surgeons, nurses and engineers. The NCR method has been futher developed to a multidisciplinary scoring system, the Patient Care Recording method (PCR), in which the total interaction between the patient and the health care provider is stated. Based on the assumption, that patients naturally devide themselves into categories of required health care. A number of important and representative indicators, each assigned a range of pointvalues are selected. The weight of each pointvalue can be controlled by the computersystem. Categories are defined for certain ranges of scores. Finally, each category is tied to information about the total needed time for the care and the treatment of the patient. This can be obtained from qualified estimates made by the staff. Validating these data and the methodological presumptions has allready been and will be done with audits or observational studies. The PCR method is easy to use and quite accurate.

2. Aim

The aim of the study was to develop a computer system, that is usable for effective planning of care for patients, staffing and departmental operations. The planning is based on the patients' need for both treatment and nursing care. At the same time the system should be usable for continuous quality improvement, production control and cost-effective analyses.

3. Method

Methodologically, the patients are categorized, based on their diagnoses, their clinical condition, and the specified level of examination, treatment and nursing care (the nursing diagnoses), into pre-determined *patient types* with a uniform course of care.

Each patient type corresponds with a *model plan* in the computer system, as shown in *Figure 2*, describing the expected resources needed. This estimate in turn is based on both the Patient Care Recording method and the estimated time for specified activities. The model plan is used in planning the time and course of the hospitalization.

The patient plan is the modified model plan for the actual patient taking into account the actual condition of the patient and describing in detail the course of treatment and nursing care. Both the model plan and the patient plan are constructed of *sub plans* specifying minor parts of the total course and the level of involvement for selected resources.

The sub plan states the patient's estimated need for resources in hours, number, costs, activities such as monitoring, level of observation, examination, treatment, level of quality standards and type of resources such as bed, room, physician, surgeon, nurse and physiotherapist.

Each patient's hospital stay is based on a defined level of standards for quality in nursing, treatment as well as in examination.

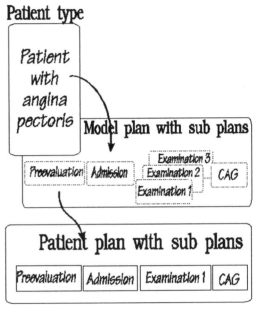

Figure 2: The PARRIS method.

A questionnaire was used to investigate staff members' expectations, knowledge and qualifications in using computer systems as a basis for developing PARRIS as well as for predicting the level of education needed for a succeessful implementation. A second questionnaire will be carried out primo 1994 to evaluate the implementation of PARRIS and the staff members' perceptions of the system as a part of the validation activities.

4. Demands and utility

Technically our demands for the computer system are: **1.** easy to use, **2.** general in structure and applicable to various clinical specialities, **3.** flexible in adjustment to both patientrelated and general changes, **4.** capable of estimating the resources needed depending on a predefined standard of treatment and nursing, **5.** capable of documenting the actual level of treatment and nursing, showing the quality of work compared to the pre-defined level, and **6.** PC-based with graphic user interface.

PARRIS' utility includes: **1.** d*epartmental planning* such as daily intake and time of hospitalization, **2.** *clinical planning* such as calculating the number of staff members needed according to the patient's level of nursing and management, **3.** *continuous quality improvement* as a result of research, **4.** *evaluation of the department's productivity* and **5.** *deviation reports* from the estimated patient plan showing causalities such as waiting times or increasing costs.

5. Relevance

Presently several recording systems have been developed for the management of nursing and treatment separately [5,6,7]. In the US such systems for daily use are common. These systems register either the nursing activities, the level of treatment or the patient's condition according to the severity of registered illness, calculating the costs as well as the quality standard [8,9].

Since the 1950's nursing activities and the level of nursing activities in Denmark have been recorded only used for nursing projects and therefor only for short periods [10,11]. The execution of continuous recording of nursing activities and nursing care, as a daily activity, depends on the complexity of the chosen system, the purpose of recording activities as well as whether usable computer systems are available. No study describes registration systems for the above mentioned topics totally.

6. Results

6.1 The questionnaire

Seventy-six percent of the staff members reported, that they uses or had been using computer systems. However sixty-six percent described their level of competence as low or very low. The level of competence increased with the time the computer system had been used. The staff members attitudes towards computer systems were generally very positive (70 %). Only one percent held a directly negative attitude. Based on these results, an educational program for the staff members was developed.

6.2 Using PARRIS

Based on the informations from the reference from the general practitioner the patient type is selected, such as *coronary evaluation*. The corresponding model plan in the EDP-system is selected at the same time showing the total calculated amount of resources, i.e. the resource profile for this patienttype. The model plan is used as a means of planning the course of hospitalization and depends for example, on the available capacity in the Cardiologic Laboratory, the availability of free beds and the staffing availability considering for example, congress participation and holidays. Coronary arteriography (CAG) is booked day number 2, special observation during total 6h post-CAG immobilization must be performed, discharge will be at day number 3, and time in the out-patient-clinic is booked for day number 10 to inform the patient about the results.

The sub plans in *coronary evaluation* represent in detail these pre-defined, multi-disciplinary activities in groupings such as *admission*, *routine examination*, *Coronary Arteriography (CAG)*, *results*, *medical treatment/ Coronary Artery By-Pass Grafting (CABG)*.

The resource profile originates from the contents of these sub plans and is calculated either in PCR scores or from the sum of well defined activities such as CAG. Though different in origin the final denomination, however, will be similar for the two methods, in that the PCR results are converted to a meassurement of time.

Upon the patient's admission, the model plan is individualized thereby forming the patient plan by futher detailing the choice and contents of the sub plans based on the informations given. For example, whether the patient is self-reliant, or on additional examinations needed, or if the patient's condition deteriorats. The course of the patient plan may currently be adjusted depending on any changes or any new information that appears. At discharge the general practitioner is informed through the electronic mail system.

Retrospectively it will be possible to point out patient related complications and bottle-necks such as waiting time in the X-Ray department, and to document the total productivity and quality of nursing care and treatment. PARRIS thus provides a tool for direct visual linking between care, quality, outcomes and costs.

7. Discussion

PARRIS' developement began in January 1993 and will be ready for departmental use in January 1994. The results will therefore be presented in detail. The PCR scoring system was initially developed and tested for nursing care. Whether it will be useable as means of estimating the needed resources multidisciplinary be investigated as part of validation activities. The validation activities will show acceptance, effectiveness, accuracy, adequacy and utility of PARRIS.

8. Conclusion

PARRIS is expected to provide a useful tool for planning and departmental administration ensuring a high level of productivity and making continuous quality improvement possible. The system will be capable of showing patients´ need for both nursing and treatment totally, assuming a certain level of quality. PARRIS is applicable in daily clinical planning, patient- and staff administration, administrative planning, productivity control and deviation reporting. Hereby, a platform for continuous quality improvement is established. We view PARRIS as an initial approach to a computer based patient and nursing record can be established as *one united* multidisciplinary patient record.

9. References

[1] Leavitt HJ. Organizational changes - structure, technology and personal methods (Danish translation). In: Borum F. EDB, arbejdsmiljø og virksomhedsdemokrati. Nyt fra Samfundsvidenskaberne. Aaby 1977: 21-31.

[2] Hjortsø E, Buch T, Ryding J, Lundstrøm K, Bartram P, Dragsted L & Qvist J. The nursing care recording system. A preliminary study of a system for assessment of nursing care demands in the ICU. *Acta Anaestesiol. Scand* 1992, 36: 610-614.

[3] Buch TF. Patient Classification Systems in Critical Care. The Nursing Care Recording System (NCR). Presented at the 6th Biennial Conference in Workgroup of European Nurse Researchers, Madrid 1992.

[4] Buch TF, Hellström C, Hjortsø E. (in review) Validitetskontrol af Nursing Care Recording systemet. Kan "fagligt skøn" anvendes i et registreringssystem ? (English Summary). In proceeding for accept to *Vård i Norden.*

[5] Greenberg AG, Douglas K, McClure BA et all. *Nursing Intervention Scoring System: a concept for management, research and communication.* Lecture Notes in Medical Informatics 1978, 1: 729-738.

[6] Cullen DJ, Civetta JM, Briggs BA, Ferrara LC. Therapeutic Intervention Scorring System: a method for quantitative comparison of patient score. *Crit Care Med* 1979, 2: 57-60. Update: *Crit Care Med* 1983, 11: 1-3.

[7] Knaus WA, Zimmerman JE, Wagner DP, Draper EA, Lawrence DE. APACHE - Acute Physiology and Chronical Health Evaluation: a physiologically based classification system. *Crit Care Med* 1981. 9: 591-597 APACHE II. *Crit Care Med* 1985. 13: 818-829.

[8] RUSH Medicus classification and quality assuring systems and
[9] San Joachin classification system **In:** Dørum & Østergård-Nielsen: Evaluering af Plejetyngdemålings- og Patientklassifikationssystemer, (English Summary). Dansk Sygeplejeråd 1987.

[10] Hee I. *Plejetyngdemåling.* København, Dansk Sygeplejeråd 1985

[11] Burgaard J. Afdelingsinformationssystemet. Hvidovre Hospital, University Hospital, Copenhagen 1990

STANDARDS

C. Classifications

Nursing Informatics: An International Overview for Nursing in a Technological Era
S.J. Grobe and E.S.P. Pluyter-Wenting, eds.

The Classification of Nursing Interventions for Persons Living with AIDS

Holzemer WL Henry SB Reilly CA and Miller T

Department of Mental Health, Community and Administrative Nursing, University of California, San Francisco, CA 94143-0608

Although existing information technology is capable of processing large volumes of nursing data, the lack of a common taxonomy limits the usefulness of the technology for both documentation of care and decision support. The need to link patient problems and nursing interventions with patient outcomes has been recognized by many nursing leaders, yet the lack of accepted taxonomies in nursing has severely constrained the ability of the profession to accomplish this task. This study was conducted as part of a larger study examining the quality of nursing care of persons living with AIDS (PLWAs) by describing the relationships between patient problems, nursing interventions, and patient outcomes. This study presents nursing activities identified from four data sources: patient and nurse interviews, intershift report, and the patient's chart. The development of taxonomies and classification systems hold significant promise for examining relationships between patient problems, nursing interventions, and patient outcomes.

1. Background

Two emergent trends in health care have significant implications for the development of nursing care information systems. First, the cost, quality, and outcomes of health care services have received serious attention from providers, consumers, and payers of health care services in the United States. At the federal level, the importance of research on the efficiency and effectiveness of health care services was recognized and mandated with the establishment of the Agency for Health Care Policy and Research (AHCPR) in 1989. In light of this trend, the nursing profession is faced with the difficult task of empirically demonstrating the relationships between patient problems, nursing interventions, and patient outcomes. Additionally, a study conducted by the Institute of Medicine [1] generated a major initiative to develop a computer-based patient record (CPR) which is expected to become a standard technology in health care within a decade. The IOM committee suggested that the adoption of a CPR and information management technologies are essential to the infrastructure of the nation's health care system. Research on data elements which truly explain variation in care and research on human-computer interfaces were identified as priority areas by the committee. It is imperative for the profession to identify data elements which capture the contributions of nursing care to patient outcomes and allow for the examination of the relationships between the cost, quality, and outcomes of nursing care. In order for the profession to accomplish these tasks, the importance of uniform and standardized nursing data, and the role of technology needs to be acknowledged by the nursing profession and incorporated into the practice of nursing. The profession's ability to delineate the relationships between the cost and quality of nursing care ultimately rests on the state of nursing data.

Acknowledgements: This study was supported by the "Quality of Nursing Care of Persons with AIDS:, NIH-NCNR-RO1NR02215, WL Holzemer, Principal Investigator. We thank the members of the Quality of AIDS care team and our clinical collaborators for their continued support of this project.

Although existing information technology is capable of processing large volumes of nursing data, the lack of a common taxonomy limits the usefulness of the technology for both documentation of care and decision support. The Nursing Minimum Data Set (NMDS) was developed in an attempt to meet nursing's need for uniform and standardized nursing data [2]. Four of the sixteen NMDS items are specific to nursing care and include: nursing diagnoses, interventions, and outcomes; and the intensity of nursing care. The need to link patient problems and nursing interventions with patient outcomes has been recognized by many nursing leaders, yet the lack of accepted taxonomies in nursing has severely constrained the ability of the profession to accomplish this task [2-12]. Clark and Lang [12] proposed that the International Council of Nurses should lead the development of an International Classification of Nursing Practice in order to support the processes of nursing practice and to advance the knowledge necessary for the delivery of cost-effective quality nursing care at the global level.

Significant achievements in the area of taxonomy development have been made, yet consensus on the adoption of a single taxonomy for describing patient problems, nursing interventions, and patient outcomes has not been reached. Four nursing classification systems will soon be incorporated in the National Library of Medicine Metathesaurus of the Unified Medical Language System and include: the North American Nursing Diagnosis (NANDA), the Iowa Intervention Project, the Omaha Visiting Nurse Association and the SABA Home Health Care Classification [13]. The inductively generated NANDA taxonomy has become the predominant system for classifying patient problems despite criticisms related to the internal consistency and theoretical underpinnings of the diagnoses [11, 14]. NANDA has also been submitted for possible inclusion in the World Health Organization's International Classification of Diseases (ICD-10) [15]. The Iowa Intervention Project classifies nursing interventions and is conceptualized as a complement to the NANDA taxonomy [6-7]. The Omaha Visiting Nurse Association and the SABA Home Health Care Classification provide systems for the classifications of patient problems, nursing interventions, and outcomes [16-19]. Grobe [20-22] is in the process of developing a lexicon of nursing interventions. The development of these taxonomies and classification systems hold significant promise for examining relationships between patient problems, nursing interventions, and patient outcomes.

2. Study Questions

This study was conducted as part of a larger study (NIH-NR02215) examining the quality of nursing care of persons living with AIDS (PLWAs) by describing the relationships between patient problems, nursing interventions, and patient outcomes. The specific research questions to be addressed in this study are: (1) What types of nursing activities are documented and reported for PLWAs hospitalized for *Pneumocystis carinii* pneumonia (PCP) and (2) What are the most frequently documented and reported nursing activities for PLWAs hospitalized for PCP?

3. Methods

3.1 Design and Study Sample

A prospective, repeated measures design was used to describe the quality of nursing care over the course of hospitalization, approximating admission, mid-hospitalization, and discharge; and at 3 and 6 months post-discharge. 201 AIDS patients with PCP were enrolled in the study from three hospitals in San Francisco. The majority of the patients were hospitalized for their first episode of PCP. The sample was predominantly Caucasian, with a mean age of 38, and sexual practice reported as the source of infection.

3.2 Study Procedure

Nursing activities were obtained from interviews with patients, interviews with nurses, a recording of nursing activities reported during intershift report and through a chart audit of the nursing care plan, the kardex, the activity record, and the nurses' notes. All interviews and data collection activities were conducted by trained nurse research assistants (RAs). During the patient interview, the patient was asked to identify 3 or 4 major problems and how the nurse was helping them to meet these problems. During the interview with the patient's nurse, the nurse was asked to identify the patient's 3 or 4 major problems and what the nurse was doing about these particular problems. The nursing activities identified in intershift report were recorded manually. The RAs recorded all nursing activities identified in the patients chart. At 3 and 6 months post-hospitalization, the patients were interviewed at an outpatient clinic. All nursing activities were recorded verbatim. Nursing activities collected from the four data sources were entered into a relational database, Paradox, for coding and analysis.

4. Results

To date, a total of 21,492 nursing activities have been coded by a nurse RA (Table 1). A classification scheme for nursing activities has been developed and is in the process of being refined. The nursing activities are being recoded with the revised classification system. This study will report on the manner in which nursing activities were classified and will report on the frequency that these activities were documented or reported.

Table 1
Frequency of nursing activities reported by time and data source

Data Source	Time 1	Time 2	Time 3	Time 4	Time 5
Patient Interview	566	411	254	37	43
Nurse Interview	1,077	737	439		
Intershift Report	735	559	359		
Chart Audit	6,832	5,854	4,039		
Total	9,210	7,561	5,091	37	43

5. Discussion

In the years ahead, the nursing profession must struggle to find a balance between standardizing nursing data, preserving the uniqueness of nursing care, and promoting innovation in the development of nursing knowledge. A uniform language for describing patient problems, nursing interventions, and patient outcomes of nursing care is required in order to develop nursing care information systems. The development of various taxonomies and classification systems provide a mechanism for standardizing the language used to describe nursing practice. The eventual adoption of a uniform taxonomy poses significant challenges and will require a concerted effort. Criteria for the selection of uniform taxonomies will need to be defined and significant compromises and negotiations will need to occur. In this process, Mass, Hard, and Craft [23] advise us to guard against the uncritical use of preexisting lists of patient data elements, as nurses may fail to observe indicators of a phenomenon truly experienced by the patient. Additionally, the classification of patient problems, nursing interventions, and patient outcomes needs to achieve conceptual congruency in order to for any relationships between them to be tested [9].

The profession must also consider the global research and development efforts in these areas. The CPR committee recommended that the relationship between the structure of patient records and the quality of patient care warranted further exploration and that specific elements of the patient records which contribute to patient care outcomes need to be identified [1]. Nursing interventions would seem to make a significant contribution to various patient care outcomes. A uniform taxonomy of nursing interventions would allow large scale studies to be conducted which examine the effect of nursing interventions on patient outcomes and have the potential to increase the quality of care and contribute to the development and revision of standards of care. International efforts to standardize and classify health data need to be supported and encouraged.

690

Nurse scientists, nurse educators, nurse administrators, and nurse clinicians need to make a collective effort to incorporate technology into the practice of nursing. The advancement of the practice of nursing largely depends on nursing's ability to document the effectiveness and efficiency of nursing care. The study Group of Nursing Information Systems [24] posed that the foundation of professional nursing is based, in part, on the documentation of its activities. In the absence of adequate and systematic documentation, the nursing profession will continue to face major obstacles in its attempts to advance nursing knowledge, to develop nursing practice, and to improve patient care. The profession's ability to delineate the relationships between the cost and quality of nursing care ultimately rests on the state of nursing data.

6. References

[1] Institute of Medicine. The computer-based patient record: An essential technology for health care. Washington, DC: National Academy Press, 1991.

[2] Werley HH and Lang NM. The consensually derived nursing minimum data set: Elements and definitions. *Identification of the Nursing Minimum Data Set. HH Werley and NM Lang (eds). New York: Springer 1988:402-413.*

[3] Lang NM, and Clinton JF. Quality assurance-the idea and its development in the United States. In:*Measuring the quality of care.* LD Willis and ME Linwood (eds). Edinburg: Churchill Livingston 1984:69-98.

[4] Lang NM, and Marek KD. The classification of patient outcomes. *J Prof Nurs* 1990, 158-163.

[5] Marek KD. Outcome measurement in nursing. *J Nurs Qual Assur* 1989, 4:1-9.

[6] McCloskey JC, Bulechek GM, Cohen MZ, Craft MJ, Crossley JD, Denehy JA, Glick OJ, Druckeberg T, Maas M, Prophet CM, and Tripp-Reimer T. Classification of nursing interventions. *J Prof Nurs* 1990, 6:151-157.

[7] Bulecheck GM, and McCloskey JC. *Nursing interventions: Essential nursing treatments.* Philadelphia, PA: WB Saunders, 1992.

[8] McCormick KA. The urgency of establishing international uniformity of data. In:*Nursing Informatics 91: Proceedings of the Fourth International Conference on Nursing Use of Computers and Information Science.* EJS Hovenga, KJ Hannah, KA McCormick, and JS Ronald (eds). Berlin: Springer-Verlag 1991:77-81.

[9] Holzemer WL. Quality and cost of nursing care is any body out there listening? *Nurs Health Care* 1990, 11:412-415.

[10] Graves JR, and Corcoran S. The study of nursing informatics. *Image* 1989, 21:227-231.

[11] Ozbolt J, Abraham IL, and Schultz S. Nursing information systems. In:*Medical Informatics: Computer Applications in Health Care.* EH Shortliffe and LE Perreault (eds). Menlo Park, CA: Addison-Wesley 1990:244-272.

[12] Clark J and Lang N. Nursing's next advance: An international classification for nursing practice. *Int Nurs Rev* 1992, 39:109-112, 128.

[13] American Nurses' Association. Nursing classifications recognized by the National Library of Medicine. *Am Nurse* 1993, March:9.

[14] McCormick KA. Nursing diagnosis and computers. In:*Clinical Judgement and Decision Making.* KJ Hannah, M Reiner, WC Mills, and S Letorneau (eds). New York: Wiley 1987:534-539.

[15] Fitzpatrick JJ, Kerr ME, Saba VK, Hoskins LM, Hurley ME, Mills WC, Rottkamp BC, Warren JJ, and Carpentino LJ. Translating nursing diagnosis into ICD Code. *Am J Nurs* 1989, 89:493-495.

[16] Martin KS and Sheet NJ. The Omaha System: A community health nursing data management model. In:*MEDINFO 92*. KC Lun, P Degoulet, TE Piemme, and O Rienhoff (eds). North-Holland: Elsevier Science Publishers B.V. 1992:1036-1040.

[17] Martin KS and Sheet NJ. *The Omaha System: Applications for community health nursing.* Philadelphia: WB Saunders 1992.

[18] Saba VK. Classification schemes for nursing information systems. In:*Proceedings of nursing and computers: Third international symposium on nursing use of computers and information science.* N Daly and KJ Hannah (eds). St. Louis: CV Mosby 1988:184-193.

[19] Saba VK, and Zuckerman AE. A home health care classification system. In:*MEDINFO 92.* KC Lun, P Degoulet, TE Piemme, and O Rienhoff (eds). North-Holland:Elsevier Science Publishers B.V. 1992:344-348.

[20] Grobe SJ. Nursing intervention lexicon and taxonomy study: Language and classification methods. ANS *Adv Nurs Sci* 1990, 13:22-34.

[21] Grobe SJ. Nursing intervention lexicon and taxonomy: Methodological Aspects. In:*Nursing Informatics 91: Proceedings of the Fourth International Conference on Nursing Use of Computers and Information Science.* EJS Hovenga, KJ Hannah, KA McCormick, and JS Ronald (eds). Berlin: Springer-Verlag 1991:126-131.

[22] Grobe SJ. Nursing intervention lexicon and taxonomy preliminary categorization. In:*MEDINFO 92.* KC Lun, P Degoulet, TE Piemme, and O Rienhoff (eds). North-Holland:Elsevier Science Publishers B.V. 1992:981-986.

[23] Mass ML, Hardy MA and Craft M. Some methodologic considerations in nursing diagnosis research. *Nurs Diagn 1990, 1:24-30.*

[24] Study Group on Nursing Information Systems. Computerized nursing information systems: An urgent need. Res Nurs Health 1983, 6:101-105.

© 1994 Elsevier Science B.V. All rights reserved.
Nursing Informatics: An International Overview for Nursing in a Technological Era
S.J. Grobe and E.S.P. Pluyter-Wenting, eds.

Nursing Interventions Classification (NIC)

Prophet CM

Department of Nursing, University of Iowa Hospitals and Clinics, 200 Hawkins Drive, Iowa City, Iowa, USA

While the nursing profession has made progress in the establishment of the Nursing Minimum Data Set (NMDS) and nursing diagnoses, nursing interventions have been poorly delineated. Formulated in May, 1987, a ten-member research team at The University of Iowa has defined and labeled 336 nursing treatments and is describing the relationships among these treatments. This Nursing Interventions Classification (NIC) is needed for at least eight reasons: (1) standardized nursing nomenclature, (2) depiction of the linkages among nursing diagnoses, nursing interventions, and nurse-sensitive patient outcomes, (3) development of Nursing Information Systems (NIS), (4) nursing clinical decision making, (5) determination of the costs of nursing services, (6) nursing resource planning, (7) description of the unique function of nursing, and (8) articulation with other health care classification systems.

The development of NIC involves five sequential, interactive research steps: (1) resolution of conceptual and methodological issues of taxonomy development, (2) initial list of nursing interventions, (3) revision of the intervention list and defining activities by means of expert survey and focus group processes, (4) arrangement of intervention list in initial taxonomic structure and articulation of rules and principles, and (5) validation of intervention labels, defining activities and taxonomy. In system development and enhancement, NIC will assist nurses and systems analysts to create NISs compatible with each other as well as with other health care information systems.

1. Introduction

The development of information systems for patient care and the capture, examination, and comparison of health data locally, nationally, and internationally have been severely hampered by the lack of a standardized, uniform nursing data base. An extremely important -- yet poorly defined -- segment of this nursing data base is nursing interventions.

A research team, led by Drs. Joanne McCloskey and Gloria Bulechek, was formulated in May, 1987 at the University of Iowa, to focus upon the classification and taxonomy of nursing interventions. Seven faculty members and one systems programmer in the College of Nursing, and two nursing administrators in the Department of Nursing at The University of Iowa Hospitals and Clinics are members of the Iowa Intervention Project. Several statisticians, consultants, and nursing experts advise the research team. The most recent two-day meeting with the entire consultant and advisory committee was held in March, 1993. This research was assisted by a grant from the National Center for Nursing Research (R01 NR02099).

2. Nursing Minimum Data Set (NMDS)

The nursing profession has made excellent progress in the clarification of nursing data elements. As espoused by Harriet Werley and colleagues, the Nursing Minimum Data Set (NMDS) has specified the nursing care elements of nursing diagnoses, nursing interventions, nursing outcomes, and the intensity of nursing care [1, 2].

As described by the North American Nursing Diagnosis Association (NANDA), nursing diagnoses have been tested and detail the first element of the NMDS. In terms of the second element, although nurses have compiled countless lists of discrete nursing actions and several classification schemata of nursing care categories, nursing interventions have heretofore not been well delineated.

The third nursing care element -- nursing outcomes -- is also not well described or categorized. Currently, a research team at the University of Iowa is investigating nurse-sensitive patient outcomes. The intensity of nursing care -- the fourth element of the NMDS -- is captured in multiple patient classification and acuity systems. Some of these nursing care elements are patient- or client-centered whereas others are nurse-focused. For example, the phenomenon of concern in nursing diagnosis is patient or client behavior. In contrast, nurse behavior is the phenomenon of concern with nursing interventions.

3. Nurse Activity Types

In examining nurse behavior, the research team identified seven types of nurse activities: (1) assessment activities to identify a nursing diagnosis, (2) assessment activities to gather data for physician's identification of a medical diagnosis, (3) nurse-initiated treatments in response to nursing diagnosis, (4) physician-initiated treatments in response to medical diagnosis, (5) daily essential functions, (6) evaluation of patient outcomes, and (7) administrative and indirect care. Of these seven types of nurse activities conducted by nurses for the benefit of patients and clients, which ones qualify as nursing interventions?

Since nursing interventions are implemented post-diagnosis, both types of assessment activities cannot be considered interventions. While critical to the determination of care effectiveness, outcome evaluation occurs even later -- post-implementation of the nursing interventions. Administrative and indirect care, although requisite in all care delivery systems, do not involve the direct treatment of the client or patient.

Therefore, the definition of a nursing intervention is "any direct care treatment that a nurse performs on behalf of a client. These treatments include nurse-initiated treatments for nursing diagnoses, physician-initiated treatments for medical diagnoses, and performance of daily essential functions for clients who cannot do these" [3].

Examples of nurse-initiated treatments are: patient contracting, counseling, reminiscence therapy, preparatory sensory information, pain management, bathing, oral hygiene promotion, feeding, positioning, and pre-operative teaching. Physician-initiated treatments include but are not limited to medication administration, electrolyte management and intravenous therapy.

Daily essential functions have been differentiated from activities of daily living (ADLs). If a client/patient is unable to perform ADLs, the nurse would initiate treatments in response to the identified nursing diagnoses of self-care deficit. However, daily essential functions such as bedmaking, equipment management, mail handling and telephone communication, may need to be carried out by the nurse irrespective of the patient's nursing or medical diagnoses.

4. Reasons for Classification

A classification of nursing interventions is needed for at least eight reasons. First, nursing must standardize the nomenclature of nursing treatments to better articulate the activities that nurses conduct on behalf of clients/patients. Multiple terms are used to communicate nurses' work and standardization of terms is required to facilitate any efforts to define nursing practice.

Second, linkages among nursing diagnoses, nursing interventions and outcomes must be described. The standardized NANDA-approved nursing diagnoses have delineated the client/patient conditions that nurses identify. Similarly, a classification of nursing interventions defines the treatments that nurses implement on behalf of clients/patients. Finally, a classification of outcomes provides a description of client/patient states to which nursing interventions are directed. Clearly articulated classification schemata allow a depiction of the linkages between and among these variables and facilitate nursing effectiveness research.

Three, the development of automated nursing information systems has been hindered by the lack of a standardized language and categories of nursing knowledge. A classification scheme for nursing interventions, complementary to the nursing diagnosis taxonomy, yields not only a logical structure but also well-defined nursing intervention content.

Four, a classification of nursing interventions enhances nursing education of clinical decision making. Nursing students and nurses, after analyzing patient data and identifying nursing diagnoses, can select and implement the nursing interventions determined through nursing research to be most efficacious for the patient population.

Five, efforts to "cost out" nursing services have been difficult due to the use of a wide variety of non-standardization tools, primarily patient classification systems. In order to ascertain nursing care costs based upon nursing treatments, a classification of nursing interventions is required. With the determination of nursing intervention costs, reimbursement for nursing care rendered is feasible.

Six, the identification of nursing costs derived from a classification of nursing interventions facilitates both the evaluation of cost-effective nursing interventions as well as the ability to plan for the human and material resources needed to deliver nursing interventions.

Seven, although registered nurses number 2.1 million, the profession of nursing remains enigmatic and invisible. By means of a classification of nursing interventions, the unique function of nursing will be crystallized through the depiction of "what nurses do."

Eight, the classification of nursing interventions must articulate with other health care classification systems. Standardized health care classification systems have been available for reimbursement, research and administrative purposes for many years; for example, Uniform Minimum Health Data Sets (UMHDS), Uniform Hospital Discharge Data Set (UHDDS), International Classification of Disease (ICD), and The Current Procedural Terminology (CPT). Nursing care is not included in these data sets; hence, the development of the Nursing Minimum Data Set (NMDS) and the classification of nursing interventions.

5. Research Questions and Phases

Supported by the many reasons for a classification of nursing interventions, the research team formulated two research questions: (1) What are nursing interventions? and (2) How are nursing interventions related or classified?

The Iowa research project was conducted in two phases: (1) classification and (2) taxonomy. The classification of nursing interventions is the ordering or arranging of nursing activities into groups on the basis of their relationships and the assigning of intervention labels to these groups. In contrast, the taxonomy of nursing interventions is the systematic organization of the intervention labels into what can be considered a conceptual framework with clearly articulated rules and principles for classification. In the phases identified for the taxonomy of nursing interventions, five sequential and interactive research steps have been completed. Phase I -- classification - involved Steps 1 to 3 while Phase II -- Steps 4 and 5 -- focused upon taxonomy.

6. Nursing Interventions Classification

The first research step is the identification and resolution of the conceptual and methodological issues involved in taxonomy development. Step one was accomplished in 1988. Step two is the generation of the initial list of nursing interventions. In this step, hundreds of nursing activities were obtained from nursing textbooks, care planning guides and automated nursing information systems. The research team performed eight content analysis exercises to create a list of approximately 400 intervention labels. In step three, the intervention list and defining activities were revised by means of expert survey and focus group processes. Final refinement and editing were completed by the research team.

For the expert survey process in step three, a two-round Delphi questionnaire was sent to Master's-prepared nurses who are certified in particular specialty areas. Each questionnaire contained selected intervention labels, definitions and associated activities. The respondents rated the extent to which the associated activities are characteristic of the intervention label and suggested revisions to the definition and any additional associated activities.

To establish content validity for the interventions, an adaptation of Fehring's methodology was used to calculate weighted ratios [4]. Activities with ratios greater than .80 were considered critical whereas activities with ratios less than .50 were discarded. Finally, an Intervention Content Validity score (ICV) was obtained for each intervention by summing individual activity ratios and averaging the results.

By means of these expert surveys, eighty-seven nursing intervention labels were created and validated. The June 1992 volume of Nursing Clinics of North America reports on this series of national surveys which involved responses from 483 nurse experts on the content of specific nursing interventions [5].

The alternate process in step three -- focus group -- was used for the remainder of the nursing interventions. Initially, a research team member prepared a nursing intervention label, definition and associated activities through a database search and literature review. Following consultation with clinical experts and revision by a small group of core team members, the author presented the content to the entire research team for refinement. While this method did not provide Intervention Content Validity scores (ICVs), the resulting nursing intervention label is well-defined with a comprehensive list of associated nursing activities.

The report of the first phase of the project--entitled <u>Nursing Interventions Classification (NIC)</u>--was published in May, 1992. NIC includes a summary of the research process -- steps one through three -- to create this standardized nursing language [6]. Following the research summary, <u>NIC</u> provides an alphabetical list of 336 nursing interventions. Each nursing intervention has a concept label, a definition, a set of implementation activities, and a brief list of background readings. Additionally, an comprehensive index aids the nurse in accessing the nursing intervention by a cross-listing of familiar terms.

7. Nursing Intervention Taxonomy

The research team has also completed the second major phase of the research: the development of a taxonomic structure to support the classification. In step four, the complete list of nursing intervention labels was placed in an initial taxonomic structure and rules and principles governing the taxonomic structure were articulated. The nursing interventions were ordered in relationship to one another on the basis of abstractness and similarity.

To generate the initial similarity ratings, each member of the research team sorted the nursing intervention labels into related groups with a maximum of twenty-five categories. The data from these sortings were analyzed using hierarchical clustering to determine the number of raters who placed any two interventions into the same group. Hierarchical cluster analysis groups objects into successively larger clusters on the basis of their similarities [7, 8]. As a result of this analysis, twenty-seven preliminary clusters of interventions emerged.

In step five, the validation of the intervention labels, defining activities, and taxonomy occurred wherein clinical nursing experts rated the similarities of the intervention labels. In this step, the research team, as a group, rated the individually identified clusters for internal validity. Multidimensional scaling and hierarchical cluster analysis were performed on these expert ratings to derive the taxonomy of nursing interventions.

In order to encourage further clinical review and validation of NIC, a review form is included in the book. Additionally, in May, 1992, a questionnaire soliciting feedback regarding NIC was distributed to the clinical nursing specialty organizations participating in the American Nurses' Association Committee on Nursing Practice Standards and Guidelines.

As a result of steps four and five, the taxonomy of nursing interventions has been established. The 336 original and 21 new nursing interventions were sorted into twenty-six classes. These twenty-six classes were subsumed by six domains, the most abstract level of the three-tiered taxonomy.

8. Unified Language Systems

By 1993, The American Nurses' Association endorsed NIC as one of four classification schemata for inclusion in the proposed Unified Nursing Language System [9]. The other schemata are: North American Nursing Diagnosis Association (NANDA) Taxonomy I, Home Health Care Classification developed at Georgetown [10], and the Omaha System [11]. Using computer-based interactive software, Grobe has examined intervention statements used by nurses in order to establish and validate a nursing intervention lexicon and taxonomy [12].

Moreover, by January 1993, the 336 nursing intervention labels of NIC were included as preferred terms in the metathesaurus for the Unified Medical Language System (UMLS) of the National Library of Medicine. The UMLS supplies information that computer programs can use to interact with users to interpret or refine questions, to identify relevant data bases and to convert users' terms into a vocabulary used by information sources.

9. Summary

For the many reasons cited, a classification of nursing interventions is needed not only by the nursing profession but also by other health care professionals and the health care industry. NIC will assist nurses and system analysts to create nursing information systems compatible with each other as well as with other health care information systems. Nursing Interventions Classification will provide the structure and content to define nursing interventions as identified in the NMDS and facilitate the achievement of a shared data base of nursing knowledge.

10. References

[1] Werley HH and Lang NM. *Identification of the Nursing Minimum Data Set.* New York: Springer Pub. Co. 1988.

[2] Werley HH, Lang NM and Westlake SK. The Nursing Minimum Data Set Conference - Executive Summary. *J Prof Nurs* 1986, 2(4):217-224.

[3] McCloskey JC, Bulechek GM, Cohen MZ, Craft MJ, Crossley JD, Denehy JA, Glick OJ, Kruckeberg T, Maas M, Prophet CM and Tripp-Reimer T. Classification of Nursing Interventions. *J Prof Nurs* 1990, 6(3):151.

[4] Fehring RJ. Validating Diagnostic Labels: Standardized Methodology. In: CLASSIFICATION OF NURSING DIAGNOSES '86. Hurley ME (ed). St. Louis: CV Mosby, 1986.

[5] Bulechek GM and McCloskey JC. Symposium on Nursing Interventions. *Nurs Clin North Am.* Philadelphia: W.B. Saunders, 1992.

[6] Iowa Intervention Project. *Nursing Interventions Classification (NIC).* St. Louis: Mosby-Year Book. 1992.

[7] Everitt B. *Cluster Analysis.* London: Heinemann, 1974.

[8] Sokal RR. Classification: Purposes, Principles, Progress, Prospects. *Science* 1974, 185:1115-1123.

[9] American Nurses' Association. *Databases to Support Nursing Practice.* Washington, DC: American Nurses' Association. 1993.

[10] Saba VK, O'Hare A, Zuckerman AE, Boondas J, Levine E and Oatway DM. A Nursing Intervention Taxonomy for Home Health Care. *Nurs Health Care* 1991, 12(6):296-299.

[11] Martin KS and Sheet NJ. *The Omaha System: A Pocket Guide for Community Health Nursing.* Philadelphia: W.B. Saunders, 1992.

[12] Grobe SJ. A Nursing Intervention Lexicon and Taxonomy: Methodological Aspects. In: NURSING INFORMATICS '91. Hovenga EJS, Hannah KJ, McCormick KA and Ronald JS (eds). New York: Springer-Verlag, 1991: 126-131.

Nursing Informatics: An International Overview for Nursing in a Technological Era
S.J. Grobe and E.S.P. Pluyter-Wenting, eds.

A Home Health Classification Method

Saba VK[a]

[a]Georgetown University School of Nursing, Washington, DC 20007

A clinically sound and statistically significant Preliminary Home Health Classification Method (HHCM) has been developed from a study conducted at the Georgetown University School of Nursing. It consists of: four patient care models (nursing, medical, functional status, and socio-demographic); an assessment instrument; a scoring methodology; and a process for predicting resource use and measuring outcomes. It will predict home visits by nurses and/or all providers for 30 day intervals during an episode of home health care.

I. Background

With the enactment of Medicare and Medicaid legislation in 1965, the care to the elderly sick at home changed drastically in the United States. The legislation provided payment for home health care services to those recipients eligible for care, who previously could not afford services. As a result, the home health industry grew rapidly. The number of home health agencies (HHAs) increased five-fold from 1,275 in 1966 to 6,129 in 1992; the number of patients served grew from almost half a million to over 1.5 million; and the costs grew from less than $50 million to over 11.8 billion in 1987 for home care [1].

In the 1980's other legislative events also increased the need for home care. Changes in the requirements for certification by agencies and the removal on the limit of home visits also expanded services. Further, the adoption of reimbursement for diagnosis related groups (DRGs) encouraged earlier discharge from hospitals of patients "sicker and quicker" to care in their homes [2].

In 1987 the Omnibus Budget Reconciliation Act (OBRA-87) was passed adding new burdens on HHAs, in order to control quality and cost. The law required that the HHAs providing services must have a clinical record which: (a) is prepared in accordance with accepted professional standards; (b) includes a plan of care; (c) provides cost-effective care; and (d) identifies patient care outcomes in measurable terms [3].

2. Research Method

These legislative changes and requirements led to the Home Care Classification Study (1987-1991) conducted at Georgetown University School of Nursing and funded by the federal government. The major goal of the Study was to develop a method to assess and classify the acuity of home health Medicare patients in order to predict their need for nursing and other home care services; as well as measure outcomes of care. To accomplish this goal, data on resource use correlated with a battery of medical diagnostic, functional status and socio-demographic variables were collected using a specially designed Abstract Data Collection Form [4,5].

The data were obtained from 8,840 discharged Medicare patients from 646 sample agencies, which were randomly stratified by staff size, type of ownership, and geographic location. Data on an array of assessment and service variables, number and type of home care visits, and outcomes were collected retrospectively on each patient for an entire episode of care, from admission to discharge.

The research produced a great deal of new information on the characteristics of home health agencies, patients, and services, including length and volume of visits. These data were also analyzed to identify the variables that predicted resource use and led to the development of the HHCM. A brief summary of the major findings follows:

3. Descriptive Findings

3.1 Home Health Agencies/Patients

The sample agencies offered an array of home health services, the major service being skilled nursing care. The nurses not only provided nursing care, but also managed services offered by other providers: physical therapists, occupational therapists, speech therapists, medical social workers, and home health aides.

The Medicare patients were predominantly elderly, white, middle class females, married or widowed, and living in their own homes with an available caregiver. Most (93.8%) were 65 years of age or older, and more than half were at least 75 years old, as would be expected in a population of Medicare patients. The majority of patients were mentally oriented and able to comprehend and communicate adequately.

3.2 Length of the Episode/Visits

The analysis of episodes of home health care identified three distinct episodes of care intervals: short term patients with less than 30 days (50%), intermediate patients with between 30 to 120 days (43%), and long term, with over 120 days (7%). The number of home visits differed for these three intervals; the short term patients received 5.8 nursing visits, whereas the intermediate and long term patients received 9.3 visits.

3.3 Medical Diagnoses/Surgical Procedures

All Medicare patients need at least **one** medical condition for admission. The most frequent medical diagnoses and surgical procedures were Congestive Heart Failure (5.6%) and Cerebral Vascular Accident (3.8%), and Orthopedic Surgery (1.4%).

3.4 Nursing Diagnoses/Interventions

The study also identified 40,361 nursing diagnoses/ patient problems and 73,529 nursing interventions, which were coded using Saba's newly developed taxonomies. On the average **three** nursing diagnoses/ problems and **five** nursing interventions were reported for an episode of care. The three most frequently reported nursing diagnoses were medication knowledge deficit (23.0%), physical mobility impairment (22.3%), and cardiac output alteration (20.6%); whereas the nursing interventions were medication administration (46.4%), cardiopulmonary care (36.1%), and nutrition care (30.7%).

4. Predictive Analysis

The major analytical efforts consisted of developing statistical models that related the independent variables to measures of resource use (dependent variables). The models were statistically tested using linear regression and analysis of variance (ANOVA). They were computed in order to evaluate the predictive power of the independent variables singly and in combination [6]. The major findings were: (a) the nursing intervention model was the best predictor of nursing visits; (b) nursing diagnosis and nursing intervention combined model was the second best predictor; (c) medical diagnosis and surgical procedure models had limited predictive power; and (d) socio-demographic and functional status models had little or no predictive power.

5. Preliminary Home Health Classification Method

A clinically sound and statistically significant Preliminary Home Health Classification Method was developed from the data analysis. The scoring methodology proved the predictive ability to be reasonably accurate for first 30 days of care within an episode of home health care. The Method consists of: (a) four patient assessment models: nursing, medical, functional status, and socio-demographic (b) an assessment instrument, (c) a scoring methodology, and (d) a process for predicting resource use as well as measuring outcomes.

5.1 Conceptual Framework

The HHCM consists of four patient assessment models using the Nursing Assessment Model to operationalize it. The conceptual framework is based on the nursing process proposed by the American Nurses Association (ANA), as the framework for clinical nursing practice. It consists of six levels of care: assessment, diagnosis, outcome identification, planning, implementation, and evaluation [7].

Table 1.
Standards of Care

Assessment:	Collects patient health data
Diagnosis:	Analyzes assessment health data to determine diagnosis
Outcome:	Identifies expected outcomes of patients derived from nursing diagnosis
Planning:	Develops plan of care and prescribes interventions to attain expected **outcomes**
Implementation:	Implements the intervention (types) as identified in the plan of care
Evaluation:	Evaluates the attainment of actual outcomes

5.2 Nursing Assessment Model

The Nursing Assessment Model consists of 20 Home Health Components, 145 Nursing Diagnoses, 3 Expected Outcome/ Goals (Improved, Stabilized, and Deteriorated), 160 Nursing Interventions, and 4 Types of Intervention Actions (Assess, Direct Care, Teach, Manage) [8].

Assessment→	Diagnosis→	Outcome→	Planning→	Implementation→	Evaluation
Home Health Components (20)	Nursing Diagnosis (145)	Expected Outcome (3)	Nursing Intervention (160)	Type action (4)	Actual outcome (3)

Figure 1. Conceptual Framework: Nursing Assessment Model

5.2.1 Home Health Components: The 20 home health components provide the structure for the Nursing Assessment Model to measure four sets of variables related to the nursing process. They are used to map and link patterns of nursing process levels to resource use and outcomes. A home health component is a cluster of elements that represent a health, functional, behavioral, or physiological home health care pattern. The four sets of nursing variables follow.

Table 2.
Twenty Components of Home Health Care

1.	Activity	11.	Physical Regulation
2.	Bowel Elimination	12.	Respiratory
3.	Cardiac	13.	Role Relationship
4.	Cognitive	14.	Safety
5.	Coping	15.	Self-Care
6.	Fluid Volume	16.	Self-Concept
7.	Health Behavior	17.	Sensory
8.	Medication	18.	Tissue/Skin Integrity
9.	Metabolic	19.	Tissue Profusion
10.	Nutritional	20.	Urinary Elimination

5.2.2 Nursing Diagnoses: The Classification of 145 Home Health Nursing Diagnoses, categorized by 20 home health components, is used to assess the patient and the reason for home health care. A nursing diagnosis, the cornerstone of the nursing process, a clinical judgement about the patient's response to actual or potential health problems. Nursing diagnoses provide the basis for selection of nursing interventions to achieve outcomes for which the nursing is accountable [9].

5.2.3 Expected Outcome/Goal: Three types of expected outcomes goals are used--improved, stabilized, or deteriorated--to code the patient's expected outcome goal for each nursing diagnosis.

5.2.4 Nursing Interventions: The Classification of 166 Home Health Nursing Interventions also categorized by the 20 home health components is used to code all nursing services provided. A nursing intervention is a single home health nursing service, significant treatment, or activity designed to achieve a patient outcome for a medical and/or nursing diagnosis for which the nurse is accountable.

5.2.5 Type of Intervention/Action: Four types of nursing intervention actions are used-- assess, direct care, teach, or manage--to code each nursing intervention, a type of activity (cognitive or physical).

5.2.6 Evaluation/Actual Outcome: At an predetermined time interval the evaluation of care is measured by comparing the expected outcome goal for each nursing diagnosis with the actual outcome.

5.3 Medical Assessment Model

Twenty mutually exclusive groups are used to code the primary medical diagnosis or surgical procedure, identified by a physician, as the medical condition (reason) for admitting a patient to home health care.

5.4 Functional Status Assessment Model

A nine item Activities of Daily Living (ADL) scale is used to measure the patient's ability to perform the activities of daily living. The levels of independence for each activity are measures as: independent, needs assistance, and dependent.

5.5 Socio-demographic Assessment Model

A set of ten variables are used to measure the patient's demographic and social support variables.

6. Assessment Instrument

An instrument designed to collect the assessment variables on admission, at 30 day intervals, when a change in status occurs, and/or on discharge.

7. Scoring Methodology

The measures of resource use consist of number of home visits, by nurses and by all providers; and length of the episode of care, for 30 days intervals during an episode of care. The scores are based on a workload study conducted by the agency to establish the predictors.

8. Conclusion

In summary, the Preliminary Home Health Classification Method will provide a new method for predicting resource use and measuring outcomes based on a nursing model. It uses Saba's taxonomies which provide 20 home health components as the framework needed to develop patterns of home health care based on the nursing diagnosis. The taxonomies can provide a standardized terminology for documenting home health, codes, and statistics needed for determining costs of care.

9. References

[1] National Association for Home Care. Basic Statistics About Home Care 1992. *NAHC Fact Sheet.* Washington, DC: NAHC, 1992.

[2] Wood J. The Effects of Cost-Containment on Home Health Agencies. *Home Health Care Quarterly*, 1985-85, 6(4), 59-79.

[3] National Association for Home Care. *Homecare: Omnibus Budget Reconciliation Act of 1987 (OBRA'87).* Public Law 100-203. Washington, DC: NAHC, 1987.

[4] Saba VK. Home Health Care Classification. *Caring* May 1992, 10(5), 58-60.

[5] Saba VK. *Home Health Care Classification Project.* Washington, DC: Georgetown University School of Nursing (NTIS # PB92-177013/AS), 1991.

[6] Saba VK, and Zuckerman AE. A New Home Health Care Classification Method. *Caring* 1992, 10(10), 27-34.

[7] American Nurses Association. *Standards of Clinical Nursing Practice.* Kansas City, MO: ANA, 1991.

[8] Saba VK. The Classification of Home Health Care Nursing Diagnoses and Interventions. *Caring*, March 1992, 10(3), 50-57.

[9] North American Nursing Diagnosis Association, *Taxonomy I: Revised* St. Louis, MO: NANDA, 1990.

STANDARDS

D. Technology assessments; guideline development

Nursing Informatics: An International Overview for Nursing in a Technological Era
S.J. Grobe and E.S.P. Pluyter-Wenting, eds.

Evaluating Information Support For Guideline Development

McQueen L and McCormick K and Hudgings C

*Office of the Forum for Quality and Effectiveness in Health Care, 6000 Executive Boulevard, Suite 310
Rockville, MD 20852*

The Agency for Health Care Policy and Research (AHCPR) has taken a leadership role in the establishment of a new program to develop, periodically review, update and evaluate clinical practice guidelines. The Director and Senior Health Care Policy Analysts responsible for managing the development of AHCPR-supported guidelines recognize the importance of the appropriate use of information technology in both the development of guidelines and in the management of this complex and important program. This paper will provide an overview of the way in which computers facilitate the management decisions which have led to appropriate applications of technology. The scarcity of publications in the nursing literature related to computer applications in guideline development has motivated this study. It will also describe additional resources that could facilitate communications in guideline writing.

1. Background

In November, 1989, Congress amended the Public Health Service Act to create the Agency for Health Care Policy and Research (AHCPR) in order to promote the quality, appropriateness and effectiveness of health care services and to improve access to these services. The strong emphasis on outcomes and effectiveness research led to the initiation of many creative new projects designed to promote the quality of health care in the United States. One of the most innovative ideas to reach fruition was the creation of a program to facilitate the public-private creation of clinical practice guidelines.

Within AHCPR, the Office of the Forum for Quality and Effectiveness in Health Care (the Forum) has primary responsibility for facilitating the development, periodic review, update and evaluation of guidelines and the medical review criteria, standards of quality and performance measures related to the guidelines. Guidelines are defined by the Institute of Medicine as, "systematically developed statements which assist practitioner and patient decisions about appropriate health care for specific conditions" (1990), and are based on the analysis of relevant published scientific data relevant to the topic. Current interest in guideline development has soared in recent years and more than 1500 guidelines are currently being produced or updated by professional associations or other groups in the United States. This trend is expected to continue as outcomes and health services research gain increasing attention in the health care reform agenda.

The Forum presently manages the development, review, update and evaluation of twenty-three guidelines by multidisciplinary panels of experts and health care consumers charged by Congress to review the scientific evidence related to their topic. Some AHCPR-supported panels are coordinated through contracts, while others are coordinated directly by AHCPR. Medical review criteria, standards of quality and performance measures for each guideline are also developed, updated and evaluated. The instigation and management of this ambitious program would be impossible except for appropriate uses of various technologies, including the personal computer. The importance of information planning and support has been recognized from the beginning, as technology is used to maximize the efficiency of guideline development and production.

Nurses play key leadership roles in all aspects of AHCPR-supported guideline development. Nurses serve as panel members or chairs on all AHCPR-supported guideline panels, and as projects officers, directing guideline development for AHCPR.

The complexity imposed by the AHCPR methodology require that all available supports be given to each panel and that efficiency be constantly monitored and promoted. In addition to the guideline itself, each panel produces four other documents, totaling more than 1200 pages, during the 12-18 months allotted for initial development. These five guideline products are developed after extensive literature searches are conducted and the scientific evidence is amassed from relevant published literature related to the topic. Each panel is also required to conduct an open meeting for the public, peer and pilot review the draft documents, and consider cost impact to their recommendations. The amount of data collected and the speed and sophistication required for complex analysis during the short development time demands that resources be planned and expended carefully.

Personal computers were implemented in ways which optimize both the quality of the final product and the management of the complex processes involved in guideline development. The Forum Director and the Senior Health Policy Analysts who manage the guideline panels recognized from the beginning that the ambitious schedule would be impossible unless every aspect of project management were made as efficient and effective as possible. Direction regarding the appropriate uses of technology is one of the many ways AHCPR supports the needs of each panel.

Management decisions made while planning the information support for the panels were influenced by the reports in the literature. Since there are no citations in the nursing literature directly related to computer applications for the management of guideline development, the international literature related to information systems and guideline development was generalized while planning the implementation of the information system support needed for guideline development. Publications related to clinical practice guidelines by Gardner[1] (1992), Musen[2] (1992) and others were considered, in addition to the nursing and other scientific literature related to decision-support and information system management (McCormick[3] 1991; Suwa[4] 1982; Petrucci[5] 1992; Bloom[6] 1987; Okada[7] 1988).

Based on these and other publications, the information support was planned to provide fast and effective technology, while planning resource expenditures carefully. The complexity of the guideline development process and the guideline documents themselves provided the incentive to simplify the requirements for the end-users, guard against any excess implementations, while providing the capability to generate all of the needed applications and communications. A management decision was also made to frequently evaluate the end-user satisfaction, and use the feedback to change and upgrade the system on a regular basis.

2. System Description

Hardware, software, and professional support is provided by AHCPR for each guideline panel. IBM compatible 486 computers are provided to the co-chairs of each panel, and are used by the methodologist, writer/editor and others developing each guideline. Although the 500 experts and consumers now serving as panel member and chairs have personal preference for the software needed, the Forum has found standardization of some of the software between panels to be essential, while allowing for flexibility and personal preference for other applications. The consistent use of some identical software between panels assures that all documents can readily be converted to electronic media for on-line dissemination and reduces the difficulties and delays associated with the preparation of manuscripts and camera-ready copy for each of the five guideline documents printed during the intense production phase. Wordperfect 5.1 is used for all content and the production of tables, and Harvard Graphics is used for all figures. Pro-Cite 3.5 is used to input, manage, organize and format the references and bibliographic information used in developing the guidelines products. The bibliographic information for each reference is entered as a record in the Pro-Cite database either by manual entries or importation from other on-line databases. Since each panel reviews up to 100,000 abstracts and 1000 full-text articles, the consistent maintenance of the Pro-Cite database is crucial to the management of the literature. The MacFlow program is used for algorithm development. Procomm Plus, Grateful Med, Lotus 123, and utilities packages are also provided. Although on-line support is included with several of the packages, the Forum provides additional user support as needed. The Forum provides the education necessary to assist all users and to update the systems to accommodate individual needs.

For some applications, the Forum has assisted users to design systems which not only include the standardized software, but also incorporate personal preference for other, additional programs. Several panels, for example, use different relational database, spreadsheet, and statistical analysis software packages. Whenever the use of a different software package promotes the efficiency of guideline development, efforts are made to accommodate these preferences.

AHCPR has balanced individual preferences with the need for all panels to use similar software which readily allows for the creation of products which meet specified formats. Panel chairs are frequently asked to provide feedback about the system and to communicate additional needs to the Forum. Verbal and written interviews directly related to use and satisfaction are routinely administered and discussions regarding computerization are included in management meetings. A database on a commercial relational software package is maintained at the Forum for this purpose. The feedback is used when planning who to best meet the on-going needs of the panels. The end-user satisfaction with the required software is of primary concern and on-going evaluations are made, particularly for Pro-Cite. Based on the feedback received, the system has evolved and improved over time. Additional software and hardware standards are added, after they are tested by individual panels. For example, the routine use of fax-modems is now being tested and may become a standard means of communication between the panel chairs, members, consultants, AHCPR and the methodologist. Two other panels are pilot testing the use of a network in which all panel members can more easily communicate and transfer information.

The Forum has created centralized computer systems to compliment the systems used by individual panels. Two large administrative databases allow the Forum to compare data related to the functions and management of the twenty-three panels now working to develop or update clinical practice guidelines. The information gained from these databases allows for the evaluation of existing strategies and the analysis of costs, thereby promoting efficient guideline development.

The systems described above to support guideline development are one part of the overall plan created by the Forum for using personal computers as a workstation. Figure 1 shows the model of using computers during development, dissemination, and evaluation. This model illustrates how the computer output for bibliographic citations, full text retrieval, CD-Rom, networks, and expert systems during evaluation, eventually provides feedback for guidelines updated on a regular schedule after release.

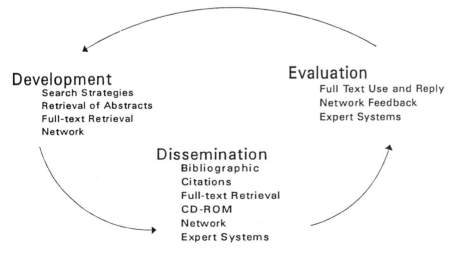

Figure 1. FEEDBACK FOR GUIDELINES

708

3. Conclusions

Nurses at AHCPR have planned implemented, managed, and evaluated the use of personal computers to facilitate the development and update of clinical practice guidelines. The scarcity of published nursing literature on computer applications associated with guidelines motivated these nurses to publish their findings. IBM compatible 486 personal computers equipped with WordPerfect 5.1, Harvard Graphics, Pro-Cite, procomm Plus, Grateful Med and other software are supplied to each panel and user support is provided as necessary. This technology is used as each panel reviews extensive literature searches and produces five scientific documents in twelve to eighteen months. The appropriate use of technology for this project has occurred due to careful planning efficient and effective use of resources, provision of sufficient end-user support, evaluation of the system, and revision or expansion of the system over time. Communication and on-going adaptations to the needs of the users has resulted in the creation of a system which promotes the final goal of guideline development.

4. References

Book:
[1]Gardner E. (1992). *Putting guidelines into practice.* Modern Healthcare 1992, September: 24-26.

Book:
[2]Musen A, Tu S and Shahar Y. (1992). *A Problem-solving model for protocol-based care:from eoncocin to eon. Proceedings of Medinfo 92,* Amsterdam:Elsevier Publishing September: 6-9.

Book:
[3]McCormick KA. (1991). *Future data needs for quality of care monitoring, DRG considerations, reimbursement and outcome measurement.* IMAGE:The Journal of Scholarship, 23,4-7,1991.

Book:
[4]Suwa M, Scott AC, and Shortliffe EH. (1982). *An approach to verifying completeness and consistency in a rule-based expert system;* AI Magazine (US);3(4),16-21.

Book:
[5]Petrucci K, Jacox A, McCormick K, Parks P, Kjerulff K, Baldwin B, and Petrucci P. (1992). *Evaluating the appropriateness of a nurse expert system's patient assessment;* Computers in Nursing 10(6),243-249.

Book:
[6]Bloom C, and Salano F. (1987). *A nurse expert system to assign nursing diagnosis.* Computers in Nursing, 5(4),140-145.

Book:
[7]Okada J and Okada O. (1988). *Prolog-based system for nursing staff schedule implemented on a personal computer;* Computers in Biomedical Research, 21(1),53-56.

Article:

Field MJ, and Lohr RN (editors) (1990). *Clinical Practice Guidelines:Directions for a New Program* . Institute of Medicine Report, National Academy Press.

Article:

Hadorn DC, McCormick KA and Diokno A. (1992). *An annotated approach to clinical guideline development.* Journal of the American Medical Association, 267(24).

Nursing Informatics: An International Overview for Nursing in a Technological Era
S.J. Grobe and E.S.P. Pluyter-Wenting, eds.

A Data Model for an Automated Nursing Tool to Support Integrated Rapid Care Planning in a Multiple Patient Assignment

Lange L L and Rossi J A

*Clinical Nursing Informatics Program, College of Nursing, University of Utah,
25 S. Medical Drive, Salt Lake City, Utah 84112, USA*

Integrated rapid care planning (IRCP) is the process of designing a set of nursing care activities for multiple patients to be accomplished during a single work shift or episode of care. Although the written nursing care plan is the technology that supports traditional nursing care planning, technology to support IRCP has received minimal attention from vendors or in the literature. Nurses' personal shift worksheets were considered as the existing technology that supports IRCP. Content of nurses' worksheets and their plans for care in a multiple patient assignment were used to derive the proposed data model.

1. Introduction

We will describe a long-term research program that has the following aims: to describe the process of integrated rapid care planning (IRCP), to identify information requirements of the process, to describe existing information management tools used to support IRCP, and to build and evaluate the effects of automated systems to meet those requirements. Work completed to date includes a description of staff nurses' supplemental information-seeking activities [1], identification and analysis of clinical nurses' beginning-of-shift planning processes [2], and description and analysis of one information management tool, the nurses' shift worksheet. In this paper, we will describe our analysis of shift worksheets and propose a data model to support a computerized tool for integrated rapid care planning. The objectives of the study were (1) to identify and describe the content of nurses' shift worksheets, and (2) to identify data elements and derive a data model for a computerized tool for integrated rapid care planning by nurses.

2. Background

2.1 Classification Systems for Nursing Care

In 1986, Werley [3] proposed the development of a Nursing Minimum Data Set (NMDS) that would establish agreement on the concepts used to describe nursing phenomena. This effort would require identifying uniform definitions for nursing diagnoses, nursing interventions, nursing outcomes, and intensity of nursing care. Not only would the NMDS assist nurses in communicating their unique practice domain but it would facilitate the encoding and storage of large amounts of nursing data in computerized databases.

Bulechek and McCloskey [4], who direct the Classification of Nursing Interventions research team at the University of Iowa, define a nursing intervention as: "any direct care treatment that a nurse performs on behalf of a client, which includes nurse-initiated treatments, physician-initiated treatments, and performance of daily essential functions" [4, p. 290]. An inductive research method was used to identify intervention labels, group discrete nursing activities, and attach a conceptual label. Input from nurse experts was solicited to group the 134 labels into a standardized language. Identifying and classifying intervention labels is the first phase of their research; organizing labels into a conceptual framework that will lead to a taxonomy will be the second stage.

The work toward identifying standardized language for nursing is critical to subsequent development of computerized tools that support nursing practice. However, to date the various taxonomies have not been integrated in a clinically applied tool. It would seem that classification schemes and taxonomies will be useful as categories within a data model, but that both higher- and lower-level categories will be needed in a system that supports the rapid care planning process. Specifically, at a higher level, the data model must reflect the subprocesses within the care planning process, and at a lower level it must include "atomic-level" terms that unambiguously reflect clinical phenomena. In the present paper, we address the higher-level data model, which, we believe, must incorporate organizational and environmental contexts that impose requirements on the implementation of interventions. Nurses practice in multidisciplinary settings and they provide nursing care within the time-capsule of a single shift. Nurses usually care for more than one patient. And finally, a significant percentage of patient care stems from interdependent and dependent nursing functions.

2.2 Traditional Nursing Care Planning

For more than 50 years, the written care plan has been promoted as the technology to support and verify traditional nursing care planning [5]. Traditional nursing care planning follows a systematic and deliberate process of collecting and analyzing data; setting priorities among nursing diagnoses, stating goals, in terms of measurable patient outcomes, and selecting nursing interventions to meet the goals. Unlike the spontaneous and sometimes intuitive process of IRCP, traditional nursing care planning is a thoughtful, reflective activity that culminates in a carefully written plan of care. Written care plans are developed for individual patients, and, typically, they are limited to independent nursing functions [6].

In recent years, considerable attention and effort have been given to automating traditional nursing care planning technology. For example, a search of *Cumulative Index to Nursing and Allied Health Literature* identified 30 articles published since 1983 related to computerized nursing care plans. The July, 1992, issue of *Nursing Management* listed more than 40 vendors who market computerized nursing care planning programs. However, the positive effect of written care plans, computerized or manually developed, remains unproven [7, 8]

2.3 Integrated Rapid Care Planning

Integrated rapid care planning (IRCP) is the process of designing a set of nursing care activities for multiple patients to be accomplished during a single work shift or episode of care. IRCP is distinguished from traditional care planning in that it (1) is done under conditions of clinical urgency, (2) is done with the expectation of immediate action, (3) involves organizing care and setting priorities for multiple patients, and (4) requires incorporation of interdependent and dependent nursing actions. IRCP involves the processes of clinical judgement -- observation, inference, and decision-making [9] -- concerning a group of assigned patients. It requires skill in using information created by other providers, in being aware of actions of other providers and how those actions impact one's own plan of work. Finally, and perhaps most complex of all, it requires the ability to integrate information about multiple patients into a seamless plan that allows everything to get done on time, and without error.

Technology to support integrated rapid care planning has received minimal attention from vendors or in the literature. Hinson, Silva, and Clapp [10] described an automated system that integrated the treatment Kardex, nursing care plan, and nurse's notes into a one-page printout for each patient. Called the Patient Care Profile, the form provided a comprehensive picture of the nursing care requirements for a single patient on a single shift. Nurses could write notes directly on the form, which was filed as a permanent record in the patient's chart at the end of each shift. Updates were made during the shift by hand-writing information on printed profiles and by entering the new information into the computerized profile for use during subsequent shifts. Data from Patient Care Profiles were available for use by the patient classification system and for DRG-related administrative studies. Hujcs [11] described the development of an integrated charge nurse report from data existing in a computerized hospital information system. For each ICU patient, the report lists identifying data, current IV infusions, vasopressors, arterial blood gas reports, ventilator status, Glasgow Coma Score, and level of consciousness. The aim of the report is to reduce time required by charge nurses to collect data and report on patient status at the end of each shift.

We believe that one technology presently used to support IRCP is the nurse's shift worksheet. Despite the enduring use of shift worksheets by nurses, we could locate no reported studies of worksheet structure, content, or function. The worksheet is usually initiated during shift report and serves as the basis for planning, scheduling, and documenting patient care throughout the coming shift. Nurses use worksheets to integrate data from the Kardex, the medication schedule, medical orders and progress notes, nurses' notes, and shift report and to create a plan of care activities for all assigned patients during the shift. In effect, the personal shift worksheet is a representation of available information about patients and plans for patient care.

2.4 Conceptual Framework

Information processing theory [12] was used to develop the conceptual framework for the study. The theory suggests that problem solving occurs within an information processing system, which is composed of long term

712

memory (LTM), short term memory (STM), and effectors and receptors which communicate with the environment. Problem solving is assumed to involve manipulation of task-oriented symbols within STM, in a problem space that is an internal representation of the task environment. A third type of memory, external memory (EM), may be constructed to augment the limited capacity of STM.

Human problem solving behavior is determined by the demands of the task environment and the psychology of the problem solver. Problem solving behavior is constrained by limitations on human memory structures. LTM has a large, perhaps infinite, storage capacity, but STM capacity is much smaller, varying from two to nine symbol structures, or chunks. Items in STM are available for immediate processing, but its limited capacity means that only a very few, perhaps not more than two, chunks can be retained if the processing task is interrupted. Both LTM and STM capacity and read-write times are related to meaning and similarity of chunks, and to environmental distractions.

In our research program, the process of developing integrated rapid care plans for multiple patients is the problem solving task of interest. IRCP is assumed to occur as manipulation of task-related symbols within STM and LTM. Performance of IRCP should be enhanced when LTM contains symbol structures, or knowledge, relevant to the task, and performance should be limited by distractions that cause competition for space within the limited capacity of STM. The nurse's shift worksheet has an effect on IRCP performance as an EM device that is used to augment STM capacity.

2.5 Summary of Background

In summary, the written nursing care plan is the principal technology advocated to support nursing care planning. However, the written care plan provides minimal support for the process of IRCP for a multiple patient assignment. IRCP is an information process in which the nurse's shift worksheet is used as an external memory device to enhance performance. Although considerable work has been done to develop language systems for nursing interventions and other nursing processes, these systems have not yet been integrated and applied in a computerized tool that reflects the clinical reality of hospital-based nursing practice. The aim of the present study is to lay the groundwork for the development of such a tool.

3. Methods

3.1 Sample

The sample was comprised of 12 registered nurses (RNs) who had worked full-time for at least one year on one of four medical-surgical units at a teaching hospital in the western United States. The subjects averaged 35 years of age, 9 years as RNs, and 6 years on their present units. Most were baccalaureate graduates and only one also had a master's degree in nursing. The number of patients assigned to subjects ranged from 1 to 4 (mean = 2.8, SD = .72). Over all the units, the patient census on days when data were collected averaged 26.0 (SD = 6.87), the patient acuity averaged 3.4 on a 5-point scale (SD = .27), and the number of direct care staff averaged 9.0 (SD = 1.76). Even though each unit had a specialty designation (cardiovascular, orthopedic, oncology, and general surgery), all units usually had all types of medical and surgical patients in addition to patients in the specialty area. A total of 33 patients was assigned to the 12 subjects during the data collection period. Patients' length of present hospitalization ranged from an average of 4 days on the cardiovascular unit to 19 days on the oncology unit, which included a bone marrow transplant sub-unit.

3.2 Data Collection and Analysis

Data for the present study consisted of subjects' shift worksheets. Each subject was observed before, during, and for one hour after morning shift report to determine how an when worksheets were developed and supplemental information-seeking behaviors. A photocopy was made of each worksheet immediately after shift report and each subject was interviewed to determine what plans the subject had made for assigned patients. Detailed findings from the interviews have been reported elsewhere [2].

A worksheet data unit was defined as a word or phrase that could have meaning from a clinical perspective. Meaning was determined in part by context and by location on the worksheet. Data units were extracted from worksheets by a nursing graduate student who also worked as a clinician in the hospital where data were collected. The data were entered into a computerized database for coding and analysis. Data units were first coded according to subject, patient, and worksheet heading (if any). Next, the data were grouped into categories according to the type of elementary-level content they represented. The elementary-level categories were then aggregated into higher-level groups which were used to construct an entity-relationship data model. Two nurse researchers independently coded the elements at each data level, and achieved agreement of 95% or better at each level.

4. Results

4.1 The Content of Nurses' Personal Shift Worksheets

In all, 497 data elements were identified from the 12 worksheets (mean = 41.4, SD = 17.3). From the raw data, 26 elementary-level categories were derived. Ten elementary-level categories had frequencies of 20 or more: signs and symptoms (n=70), medical diagnosis (n=48), vital signs (n=47), diet (n=35), IVs (n=35), medications (n=32), medical service or physician name (n=29), intake and output (n=25), and laboratory tests (n=21).

The elementary-level data had both content and time dimensions, and both dimensions yielded several higher-level categories. Higher-level content categories included contextual identifiers, observations and assessments, and future care events. Within the contextual identifier category were such elementary-level data as patient's name, age, diagnosis, room number, and allergies. Observation-and-assessment-level data included signs and symptoms, vital signs, and diagnostic test results. Planned-care-event-level data included activities such as monitoring intake and output, medications, changing dressings, oxygen therapy, specimens to be collected, and discharge planning. In the time dimension, elements were categoized as past, existing, or future conditions or events. Future care events were further categorized as not scheduled or PRN, scheduled by the nurse, or scheduled by other (eg, surgery or medications).

4.2 Data Model for Integrated Rapid Care Planning

IRCP concerns all activities the nurse expects to accomplish for multiple assigned patients within a work shift. As reported elsewhere [2], IRCP process involves three major processes: Setting the Context, Reviewing Information, and Making Plans. IRCP involves coordinating care among the assigned patients, as well as between patients and environmental constraints. By integrating findings about the process of IRCP derived from interviews of subjects with findings about the content of shift worksheets, it is possible to propose a data model for the IRCP process. Each planned care activity can be described by answering five questions: (1) What activity is planned? (2) What actions are required? (3) Who is involved in the activity? (4) When is it to be done? (5) What follow-up is needed?

For example, the planned activity might be patient teaching; the required actions would be to assess the patient's knowledge, assemble materials, and conduct the teaching; the persons involved could be the nurse, the patient, and a family member; the time when teaching is to be done would be scheduled by the nurse; and the follow-up would be to report the teaching by documenting it in the medical record and to make a new plan to evaluate the teaching at a later time. Another planned activity might be to administer a pre-operative medication; the action required would be to determine the drug to be given, the dose, and the time; the nurse and the patient would be involved; the administration time might be scheduled by the physician, or it might be "on-call;" and the follow-up would be to document the action in the medical record. Figure 1 illustrates an entity-relationship model for rapid care planning.

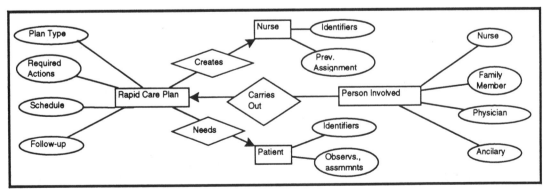

Figure 1. Entity-relationship model for rapid care planning

714

5. Discussion

The findings of the study present a description of an information management tool used by nurses in medical-surgical clinical settings. On the basis of personal experience and conversations with colleagues, we suspect that the shift worksheet is used by most nurses in most acute care settings, yet it has received no attention in the literature or from computer system vendors.

We suggest that the shift worksheet serves as an external memory device to augment short term memory during the rapid care planning process. It contains detailed information about activities the nurse intends to accomplish during a work shift. The content focus of the worksheet is heavily weighted toward interdependent and dependent nursing actions, perhaps because such time-linked, required activities are processed in short term memory. In contrast, independent nursing action plans are more likely to be constructed from knowledge existing in long term memory, thus no external memory device is needed to augment such planning.

We have proposed a data model that might be incorporated into a computerized shift worksheet. The model consists of patient-related entities and entities that describe the rapid care planning process. Contextual identifiers describe enduring characteristics of patients, such as age, room number, and medical diagnosis. Observation and assessments describe dynamic characteristics such as vital signs, laboratory test results, and signs and symptoms. Rapid care plans are described by five entities: type of plan, required actions, persons involved in the action, schedule for the plan, and follow-up actions. The model is parsimonious and can be used in a relational database design.

Future studies will be designed to test the adequacy of the model as a database design to support rapid care planning in a medical-surgical clinical environment.

6. References

[1] Lange LL. Information Processing and Information Seeking by Nurses During Beginning-of-Shift Activities. In Frisse M E (Ed.). *Proc 16th SCAMC*, McGraw-Hill 1992; 317-321.

[2] Lange LL. Information Processing and Management by Nurses during Beginning-of-Shift Activities. *Research in Nursing and Health* 1993. (under review).

[3] Werley HH and Lang N. *Identification of the Nursing Minimum Data Set.* Springer 1986.

[4] Bulechek GM and McCloskey JC. Defining and Validating Nursing Interventions. *Nurs Clin N A* 1992, 27:289-97.

[5] Henderson V. On Nursing Care Plans and Their History. *Nurs Outlook* 1973, 21: 378-379.

[6] McFarland GK and McFarlane EA. *Nursing Diagnosis & Intervention: Planning for Patient Care.* CV Mosby 1989.

[7] Holzemer WL and Henry SB. Computer-supported Versus Manually-generated Nursing Care Plans: A Comparison of Patient Problems, Nursing Interventions, and AIDS Patient Outcomes. *Comp Nurs* 1992; 10:19-24.

[8] Aidroos N. Use and Effectiveness of Psychiatric nursing care plans. *J Adv Nurs;* 16:177-181.

[9] Kelly K. Clinical Inference in Nursing: I. A Nurse's Viewpoint. *Nurs Research* 1966. 15:23-25.

[10] Hinson I, Silva N and Clapp P. An Automated Kardex and Care Plan. *Nurs Management* 1984; 15:11:35-43.

[11] Hujcs M. Utilizing Computer Integration to Assist Nursing. R. A. Miller (Ed.) *Proc 14th SCAMC*, IEEE Computer Society Press.1990; 894-897.

[12] Newell A and Simon H. *Human Problem Solving.* Prentice-Hall 1972.

Nursing Informatics: An International Overview for Nursing in a Technological Era
S.J. Grobe and E.S.P. Pluyter-Wenting, eds.

Technology Assessment of an Integrated Nursing Information System in three Dutch Hospitals

Van Gennip E M S J[a], Klaassen-Leil C C[b], Stokman R A M[c], Van Valkenburg R K J[d]

[a]BAZIS Central Development and Support Group Hospital Information System, Leiden, The Netherlands

[b]Free University Hospital, Amsterdam, The Netherlands

[c]Psychiatric Hospital "Reinier van Arkel", Vught, The Netherlands

[d]St. Antonius Hospital, Nieuwegein, The Netherlands

Nursing Information Systems promise to reduce the time needed for administration and communication at a nursing ward, to improve quality of documentation and hence that of nursing care, and also to improve nurses job satisfaction. In a joint effort, three Dutch Hospitals, together with the BAZIS foundation, are undertaking a technology assessment of the Integrated Nursing Information System (VISION) which is part of the BAZIS Hospital Information System. The study is carried out between June 1992 and April 1994, and is supported by the Dutch Ministry of Welfare Health and Culture. Its aim is to analyze the effects of VISION in three different environments. This paper presents the study set-up and first results.

1. Research objectives

Nursing Information Systems (NIS) support the process of care delivery as well as the general operation at a nursing ward. They may cause a major reduction in workload related to administration and communication [1, 2, 3]. Moreover the systems may improve the quality of documentation, nursing care and job satisfaction [1, 2, 4].

Nursing information systems can be stand-alone, linked to a Hospital Information System, or can be developed as an integrated part within an existing Hospital Information System. Full integration of the system promises the most benefits, as it prevents retyping of data, and gives the best possibilities for access of data and communication with other parts of the hospital [4].

In the Netherlands an Integrated Nursing Information System (VISION) is being developed as integrated part of the BAZIS Hospital Information System (HIS). The BAZIS HIS consists of a great number of modules

[5]. It is being used now by over 45 Dutch hospitals. The development of its modules devoted to support nursing care, i.e. its *Integrated Nursing Information System* (VISION), started early 1987. The first modules of VISION were introduced at a pilot ward of the Leiden University Hospital. Since 1987 the system has been extended gradually; most recently by the module "Careplan". The development continues.

Early 1992, three other "BAZIS" hospitals decided to implement parts of VISION : a university hospital (Free University Hospital, Amsterdam) a general hospital (St. Antonius Hospital, Nieuwegein) and a psychiatric hospital (Reinier van Arkel, Vught). This provided an opportunitity to analyze costs and benefits of the system in three new and different environments. In a joint effort, the three hospitals and the BAZIS foundation are undertaking a technology assessment of the system. The assessment is financially supported by the Dutch Ministry of Welfare, Health and Culture.

The key questions in this study are:

1   Can VISION reduce the workload at nursing wards?
2   Can it increase functionality of nursing care?
3   Can it support quality assurance?
4   Does the system contribute to improved job satisfaction?
5   What are the costs of the system and how will these develop over time?

The aim of the assessment is to provide, where possible in quantitative measures, data on the effects of VISION in three typical Dutch nursing wards. It's results will be the basis for guidelines for other Dutch hospitals that are considering implementation of Nursing Information Systems. Moreover, a software tool will be developed that will allow hospital managers to estimate the financial implications of implementing the system in their hospital. The study started June 1992 and will be completed April 1994. This paper presents the study methodology, as well as its first, preliminary results.

2. Methods

2.1 Study-design

The assessment is set up as a pre-post study, using experimental and control groups. This implies that in each of the three hospitals, two wards are involved: a ward at which VISION is implemented (the experimental ward) and a ward at which during the course of the study no VISION parts are installed (the control ward). The control wards are very similar to the experimental wards in size, specialty and management. They are included in the study to be able to correct for variables independent from the implementation of the system. In both experimental and control ward pre- and post-measurements are carried out. The before measurements have been completed; the after measurements are planned to take place between September and November 1993.

The experimental and control groups in one hospital are very similar. There are however differences between the hospitals:

-    in specialty: for the Free University Hospital Amsterdam (FUHA) two surgery wards are selected, for the St. Antonius Hospital (SAH) two internal medicine wards, and for the Psychiatric Hospital Reinier van Arkel (RVA) two "double-handicapped" wards;
-    in working methods: in the RVA wards careplans are being made for each patient; this is not done in the other hospitals wards;
-    in the number of terminals used: one at every bed (FUHA), one in each room (SAH), one/two at the ward (RVA);
-    in use of HIS functions before VISION implementation and in the extent in which VISION modules are implemented in the course of the study. Table 1 lists the use of HIS functions at the experimental and control wards for each hospital during the post-measurements.

Table 1
Use of HIS functions in control (C) wards and experimental (E) wards in post measurements in the Free University Hospital (FUHA), the Sint Antonius Hospital (SAH) and the psychiatric hospital Reinier van Arkel (RVA).

HIS functions	FUHA		SAH		RVA	
	C	E	C	E	C	E
Appointment making	X	X		X		
Kitchen (e.g. meal ordering)	X	X				
Patient classification	X	X				
Patient adm. data	X	X	X	X	X	X
Patient med. data	X	X				
Electronic mail	X	X		X	X	X
Nurse scheduling		X		X		
Stock management	X	X				
VISION vital signs		X		X		X
VISION care planning		X				X
VISION workplan		X		X		X
VISION reporting		X		X		
Handbooks	X	X		X	X	X

Because of these differences, general conclusions and guidelines on possible costs and benefits for other wards/hospitals and for other implementations may be qualitative rather than quantitative.

The same tools and data collection methods are used in all three hospitals, in both the experimental and control wards, to facilitate comparison of results. In order to be able to identify differences between pre- and post measurement which are caused by differences in workload rather than by VISION, data on a number of workload related variables are collected:

- patient classification (San Joaquin) is carried out at each ward, both during pre- and post-measurement
- data on staffing during pre and post measurement
- data on changes independent of VISION implementation (e.g. change of procedures/equipment) between pre and post-measurement.

2.2 Workload

To assess the effects of the system on the nursing workload, a worksampling study is carried out in each experimental and control ward, for 8 dayshifts, 3 evening shifts and 3 nightshifts. These measurements are done both before and after implementation. Twenty different types of activities are distinguished, which are subdivided in activities related to written information, to communication, to nursing care and "overhead". Moreover it is possible to distinguish between direct and indirect care related activities. In rounds of, on average 8 minutes, all members of the permanent staff of a ward are scored. We distinguish in all wards at least management, nurses, student-nurses, and secretaries.

2.3 Effectiveness and quality assurance

As internal guidelines on documentation and communication vary between the hospitals, they define "quality" of documentation and communication differently. Despite these differences, a universal "quality" tool was developed, in order to test the effect of the system on the functionality and quality assurance. This tool is based on "quality criteria", which have been developed for General Hospitals in the Netherlands [6]. These include e.g. criteria on completeness of information, timely documentation, the number of sources needed to retrieve information etc. In each of the wards, a test is carried out for these criteria for at least five patients. Data are collected in interviews with managers, responsible nurses and by analysis of nursing files. The test is carried out twice for every ward, by two independent researchers (nurses) both before and after implementation.

2.4 Job satisfaction

Jobsatisfaction includes aspects as "intent to stay", "satisfaction in task requirements". "satisfaction in interactions". In order to test effects on job satisfaction, a questionnaire is being developed, based on existing tools such as [7].

2.5 Costs

The costs of the system are analyzed separately in each hospital. In the cost analysis costs of hardware, software, and support are distinguished. As VISION makes part of an integrated HIS, central costs of the information system are taken into account too. The principles of the cost model are described in [8, 9].

3. First results compared with other studies

This study is the first study in the Netherlands which aims to assess effects of a Nursing Information System at general wards. Only for a NIS implemented at an Intensive Care Unit, an earlier Dutch study is available [3]. In that study it has been demonstrated by worksampling that NIS decreased the amount of time spent on information handling and increased the time spent on direct care.

In the US there have been more studies of the effects of NIS, both for ICU and for general wards. Using worksampling methods, it was found that an ICU NIS reduced time spent on administrative tasks by 21.8%, on documentation by 36.6%, and on informal consultation by 46% [1]. In a General Hospital it was found that the average time taken by each nurse to report during each shift for each patient has been reduced from 11 minutes to 6 minutes [2].

Our pre-measurements indicate that in the wards under study, the permanent staff spends on average 15% of their time on dealing with written information and about 20% on communication. These figures are relatively low as compared to US data. Early US studies indicate that 35-40% of the hospital nurse's time is spent on handling information, whereas currently "in some clinical areas total nursing time devoted to information handling may exceed 50%" [10]. This may be explained by the fact that the administrative tasks of US nurses might be more extensive as compared to these of nurses in the Netherlands, due to e.g. risks for liability claims. As a result the potential time savings by Nursing Information Systems in Dutch hospitals may be less than those reported for US hospitals. Still, early experiences in the current study show that VISION may also provide significant time savings in the Netherlands, especially in its support of the use of careplans. Early experiences in the psychiatric hospital Reinier van Arkel indicate that VISION reduces the time needed to make a new individual careplan and to maintain it significantly.

With regard to effects on quality, US studies suggest that NIS make documentation better, more readable, with information in predictable places and more complete because of prompts and more timely [1, 2, 4]. Moreover it has been suggested that NIS improve quality of care, because the computer prompts the nurses as to what to look for and what to do [1, 4] and because nurses spend more time with patients [1, 4]. It is too early yet to conclude whether these benefits can also be achieved in the wards involved in our study. Early results however indicate that VISION improves quality of documentation. For instance VISION has greatly improved the accuracy of "fluid balances" in the Free University Hospital.

In an early estimation, the costs of VISION are calculated at Dfl. 1650 (1 Dfl = ca US $ 1.80) per year per terminal [8], in a hospital wide implementation, assuming terminals at the bedside. US estimates range from $ 2000 to $ 10,000 per terminal [11][1]. The costs of VISION may be relatively low, as it uses simple terminals, and because the costs of development of the BAZIS HIS are shared by a large number of hospitals. A cost comparison should however also take into account functionality of various NISs and the nature of implementation. In the current study, it will be investigated how the costs of VISION vary for different implementations (e.g. terminals at each bedside or not).

This paper gives an overview of the set-up of the study only. Its first preliminary results are compared to literature data. During the conference, the full results of the study will be available.

4. References

[1]   Allen D, Davis M. Clinical Information Systems Impact on the Intensive Care Unit. Report study. March 1991. Lutheran Hospital La Crosse, Wisconsin, USA.

[2]   Peth C Prendergast M Hennessy J Dunford R Brennan L. Who needs bedside terminals? *Healthcare informatics* May 1992: 70-72.

[3]   Frieling S. Computers in de verpleging: de derde hand aan bed. Een empirisch onderzoek. Report study 1991. University of Limburg, The Netherlands

[4]   Knickman J Kovner C Hendrickson G Finkler S. An evaluation of the new jersey nursing incentive reimbursement awards program. Final Report, 1992, The Health Research Program, New York University.

[5]   Bakker A R. An integrated hospital information system in the Netherlands *Clin Comput* 7(2) 1990: 91-97.

[6]   Visser G, Hollands L. De Bekker J. Van Bergen B: *Beslagen ten eis*. De Tijdstroom 1992

[7]   Stamps P, Piedmonte E. *Nurses and work satisfaction -- An Index for Measurement*. Ann Arbor, MI: Health Administration Press 1986

[8]   Bakker A R, Van Gennip E M S J, Roelofs W: Bedside Nursing Information Systems; Quantities Costs In: *Nursing Informatics 1991* Hovenga E.J.S. e.a. (eds). Springer Verlag, Berlin 1991: 398-407.

---

[1] These are probably purchase costs and not costs per year (amortizated). The publication is not fully clear on this.

720

[9]   Van Gennip E M S J Willemsen W, Nieman H B J Bakker A R Van der Loo R P How to assess cost-effectiveness of HIS-applications? In: *MEDINFO '92* Lun K.C. e.a. (eds) Elsevier Science Publishers, North Holland 1992: 1209-1215.

[10]   McHugh M L: Nursing Systems: the next generation *Healthcare informatics* April 1992: 38-42

[11]   Bauer A. AHA Study Defines Bedside Terminal Issues. *Healthcare Informatics* May 1992: 74-79.

PANELS

© 1994 Elsevier Science B.V. All rights reserved.
Nursing Informatics: An International Overview for Nursing in a Technological Era
S.J. Grobe and E.S.P. Pluyter-Wenting, eds.

Collaborative Approaches to Stimulate Nursing Informatics Research in the Practice Setting: A Panel Presentation

Alt-White AC[a] McDermott S[a] and Panniers TL[b] for Spranzo LG[c]

[a]Nursing Service, VA Medical Center, 50 Irving Street, NW, Washington, DC 20422

[b]School of Nursing, University of Maryland, Baltimore, MD 21201, [c] Deceased

Nursing informatics is a newly recognized specialty by the American Nurses Association. Research will be a critical element in the development and recognition of this as a knowledge based practice specialty. One way to facilitate research is through collaboration between researchers and clinicians in both practice and academic settings. In collaborative endeavors it is important to keep in mind Lancaster's six C's of collaborative research: contribution, communication, commitment, consensus, compatibility, and credit.[1] Another important issue which needs to be addressed is trust.[2,3] Using a case study approach and the Goode et al system theory model for using new research based knowledge[4] this panel provides an analysis of the realities of establishing collaborative approaches to promote nursing informatics research in a practice setting. Three perspectives are presented including a nurse researcher and a nursing informatics specialist in a practice setting, and an academically-based nurse researcher. The panel members define and describe their roles, the relationship of one role to the others, the strategies used to develop and implement research in the practice setting, benefits and outcomes of collaboration, and the future of collaboration in nursing informatics research.

1. Objectives of the Panel

The objectives of the panel are to a) describe the role of the clinical nurse researcher, nursing informatics specialist and academic nurse researcher in establishing and sustaining collaborative research in nursing and healthcare informatics; b) identify the benefits and limitations of collaborative research and the essential strategies to facilitate successful collaboration, and c) discuss specific areas in nursing and healthcare informatics that would benefit collaborative research approaches.

2. Panel Presentations

2.1 The Clinical Nurse Researcher

One role of the nurse researcher in the clinical setting is developing and conducting research which has an effect on nursing practice. Frequently much of the clinical nurse researcher's role is collaboration- either a multidisciplinary focus or working with staff to explore an area of interest or concern. Because the role of the clinical nurse researcher is not the norm for most medical centers and, when it does exist, consists of a staff of one, the researcher may find that there is neither the time nor expertise to handle all the research which may originate from within the organization. One solution may be for the clinical researcher to seek out and facilitate linkages with researchers external to the medical center who are interested in either working alone or in collaboration with nursing staff, thereby developing networks and strengthening collaboration.[5]

In our health care setting we have fostered a relationship with an academically based nursing informatics researcher. Many factors contribute to the success of this and any collaborative effort. To begin, the organizational environment must be receptive to someone outside of their system. Next, the clinical researcher is responsible for expediting the passage of the proposal through the institutional review process. Since just about all healthcare institutions require institutional review the researcher from outside the system will need to be familiar with the basic process. The clinically based researcher, however, becomes a critical link in explaining the particulars and peculiarities of the process in that institution and expediting this usually lengthy process. Throughout any of the collaborative process the clinical researcher maintains contact with the academic researcher, and maintains relationships among the contact person for the academic in the institution (e.g., informatics specialist), clinical nursing staff and administration.

2.2 The Nursing Informatics Specialist Role

Nursing informatics specialists who develop, test, implement, and evaluate computer systems may be interested in conducting research. Yet, the time and skills to complete quality studies may be insufficient. Collaboration with a clinical nurse researcher and an academically-based researcher provides opportunities for practice-based nursing informatics specialists to participate in well-designed nursing research. Developing a collaborative research program requires a long-term commitment.[6] While numerous limitations and benefits occur with such collaboration, overall satisfaction from the contributions made to nursing research and professional development is realized. Limitations include maintaining a mutually agreeable time frame for the study and for other competing implementations. Additionally, maintaining commitment to the study as designed may mean forgoing usual control over an implementation. The nursing informatics specialist can contribute to overcoming these limitations by being able to predict and exercise authority regarding current and potential projects. Benefits include gaining a broadened research perspective relative to the development and implementation of systems, documenting the results from computerization of the nursing process and using the results to complete the quality improvement cycle. In addition, by working collaboratively there is the greater likelihood of completing the project, having the satisfaction of working with like-minded colleagues, and obtaining visibility through publications and presentations. Recommendations for system enhancements systems are specifically identified and communicated to appropriate members of the organization so that changes occur to benefit nursing.

2.3 The Academically-Based Nurse Researcher Role

Increasingly, the laboratory of studies in nursing informatics will take place in the real-world of the nurse user. For the academically-based researcher with an emphasis in nursing informatics, bridging the gap between academia and the practice setting creates rewards that go beyond the completion of the research project. The academic's role and strategies are to promote a shared research emphasis with those in a practice setting in order to advance the study of nursing informatics. Communicating, illustrating and demonstrating the research process, in understandable terms, is essential to those in the practice setting. Also needed are strategies of persuasion, assertiveness and active participation on the part of the academic for promoting research that can be prioritized in accordance with the organization's need for application of the findings. The incorporation of information systems into nursing practice is fraught with many difficulties including delays in implementation, high labor intensity and unanticipated effects. The academic's flexibility, willingness to compromise and links with additional academically-based and funding resources can be essential ingredients for building alliances that sustain the research endeavor without compromising either the integrity of the research or the benefits that can be derived for the organizational setting.[7,8] Other benefits derived by the academic includes mentoring staff to develop and implement informatic studies pertinent to a particular area of clinical practice.

2.4 Summary

There are many areas appropriate for collaborative research in nursing informatics. Included are formative and summative evaluations of implementation, training and user involvement; organizational factors and the impact of computerization; patient education using computerized programs; and the use and effectiveness of data/information sources in the delivery of nursing care.

Major benefits derived from a collaborative relationship are exploring a new area of research, building a base from which further studies and funding are generated, and participants gaining additional expertise from their association with one other. A collaborative model also provides the opportunity for professionals to work in concert to accomplish what they would be unable to do working alone. This has been true in our case. Prior to an academic researcher joining us in 1990, we had decided to focus on informatics as an area of research for the nursing service at our medical center. We had just received a small grant from Hewlett Packard to evaluate the patient monitoring and clinical information systems that were to be installed in our Medical Intensive Care Unit (MICU). Shortly thereafter, an academic researcher, Dr Spranzo came to do her project. In both instances considerable negotiation took place between the vendor or Dr Spranzo and the nurse researcher, and with others such as the nursing informatics specialist or the MICU head nurse.

Informatics research is useful from both the practice and research perspective. The research process imposes logical preciseness and empirical validity to the practice focus of an existing problem or area of interest and applying the results to the real life situation.

References

[1] Lancaster J. The Perils and Joys of Collaborative Research. *Nurs Outlook* 1985, 33:2231-232, 238.

[2] Beckstrand J and McBride A. How to Form a Research Interest Group. *Nurs Outlook* 1990, 38:168-171.

[3] Ventura M,Crosby F,Finnick M and Feldman M. Increasing Productivity by Developing Alliances. *NursingConnections* 1991, 4:15-21.

[4] Goode C,Lovett M,Hayes J and Butcher L. Use of Research Based Knowledge in Clinical Practice. *J Nurs Adm* 1987, 17: 10-18.

[5] Smeltzer C and Hinshaw A. Research: Clinical Integration for Excellent Patient Care. *Nurse Manage* 1988, 19;38-40.

[6] Lenz E. Developing a Focused Research Effort. *Nurs Outlook* 1987, 35:60-64.

[7] Singleton EK,Edmunds MW,Rapson M and Steele S. An experience in Collaborative Research. *Nurs Outlook* 1982, 30:395-401.

[8] Toussie-Weingarten C,Baker K and Manning W. Meeting Education and Practice Objectives Through Clinical Research Collaboration: The Nursing Research Parent Project. *Top Clin Nurs* 1985, 7:54-62.

Nursing Informatics: An International Overview for Nursing in a Technological Era
S.J. Grobe and E.S.P. Pluyter-Wenting, eds.

726

Nursing Informatics Synthesis Within a Graduate Program: Nursing Administration Specialization

Aroian J[a] Heller P[b] Breton O[c] and Lawless K[d]

[a]Faculty and Coordinator, Nursing Administration Specialization, Northeastern University, 360 Huntington Avenue, Boston, Massachusetts, 02115

[b]Adjunct Faculty of Nursing, Northeastern University, Senior Manager, Ernst & Young, 200 Clarendon Street, Boston, Massachusetts, 02116

[c]Faculty of Nursing, Northeastern University, 360 Huntington Avenue, Boston, Massachusetts, 02115

[d]Former Graduate Student at Northeastern University, Nurse Manager, New England Rehabilitation Hospital, 2 Rehabilitation Way, Woburn, Massachusetts 01801

Health Care Technology is exploding. Contemporary nurse administrators (managers and executives) are in key leadership positions as a part of the decision making teams at all levels of health care institutions to markedly influence total quality management and economics in relation to clinical and information technology. In order to prepare nurse administrators to carry out this expanded role function, a curriculum thread composed of two course offerings with an experiential component was developed and offered concurrently during Nursing Administration students' two quarters of practicum experience. The panel describes a partnership approach that faculty and graduate students at Northeastern University Graduate School of Nursing engaged in with a senior nurse manager consultant from Ernst & Young. The techniques utilized in planning, designing, implementing and evaluating this curriculum currently in place are discussed. Faculty, consultant and student perceptions are examined. Nursing Informatics synthesis may be a systematic process whereby nursing administrators can learn to effectively and efficiently use Information Systems in nursing and health care for strategic planning and innovative decision making within their expanded role function in health care institutions.

1. The Academic Partners Perspective

At the annual Administration Advisory meeting for the new nursing administration specialization at the College of Nursing at Northeastern University, the committee, comprised of nursing executives from affiliating agencies, faculty and students, identified nursing informatics as an area of increasing importance in the administration specialization curriculum. The offering proposed a challenge for faculty for two reasons: hiring an expert from the industry was cost prohibitive and practicum sites at major teaching hospitals and community agencies revealed only a beginning capability for INFORMATICS and computer technology. The challenge was in identifying someone who had both command of the content area and also the contacts to provide the comprehensive learning approach the faculty were seeking.

Fortunately, one of the administration students identified as her practicum goal, "to study the role of the nurse manager as a consultant to a high technology firm". The administration Graduate Coordinator accompanied the student to interview for a practicum placement in the consultant management firm of Ernst & Young with a Senior

Manager as her preceptor. The Senior Manager is a master's prepared nurse who has extensive experience in the planning, development and implementation of Hospital Information Systems in a variety of settings. As we discussed the Nursing Administration program, it became apparent that the Senior Manager was highly qualified and very interested in teaching the informatics component in Northeastern's Masters program. She was invited to come to campus to participate in developing the informatics course.

The first meeting was a brainstorming session about the proposed course content and teaching methodology. The outcome of this meeting was a reformulation of thinking. Instead of offering one course in informatics, the faculty decided to restructure the practicum experience (a three course sequence) to include a didactic portion with a demonstration laboratory devoted to learning about nursing informatics and health care computerization. In order to implement this plan, the faculty needed approval from the Graduate Curriculum Committee and administration.

To expedite the process, the senior manager suggested she write a proposal to formalize the relationship between Ernst & Young and Northeastern University College of Nursing. Thus a teaching/consulting "partnership" was born.

All agreed that the curriculum goal was to introduce nursing informatics into the Nursing Administration program to prepare students to effectively and efficiently use Information Systems in nursing for strategic planning, sound decision making and innovative management in nursing service delivery within their role as managers/clinical specialists in advanced nursing practice.

The next step was for faculty to look at how this content fit into the overall Master's curriculum. They considered both the organizing concepts (knowledge, competence, role) for the Master's program as a whole, and the Manager As Developer Model for the Administration specialization in particular. The fit was congruent on both counts.

Beneficial outcomes of the partnership for the College included state-of-the-art curriculum and instruction in nursing informatics and technology; faculty development tailored to the needs of the program; an expert instructor who has the resources to secure vendor demonstrations and software applications from the leaders in the field; instant credibility with students for a new program offering; assistance with timely development and implementation of the program; development of teaching aids and other curricular materials; and establishment of an excellent working relationship with a major consulting firm of national renown.

2. The Consultant Firm's Perspective

Ernst & Young was pleased to assist Northeastern University Graduate School of Nursing with the development and instruction of a Nursing Informatics course.

We were confident that a successful outcome could be accomplished, and knew that in order to be successful, the following ingredients must be in place from the consulting firm:

2.1 The understanding of the impact of technology on the nursing profession. As the use of information technology in health care continues to grow, so too will the application of such technology in the practice of nursing. Numerous implementation engagement experiences had given us an understanding of nursing systems from the clinical, business and technical points of view.

2.2 An approach to designing a nursing informatics curriculum that is based on a pragmatic view of currently available nursing information systems technology and the evolving technologies the graduate nurse may confront in the future.

We used our knowledge of the industry to identify appropriate topics and issues in clinical nursing, nursing management and nursing research that are supported by information technology.

As a result of this process, we have developed a strategic approach that the University has incorporated into their vision of the nursing informatics curriculum. Topics included nursing care delivery models and information needs, the potential for nursing information systems, planning, selecting and implementation of hospital information systems and decision support/expert systems capabilities. Nursing informatics professionals from the large Boston teaching hospitals allowed the students to spend a day to appreciate the challenges they all face in the real world of implementing these types of systems.

We also assumed the role as practicum preceptor for graduate students who desired to study the role of a nurse manager in an information technology consulting firm.

3. The Faculty Perspective

As with any new initiative, early involvement can create a very positive response. The College of Nursing faculty were given the opportunity to register for the new course offerings in nursing informatics. The expectation was that once the commitment was made, faculty would attend both courses over twenty weeks. Continuing education credit was awarded at the end of each course.

At the time of the first course offering, many faculty had been using computers for a number of years in a variety of settings. At our university, each nursing faculty has had a computer in her office for the past three years. We were fortunate as a college to be one of the first to acquire an interactive video system. A cluster of computers had been in place in the Nursing Laboratory for a number of years. The information presented in the informatics course added new perspectives to the faculty's knowledge of the nursing profession's involvement in computerization. The feedback on evaluation of the new courses was very positive.

Operationalizing the informatics offerings after the first year has been a smooth transition. The responsibility for teaching the courses was delegated to one of the nursing faculty who had implemented computer assisted instruction for our nursing courses and also developed expertise with a variety of computer technologies during her tenure as coordinator of the Nursing Laboratory. As one of the faculty who completed the two nursing informatics courses, she was eager to meet this new challenge.

In addition to the above courses, a new informatics course is being offered for our newly approved RN-MSN program. Graduate students in the non-administration specialization and undergraduate junior and senior students are encouraged to take the course.

We have been fortunate in continuing our collaboration with the nursing consultant who also serves as adjunct faculty in the College of Nursing. The ongoing relationship has afforded us continued access to key people involved in hospital information systems in a variety of settings as guest speakers for some of our classes.

The instruction for the experiential component of the practicum has been taught by the staff of the university's Division of Academic Computing. The classes are held in state-of-the-art university computer labs that are specifically designed for teaching. The objectives are clearly articulated with each instructor in order to facilitate the students' competency achievement.

The development of informatics content in the curriculum continues to be a very exciting and enriching experience for all involved.

4. Learning Outcomes: The Student Perspective

The Nursing Informatics courses offered in the Nursing Administration program at Northeastern University have provided fledgling nurse managers and nurse administrators with understanding of the critical import of Information Systems (IS) in today's health care arena. The IS emphasis demonstrated how it directly impacts and shapes practice in ways that are cost-effective and improve the overall quality of patient care. It also revealed how the role of the nurse manager or executive is enhanced when management information systems are utilized.

An integral component of this course involved education relative to planning, implementation and management, and enhancement of IS in health care settings. It is clear that, from the outset, nursing must play a central role in each phase of the procurement and maintenance process. With a germane background in administrative theory, students are well-prepared to assume significant roles as project leaders in this domain.

Incorporated into the course curriculum are opportunities for students to observe proprietary vendor demonstrations, to interact with industry experts, to learn the dynamics of system architectures, and to explore the latest in technological innovation in healthcare. Course completion requires assessment of an organization's existing IS functionality along with development of a Request for Proposal (RFP) for certain modules of a nursing system. Lastly, course coordinators facilitated students spending a day shadowing(interviewing nursing IS personnel in various institutions in order to more accurately understand the variety of roles that nurses can play in hospital IS.

Having completed these nursing administration course offerings, I was inspired to pursue further learning in the field of nursing informatics, hence I completed a Directed Study under the guidance of the Nursing Information Systems Manager at Brigham & Women's Hospital in Boston. Throughout this experience, I was able to transfer knowledge gleaned from the classroom setting to a practice environment and to concretely examine the role that nursing plays in the development of IS. Further, by way of an engineering elective, I have expanded my IS learning outside of the nursing field in order to gain broader insight into the business of corporate IS planning and management. Through case study analysis, students learn how the use of sound IS business strategies can effectively and efficiently direct an entire corporation's success. To achieve a full understanding of the intricacies of nursing management information systems, I am also planning another directed study whereby I might examine the availability and use of these important management tools in healthcare.

Given this well-rounded body of knowledge in the Nursing Informatics domain, I am now beginning to explore career opportunities focusing on Information Systems in healthcare. With a solid foundation in nursing administration and a strong understanding of the organizational benefits and functionality of nursing informatics, I am empowered to realize my goal as a specialist in this burgeoning field.

Mobile Pen-based Technology as the Interface
of a Clinical Information System:
A Panel Presentation

Graves J R [ab] Fehlauer C S [ab] Gillis P A [ac] Booth H [ab] Vaux C [ad] and Soller J [ab]

[a]*Geriatric Research, Education, and Clinical Center, Veterans Affairs Medical Center, 500 Foothill Blvd, Salt Lake City, Utah.*

[b]*University of Utah, Salt Lake City, Utah.*

[c]*Bell Atlantic Healthcare Systems, Peachtree'Dunwoody Rd., Atlanta, Georgia*

[d]*Mercy Medical Center, Redding, California.*

Pen-based technology has been used by the Salt Lake VAMC GRECC [1] informatics research group to serve two purposes: a) to house an instrument devised to evaluate the nursing practice behaviors before and after introduction of various informatics "treatments" in a prospective informatics intervention study and b) to serve as the interface device of a new "clinical information system."As interesting as the technology is, the technology is not the "point." The point is still patient care, nursing practice, and clinical decision support. In this panel, we will look at how this technology facilitates nursing as we discuss a) the reasons for selecting this technology relative to the ability of the technology to support data input to a clinical database using atomic-level definitions of nursing data,b) the ability of the technology to support retrieval of entered information, and c) the ability of the technology to support acquisition of data to build the knowledge of nursing.

1.0. Study Design

...The interdisciplinary research program from which this work stemmed is designed to develop, implement, and evaluate several informatics treatments to improve quality of care of elderly patients by improving the identification and prediction of delirium. The experimental design can be represented as a 7 x 100 (Treatment x Time) interrupted time series factorial design. The treatments will occur over three years in the following sequence: Baseline A, Expert only, Expert and Iliad, Iliad only, Baseline B, Iliad only, Baseline

B.   The treatments being compared are: (a) current standard practice and charting   (Baseline A), (b) standard practice and charting after introduction of improved charting methods (Baseline B), (c) house staff identification of delirium after introduction of an expert diagnostic system for delirium (Iliad[a]) and, (d) a "gold standard expert observer" of delirium (a nurse specialist). The mobile pen-based computer with the newly developed clinical nursing information system serves as Baseline B. The mobile penbased computer with the nursing practice profile instrument is used before and after introduction of the Baseline B CNIS to measure effect on practice patterns.

The work reported in this paper is a part of the informatics research being done by the GRECC [2]. Thus far, nursing has had a major role in: a) design of a computer-based application to describe nursing practice characteristics before and after introduction of the new technology; b) designing and building the research and clinical database to manage all the data for the project, including all assessment and observation data recorded; and c) designing the interface of a state-of-the-art computerized clinician workbook that we use not only as a data collection/charting tool, but also to retrieve patient data needed for point of care real-time decision making.

2.0 Technology Evaluaton

To evaluate the effect of the pen-based mobile computer technololgy on nursing practice, a nursing activities profile (NAP) program was developed on the same platform. This method of assessing the effect of the technology on practice activities was the concept of the physician principal investigator of the study. This program was developed by a clinical nurse specialist, a programmer and nurse informaticists. The mobile pen-based technology allows real-time tracking of nurse activities and locations on the geriatric unit, which is the pilot site for the patient assessment tool (PAT).

Field testing was performed to evaluate the data elements and concepts of the initial design.   The initial testing revealed an inadequate selection of data elements as well as the inability to properly track and separate activities by time due to inadequate stop and start tags. Additionally, it was realized that nurses engaged in simultaneous activities, and that occasionally timing needed to start before the observer could identify the activity completely. Multiple trials and revisions were necessary before the finalized version was ready for data collection.

2.1. Evaluation Design

The NAP interface design allows an observer to quickly record the location and activity of the nurse. A map of the ward is displayed on screen, alongside 140 individual nursing activity selections. These activities are subgroups of activities such as assessment, interventions, and documentation. A single nurse is tracked by the observer continuously throughout an eight hour shift. During that time, the location of the nurse being observed is selected by the observer touching the pen on the appropriate map site. Activities are then selected as initiated and can be deselected individually or in multiples as completed. A validation step is performed after a prompt which is displayed every 15 entries. This allows for intra-rater reliability testing with the subject as a control. The rater asks the subject "What are you doing at this moment?" and the response is entered verbatim in free text. As this is the only required verbal exchange between rater and subject, there is minimal disruption of work flow. The output file produced includes nurse code number, time, location, current activities and incremental count of activities. Although this program was designed to track many nursing activities, for this study we are focusing on information processing. The database was constructed to allow us to answer questions such as:

- where did the nurses perform their documentation and information retrieval activities?
- which existing hospital computer programs were accessed?
- what is the frequency, duration, and location of specific activities during a specific time period?
- what activities occurred concurrently?

The application is unique as compared to traditional work sampling and self-report methods in that it:

- is completely paper less until after the statistical analysis.
- allows for recording continuous and simultaneous nursing activities throughout an entire shift

The NAP development process served as a guide to design of the larger application for patient assessment. The traditional system development life cycle was modified to our clinical informatics approach. The unique nature of clinical information requires that clinicians, trained in the processing of clinical information, are key development team members so that the data can be collected and retrieved in a manner useful for real time clinical decision making and research purposes.

3.0. Prototype

A prototype for the patient assessment tool had been created by a computer scientist working with nursing administrative personnel. This contained many elements and structures from a nursing assessment program being developed for the decentralized hospital computer program (DHCP) of the Veterans Administration Medical Centers. A clinical nurse specialist and a nursing informaticist were hired to redesign the database and prototype for implementation on an acute care geriatrics medical unit. Multiple attempts were made to redesign the initial mobile computer prototype, however, the interfac was found to be hierarchical and not congruent with the usual nursing work flow. As well, the database did not contain elements at the atomic level necessary for a real-time decision support system. Atomic level data is the lowest level to which an observation can be reduced and retain clinical significance. These atomic level elements can be combined in meaningful ways by multiple clinicians to create patient specific information, and has the potential for further analysis and knowledge generation.

3.1. Data Elements

The 1500 data elements used in the PAT were selected after a careful review of existing paper forms, policies and procedures, user requests, and clinical references. To promote database integrity , no default nor forced data entries were included other than date and time of entry. It is our belief that default entries may promote erroneous data, and the pen based technology allows for rapid selection of appropriate observation elements.

3.2. Interface

Interface design for the PAT, including content and functionality, followed a nursing model for patient assessment. Data entry methods include selection of assessment variables (controlled vocabulary) by a) touch selection using an electronic pen, b) "typing" free text entries on an on-screen keyboard, and c) on-screen handwriting which has limited functionality to date as the technology has not as yet developed to the level of accuracy and speed necessary for clinical applications. Validity checking and data comparison alert the user to change in patient condition and out-of-normal range entries.

3.3. Screen Design

The screens were designed following principles of form and function as well as visual aesthetics. In that screen size of the computer model to be used in implementation is approximately 5 x 7 inches, considerations such as font size and type, groupings, and white space were carefully evaluated. Navigation between screens is intuitive and shallow; the user cannot become lost in multiple embedded screens. The user enters a screen by selecting a body system or common nursing activity from the main menu. Further screen links are automated, with navigation inherent in the design.

3.4. Evaluation

Initial screen designs were evaluated by the users and revisions made as requested. Multiple field tests were conducted to polish the controlled vocabulary and format. Developers assured that data elements included not only those currently used by nurses to describe patient assessments and psychosocial and behavioral observations but also data from selected delirium diagnosis scales and classification systems, including DSM-III, which were required for the research study for which the program was designed.

4.0. Training

Training in use of the PAT will be scheduled prior to summer 1993 implementation. Learning the functionality of the program takes as little as 15 minutes. Becoming accustomed to individual screen elements will require more time. Short training time is a distinct advantage when time is such a valuable commodity. The pen based computer design allows an easy point and touch method of data entry, a major factor in the minimal training time. The familiar pen usage is not as intimidating as other computer systems to those who have not had prior computer experience, thereby minimizing the resistance to change.
Evaluation of the technology and its effect on medical and nursing decisions and practice will not be completed for a year after implementation. Initial studies for the pre-implementation phase have revealed that 21% of all nursing activities initiated on an eight hour shift are related to documentation and information retrieval. The time involved to carry out those activities has not been evaluated at this time. In order to analyze the change in activities the actual time spent in information processing will be studied. Chart audits will be conducted to evaluate completeness and legibility of nursing entries. User surveys will be distributed and analyzed to determine the users satisfaction with the technology and their perceptions as to the effect of the system on charting practices.

References

[1,2]   Salt Lake City Veterans Affairs Medical Center Geriatric Research, Education and Clinical Center.

Nursing Informatics: An International Overview for Nursing in a Technological Era
S.J. Grobe and E.S.P. Pluyter-Wenting, eds.

734

The Nursing Information System Software Utilizing Penpad Technology Pilot Project

Vasquez M[a] Lemke S[b] Ploessl J[b]

[a]*Health Care Expert Systems, Inc., 1025 Ashworth Road Suite 420, West Des Moines, Iowa 50265*

[b]*Iowa Methodist Medical Center, 1200 Pleasant Street, Des Moines, Iowa, 50309*

This presentation will outline and discuss the findings of a pilot project which was completed in the summer of 1992 at Iowa Methodist Medical Center in Des Moines, Iowa. The project was completed on a 35 bed Neurosurgical/Neurology nursing unit.

The changing environment of health care has lead to changing documentation requirements for nursing and other health care providers. Factors such as ever changing advanced technology, increasingly acute patients and requirements from insurers has influenced us into closely scrutinizing bedside information systems. Systems that allow data input and information access at the point of care, face to face with the patient, seem to offer the greatest long term benefit. Based on these types of trends, we chose to initiate a pilot project utilizing an existing software package on a different input and display device called the penpad. This hardware technology is currently being used in different business areas but there has not been much utilization in the health care arena.

The goals of the pilot include evaluating the Nursing Information System software performance and the integration of a penpad data input/display device. Other goals include evaluating the penpad as an alternative to bedside terminals, evaluating the effect of the penpad and the software on the clinicians and their practice.

We will discuss the benchmarks that were utilized to obtain these goals. They include a time study, an evaluation of overtime charting activities, a clinical nurses' attitude survey, a quality charting evaluation and the amount of the chart that this system could automate for our hospital.

1. Introduction

Advances in computer technology offer many opportunities for the health care arena. It is being realized by administrators, managers and health care providers that the future holds more and more applications involving computer systems. We are able to acknowledge the benefits computer systems offer in education, research and more so today, in clinical care. Computer systems offer us the opportunity to better utilize our current resources. The changing health care environment leads us to investigate how we can appropriately use computer systems and use them in a way that will allow us the most benefit.

Factors such as advanced technology, increasingly acute patients who require more care and assessment and requirements from insurers has made us closely scrutinize our current processes of documentation for nurses, physicians and other health care providers. We have identified documentation practices as an area where the benefits of implementation of a computer system will be realized in cost savings and quality issues.

Our current system of documentation is cumbersome and paper intensive. We utilize approximately 10 different forms ranging from two different admission assessments (one for hospital stays less than 72 hours and one for a regular admission), to various flowsheets used for specific documentation or based on individual unit preference, to nursing progress notes, to medication records. Because of the fragmentation of the documentation on the various forms, it is difficult to ascertain a clear picture of the patients condition and improvements or lack of improvements in their condition.

In our current system of documentation, duplication of data and access to data are real issues. Nurses, at the beginning of their shift, complete their daily worklist from information they obtain from the patient's Kardex and from the previous shift report. The worklist is carried with them throughout the day and patient data is noted on their worklists. The nurses will then transcribe data from their worklists to the patients medical record (chart) at time periods during their shift when they have the time or charting occurs at the end of the shift and overtime accrues. The data that the nurses gather is not available to other health care providers until the nurse transcribes it onto the chart. Health care providers who want access to current shift data on a specific patient have to locate the appropriate nurse for this information.

2. Benchmarks of the Pilot Project

Standards of care for completion of the medical record, Kardex, and care plans have been developed by our institution and these standards are audited by staff nurses on a monthly basis. We will use these standards as a benchmark tool to evaluate the completeness and appropriateness of our charting as well as the completeness of the patient Kardex and nursing care plan. We evaluated the studies that were completed prior to the beginning of the pilot, from January 1992 to May 1992, and found that even though we were meeting the target we had set for acceptable compliance to the standards, we had room for improvement in certain areas. The audits showed that we were in compliance with the standards 92% of the time as related to the chart or medical record, 91.8% of the time as related to the patient Kardex, and 85% of the time as related to the nursing care plans (averages over the 6 month period). In closer evaluation of the data, we discovered certain individual parameters that will be looked at closely for improved compliance with computerized documentation. These parameters focus on specific areas that should be assessed and documented on specific patient populations as defined in our clinical criteria.

One of the benefits we identified for using the computerized documentation system was to decrease the amount of overtime spent charting by 50%. We have estimated, based on our audits, that approximately 90% of our overtime is related to charting.

The pilot project, based on the nursing evaluations, was considered positive and successful. Many of the success measures that were identified were unable to be evaluated at the end of the pilot because of the abbreviated number of functions automated during the project, however, as we continue the project and automate additional functions, we will complete these measures. Informal evaluation, based on comments by the nursing staff and acceptance of the new method of documentation utilizing computers, does support the successfulness of the project. Nurses perceived that charting utilizing the penpad computer was faster and that, in turn, allowed them more time at the bedside for direct patient care. During the pilot, patients also expressed interest in the new technology and had positive comments regarding the computers and utilizing these at the bedside.

One of the benchmarks utilized to evaluate the pilot project was an attitude survey which was given to the nurses after the pilot. The survey was developed before the pilot and included 17 questions. The questions addressed the change in the charting process utilizing the pen unit and the software acceptance. An additional eight questions addressed the pen unit hardware and the upload and download (communication) process. The Likert statement responses included strongly agree, agree, uncertain, disagree and strongly disagree. There were eight negative statements and eight positive statements.

We had 18 nurses return their surveys out of a total of 33 nurses who utilized the system. The nurses sent the surveys directly to our management engineering department who tallied the results. The survey was given to the nurses within three weeks after the completion of the pilot. We felt their overall opinion of the pilot, the change in the charting process and the pen unit hardware was positive.

An additional benchmark utilized to evaluate the effectiveness of the pilot included a work sampling study. We did this work sampling study before the pilot was started. We had anticipated doing a repeated study after the pilot but we felt we needed to automate more than two nursing documentation forms in order to realize a significant change. Given the resources necessary for an accurate work sampling study and the importance of this benchmark, we decided to repeat it after our implementation of additional nursing documentation forms on the pen unit.

Our pre-pilot work sampling study was completed with five different nurse observers who were educated on the use of a work sampling tool. The tool broke out the nursing activities into six major sections; direct patient care, transporting activities, nurse collecting lab samples, personal/fatigue, delay and a documentation section. The documentation section was broken down into the 19 major documentation form types. Overall, the nurses spent 25.3% of their typical work day doing documentation. Of that 25.3%, the majority of time is spent on flowsheets, orders and medication documentation.

3. Penpad Technology

A pen unit is essentially very similar to the hardware necessary for a laptop personal computer [1]. They run under the major operating systems or a proprietary operating system. The major operating systems include Windows for Pen, Penpoint, PenDOS, PenRight! and PenPal. The microprocessor can range from the 8086 to the 80486 family. The storage media can range from hard disk, nonvolatile RAM or memory chips that preserve their contents [1]. Many units have the standard parallel, serial ports and keyboard ports which can be utilized to connect to peripheral devices or printers. The screen serves as the display and the input device. The screen has a digitizer underneath which interprets the action of the pen. The pen can resemble a ballpoint or a stylus attached to the pen unit [1]. As the user touches the screen with the pen, it acts like a mouse, selecting the item you press the pen against. The systems all have handwriting (printing only) recognition which is still not 100% interpretive [2]. Each pen unit has software on the device which enables training the unit to recognize a set of hand written characters and numbers. Training the system to individuals' handwriting styles does enhance the recognition capabilities, however we found that people change their handwriting techniques over time and when in a hurry it can create problems. We plan on using word phrase selection instead or handwriting as much as possible.

There are approximately ten pen tablet vendors on the market at the writing of this paper. Some of these include GRiD Systems Corp., IBM Corp., NCR Corp., Fujitsu, PI-Systems Corp., Tusk, Momenta Corp., Microslate, Samsung and Data Entry Systems. The prices of the pen tablets can run from $2,000 dollars to $5,000 dollars per unit depending on the model, processor, hard disk and memory.

Penpad units have had significant publicity and advocacy within the computer industry over the last 2-3 years since their debut. The computer industry experts have followed the sales of penpad units. Most of these experts agree that penpad technology will grow within the vertical market and applications [2]. At first penpads were believed to have wide spread use within the horizontal markets and applications such as word processing or spreadsheets [2]. The health care industry is a prime example of a vertical market with a specific application. Nurses are one of the may "mobile" workers that can benefit from penpads. Many nurses chart as they move around the patient's room or in the hallway. For the above reasons, we felt it was beneficial to do a pilot with the penpad technology as alternative to bedside terminal in our nursing units.

4. Implementation of the Pen Pad Pilot

The pilot was started May 27, 1992 with training of all nursing staff and unit clerks on the neurosurgical/neurology unit for 2-3 weeks on the first pen unit trialed. The training of each unit clerk took 1/2 hour and nurses took one hour. There was some additional training needed as we brought in the other two pen units but this took less than an hour and was necessary mainly for hardware and upload/download difference. The until clerks downloaded the latest nursing data to the file server and at the same time, uploaded the patient census at the change of the shift. The file server was a 486 personal computer that was connected to a wide area ethernet so we could access the software on other terminals. The printing of the reports was done locally from the personal computer. The unit clerks did not enter any data on the penpads. They did however, update the census with the patient names and 12 digit account numbers that were taken off the mainframe system. We did not have an ADT interface to the software during the pilot but we plan to have this once we continue the project. The nurses did dual charting (on their worklist and the penpad) until all testing was completed. We did testing to ensure correct data on the file server and pen units for at least three weeks. We did utilize the reports from the system during the testing.

We started with the night nurses completing their vitals and neuro flowsheet data on the pen unit and they sent that information to the file server for print outs at the end of their shift through a RS232 connection. We brought on the evening shift and day shifts within 2-4 weeks after the night shift. Each pen unit was trailed for approximately 4-6 weeks.

Three penpad vendors were used during the pilot using the same forms developed in three different programming languages. They were:

PI Systems-forms were created in PI SDK development environment running a proprietary operating system.
Fujitsu-forms were created in PenPAL running PenDOS.
NCR 3125-forms created in Pen Windows using Visual Basic.

The PACE Nursing Information System is a UNIX based nursing bedside charting system originally designed to use terminal or personal computer keyboard devices as data input devices. This pilot replaced the keyboard devices with penpad technology. After the pilot acceptance, it was determined that to take full advantage of the PACE Nursing Information System flexibility, the penpads would use terminal emulation using spread spectrum communications to update the central charting system. This would allow flowsheet and other form changes to be made quickly without having to update and manage screen and version integrity with each penpad. The pilot started May 27, 1992 and ended September 11, 1992.

5. Evaluation of Pilot-Summary

We are fast moving from an age where the electronic medical record was a curious dream of the future to an age where electronic collection and transmission of data is an expected method of doing business; from an age where physicians and other health care professionals were leery and uncomfortable with computers to an age where they are not only comfortable with them, but are expecting the technological advances they provide. There is no serious question to the value of an electronic medical record, only decisions as to the methods and means to accomplish it.

The question for many hospitals over the last 5-10 years is "should we put terminals at the bedside"? The concept of capturing the data at the point of care made good sense. However, concerns arise as to where do you put this terminal in an already crowded room and how do you justify this high expense in hardware which may be used 20-30% of the eight hour shift? Charting at the bedside can save nurses charting time at the end of the shift. Our nurses, 89%, felt that penpads would help them chart at the bedside and 72% felt that charting at the bedside would save them time.

Penpads will continue to drop in cost as the personal computers did once the market matured. Giving each nurse a penpad to use would significantly cut the cost of the hardware. The pen units could be shared with other ancillary personnel when not being used. Dumb terminals at the bedside might seem cheap now but they have limited useful life outside the patient's room. Penpads will soon be priced close to a dumb terminal and the ratio will be less than the number required for each patient room. The penpad is also intuitive to use, it is very similar to pen and paper and requires less training time than a keyboard application. Of our nurses, 83% preferred the pen unit over a keyboard from our survey. The penpads also allow multiple care providers access to "one" chart similar to bedside terminals. Of our nurses, 61% felt that the chart would be more accessible to other healthcare providers with the pen units.

The penpad technology is rapidly changing. Many people are waiting for the technology to stabilize before attempting to try the units. We would strongly recommend a pilot utilizing this technology. Health care information today is in a state of disorganization, non standardization and inaccessibility. Pen units help get our information in the necessary digitized format as we sort through the many "process" issues as to what data we really want and need. Once digitized and standardized, the inefficiencies of the health care industry can decrease and with that comes a decrease in the cost of health care. We will be able to input the data with ease and avoid duplicate documentation and at the same time easily manipulate and retrieve this data. In summary, the pilot project has showed us many benefits as we continue our penpad utilization in automation our medical record.

6. References

[1]Hardaker M. Back to the Future. *Windows User* July 1992. 73-86.

[2]Barr C. Pen *P.C Magazine* 1992. 11:175-201.

Nursing Informatics: An International Overview for Nursing in a Technological Era
S.J. Grobe and E.S.P. Pluyter-Wenting, eds.

738

Computerization of Management Decision Support Data

McMahon L[a] Kraft MR[b] and Vance B[c]

[a]Chief, Nursing Service, Veterans Affairs Medical Center, Providence, RI

[b]Associate Chief, Nursing Service, Veterans Affairs Medical Center, Hines, IL

[c]Chief, Nursing Service, Veterans Affairs Medical Center, Atlanta, GA

The Department of Veterans Affairs (DVA) Decentralized Hospital Computer Program (DHCP) is a comprehensive integrated hospital information system with a nursing component.[1] The modular design of the nursing content allows for computerization of clinical, administrative, research, and education data.

Data elements for content areas were developed and prioritized by a VA special interest users group (SIUG) with national representation. Nursing program design specifications identified the need for accurate and timely information to support management decisions and resource allocation. As the administrative modules of the nursing package come on-line, elements which link personnel data, fiscal information, patient acuity, and actual versus required staffing are available to nurse managers and nursing service administrators.

A recruitment software package links to the personnel data base which includes demographic and professional information. Tracking systems generate reports on patient classification, earned versus actual patient care hours, quality assurance, productivity data, and cost data. Actual payroll data provides cost information for earned days off, overtime, differentials, and cumulative FTEE as well as regular hours/dollars per patient day. On-line data and the associated report capabilities are used to support the nursing service and nursing unit budgetary process.

The panel presentation will address package elements, functionality, and current and projected applications to nursing management decision support.

1. Computerization of Management Decision Support Data

The Department of Veterans Affairs (DVA) Decentralized Hospital Computer Program (DHCP) is a comprehensive integrated hospital information system that does include a nursing component. The modular design of the DHCP nursing package allows for computerization of clinical, administrative, research, education, and quality improvement data.

Data elements and package functionality for each of the nursing modules were designed and prioritized by DVA nursing special interest users groups (SIUGS) with national representation. As software was completed it was sent to ALPHA and BETA test sites and then underwent external verification before final release.

Nursing administrative SIUG members working on design specifications identified the need for accurate and timely information for resource allocation and other management decisions. As the modules of the administrative nursing package have come on line, nurse managers and nursing service administrators have gained ready access to personnel data, payroll and other fiscal information, patient census and acuity data, on-duty staffing figures and productivity reports.

1.1 Personnel Data

The nursing personnel data base includes individual demographics, educational preparation, work experience, licensure, certification, credentialing, and payroll information. This data is available on a "need-to-know" basis with unit personnel data available to the unit nursing manager and clinical section/division and total nursing service data available to second and third level nurse administrators. Employees can review their own data base on a "read only" basis.

1.2 Patient Classification

Patient census information and daily classification information which reflects patient acuity and determines related staffing needs is available on-line for daily and shift by shift staffing. In addition, this data, over time, produces acuity trending reports for the budgetary process.

1.3 Man-hours

Actual on duty staffing hours are entered in the man-hour package which distinguishes between direct and indirect care hours. Indirect hours are further broken down to identify hours for orientation, education, administrative duties, and other activities, i.e. union business.

1.4 Workload Statistics

The data from the patient classification and man-hour files is utilized for the generation of the workload productivity report. This report compares budgeted and recommended staffing to actual staffing and produces a productivity report for each tour of duty or for each 24 hour period. These reports can be produced by shift, day, week, month or quarter and have proved to be a useful tool for review of staffing during the JCAHO survey process.

1.5 Fiscal Information

On-line payroll data can produce unit, section and service cost information for hours worked, earned time off, leave usage, overtime, holidays, and differentials for weekends and off-tours. The integration of fiscal data with patient census/acuity data produces the cost/hours per patient day. This information is valuable in the unit based budgeting process. In addition to the production of administrative reports, the computerized payroll data base allows all employees access to their personal annual and sick leave balances. They may also request leave via the computer.

1.6 Recruitment

Software specifications for the recruitment/retention data base will allow required application information to be put on-line by the candidate or by support personnel. Results of the interview process will be documented on line. When a candidate moves to a hire status this information will be transferred into the nurse staff files and the permanent personnel data base thus avoiding duplicate entry. At any time within the recruitment/hire process the status of any candidate will be immediately available. Report capability includes all the mandatory VA recruitment and retention reports.

2. Panel Presentation

The objectives of the panel presentation are: a) to describe a comprehensive integrated hospital information system that includes a nursing component, b) to discuss the process used to develop and prioritize the data elements for content areas, c) to describe the modules of the administrative nursing package: personnel data, patient classification, man-hours, workload statistics, fiscal information and recruitment and d) to discuss the application of the package to nursing management decision support.

Achievement of the objectives will be facilitated by addressing the following questions: a) what levels of nursing staff involvement are required to develop a comprehensive information system with a nursing component, b) what additional elements would be useful in each of the modules, c) what lessons have been learned that would assist others in planning and designing a similar system, d) how adaptable are the data elements for use in an ambulatory or primary care setting and e) what enhancements are anticipated and/or desired?

3. Summary

The integration of each of these modules produces a powerful support system for nurse managers within the VA health care system which includes 172 medical centers, 229 outpatient clinics, 122 nursing homes, and 27 domicillaries. [2] As each facility implements the Nursing package modules, the resulting data base provides valuable information to support local management decisions and allows system-wide comparisons of effectiveness across institutions.

740

Huber and others[3] from the University of Iowa have identified 18 elements for a Nursing Management Minimum Data Set (NMMDS) representing core data elements that help nurse managers make sound decisions. With no knowledge of the Iowa development project, the development of the DVA DHCP management support system included 13 of the 18 elements of the NMMDS. Some of the missing elements were related to cost reimbursement issues which are not significant in the VA system.

4. References

[1] Dept of Veterans Affairs, Veterans Health Serv and Res Adm, Med Information Resources Management Office, *Decentralized Hospital Computer Program.* Washington: Information Systems Center, October 1990.

[2] Dayhoff R and Maloney D. Exchange of Veterans Affairs Medical Data Using National and Local Networks. *Ann N Y Acad Sci,* 1992.

[3] Huber, D et al. A Nursing Management Minimum Data Set. *J Nurs Adm,* Vol. 22, No. 7/8, July-August, 1992, 35-40.

Nursing Informatics: An International Overview for Nursing in a Technological Era
S.J. Grobe and E.S.P. Pluyter-Wenting, eds.

An Integrated Clinical Nursing Package Within the Department of Veterans Affairs Medical Facilities

Vance B[a] Swenson J[b] Gilleran J[c] Smart S[d] and Claflin N[e]

[a]Chief, Nursing Service, VA Medical Center, Atlanta, Georgia

[b]VA Medical Center, San Francisco, California

[c]VA Medical Center, Hines, Illinois

[d]VA Medical Center, Sheridan, Wyoming

[e]VA Medical Center, Phoenix, Arizona

Hospital information systems have the potential for improving quality and cost effectiveness of health care. Predictions for the year 2000 have included clinical information systems as a requirement for achieving the best patient outcomes. Since the mid 1980's the Department of Veterans Affairs (VA), the largest health care system in the free world, has been developing a comprehensive hospital computer program linking clinical and administrative requirements to patient care. The long range goal is a computerized patient record.

Nurses in clinical practice, education, and research have assumed a vital role in the development and implementation of the VA Integrated Health Care Information System. A group of nurses with expert knowledge in clinical nursing specialties developed the specifications for automating clinical nursing information. The computerization of nursing information has the purpose of enhancing the processing and improving the quality of information used in providing patient care. There was consensus regarding the influence of the nursing process on the design of the software package. Functional Health patterns provided the framework for the assessment module and nursing diagnosis the entry point for the care plans module. The program was designed to be sufficiently flexible to accommodate any theoretical framework directing nursing practice in individual Veterans Affairs Medical Center Nursing Services.

The innovative aspects of the nursing software include a total integration with the hospital information system and nursing clinical requirements as the base for the program's structure. The integrated clinical nursing package has several modules: Initial Patient Assessment, Patient Plan of Care, Clinical Observation Measurements, Progress Transfer Discharge Notes, Quality Improvement and Education.

1.0 Objectives:

1. Describe components of the VA Clinical Nursing Information System.
   a. Initial Patient Assessment
   b. Patient Plan of Care
   c. Clinical Observation/Measurements
   d. Documentation
2. Demonstrate the relationship of the clinical care modules to Quality Improvement monitoring.
3. Describe mechanisms for maintaining computerized educational records.

2.0 Clinical Module Of Decentralized Hospital Computer Program (DHCP) Nursing

2.1 Initial Patient Assessment

This module contains the admission assessment which can be tailored by each VA facility to meet specific needs. It is consistent with the format used for other forms of electronic nursing documentation including the patient plan of care, progress notes, discharge notes, transfer note, and shift assessment.

2.2 Patient Plan of Care

This component contains standardized care plans and guidelines that can be modified by each VA facility to meet their needs. Further, patient care plans can be generated to include data on patient problems, patient goals/expected outcomes, interventions/orders, dates of problem evaluation/resolution, target dates for accomplishing goals, defining characteristics, etiologies, related risk factors, and related problems. The data in the care plan software uses a shared data base with the assessment software. The Patient Plan of Care software component supports standards of nursing care and practice as identified by each VA facility. The developers of this module are currently improving its functionality for interdisciplinary implementation. This will allow all disciplines the ability to enter their respective data on a fully integrated patient plan of care.

2.3 Clinical Observation/Measurement

This software has been designed for patient vitals/measurements, intake and output monitoring, intravenous fluid monitoring and care, as well as ongoing physical and psychosocial patient assessment in the form of shift assessments. Many of the clinical observation/measurement software programs are also available to other disciplines to document their clinical observations and measurements. For example, Dieticians have use of the vitals/measurements software to record patient's height and weight;. The component also contains options for producing patient assignment worksheets, end of shift reports, ward census reports, nursing inquiries on individual patients, patient care flow sheets, graphic displays, and summaries. These options integrate data from the various clinical software programs into useful tools for direct nursing care delivery.

2.4 Progress, Transfer, and Discharge Notes

This component provides each VA facility with standard nursing notes which are tailored to meet individual facility needs. It allows nurses to record interward transfer notes, discharge and other progress notes electronically by pulling from an established on-line database. The clinical module of the Nursing DHCP software promotes sound clinical practice and clinical competency by providing nurses and other health care providers with the necessary computer tools to perform their clinical functions.

2.5 Education

The purpose of the Education Package is to track the proficiency and competency requirement for individual staff members as well as groups of staff. The package is accessible to all disciplines of the medical center and is fully integrated within the total computer system while maintaining the individual integrity of the service-specific requirements. Mandatory annual reviews, attendance at continuing education activities, and attendance at ward/unit level inservice reports are available for a service, a ward, or an individual. The data can be entered and retrieved, both centrally and at the individual person/unit level. These reports can be sorted by a variety of date parameters. Deficiency reports are available when a mandatory class has not been completed. This option is particularly useful in the administration and documentation, of compliance with internal and external review organizations' requirements for documenting nurse competency.

2.6 Quality Improvement

The Quality Improvement (QI) module of the Nursing Package is designed to support the members of the nursing staff in unit-based and interdisciplinary quality improvement activities.

The QI Summary covers all JCAHO requirements for quality improvement. Each unit or nursing service enters data for assigned responsibility, scope of care, and key functions. Nursing standards of care and practice are integrated with the Nursing Care Plan module. Standards of Care are pulled from expected outcomes; standards of practice are pulled from nursing interventions.

Data is entered for data source, sample, size, methodology, frequency, and monitoring period. The survey statistics are pulled from the Survey Generator, a data entry/statistical package. Each indicator is identified individually; with data entered for type of indicator, numerator, denominator, definition of terms, rationale, and method of determining variance. For each indicator, recommendations are made, including who will take action, who/what is expected to change, when actions were taken, and evaluation of effectiveness of actions. Communication is clearly identified, with receiver of results. References are included. A separate option can be used for impact or any other information that may be needed.

The Survey Generator is a data entry package that allows surveys or questionnaires to be developed. The developer can choose from multiple choice, true/false, yes/no, sorting by header, or free test for responses. When data are entered, the program provides a summary of statistics. The tool can be sorted by demographics. For example, the patient and/or nurse entering the data can be entered. This information is integrated with the User file and Patient files in DHCP. The survey generator can be used by all services in the hospital and is ideal for interdisciplinary indicators. The survey generator can be used for multi-site indicators and will provide data by facility and in aggregate.

The Incident Reporting package is used by nurses and other health care professionals for all incident reports. Data can be entered by nurses on individual units. Data are aggregated in the Quality Management office and disseminated back to nursing units, and can be transmitted to regional and VA Central Office.

Finally, the QI module for the nursing package includes several help sections, with examples of aspects of care/key functions, sample QI plan, sample hospital plan for providing nursing care, sample standards of care and practice, and sample indicators.

3.0 Summary/Integration

A clinical information system for Nursing, although vitally important, is just "one piece" of the desired automated clinical record. Data should be input only once and then be available to whomever needs it, regardless of package. Until 1988 the Department of Veterans Affairs (VA) developed its software to meet the needs of administration, fiscal and specific clinical services. All developed software used a uniform set of tools for file construction, security and menu management. All software had to be able to operate on a variety of hardware platforms, be modular in design, vendor independent, adhere to current HL7 standards and flexible enough to meet the unique needs found in 171 hospitals, 357 outpatient clinics, 128 nursing homes and 35 domiciliaries. At that time a few data fields, Patient Demographics, were shared between packages. But, this was not the norm, since developers at 7 different Information System Centers (ISCs) were required to be constantly aware of current, past and future developments. Sharing agreements were pursued when a needed data field was identified. Many fields were unknowingly duplicated in a desire to implement the specifications identified by the expert panels. A good example was allergy tracking, a priority of all clinical services. This data field was found in Dietetics, Nursing, Pharmacy and Medical Information Services software.

In 1988, a VA planning committee identified applications that integrate patient data for clinical care as the biggest development priority for the VA. A small multi-disciplinary group with support from all ISCs, was given the task to begin automating the clinical record. The group readily identified the need for users to have the capability for easy retrieval of information concerning their patients without regard for the technical intricacies.

The first General Medical Record (GMR) package developed using this patient centered criteria, was the Health Summary. The initial target consumers were the patients and clinicians in the outpatient clinic areas. However,this package soon became extremely valuable to the clinicians and the treating of patients in the hospital. The Health Summary is a generic tool that generates a report by integrating currently available clinical data residing the VA Hospital Information System. Clinicians can customize their reports, review them on the screen or use a printed

744

software, that has been totally integrated and is available to all clinicians follows.

3.1 Allergy/Adverse Reaction
Software that allows verification of both historical and observed reactions; tracks sign/symptoms, allows generation of Food and Drug Administration - Adverse Drug Reaction (FDA-ADR) report.

3.2 Order Entry/Results Reporting
A package that supports physician order entry; electronic signature; order sets; personal and team patient lists; incorporated Health Summary (HS), alerts/notifications, consults and progress notes.

3.3 Progress Notes
Software used to generate patient crisis notes, clinical warnings and advanced directives.

3.4 Problem List
A module that is designed to be generic and used by all disciplines. Nursing Diagnosis/Patient Problems can be extracted from those identified on the Care Plan.

3.5 Generic Text Generator
A utility that builds blocks of text from coded documents using a menu-driven data entry mechanism. Examples of it's usage include, Nursing Care Plan, Assessment Took Mental Health Treatment Plan, History and Physical, and Progress Notes

VA developed expert systems/decision support tools are under continuous development. The Department of Veterans Affairs has a commitment to provide to it's customers (nurses, physicians and other clinicians) quality information for improved patient care services.

4. References

Barry, C., & Gibbons, L. (February 1990). Information Systems Technology: Barriers and Challenges to Implementation. JONA, 20:40-42.

Behrenbecky, J. etal. (1990) Strategic Planning for a Nursing Information System in the Hospital Setting. Computers in Nursing , 8:236-242.

McLaughlin, K. etal (1990). Shaping the Future: The Marriage of Nursing Theory and Informatics. Computers in Nursing, 8:174-179.

Patterson, C. Quality Assurance Control, and Monitoring the Future Role of Information technology From the Joint Commission Perspective. Computers in Nursing, 8:105-110.

Nursing Informatics: An International Overview for Nursing in a Technological Era
S.J. Grobe and E.S.P. Pluyter-Wenting, eds.

Comprehensive Perspectives on Clinical Information Systems Implementation

Hall PD[a] Button PS[a] Joy JA[a] Edwards WH[a] and Sturd PH [b]

[a] *Dartmouth-Hitchcock Medical Center, Lebanon, NH 03756*

[b] *Cerner Corporation, 2800 Rockcreek Parkway, Kansas City, MO 64117*

The purpose of this panel presentation is to analyze key strategies that impact all phases of Clinical Information Systems (CIS) implementation, from planning to go-live. The authors' experience as co-development partners for the design and implementation of provider documentation and physician order entry functionality at a 420 bed tertiary care medical center will provide the background for the information presented.

Strategies to be discussed will include: consideration of the planning phase as the first building block of the implementation process, and of subsequent phases as incremental steps towards implementation; utilization of a team approach; the importance of communications; extensive and user involvement throughout the process, with a particular focus on physician involvement and the ambitious goal of direct order entry by physicians; and attention to technical issues by non-technical staff. Objectives of the presentation include:

• Identification of key concepts that impact successful CIS Implementation
• Examination of the use of these strategies in one implementation process
• Exploration of ways to include end user physicians, nurses, and others, in the development and implementation process

The panel participants are members of a project team that has undertaken the implementation, and in some aspects, the co-development, of a clinical information system (CIS) that will ultimately include physician order entry, multidisciplinary care planning and documentation, laboratory, pharmacy, respiratory therapy, and a chart browsing function, integrated with pre-existing systems for finance, ADT, scheduling, radiology, and additional clinical functions.

1. Building Blocks of the Implementation Process

The first key strategy to be considered is the importance of considering the planning phase as the cornerstone of the implementation process. Every activity and contact can be seen as an opportunity to share information and garner support for automation efforts. Inviting department directors, a wide spectrum of nurses and physicians, and administrators to informational meetings and vendor demos during the planning and selection process will assure a widespread awareness of plans for the future. Continued regular contacts with these extended groups facilitates later functional review and database work.

Similarly, other tasks addressed early on will serve as the basis for work undertaken in later phases. It is important to define a vision and identify goals during the planning process, both of which will serve to give direction to the project and provide a touchstone for project evaluation. A more concrete example of avoiding redundant effort is the evolution of a document from a simple list of desired functionality to a Request for Proposal to a vendor evaluation and finally to a detailed points specification for software design and review. The importance of maintaining complete documentation of the process and tasks accomplished becomes evident when considering this strategy of building on prior phases and tasks. Further examples of building on prior work will be seen in the sections on communications and user involvement.

2. The Project Team

The development and implementation work has been undertaken by a project team, including nurses, physicians, Information Services, Respiratory Therapy, Laboratory, Pharmacy, other ancillaries, and Medical Records and Risk Management on an ad hoc basis. Close collaboration with a vendor on many different aspects of the system expands the concept of the project team even further, to encompass two very different organizations, geographically distant, but with a common goal and vision.

Building a sense of team can be a challenge, and is well worth the investment of some time and money. We spent two and a half days at a teambuilding program, working together on problem solving and group challenges, and establishing relationships outside the traditional workplace. This proved to be a valuable step in cementing our team, and we often refer back to the lessons learned there. Some of the challenges and rewards of the team approach will be further discussed related to communications, technical aspects, and from the vendor perspective. The team concept has been an important strategy for promoting ownership of the system, and for assuring that it will meet the needs of all users in providing quality patient care.

3. Communications

Communication was a third key implementation strategy in this co-development project. The assumption underlying significant investment of time and energy in various communication efforts was the belief that a project team comprised of informed participants functions more effectively. Pro-active communication about project plans, progress and problem solving decreases the likelihood of confusion and diversion of resources to correct misinformation. This assumption is certainly not revolutionary. Our experience, however, was that actually incorporating predefined communications in our operations was quite challenging. The difficulty appeared to be related to the up front organization required to comply with our overall communication plan, as well as some team members' natural aversion to the basic preventive, rational nature of the communication plan.

The actual communication plan for the project was developed during the initial several months of the multi-year project. The project team monitored compliance with the plan monthly and reported to the Executive Committee. Also, the team evaluated the plan itself annually and made revisions based on evaluation results.

The plan itself was comprised of specific structured communication activities in each of the following categories: project documentation, executive level communication, project operations' communication, DHMC broad organizational communication, and implementation of specific communication technologies.

4. End User Involvement

The involvement of end users was definitely one of the strategies emphasized in this project. Based on review of the literature and networking with other organizations, vendors, and consultants, the project team developed a strong sense that problems with other systems were related to design that did not incorporate the end users' perspective and lack of buy-in by users. Therefore, as part of the development of the initial vendor selection process, a nursing user group was established. The group included staff nurse representation from every nursing unit, as well as a few representatives of leadership roles. In every phase of the project, the team has provided the appropriate education or orientation for that phase to the User Group members. The user group members have then participated as key resources in each phase. The input of this group is considered one of the most significant in shaping decision-making.

Many group members have participated for the whole life of the project and are now well-educated, strongly invested participants in our project. They often initiate unit-based CIS project activities to assure their staff nurse colleagues are informed and getting ready for implementation.

As the project progressed, the concept of end user involvement was extended to include a broad representation of more nursing staff, secretaries, physicians, respiratory therapists, social workers, and others in focus groups, workflow sessions and unit based user groups.

5. Physician Order Entry and Involvement

Direct order entry by physicians into a computer system, and the benefits to be reaped from such a system, have been high intensity topics in health care for many years. Until fairly recently, though, physicians themselves have apparently taken a wait and see attitude about clinical computer systems. As a result their input has often been neglected. Unfortunately, as experienced system implementation specialists have noted, end user input is critical to the ultimate success of the clinical computing change process.

There are a variety of reasons for the apparent disconnect between medical software developers and physicians: autonomy of practice and variety of approaches to clinical information; complicated legal nature of clinical software; high cost of software development with a questionable market; and probably the most compelling, the intense focus of the clinical provider on direct patient care concerns (leading to an apparent lack of interest in development and use of clinical systems). At the Dartmouth-

Hitchcock Medical Center once these constraints of physician involvement in clinical software development were defined, the full-time staff was focused on managing the project work within those constraints.

The Medical Center, committed from the beginning to direct user involvement in software design, paid a core team of physicians to offer guidance to our co-development partner on the basic design of the system for physician use. During development of the foundation of the system, the full-time project team acknowledged the professional demands of the physician group and tested software independently as it was revised. It was, therefore, very important that the support team had clinical expertise, and in fact all team members were practitioners of one of several clinical disciplines. As the team evolved, a systematic process of reviewing and testing software, presenting problems, questions, and issues for review by the physician group in short intense sessions was developed as the most economical means of getting non-trivial input from the physician users. Staff often brainstormed alternatives and prepared extensively for meetings to facilitate decision making by the physician team.

Once the fundamentals of the order management system were in place we felt it necessary to broaden input from physicians as we began to fine-tune system functions. Because we understood the need to balance the physicians' primary patient care role with the needs of the project to get non-trivial input from the broadest possible physician base, we used the concept of Focus Groups. Our version employed the concept in its purest sense, very short meetings with very narrow objectives. Since physician to physician dialogue was considered key, the physician core group took complete responsibility for development of the content and presentation of these meetings.

The meetings, which were conducted for one hour, once a month, beginning about one year prior to implementation of the system, were very effective. Key to the effectiveness was a strategy of offering additional opportunity for project activity. During the initial meetings of the Focus Groups, we made clear that any physician who wished to have more involvement with the project and the team was welcome to attend meetings or visit the testing lab. The official Focus Groups, however, would be confined to specific topics and agenda items. With clear statement of the individual Focus Group objectives we were able to keep discussion narrowed effectively at hand to the topics. Other groups, as a function of their role in the Medical Center, were invited and eventually assumed leadership in specific areas of development. The Pharmacy and Therapeutics Committee and Medical Records Committee for instance were engaged early on in the process and increasingly took responsibility for protocols and policies related to the implementation.

Assuring software flexibility and customization was another strategy we used successfully. This had significant impact on our ability to effectively address differences in the way various practitioners approach order management, and addresses another of the key reasons why physician use of computers for order entry has been delayed.

6. Technical Issues

As clinical departments begin to implement the increasingly available clinical systems, their focus is naturally on the functionalities the systems provide for clinicians. While this focus is appropriate, it is important that clinical departments plan a way to address the technical issues that are concomitant with implementing clinical systems. The phrase "technical issues" is often used to refer to a wide range of system issues. In this discussion it is used in particular reference to system networks, peripheral devices, CPU, disk space, memory requirements and implications of database decisions. Though there are many approaches that can be used to navigate the difficult issues surrounding these topics, the following three strategies can be easily and effectively implemented. The first two of the following strategies should be initiated during the selection phase of the project.

1. Include an individual on the project team with a background in technical issues. Even if you are implementing your system with the help of an internal information systems department, the inclusion on the project team of individuals skilled in technical issues but also familiar with the implications on computer use in the clinical areas is recommended. A team member with these qualifications will provide a dimension of understanding that is difficult for consultants to provide as you work through some of the difficult issues.

2. Identify individuals within your institution with experience in specific areas. There are often "experts" tucked away within an institution, in clinical, ancillary, information services and other areas. By using formal meetings with department directors and informal interpersonal networks, project teams can tap into a rich resource at a minimum expense and can promote the collaborative spirit key to good clinical systems.

3. Select a vendor with proven experience in implementation and support of efficient systems. There are often many options available to a hospital when they begin to build their database, and the database builders need to be aware of the potential impact of the choices available. The responsibility for this role rests mainly with the vendor representative. It is their job to clearly define the options available and their respective impact. The vendor's ability to provide this information will be a function of their experience in the industry and their familiarity with your institution's approach. The impact of this type of guidance on your production system's performance, in response time, CPU and disk space usage, and ease of use will vary with different vendors, but because it can be significant, prospective purchasers of information systems should evaluate vendors' ability to provide this service. Without guidance it is often easy for an institution to make database decisions that would have serious disk space or other implications unforeseen by clinical project team members.

748

7. Summary

The success of a comprehensive clinical systems implementation depends on many factors. The timeframes for such projects are often prolonged, and the process can potentially become both fragmented and frustrating. The strategies presented represent some of the ways we found valuable in managing such a complex undertaking. Each of these approaches contributed to assuring the outcome of a system that will serve as an effective tool for clinicians in their provision of quality patient care.

Nursing Informatics: An International Overview for Nursing in a Technological Era
S.J. Grobe and E.S.P. Pluyter-Wenting, eds.

Security and confidentiality forum:
Changing the future

Barber B[a] Marr PB[b] Hovenga EJS[c] and Gerdin-Yelger U[d]

[a]*Information Management Centre, Birmingham, UK*

[b]*Director, Hospital Information Systems, New York University Medical Center, New York, NY*

[c]*Evelyn J. Hovenga & Associates Pty Ltd, Queensland, Australia*

[d]*Stockholm County Council, Stockholm, Sweden*

The rapid increase in the use of Information Systems within the Health Care Environment is having a profound effect on the way in which Health Care is delivered. Almost all activities have some aspects of their work handled with the aid of various types of Information System and the use of these systems is impacting even closer on the crucial issues of patient care. The basics of "Computer Hygiene" need to be taught to all so that they become aware of the fundamental requirements for the safe operation and use of Information systems in Health Care. There is no need to turn everyone into security specialists but everyone needs to understand what is safe practice and what could be potentially dangerous. Members of the Forum will be invited to make a ten minute presentation on the key issues as a prelude to the Forum discussion.

1. Objectives of the Panel

1. To Raise the Awareness of Security Issues in the Health Care Environment
2. To Examine the Security of Health Care Treatment Systems
3. To Consider the Training required by Nurses in Security
4. To Interpret the Professional Requirements of Confidentiality in Computer Systems

2. Topics for Consideration

1. Know country's legal requirements regarding medical confidentiality and data protection
2. Know procedures for safe use of systems used
3. Know organisation's security and data protection requirements
4. Use only authorised and tested software
5. Practice basic physical security
6. Practice safe password management
7. Avoid all unnecessary disclosure of medical information
8. Ensure accuracy of information input
9. Check information output as reasonable
10. Take regular back-up copies of information
11. Participate in plan for disasters
12. Avoid smoking in critical areas
13. Be security conscious - insecure information systems can damage your patients

3. Questions for discussion

How far are the nursing users of information systems aware of the requirements of computer hygiene? What steps need to be taken to support a greater awareness of the issues?

Nursing Informatics: An International Overview for Nursing in a Technological Era
S.J. Grobe and E.S.P. Pluyter-Wenting, eds.

Telematics for health care in the European Union

Mortensen R[a] Mantas J[b] Manuela M[c] Sermeus W[d] Nielsen GH[e] and McAvinue E[f]

[a]Director, Danish Institute for Health and Nursing Research, Fensmarksgade 3, DK-2200 Copenhagen N, Denmark

[b]Professor, University of Athens, Laboratory of Health Informatics, Athens, Greece

[c]Chief Nurse, Hospital da Universidade de Coimbra, Cirurgia Maxilo-Facil, Coimbra, Portugal

[d]Professor, Centre for Health Services Research and Nursing K.U. L:euven, Belgium

[e]Research Manager, Danish Institute for Health and Nursing Research, Fensmarksgade 3, Copenhagen N, Denmark

[f]Head of School for Nursing, Uni-Kilnikum-Ulm, Krankenhausweg 3, Ulm, Germany

1. Background

The R&D programme of the European Union (EU) called Advanced Informatics in Medicine (AIM) has in Europe become a kind of focal point for transnational developments in health care informatics, including European initiatives to develop standards and minimum data sets. The AIM programme has supported a series of projects concerned with both standards in health care, e.g. Standardization in Europe on Semantical Aspects of Medicine (SESAME), and the definition of transnational hospital minimum data sets in Europe, e.g. Hospital Comparison (HOSCOM).

The AIM programme also played a role, when the European Standardization Committee (CEN) in April 1990 established Technical Committee number 251 (TC 251) in order to develop standards in health care informatics. TC 251 consists of 5 working groups: 1) Health Care Information Modelling and Electronic Patient Record, 2) Health Care Terminology, Coding Systems and Knowledge Bases, 3) Medical Imaging and Multimedia, Communication with Medical Devices, 4) Health care security, Privacy, Quality and Safety, and 5) Standards for Intermittently Connected Devices. The working group structure has been "mirrored" by the relevant standardization bodies on national level in Europe and by the Health Care Informatics Standards Planning Panel (HISPP) in the USA.

In response to nurses wish to be part of the growing European health care informatics community the AIM office in 1991 launched TELENURSING, a so-called concerted action with the full title: A Concerted Action on European Classifications for Nursing Practice with special regard to Patient Problems/Nursing Diagnoses, Nursing Interventions and Outcomes.

2. Objectives

The overall objectives of TELENURSING can be summarized as follows:

2.1. To create a European Platform for nurses interested in classifications of patient problems/nursing diagnoses, interventions and outcomes and minimum data sets taking into account modern information technology.

2.2. To create European network of nurses interested in health care informatics and willing to participate in AIM consortia.

2.3. To create awareness among nurses of standardization efforts in health care informatics, e.g. CEN/TC/251 with regard to items of TELENURSING: Definition (Terminology) coding and classification.

2.4. To link the technical approach of CEN/TC/251 with the professional approach of WHO and ICN with regard to developments of classifications in health care.

3. Approach

In order to achieve these objectives TELENURSING will carry out three activities, namely:

3.1. Distribution and collection of TELENURSING questionnaire with three dimensions:

3.1a. a professional dimension: The nursing Process
  3.1b. a technical dimension: Documentation, Definition, Coding, Classification, Standardization, Nursing Minimum Data Sets and finally
  3.1c. a decisional dimension: From national to ward level,
3.2. Development of TELENURSING proposal for European Standard Data Sheet including examples of essential nursing care data:
  3.2a. patient problems/nursing diagnoses in order to describe diversity of patient population from a nursing point of view
  3.2b. nursing interventions in order to describe variability of practice patterns in nursing and finally
  3.2c. patient outcomes in order to describe clinical quality of nursing care and
3.3. Collection of data according to European Standard Data Sheet and creation of computerized "mini"-European Nursing Health Data Base according to structure of European Standard Data Sheet.

4. Results

Results of the TELENURSING questionnaire clearly demonstrates, that nurses in Europe are interested in initiatives to develop standards and nursing minimum data sets.

In the following countries, nurses and nurse researchers are actively engaged in initiatives of relevance to the development of standards and minimum data sets in nursing: Belgium, Denmark, Italy, Ireland, Netherlands, Portugal, Sweden, and UK.

5. Next step

TELENURSING hopes as part of the concerted action in Europe to achieve the development of standards and a Minimum Data Set of Essential Nursing Care Data to be collected for a Euro-Nursing Health Data Base!

Standardization in health care informatics is therefore not a goal in itself. The idea of TELENURSING as a European Concerted Action is to promote standardization of definitions, classifications, and coding of data in order to further the development of internationally comparable minimum data sets in nursing based upon uniform definitions of data items.

Real use of standards and minimum data sets is believed to improve availability, quality and comparability. By thus collecting real data on a small scale level TELENURSING hopes to create a learning and educational process to obtain a progressive better uniformity and comparability of essential nursing care data in Europe allowing comparisons between and inside European countries of data for the purpose of monitoring the efficiency of nursing care.

6. Implications

TELENURSING has, however, a wider perspective. Among the many aspects covered by the WHO's wide definition of the term "health" as "a complete state of physical, mental and social well-being" are aspects of health related to nursing. In order to highlight nurses contribution to the regional target of "health for all by the year 2000" WHO/EURO in 1981 initiated the multinational study "Peoples Need for Nursing Care" involving 11 European countries.

Peoples Need for Nursing Care can be regarded as the first attempt on a European level to define and collect information on aspects of physical, mental and social well-being related to nursing. At the same time the study was an attempt to supplement traditional health indicators of mortality and morbidity with measurable health indicators related to nursing.

WHO/EURO has recently (1993) proposed, that a national strategy on Continuous Quality Development should include development of adequate information systems based upon key basic minimum data sets comprising good clinical health indicators. It goes without saying, that development of adequate information systems measuring progress towards health for all by the year 2000 must include indicators of aspects of health, i.e. aspects of physical, mental and social well-being, related to nursing! In other words: Adequate information systems must include internationally comparable basic nursing minimum data sets based upon internationally comparable clinical indicators of aspects of health related to nursing.

TELENURSING is a small scale attempt to define and collect information on aspects of physical, mental and social well-being related to nursing. In a sense the idea of TELENURSING is to supplement traditional health indicators of mortality and morbidity with measurable health indicators related to nursing.

In a wider perspective TELENURSING therefore is a step towards data development for computerized nursing effectiveness research in Europe based upon clinical outcome indicators measuring essential aspects of health related to nursing.

7. How can nurses in Europe from a practical point of view

7.1.   Strengthen and coordinate their influence on the <u>standardization</u> efforts in health care informatics (e.g. CEN/TC/251) with regard to definitions and codings of nursing terminology related to the International Classification for Nursing Practice (ICNP) being developed by the international Council of Nurses (ICN)?

7.2.   Strengthen and coordinate their efforts to define, collect and analyze internationally comparable basic <u>minimum data sets</u> as envisioned by e.g. WHO/EURO in order to measure indicators of aspects of health, i.e. aspects of physical, mental and social well-being of patients, related to nursing using the EU R&D programme Advanced Informatics in Medicine (AIM)?

POSTERS

Nursing Informatics: An International Overview for Nursing in a Technological Era
S.J. Grobe and E.S.P. Pluyter-Wenting, eds.

Informatics in a nursing curriculum: Assessing attitudes.

Bostock EA and Hardy JL

School of Nursing and Human Movement, Australian Catholic University (NSW) 40 Edward Street, North Sydney, NSW 2060 Australia

Nurses' requirements in relation to education have changed with the advances occurring in technology and specifically with the introduction of computing technology in health care facilities. The Nursing Department of The Australian Catholic University (NSW), Sydney, Australia, acknowledged the need to prepare nurses for the technological advances of the workplace and introduced Computing and Nursing Informatics into the curriculum in 1992.

1. Introduction

The promotion of positive attitudes of nurses toward the use of automated information systems are as important as the technology itself. If nurses do not believe that the computer system will help them in the delivery of patient care, or enhance their educational goals, they will not use it [1]. It is therefore essential to measure and evaluate nurses attitudes to computers and nursing informatics.

The Nursing Studies unit integrated Nursing Research, Computing and Nursing Informatics as a year long subject taught to first year nursing undergraduate students. The unit was perceived by the researchers as being dynamic and providing an opportunity to plan, act, observe, reflect and evaluate in a manner consistent with the model offered by Action Research. The structure of the unit was designed after reviewing the literature and consulting with peers. A framework of Action Research was employed to gather information. Two evaluation instruments were employed; a 10 Item Questionnaire using a 4 point Likert scale and Focus Group Interviews.

2. Poster goals

The poster will (1) summarise the development of the course design (2) describe the methods of assessing student attitudes to a Nursing Informatics program and (3) present the findings of the study.

3. References

[1] Schwirian PM, Malone JA, Stone VJ, Nunley B and Francisco T. Computers in nursing practice: A comparison of the attitudes of nurses and nursing students. *Comp Nurs* 1989, 7: 168-177.

Nursing Informatics: An International Overview for Nursing in a Technological Era
S.J. Grobe and E.S.P. Pluyter-Wenting, eds.

A Health Education Program for the Elderly in Their Homes Provided by ADN Students with Notebook Computers

Cooper C, Gerth S, Hamilton L, Lewis K, and Randolph J

Faculty Members, School of Nursing , Parkland College. 2400 W. Bradley. Champaign, Il. 61821

1. Purpose

The purpose of this project is to examine the effect of Associate Degree Nursing students' use of notebook computers and a specific nutritional software package to structure health teaching provided to frail elderly clients in their homes. The two hypothesis being tested are:

1. Students who utilize a computer software package with their client for the nutritional assessment and teaching assignment will provide more information than students who rely on non- computer based reference materials and resources.

2. Frail elderly clients will improve their nutritional intake when the student utilizes the structure of a computer software package rather than rely on written references and resources.

2. Methodology

Clients are the frail elderly with a score above 21 on the Mini-Mental-State Examination(MMSE) assigned to students by a social service agency with whom Parkland College collaborates to provide a student practicum. Frail elderly clients assigned to the treatment group will utilize a notebook computer to analyze a written dietary record. The student and the client in the home setting will review the dietary analysis and identify foods to improve nutritional status using a nutrition software package. Four weeks after the computer assisted instruction the student and the client will use the nutritional software package to analyze and identify any change in the clients' dietary patterns. The control group will follow the same procedure except that, instead of using the identified computer software package, students will analyze their client's dietary log using a paper and pencil procedure learned and used in a prior course. The student will use written resource materials for analysis and teaching regarding client's nutritional status.

3. Data Analysis

The hypotheses will be tested using a T-Test aimed at the detection of any significant differences between the amount of information given(Hypothesis 1) and the learning outcomes as measured by changes in the clients dietary patterns (Hypothesis 2) when the structured is compared to the unstructured treatments.

Nursing Informatics: An International Overview for Nursing in a Technological Era
S.J. Grobe and E.S.P. Pluyter-Wenting, eds.

An Author Co-Citation Analysis of Published Maternal and Child Health Nursing Research from 1986-1990

D'Auria J P

Assistant Professor of Nursing, Dept of Health of Women & Children, The University of North Carolina at Chapel Hill, Chapel Hill, North Carolina 27599-7460, USA.

Author co-citation analysis (ACA) is a bibliometric strategy for generating visual representations of the scholarly evolution of an emerging disciplinary field using its published literature. Descriptive and/or multivariate statistical strategies may be used to identify prominant individuals cited in published research literature and the range of influence they are having in the emergence of a new field. The purpose of this study was to explore and describe the evolving intellectual structure of the scholarly community in the maternal and child health nursing (MCN) subfield as represented in the citation patterns of published nursing research from 1976-1990. Due to the emergent nature of MCN research literature, an ACA was conducted using frequently cited and co-cited primary nurses and nonnurse authors from 1986-1990. The unit of analysis is the body of works *(oeurve)* by an individual author. Authors whose works are seen as related are jointly cited (co-cited) in subsequent research documents. The frequency of co-citation provides evidence of a relationship between two works as judged by nurse researchers who published in the scientific literature being investigated. Prior research in other disciplinary fields have supported that authors who cluster together represent an effective way to retrieve information when paired in author searches.

This study is the first ACA conducted with the nursing literature. A citation index was constructed using cited nurse and nonnurse authors ($\underline{N}$ = 2703) from 187 MCN research articles in *Journal of Advanced Nursing (JAN), Nursing Research (NR), Research in Nursing & Health (RINAH)*, and *Western Journal of Nursing Research (WJNR)* from 1986-1990. Data were collected from Social SCISEARCH® with the exception of WJNR which was manually entered. An analytic database of authors cited 14 or more times from 1986-1990 was created. In both cases, an insufficient number of authors met the criteria for multivariate analysis. The first author set included all primary nurses and nonnurse authors who were cited 14 or more times by MCN researchers publishing from 1986-1990. Co-cited author pairs were compiled and co-citation frequencies were counted. Cocitation summary statistics were reported and analyzed for the co-cited authors with a mean co-citation frequency of 2 or more over the 5 year period. Due to the low occurrence of co-citation among scholars in the first author set, a second author set was selected using only primary nurse authors. There was a generally low consensus among citing nurse author's in the referencing of authors' works as well as the perceptions of relationships (co-citations) of authors' works in the MCN subfield. Data supported the emergence of an embryonic network of MCN scholars with citation histories and co-citations specificially in the research specialty area focused on maternal behavior during the prenatal, postpartum, and/or infancy periods. Further features of nursing science in the MCN subfield were not visible using citation data.

The results of this bibliometric analysis support the value of applying alternative research methodologies to the published literature in the field of nursing. Rigorous and systematic bibliometric research of citation data will contribute working models of the development of nursing science which can be used to evaluate scientific progress in the field of nursing. This research may increase the visibility of scientific information and facilitate the networking of scientists and research information in the field of nursing. Further studies are needed to validate the assumptions of ACA in the nursing literature. Contextual analyses and keyword analyses of related (co-cited) authors' work would provide insight into the communication patterns of nurse scholars and suggest ways to enhance the dissemination of scientific communication and prevent the loss of knowledge being developed in the MCN subfield More importantly, bibliometric studies may provide alternative views of the evolution of nursing knowledge, thus, opening up new avenues for debate and hypothesis generation among scholars in regard to the evolution of nursing science.

Identifying the information usage patterns of a diverse nursing population

Pravikoff DS and Hillson SB

CINAHL Information Systems, Glendale Adventist Medical Center, 1509 Wilson Terrace, Glendale, California 91209, United States of America

This poster presentation describes the way in which diverse segments of the nursing population meet their information needs. Its specific purpose is to compare both information needs and information access in nursing students, nurse clinicians, nurse executives, faculty and researchers attending various informational conferences or belonging to a wide range of nursing specialty groups.

The questionnaire asked specifically how often these nurses consulted information resources, what sources were used, whether computers were accessed, whether the nurses utilized various on-line and/or CD-ROM products, and how satisfied they were with the information obtained. The study period spanned the years 1989 to 1993.

Specific information on computer familiarity and participation in nursing research, journals most frequently accessed, and barriers to accessing information will be presented. Relationships, if any, between these and other variables and demographic data will be discussed. Comparisons will be made between the various nursing groups.

Based on the results of this research, steps will be recommended to assist professional nurses to use information in the most effective way possible.

© 1994 Elsevier Science B.V. All rights reserved.
Nursing Informatics: An International Overview for Nursing in a Technological Era
S.J. Grobe and E.S.P. Pluyter-Wenting, eds.

759

Benefit analysis of implementing a bedside terminal computerized system

Gallien-Patterson Q

VA West Side Medical Center, Chicago, IL, 60612

1. Introduction

Computerized patient care systems have become available to health caregivers in most hospitals from a central location. This type of access prohibits prompt updating and retrieving of patient information. In general, bedside monitoring is a concept which augments or enhances centralized patient care systems with bedside terminals placed at the point-of-care (POC), the patient's bedside or treatment site. This is a study designed to examine the benefits of implementing a bedside monitoring (POC), system on a typical patient care ward of a Veteran Health Service Medical Center. POC systems were introduced primarily to capture immediately observed patient data. Facilitating timely monitoring of patient data assures more informed clinical making decisions by nurses, according to Herring [1]. Denger [2] reports other perceived benefits to include reduced nurse overtime, retaining/attracting nursing staff, better accounting of clinical costs, reducing patient length of stay, liability reduction, and standardization of patient care.

The approach and technology used in choosing and implementing a POC system is based on the type of care provided to the patient, the structural environment, and the complexity of the tasks or activities performed. Devices used in a POC system can vary from fixed to portable or a combination.

2. Methodology

This study was conducted for approximately one year (June 1991-September 1992). Two tools were developed; one to assess staffs' perceptions and another to measure time required by nurses to perform and document care for selected nursing procedures, i.e., admissions, vital signs, intake and output, developing and revising care plans and end-of-shift reporting. The tool to assess the nursing staffs' perceptions was a pen and pencil test administered to all nursing staff working on the ward both prior to and after initiation of project. Due to time and personnel constraints, this study focused on the nurse's role, however it was felt that informal data collection on other caregivers could be used to direct future studies.

3. Conclusions

The implementation of a point-of-care system has provided the Veteran Health Administration with a prototype POC model. When all factors are examined there appears to be evidence to support implementation. The nursing staff was optimistic about the concept of POC; 69% pre-installation and 100% post-installation. It was felt both pre and post installation that bedside terminals would increase nurse productivity, improve accuracy/legibility and quality of documentation, increase accessibility of patient data, and improve information gathering/retrieval (100%). 77% of staff felt that they would make a quick adjustment to POC pre-installation as compared to 100% post-installation, indicating that the system is user-friendly. Stationary terminals were preferred, 53% pre-installation and 100% post-installation.

A comparison of Pre and Post POC data from a time and motion study showed a decrease in the amount of time needed to perform selected nursing procedures. Overall a total of 13.5 minutes/patient potential time savings was realized with the POC computerized system.

4. References

[1] Herring D. A Closer Look at Bedside Terminals. *Nurs Manag* 1990, 7: 54-61.
[2] Denger S and et al. Implementing an Integrated Clinical Information System. *Jour of Nurs Admin*, 1992, 8(12) 28-34.

Nursing Informatics: An International Overview for Nursing in a Technological Era
S.J. Grobe and E.S.P. Pluyter-Wenting, eds.

Role of computers in nursing research

Grzankowski J

State University of New York at Buffalo; Buffalo, NY 14211

1. Introduction

Nursing research, as with any other type of research, entails the collection and evaluation of a large volume of data. The computer has made significant contributions to this process. This assistance is examined in relation to the five phases of the research process: assessment, planning, implementation, and evaluation.

2. Assessment

Some data banks available for use in the assessment phase are CINAHL, Medline, ERIC, and SUPERINDEX. These data banks can review present citations and abstracts on pertinent topics, help delimit the problem, identify theory and variables, and help the researcher formulate his/her hypothesis.

3. Planning and implementation

Questions to consider when entering the planning phase such as selecting a research design, specifying a population, as well as conducting a pilot study, and assisting in the collection of research data are tasks which the computer is capable of. Software can help the researcher in both descriptive and inferential statistics and reports. Some thoughts on computer simulation to consider are its ability to overcome methodological limitations while still maintaining validity.

4. Evaluation

The advantages of word processing software in presenting a comprehensive report are part of the evaluation phase. The software available helps to present the data in both text and graphic form. The use of e-mail, networks, and lightweight disks allow for the inexpensive and quick distribution of research findings.

5. Legal & ethical considerations

The legal and ethical considerations regarding patient confidentiality are professional codes of ethics, common law, and specific computer access laws with references to statutes which currently cover information accessibility and policies regarding computer operators' privileges and responsibilities.

Nursing Informatics: An International Overview for Nursing in a Technological Era
S.J. Grobe and E.S.P. Pluyter-Wenting, eds.

761

"Touching the Patient Through the Science of Technology: The Clinical Perspective"

Lehmkuhl, Diana, R.N., M.E.D.[a]; Harsanyi, Bennie E., R.N., Ed.D.,[b]
Hott, Roger, R.N., M.M.[c]; McGeehan, Lisa, M.B.A.[d]

[a,b,c,d,] SMS, 51 Valley Stream Parkway, Malvern, PA 19355

We as nurses must touch technology in order to touch our patients with quality care derived from the translation of data into information and ultimately into clinical knowledge. As nursing care has evolved, the demands for the integration of complex data from diverse sources across episodes of care, institutional and organizational boundaries, and windows of time have also evolved. The pursuit of technology to deliver this quality care has also escalated. This poster presents the current and future technology available to address the relevant health care industry trends and resulting business and clinical issues regarding nursing care delivery.

A model illustrating the health care industry trends, associated nursing care delivery issues, and the technological options will be used to address six major areas currently being challenged and impacting nursing care delivery. These areas include organizational structures, management approaches, health care roles, consumers' perceptions of quality, delivery practices, and evaluation of care delivery. For example, the trend towards managed care has resulted in a business issue of a cost/profitability analysis across the health care continuum. The relevant clinical issue is the delivery of cost-effective therapeutic options resulting in predictable patient outcomes. The technological solution includes automated case management, integrated relational data bases, expert care rules, and decision support technology. The trends toward organizational restructuring results in a business issue of performance analysis across the health care enterprise and continuum of care. The clinical issue is the required access by multi-disciplinary care providers to comprehensive and integrated patient centered information. The technological solution includes open system architecture and the electronic patient record including medical and document imaging. A major trend is consumer satisfaction which includes the business issue of marketing health care services ranging from wellness and prevention to home health care. The clinical issue is education of the consumer and the inclusion of the consumer in his/her health care decision making. The technological solution includes the availability of online patient centered data, support for diverse data entry and access options, and multimedia patient education tools. The trend towards continual quality improvement requires a strategic business focus. The clinical issue is continual refinement of treatment options, patient centered delivery processes, and outcome evaluation. The technology includes computerized protocols, standards, taxonomies, and outcome relational data bases for internal and external clinical comparisons.

Nursing Informatics: An International Overview for Nursing in a Technological Era
S.J. Grobe and E.S.P. Pluyter-Wenting, eds.

762

Traditional and non-traditional baccalaureate nursing students and attitude toward computer-based video instruction

Hassett M R[a] Hassett C M[b] and Koerner D K[a]

[a]Dept of Nursing, Fort Hays State University, 600 Park St, Hays, KS 67601-4099 USA

[b]Dept of Computer Information Systems & Quantitative Methods, Fort Hays State University, 600 Park St, Hays, KS 67601-4099 USA

1. Introduction

This exploratory descriptive investigation examined whether differences existed among traditional and non-traditional baccalaureate nursing student subjects who used a Computer-Based Video Instruction (CBVI) program with learner control options. Mruk [1] found that individualized instruction rather than heavy formal structure created a more effective learning environment for non-traditional learners. The theoretical framework included Gagne's conditions of learning [2]. A sample of volunteer students from four groups ($\underline{N}$ = 82) was recruited.

2. Tools

Tools used were: computer-based Screening Pretest (SP); CBVI program with learner control options and Embedded Content Questions (ECQ); and a computer-based Adjective Rating Scale (ARS). Acceptable reliability and validity data were established. The study examined differences by traditional (24 and younger) and non-traditional (25 and older) subjects on: ARS scores, learner control choices, and test scores.

3. Data

The SP showed a relatively high level of previous knowledge ($\underline{M}$ = 70%). Both traditional ($\underline{n}$ = 54) and non-traditional ($\underline{n}$ = 28) subjects indicated positive attitudes toward CBVI, a 12% increase in scores was found following the computer-based content, and learner control choices were commonly not made. An interesting, though not significant result (*chi square*, $\underline{p}$ = .08), showed a clear tendency to see more information when that choice was available ($\underline{n}$ = 36, 44%). A greater percentage of non-traditionals chose this and they scored 4% higher on ECQ.

4. Conclusions

This investigation indicated that CBVI can be effective and acceptable learning method for both traditional and non-traditional baccalaureate nursing students. Findings are similar to those of a previous study conducted in 1989 with the same CBVI program [3], this time using a larger sample and adding non-traditionals.

5. References

[1]   Mruk, CJ. Teaching Adult Learners Basic Computer Skills: A New Look at Age, Sex, and Motivational Factors. *Colleg Microcomputer* 1987, 5:294-300.
[2]   Gagne, RM. *The Conditions of Learning and Theory of Instruction* (4th ed.). New York: Holt, Rinehart and Winston, 1985.
[3]   Hassett, MR. Differences in Attitude Toward Computer-Based Video Instruction and Learner Control Choices Made by Baccalaureate Nursing Students of Sensing and Intuitive Psychological Type (Doctoral dissertation, The University of Texas at Austin, 1990). *Diss Abstr Internl* 1991, 51: 4277-B.

© 1994 Elsevier Science B.V. All rights reserved.
Nursing Informatics: An International Overview for Nursing in a Technological Era
S.J. Grobe and E.S.P. Pluyter-Wenting, eds.

Communication Networks: A Tool for Nurse Researchers

Holtzclaw B J

Office of Research, School of Nursing, University of Texas Health Science Center at San Antonio, 7703 Floyd Curl Drive, San Antonio, Texas 78284-7947

Nurse researchers need access to the latest in nursing knowledge to plan proposals and publish relevant manuscripts. While some of this knowledge is published and available through traditional library networks an indexes, a considerable amount is evolving or awaiting publication. Researchers remain on the cutting edge of their science by direct contact with other investigators. They provide methodological, theoretical, and clinical consultations, collaborate on studies, and share findings with one another. Needs for such interchange are often so urgent, complex, and geographically extensive that conventional mail or telephone communication is expensive in cost and convenience. Computer linked communication networks and electronic mail (e-mail) offer diverse resources for the nurse researcher with systems that may already be in place. The mainframe computer has long the statistical workhorse of research-active faculty. Yet, surprisingly few have taken advantage of the computer's capability for accessing networks. Once a user account is established at a participating institution, there is no cost for communicating with other network users anywhere in the world.

Several worldwide network systems connect computers in academic and research settings but most universities use BITNET (Because It's Time Network) and Internet. To use these networks, one gains access through a designated "host" institution that subscribes to the service. The subscribing institution, in turn, allow individual users to use the network. Universities vary in support of network use: some charging faculty nothing, while others bill for time and file storage. Once the account is established, the user has access to other network users anywhere in the world. Networks offer multiple services to the nurse researcher: 1) free long-distance communication, 2) the option of writing and transmitting messages in a single operation, 3) 24 hours a day service, 4) message storage for the recipient, 5) access to electronic newsletters, journals, or libraries, and 6) document transfer capability to others on the electronic network. Services are as close as the user's terminal or modem-linked personal computer (PC).

Sigma Theta Tau, International, is pioneering network use through their Virginia Henderson International Nursing Library (INL) system accessible through Internet and their network-linked electronic journal, *The Online Journal of Knowledge Synthesis for Nursing* launched at the 1994 Sigma Theta Tau International biennial convention. Networks provide National or regional research associations excellent means for communicating calls for abstracts, reports, or notices. Some organizations foster this communication by special sessions on network use at their research conferences. Another route for disseminating research information is the *listserver*, a news service to which individuals subscribe and communicate through a membership distribution list. E-mail is likely to play a more important part in all NIH and federal document dispersal in the future because of its obvious cost savings. The *NIH Guide for Grants and Contracts* is already accessible through Internet.

Obviously the communication network is only effective if it is used. To access a wide cluster of colleagues or consultants, there must be a wide circle of network users. Research directors in academic and clinical settings are in excellent positions to demystify use of computer networks and develop networks between researchers and research consumers. This scenario includes the nurse in the clinical setting bringing patient-care problems to the research network for discussion and assessment of the current state of the science with nurses and researchers in other settings. Researchers in academic settings come to the network for reality checks and input into research proposals and to share findings. As the network grows, the circle of users and the scope of expertise and knowledge increases.

Growing use of computer networks by research colleagues will lead to new innovations in their use and the future for this mode of communication appears bright. Use of electronic communications networks for nurse researchers provides efficient, cost-effective and relatively simple ways for keeping current, sharing information, and improving the state of the science.

Nursing Informatics: An International Overview for Nursing in a Technological Era
S.J. Grobe and E.S.P. Pluyter-Wenting, eds.

Computer Applications to Stimulate Critical Thinking

Hribar, K.

Clinical Nurse Specialist, University Hospitals of Cleveland, Cleveland, Ohio

1.   Critical Thinking

Nursing is a science of ever increasing complexities. New technologies have increased the quantity of data collected on a single patient to overwhelming volumes of facts. The nurse managing patient care needs to synthesize and process a vast array of data. This process of collecting data, evaluating data and making clinical care decisions or judgements is the critical thinking process in clinical nursing practice.

The stress of responsibility for the results of actual clinical care decisions often overwhelms students and new nurses. The inexperienced practitioner finds him or herself unwilling to take a risk; one which might also put the patient at risk. The challenge of clinical nursing education becomes that of providing early opportunities to practice critical thinking skills and build a background of experiences in an environment less threatening than the actual patient care setting.

2.   Applications

One of the most adaptable means of building such experiences is through the use of computer simulations. The *TLC General Hospital* is one such program. This practice clinical information system provides complete clinical data records for various simulated patients. Data is provided on medications, orders, tests, charting, virtually every imaginable component of a patient's paper chart. Because of the realistically vast amount of data available on each patient, students can practice reviewing data for significance and making clinical judgements based on the data presented. Unlike in a simple instructor designed patient case study, there are no prompts as to what type of data is most significant. The practitioner must evaluate and judge...and learn in the process while building experiences in clinical decision making.

While the TLC program provides a vast bank of patient data, the true value in utilizing such a system comes from the design of the decision-making applications. Assignments may be as simple as adding an intervention to the careplan or prioritizing the nursing activities. Because the program is not interactive, hypothetical patient responses need to be generated by the preceptor or instructor. Expert feedback is vital for learners to discover the consequences of their patient care decisions.

The use of interactive video programs moves the computer simulation of critical thinking to a more experiential level. In an interactive video disc program like AJN's *Care of the Elderly COPD Patient*, the learner is presented with more sensory data. Sights and sounds simulate a realistic clinical presentation. Questions guide the student through the experience. The student is prompted through data collection and questioned on appropriate clinical decisions. Immediate feedback is offered for correct or incorrect responses. The realism of the presentations challenging the viewer, and encourages continued the success in critical thinking by the practice of clinical decision making skills.

Nursing Informatics: An International Overview for Nursing in a Technological Era
S.J. Grobe and E.S.P. Pluyter-Wenting, eds.

765

Developing a new paradigm for nursing documentation

Ireson C L [a] and Velotta C L [b]

[a] Dept of Nursing, University of Kentucky Hospital, 800 Rose Street, Lexington, Kentucky, USA

[b] Dept of Information Management, University of Kentucky, 800 Rose Street, Lexinton, Kentucky, USA

Two major factors influence new paradigms structuring documentation of the nursing process: (a) the need to consider the incremental needs of the patient when planning and documenting care (b) the role of a computer system to facilitate the structure of documentation.

The care plan is the best known and most widely used schema for organizing the collection and storage of nursing data [1]. It provides space for nursing diagnosis, expected patient outcomes, and interventions. The evaluation component, however, has no defined location. Consequently, nurses give more attention to documenting the assessment and intervention components of the nursing process than to evaluating the effects of nursing care.

Structuring evaluation as a decision tree by breaking desired patient outcomes into subgoals improved nurses' ability to evaluate patient progress, thus should contribute to outcome attainment. This labor intensive function, when done manually, does not prompt the nurse to consider whether the interactions with the patient and the patient's response were congruent with the intended plan of care. Traditional nursing care plans function in a linear decision making mode connecting nursing diagnoses to expected patient outcomes. In contrast, expert decision makers use pattern recognition to break complex problems into smaller parts. Similarly, structuring subgoals to allow for continual evaluation supports the iterative process necessary for validation and /or revision of the care plan to reach desired outcome goals.

Once a care plan with incremental subgoals has been formulated, two challenges remain to operationalize the planning tool. First, the predetermined interventions must be actualized in the context of the daily workload. Then, the effect of the interventions on the patient outcomes must be analyzed. Automated systems can engage the nurse in cognitive processes that direct decisions toward intended outcomes or assist in making adjustments that meet the patient's needs. Computerized patient records are not superior to manual records in reaching outcomes since they merely replicate traditional charting methods [2]. Advanced nursing systems must use a model that reflect cognitive strategies used by experts.

References

[1] Grier, MR. Information Processing in Nursing Practice. *Annu Rev Nurs Res* 1984, 2: 265-287.
[2] Holzemer, WL and Henry SB. Computer-supported Versus Manually-generated Nursing Care Plans. *Comput Nurs* 1991, 10:19-24.

Nursing Informatics: An International Overview for Nursing in a Technological Era
S.J. Grobe and E.S.P. Pluyter-Wenting, eds.

A Qualitative Look at Interactive Video From the Nursing Student's Perspective

McGonigle D[a] Wedge K[b] Bricker P[c] and Quigley A[d]

[a]*School of Nursing, Penn State University, University Park, PA 16802-6508 USA*

[b]*School of Nursing, University of Pittsburgh, Pittsburgh, PA 15261 USA*

[c]*Doctoral Candidate, School of Nursing, University of Pittsburgh, Pittsburgh, PA 15261 USA*

[d]*Adult Education, Penn State University, Monroeville, PA 15146 USA*

1. Introduction

The conceptual framework for this research project arises from Knowles' [1] theory of andragogy that both empowers the learner's selection of relevant content and enhances self-directedness. Andragogical, or adult learning, principles apply to nursing students; as adults, they build on and relate to past experiences they have encountered. The purpose of this qualitative descriptive study is to determine the extent of the andragogical effectiveness of interactive video from the learner's perspective. This study will provide learner-based information that nurse educators need in order to assess the integration of interactive video into nursing education.

2. Sample

This opportunistic and purposeful sample will consist of six generic nursing students from the University of Pittsburgh and six registered nurse students returning for their baccalaureate degrees at Penn State University. In addition, one generic nursing student and one registered nurse student will participate in the pilot phase of this study.

3. Method

This study will be carried out by means of one semi-structured interview consisting of open-ended questions to explore the perceptions of nursing students using interactive video. Each participant will complete the interactive video program, *Perinatal Family Care* and be interviewed within two weeks of completion.

4. Findings

This project is in process and the findings will be presented at the Symposium.

5. References

[1]   Knowles, M. *Andragogy in Action*. San Francisco: Jossey-Bass, 1984.

Environmental Model for the Identification and Prioritization of Nursing Applications

Nagle L M Meadwell K Cechetto B

Nursing Informatics Program, Gerald P. Turner Department of Nursing, Mount Sinai Hospital,
600 University Avenue, Toronto, Ontario CANADA M5G 1X5

A majority of health care settings have opted for multi-modular, single vendor software solutions for clinical and administrative applications. Yet some organizations have opted for non-modular, multi-vendor solutions for the same information management functions. Either approach necessitates decision-making related to the selection and implementation of each system component. This paper describes an environmental model developed by a nursing department which has chosen the multi-vendor approach to managing nursing information. The model addresses the identification of potential applications of information technology and the prioritization of these applications within the context of the departmental, professional, and political environments of an organization. Advancing the development and adoption of information technologies within any organization will be largely governed by a myriad of internal and external environmental factors. In the process of identifying and prioritizing applications, criteria for product and post-implementation evaluation are logically generated. The model clearly supports the dynamic nature of nursing and illustrates the inherent value of a holistic, environmental approach in considering the adoption of information technology.

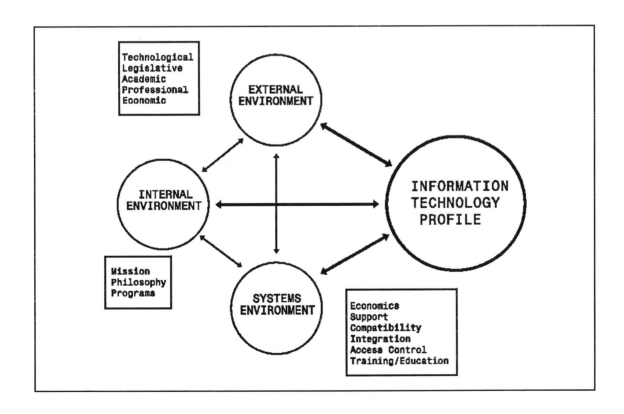

© 1994 Elsevier Science B.V. All rights reserved.
Nursing Informatics: An International Overview for Nursing in a Technological Era
S.J. Grobe and E.S.P. Pluyter-Wenting, eds.

Successful implementation of computer-assisted instruction (CAI)

Perciful EG

Associate Professor, Nursing Department, West Chester University, Church Street, West Chester, Pennsylvania, United States

Quality assurance and cost containment are words echoed throughout the world today. Implementing computer technology is expensive. Sharing information that increases the likelihood of success is therefore imperative. The purpose of this study was to describe the factors associated with successful implementation of CAI. Lewin's concept of planned change provided the framework for this ex post facto correlational study. The purposively selected sample of baccalaureate nursing programs (N=77) had received grant money from the Helene Fuld Health Trust to implement computer technology. Data were provided by nurse faculty (N=278).

Data collection method was a mail survey with findings based upon a 51% response rate. The survey included: a demographic form, the Planning and Implementing Phases for CAI (PIP-CAI), the Successful Implementation of CAI (SI-CAI) [1], and the Attitude Toward CAI [2]. A content validity index of .81 for the PIP-CAI and, .79 for the SI-CAI was established by a panel of eight experts in nursing and computers. Cronbach's reliability coefficient for the PIP-CAI was .91 with a sample of 278 nurse faculty. Both the Attitude Toward CAI and the SI-CAI had alpha coefficients of .88. The potential range in scores for the SI-CAI including the addition of a scaled score derived from the Attitude Toward CAI was from 24 to 120. A cutoff score of greater than 77 was used to indicate the presence of increasing degrees of successful implementation of CAI.

Data analysis included descriptive statistics, correlation correlation coefficients, and ANOVA. Findings revealed that 39 of the 77 nursing programs in the sample (50.6%) had achieved success with the implementation of CAI. Analysis of variance showed no significant ($p<05$) difference between those schools scoring lower degrees of success (scores of 77 or lower), and those schools scoring higher degrees of success (scores greater than 77), with respect to four demographic variables (size of the institution according to the number of FTE students, number of computers within the institution for student use, number of computers within the nursing building(s) for student use, and the number of different software programs owned by the nursing programs). Study findings also suggested that successful implementation of CAI is not associated with the length of either the planning or implementing phases.

Eight factors comprising the predictor variable, planned change, were entered into a stepwise multiple regression to examine their contribution to the prediction of the degree of successful implementation of CAI. The eight factors, consisting of four factors present during both the planning and implementing phases, include: administrative support, resources, faculty support, and faculty participation. Faculty support during the implementation phase entered on the first step ($R=.58$, $p<.0001$). Resources during the implementation phase entered on the second step ($R=.65$, $p<.01$). The final factor entered was administrative support during the planning phase ($R=.68$, $p<.05$). The amount of variance in successful implementation of CAI explained by these three factors was 46.5%. In conclusion, efforts to assist with the planned implementation of CAI within nursing education need to focus on acquiring administrative support during the planning phase and maintaining faculty support and adequate resources throughout the implementation.

1. References

[1] Perciful EG. The relationship between planned change and successful implementation of computer-assisted instruction (CAI) as perceived by nurse faculty. *Dissertation Abstracts International* 1991, 52: 25504B. (University Microfilms No. 91-29261).

[2] Allen LR. Measuring attitude toward computer assisted instruction: The development of a semantic differential tool. *Comput Nurs* 1986, 4: 144-151.

© 1994 Elsevier Science B.V. All rights reserved.
Nursing Informatics: An International Overview for Nursing in a Technological Era
S.J. Grobe and E.S.P. Pluyter-Wenting, eds.

The Evaluation Of A Planned Process For Facilitating The Use of Nursing Informatics In a Nursing Curriculum

Rossel C L

College of Nursing, Lewis University, RT 53, Romeoville, IL 60441 USA

1. Introduction

This evaluation research examined outcomes of the use of Nursing Informatics in the nursing curriculum at both the Baccalaureate and Master's level and attempted to elucidate the potential future of the nursing computer lab within that context. During the 1992-1993 and 1993-1994 school years, the following data were collected: 1. survey of second semester sophomore students to determine level of computer experience; 2. survey of graduate students who had completed the *Nursing Infomatics* course for evidence of change; 3. content analysis of the Baccalaureate course syllabi for inclusion of Computer Assisted Instruction (CAI) as a teaching methodology and listing of CAI titles in the Activity column; 4. comparison of use of Nursing Informatics applications in the graduate program between the spring of 1992 and spring of 1994; 5. survey of computer lab use; 6. survey of faculty regarding present and potential educational uses of computers; and 7. trace the evolving process of the computerization of the University at large and its impact on the College of Nursing.

2. Tools

The tools used were developed by the researcher and reviewed by an expert in the field of instrument development. The tool used with the sophomore students to determine level of computer experience and the tool used with graduate students who had completed the *Nursing Infomatics* course were piloted tested. Test-retest reliability and content validity were acceptable.

3. Findings

Most of the 87 sophomore students had used a computer to search the literature and write a paper. However, none of had any knowledge or experience with CAI and/or interactive video. Of the 70 graduate students, 97% reported that they felt more comfortable using a computer and used a computer more at work. Graduates also expressed more confidence in their ability to independently problem-solve questions about software applications. Most of the students used the CAI or interactive video when it was required by the instructor. When a structured application was developed by the instructor, use increased to 100%. CAI that was listed as optional was seldom used. Content analysis of the course syllabi indicated that about half listed the available CAI and interactive video. These findings helped faculty identify the need to link the use of CAI directly to course objectives and to list the experience as *required*. For the graduate courses, in the spring of 1992, only N555-Nursing Informatics was related to the use of computer technology in nursing. By the Spring of 1994, applications and software had been integrated into most of the courses. Graduate student demonstration of ability to use Nursing Informatics was identified as a desirable goal but has yet to be defined. Faculty's vision of future uses included a link with clinical agencies for orientation to the agency's documentation system. The 20 faculty responding reported that learning objectives that would incorporate computer technology should be integrated into each of the nursing clinical courses. Todate, about half of the courses include these objectives.

© 1994 Elsevier Science B.V. All rights reserved.
Nursing Informatics: An International Overview for Nursing in a Technological Era
S.J. Grobe and E.S.P. Pluyter-Wenting, eds.

A Clinical Approach to the Development of a Nursing Data Set

Workman LL[a] and Dool JB[b]

[a]*Deptartment of Patient Care Services, University of Cincinnati Hospital, 234 Goodman, Cincinnati OH 24567*

[b]*Deptartment of Patient Care Services, University of Cincinnati Hospital, 234 Goodman, Cincinnati OH 24567*

The Nursing Minimum Data Set (NMDS), its components, and application to nursing practice have been described in the literature as a standardized process which can be used to regularly collect essential and comparable core nursing data across settings.[1] According to Werley et al,[1] the elements of the NMDS include: Nursing Care Elements; Patient or Client Demographic Elements; and Service Elements. The collection and analysis of data around these elements and subelements provided nurses the information needed to compare care and outcomes across populations, settings, geographic areas, and time. This data can further be used to determine nursing resources needed and to evaluate effectiveness and efficiency of nursing care delivery. The purpose of this project was to develop a comprehensive nursing data set which would organize patient related health characteristics, nursing diagnoses, nursing interventions, and patient outcomes. In keeping with the need for a standardized data set in nursing as defined by Werley and Lang,[1] a project was undertaken at a major university health sciences center to develop a computerized nursing data set (NDS). This project was viewed as consistent with the American Nurses Association database initiative.

Phase I of this project involved the development of patient care standards. The organizing framework used was the Oncology Nursing Society standards[2] from which 11 functional categories: Health Promotion, Information, Coping and Cognition, Comfort and Sleep, Nutrition, Protective Mechanisms, Mobility, Elimination, Reproduction/Sexuality, Ventilation, and Circulation were identified. Using these 11 functional categories, patient outcome standards were developed for the 3 clinical nursing areas: acute care, critical care, and ambulatory/community care. Establishment of outcome standards across settings was directed at enhancement of care continuity.

In Phase II, Carpenito's[3] nursing diagnostic categories provided structure for the identification of related clinical factors, medical conditions (DRGs), nursing interventions, and patient outcomes. Next, using McCloskey and Bulechek's[4] text as a primary reference, all nursing interventions related to each of the nursing diagnoses were reviewed and validated. Nursing actions identified by McCloskey and Bulechek were further differentiated as nursing assessment activities or as nursing interventions. This activity was viewed as critical in the delineation of independent from dependent nursing actions within the NDS. To accomplish the project goal, 11 clinical nursing groups whose clinical expertise corresponded with the defined functional categories were established. Group membership consisted of 105 nurses from all clinical areas.

Phase III of the project focused on data analysis. In this phase all materials developed were circulated among all clinical groups for verification and/or inclusion of clinical findings, related factors, DRGs, nursing diagnoses, and nursing interventions appropriate to each clinical specialty. The outcome of the process was the development of a comprehensive set of data related to each of the nursing diagnostic categories. Content validity was established using content experts.

References

[1] Werley HH and Lang NM (eds.). *Identification of the nursing minimum data set*. New York: Springer Publishing Co., 1988.

[2] *Standards of Oncology Nursing Practice* (1987). Kansas City: American Nurses Association and Oncology Nurses Society, 1987.

[3] Carpenito LJ. *Handbook of Nursing Diagnosis* (4th ed.). Philadelphia: J.B. Lippincott Co., 1991.

[4] McCloskey JC and Bulechek GM (eds.). *Nursing Interventions Classification (NIC)*. St. Louis: Mosby-Year Book, Inc., 1992.

© 1994 Elsevier Science B.V. All rights reserved.
Nursing Informatics: An International Overview for Nursing in a Technological Era
S.J. Grobe and E.S.P. Pluyter-Wenting, eds.

An Analysis of a Four Year Undergraduate Nursing Informatics Curriculum on Student Perceptions of Nursing Informatics

Travis L L[a] and Hoehn B[b]

[a]Frances Payne Bolton School of Nursing, Case Western Reserve University, 10900 Euclid Avenue, Cleveland, Ohio, 44106-4904.

[b]KPMG Peat Marwick, 345 Park Avenue, New York, New York, 10154.

In Fall 1990, the Frances Payne Bolton (FPB) School of Nursing formed a consortium with three major teaching centers, the Cleveland Clinic Foundation, MetroHealth Medical Center and the University Hospitals of Cleveland, to launch a new undergraduate program in Nursing. The program was designed to incorporate the best educational opportunities of collegiate preparation with those traditionally associated with the hospital-based diploma schools of nursing. A unique aspect of this program, differentiating it from other BSN programs, is the innovative inclusion of nursing informatics integrated throughout the four year curriculum. This informatics coursework provides the student with a pragmatic view of the available state-of-the-art technologies of the present and the potential technologies they will confront in the future. It is designed to complement the student's clinical as well as nursing science class work.[1] As evidence of the school's commitment to nursing informatics, the informatic coursework is required by all students for graduation from the BSN program.

The first class to complete this curriculum will graduate in the Spring of 1994. This paper will present the findings of a longitudinal study initiated at the start of the 1990 freshman course and conducted throughout the four year roll out of the Nursing Informatics track. We will discuss the students' initial perceptions of automation and how they have evolved over the course of the program.[2,3] We will also examine how their final perceptions compare with graduate nurses currently practicing in both automated and non-automated clinical environments.[4] It is our belief that these students will be their institutions' leaders and active participants in future nursing automation efforts. We will discuss our plans to track this class' career progression at predetermined intervals in an effort to identify their roles in nursing information systems projects and their evaluation of preparedness to assume this responsibility.

[1] National Center for Nursing Research. *Nursing Informatics: Enhancing Patient Care*. Bethesda, MD: U.S. Dept. of Health and Human Services, U.S. Public Health Services, National Institutes of Health, 1993.

[2] McConell, E A, O'Shea, S S and Kirchhoff, K T (1989). RN Attitudes Toward Computers. *Nursing Management* 1989, *20*(7): 36-40.

[3] Travis, L L and Youngblut, J. Supporting patient centered computing through an undergraduate nursing informatics curriculum: Stage III. In: *Proceedings of the Seventeenth Annual Symposium on Computer Applications in Medical Care*. Charles Safran (ed). New York: McGraw-Hill, 1993: 757-761.

[4] Sparks, S M. *Computer Based Education in Nursing*. Bethesda, MD: U.S. Dept. of Health and Human Services, National Institutes of Health, National Library of Medicine, 1990.

Nursing Informatics: An International Overview for Nursing in a Technological Era
S.J. Grobe and E.S.P. Pluyter-Wenting, eds.

772

Evaluation of Interactive Videodisc Simulations Designed for Nursing to Determine Their Ability to Provide Problem Solving Practice Based on the Use of the Nursing Process

Klaassens E L

Department of Nursing, Trinity Christian College, 6601 West College Drive, Palos Heights, Illinois 60463

1. Purpose of the Study

There is a dearth of research relating interactive videodiscs (IVD) to problem solving based on current literature both in America and internationally. This study was undertaken to test the claim that IVD simulations provide adequate practice of problem-solving for nursing students. The theoretical framework was the nursing process and the method of evaluation was computer program modeling [1].

2. Methods

An evaluation tool was designed that incorporated subcomponents of the steps of the nursing process as discrete cognitive elements to evaluate [2]. The tool was used by thirty three baccalaureate nurse educators who viewed one of four of the most commonly used IVD computer simulations designed for nursing. Evaluation was based on a likert scale of 1-4, 4 being strong agreement and 1 strong disagreement that a subcomponent was present. The data were analyzed and adequacy for practice was determined by at least 75% inclusion with a mean of 3.0.

3. Results and Discussion

Based on the results of the study, it was concluded that three of the four IVD simulations could be rated adequate for problem-solving practice. A related finding was that the majority of nurse educators perceived IVD as useful for instruction and problem solving.

Implications for nurse educators include a recommendation to thoroughly evaluate each IVD for adequacy as a problem solving teaching strategy before adoption using a tool such as the one designed for this study. Implications for students include a recommendation to use IVD not only for information or entertainment, but as a practice instrument for solving simulated client problems. Implications for IVD developers was to use a team approach to include nurse educators to assure that the IVDs conform to curricular objectives. It was strongly recommended that further research be conducted to systematically evaluate each nursing IVD computer simulation to determine its worth and usefulness as a problem-solving teaching strategy.

[1] Borich G and Jemelca R. *Programs and Systems: An Evaluation Perspective.* New York: Academic Press, 1982.

[2] Grobe S. Computer Assisted Instruction: An Alternative. *Comput Nurs 1984, 2: 92-97.*

Nursing Informatics: An International Overview for Nursing in a Technological Era
S.J. Grobe and E.S.P. Pluyter-Wenting, eds.

Evaluation of the effect of a computer orientation program on new nurse employee's attitudes to computerization

Gore ML, Persaud D and Dawe U

Department of Staff Development, Informatics, and Patient Education, Calgary General Hospital, Peter Lougheed Centre, 3500-26 Avenue NE, Calgary, Alberta, Canada, TIY 6J4

1. Introduction

This quasi-experimental study with a repeated measures analysis examined the effect of a computer orientation program on nurses' attitudes towards computerization. Thomas [1] stated that resistance to computing in nursing results from inadequate experience, lack of exposure, or unfavourable attitudes towards technology. A sample of 67 staff nurses from the orientation program was examined.

2. Tools

Two instruments were used to collect data from new staff nurses. The participants were measured prior to computer orientation, immediately following computer training and again after 3 months on the nursing unit. The instruments developed by Stonge and Brodt [2] and Thomas [3] were used to measure attitudes to computers in nursing practice. Both instruments are Likert type scales with five response categories. Stronge & Brodts' tool contained 20 items, whereas, Thomas's tool contained a two 30 item questionnaire.

3. Data

Paired t-test analysis of the Thomas' tool demonstrated a significant difference between the mean scores after computer orientation and at a 3-month re-test period. A paired t-test analysis of the Stronge and Brodt tool, with similar testing as Thomas' tool, demonstrated no significant difference between mean scores. The data suggests that two measures of attitude changed significantly following 12 hours of orientation.

4. Conclusion

The findings suggest that most staff nurses were relatively positive in their attitude toward computerization. The data suggests that two measures of attitude changed significantly following the twelve hours of computer orientation. The results of the study indicate that the majority of nurses are quite positive to computerization but with increased information regarding the utilization of computerization, their attitude would be somewhat higher. Assessment of attitude is an integral part of the implementation of a HIS.

5. References

[1] Thomas B. A survey of computers in nursing. *Comput Nurs* 1985, 3: 173-179.

[2] Stronge JH and Brodt A. Assessment of nurses' attitudes toward computerization. *Comput Nurs* 1985, 3: 154-158.

[3] Thomas B. Development of an instrument to assess attitudes toward computing in nursing. *Comput Nurs* 1988, 6(3): 122-127.

Nursing Informatics: An International Overview for Nursing in a Technological Era
S.J. Grobe and E.S.P. Pluyter-Wenting, eds.

774

Testing a Model for Systematic Multidisciplinary Documentation in Stroke Care

Hamrin E [a] Boberg K [b] Ehnfors M [c] Fredriksson H [b] and Thunberg M [a]

[a]Department of Caring Sciences, Faculty of Health Sciences, S 581 85 Linköping, Sweden.
[b]Department of Neurology, University Hospital, S 581 85 Linköping, Sweden.
[c]Örebro College for the Health Professions, Box 1323, S 701 13 Örebro, Sweden.

1. Introduction

The aim of the present study was primarily to develop a model which could be used for databased documentation in acute stroke care.

2. Methods

In the spring of 1991, records of patients with acute stroke at the Department of Neurology in the University Hospital of Linköping were screened for notes made by RNs, PTs and OTs. The examination was made using the VIPS model, developed by Ehnfors and coworkers in 1991. Seventy-seven records from two wards, representing all discharged patients during a two month period, were investigated. Ward A was a stroke ward with 16 beds and ward B, a general neurological ward with 30 beds. During 1992 a multidisciplinary documentation was developed primarily in ward A and the VIPS model was used in that ward as the basis for nursing documentation from the autumn, 1992. Also, an "IVP program" software was tested in ward A for one month in the autumn of 1992. A new evaluation concerning the documentation was performed using the VIPS model on patients discharged from the same wards during two months (spring 1993), 60 records in all. Three computerized records from ward A were also examined.

3. Results

Mainly, the results from the spring of 1993 and the computerized program (autumn 1992) will be reported on. Comparing wards A and B, there was a significant difference between the wards concerning notes on Nursing Status, where the RNs, PTs and OTs in ward A had kept notes more frequently. The nurses in ward B had made more notes on Nursing Intervention. The nurses in ward A had made more frequent notes on Nursing Outcome and Discharge Notes, while notes on the Nursing Diagnosis and Goals were very poor in both wards. The PTs and the OTs, especially in ward A, kept more frequent documentation than their colleagues in ward B in most of the key words. Evaluating the pilot study on computerized documentation from autumn 1992, one can see a major increase in the nursing notes on Diagnoses, Goals and Outcome, where the computer program has been a help in using the nursing process in full.

4. Conclusion

The VIPS model is an effective way of systematising documentation in multidisciplinary stroke care. The model can be used also as a basis for documentation and computerization. However, the registered nurses need continuous training in using the whole nursing process.

5. References

[1]   Ehnfors M, Thorell-Ekstrand I and Ehrenberg A. Towards basic nursing information in patient records. *Vård i Norden* 1991, 21(3/4):12-31.

Nursing Informatics: An International Overview for Nursing in a Technological Era
S.J. Grobe and E.S.P. Pluyter-Wenting, eds.

Test of the first Swedish Nursing Information System with an Index of Key Words

Karlsson I [a,b] Persson C [a,b] Franzén B [a,b] Peterzén U [b] and Stoltz-Lövgren M [b]

[a]Div of Heart/Lungtranspl, [b]Dept of Heart/Lung Diseases, Sahlgrenska Hospital, 413 45 Gothenburg, Sweden.

1. Introduction

Swedish nurses have a long and strong tradition of oral reports of nursing care. There is a lack of written communication and the consequences are that today's nursing records usually are one-sided medically oriented, unstructured, sometimes unreadable and often non existant [1]. For these reasons a documentation system based on standards and a common terminology, which is applicable both nationally and internationally is necessary.

The aim of this ongoing study is to evaluate the clinical value of the VIPS model [2] which embraces four basic concepts in nursing: Well-being, Integrity, Prevention and Safety, following the nursing process, built on keywords and computerised [3]. The effects may be: Increased patient safety, possibility to conduct quality assurance, increased consciousness about nursing responsibility and increased efficiency about how the nursing care is performed.

2. Methods

Study methods included review of previous nursing records (N=50). Two questionnaires will be used: one concerning nurses' definitions of their profession and one concerning their opinions of the essential in nursing documentation (N=135). Time-study methods will be used to collect information on nursing report time. Education and introduction of the VIPS model/computer program has already been completed through a three-day course. This evaluation will start in January 1994.

3. Results and discussion

Preliminary results indicate that fewer than 20% of the nurses considers documentation as an area of concern. Review of the records also demonstrates that the notes primarily contain medically oriented data and that outcomes from nursing interventions exist in only a few cases. The average report-time/day, at the Division of Heart/Lung transplantation, was 2 h and 24 min, occupying an average of 27 persons/day. Important nursing information is passed on orally, which is a vulnerable and ineffective system, and has a potential risk for patients. After the introduction of the VIPS model, the nursing process is documented to a large extent, and a diagnostic reasoning is thought to be in progress.

However, a language based classification system such as VIPS, is thought to have considerable significance for quality of nursing, for development of knowledge, as a base for research and for giving access to stored nursing textual data in today's increasing use of computers, in clinical practice [4,5,6]. Finally, well documented nursing care is a condition for quality assurance [7], and a necessity for the patient's safety.

4. References

[1] Kreuger Wilson C. Quality-driven information systems: A time to act. *J Nurs Qual* 1992, 7:7-15.
[2] Ehnfors M et al. Towards Basic Nursing Information in Patient Records. *Vård i Norden* 1991, 11:12-31.
[3] SPRI (The Swedish Planning and Rationalization Institute for the Health and Social Services). Att dokumentera omvårdnad med hjälp av dator. Delrapport Spri-projekt 13104, 1992.
[4] Donabedian A. Evaluating the quality of medical care. Milbank Memorial Fund Q, 1966: 4:166-206.
[5] Devine E and Werley H. Test of the Nursing Minimum Data Set: Availability of Data and Reliability. *Nurs Res* 1988, 11:97-104.
[6] Grobe S. Nursing intervention lexicon and taxonomy study: Language and classification methods. *Adv Nurs Sci* 1990, 13:22-33.
[7] Donabedian A. Criteria and Standards for Quality Assessment and Monitoring.*Quality Rev Bull* 1986,12:99-108.

Nursing Informatics: An International Overview for Nursing in a Technological Era
S.J. Grobe and E.S.P. Pluyter-Wenting, eds.

776

In the direction of an integrated nursing information system

Vallina M[a] and Falero S[b]

[a]*Information System & Computer Manager, Hospital Rio Hortega, Valladolid SPAIN*

[b]*School of Nursing, Ferrol University, Nursing Direction Staff, Hospital Arquitecto Marcide, Ferrol SPAIN*

Computer Science, understood as automatic treatment of information, is a tool that allows us to obtain, by means of processes about scattered data, connected information as support for research and decision making. In this view we need to establish the reasons by which the importance of the Information Systems grows exponentially in Health Care. First of all we shall face the expectations on social demands about specialized assistance in Hospitals. Citizens are more and more informed and request sympathetic and personalized assistance, supported by the appropiate technology. Our organizational structures are also involved in an environment of greater complexity, with a highly specialized level. This requires informed professionals who understand Information Technology. On the other hand we have to take into account that limited resources are available. Because of these circumstances it is necessary to review the initial definition. Until now Computer Science has been a tool, from now on and looking into the future Computer Science in Healh Care should be understood as : *Strategic Plan Support for the technologic challenges implied by the limited resources management in a complex organizational structure.*

Thus, we have to create an objective upon the following grounds: (a) Single data are not good enough, we need information; (b) Technologic and organizational changes are running at full speed. It is also necessary to consider the following : (a) Information tasks must be performed in the most suitable place for the user; (b) Increasing productivity and cost reduction should be achieved by means of full information decisions, thus realizing significant savings; (c) Individual autonomy must be balanced by team work integration and team work connection; (d) Information must be available at both the Organization and Management level.

One of the most powerful grounds of Hospital Information Systems (HIS) is the whole integration of nursing activities. The four priority areas that need system design are : (a) Shifts and Personnel Planning System; (b) Indirect Assistance Task System; (c) Standard Care Planning System; (d) Inventory Control and Management The aim of Shifts and Personnel system is the criteria standarization for nurses distribution, with significant time savings and supression of mistakes due to the presence of personnel plan in the system. In this way we will be able to select the most adequate distribution of nursing personnel for patient care. The aim of the Indirect Assistance Task System is to solve the relation between the remaining Hospital Departments, dealing with such aspects as patient location, administration circuit, and electronic mail. The Standard Care Planning System is the most important Nursing Information System. The system will be supported by a Care Planning Data Base. This care plan will be related to the patient necessities, diseases an care levels and it will also generate a standarized catalogue of daily activities. The system will allow a evaluation of the planned and used resources. The aim of the Inventory Control and Management System is to obtain whole data on-line, as regards the stocks comsumption in any plant or Hospital unit. By using technologies as bar code we plan to manage to advance in the establishment of a ratio per patient and/or disease. The system also will allow an automatic stocks restoring, which will be implemented by an inner contract between each plant and the Hospital General Store. A third advantage of the program is that it activates an alarm system which allows the management of deviations and the prevention of any running out of a given item.

During 1.994, at least ten hospitals in Spain are developing nursing information systems in this way with a total integration data on-line objective.

Nursing Informatics: An International Overview for Nursing in a Technological Era
S.J. Grobe and E.S.P. Pluyter-Wenting, eds.

Hospital-University partnership in information management

Hilgenberg CS[a] and Damery LC[b]

[a]School of Nursing, Millikin University, 1184 W Main St, Decatur, IL 62522

[b]Specialist Medical Information System, St. Mary's Hospital, 1800 E Lake Shore Drive, Decatur, IL 62521

1. Introduction

The need for a cooperative partnership between nursing practice and nursing education is becoming more evident in order to prepare graduates who can assume the responsibilities of today's professional nurse [1]. Few nursing graduates are prepared to use the computer as a tool for managing information and improving patient care [2]. Orientation to the hospital information system (HIS) by the employer compounds the stress of reality shock for the graduate and adds to the cost of orientation for the institution.

2. Summary of Case Study

A hospital clinical site initiated an agreement with a local baccalaureate nursing program to provide on-campus experience with HIS. Among the hospital's goals were to ease the entry process for the new professional and to reduce the nurses' orientation needs associated with automated information systems. Via a remote terminal nursing students utilized the hospital's practice database for assignments designed to lay the foundation for future information management responsibilities.

3. Evaluation

After two years of implementation, reactions of hospital staff, students, and nursing faculty have been favorable. Preliminary evaluations by orientation staff indicated that students with this experience demonstrate more positive attitudes and greater confidence in using the computer as a tool in patient care. The partnership improved dialog and strengthened the relationship between the hospital and the school of nursing and helped fulfill the hospital's mission in community involvement.

4. References

[1] Bevis EO. Alliance for destiny: Education and practice. *Nurs Manag* 1993, 24:56-61.

[2] Lawless KA. Nursing informatics as a needed emphasis in graduate nursing administration education: The student perspective. *Comp Nurs* 1993, 11:263-267.

GRADUATE STUDENTS POSTERS

Nursing Informatics: An International Overview for Nursing in a Technological Era
S.J. Grobe and E.S.P. Pluyter-Wenting, eds.

Infection Control Surveillance Database Systems Analysis and Design:
A Nursing Informatics Approach

Hodges R S

Sponsor: Dr. Cheryl B. Thompson, PhD., Dept. of Nursing Informatics, University of Utah, College of Nursing, 25 North Medical Drive, Salt Lake City, UT 84112, U.S.A.

** The opinions or assertations contained herein are the private views of the author and are not to be construed as official or reflecting the views of the Department of the Army or the Department of Defense**

1. Objectives

The objective of this project is to do a systems analysis and design for an infection control surveillance database for the infection control nurse at Tripler Army Medical Center, Hawaii. This project will focus on interfacing with the current Hospital Information System to gather the data and information necessary to conduct surveillance and develop the required reports.

2. Background and Significance

Infection control surveillance systems need to provide useful information to the infection control practioner and committee in the least amount of time[1]. Computers assist infection control in gathering the raw data needed for surveillance and performing data analysis to turn that data into useful information[2]. Clinical data collected by this application could eventually be used to determine the effects of infection control surveillance and interventions on patient outcomes.

3. Setting

This project will be conducted at Tripler Army Medical Center (TAMC), Hawaii. The current infection control surveillance system uses four computer programs or systems at three separate locations.

4. Methods and Procedures

The systems development life cycle (SDLC) [3] will be used in the analysis and design of this database. The database design will utilize a data driven approach for relational database[5] development, by determining the data requirements and then developing a conceptual, a logical, and finally a physical design for the database. An entity-relationship diagram will be developed to assist in the database design and to communicate the design to the end users.

5. Current Status

This project is in the system analysis phase of the SDLC. Final design will be completed by 20 May, 1994.

6. References

[1] Castle M. *Infection Control: Principles and Practice.* New York: Wiley, 1980.
[2] Reagan DR. Computer Use in Infection Control. In: Prevention and Control of Nosocomial Infections. Wenzel, RP(ed). Baltimore: Williams & Wilkins, 1993: 981-992.
[3] Whitten J, Bentley L and Barlow V. *Systems Analysis & Design Methods.* Boston: Irwin,1989.
[4] Batini C, Ceri S and Navathe SB. *Conceptual Database Design. An Entity-Relationship Approach.* Redwood City, CA: The Benjamin/Cummings Publishing Company, Inc.: 1992.

Nursing Informatics: An International Overview for Nursing in a Technological Era
S.J. Grobe and E.S.P. Pluyter-Wenting, eds.

The nomenclatures and classifications of nursing practice in Finland: Methodological questions

Halttunen A

Doctoral Student; Faculty Sponsor: Katri Vehviläinen-Julkunen, Department of Nursing Science, Kuopio University, P.O. Box 1627, 70211 Kuoplo Finland.

1. Background

In Finland, as well as in different countries, the urgency to develop nomenclatures and classifications for nursing practice has occurred. Today, the lack of common concepts and unified language is a very big problem in nursing [1]. The attempts to find out the impact of nursing services, and capture the core of nursing have no success without the common tools; nomenclatures and classifications with their clear terms. These tools are also necessary for the development of nursing information systems [2]. Nursing information systems and data bases which include the content of nursing facilitate the profession to take care of patients with high quality and guarantee the continuity of nursing services.

2. Data

The objective of nomenclature projects, started 1991 and 1993 in Finland, is to collect the data from nursing practice, analyze the data and formulate the nomenclature for nursing practice. The data collection in 1991 included descriptions of nursing activities (n=340) at five hospitals. In 1993 the data were collected at one hospital, in five different wards. The both periods of data collection included three weeks. In the research process some methodological problems have appeared: The questions are; how to classify the data and which are the suitable methods to validate the individual data. The planned research methods are; content analysis of data and Delphi-technique.

3. Conclusion

The attempt to formulate the nomenclatures in different countries is strongly going on [3]. Because it is important to match the results also internationally, the discussion of research methods is necessary. The discussion could be suitable forum to exchange the ideas, and the advanced effort for the investigators is obvious.

4. References

[1] McCormick KA. A Unified Nursing Language System. In *Nursing Informatics: Where caring and technology meet*, eds. Ball MJ, Hannah KJ, Gerdin-Jelger U and Peterson H. New York: Springer-Verlag, 1988: 167-178.

[2] Zielstorff RD, Hudgings CL, Grobe SJ. *Next-Generation Nursing Information Systems, Essential Characteristics for Professional Practice.* American Nurses Publishing. Washington DC, 1993.

[3] International Council of Nurses: *Nursing's Next Advance: An International Classification for Nursing Practice (ICNP).* ICN Headquarters Geneva, Switzerland, October 1993.

Nursing Informatics: An International Overview for Nursing in a Technological Era
S.J. Grobe and E.S.P. Pluyter-Wenting, eds.   783

Nursing informatics and nursing education:
Development of an integrative model

Saranto K

Doctoral Student; Faculty Sponsor: Helena Leino-Kilpi, Associate Professor, University of Turku Department of Nursing, SF 20720 Turku, Finland

1. Objective

The objective of the project is to develop a model for teaching nursing informatics in basic nursing education.

2. Background and Significance

Information technology is used in every university and regional hospital and in advanced health care centers in Finland. The lack of continuing education and training in computers, however, prevents nurses from utilizing the systems in the hospitals.

In the Finnish nursing curriculum the information technology has a very insignificant place. The elementary knowledge about microcomputers and information technology is taught in the basic training. The students are able to use word processing and they are familiar with legality including data security in hospitals.

There is no existing model for teaching nursing informatics in Finland. So, by creating and testing a model of teaching nursing informatics, the project will enhance the utilization of nursing informatics.

3. Setting and environment

The project is conducted in the Finnish nurse education system and it is a part of a wider project: "The quality and outcomes of nursing education."

The project consists of three phases from 1993 to 1998. In the first phase, the purpose is to find out the stage of knowledge of information technology needed by nurses. In the second phase, a measuring instrument will be formulated. In the third phase, an educational intervention will be carried out in nursing education.

4. Methods and procedures

In the first phase, the delphi-technique and survey will be used. The members of the panel are chosen from four specialists' groups: Nurse educator, student, clinical nurse specialist and patient. In the second phase, the measuring instrument will be created based on the survey. In the third phase, an intervention study in one nursing college will be carried out.

5. Current status

In Fall 1993 the project is in the first phase. The second phase will start in Spring 1994. The third phase will start in Fall 1995.

The first phase will be presented in this poster.

Nursing Informatics: An International Overview for Nursing in a Technological Era
S.J. Grobe and E.S.P. Pluyter-Wenting, eds.

784

Criteria for an ideal information system for the school of nursing

Joslin S Henry E and Prin P

Doctoral Students; Faculty Sponsor: Carole Gassert, Faculty, University of Maryland at Baltimore, School of Nursing, 655 W. Lombard St., Baltimore, MD 21201

1. Objective

This poster presents a request for proposal (RFP) project which was done as a requirement for a graduate nursing informatics class. The first objective of the project was to determine faculty information needs for an ideal information system. The second objective was to justify the system by presenting a cost benefit analysis.

2. Background and significance

Research describing nursing faculty's use of computer technology is limited. Most studies of computers in nursing academia have focused on students and the use of computer assisted instruction, or attitudes towards computers. While research findings provide direction for teaching strategies that incorporate computers, they do not address the information system (IS) needs of faculty to attain these strategies.

3. Setting and environment

The setting for this project was the University of Maryland at Baltimore, School of Nursing. This school is one of six professional schools located on the Health Sciences Campus. The school offers BSN, MS, Ph.D. degree programs on multiple campuses throughout the state. Approximately 1000 students are enrolled in this school which has 150 faculty. Although most faculty have access to desktop computers, an integrated faculty information system does not presently exist.

4. Methods and procedures

Several methods were used to determine faculty IS needs: electronic mail survey, faculty interviews and conferences with IS staff. Based on the results of these methods a Request for Proposal was developed. A cost benefit analysis was created to theoretically justify the proposed system.

5. Current status of the project

A three component system was proposed. The first component was an Educational Information System (EIS) which would be used to manage student data. The second component, a Clinical Information System (CIS), would provide a nursing knowledge database to be used for nursing practice, inservices and education. Lastly, a Faculty Administrative Support System (FASS) which would provide information relating to administrative support functions was included. The cost benefit analysis indicated recovery of initial investment within three years.

Nursing Informatics: An International Overview for Nursing in a Technological Era
S.J. Grobe and E.S.P. Pluyter-Wenting, eds.

The use of the Nursing Severity Index for the prediction of mortality and length of stay in AIDS patients hospitalized for <u>Pneumocystis carinii</u> pneumonia

Dolter KJ

Doctoral Student; Faculty Sponsor: Suzanne Bakken Henry, University of California, San Francisco, CA 94143 USA

1. Introduction

Severity of illness measures (SOIM) such as MedisGroups and Apache III are utilized to adjust for variation in health status which otherwise might obscure the effects of nursing or medical interventions. A more recently developed SOIM based on nursing diagnoses (ND), the Nursing Severity Index or NSI [1]., differs from these other methods in that it includes domains of health other than the physiologic. The NSI, a score obtained by totalling the number of 34 NDs present on the admission of a patient to the hospital, was found to significantly predict in-hospital mortality and length of stay in a large Midwestern sample (N=7302) and to add to the ability of MedisGroups to predict mortality and length of stay. The measure was developed using a computerized ND database. After formal training to standardize their use of ND, nurses recorded the presence or absence of 61 NDs within 48 hours of patient admission using a light sensitive pen for barcode data entry on a hand held computer terminal. The purpose of this analysis was to determine the ability of the NSI to predict length of stay and mortality under circumstances in which there was no systematic computerized listing of ND or standardized training in the use of ND.

2. Methods

A secondary analysis was conducted using data generated by the first phase of a study (NR02215, W.L. Holzemer, P.I.) examining linkages among patient problems, nursing interventions, and patient outcomes in persons living with AIDS (PLWAs) hospitalized for <u>Pneumocystis carinii</u> pneumonia (n=156). Since ND was not utilized consistently by nurses in the sample, a listing of patient problems identified by nurse report, intershift report, nursing care plan, patient activity record, or Kardex was entered into a Paradox database. An NSI was computed for each patient after the identified patient problems were coded into one of the 34 NDs comprising the index.

3. Results

Descriptive statistics for the NSI for this sample are range 0-9, mean 3.0, and standard deviation 1.8. These contrast with the NSI statistics from the original study, range 0-34 and mean 7.3. Correlations between the NSI and length of stay (r=.05, p=.53), in-hospital mortality (r=-.09, p=.27), mortality at 3 months (r=-.14, p=.10), or mortality at six months (r=.05, p=.53) demonstrated no associations.

4. Discussion

Reasons for the NSI's lack of predictive ability for length of stay and mortality in t'is study possibly relate first, to the lack of a ND data entry system which would facilitate full and systematic consideration of all 34 NDs and second, to the homogeneity of t'e sample. A major limitation of the analysis is the application of the NSI to data not collected for that purpose. Recommendation is for further study of the NSI in more varied and larger samples.

5. References

[1] Rosenthal GE, et al. Development and validation of the Nursing Severity Index. *Medical Care* 1992, 30: 1127-1141.

Nursing Informatics: An International Overview for Nursing in a Technological Era
S.J. Grobe and E.S.P. Pluyter-Wenting, eds.

786

Dysplasia clinic database

Randell CL

Masters Student; Faculty Sponsor: Suzanne Bakken Henry, School of Nursing, University of California, San Francisco, CA 94143 USA

1. Introduction

The personnel in the Obstetrical/Gynecological Clinic are responsible for tracking of dysplasia patients. These patients are at risk for cervical cancer, and are required to have biopsy and colposcopy testing every three months for a year. As the dysplasia population increased, problems developed with manually tracking these patients. To streamline procedures, a database program was developed using Paradox 4.0

Paradox was chosen over other databases for several reasons. First, the program is easy to use in terms of database development and daily queries. In addition, the vendor provides excellent technical support. The relational capabilities of Paradox make linkages among tables simple. The program also has the capability of producing a variety of reports and mailing labels. The reports are easily tailored to meet individual needs.

2. Methods/procedure

The dysplasia database contains the patient's name, age, social security number, address, telephone numbers (both home and business), physician name, date of last visit, date of next required visit, records location, physical examination findings, biopsy results, and dates of patient notification letters. Records are sorted either alphabetically by last name, social security number, or chronologically by date of next required visit. These various sorting methods allow for easy location of individual patient records, and quick identification of patients needing immediate follow-up letters. The database, which now contains over 400 patient records, is maintained by the nursing personnel in the clinic.

The staff committed themselves to a major initial time investment when they agree to create and maintain the database. The actual creation of the database required only three to five hours. However, entering the initial data for over 300 patients was labor intensive and was done over several months by the clinic's registered nurse. Now individual records are updated in less than three minutes, half the amount of time it often took jut to find the old handwritten dysplasia cards.

3. Results

This system offers several advantages over the manual procedures. Individual reports containing dysplasia data and pertinent medical history are printed the day before dysplasia appointments, giving providers valuable information even in the absence of the medical record. Staff time is saved since they are no longer responsible for maintaining the 5x8 cards that were easily lost or misfiled. In addition, once records are sorted by "next required visit", all patients needing immediate follow-up ar identified at the push of a button. The database can then generate mailing labels again saving time. Most importantly, the computerized system ensures that all patients are notified of their follow-up appointments.

4. References

[1] *Paradox, User's Guide (2nd ed.).* Scotts Valley, CA: Borland, 1992.

Nursing Informatics: An International Overview for Nursing in a Technological Era
S.J. Grobe and E.S.P. Pluyter-Wenting, eds.

Type of data collected by experienced and inexperienced critical care nurses managing computer-simulated tachydysrhythmias

Kim HJ

Doctoral Student; Faculty Sponsor: Suzanne Bakken Henry, Department of Nursing, University of California, San Francisco, 500 Parnassus Ave, CA 94143-0602

1. Introduction

Research studies on clinical decision making in nursing have demonstrated differences between inexperienced and experienced nurses in the areas of cue recognition, diagnosis, and care planning. The purpose of this study was to determine if inexperienced and experienced critical care nurses varied in the type of data collected prior to intervention. The sample (N=68) had a mean age of 34.2 years with 9.4 nursing experience and 5.8 years critical care experience.

2. Tools

Tach-Man is a computer program that generates interactive simulations related to the management of tachydysrhythmias. Each critical care nurse completed the same versions of atrial flutter and ventricular tachycardia. The amount and type of data collected prior to intervention was manually tracked during the simulation. Types of data available were: current complaint, past medical history, medications, medication allergies, arterial blood gas results, electrolytes results, chest x-ray results, and physical exam findings.

3. Data

The most frequently collected type of data were current complaint (51%), physical exam (25%), and medications (18%). There were no significant differences between nurses with less than one year of nursing experience and one year or more of nursing experience on the type of data collected prior to intervention or definitive intervention in the two simulations. However, nurses with less than one year of critical care experience were more likely to collect physical exam data in both the atrial flutter (p=.03) and ventricular tachycardia (p=.0001) prior to definitive intervention. Significant differences were found between the type of data collected for atrial flutter and ventricular tachycardia. More data related to history was collected prior to the first intervention (p=.002) and prior to definitive intervention (p=.003) for the atrial flutter than the ventricular tachycardia.

4. Conclusions

There were some differences in the frequencies of types of data collected between inexperienced and experienced critical care nurses and between the two types of dysrhythmias providing support for previous research studies indicating that both the nature of the task and the experience of the decision maker with the task affect the process of clinical decision making. Future research is needed to examine differences in decision making in actual clinical practice.

5. References

[1] Benner P. *From novice to expert: Power and excellence in nursing practice.* Palo Alto: Addison-Wesley, 1984

[2] Corcoran S. Planning by expert nurses in cases of varying complexity. *Res Nurs Health* 1986, 9: 155-162

Nursing Informatics: An International Overview for Nursing in a Technological Era
S.J. Grobe and E.S.P. Pluyter-Wenting, eds.

The assessment of symptomatology: Examining methods and outcomes

Reilly CA

Doctoral Student; Faculty Sponsor: William L. Holzemer, University of California, San Francisco

1. Introduction

The efficiency and effectiveness of health care services has become an area of national importance. Health care professionals must begin to empirically demonstrate the contributions of the care provided to patient outcomes. As symptoms are the most common reason that people seek health care and nurses play a vital role in symptom management, examining the effect of nursing interventions on symptom status is one strategy for assessing the impact of nursing care on patient outcomes. In order to effectively assess and manage symptoms, to examine the impact of nursing interventions, and to conduct research across settings and populations, it is necessary to routinely measure symptoms from the patient's perspective. Having patients assess their symptoms would increase involvement in their care, would provide valid and trended data on symptom status, and could guide nursing interventions aimed at symptom management. These effects may increase patient satisfaction with their health care. Research which explores the relationships between nursing interventions, symptom status, and patient outcomes could make significant contributions to various facets of the health care system. In the assessment of patient symptoms, the use of computer-based tools provides a method for the automated trending of symptoms.

2. Specific aims

The specific aims of this study, which is currently in progress, ar to determine whether or not the routine assessment of symptom status contributes to variations in patient outcomes, to determine whether or not the routine assessment of symptom status influences symptom management, and to determine patient preferences for documenting symptom status with two computer-based methods.

3. Study sample

The population of interest in this study includes all patients hospitalized in an acute care facility. A convenience sample will include patients who are at least 18-years-old, who can read English, and are newly admitted to an acute care hospital. Exclusion criteria include patients with documented cognitive impairment, patients admitted to an intensive care unit, or patients with loss of consciousness.

4. Methods and procedures

A cohort design in which treatment partitioning is possible will be used in this study. The independent variables include the implementation of two methods for documenting symptom intensity, frequency, and distress: a pen-based computer and a multimedia computer-based program. The two documentation systems will contain the same self-report measure of symptom status. The dependent variables include patient satisfaction with car, patient preference regarding type of documentation method, the documentation of symptoms, the documentation of symptom management interventions by health care providers, the symptom status of the patient, and length of stay. Patients in the control group will complete the instruments which measure the dependent variables at admission and discharge, and will receive the usual care. A later cohort of patients, from the same unit, will constitute the treatment group. This cohort will follow the same study protocol and will also document symptom status on a daily basis. for two days, patients will use one of the computer-based methods to document symptom status and on the third day will switch to the other method. A hard copy of the patient's symptom status, which trends the course of symptoms over time, will be placed in the patient record and with standard flow sheets.

Nursing Informatics: An International Overview for Nursing in a Technological Era
S.J. Grobe and E.S.P. Pluyter-Wenting, eds.

Bedside terminals: Cost-benefit analysis

Driver LC

Graduate Student; Faculty Sponsor: Kay Hodson, Ball State University, Muncie, IN 47306

1. Introduction

The immense amount of data a hospital generates requires a computer system that can process information in an efficient manner. Data processing systems by improving efficiency can produce a savings of thousands of dollars. Hospital information systems were first utilized for financial accounting and have progressed into the age of informatics. Bedside terminals are an approach to data entry that is maximally effective, due to capture at the point of care, to meet the challenges facing nursing today.

2. Purpose

The purpose of this evaluation research study is to determine if bedside terminals are justifiable though a cost-benefit analysis. Many authors suggest the use of a cost-benefit analysis to justify the purchase of bedside terminals [1-3]. Cost-benefits analysis was done to determine whether the benefits outweigh the costs involved in implementing a bedside terminal system.

The General Systems Theory, formulated by Ludwig von Betalanaffy in the late 1920's, was the theoretical framework used for this study. This framework was chosen due to the complexity of the healthcare system. Nurse administrators must have a sound theoretical base on which to evaluate decisions.

3. Tool

A non-standardized checklist of factors was developed from the literature review to evaluate the associated costs related to bedside terminals. These factors included; patient census, acuity, lost charges, reimbursement denials, and medication errors. Interrater reliability was established by a panel of three experts on cost-benefit analysis. Content validity was established by a review of the factors on the checklist by a panel of Nurse Managers with experience in computer systems and cost-benefit analysis.

4. Setting

A convenience sample of one medical nursing unit from a large midwestern metropolitan hospital was chosen for data collection. The unit is typical with a stable census and staffing pattern. One month of data will be evaluated for this study.

All participants were notified of rights as human subjects and the confidentiality of this study. A cover letter informed subjects of procedures, risks, and benefits. Ball State University's Institutional Review Board granted permission to conduct the study.

Data will be obtained from financial reports and nursing management interviews. Based on the literature, monetary values will be arbitrarily assigned to the factors. Costs will be assigned based on projected figures for bedside terminal implementation in 1993 obtained from the literature.

5. References

[1] Andrew, WF. Special Report: *Bedside/Point-of-care Information Systems*. Winter Haven, FL: W.F. Andrew and Associates, 1992.
[2] Holmes, B. The impact of clinical information systems on the future of nursing. *Imprint* 1990, 37: 39-40.
[3] Korpman, RA. Patient care automation: the future is now Part 6. Does reality live up to the promise? *Nurs Econ* 1991, 9: 24-27

© 1994 Elsevier Science B.V. All rights reserved.
Nursing Informatics: An International Overview for Nursing in a Technological Era
S.J. Grobe and E.S.P. Pluyter-Wenting, eds.

790

Diffusion of innovation: The adoption of information technology by school nurses

Bergren MD

DNS Candidate; Faculty Sponsor: Judith S. Ronald, School of Nursing, University at Buffalo, 115 Kimball Tower, Buffalo, NY 14214

1. Objective

This poster presents a follow up study of information technology diffusion among school nurses. The lack of computerization within the school nurse population presented an opportunity to prospectively study Rogers' Diffusion of Innovation Theory [1]. The purpose of the follow up study is to identify the pattern and rate of the adoption of information technology in school health.

2. Background

Using manual record keeping, data compiled to create a student health record results in a collection of dozens of pieces of paper. These data cannot be efficiently retrieved, aggregated, and analyzed. As a result, student health needs remain unidentified. Despite the promise of technology to meet these needs, school nurses have been slow to adopt computerization into the health office.

3. Setting

This inquiry builds upon a previous study conducted by this investigator which examined the knowledge and attitudes of school nurses' toward computers [2]. The study found the subjects possessed a low level of computer knowledge. However, they held positive attitudes toward computers and perceived computerization to have a relative advantage over present practice. The subjects in the study had yet to adopt information technology into the health office.

4. Methodology

The original subjects were randomly selected from the roster of the Western New York Association of School Nurses. In the follow up study, data are being collected from the original 40 subjects via semi-structured telephone interviews. The interview schedule includes demographic information, information technology use, and variables proposed to influence the innovation decision.

5. Data analysis

Data analysis will be performed in early 1994. Multiple regression will estimate the amount of variability in adoption attributable to selected variables deemed relevant by the theory. The variables which significantly influence the adoption of information technology can provide the focus for technology-oriented intervention strategies within the school nurse population.

6. References

[1] Rogers, EM. *Diffusion of innovation*. New York: The Free Press, 1983.
[2] Bergren, MD. School nurses' knowledge and attitude towards computers. (Unpublished Masters Project, University at Buffalo, State University of New York, 1992).
[3] Korpman, RA. Patient care automation: the future is now Part 6. Does reality live up to the promise? *Nurs Econ* 1991, 9: 24027

© 1994 Elsevier Science B.V. All rights reserved.
Nursing Informatics: An International Overview for Nursing in a Technological Era
S.J. Grobe and E.S.P. Pluyter-Wenting, eds.

International electronic collaborative research: One participant's experience

Erdley WS

DNS student; Faculty Sponsor: Judith S. Ronald, School of Nursing, University at Buffalo, Kimball Tower, Buffalo, NY 14214

1. Objective

This poster reports the author's experience as a member of an international collaborative research project team that conducted research on the Internet about the Internet. The purpose of the poster is to briefly describe the study and compare the author's experience with traditional research process.

2. Summary of the research project

The purpose of the research project was to examine a representative sample of messages across different networks using content analysis methodology. Messages for the study were randomly selected from Bitnet, CompuServ and Usenet networks and then coded by different members of the research team. Sample messages were examined for emotion, nature, structure, quality, and group impact. Message analysis was done by project Coordinators using Krippendorf's comparative content methodology [1]. Secondary analysis of data will be conducted by individual research team members.

3. Comparison of traditional and electronic collaborative research processes

Traditional research process uses a five-step approach of problem definition, hypotheses, testing, analysis, and reporting of results. This research project followed this approach in a broad sense. Project Coordinators are a university faculty member from Israel and a doctoral student from Australia. Team members were recruited through world wide email postings. All communication among team members used email and a private listserve. Copyright, ethics, and sampling policies were discussed by the Coordinators and committees compose of research team members. Suggestions of committee members and the Coordinators about policies were shared with all members of the research team, discussed, and then ratified by group vote using electronic communication.

4. Significance and potential for nursing

The use of computer-mediated communication for collaborative research creates advantages and challenges for nursing. Advantages to using computer mediated communication include timely communication between participants and collaboration with researchers from different countries and disciplines. Issues and challenges include limits of data exchange, ethics of studying electronic messages, sampling procedures, and recruitment of subjects and research team members.

5. References

[1] Krippendorf, K. *Content analysis*. California: Sage, 1980.

Nursing Informatics: An International Overview for Nursing in a Technological Era
S.J. Grobe and E.S.P. Pluyter-Wenting, eds.

792

Information technology support for CQI: Continuing development of a nursing quality assurance/improvement information system

Gugerty B

Doctoral Student; Faculty Sponsor: Judith S. Ronald, School of Nursing, University of Buffalo, 1030 Kimball Tower, 3435 Main Street, Buffalo, NY 14214 USA

1. Background

The transformation of Quality Assurance to Continuous Quality Improvement (CQI) is a significant trend in nursing and healthcare. Pay guarantors and regulators require agencies to document Nursing CQI efforts to solve identified problems and provide a mechanism for ongoing quality improvement. This poster describes the continuing development of a successful Nursing Quality Assurance/Improvement Information System (NQA/I-IS). The system uses relational database technology to provide a powerful tool for management of large volumes of Quality Assurance/Improvement data and information. The development of the system is a three phased project. Phase I was design and construction of the Information System and Phase II was implementation, verification, and improvement of the system. The system was successfully implemented in 1992. A survey of users at the conclusion of phase II revealed high satisfaction with data entry, data management, and basic reporting capability of the system. Phase III will be migration of the system to a Medical Center Network.

2. Purpose

Despite the improvement provided by the NQA/I-IS, the changing healthcare and CQI environment now demands still greater functionality and flexibility if the system is to remain a useful tool. The Post Phase II User Survey showed a need for exporting data out of the system for use in other systems, graphics generation within the system, and data trending across several data collection periods. Examples of these three types of system outputs are a prominent feature of this poster presentation. Meeting these user needs became the objectives of a new phase of the project: Phase IIA-Improvement of Outputs of the NQA/I IS.

3. Results

Currently, exporting functionality has been implemented. Importing functionality is under development. A graphics module has been added to the system. The first graphics module prototype has been released and is being tested by end users. A revised reports module that trends information from four previous periods has been designed. Development and prototyping of this trending capability of the system is planned for early 1994.

4. Conclusions

This project demonstrates the dynamic nature of the systems development life cycle and the relationship between nursing practice and systems design and function in a Nursing QA/I context. The information needs and practice realities of the practitioners guide the development of the system. The system enables the users to transform data into information in ways that were previously unavailable. The development team plans to continue to closely monitor the effectiveness of the system in meeting the information management needs of end users. Partnership with end users in system development is essential if the system is to continue to support CQI in healthcare agencies.

Nursing Informatics: An International Overview for Nursing in a Technological Era
S.J. Grobe and E.S.P. Pluyter-Wenting, eds.

Clinical pathways request for proposal: Application of a nursing informatics model

Byrne JD Creech CA and Wark CG

Graduate Students; Faculty Sponsor: Carole A. Gassert, University of Maryland at Baltimore, School of Nursing, 655 West Lombard St, Baltimore, MD 21201-1579 USA

1. Objective

The objective of this project was to select an appropriate nursing information system through application of a nursing model and systems analysis principles. The students prepared a request for proposal for a clinical pathways information system.

2. Background

In the past decade, acute care facilities have been driven to decrease lengths of stay while maintaining or improving quality care at cost efficient rates. The University of Maryland Medical Center (UMMC) decided to implement the use of clinical pathways (CPs) to facilitate an outcomes management approach. CPs have been documented to facilitate the coordination of complex care delivery processes while improving clinical, functional, service quality, and financial outcomes.

3. Setting

UMMC, a 747-bed academic and tertiary care facility located in metropolitan Baltimore, served as the project site. This facility is part of the larger University of Maryland Medical System. Nursing Clinical Practice Coordinators orchestrated the introduction of CPs to the care delivery system. Pathways for Coronary Artery Bypass Graft surgery and Epilepsy surgery were in pilot testing at the time of the project.

4. Methods

Gassert's Model for Defining Information System Requirements served as the theoretical framework for this project and the basis for preparing the request for proposal [1]. The model suggests a means of identifying, organizing, and depicting system requirements.

5. Status

A copy of the request for proposal was submitted to the Nursing Information Systems Department upon completion of the project in May, 1993.

6. References

[1] Gassert CA. Defining nursing information system requirements: A linked model. In: Proceedings of the Thirteenth Annual Symposium of Computer Applications in Medical Care '89. Kingsland LC (ed). Los Angeles: *Computer Society Press*, 1989: 779-783.

© 1994 Elsevier Science B.V. All rights reserved.
Nursing Informatics: An International Overview for Nursing in a Technological Era
S.J. Grobe and E.S.P. Pluyter-Wenting, eds.

Evaluating the usage of an electronic bulletin board in a nursing informatics graduate program

Martin MJ

Masters Student; Faculty Sponsor: Carole A. Gassert, University of Maryland at Baltimore, School of Nursing, 655 W Lombard Street, Baltimore, Maryland 21201.

1. Objective

The purpose of this project is to evaluate the usage of the electronic bulletin board at the University of Maryland at Baltimore (UMAB) School of Nursing. The objectives are to determine the level of user satisfaction, frequency and patterns of use, conference participation, barriers to using the bulletin board, and recommendations for change. Further evaluation is needed to increase participation on the bulletin board.

2. Background

The background of the Nursing Informatic Bulletin Board System (NIBBS) was started by two Nursing Informatic graduate students as part of their seminar paper. The bulletin board was implemented in the Winter of 1992 to facilitate communication among faculty, graduates and students, and disperse information to those students who aren't frequently on campus. NIBBX is currently maintained in the UMAB's School of Nursing Informatics Lab. Access is available to current Nursing Informatic (NI) students, NI graduates and NI faculty through local or remote access.

3. Setting

The project will take place in UMAB's School of Nursing Informatics Lab. UMAB's NI program has enrolled 121 students since opening in Fall 1988. Students live in MD, VA, PA and NJ. They commute to Baltimore for some of their courses. The interdisciplinary courses are taken at one of three other campuses. Currently, there are 37 graduates through August 1993.

4. Methods/Procedures

Methods include surveying current students, graduates and faculty to obtain feedback. The survey focuses on usage and satisfaction.

5. Results

Currently, no results are reported since the project is still under development.

Nursing Informatics: An International Overview for Nursing in a Technological Era
S.J. Grobe and E.S.P. Pluyter-Wenting, eds.

Database monitoring of tuberculosis in nursing homes

Poker AM

Masters Student; Faculty Sponsor: Carole A. Gassert, University of Maryland at Baltimore, School of Nursing, 655 West Lombard Street, Baltimore, MD 21201

1. Background and significance

The resurgence of tuberculosis (TB) has been noted in the United States since the mid 1980's. Incidence of TB infections increase with age and persons over 55 years old account for 50% of the new cases. It has been found that populations residing in nursing homes are infected at a higher rate than the elder population in the community. Another contributing factor to the spread of TB infections in the nursing home is the growing number of HIV positive individuals entering nursing homes. Due to their immune suppression, these HIV positive persons are at high risk of contracting TB. The tuberculosis infected nursing home resident interacts with family and friends, various medical and social services, and thus poses an increased risk of infecting other residents and the community.

2. Purpose

The primary concern of this project is to assist in tracking of TB clients and contacts to facilitate prevention and control of the infection, thereby reducing the incidence of TB. Information tracking is a key element in the Centers for Disease Control's (CDC) strategies for dealing with tuberculosis. CDC recommendations include: patient isolation, proper ventilation, tracing the source of the infection, preventative therapy and continuous surveillance (CDC 1990).

3. Methods and procedures

A tuberculosis database in a nursing home, as a method of surveillance, would greatly assist in monitoring TB. The database would track the source of infection, promote documentation of preventative or therapeutic treatment and generate reports to proper public health facilities. Reports could be generated to identify trends and support research. The database would maintain accurate and timely data and could link nursing homes to each other. Information could be exchanged between nursing homes in the community and/or public health facilities. It is feasible to develop a national TB database of nursing home residents. The national database could be linked to an international database which would enable identifying trends, tracking and noting geographic patterns of TB in nursing home patients.

4. Results

The project is in its development phase. A test nursing home is being chosen and a needs survey executed to establish the database's entities. TB is not restricted to any given community, therefore this project could have potential local, national and global significance.

5. References

[1] Centers for Disease Control. (1990). Guidelines for preventing the transmission of tuberculosis in health-care settings, with special focus on HIV-related issues. *Morbidity and Mortality Weekly Report*, 39 (RR-17), 1-29.

Nursing Informatics: An International Overview for Nursing in a Technological Era
S.J. Grobe and E.S.P. Pluyter-Wenting, eds.

Processing information for decision making in resource management

Coleman S

Master's Student; Faculty Sponsor: Carole A. Gassert, University of Maryland, School of Nursing, Lombard Street, Baltimore, Maryland

1. Background

Decision support systems have been receiving more and more interest with the advent of the information age and the global economy. Managers, including healthcare managers are expected to keep up to date on all the various sources of information that are available. The need increases as communication technology improves at a phenomenal rate. With a glut of information it is harder to sift through and choose the data most relevant for effective decision making. Decision support systems can make this task easier, but to provide effective support a decision support system (DSS) must aid the decision maker throughout the process. The development of decision support systems has been limited by a lack of knowledge about how nurses reach a decision. Many authors have identified the need to analyze the process through which decision makers solve a problem [1, 2, 3, 4].

2. Objectives and setting

This project looks at the system currently used at the Veteran's Affairs Medical Center in Washington, DC in determining nurse staffing and resource management needs. It will evaluate a methodology for projecting nursing resources as well as providing an opportunity to identify areas for system improvement. The organization has recognized the need to meet patient care, administrative, educational, and research needs based on the medical center's as well as each individual nursing unit's patient population.

3. Methodology

To develop effective and efficient resource management, it is first necessary to understand which data elements the managers at the various levels consider important and how these managers utilize these elements to make decisions. A number of factors determines the nursing workload and are key to the quality of the decision making related to nurse staffing.

All of these factors are considered and documented on worksheets, along with a minimum unit based data set. Through verbal protocol analysis, the nurse managers decision making processes will be analyzed throughout the use of these worksheets and the data set.

4. Status

Following the analysis of data, recommendations will be made as to how best to automate the process to supplement the decision makers.

5. References

[1] Mackay JM, Barr SH and Kletke G. An Empirical Investigation of the Effects of Decision Aids on Problem-Solving Processes. *Dec Sci 1991*. 23: 648-668.
[2] Ozbolt JG. Developing Decision Support Systems for Nursing. *Comput Nurs* May/June 1987.
[3] Todd P. and Benbasat I. Process Tracing Methods in Decision Support Systems Research: Exploring the Black Box. *MIS Quart* December 1987. 493-508.
[4] Weber ES and Konsyski BR. Problem Management: Neglected Elements in Decision Support Systems. *J Manag Inf Syst* Winter 1987-88, 4. 3: 64-79.

Nursing Informatics: An International Overview for Nursing in a Technological Era
S.J. Grobe and E.S.P. Pluyter-Wenting, eds.

Expert system for management of urinary incontinence in women

Gorman RH

*Doctoral Candidate, University of Florida, PO Box 100197, College of Nursing, Gainesville, FL 32610-0197 USA
and Nursing Information Systems Coordinator, VA Medical Center, 1601 Archer Road, Gainesville, FL 32608-1197
USA. Faculty Sponsor: Molly C. Dougherty*

1. Objectives

The objectives of the study are to determine the effectiveness of an expert system on a personal computer as a means to disseminate the Agency for Health Care Policy and Research (AHCPR) guidelines for urinary incontinence, examine the use of an expert system by female consumers, and add to the body of knowledge for female consumer outcomes research.

2. Background and significance

The AHCPR, established by Congress in 1989, develops clinical practice guidelines based on expert knowledge. The practice guidelines are developed in response to identified wide variations in healthcare for specific health problems. The intent of the AHCPR is to widely disseminate the results of its research.

The AHCPR guidelines for Urinary Incontinence in Adults [1] report the incidence of urinary incontinence for noninstitutionalized persons older than 60 to be from 15 to 30 percent, with women twice as likely to have incontinent episodes. Computer technology offers a pivotal opportunity to make health information such as AHCPR urinary incontinence guidelines accessible to consumers in a personal, interactive way. The expert system is based on the domain of knowledge related to urinary incontinence in adults.

3. Setting

Participants come to an office with a personal computer, VCR, and desk. The investigator provides one of three interventions, depending on the participants' group random assignment.

4. Methods and procedures

The knowledge domain is placed in an expert system shell. The study utilizes an experimental design with the expert system, AHCPR booklet, or general video (control group) as the intervention and two outcome variable. The outcome variables are the number of urinary incontinent episodes recorded in a three day bladder diary and completion of a questionnaire on the impact of incontinence. Outcome variables are measured two weeks pre and two and six weeks post intervention. Repeated measures analysis of variances are used to determine a significant difference within subject, between subjects, and within subjects by intervention interaction for urinary incontinent episodes and impact measurements. The sample size is 90 with 30 in each group. Data collection is currently in progress.

5. References

[1] Agency for Health Care Policy and Research. Clinical practice guideline: Urinary incontinence in adults. DHHS Publication No. AHCPR 92-0038. Silver Spring, MD: AHCPR Publications Clearinghouse, 1992: 3.

© 1994 Elsevier Science B.V. All rights reserved.
Nursing Informatics: An International Overview for Nursing in a Technological Era
S.J. Grobe and E.S.P. Pluyter-Wenting, eds.

Recording and monitoring blood pressures using *Hypercard* 2.1

Heermann LK

Masters Student; Faculty Sponsor: Linda Lange, EdD., R.N., Assistant Professor and Director, Nursing Informatics Program, College of Nursing, University of Utah, 25 North Medical Drive, Salt Lake City, UT 84112, U.S.A.

1. Objective

The objective of this project is to provide an intelligent records management tool for use in monitoring blood pressures. Blood pressure entries are displayed in a table showing the trend of the blood pressure over time. Alerts are displayed for any values out of user defined limits, or extreme variations from previously recorded values.

2. Background and significance

Successive blood pressure readings are used in a wide variety of settings. In the acute care setting, blood pressure is a routine assessment and is recorded in numerical form in tables or marked on a graph. These visually display each pressure in relation to the other pressures. Knowing any upward or downward trends aids in determining when intervention is needed. Successive blood pressure records are also kept by individual patients at home to monitor hypertension, cardiac medications, and multiple other conditions.

Use of a computerized record in the hospital and outpatient setting can improve the readability of the information making it more useful. The alert system monitoring each value aids busy professionals from not overlooking early signs of hyper or hypotension. The alerts assist individual patients in determining when to contact their physician.

3. Setting

The program was developed within an introductory nursing informatics course. Setting for the project is the Nursing Informatics Laboratory at the University of Utah.

4. Methods and procedures

This program was designed using *Hypercard* 2.1 on the Apple Macintosh Operating System, Version 7.1. The program is individualized for each patient by the user setting the parameters for each alert. The program requires the keyboard entry of blood pressure values and the time the values were obtained. A table displays successive blood pressure readings with the date and time of their measurement. The table includes the time medications were taken. Alert messages are displayed only if the values entered exceed the parameters set.

5. Current status

In December 1993, a prototype was pilot tested with fellow students in the laboratory setting.

DEMONSTRATIONS

© 1994 Elsevier Science B.V. All rights reserved.
Nursing Informatics: An International Overview for Nursing in a Technological Era
S.J. Grobe and E.S.P. Pluyter-Wenting, eds.

Development of Interactive Instructional Software for Neurological Assessment Using the IBM Advanced Academic System

Bongartz C[a] Wedge K[b] and Joseph M[c]

[a]*Nursing Department, Community College of Allegheny County, 1750 Clairton Road, West Mifflin PA 15122*

[b]*Nursing Department, University of Pittsburgh, 453 B Victoria Building, Pittsburgh PA 15216*

[c]*Nursing Department, Monongahela Valley Hospital, Country Club Road, Monongahela PA 15063*

Student nurses required to learn neurological assessment skills must master a complex set of psychomotor behaviors correlated with the advanced concepts of analysis, synthesis and evaluation. These concepts are extensive and difficult for the student to accomplish in a limited laboratory period. Due to past difficulties teaching this skill, interactive instructional software was developed using the IBM Advanced Academic System and the *ToolBook* authoring system.

The objective of this demonstration is to illustrate the integration of instructional software into the classroom setting and to discuss how this can enhance nursing education. Use of the *Run Time ToolBook* software presents interested individuals with an opportunity for hands-on demonstration along with a discussion of the developmental process and techniques used.

An instructional design team consisting of an instructional designer, nurse educator and subject matter expert was involved in the development of this instructional software. The instructional designer and nurse educator collaborated with screen design, content sequencing and software programming. During development of the project, the content expert reviewed the software for content validity and applicability to hospital based education for facilitating continual learning and updating nursing knowledge.

The instructional software consists of seven 'books' or modules with each module containing four sections: 1) the neurological assessment procedure presented in a textual format, 2) the procedure presented as either a graphic or multimedia component to illustrate the psychomotor portion of the skill, 3) the possible normal and abnormal findings, and 4) a short quiz to test content retention.

Currently, this instructional software is used by students enrolled in the Associate Degree Nursing Program at the Community College of Allegheny County. The software is utilized concurrently in the classroom setting and the auto-tutorial laboratory. In the classroom, the neurological assessment is presented using a computerized projection system. This frees the faculty from paper turning and permits immediate reinforcement of psychomotor skills. Multiple projections and windowing of anatomical locations correlate the procedure with results obtained. Also, presentation from any module or section is permitted through the hypertexting capability of the *ToolBook* authoring system. In the auto-tutorial laboratory, through the use of hypertexting and clearly marked navigational buttons, the student can easily move within a module or modules. This enable the student to meet their individualized learning needs independently.

The high level of attention and interest exhibited by the students indicated their approval of this new medium for classroom use. Utilization of the Response Pads available with the Advanced Academic system enables students to take a more active role in the classroom setting. The response pads also provide monitoring of student responses and permit immediate remediation.

Nursing Informatics: An International Overview for Nursing in a Technological Era
S.J. Grobe and E.S.P. Pluyter-Wenting, eds.

Clinical Decision Making Using Computer Simulations

Conrick M[a] and Foster J[b]

[a]School of Nursing, Griffith University, Nathan, QLD, 4111, Australia.

[b]School of Nursing, Queensland University of Technology, Locked Bag No 2, Red Hill, QLD, 4059, Australia.

This demonstration will provide a brief overview of the development of the programs and allow participants to "trek" through selected clinical decision making simulations.

As an initiative of the Department of Education, Employment and Training and the Queensland University of Technology, a grant was made to the School of Nursing to develop Computer Based Education in collaboration with the Computer Based Education Facility (CBE) of the University. The programs would be used to promote clinical decision making skills in students undertaking the Bachelor of Nursing program.

The effectiveness and efficacy of the nurse's clinical decision making skill depends upon the ability of the nurse to translate nursing knowledge to nursing care. It is imperative that nursing students develop clinical decision making skills from their first entry into nursing education. To facilitate this, computer packages, which simulated client situations requiring decision making skills, were seen to be the most appropriate method of providing multiple experiences whilst negating patient risk. Concepts from the nursing process are combined with graphic design in development of these simulations to ensure interactivity and promotion of student clinical decision making process skills.

The first modules incorporated a health orientation with subsequent modules developed, moving into the acute care arena with age groups from teenagers to the elderly. Aims of the project included, emphasis being placed on process and not content, no fatalities to occur and to ensure a dynamic process. The format developed to achieve these aims incorporated the nursing process, with the ability to choose from three paths, and within these there are designated "critical elements" of the decision making process.The scoring system is quite complex with both progressive scores and scoring on critical elements, but, it also enables scoring of every screen throughout each module. Evaluating student confidence levels throughout the decision making process was also seen as critical and a "Confidometer" was developed to measure this when students were presented with a critical element.

These simulations have been used by students for over twelve months with very positive feedback, especially on gaining understanding and confidence in clinical decision making processes. An action research project on the development of the modules has been completed and published with the quantitative research project currently in progress.

Nursing Informatics: An International Overview for Nursing in a Technological Era
S.J. Grobe and E.S.P. Pluyter-Wenting, eds.

803

A day with well babies/children

Devney AM[a], Manlove LL[a], Benevich E[b] and Shipman B[c]

[a]Northern Illinois University, DeKalb, Illinois

[b]Assistant Professor of Nursing, North Park College, Chicago, Illinois

[c]Department of Health, Lake County, Waukegan, Illinois

This session will present completed sections of an interactive video program designed to teach senior nursing students and beginning public health nurses the interview and assessment skills used in the well baby clinic setting. The instructional design components emphasizing learner interaction using keyboard input with feedback will be demonstrated.

The clinical area of assessing healthy babies and young children and counseling parents regarding the maintenance of an optimum state of wellness is an exciting field. It demands the utmost of students and beginning practitioners to learn both cognitive and psychomotor skills. To learn assessment one must follow a model, use controlled vocabulary and be allowed to practice under supervision. Because of time restraints adequate practice is often missing from current training. Computer based interactive video learning environments can present students with the opportunity to learn and practice such skills in a non-threatening, non-time restrictive situation.

Baby Well is an interactive video simulation that teaches decision making, interview and physical assessment techniques in the assessment of well babies/children in a clinical setting. Students can be both observers and participants. As an observer the students may access an informational sound track and hear an expert explain the on screen assessment. As a participant the student performs an assessment using the on-line forms and access to a controlled vocabulary while viewing a real time assessment. If unsure of the application of a particular discrimination, (the difference between a eyes that were tracking or eyes that are not) the students can seek explanation in the form of a video clip example. Students then compare their assessments to those of experts. A glossary, on line help and culturally specific support have all been incorporated into this module to ensure students have the necessary support tools.

This interactive program is an example of the versatility of the technology and the ability of the "coaching skills" of the computer for learners. It permits learners of varying backgrounds the opportunity to learn, test and assess their repertoire as they approach the challenging clinical evaluation of healthy children.

1. References

[1]   Hewson M. The role of reflection in professional medical education: A conceptual change interpretation. Eric Document ED310672, 1989:28.

[2]   Levin W. Interactive video: The state of the art teaching machine. *The Computing Teacher* 1983, 11:11-17.

[3]   Pasch M. Does coaching enhance instructional thought? *J of Staff Development* 1992, V13 n3: 40-44.

[4]   Morgan R. Peer coaching in a preservice special education program. *Teacher Education and Special Education* 1992, v15 n4: 249-58.

[5]   Sweeney M and Gulino C. From variables to video disks. *Comput Nurs* 1988, 6:157-162.

© 1994 Elsevier Science B.V. All rights reserved.
Nursing Informatics: An International Overview for Nursing in a Technological Era
S.J. Grobe and E.S.P. Pluyter-Wenting, eds.

An Open Software: Uses From Classroom to Bedside

Dockray K T

1808 19th Street, Lubbock, Texas 79401

1. Introduction

Smart or pro-active software lets anyone register in a computer what one thinks, sees or does, as fast as is possible. Running in a notebook machine, one program takes common clinical abbreviations, acronyms and any other user-selected symbol string. These are translated into numerical values, single sentences or whole paragraphs of text. Recording is speeded because many entry fields are power-assisted. Patients' names are automatically verified, acronyms are self-checked and date/location descriptors appear spontaneously.

Information caches can be screened at any point during data entry to help the worker remember missing facts. If these fail, long-distance databases can be probed.

The procedures, observations and results of ward work are captured in electronic memory and are printed immediately for the chart. The data can be facsimile transmitted to remote readers and analyzed when desired.

2. Tools

Character-based records are created by computed translation of commonly-used clinical abbreviations or any other symbol string selected by the user into readable text. A relational database supports knowledge retrievals and administrative manipulations.

3. Data

One hundred thousand x-ray reports were created in an averate of one minute each with 84% fewer typing strokes. Printouts and facsimile transmissions were immediate. All entered data was retrievable for effectiveness and outcome studies. The doctor's diagnostic mistake rate was cut by half by checking his machine's pop-up memory caches or by calling long-distance databases.

Time and labor expenses were reduced 50% by automatic diagnostic codings, modem-transmission of charges to a billing system and other inventory features.

4. Conclusions

Smart software for records creation, message transmission and knowledge study is effective for one clinical worker. It seems likely that students taught with the software would have a personalized learning and applications tool that could be taken directly from classroom to the bedside.

5. References

[1] Dockray KT. An analysis of Making, Reading and Reporting Films of 100,000 Patients with Implications for Equipment Design. Proc. SPIE 1978, 152: 79-84

Nursing Informatics: An International Overview for Nursing in a Technological Era
S.J. Grobe and E.S.P. Pluyter-Wenting, eds.

A CD-ROM approach to accessing the nursing literature

Levy JR and Pravikoff SD

CINAHL Information Systems, Glendale Adventist Medical Center, 1509 Wilson Terrace, Glendale, California 91209, United States of America

This demonstration will present techniques for searching the nursing literature using state-of-the-art CD-ROM technology. The use of various search strategies will maximize search results in the shortest time possible. The demonstration will provide the audience with techniques for developing search strategies for accessing specific research topics using approved thesauri terms. The Nursing & Allied Health (CINAHL) database will be used to demonstrate these searches. Information on how to apply these techniques to other medical databases will also be addressed. Several comprehensive search topics will be featured.

A multifaceted search will familiarize the audience with the elements of search strategy development using the following steps: 1) selecting the main subject headings; 2) using Boolean search techniques to combine two or more terms; and 3) choosing appropriate subheadings. Quality filtering using limits by publication type, age groups, journal subset, or year of publication will be shown to illustrate the importance of narrowing a search.

This presentation will provide the audience with an understanding of how CD-ROM technology can be used on a daily basis to enhance education, clinical problem-solving, administrative decision-making, and research. Participants will learn how to search the literature without assistance as well as acquire information on the selection of appropriate databases and software systems for their specific uses.

Nursing Informatics: An International Overview for Nursing in a Technological Era
S.J. Grobe and E.S.P. Pluyter-Wenting, eds.

806

Demonstration of mobile pen-based technology

Graves JR[ab], Fehlauer CS[ab], Gillis PA[ac], Booth H[ab], Vaux C[ad] and Soller J[ab]

[a]*Geriatric Research, Education, and Clinical Center, Veterans Affairs Medical Center, 500 Foothill Blvd, Salt Lake City, Utah.*

[b]*University of Utah, Salt Lake City, Utah.*

[c]*Bell Atlantic Healthcare Systems, Peachtree Dunwoody Rd, Atlanta, Georgia.*

[d]*Mercy Medical Center, Redding, California.*

The purpose of this demonstration is to exhibit the pen-based hand-held device that is the mobile peripheral to the Salt Lake City VA GRECC[1] research clinical nursing information system. In practice, the peripheral device communicates with the local database server (a 486 Intell-chip MS-DOS machine) via radio waves. We will demonstrate the interface only and will use battery and/or electricity. Two major applications will be shown with the device.

The Patient Assessment Tool (PAT), which is the atomic-level clinical nursing data interface to the information system, will be shown. In addition, we will demonstrate the Nurse Activity Profile (NAP) Instrument developed on this device to evaluate changes in patterns of nursing activity before, during, and after implementation of various information system components. The profile is especially sensitive to patterns of information processing, but includes approximately 140 explicit nurse behaviors.

1. References

[1] Salt Lake City Veterans Affairs Medical Center Geriatric Research, Education and Clinical Center.

Nursing Informatics: An International Overview for Nursing in a Technological Era
S.J. Grobe and E.S.P. Pluyter-Wenting, eds.

807

The Virginia Henderson International Nursing Library

Graves J R[a]

[a] Virginia Henderson International Nursing Library, 550 West North Street, Indianapolis In, 46202 USA.

1. Description

The Virginia Henderson International Nursing Library is sponsored by Sigma Theta Tau International, the Honor Society of Nursing. It is composed of a set of knowledge and information services to support the mission of the organization which is to improve the health of all peoples by improving the scientific basis of nursing. The electronic Henderson Library is housed at the Center for Nursing Scholarship in Indianapolis. It is accessible through Internet and, soon, by telephone and modem. Hardware and software have been upgraded to accommodate a large number of simultaneous users. An acquisitions program for ensuring representativeness of the registry has been initiated in 1994. All services described below will be demonstrated.

2. Information Services

The Library currently houses a Registry of Nursing Research and Researchers. Other research information services include a database of unpublished abstracts of papers presented at research conferences and a database of STTI grants awarded, both of which are linked to the Registry of Researchers. In addition, Table of Contents databases are available for Image and Sigma Theta Tau Monographs. A Table of Contents database for Nursing Institute for Nursing Research Reports is in the planning stage.

3. Knowledge Services

The Online Journal of Knowledge Synthesis in Nursing, (OJKS) housed at and electronically printed and distributed by OCLC, is the second peer-reviewed electronic journal in the health sciences. OJKS delivers synthesized knowledge (narrative "critical review" of research) for nursing practice. The format is available in hypertext (Windows) or ASCII (MS-DOS). A Macintosh version is expected in 1994.

The Research Registry is being expanded into a Knowledge Registry. The "Survey of Nurse Researchers" currently designed to gather data needed to register nurse researchers and their research projects now includes data about the knowledge generated by completed research projects (variables studied together, the relationship studied, the finding (statistical and narrative), clinical and statistical significance). Searchers will be able to find all registered research that studied x with y with 100% sensitivity and 100% specificity. Since the knowledge itself is indexed, it can be searched directly, not indirectly using Boolean methods of access.

4. Data Services

The Library is currently investigating the feasibility of storing "retired" Research Data Sets donated by nurse researchers. These data sets will be made available online for secondary analysis and teaching purposes to qualified persons (researchers, teachers, and nursing students)

5. Conferencing Services

Online conferencing software has been bought and is being readied for general introduction Summer, 1994. This service will provide electronic conferencing organized for various types groupwork such as (a) OJKS discussion groups with authors (b) support of collaborative research work for multicenter data collection, discussion, and authoring of research reports (c) library demonstration research such as the use of electronic conferencing by clinicians and clinical experts using a case study approach, (d) an International clearinghouse for speakers, teachers and (e) virtually any conferencing that supports the generation, dissemination or utilization of nursing knowledge.

© *1994 Elsevier Science B.V. All rights reserved.*
Nursing Informatics: An International Overview for Nursing in a Technological Era
S.J. Grobe and E.S.P. Pluyter-Wenting, eds.

arcs©: A relational-knowledge computer system
that stores, manages, and models knowledge from the scientific literature

Graves J R[a]

[a] Geriatric Research Education, and Clinical Center, SLC VAMC, 500 Foothill Blvd (182) SLC UT 84148 USA

1. Introduction

In nursing, there are four central knowledge-types (empirical, ethical, esthetic, and personal) and three major sources of knowledge: clinical data, expert nurses, and the scientific literature. *arcs* was developed to store, manage and model the relational type of knowledge generated by the scientific research process (empirical knowledge-type) and usually reported in the scientific literature.

2. Description

arcs is a computer based knowledgebase management system that supports the building and maintenance of a library of research (or other relationally structured) knowledge. *arcs* consists of 4 major objects:
   a.   Builder: contains screens for direct data entry, editing, and browsing
   b.   Tracker: permits location and aggregation of knowledge in different views
   c.   Importer/Exporter: allows one to enter batch data from a SilverPlatter search, a tabular data entry form, and
        from the personal computer versions of *arcs*
   d.   Modeller: generates relational models of the contained knowledge

Research-knowledge is relational knowledge; i.e. how two or more entities in the world are related together. One of the models of such relationships is that of a directed graph [1]. A directed graph consists of a set of vertices and a set of arcs. The vertices can be used to represent any objects, such as research variables studied together: arcs represent the relationships between the objects or variables. Formally, an arc is an ordered pair of vertices (v,w). The arc (v,w) can be expressed as v ---> w   and drawn as:

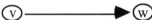

arcs takes its name from this natural model of research relationships. The relational map generated by the graphical version of *arcs* will model all of the research relationships contained in its knowledgebase between a selected focal variable and all or some variables studied with it.

There are major differences in an *arcs* model and the more familiar causal-associational models produced manually by researchers. First of all, the user may choose to model not only directional and symmetric (associational) relationships between studied variables, but also those relationships demonstrated using descriptive, difference, and complex model or "causal" statistical methods. This choice of mapping permits much more detailed information about the range and nature of the relationships being explored between linked variables. Each arc, 2 variables linked by a relationship, retains its link to its source document information. Each unique variable name can be *inspected* to see how many times it occurs in the knowledgebase and the frequency with which it is a dependent vs. independent variable. Each arc can be *inspected* to see what variables it links and important attributes of the relationship such as source, finding, significance, etc.

The relational map thus produced allows the user to easily see gaps and conflicts in a domain of knowledge as well as agreements of studies reporting knowledge between the same variable pairs. The inspectors allow smaller units of knowledge to be explicated for additional study. Relational maps generated by ARCS in several domains will be illustrated.

3. References

[1] Aho A, Hopcroft JE, Ullman JD. Data Structures and Algorithms. Reading, Mass: Addison Wesley Publishing Co, 1983.

Nursing Informatics: An International Overview for Nursing in a Technological Era
S.J. Grobe and E.S.P. Pluyter-Wenting, eds.

Teaching Graduate Students to Develop Computer Simulations

Guyton-Simmons J

School of Nursing, Medical College of Ohio, P. O. Box 10008, Toledo, Ohio 43699-0008, USA

This demonstration will teach participants to create noncued, natural-language computer simulations. The development process uses an authoring system, Druid, with IBM compatible personal computers. Graduate students who were computer novices have learned to create simulations in a few hours. Two of these simulations will be demonstrated. After viewing the simulations as a respondent, participants will view the simulations in the authoring mode. The structure and process of simulation development will be explained, using overhead screens as examples. The structure of the simulation consists of scenarios, sections, and responses. A scenario sets the scene by presenting a patient situation. Queries for additional data or actions to resolve problems are initiated by the respondent by typing on the keyboard. Responses to predicted queries or actions are developed by the author. These responses are activated by matching keywords or phrases in the query/action, giving the respondent additional data about the cause of problems or the effects of interventions. Each section contains a patient problem to be assessed or managed; successful completion is determined by activation of essential responses. Lack of activation of successful responses in a specified time period elicits a remedial response or section. The simulation is developed in an iterative manner. After the skeleton structure is developed, the simulation is compiled and given to expert clinicians. Queries are traced and the printouts used to add and refine responses. The revised form is then given to novice clinicians. Further modifications are made and responses added for incorrect and superfluous queries. The completed simulation can be easily modified to accommodate agency policies and revisions in treatment protocols.

Graduate students who developed computer simulations have increased clinical knowledge as well as learned computer skills. They used literature and other resources to clarify or confirm appropriate selection of interventions, medication dose, lab values, and other data. As expert clinicians reviewed the simulations, different ideas would emerge about what signs and symptoms were relevant to a patient problem or which interventions were appropriate. Clinical issues were discussed with peers, as well, Thus, in creating simulations the students increase their own clinical expertise while learning to develop computer simulations. They identify and translate their own clinical decision-making into a realistic computer simulation for novice learning. At the same time, the students learn strategies for teaching novices how to select relevant assessment data and appropriate interventions. They create an instructional product which can be used to teach clinical decision-making to staff or students.

Nursing Informatics: An International Overview for Nursing in a Technological Era
S.J. Grobe and E.S.P. Pluyter-Wenting, eds.

810

Interfacing Two-way Interactive Video Technology with Nursing Continuing Education

Havice P A[a] and Knowles M H[b]

[a]*Dept of Nursing, Coordinator of Continuing Education, Fort Hays State University, 600 Park Street, Hays, KS, 67601*

[b]*Dept of Nursing, Assistant Professor of Nursing, Fort Hays State University, 600 Park Street, Hays, KS, 67601*

The information age has placed international communication within the grasp of nurses everywhere. Nurses are using modern technology to enhance patient care in many ways. One such technology is two-way interactive video (TWIV). TWIV not only allows nurses to communicate with nurses in different cities, but will also facilitate communication between nurses in different countries.

Conventional methods of providing continuing education for nurses around the world has meant a great investment in time, money and resources for the presentor and the participants. TWIV provides a means of delivering educational opportunities to nurses, whether they are 5 miles or 5,000 miles away. As we enter the 21st century, TWIV technology will become increasingly more "user friendly", convenient and affordable.

This presentation will focus on the role of TWIV technology in providing continuing education for nurses around the world. Ineffective and effective teaching strategies will be presented. Segments of an actual TWIV presentation will be shown and critiqued. The utilization of different types of audio-visual equipment through TWIV will also be explored. Several studies examining the effectiveness of learning through two-way interactive video as compared to the traditional classroom setting will be mentioned.

Nurses who are informed about the newest learning technologies will be able to guide the rest of the nursing profession into the future. TWIV will allow nurses to expand their knowledge in an easily accessible way. For example, the nurse could use this new technology to access continuing education offerings, consult other professionals about case studies, provide input to manufacturers concerning product development, or discuss international nursing issues with nurses in other countries. The uses for TWIV are infinite. With the large amount of information that nurses need to access, TWIV provides a way for nurses to remain the experts on nursing.

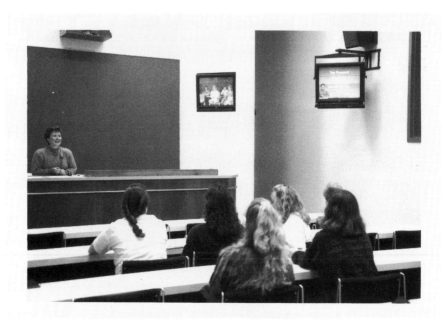

Nursing Informatics: An International Overview for Nursing in a Technological Era
S.J. Grobe and E.S.P. Pluyter-Wenting, eds.

811

WAM (Ward Activity Monitor) and WIP (WAM Information Processor): Software to help represent ward work for benefits realisation projects.

Jones B T

Department of Psychology (Nurse Information Processing Group), University of Glasgow G12 8QQ, Scotland UK

1. The Problem

Non-participatory activity monitoring has been one of the standard ways of measuring (qualitatively and quantitatively) what nurses do in wards. It is especially pertinent to IT Benefits Realisation projects (for example, those accompanying the introduction of ward-based Nursing Information Systems, particularly with care-planning modules).

Because such monitoring is terribly labour-intensive, however, it is only carried out infrequently and, therefore, often *poorly represents* contemporary ward work, defeating its very purpose. Once the data is collected, however, there is yet more labour, for it needs to be processed so that it can be used. Most who process such data know that, as a rule of thumb, for every man-shift of monitoring there is at least another man-shift needed for processing. Consequently, it is no wonder activity monitoring is reluctantly implemented.

Activity monitoring, itself, is a two-phase process: (i) activities are seen, understood and categorized (we call this *monitored)* and then (ii) they are recorded (we call this *recorded)*. It is an unfortunate feature of exercises such as this that while a single nurse can comfortably *monitor* the activities of a number of others, it is the mechanical process of *recording* this information that severely interfers with proper monitoring and, thereby, compromises the representation. Solving the representation problem is the proper role of informatics [1].

2. A solution

With the traditional approach to monitoring, too much cognitive effort needs to be diverted towards *recording* (something anybody can do) at the expense of *monitoring* (which requires the intelligent application of nursing knowledge if ward work is to be properly represented) - and this is exactly the wrong way round. WAM and WIP [2] are software tools (that take advantage of the 1980s' development in graphical user interfaces, GUI/WIMP) that we have developed for our own research and they have been designed to specifically address the two labour-intensive aspects outlined above - permitting the nurse-monitor to concentrate on what is project-important important. This helps assure the *validity* of the representation and modules within WIP also help assess its within-session statistical *reliability*.

The session will demonstrate the use of WAM and WIP and the sort of information it provides. The computer platform is Apple (anything at or above MacPlus) or IBM-compatible (anything at or above 386) and the base software is PLUS2 (cross-platform software for Apple *and* IBM-c).

WAM/WIP have been central to project of ours in the following areas: ENT, mental handicap, care of the elderly and centre-based community health. WAM/WIP can be used for either client-centered or service-centered representations.

3. References

[1] Jones, BT. Heeding, measuring, utilising - the Informatics Template: an explicit working definition for informatics. *Int J Health Inf* 1993, 2(3): 8-11.
[2] Jones, BT. and Buchanan, M. Relieving the bottlenecks in ward activity monitoring through IT. *Inf Tech Nurs* 1989, 1(2): 27-31.

Nursing Informatics: An International Overview for Nursing in a Technological Era
S.J. Grobe and E.S.P. Pluyter-Wenting, eds.

812

Computer patient simulations for pediatric nurse practitioner students

Kilmon C

*Department of Community Health/Gerontology, The University of Texas School of Nursing at Galveston, 1100
Mechanic Street, Galveston, TX 77555-1029, (409) 772-8247 FAX: (409) 772-5118*

This Macintosh program is designed to help graduate nurse practitioner students learn assessment and management of children with minor health problems. Each patient simulation case represents a child with a health problem. Following a brief introductory statement about the case, the learner has an opportunity to select appropriate historical, physical and laboratory data in order to make a diagnosis. The learner then is asked to make one or more diagnoses, develop a plan of management and compare his or her diagnosis and management plan with that proposed by the case author.

Cases are created by modifying a set of template databases so that the data in them are age-appropriate and characteristic of a given health problem. The modified databases are then linked to function as a single program. Each template database is a Hypercard stack. Three stacks (historical information, physical examination data, and laboratory data) contain information appropriate for a healthy 19 month-old child. An additional template stack contains historical information appropriate for a 15 year-old. The remaining template stacks are an introductory stack in which an explanation of the program is given, and a closing stack in which there is space for the student to enter appropriate diagnostic information, options for follow-up care, an author synopsis of the case, and a list of references for further reading.

The program will be marketed as sets of related cases and is anticipated to be useful as a form of continuing education for nurse practitioners in practice as well as in the education of nurse practitioner students. No computer experience is needed in order for students to use the program.

This program is unique in that it is designed specifically for nurse practitioners and contains a set of intervention options that reflect the practice of pediatric nurse practitioners. Health promotion, patient education, supportive services, and management of psychosocial problems are included along with management of acute illnesses. Plans for future development of the program include expansion to reflect the practice of other types of primary care nurse practitioners and development of a more general basic nursing program.

Nursing Informatics: An International Overview for Nursing in a Technological Era
S.J. Grobe and E.S.P. Pluyter-Wenting, eds.

Utilizing a computer based training program to teach nurses to use a Hospital Information System

Klebanoff J L

Hospital Information System Department, New York University Medical Center, 550 First Avenue, New York City 10016, United States

As hospital information systems become more common in healthcare facilities, they present yet another aspect of technology that a nurse must master in clinical practice. A nurse's education comprised of anatomy, physiology and nursing science must now encompass the ability to function in the computerized workplace. A comprehensive training process must be in place to support and facilitate integration of the computer into the nurse's clinical practice, as well as demonstrate the efficacy and benefits that the information provides.

This demonstration will focus on a computer based training (CBT) program utilized to train nurses in the use of a hospital information system. The CBT program is an interactive process in which the nurse-learner is guided through pathways identical to those in actual use. Cues and instructions are given on how to navigate the pathway which is self-directed and self-paced. Immediate feedback is given throughout the program regarding the participant's progress.

The CBT program focuses on taking the nurse-learner from the basic to the specific and strives to provide a working understanding of how to retrieve and enter data into a hospital information system. Utilizing the guided CBT exercises the nurse-learner acquires a fundamental understanding of system basics, data retrieval, the charting of medications, unit tests and vital signs; supply ordering, generating printouts, error correction and late data entry.

The demonstration will present advantages and disadvantages of utilizing a computer based training program versus a book/manual or lecture type learning program. Aspects of program development and administration will also be discussed. The demonstration will include the use of slides and projection of the PC-based CBT program.

© 1994 Elsevier Science B.V. All rights reserved.
Nursing Informatics: An International Overview for Nursing in a Technological Era
S.J. Grobe and E.S.P. Pluyter-Wenting, eds.

Vital signs: A comprehensive approach

McAfooes J

Nurse Educator, Fuld Institute for Technology in Nursing Education, Athens, OH.

This demonstration will show *Vital Signs: A Comprehensive Approach*, a level -III interactive video program developed by the Fuld Institute for Technology in Nursing Education. Although the program was written in English, it is possible to include text and subtitling in other languages through changes in computer programming. A portion of the program has been translated into Spanish and will be shown during the demonstration.

Nursing Informatics: An International Overview for Nursing in a Technological Era
S.J. Grobe and E.S.P. Pluyter-Wenting, eds.

815

Perinatal Family Care: A Learning Module on Intrapartal Nursing Care

McGonigle D[a] and Wedge K[b]

[a]School of Nursing, Penn State University, University Park, PA 16802-6508 USA

[b]School of Nursing, University of Pittsburgh, Pittsburgh, PA 15261 USA

Perinatal Family Care is an interactive video program that does not require extensive computer skills and is conducive to rapid learning within a safe environment. The module is comprised of 79 pages that provide the learner with information about families giving birth. Through interaction with text, graphics, and video images, the user learns about care provided to these very special families. *Perinatal Family Care* is designed to accompany the Birth Disc videodisc developed by Harriette Hartigan.

1. Introduction

This video demonstration will enable the participants to view the interactive video learning module, *Perinatal Family Care*. This presentation will review the purpose and rationale for using this interactive video program with both generic nursing students as well as returning registered nurse students. The components of the courseware and the concept of mapping and navigation will be discussed.

2. Objectives

The participants will be able to: describe the learning module in *Perinatal Family Care*, assess mapping and navigation throughout the module, and evaluate the components of the module.

3. Demonstration

The presentation will begin with a discussion of the purpose and rationale for developing the *Perinatal Family Care* module. The concept of mapping and navigation will be reviewed. The video demonstration will highlight the components of the program accessed from the MAP and the additional information available via buttons, hotwords, and scanning controls.

Nursing Informatics: An International Overview for Nursing in a Technological Era
S.J. Grobe and E.S.P. Pluyter-Wenting, eds.

AIDSNET: An innovative strategy of nursing outreach

Parietti ES and Atav AS

Binghamton University, State University of New York, Binghamton NY 13902-6000 USA

AIDSNET is a computerized health care support network that provides nursing consultation, case management, social support and AIDS related information to rural, homebound HIV+/PWAs(Persons With AIDS) living in upstate New York. Personal computers in AIDS patients' homes are connected via modems and existing telephone lines to a central computer in the Decker School of Nursing at Binghamton University. Although AIDSNET operates as a bulletin board system (BBS), it offers unique services to its users. AIDS patients in rural areas have an opportunity to access nursing experts in the care of AIDS patients for consultation, send and receive messages, and read or download information from national AIDS networks. AIDSNET is on-line 24 hours a day, 7 days a week, providing services free of charge to users. All professional services on AIDSNET are donated. Users access the system with a password and may remain anonymous if they choose.

The network was established in May of 1991 with 5 computers and modems donated by the Decker School of Nursing. These computers were installed in AIDS patients' homes, and instructions were given accessing the network. Once the network was up and running, additional PWA users, who own their own computers, were recruited to AIDSNET. As computer equipment is donated to the project, it is placed in the home of an interested homebound AIDS patient.

AIDSNET has 28-30 users, and averages 177 calls a month to the network. Content analysis of questions to the AIDSNET nurse consultant reveal that social support, illness support, treatment protocols and HIV status are predominant themes on the network.

AIDSNET has reduced the effects of social and geographic isolation of homebound PWAs in the area by providing a communications pathway to peers and professionals. The network has also increased the ability of PWAs to cope with the demands of their illness by providing access to nurse consultants who are experts in the care of AIDS patients. The success of AIDSNET has demonstrated that interactive telecomputing can revolutionize the home care of rural isolated patients by providing nursing outreach and critical access to health professionals.

AIDSNET demonstration will include on-line access to the health care support network via personal computer and modem. Services available on the system will be shown, and the audience will be able to read recent general messages sent by the nurse consultant to all users.

Nursing Informatics: An International Overview for Nursing in a Technological Era
S.J. Grobe and E.S.P. Pluyter-Wenting, eds.

IVD: Examples of how one disc achieves many goals

Price MR

The PENZANCE Professional Nursing and Health Career Enhancement Center, Columbia-Presbyterian Medical Center, 622 West 168th Street, New York 10032 USA

Department of Nursing, Teachers College Columbia University, 525 West 120th Street, New York, New York 10027 USA

Cambre & Castner (1991) found that the successful integration of interactive videodisc (IVD) technology into nursing curricula lags far behind faculty enthusiasm for the technology. In most instances, faculty use IVD as an add-on optional assignment that supplements traditional instruction. They often assign an IVD program in its totality. Many students who complete these optional add-on assignments report racing through the videodisc in linear fashion. Students do not hold themselves accountable for mastering the material on the videodisc when they know faculty will present or make the material available in a different format. Eighty-seven percent of the students surveyed report using IVD as one reads a book: beginning to end, chapter by chapter. Faculty that continue to use IVD programs in this manner will never realize the potential of this technology.

In this presentation I will address the above issues as I demonstrate how faculty use the interactive video disc program <u>Nursing Care of the Elderly Client with Chronic Obstructive Lung Disease</u>, to meet course objectives in an undergraduate, and graduate nursing program. In order to provide educationally sound learning experiences, selected portions of the program were combined with assigned readings and other instructional resources to design competency based learning modules. In the undergraduate program, faculty use these IVD modules as instructional tools to teach Chest Assessment Skills, Nursing Management of Clients on Mechanical Ventilators, Acid-Base Balance/Blood Gas Interpretation, Nursing Management of Clients with Respiratory Dysfunction, and Breathing Techniques. In the graduate program, faculty use the interactive videodisc program as an assessment or instructional tool for students who are preparing for leadership roles in advanced practice or education. IVD assignments are a required component of the course, and students are accountable for mastering the content. IVD modules are assigned as independent, team or small group anchored instructional learning experiences. The purpose and the advantages of each integration strategy are explored and the use of anchored instruction as a problem solving strategy demonstrated. An outline of the instructional tools included in the modules, and the underlying rationales for the use of these instructional aids is provided.

The interactive video program, Nursing Care of the Elderly Client with Chronic Obstructive Lung Disease, runs on the FITNE or IBM Infowindow platform.

1.   References

[1]   Camber M & Castner L. *The Status of Interactive Video Technology in Nursing Education Environments (Doctoral Dissertation, The Ohio State University, 1991).* Prepared for the Fuld Institute of Technology in Athens, Ohio.

[2]   The Cognition and Technology Group at Vanderbuilt. Anchored Instruction and its Relationship to Situated Cognition. Educational Researcher, 2-10.

Nursing Informatics: An International Overview for Nursing in a Technological Era
S.J. Grobe and E.S.P. Pluyter-Wenting, eds.

818

Multimedia Patient Case Study Simulations:
A Demonstration Illustrating Their Evaluation and Use

Rizzolo M A

Director, Interactive Technologies, American Journal of Nursing Co., 555 West 57th St., New York, NY 10019

Patient case study simulations are unique applications of multimedia technology. The combination of video, audio, graphics and the branching power of the computer permits the creation of learning experiences that have never before been possible. They can allow learners to practice patient care management and decision-making in a risk-free environment. They can provide all students with an experience caring for patients with common problems, as well as conditions that are rarely seen. Patient case study simulations can place the learner in a variety of environments. And, they can provide the ideal learning sequence by presenting a patient with a condition that matches the content that is being studied. Multimedia patient case study simulations using videodiscs, usually referred to as interactive video (IAV), have been commercially available for a few years and have received an enthusiastic reception by nurse educators. This demonstration will show selected segments from three IAV patient case study simulations:

Nursing Care of the Elderly Patient with COPD, a program that permits learners to manage the care of Mr. Presley, an elderly man with COPD and pneumonia, through four stages of his care in the hospital. It begins with his emergency admission, progresses through his respiratory arrest and care while he is on a mechanical ventilator in the intensive care unit, and follows him to his discharge.

Nursing Care of Elderly Patients with Acute Cardiac Disorders, which features two case studies: Mr. Kent a 73 year old man who has had a myocardial infarction; and Mr. Talbert, an 80 year old man with congestive heart failure. The simulations provide an opportunity for the nurse to listen to heart sounds, analyze ECG rhythms, regulate fluid and oxygen therapy and initiate emergency interventions.

Ethical Dilemmas and Legal Issues in Care of the Elderly takes the nurses who are caring for Ms. Burbank through four ethical situations and their legal implications: advance directives, use of restraints, reassignment of a nurse, and do not resuscitate orders.

Throughout the demonstration, the focus will be on the evaluation of fidelity in patient case study simulations. Fidelity refers to how closely a simulated experience imitates reality. Vignettes from the program will be used to illustrate five elements of fidelity: realism, level of decision-making, user input, feedback and record keeping, and the balance of video and text. Suggestions for use of multimedia patient case study simulations will also be discussed as the programs are demonstrated.

Nursing Informatics: An International Overview for Nursing in a Technological Era
S.J. Grobe and E.S.P. Pluyter-Wenting, eds.

Denver Free-Net Demonstration

Skiba DJ and Mirque D

*School of Nursing, University of Colorado Health Sciences Center, Campus Box C-288, 4200 E. Ninth Ave.,
Denver, CO 80262, USA*

The Denver Free-Net (DFN) is a community computing system that provides an on-line communication vehicle and a repository of information and resources for the greater Denver metropolitan region. The system is available to anyone with access to a computer with a modem and telecommunications software. The Denver Free-Net is available on a 24 hour a day basis and can be reached via the Internet.

The DFN is conceptualized as an electronic city in which users can enter buildings that are commonly found in most communities. For example, a user can enter the Health Care Building and can select from menus which contain health care resources. Within each building, users can enter rooms that represent different features of the system such as Reading Rooms, News Room, or Community Values Discussion Rooms. Users can also select menus that correspond to sub-menus such as the University of Colorado Health Sciences Center, Department of Health or the Denison Health Sciences Library. The menus of the system provide users with access to text-read only documents, text-based retrievable documents, and searchable databases.

In addition to information access and retrieval, users can use various communication mechanisms such as electronic mail services, file transfer protocols capabilities and remote login services to selected Internet systems. Communication is also enhanced by the use of Question & Answer Forums, Discussion groups available on a local, national and international levels, electronic support groups, and the CHAT function in which users can communicate in real time. These services allow the Denver Free-Net to facilitate both communication and information access.

In the Health Care Building, the Healthy People 2000 framework is used as a means to structure information in the building. Citizens can access resources in health promotion, health protection, preventive services and surveillance & data systems. Information resources and communication vehicles are established within each of the Healthy People 2000 priority areas. For example, a user can access information about consumer nutrition tips for children, leave a question about women's dietary needs or participate in a worldwide discussion group on nutrition under the Health Promotion's sub-menu for Nutrition. The Health Care Building also houses the communication mechanisms and instructional materials for distance education and traditional courses offered by the School of Nursing.

A demonstration of the Denver Free-Net will highlight the unique features of this community computing system and how it can be used as a means to deliver health care.

Nursing Informatics: An International Overview for Nursing in a Technological Era
S.J. Grobe and E.S.P. Pluyter-Wenting, eds.

820

Using Technology to Enhance Patient Care

Sweeney M A Lester J Mercer Z Reutelhuber E Koleosho O Oppermann C
Rios D and Cooper M

The University of Texas Medical Branch, Galveston, Texas 77555 U.S.A.

The University of Texas Medical Branch in Galveston has developed a series of educational programs for patients in community-based maternal-infant clinics. The Healthy Touch" Series provides instructional information on: Feeding Your Baby, Safety and Immunization , and Having A Healthy Pregnancy. The multimedia programs were developed primarily for patients, but will be revised and extended at a later date for professional level continuing education. The development and evaluation of the programs was funded by the W.K. Kellogg Foundation.

The multimedia delivery platform consists of a 486 microcomputer, a videodisc player, touch-sensitive VGA monitor, and CD-ROM drive. Computer hardware and software permit many types of visual and auditory messages to convey the instructional content while the interactive design creates a variety of choices for patients.

The first part of the demonstration shows how a bilingual technology-based program can be easily managed by patients who are technological novices and who may not have highly developed reading skills. Feeding Your Baby, provides an interactive experience in learning about nutrition by "shopping" in our specially designed 3-D grocery store. Patients initially select the language for the audio track and then receive an orientation to the program design and navigation instructions by the grocer himself. They can move through various aisles and browse through the colorful shelves which are set up with labels above each item. If learners touch the label, the name of the food item is spoken aloud. If they touch the food itself, they obtain feedback on nutrient composition and values, or the age-appropriateness of the food. Sound effects and animation make the shopping excursion enjoyable as well as instructive.

The second part of the demonstration illustrates two aspects of the safety program entitled, Home "Safe" Home. It shows how strategic decisions in the planning stages can make wise use of programming resources and graphic screens. The interactive program permits learners to choose between a "browsing" mode of moving ad lib through the rooms or a "tour" mode which is more structured. Tours include topics such as Fire Safety, Electrical Safety, Environmental Safety, and a special Grandparents tour. The skillful addition of digital video windows adds a talking, real-life tour guide, and provides for a demonstration mode in moving video. The moving video enhances and extends the instructional capability to the graphics screens and animation of the safety house.

The final part of the demonstration will show a computer-managed "interview" which is used in the program evaluation component. The bilingual interview permits the option of "hearing" the questions and answering options read aloud to accommodate patients requiring assistance with reading skills. Responses are immediately filed in digital format for retrieval in reports at a later date. Patient response to the computer-based "interviewer" will be reviewed.

Mastering clinical skills: Chest tubes

Yoder ME

Nursing Software Development, 1496 West University Heights Drive North, Flagstaff, AZ, 86001, USA

This demonstration features a computer assisted tutorial, *Mastering Clinical Skills: Chest Tubes*. This program goes beyond the basic procedure. Instruction emphasizes the skills necessary to truly manage a patient with pleural or mediastinal chest tubes. It features concepts, decision making, trouble shooting and handling emergencies for a variety of patients with chest tubes. Instructional sequences include both text and animation. The program incorporates a three-level design to met the needs of both preservice and inservice learners. The three levels are instruction, review, and testing.

Upon completion of this program, the learner will be able to:

1. Distinguish between pleural and mediastinal chest tubes.
2. Identify the purpose of each chamber in the drainage unit.
3. Recognize expected chamber action in a variety of patient situations.
4. Recognize and locate air leaks.
5. State dangerous practices to be avoided.
6. Describe common emergencies with interventions.

The program also includes a mastery test of patient situations to which the learner must apply the information learned in the program. Results of the mastery test can be printed out to provide documentation of learning achieved.

Mastering Clinical Skills: Chest Tubes runs under MS-DOS 3.0 or higher with a minimum of 256K of memory and an EGA monitor.

© 1994 Elsevier Science B.V. All rights reserved.
Nursing Informatics: An International Overview for Nursing in a Technological Era
S.J. Grobe and E.S.P. Pluyter-Wenting, eds.

822

Department of Veterans Affairs Decentralized Hospital Computer Program
for Nursing Service

Gilleran J [a] Lang B J [b] Smart S [c] and Ziacik J[d]

[a]Nursing Service (118), VA Medical Center, Hines, Illinois, 60141, USA

[b]Dept. of Veterans Affairs, Hines Information Systems Center, P.O. Box 7008, Hines, IL, 60141-7008, USA

[c]Nursing Service (118),VA Medical Center, Sheridan, Wyoming, 82801, USA

[d]Nursing Service (118),VA Medical Center, Decatur, Georgia, 30033, USA

This demonstration represents an overview of the nursing clinical and management information system
implemented in the Department of Veterans Affairs Medical Centers.

1. Introduction

Since the mid 1980's, the Department of Veterans Affairs (DVA) has developed the Decentralized Hospital
Computer Program (DHCP) Nursing software with the goal of automating the Nursing Service in all facets of its daily
operation. The software is comprised of four modules: administration, clinical, staff education and quality
management. Each module is integrated with the hospital's DHCP clinical and management information system
which operates in 167 hospitals, 229 outpatient clinics, 122 nursing homes, and 27 domiciliaries. The software is
written in ANSI M (formerly known as ANSI MUMPS).

2. Demonstration and Discussion

The content of the demonstration will cover each of the four DHCP nursing modules. Emphasis is placed on the
clinical module and its potential for providing a national nursing knowledge base and supporting decision aids.

Clinical Module: The clinical module was designed to automate the elements of the nursing process and provide
linkages to the integrated clinical record created by various DHCP applications. Software functionality supports the
planning, data entry, data retrieval and analysis of nursing care provided to the client. Problems identified through the
assessment are automatically triggered into the care plan. Patient problems, clinical alerts, and orders are reflected on
the patient care assignment worksheets and the end of shift reports which are generated from the system. Patient
progress is documented through: (i) clinical observations/ measurements functions such as vital signs, intake and
output, physical assessment; (ii) progress, transfer, and discharge notes; (iii) various patient care flowsheets; (iv)
graphic summaries; and (v) health summary. All applications are site configurable; and can be modified to comply
with various nursing care delivery models and nursing practice standards implemented at a medical facility. A text
generator utility which provides the basic programming tool for the clinical module will be discussed.

Administration Module: Provides management support to the largest service within the DVA and is integrated with
hospital and national database management information systems. Tracks employee demographics, military experience,
certification, credentials, professional experience, and work assignments to generate resource management and ad hoc
reports. The software contains an interface which transfers data from the position control module to various staff
schedulers (e.g., RES-Q RN, ANSOS, MDAX, InCharge, etc.)

Staff Education Module: Provides a management tool to document attendance at staff inservices, continuing
education and continued clinical competency offerings required by regulatory agencies and licensing boards. Cost of
program attendance is tracked and information is stored in the Personnel Accounting and Integrated Data (PAID)
software. Data is rolled up into a national database.

Quality Management Module: Contains options for data collection and reporting of administrative and clinical
monitors to survey compliance with established standards of care and practice. The software provides tools for
extracting and rank ordering patient problems and nursing interventions associated with nursing and medical diagnoses.

A Five Year Retrospective Of The HBO & Company Nurse Scholars Program

Simpson R[a] Skiba DJ[b] Ronald JS[c]

[a]*Executive Director, Nursing Affairs, HBO & Company, Atlanta, Georgia, USA.*

[b]*Associate Director, Center for Nursing Research, University of Colorado Health Sciences Center, Denver, Colorado, USA.*

[c]*Associate Professor, State University of New York at Buffalo, Buffalo, New York, USA.*

1. Description of Program

Despite the progress made in nursing education, the advancement of nursing informatics and the proliferation of information systems in hospitals and medical institutions, few faculty members in nursing schools around the world have direct experience with the development and use of information systems to facilitate nursing practice. As a result, there is a wide gap between education and service, with few nurses in academia adequately preparing nurses for the reality of nursing informatics in the workplace. This gap has made it difficult to translate "real world" clinical applications into the nursing educational realm.

In general, nursing informatics has been defined as a combination of computer science, information science and nursing science designed to assist in the management and processing of nursing data, information and knowledge to support the practice of nursing and the delivery of nursing care (Ozbolt and Graves, 1993). To bridge the gap between education and service and prepare professional nurses for the practicing in the 21st century, HBO & Company (HBOC) created a unique collaboration between corporate business interests and nursing education.

Initiated in 1989, the HBOC Nurse Scholars Program was designed to teach faculty how to *teach* nursing informatics to future generations of nursing students and to put the structures in place to better prepare students for automated clinical practice. Long-term goals included support for educating students in the use, design, implementation, and management of information systems in the clinical arena--i.e., integrating nursing informatics into core nursing curricula. The emphasis is not on "computer skills" or computer literacy, but on teaching informatics as a body of science and reorienting the teaching of nursing content given the capabilities of nursing information systems. The dissemination and diffusion of nursing informatics knowledge is expected to help nurses at all levels function as informed participants in the design, selection, implementation, use, management and evaluation of automated information systems.

Each year since its inception, the HBOC Nurse Scholars Program has provided nine nurse educators an intensive classroom and hands-on training experience designed to address the concepts and methods of automated systems. These teacher/scholars are selected one from each of the nine American Organization Nurse Executives (AONE) regions in the United States. In the past two years, one scholar from Canada and the United Kingdom have also participated; 1994 will mark the first year an Australian Nurse Scholar will participate in the program. Every September, HBO & Company contacts more than 600 deans of programs offering graduate and baccalaureate nursing degrees for nominations of scholars. The deans nominated a faculty member or members whose applications and concept papers are returned to HBOC by December. Nominees are evaluated and selected by an external advisory group from the educational and service communities. Nationally known leaders in nursing information systems from universities, healthcare institutions and businesses serve as faculty along with experts from HBO. The faculty consists of approximately 25 individuals, selected for their expertise in informatics.

The program has specified five clear objectives:

1. Analyze healthcare information systems and how they assist nurses to provide quality patient care, increase efficiency and manage shrinking resources.
2. Explore the issues for identifying information requirements for nursing.
3. Understand the principles of selection, implementation, and evaluation of healthcare information systems.

4.   Examine strategies and issues related to integrating nursing informatics into the nursing curriculum.
5.   Interact with the HBO & Company Hospital Information Systems.

1.1. The Uniqueness of a Private Sector Collaboration

The fact that the Nurse Scholars program has been conceived, implemented, managed and funded by a private sector corporation marks a new of cooperation between nursing academia and for-profit developers of healthcare information systems. The Company was careful to preserve and protect the integrity of nursing education during the formation of the project by involving respected scholars of nursing and informatics to serve as consultants on the project. The two consultants and co-developers of the program--Diane J. Skiba and Judith S. Ronald--were widely respected for having spent more than 15 years actively promoting the integration of nursing informatics into the nursing curriculum. Both consultants also served as original charter members of the National League for Nursing's (NLN) Council for Nursing Informatics. Roy L. Simpson, HBO & Company's Executive Director of Nursing Affairs is a nursing leader who was also an original charter member of the NLN Council for Nursing Informatics; Simpson served as HBOC's internal guiding force for the program.

HBO & Company is a publicly-held American company based in Atlanta, Georgia. It is listed on the NASDAQ as HBO. The Company was formed in 1970 as a hospital information systems supplier and has emerged nearly 15 years later as a leader in the field, with $275 million in annual sales. HBOC houses two main product lines-- software that operates within an IBM mainframe environment for larger hospitals or teaching centers (450+ beds), and software that operates on minicomputer platforms such as Data General and Digital Equipment Corporation (DEC) systems for mid-sized hospitals. Both product lines include clinical management or information systems, financial systems, decision-support systems and executive information systems.

Since the Company straddled the market in terms of delivering both mainframe and mini-computer/networked systems, it was able to incorporate the practical realities, differences and similarities of each hardware platform into the Nurse Scholars curriculum. The goal was to expose nurse scholars to a "live" interactive environment featuring each platform so that objective observations could be made about performance variables and functional similarities and differences. The hands-on experience removes the barrier of theoretical discourses and allows faculty members to experience first-hand precisely what their students will experience as a requisite once they graduate and move into practicing in the current and future automated practice environments.

3. The Curriculum

The distinction of the HBOC Nurse Scholars Program is that it incorporates a realistic and practical approach to informatics curriculum but, more importantly, also emphasizes creativity within use, management, selection, development and evaluation of nursing information systems. The idea is that it is not enough to teach computer basics nor even mandate the science as a core requisite. Data and the mechanics of its storage and transference is virtually useless until it is recast as usable information.

The curriculum of the program therefore emphasizes the importance of instructing future nurses on the methods and necessity for extracting and synthesizing information, which has become paramount in today's automated patient care environment. As such, the broad content areas of the program include:

o   An overview of nursing informatics taking into account the historical perspective and the evaluation process.
o   Basic concepts of automated healthcare information systems, including definitions, design goals and security issues.
o   Alternate approaches to system development.
o   Evaluation criteria for various system approaches.
o   The various information systems within the hospital system that support specific clinical, administrative and management functions.
o   The life cycle of the hospital information system (HIS) or nursing information system (NIS), including the research and feasibility evaluation process, the selection process, implementation and maintenance of systems, and ongoing evaluation of installed systems.
o   Research issues, including nurses information needs, effectiveness of nursing information systems, the nursing decision-making process, and the impact on organization, patient care and nursing care practice.

o   Curriculum issues related to the integration of nursing informatics into the undergraduate/graduate nursing curriculum; objectives, resources, content, placement, and learning activities.
o   Introduction to HBO & Company's HIS systems--mainframe and minicomputer based.

Formal and informal discussions, lectures and hands-on practice sessions with "live" information systems serve as the focus for the educational program. In addition to the above topics, the Nurse Scholars faculty also identify issues that serve as barriers to the advancement of information systems that will support nursing practice. One key barrier, for example, is the lack of nursing taxonomy and lexicon. Faculty and nurse scholars, for example, will discuss the implications of Graves and Ozbolt's (1993) observation that it is the absence of codified data that has inhibited the inclusion of nursing information in the various discharge abstract databases on which health policy decisions are increasingly based.

The goals and objectives of the program have remained essentially the same since the program's inception. However, specific content to meet the goals and objectives has been modified in response to developments in the field of healthcare informatics and feedback from the Scholars. For example, technical advancements have resulted in increased emphasis on workstations, networks and distributed systems. In the application areas, more time is spent discussing actual and potential data sets provided by different information systems, how these data sets can be used by nurses to assist in clinical and administrative decision-making, and increased consideration of the impact of information technology from psycho-social, ethical, legal and professional perspectives. In addition, the focus of nursing information system evaluation has shifted from a pure research perspective to an application orientation. Curriculum issues have expanded beyond the integration of nursing informatics into the curriculum to the exploration of curriculum changes needed to prepare nursing students to work with the computer as a partner in their professional practice. In response to changing healthcare environments, the faculty also review with nurse scholars the impact of American health care reform initiatives on the development and use of information systems to manage clinical, administrative and financial data.

Throughout the program, each scholar receives teaching materials that can be integrated directly into the scholar's own academic program including objectives, content outline, bibliography, a textbook, several monographs, a set of generic slides, and demonstration disks. These materials serve as a base from which scholars can build their own educational programs and initiatives to share with nursing students and colleagues.

4. Impact of Program

The HBOC Nurse Scholars Program has had tremendous impact on a number of constituencies, including the Company as an institution, to nursing education and to participants (Nurse Scholars).

4.1 The Impact on HBO & Company

From the outset, the Company was committed to creating a program that benefited nurse educators; it has stuck closely to its goals of avoiding any hint that it was trying to "sell" its systems or solutions. After five years of success, HBO has determined that it has benefited from an opening up of markets as the Company gains exposure to academic institutions throughout North America and England. In addition, the creation, sponsorship and funding of the entire program it has given the company's internal sales and account management personnel the ability to demonstrate to the nursing practice and academic community the Company's commitment to nursing *without the direct expectation of profit*.

In addition, the Company benefits from a more educated consumer; HBO understands that future generations of nursing graduates will one day be in a position to select a hospital information system or nursing information system for their own institutions. The Company considers this education an "investment" in its future.

Finally, HBO has benefited from the program by enjoying an increase in name recognition among the nursing community. The HBO Nurse Scholars Program is widely recognized and respected as an important means to promote and encourage the advancement of nursing informatics; the Company's association with this admirable goal has considerably increased its visibility in the nursing community.

In addition to the Nurse Scholars Program, the Company has demonstrated its commitment to the nursing profession by creating a Nursing Advisory Panel. Conceived in the same year the Scholars program was initiated (1989), the Nursing Advisory council was put in place to help the Company define strategic plans for future nursing systems and to review high-level clinical system design strategies. This Nursing Advisory Panel or "think tank" of national recognized nursing experts also advises the Company on such issues as development of selection criteria for the Nurse Scholars Program as well as with the evaluation of international markets for clinical systems.

4.2 The Impact on Nursing Education

The HBOC Nurse Scholars Program has influenced the area of informatics in nursing education. First and foremost, the program helped to create a critical mass of educators who have critically analyzed what concepts and knowledge is required for a course in nursing informatics. While many educators have taught courses prior to the Scholars Program, most have acknowledged that the courses focused on computer literacy and did not contain the depth and breadth of nursing informatics. This critical mass has also reflected upon their individual school of nursing's curriculum and how the curriculum needs to be changed to reflect the changing clinical environment. The educators have also seen a glimpse of the future and are rethinking the teaching-learning process. An additional impact is that these faculty are geographically dispersed, ensuring that all the talents are not centered in one Mecca.

Second, a network has evolved among the Scholars. The network has provided multiple opportunities for sharing and providing consultations to each other's schools. One example is the creation of a faculty development series that three Scholars created across their respective schools. The work from this collaboration resulted in the writing of a textbook eventually published by the National League for Nursing. The Scholars call upon each other for consultations and help each other in the development of courses and instructional materials. In one cohort, one scholar has worked with two other schools to expand their informatics curriculum. The networks have crossed cohorts and have fostered numerous collaborative projects.

Third, Scholars have assumed leadership roles in nursing informatics. These roles include: post doctoral study, committee and board membership in a variety of national nursing organizations, and participation in invitational conferences and summits.

Fourth, the program has provided numerous opportunities for the Scholars to use their knowledge of information systems. Many scholars have given presentations at national and international conferences. The Scholars have also called up on many of the HBOC staff and lecturers to talk at their schools. Several faculty have joint appointments in academia and in service as a result of their participation in the HBOC Nurse Scholars Program.

In summary, the HBOC Nurse Scholars Program has created a critical mass of educators across the United States knowledgeable in the area of informatics who are in turn sharing their knowledge with the greater nursing community.

4.3 The Impact on Nurse Scholars

Evaluation of results has played a key role in the program since its inception. The goal is to obtain feedback from various constituent groups and to provide information for continuous improvement on course curriculum, teaching materials, applicability to specific scholar curriculums and overall feedback about the structure and implementation of the program. Scholars are asked to review the quality of the program and how effectively the program met identified goals. In addition, participating scholars are contacted after the program for post-assessment follow-ups.

Results of the post-assessments continue to be positive. Results from participation in the Program include attendance in postdoctoral programs in informatics, strengthening of undergraduate and masters-level informatics courses, elections to professional organizations related to informatics and the design of faculty development and/or enrichment programs by several of the scholars. To share some of the results, we found anecdotal discourse on the success of the program is by far the strongest evidence of its effectiveness. HBO & Company, through interviews, has amassed the following input and information from participating Scholars:

Suzanne Henry, a 1990 Scholar, was awarded a post-doctorate fellowship at Stanford University. Another 1990 Scholar, Ramona Nelson from the University of Pittsburgh, was elected to the Executive Committee of the National League for Nursing Council of Nursing Informatics.

Richard Redman, PhD, RN, assistant professor at the University of Michigan and Nurse Scholar in 1990 used the information he learned and the expertise he gained to act as a vocal member of the selection committee in choosing an information system for the medical center. "The Nurse Scholar's Program gave me the knowledge base I needed to help make an informed decision on a system," he asserts. Of the program, Redman says he "was especially pleased with its practical focus. Whereas a standard computer class deals mostly with analysis and word processing, this program focused on the nursing practice as it exists in today's hospital." He also comments that the "program was like a mini-sabbatical. It was exciting to mix with people actually in the industry."

Another 1990 Scholar, Nancy M. Longcrier, assistant professor at Clemson University, Clemson, South Carolina, reports that she rewrote her syllabus to incorporate material from the Nurse Scholars Program into her curriculum. "When I came back from the seminar, there were so many new things to teach that I had to have my students choose the things they most wanted to cover in the few weeks we had left in the school year."

Betty Paulanka, Ed.D., RN, of the University of Delaware College of Nursing, says of her 1991 program participation that such an intense learning experience inspires and challenges participants to educate their colleagues and students when they return to their respective schools. "In the past, I tended to get all excited about the potential of nursing information systems during a workshop," Paulanka notes. "Then I went back to the 'real world' and the importance and urgency faded away. Now I realize that I can't let this knowledge go by the wayside."

Scholar Bunny J. Pozehl, PhD, RN, of the University of Nebraska Medical Center in Omaha, says she came to the 1991 Nurse Scholars Program expecting to augment her "basic course" in nursing informatics--taught as an elective for undergraduates, but came away with a different perspective: "I came away with so much more in terms of where nursing is and where we need to go," she points out. "I came away with the realization that I have a big mission ahead of me."

As a result of her 1992 Nurse Scholars experience, Ida Androwich, PhD, RN, associate professor, Niehoff School of Nursing, Loyola University of Chicago, says she is considering restructuring the school's entire informatics course offerings. In addition, she also became involved in the "planning stages for a summer institute on nursing informatics for faculty in the Midwest" thanks to the program.

Nurse Scholar Cassy Pollack, PhD, RN, chairperson of the nursing systems in the policy and community health division of Yale University in Connecticut, says she brought a limited background in informatics to her participation in the 1993 program, but also a healthy dose of skepticism. "I expected to learn a lot but in reality to be bored a little, too," she says. "I wasn't. The program was phenomenally valuable and stimulating." Pollack is involved in developed an informatics course "to help students develop a process of critical thinking [which] involves teach them how to take data and convert it into information so that they can make informed and appropriate decisions needed for leadership."

5. Summary

The HBO & Company Nurse Scholars program continues to evolve as a pioneering model for facilitating a bridge between nursing education and nursing practice, academia and the corporate sector. Since 1989, [insert number] of faculty from the United States, Canada and the United Kingdom have participated in the Nurse Scholars Program with the clear goal of disseminating the knowledge of nursing informatics throughout the nursing community--i.e., students, faculty, practitioners and administrators. The dissemination and diffusion of nursing informatics knowledge is expected to help nurses at all levels function as informed participants in the design, selection, implementation and evaluation of automated systems well into the 21st century.

6. References

[1] Ozbolt, J.G and Graves, J.R. Clinical Nursing Informatics--Developing Tools for Knowledge Workers. *Nurs Clin North Am* 1993, 28: 407-425.

[2] Skiba, D. J., Simpson, R.L. and Ronald, J.S. HealthQuest/HBO Nurse Scholars Program: A Corporate Partnership With Nursing Education in *Computer Applications in Nursing Education and Practice*, Arnold, J. and Pearson, G. (eds). National League for Nursing, New York, 1992: 224-235.

[3] Simpson, R.L. Closing the Gap Between School and Service. *Nurs Mngr*, November, 1990: 14-15.

Nursing Informatics: An International Overview for Nursing in a Technological Era
S.J. Grobe and E.S.P. Pluyter-Wenting, eds.

828

Allergy/Adverse Reaction Tracking Program:
Reversing the Process from Bedside to Computer

Slonaker P S[a] Gordon D G[b] and Milfajt R[c]

[a]Nursing ADP Coordinator, Dayton Veterans Affairs Medical Center, 4100 West Third Street, Dayton Ohio 45428

[b]Clinical Coordinator, Dayton Veterans Affairs Medical Center, 4100 West Third Street, Dayton Ohio 45428

[c]Project Manager Software Development, Information Systems Center, Hines, Illinois 60141

Manubay's Laws for Programmers[1] states, "Users don't know what they really want, but they know for certain what they don't want." Therein lies the focus of this paper. Too many times software programs are written by programmers under the direction of developers who feel they are in touch with the perceived needs of the computer system users. A need to track allergies was identified by the Department of Veterans Affairs. A multi-disciplinary group was appointed to identify user needs and develop a computer program. After a plan was developed, it was submitted to computer programmers. The finished program was presented to alpha and beta test sites for evaluation. End users provided immense, valuable feedback. The program was fundamentally altered in response to users comments. The program continues to be revised and re-submitted to alpha and beta test sites.

1.0 Introduction

The Department of Veterans Affairs (VA) Chicago Information Systems Center (ISC) embarked on developing a national Allergy/Adverse Reaction Tracking program (AART). A group called a Clinical Applications Resource Group (CARG), which consists of VA physicians and clinicians, determined a national need to track allergies. This group then established an allergy expert panel which consisted of a nurse, two pharmacists, a dietician, a radiologist, a physician, a chief of Medical Administration Service (MAS) and an allergist. The purpose of the program was to create a national allergy tracking system and facilitate compliance with new Joint Commission for Accreditation Healthcare Organizations (JCAHO) requirements.

The expert panel first established what the VA was already using to track allergies. The system was evaluated for advantages and disadvantages. Additional information deemed pertinent was included in the program specifications. Planning encompassed the theoretical role assigned various health care workers. Originally, unit clerks, nurses, and physicians would have the primary data entry role. Dietetics could enter and verify food allergies and delete food preferences (food preferences were handled in the dietary program). The pharmacist would have the responsibility of verifying allergies. The process of verification of an allergy/adverse reaction is one that ensures the correctness of the data. The verifiers, who may be Clinical Pharmacists, Dieticians, and other clinical personnel, are designated by the specific VAMCs where they are employed. They compare patient data: i.e. laboratory results, medications patient ingested, signs and symptoms, and descriptions of patient's reaction. This data is entered into a specific verification program that calculates the likelihood of a True Allergy versus an Adverse Reaction through the use of an FDA algorithm.

2.0 Design

In February of 1991, a programmer/developer was assigned to the project and began to develop a tracking program for all VA facilities. The design phase involved two programmers for four weeks. Six additional weeks were required by two programmers to complete the coding phase. Approximately three months were required to prepare the program for site testing. After the program was developed, 8 Alpha and Beta test sites were selected. The role of an Alpha test site is to use the program, identify flaws, and provide feedback. A Beta test site continues site testing and suggests necessary program changes as needed. The Dayton and Hines Veterans Affairs Medical Centers (VAMC) were selected as Alpha test sites.

The new program, Version 2.0, arrived and was installed May, 1991 in the test account. The test account is a trial environment that is intended to reflect the actual computer functioning but uses bogus data. Initial feedback came from service Automated Data Processing Application Coordinators (ADPAC). The role of the ADPAC is to manage and maintain software and to educate and update users. Participating ADPAC's at Dayton were from MAS, Dietetics, Pharmacy and Nursing. An Alpha and Beta test site conference call was established bi-monthly to provide the expert panel and programmers/designers feedback. Problems were identified and suggested corrective actions identified. To correct flaws, a 'patch' was generated. A patch is a short set of instructions intended to revise the programming code.

3.0 Implementation

Vague guidelines were provided as to who should enter the allergies, or what role each affected service should have. A committee was formed that included a representative from Information Resource Management (IRM) and ADPAC's from Pharmacy, Dietetics, Nursing, and MAS. Following many discussions, a plan for entering allergy/adverse reaction data was developed.

For inpatients, unit clerks at the admissions desk were designated to initially enter historical allergies in the computer. They also marked the identification arm band with an allergy alert red dot. Unit clerks on each ward would review the allergies, mark the chart and enter any missing information into the computer. Registered nurses were responsible for entering any additional allergies discovered while obtaining the nursing admission assessment. Clinically observed allergic or adverse reactions were also entered by the patient's supervising nurse. If a unit clerk was not available, the nurse assumed her/his responsibilities for entering data into the computer.

After the initial data entry of an observed allergy or adverse reaction, the program would send a notification to the facility's clinical pharmacist. The clinical pharmacist would review the data for drug-drug, drug-food or drug-other interactions. Upon establishing a viable allergy or adverse reaction, the pharmacist would verify it in the computer.

Dietetics, pharmacy, MAS, and nursing began training end users in June 1991. Nursing quickly developed a simple training manual demonstrating how to enter historical and observed allergies/adverse reactions. The manual was advanced to all services involved. The Allergy/Adverse reaction was added to nursing's new employee orientation and additional allergy classes were offered to existing employees. Training also occasionally occurred on the nursing ward as necessary.

4.0 Evaluation

Feedback about the program was solicited and evaluated following each class session. Several classes were conducted in the same conference room where the bi-monthly Allergy/Adverse Reaction Tracking conference calls for Alpha and Beta test sites were held. This provided a unique avenue for feedback. Most of the nurses that participated were experienced VA nurses. Alpha and Beta sites evaluation and dialogue about the program stimulated additional suggestions and constructive criticisms of the program. A number of changes were suggested by nursing, 10 were actually integrated into the program. Several suggestions involved nuances in language interpretation between the developers and that of the nursing staff. Changes in the package include: (See Table 1)

1. <CR> - Users did not know this symbol means carriage return and suggested "push return to continue" as an alternative.
2. Observed comments (an area where the users could type text) were required before the program asked for

the signs and symptoms of the allergic reaction. If the user was not familiar with the program, signs and symptoms were entered in both comments and signs and symptoms fields.

3. The print output entailed an extensive, descriptive printed form. Nurses using the program found it very cumbersome to decipher. A simple list of verified allergies was requested. Multiple print options were created: a food allergy only option, a drug allergy only option and a simple verified allergy list.

4. The original data entry option was entitled "Select Allergy/Adverse Reaction". Staff felt that an allergy was the result of the patient's reaction to an allergen. The default was changed to Enter the name of the Allergen:

5. The "Select Allergy/Adverse Reaction//" default prompt was interpreted by staff as an event that had already occurred. The default was changed to "Enter Allergy/Adverse Reaction//".

6. A standard abbreviation used by nurses in clinical practice is SOB (Shortness of Breath). This was not included in the Signs & Symptoms File. If SOB was entered at the Other: default, the program prompted "Not in the signs/symptoms file. Would you like to add it?" Requests by staff to add to the Signs and Symptoms file was acknowledged and is now included.

7. Along with medical abbreviations, the program would allow the entry of PCN for penicillin at the reaction entry prompt, but would not allow PCN when specifying an allergen to print. This problem was later addressed by pointing the program to the National Drug file.

8. The program would not allow for the entry of an observed non-drug reaction. This was altered so any observed allergy/adverse reaction could be entered. A prompt was inserted to select drug, food or other.

9. After entering the data associated with an observed reaction, a treatment and test field appeared. Originally the field reviewed all test and treatments the day before and the day after the observed reaction. The user was unable to control the date ranges that were displayed, and unable to get out of the circular programming without using a "^" to escape. The program was altered to facilitate flow through this area. At this time, the treatment and test display remained in the program.

10. While training during a conference call, an end user asked a very valid question. "Why is there no place to enter the signs and symptoms of a historical allergy?" The user went on to point out when doing an assessment, this was an obvious question to ask. This suggestion was addressed, but not until the version 3.0 of the program.

11. Another problem identified was the accidental entry of reactions. When the user typed in the first few letters of a substance, the computer would suggest what it thought the user meant. For example if SUL was entered, the computer could respond SULFITES OK? YES//. If the user had meant SOL, they could type in "^" to escape the function. The program would enter sulfites as a reaction regardless. The program was altered to prevent additional records when the user attempted to exit a prompt without entering data.

12. A large number of common substances were not included in the data base the program referenced. For example: NutraSweet, saccharin, nitrates and citric acid were not available for selection. Since this was identified, the program now references the National Drug file.

13. After entering a reaction, the program would return to the PATIENT NAME: prompt instead of asking if there were more reactions to be entered. Re-entering a patient name was time consuming. The program was altered to return to the Enter Allergen: prompt and, if the user simply pushed return, the program would return to PATIENT NAME:. A second return would return the user to the main Allergy/Adverse Reaction Tracking menu.

4.1 Table

Table 1
Program Flow Allergy/Adverse Reaction Tracking Program 2.2 as Released to Alpha and Beta Sites

---

1 Enter/Edit Patient Allergy/Adverse Reaction Data
2 Allergy/Adverse Reaction Print Menu
3 Date/Time Chart and ID Band Marked Edit
Select Allergy/Adverse Reaction Tracking System Option: **1<CR>**

Table 1
Program Flow Allergy/Adverse Reaction Tracking Program 2.2 as Released to Alpha and Beta Sites

---

Select PATIENT NAME: **M7890**   MOUSE,MICKEY

Select Allergy/Adverse Reaction: **AMPH<CR>**
  AMPICILLIN   OK? YES// **N<CR>**
    1.   AMPHETAMINE
    2.   AMPHETAMINE ADIPATE
    3.   AMPHETAMINE ASPARTATE
    4.   AMPHETAMINE RESIN COMPLEX
    5.   AMPHETAMINE SULFATE
    6.   AMPHOTERICIN B
TYPE '' TO STOP, OR
CHOOSE 1-6: **6<CR>**
  AMPHOTERICIN B   OK? YES// **<CR>**

(O)bserved or (H)istorical Allergy/Adverse Reaction: **O<CR>**

COMMENTS ON OBSERVED DATA:
  1> **<CR>**

DATE/TIME OBSERVED: **T@10AM** (FEB 12, 1991@10:00)
OBSERVER: PETIT,YVENS// **<CR>**
DATE/TIME MD NOTIFIED: **T@10:10** (FEB 12, 1991@10:10)

No Signs/symptoms have been specified. Please add some now.
The following are the top ten most common signs/symptoms
  1. RASH   7. HIVES
  2. ASTHMA   8. DRY MOUTH
  3. HYPOTENSION   9. DRY NOSE
  4. DROWSINESS   10. ANXIETY
  5. NAUSEA, VOMITING   11. OTHER SIGN/SYMPTOM
  6. DIARRHEA
Enter from the list above: **1,11<CR>**
Enter OTHER SIGN/SYMPTOM: **SHORTNESS OF BREATH**
SHORTNESS OF BREATH   OK? YES// **<CR>**
Would you like to add another sign/symptom? NO// **<CR>**
The following is the list of reported signs/symptoms for this reaction
1   RASH
2   SHORTNESS OF BREATH
Enter Action: **? <CR>**
    ENTER AN A TO ADD SIGNS/SYMPTOMS TO THIS LIST,
    OR D TO DELETE SIGNS/SYMPTOMS FORM THIS LIST,
    OR <CR> TO ACCEPT THIS LIST OF SIGNS/SYMPTOMS.
Enter Action: **<CR>**

Select Date/Time Range to View Tx/Tests
View previous TX/Tests from: Jan 11, 1991@10:00// **<CR>**
To: Jan 13, 1991@10:00// **<CR>**
(Information is displayed in reference to drugs, to lab values, to radiology tests and to outpatient prescriptions)

Table 1

Program Flow Allergy/Adverse Reaction Tracking Program 2.2 as Released to Alpha and Beta Sites

---

Select Action: **<CR>**
Select DATE/TIME CHART MARKED: **N<CR>** FEB 12, 1991@11:17
Select DATE/TIME ID BAND MARKED: **N<CR>** FEB 12, 1991@11:17
    (Entered data is displayed)

Would you like to sign off on this allergy/adverse reaction? **Y<CR>**

Select PATIENT NAME: **<CR>**

In September, 1991, the revised program, Version 2.2, was installed into production. Production refers to the live account that uses actual patient data. Evaluation continued by all participating sites. Numerous suggestions continued to be voiced to the programmers. One such concern was the misspelling of allergen.

The Alpha and Beta site calls ceased in late September. Further suggestions were directed though Electronic Enhancement and Error Reporting (E3R's). E3R's are a simple method used to make suggestions by electronic mail. The staff have access to this avenue through their perspective ADPAC. The suggestions are funnelled through the expert allergy panel. The panel prioritized the recommendations and designated which suggestions should be included in the next version of the program. The Dayton VAMC continues to be an Alpha test site and is currently evaluating the second major release, Version 3.0, of the program.

5.0 Summary

Developing a package that meets users' needs requires defining the problems, evaluating the needs, and designing the software to handle the problem. Teague and Pidgeon[2] describe this process as the software development life cycle. They define eight phases that take place: identify user needs, establish user requirements, determine hardware and software environment, design the system, develop system acceptance test, construct the system, integrate the system with using organization, and operate, modify and enhance the system. A modified version of this paradigm was followed in designing the Allergy/Adverse Reaction software. The hardware and basic system software were already in place. The Decentralized Hospital Computer Program (DHCP) is the basic Department of Veterans Affairs Medical Centers controlling program. It provides an integrated data base for all services to enter or retrieve patient data. This allows for modular designed programs to be added. The Alpha and Beta test sites actually are involved with developing system acceptance tests and constructing the system. This is accomplished through testing the database in a practice environment. Staff from all of the participating services evaluated the AART program first in a test environment, where a number of "bugs" were modified, and in a live environment. Staff from the various services suggested changes that were also incorporated into the program. After Alpha/Beta testing, the program was released for VAMC system use. The eighth phase (Operate, modify and enhance the system) is a continuing process with the recent release of Version 3.0 of the Allergy/Adverse Reaction Tracking Program.

6.0 References

[1]Manubay's Laws for Programmers. *LAWS OF COMPUTING*, December 1992: Electronic Mail
[2]Teague L., and Pidgeon C. *Structured Analysis Methods for Computer Information Systems*, 1984: Chicago,ILL: Science Research Associates, Inc.

INDEX OF AUTHORS

SUBJECT INDEX